COMMUNITY HEALTH NURSING: KEEPING THE PUBLIC HEALTHY

COMMUNITY HEALTH NURSING: KEEPING THE PUBLIC HEALTHY

LINDA L. JARVIS, M.S.N., R.N.

**ASSISTANT PROFESSOR
BOSTON UNIVERSITY
SCHOOL OF NURSING
BOSTON, MASSACHUSETTS**

 F. A. DAVIS COMPANY•Philadelphia

Library of Congress Cataloging in Publication Data
Main entry under title:

Community health nursing:
  Keeping the public healthy

  Includes bibliographies and index.
  1. Community health nursing. I. Jarvis, Linda L.
[DNLM: 1. Community health nursing. WY106 J38k]
RT98.K43   610.73′43   80-16953
ISBN 0-8036-4925-8

This book is dedicated with love and appreciation to my Dad and Mom, Frank and Louise Jarvis

PREFACE

This text has been developed for students and practitioners in community health nursing. Through observation and discussion with students and clients and interaction and debate/discussion with peers and colleagues, the form and structure of this text eventually evolved. It is my intent to reflect the many recent dynamic changes experienced by society, the health care field, and community health nursing.

The text is divided into seven major units: *Health Care in the Community* provides an overview of what the community is; the health-care delivery system; the political, legislative, and financial status of health care; education; and the tools and resources available to the community health nurse. *Community Health Nursing Roles* are examined in detail providing the reader with insight into the preparation, scope of service, and impact each role can have on health care. Areas covered include ambulatory care; occupational, school, and public health; home care; midwifery; gerontology; and continuing care. *Diseases Affecting Community Health* identifies specific diseases, their etiologies, treatment and prognosis, and their effect on individuals and groups. *Mental Health Issues*, such as family crises and drug and alcohol abuse, and *Social Issues*, such as nutrition and death and dying, examine the effect these issues have on community health. *Environmental Issues*, including air, water, and noise pollution; waste disposal; and radiation are explored as priority problems affecting community health. *Personal Experiences in Community Health Nursing Roles* presents an individualized perspective of specific nursing roles and provides the reader an opportunity to analyze and critique various roles and responsibilities. Terminology is defined within the content of each chapter.

In depth exploration of these topics should sensitize the reader to the need for concern by community health nurses, the scope of the role or problem, and the steps to be taken to modify or remove the impact on the population. Community health nursing can expand its effect only as the nurses working in the field become aware of the need, means, and potential for providing direct and indirect nursing services. The aim of this text is to provide that awareness.

Linda L. Jarvis

ACKNOWLEDGMENTS

Many people have been instrumental in the completion of this endeavor. As I review the past several months of writing activity, I am impressed with how smoothly the process actually worked. The people who have been involved directly and indirectly are many. My deep gratitude is extended to each.

In particular, I wish to thank the contributors whose enthusiasm and support made the text possible; the editors and staff of the F.A. Davis Company; and the typists, Terry Lundbohm, Janet Youkeles, and Diane O'Brien.

My family and friends by providing support, encouragement and coffee also helped make this book a reality. My efforts to acknowledge their input will always prove inadequate.

I would like to especially thank all the students I have had the privilege to know. They have taught me about teaching, learning, and flexibility, which has directly shaped my thinking, approach, and understanding of education and students.

LLJ

CONTRIBUTORS

MARGARET REGISTER BEAN, M.N., M.S., R.N.
Public Health Nursing Consultant, Team Evaluation Center, Inc., Tennessee State Health Department, Chattanooga, Tennessee

BARBARA B. BECKER, M.S., A.N.P., R.N.
Supervisor, Serving Seniors Program, Denver Visiting Nurse Service, Denver, Colorado

JANICE STEVENSON BERNS, M.S.N., R.N.
Instructor, Boston University, School of Nursing, Boston, Massachusetts

VIRGINIA TROTTER BETTS, M.S.N., J.D., R.N.
Associate Professor, Psychiatric Mental Health Nursing, Vanderbilt University, Nashville, Tennessee

LYNNE BIGELOW, M.S., R.N.
Beth Israel Hospital Home Care Program, Boston, Massachusetts

CAROL ANN BINGHAM, M.S.N., R.N.
Washington Home Hospice Unit Leader, Washington, D.C.

NANCY BINNER, M.P.H., R.N.
Uphams Corner Home Care Program, Dorchester, Massachusetts

ROBERT D. BRUCE
Consultant in Noise Control Engineering, Bolt, Beranck, & Newman, Inc., Cambridge, Massachusetts

GWENDOLYN BUCHANAN, M.S.N., R.N.
Volunteer Faculty, Assistant Professor, Oklahoma University, College of Nursing; Assistant Chief Nursing Service, Surgery and Ambulatory Care, Veterans Administration Medical Center, Oklahoma City, Oklahoma

GERI C. BUDESHEIM, M.N., R.N.
Assistant Professor, Medical and Surgical Nursing, University of Kansas College of Health Sciences, School of Nursing, Kansas City, Kansas

EMIL THEODORE CHANLETT, M.S.P.H., M.S.S.E.
Professor of Sanitary Engineering, Department of Environmental Science and Engineering, University of North Carolina, School of Public Health, Chapel Hill, North Carolina

MARYROSE CONDON, M.S., R.N.
Guest Lecturer, Northeastern University, School of Nursing, Pediatric Nurse Practitioner Program; Clinical Specialist, Tufts New England Medical Center, Boston Floating Hospital, Pediatric Cardiology Department, Boston, Massachusetts

JAMES CROOK, Ph.D.
Senior Sanitary Engineer, State of California, Department of Health Services, Sanitary Engineering Section, Berkeley, California

LOUISE DAUGHERTY, M.S.N., R.N.
Nurse Coordinator, Ambulatory Care, American Lake VAMC, Tacoma, Washington

PATRICIA M. DiSABATINO, M.S., R.N.
Instructor, Temple University, College of Allied Health Professions, Department of Nursing, Philadelphia, Pennsylvania

SISTER ROSEMARY DONLEY, Ph.D., R.N.
Associate Professor and Dean, Catholic University of America, School of Nursing, Washington, D.C.

SUE DRISCOLL, M.S., R.N.
Instructor, University of Wisconsin, School of Nursing; Clinical Nurse Specialist, Pulmonary Disease, University of Wisconsin Hospital and Clinics, Madison, Wisconsin

LINDA DUMAS, M.A., M.S.N., R.N.
Instructor, Boston University, School of Nursing, Boston, Massachusetts

BEVERLY MEDEIROS GALLAGHER, M.S.N., R.N.
Instructor, Boston University, School of Nursing, Boston, Massachusetts

PAULA GANNON, B.S., R.N.
Continuing Care Nurse, Tufts New England Medical Center, Boston, Massachusetts

PHEBE GOLDMAN, B.S.N., P.H.N., R.N.
Field Supervisor, Denver Visiting Nurse Service, Denver, Colorado

PHYLLIS J. GOODHUE, M.S., R.N.
Continuing Care Coordinator, Affiliated Hospitals Center, Peter Bent Brigham Division, Boston, Massachusetts

DIANA GUTHRIE, M.S.P.H., R.N., F.A.A.N.
Diabetes Nurse Specialist, Assistant Professor, University of Kansas, School of Medicine; Adjunct Faculty, Wichita State University, Wichita, Kansas

RICHARD GUTHRIE, M.D., F.A.A.P.
Pediatric Endocrinologist and Diabetologist, Professor and Chairman, Department of Pediatrics, University of Kansas, School of Medicine, Wichita, Kansas

LEANNE P. HALFMAN, M.S., S.N.P., R.N.
School Nurse Practitioner Coordinator, Gary Community School Corporation, Gary, Indiana

MARGARET SMITH HAMILTON, M.S., R.N.
Instructor, Psychiatric Nursing, Boston College, Boston, Massachusetts

FREDDA HERZ, Ph.D., R.N.
Assistant Professor and Coordinator of the Graduate Program in Primary Care Nursing, Child and Adolescent Mental Health, H. H. Lehman College, Department of Nursing, New York, New York

LINDA L. JARVIS, M.S.N., R.N.
Assistant Professor, Boston University, School of Nursing, Boston, Massachusetts

MAXENE JOHNSTON, M.A., R.N.
Director, Ambulatory Nursing, Childrens Hospital of Los Angeles, Los Angeles, California

EILEEN KIRK, M.S., R.N.
Uphams Corner Home Care Program, Dorchester, Massachusetts

JOAN STACK KOVACH, M.S., R.N.
Clinical Supervisor, Boston University Graduate School, Psychiatric-Mental Health Nursing; Psychiatric Nurse Clinical Specialist, Children's Hospital Medical Center, Department of Psychiatry, Boston, Massachusetts

THERESE G. LAWLER, M.S.N., R.N.
Doctoral Student, North Carolina State University; Associate Professor, East Carolina University, School of Nursing, Greenville; Adjunct Assistant Professor, University of North Carolina, School of Public Health, Chapel Hill, North Carolina.

MARILYN B. MAJOR, M.P.H., R.N.
Assistant Professor, University of Michigan, School of Nursing, Ann Arbor, Michigan

BARBARA JO McGRATH, M.N., R.N.
Director of Nursing Education, Fayetteville Area Health Education Center, Fayetteville; Clinical Assistant Professor, Duke University Medical Center, School of Nursing, Durham, North Carolina

THALIA METALIDES, M.S., R.D.
Nutritionist, Ambulatory Services, Children's Hospital Medical Center, Boston, Massachusetts

JOAN E. MULLIGAN, Ph.D., C.N.M.
Associate Professor, University of Wisconsin-Madison, School of Nursing, Graduate Program and College of Letters and Science, Program in Women's Studies, Madison, Wisconsin

SALLY M. O'NEIL, Ph.D., R.N.
Professor and Chairperson, University of Washington, Department of Maternal and Child Nursing, Seattle, Washington

PARKER C. REIST, Sc.D., S.M. in Hyg.

Professor of Air and Industrial Hygiene, University of North Carolina, School of Public Health, Department of Environmental Science and Engineering, Chapel Hill, North Carolina

NICKI MORINA RICHARDS, M.S., R.N.

Instructor, Boston University, School of Nursing, Boston, Massachusetts

SHARON SCHINDLER RISING, M.S.N., C.N.M., R.N.

Assistant Professor of Nursing and Obstetrics/Gynecology, University of Minnesota, School of Nursing, School of Medicine; Director, Childbearing-Childrearing Center, University of Minnesota Hospitals, Minneapolis, Minnesota

ANNE WETZEL SALETTA, M.S.N., R.N.

Instructor, Community Health Nursing, Vanderbilt University, Nashville, Tennessee

MARY SCANLON, M.Ed., C.O.H.N., R.N.

Visiting Nurse Practitioner, The Gillette Company, Safety Razor Division, Boston, Massachusetts

CAROL A. SILBERSTEIN, M.Ed., R.N.

University of Cincinnati, School of Nursing, Cincinnati, Ohio

EDWARD BERNARD SILBERSTEIN, M.D.

Professor of Radiology and Associate Professor of Medicine, University of Cincinnati, College of Medicine; Associate Director, Radioisotope Laboratory, Cincinnati General Hospital; Chief, Nuclear Medicine Service, Cincinnati Veterans Administration Medical Center, Cincinnati, Ohio

MARGARET MATTHEWS SLOCUM, M.S., R.N.

Formerly, Nursing Instructor, Boston University, School of Nursing, Boston, Massachusetts

DAVID P. SPATH, Ph.D.

Senior Sanitary Engineer, State of California, Department of Health Services, Sanitary Engineering Section, Berkeley, California

MARION G. SPENCER, M.S., C.A.G.S., R.N.

Associate Professor, Department of Gerontological Nursing, Boston University, School of Nursing, Boston, Massachusetts

MARILYN L. STEMBER, Ph.D., R.N.

Associate Professor of Nursing and Sociology, University of Colorado, Health Sciences Center, Denver, Colorado

MACKEY P. TORBETT, Ph.D., R.N.

Associate Professor, Medical and Surgical Nursing, University of Kansas, College of Health Sciences, School of Nursing, Kansas City, Kansas

LAURA NELSON TRENT, B.S.N., R.N.

Staff Nurse, Metropolitan Health Department, Nashville and Davidson Counties, Nashville, Tennessee

ROSALYN JONES WATTS, M.S.N., R.N.

Assistant Professor, University of Pennsylvania, School of Nursing, Philadelphia, Pennsylvania

CONTENTS

UNIT I.   HEALTH CARE IN THE COMMUNITY   1

   1.   INTRODUCTION   3
Linda L. Jarvis, M.S.N., R.N.

   2.   COMMUNITY   5
Linda L. Jarvis, M.S.N., R.N., and
Linda G. Dumas, M.A., M.S.N., R.N.

   3.   HEALTH AND ILLNESS   25
Linda L. Jarvis, M.S.N., R.N.

   4.   COMMUNITY HEALTH NURSING   39
Linda L. Jarvis, M.S.N., R.N.

   5.   HEALTH CARE DELIVERY SYSTEM   53
Linda L. Jarvis, M.S.N., R.N.

   6.   POLITICS AND PRACTITIONERS   69
Maxene Johnston, M.A., R.N.

   7.   HEALTH CARE LEGISLATION AND FINANCING   83
Sister Rosemary Donley, Ph.D., R.N.

8. **HEALTH EDUCATION IN COMMUNITY HEALTH NURSING**   93
Linda L. Jarvis, M.S.N., R.N.

9. **TOOLS AND RESOURCES FOR THE COMMUNITY HEALTH NURSE**   101
Linda L. Jarvis, M.S.N., R.N.

UNIT II.   COMMUNITY HEALTH NURSING ROLES   111

10. **NURSING ROLE IN AMBULATORY CARE**   113
Louise G. Daugherty, M.S.N., R.N., and
Gwendolyn J. Buchanan, M.S.N., R.N.

11. **NURSING ROLE IN OCCUPATIONAL HEALTH**   123
Carol A. Silberstein, M.Ed., R.N.

12. **NURSING ROLE IN SCHOOL HEALTH**   141
Marilyn L. Stember, Ph.D., R.N.

13. **NURSING ROLE IN PUBLIC HEALTH**   175
Marilyn B. Major, M.P.H., R.N.

14. **NURSING ROLE IN HOME HEALTH CARE**   199
Beverly Medeiros Gallagher, M.S.N., R.N.

15. **NURSING ROLE IN EDUCATION**   219
Linda L. Jarvis, M.S.N., R.N.

16. **NURSING ROLE IN MIDWIFERY**   239
Joan E. Mulligan, Ph.D., C.N.M.

17. **NURSING ROLE IN DEVELOPMENTAL DISABILITIES**   257
Margaret Register Bean, M.N., M.S., R.N.

18. **NURSING ROLE IN GERONTOLOGY**   295
Marian G. Spencer, M.S., C.A.G.S., R.N.

19. **NURSING ROLE IN COMMUNITY MENTAL HEALTH**   319
Janice Stevenson Berns, M.S.N., R.N., and
Margaret Smith Hamilton, M.S., R.N.

20. **NURSING ROLE IN CONTINUING CARE**   355
Phyllis J. Goodhue, M.S., R.N.

UNIT III.   MAJOR DISEASES AFFECTING COMMUNITY HEALTH   369

21. **CARDIAC AND CIRCULATORY DISEASES**   371
Rosalyn Jones Watts, M.S.N., R.N.

22. **CANCER**   393
Carol Ann Bingham, M.S.N., R.N.

23. **DIABETES MELLITUS**   **423**
Diana W. Guthrie, M.S.P.H., R.N., F.A.A.N., and
Richard A. Guthrie, M.D., F.A.A.P.

24. **INFECTIOUS DISEASES**   **451**
Nicki Morina Richards, M.S., R.N.

25. **CHRONIC OBSTRUCTIVE LUNG DISEASE**   **475**
Sue Driscoll, M.S., R.N.

26. **ARTHRITIS**   **497**
Mackey P. Torbett, Ph.D., R.N., and
Geri C. Budesheim, M.N., R.N.

UNIT IV.   **MAJOR MENTAL HEALTH ISSUES AFFECTING COMMUNITY HEALTH**   **519**

27. **FAMILY CRISES AND EMOTIONAL DISORDERS**   **521**
Fredda Herz, Ph.D., R.N.

28. **SUBSTANCE ABUSE: DRUGS AND ALCOHOL**   **537**
Virginia Trotter Betts, M.S.N., J.D., R.N., and
Anne Wetzel Saletta, M.S.N., R.N.

29. **VICTIMOLOGY**   **555**
Patricia M. DiSabatino, M.S., R.N.

UNIT V.   **MAJOR SOCIAL ISSUES AFFECTING COMMUNITY HEALTH**   **567**

30. **COMMUNITY NUTRITION**   **569**
Thalia Metalides, M.S., R.D.

31. **DISABILITIES**   **603**
Linda L. Jarvis, M.S.N., R.N.

32. **GRIEF, DYING AND DEATH**   **611**
Linda L. Jarvis, M.S.N., R.N.

UNIT VI.   **MAJOR ENVIRONMENTAL ISSUES AFFECTING COMMUNITY HEALTH**   **621**

33. **POPULATION ISSUES**   **623**
Linda L. Jarvis, M.S.N., R.N.

34. **SAFETY AND ACCIDENTS**   **631**
Linda L. Jarvis, M.S.N., R.N.

35. **AIR POLLUTION**   **637**
Parker C. Reist, Sc.D., S.M. in Hyg.

36. **NOISE POLLUTION**   **647**
Robert D. Bruce, S.M. Elec. Eng., E.E.

37. **WATER POLLUTION**   **659**
David P. Spath, Ph.D. and James Crook, Ph.D.

38. **SOLID WASTE MANAGEMENT**   **667**
Emil T. Chanlett, M.S.P.H., M.S.S.E

39. **IONIZING RADIATION AND COMMUNITY HEALTH**   **681**
Carol A. Silberstein, M.Ed., R.N., and
Edward D. Silberstein, M.D.

UNIT VII.   **PERSONAL EXPERIENCES IN COMMUNITY HEALTH NURSING ROLES**   **693**

40. **AMBULATORY CLINICAL ROLE STUDY**   **695**
Maryrose Condon, M.S., R.N.

41. **OCCUPATIONAL NURSING CLINICAL ROLE STUDY**   **701**
Mary E. Scanlon, M.Ed., C.O.H.N., R.N.

42. **SCHOOL NURSE PRACTITIONER**   **709**
Leanne P. Halfman, M.S., S.N.P., R.N.

43. **PUBLIC HEALTH NURSING CLINICAL ROLE STUDY**   **731**
Laura Nelson Trent, B.S.N., R.N.

44. **COMMUNITY HEALTH NURSING: ONE NURSE'S PRACTICE**   **741**
Barbara B. Becker, M.S., A.N.P., R.N.

45. **COMMUNITY HEALTH NURSING: A PERSONAL PERSPECTIVE**   **751**
Phebe Goldman, B.S.N., P.H.N., R.N.

46. **THE AHEC NURSE AS A COMMUNITY EDUCATOR**   **761**
Barbara Jo McGrath, M.N., R.N., and
Therese G. Lawler, M.S.N., R.N.

47. **A PREVENTIVE HEALTH PROGRAM FOR LOW INCOME WOMEN**   **795**
Margaret Matthews Slocum, M.S., R.N.

48. **NURSE-MIDWIVES IN ACTION AT THE CHILDBEARING-CHILDREARING CENTER**   **811**
Sharon Schindler Rising, M.S.N., C.N.M., R.N.

49. **INDEPENDENT NURSING PRACTICE IN DEVELOPMENTAL DISABILITIES**   **825**
Sally M. O'Neil, Ph.D., R.N.

50. **GERONTOLOGY CLINICAL ROLE STUDY**   **837**
Lynne Bigelow, M.S., R.N., Nancy Binner, M.P.H., R.N., and
Eileen Kirk, M.S., R.N.

51. **COMMUNITY MENTAL HEALTH CLINICAL ROLE STUDY**   **861**
Joan Stack Kovach, M.S., R.N.

52. **CONTINUING CARE CLINICAL ROLE STUDY**   **877**
Paula Gannon, B.S., R.N.

INDEX   **883**

UNIT I
HEALTH CARE
IN THE COMMUNITY

The practice of community health nursing requires a wide knowledge base. The community environment, health and illness attitudes and behaviors of the target population(s) and an understanding of the health care delivery system at the local, state and federal level will provide an operational base from which the community health nurse can work. In addition, the nurse will need to be sensitive to political, legislative and financial issues which impact on the care sought and received by the consumer. Health education approaches and various tools and resources will aid in the delivery of quality nursing care.

The theoretical and philosophical base from which the community health nurse works will provide the foundation for further role definition and growth. Community health nursing is based on various nursing theories with major goals of health promotion and maintenance and healthful living practices directed toward specified aggregates.

The chapters in this unit are designed to provide a foundation of knowledge about community health nursing and the various factors which must be considered when planning community health nursing care for the individual, family or general community. It is the basis for the development of the following units.

CHAPTER 1

INTRODUCTION

LINDA L. JARVIS, M.S.N., R.N.

This book has been designed for the baccalaureate nursing student and the beginning community health nurse. For the baccalaureate student, it will provide a wide base of community health nursing theory. For the beginning practitioner, it will serve to reinforce past learning and provide input into various community health roles and responsibilities.

To this end, a large segment of the book has been devoted to specific community health nursing roles. All speciality nursing roles address a particular aggregate designated by age, condition, and/or geography. Since target groups are the recipients of community health services, we have selected a wide cross section of target groups to show the scope of community health nursing. This has been done by providing the reader with a review of the historical development of the role, an explanation of educational and clinical preparation, an overview of the scope of services provided by nurses in these settings and legal and legislative considerations. This information is provided early in the book and is followed in the last unit of the text by clinical role studies by nurses working in these speciality areas.

The first unit of the text explores the concept of community health nursing, health care delivery in the United States, health education, tools and resources useful in providing community nursing services, and legislation and financing of health care. These issues are of direct concern to all nurses, but particularly influence the community health nurse as she or he attempts to provide services to diverse groups.

Because of the many environmental, disease, social, and mental issues affecting our society, space has been provided for exploration of some of these concerns. It is becoming increasingly clear that community health nurses need a broad base of data as well as sensitivity and sophistication toward the various environmental, social, mental, and disease conditions that influence the health status of different population groups. The prevention of disease and the promotion of health has become a complicated process requiring the cooperation of many professional groups. This is no longer the sole responsibility of the health department but, rather, the combined responsibility of health care professionals, educators at all levels from elementary school to college, occupational groups, environmentalists, and various social and mental health groups and organizations.

Community health nursing has been expanding in the scope of its services. Always concerned with the health status of various groups, the speciality has moved from a primary base of the traditional public health and visiting nurse into such areas as midwifery, occupational health, gerontology, school nursing, education, developmental disabilities, community mental health, continuing care, and ambulatory care. Work sites include institutions, clinics, housing projects, health departments, factories, and offices as health needs are identified. The reader is encouraged to explore the variety of community health nursing activities carried on in the community.

The degree to which a nurse in the community can provide a wide range of services will depend in large part on her knowledge of the community in which she works, the kind and quality of services and resources available to the citizen group under her care, and her ability to work through and within the health care delivery system. If the system can be overwhelming to the professional health care provider, how much more so for the consumer. The acquisition of knowledge and skills necessary to provide community health nursing care is a dynamic, on-going process which continues throughout the career of the nurse. Changes are sometimes made quickly and trends for service to particular groups may need prompt attention in order to obtain funds and support for their implementation. Political savvy is imperative. As the society becomes more complicated, the need for political astuteness is critical as one provides nursing services through the system. Care must be taken to analyze the power structure and find ways to work through it.

This book represents the thoughts, efforts, and knowledge of the many contributors. Each was chosen because of special skill and knowledge in a particular area. The diversity of topics was chosen because of observed need of students to be exposed to such information. To this end, readers are encouraged to explore topics of particular interest in more depth. The nurse in the community faces many challenges in the provision of nursing care. Opportunities for meeting community health care needs and problems vary but are directly related to the knowledge, skills, sensitivity, and creativity of the nurse. It is hoped that this text will stimulate and encourage the nurse in the practice of community health nursing.

CHAPTER 2
COMMUNITY

LINDA L. JARVIS, M.S.N., R.N., AND
LINDA G. DUMAS, M.A., M.S.N., R.N.

One of the greatest challenges facing the community health nurse is a comprehensive knowledge and understanding of the community in which he or she works. This knowledge provides a basis from which the nurse will plan and deliver health care. In addition, the incorporation of interdisciplinary health services is dependent upon a knowledge of community resources. There is ambiguity in many of the definitions of community, and it may be due in part to the nature of community as an integral part of everyday life. This chapter will identify selected definitions of community and will focus on some of the issues which are of concern to community members.

DEFINITION OF COMMUNITY

The diversity of ideas about what constitutes a community is exemplified in the following definitions. Basic to all is the concept of groups, but the interactions which define their communal nature range wide in scope. Community. . .

"includes a group of people who have common health interests and needs which they can identify or be helped to identify."[1]

"is patterned interaction within a domain of individuals seeking to achieve security and physical safety, to derive support in times of stress and to gain selfhood and significance throughout the life cycle."[2]

5

"can be viewed as a place, as a social system and as a collection of people."[3]

"is made up of many groups who serve as channels of communication, audiences, and sounding boards."[4]

"is a group of people living in the same locality and under the same government; the district or locality in which they live; a social group or class having common interests."[5]

The commonality in all the above descriptions of community is people. There can be no community without people; individuals give character and set parameters to communities. It is important to realize that one is a member of many communities at the same time. A central focus of interest often determines specific community characteristics. Such foci may be geographic boundaries, educational status, culture, ethnicity, occupation, political structures, and socioeconomic status.

Community boundaries may be defined on a continuum ranging from simple to complex. The neighborhood where one lives is a community. Another community may be the larger structure of the town, city, or county. The overall structure is the state which constitutes the national and international frameworks (Fig. 2-1). Each of these geographic units is directly influenced by parameters such as rivers, mountains, mineral deposits, railroads, highways, factories, plains, and temperatures. All of these factors impact on the structure of a community.

For example, if coal deposits are located in an area, they will provide a source of revenue which will affect the economy and the population density of the surrounding communities. As long as resources are present, with the feasibility of accessible methods

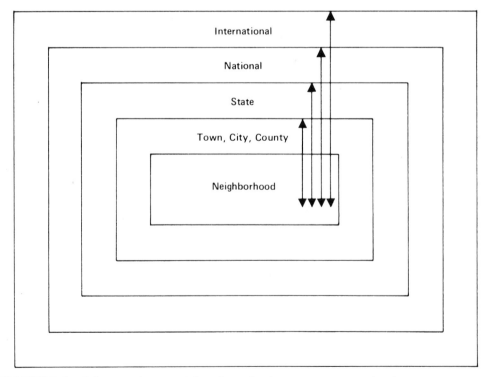

FIGURE 2-1. Schematic drawing of the relationship between community levels.

for mining, people will remain in the area to live, work, and raise families. Another example may be large water resources such as lakes, rivers, or the sea. Such resources provide economic options via fishing, trade routes, and/or recreational opportunities. As opportunities increase in diversity, so do the interests and characteristics of the populations comprising the communities. A dearth of natural, man-made, or economic resources will also impact on the character of a community. Inaccessibility to an area leads to a reduction in migration or movement in and out of an area. Such communities experience minimal social, political, or economic change.

In summary, physical community boundaries exist in many forms. They may be streets, railroads, rivers, or numerous other natural and man-made borders. Whatever the form, each will give structure to a community and may directly influence the economic and social characteristics of an area.

While the physical and geographic parameters define and separate communities, it is the characteristics of the people which give a community its uniqueness. An example is culture. Culture is a major influence in every community. It is evidenced in the norms, values, religious practices, educational expectations, and occupations of community members. Leininger speaks clearly to the importance of knowing the cultural characteristics of the population with whom one works.[6] Knowledge of cultural influences enables a person to understand and evaluate the behavior of others who hold belief systems that are different from ones own.

In discussing the characteristics of the community, Klein speaks of the community's view of itself—the perceptions which people have of themselves, the norms or values which guide their actions, and the ways in which people live their lives in their particular settings. She goes on to say that in understanding any community, it is important to know the power structure and the communication channels which exist.[7] Equipped with such knowledge, one is able to identify resources which can be of value in a plan or design, and give momentum to the implementation and subsequent change.

In this discussion, the emphasis has primarily been on the community as a defined geographic group. This is a dominant determinant, but as such provides a narrow view of the community concept. Sanders' perspective of community as a place, a social system, and a group of people allows for the concept to be used for a variety of settings, interests, and group members.[3] The remainder of this section will illustrate the broadened meaning of community with several common examples.

The institution of the school constitutes a large community. The members of the community may be subdivided into units based on grade levels, educational interests, or age. Their common interest is the acquisition of knowledge, and concerns are focused on issues such as competency of instructors, adequacy of physical facilities, funding, and opportunities for future employment.

Another community may be an occupational group. This group may be seen holistically, as the overall work force, or studied on the micro level by the specific occupations *within* the work force. Such groups may be blue collar, white collar, or professional workers. Commonalities within the groups may be class interests, financial security, and the social structure of the work place.

Church, civic, political, and service groups may also constitute communities. Shared concerns focus on the goals and objectives of the organizations, and communal ties may be strengthened by the extent of social interaction involved in meeting organizational needs. An excellent example of a political community is the party structure.

In summary, people are members of more than one community at a time. In identifying the communities to which a client belongs, the nurse formulates a data base consisting of the beliefs, norms, and overall support systems of that individual and his or her family.

POPULATION

Populations are integrally related to communities but the concepts are not one and the same. In the following section, discussion will focus on a definition of populations using high risk status as an example of special interest to health service workers. Demography, or the study of populations, will be examined to provide the student with a framework for understanding common terminology and the significance of rates.

Population Characteristics

In the definition, study, and analysis of populations, several common parameters are used. Thomlinson writes,

"population study involves the number and variety of people in an area and the changes in this number and variety. Population analysis consists of: 1) acquiring basic information concerning population distribution, characteristics and changes; 2) explaining the causes of changes in these basic facts; and 3) analyzing anticipated consequences of probable future changes."[8]

The key words in the study and analysis of populations are the *descriptions* of change, the *reasons* why change has occurred, and the projected *outcomes* of such change. A discussion of these factors will be prefaced by a definition of the concept of populations.

Definition of Populations

"A population is an aggregate of disparate items or individuals each one of which conforms to a given definition, retains an identity with the passage of time and exists only during a finite interval. An individual enters a population or is 'born' when it first conforms to the definition which identifies the population; it leaves the population, or 'dies' when it ceases to conform with its definition."[9]

Populations are identified by biologic and social characteristics. The biologic are ascribed or inborn, and the social are acquired.[8] Examples of biologic characteristics are age, sex, and race. They are the basic properties of human beings and profoundly influence fertility, marriage, mortality, and migration.[8] Social, or achieved characteristics relate to socioeconomic status, marital status, occupation, education, religion, and culture. It is important to understand the interrelatedness of biologic and social variables, for their combinations reflect the parameters which distinguish communities and contribute to their uniqueness.

An individual may be a member of several communities and also a member of more than one population. For example, a black woman may live in a neighborhood, be a member of the nursing profession, and be a wife and mother. Can you distinguish which characteristics differentiate population and community? It is difficult and the two may overlap, but the important point to remember is that an individual is only a member of a population while he or she *shares* the variable of interest with the other members.

As an illustration of this point, consider the biologic variable of age. From infancy to old age, an individual will enter and leave various populations. A baby is a member of the population of infants until she is a year old. At that time, the child leaves the infant population and enters a group defined by childhood. When the child becomes an adolescent, she leaves behind the population of children. As this individual moves through life, she will always belong to a population defined by the criterion of age. Another population to which this person will belong for a lifetime will be defined by sex.

As an example of populations designated by *combinations* of social and biologic variables, the discussion will focus on populations at risk. This will direct the focus to health and illustrate the integral relationship between environmental and biologic characteristics.

An Overview of At-Risk Characteristics

In the study of populations, indices of risk factors are used to describe and classify the variables which increase the vulnerability of an individual or a group to illness and illness inducing behaviors. Historically, at-risk indices were emergents of the disease model of illness. This model predominated in times when communicable diseases were ravaging populations throughout the world. In the early nineteenth century there was a significant decline in the incidence of infectious diseases, but prior to this time illness and death were the primary measures of the health status of populations.

The model of the illness-health continuum emerged when medicine recognized that environmental and psychological factors were assuming dominant roles in illness experiences. The current emphasis in health care is on health maintenance, health promotion, and prevention of illness inducing behaviors. The integral relationships between culture and at risk behaviors is finally receiving its overdue recognition. [10]

When an illness model predominates, medical interventions occur after the fact. Attention is given only after someone becomes ill. Examples of this focus range from pneumonias and tuberculosis to low birth weight infants, women exposed to rubella during early pregnancy, and the disabling effects of accidents, heart disease, and stroke. Common to all is the occurrence of an *event prior* to intervention. At-risk indices and biologic characteristics are one and the same.

Members of twentieth century society have witnessed an increasing recognition and acceptance of the biosocial or environmental model of health and illness. Such a model more effectively meets the needs imposed by the social problems we share today. Every individual, regardless of class, race, or occupation, is exposed to multiple risks during his lifetime. Risks are interrelated and of psychological, environmental, and biologic origin. Psychological risks may relate to developmental or situational events occurring in the life cycle. Examples range across a continuum beginning with infancy and ending with old age. The infant who struggles for homeostasis with the environment becomes the toddler who is curious about the world. The child grows into an adolescent in search of identity. The high numbers of accidents, suicides, and disabilities in these populations attest to their at-risk status. Developmental and situational crises characterize the lives of people in the middle years and old age. Such crises may reflect dissatisfaction with the ways in which one has conducted his life, and, in later years, culminate in poverty and social isolation. All age groups are illustrative of the social, biologic, and psychological variables interplaying in at-risk behaviors. [11]

Occupational groups are another example of populations at risk. Unemployment is a major problem of social significance, often, but not always, class related. Safety hazards in work settings are other factors, ranging from environmental effects in factory settings to the stressors encountered in the office bureaucracies. All may lead to heart disease, hypertension, cancer, and alcoholism. In the assessment of at-risk variables, it is important to recognize the *potential* for the occurrence of an illness or disruptive event, for health promotion is far easier to attain than restoration from serious illness or disability.

At-risk variables occur along the socioeconomic continuum. The stressors of poverty are at one end, with the stressors of excessive competition for economic and social rewards at the other. In between the two poles are the numerous differentials associated with combinations of both ways of life. Certain persons are more vulnerable than others, and it should be remembered that multiple factors assume dominant roles in the susceptibility of individuals and groups to illness or poor health. The point to be emphasized is that *every* individual is at risk. However, differentials lead one to conclude that some are more at risk than others.

In summary, mortality and morbidity rates continue to be striking parameters of American health. They point to dominant health problems—what they are, who they most frequently affect, and the difficulties involved in prevention. In contemporary society pervasive problems associated with environmental adaptation in a highly advanced technologic age have posed health problems to all groups which are socially, psychologically, and biologically interrelated. We can no longer focus on problem-specific interventions. Health workers are examining the long term nature of health and illness.

The Rates: Mortality, Morbidity, and Fertility

Using the example of at-risk groups as a frame of reference, the discussion will now be directed to the method of studying populations. The method is called demography, and demographers are concerned with three variables: births, deaths, and migration. Demography is a descriptive and quantitative method which focuses on the characteristics of populations. Demographic data are used on both macro and micro levels of analysis. The macro level is concerned with the larger social structure, while the micro level focuses on the analysis of individuals and the variations in groups or communities to which they belong.[8]

For example, in the analysis of health care in the United States, macrodemographers are interested in the structural characteristics of the health system. Some of the variables examined are 1) cost, including mechanisms of third party payment, 2) the utilization of health services, and 3) the overall accessibility and availability of health care to groups in rural and inner city areas. Microdemographers focus on the description and analysis of the help-seeking behaviors and patterns of decision making by individuals and families. Comparative analyses may be made between the various racial and socioeconomic groups. Other comparisons may relate to age and sex specific variables. Questions of overriding interest are: "What are the deterrents to help-seeking behaviors?" "How do such behaviors influence the numbers and types of individuals comprising the various populations?"

Demographic data are collected in several ways. In general, the data that describe the overall profile of United States populations are collected by the census, sample surveys, and vital statistics. Vital statistics include the registration of births, deaths, marriages, divorces, and diseases.[8] The Department of Health, Education and Welfare, the Department of Commerce, and the Public Health Service are examples of agencies which assist in the data collection.[8] Hauser writes,

"As a science, demography is not a unitary field . . . demography not only combines the interests of a number of separate scientific disciplines, but it also straddles the natural and social sciences." [12]

In this section, the example used in the discussion of rates will be epidemiology or the study of the occurrence of disease in a population. [13] It should be remembered that epidemiology is only one example of the demographic method. Other types of demographic data include measurement of the social, economic, or age/sex differentials in populations.

A basic measure in epidemiology is a count of the number of persons in a group being studied who have the characteristic of interest, usually a disease. In order for a count of persons in a group to be meaningful, it must be seen in proportion to the total number in the group being studied. A proportion is a fraction, with the numerator being the number of persons who have the variable of interest. The denominator is the total number of persons in the population being studied. [13] As an example, assume you wish to investigate the incidence of hypertension in a group of men, 40 to 45 years old. If there are 10 persons in the group with hypertension, and 40 persons in the total group being studied, the proportion of rate would be 10/40 or 25 percent. The number 10 would not be descriptive if you did not include the total number of persons in the group. Note the difference between 10/40, 10/400, and 10/4000. Analysis of these rates would have strikingly different implications.

Rates generally involve a time relationship. The most common *morbidity* or *illness* rates are incidence and prevalence. *Incidence* refers to the process of illness developing over a period of time, usually one year. *Prevalence* describes a group at a certain point in time; [13] it describes an event. The temporal frame may be one day, such as the first day in the life of a group of neonates or in the first postpartal day of the mothers.

The *mortality* rate refers to the number of *deaths* over a period of time. Again, the frame of reference is usually a one year period. *Mortality differentials* refer to the differences in the death rates between populations. Table 2-1 shows the proportions used for the most common rates in the study of groups. With comparisons of mortality/morbidity rates, researchers obtain data which are descriptive of the relationships between health, illness, and death within differential populations in the United States. The study of mortality and its relationship to population size, composition, and change has a central place in population research. [8]

Prior to the eighteenth century, the United States mortality rate was at the level of the rates in underdeveloped nations today. A striking decline in mortality was reflected in the eighteenth and early nineteenth centuries. [14] It is interesting that the decline occurred prior to significant advances in medical technology. The major influence for change in the United States death rate was improvement in living conditions through social reform. Matras writes of several major factors: rising levels of living with improved nutrition, hygienic changes through sanitation reforms, and the lowered incidence of communicable disease. [14] In the twentieth century, a second important phenomenon occurred: mortality and morbidity differentials reflected changes in the concepts of health, illness, and death as they assumed new political, moral, and social meanings. The relationships between a highly technologic environment and chronic illness became a dominant focus of the health delivery system.

Historically, population changes are reflective of two major factors influencing mortality control: 1) the exposure to the hazards that lead to death and 2) the quality and acces-

TABLE 2-1.   Common rates used in the study of populations*

I. Morbidity or illness rates

Prevalence rate
(a condition exists)
$$= \frac{\text{No. of persons having a disease}}{\text{Total No. of persons in group being studied}} \quad \begin{array}{l}\text{Per}\\ \text{unit}\\ \text{time}\end{array}$$

Incidence rate
(a condition will develop)
$$= \frac{\text{No. of persons developing a disease}}{\text{Total No. of persons at risk}} \quad \begin{array}{l}\text{Per}\\ \text{unit}\\ \text{time}\end{array}$$

II. Mortality or death rate
$$= \frac{\text{No. of persons dying due to a particular cause or all causes}}{\text{Total number in group}} \quad \begin{array}{l}\text{Per}\\ \text{unit}\\ \text{time}\end{array}$$

Age specific† mortality rate
$$= \frac{\text{No. of persons dying in a particular age group}}{\text{Total No. in same age group}} \quad \begin{array}{l}\text{Per}\\ \text{unit}\\ \text{time}\end{array}$$

III. Crude birth rate‡
(fertility rate)
$$= \frac{\text{Number of births}}{\text{1000 females}} \quad \begin{array}{l}\text{Per}\\ \text{unit}\\ \text{time}\end{array}$$

---

*Compiled from Friedman, Gary D.: *Primer of Epidemiology,* McGraw-Hill, New York, 1974, pp. 7–12.
†Mortality or morbidity rates may be specific for a number of variables such as age, sex, occupation, socioeconomic status, or disease.
‡Unreliable reporting methods may contribute to misleading numbers in this index.

sibility to the treatment of such hazards. [14] The exposure to hazards differs for urban and rural areas, minority and white groups, blue collar and professional occupations, and poverty and affluence. Matras writes of two separate social processes in health care:

> "the first distributes individuals in the society in a manner that exposes them differently to the risks of disease and injury; and the second institutionalizes treatment and care facilities and medical technologies in such a way that they are differentially accessible to different population subgroups." [14]

His points are salient ones, and they direct attention to a stratification in health care which is not easily admitted to in a society that perceives itself to be egalitarian. In your assessment of populations you will need to consider both individual help-seeking be-haviors *and* the structural deterrents to them within the health system. Critical attention to health services and their effectiveness in meeting population needs at the local levels may make a difference in the facilitation of change and in the eventual eradication of the disparate mortality differentials.

The morbidity (illness) rates were once indices of communicable diseases. After having read the section on at-risk populations, you can see that there has been a dramatic shift in the focus of health care in the United States.

> "Morbidity, or the study of illness, is important for four reasons: 1) periods of sickness are likely to involve absence from work and a resultant interference with national pro-

ductivity and family solvency; 2) hospitalization involves economic losses for the individual and his society; 3) the anguish and preoccupation with illness and pain and the fear of bereavement are matters of serious concern even to those who do not experience them; and 4) the social functions and dysfunctions of sickness are integral to the cohesion or disruption of the group."[8]

As technology and medicine have influenced the prolongation of life, many of the illnesses that are most prevalent in society today are no longer fatal. Serious diseases that were once significant factors in the mortality rates are now being controlled. Unfortunately, chronic illness has become a part of everyday life for millions of Americans.

Today, the psychological suffering, physical disabilities, and the economic losses resulting from chornic illnesses are unparalleled. Target populations such as the elderly and those with chronic degenerative diseases are being increasingly identified. A primary objective in their health care is to prevent institutionalization for as long as possible. Hospitals should not be occupied by the chronically ill on a long term basis. Such an event is a depersonalizing experience and causes havoc in the lives of many families. Until there are major structural changes in the health system, the economic and psychologic burdens on health care recipients will remain as they are today.

In summary, the biologic-social continuum of chronic illness presents multifaceted problems to health caretakers. Goals are twofold: 1) to motivate people to take better care of themselves and 2) to mandate government regulations which will protect members of society from the unwarranted influences that lead to illness and disability.

NEW DIRECTIONS IN FERTILITY DIFFERENTIALS

Fertility or the birth rate of a population is the second major determinant in the structure of populations and in demography. Rates similar to those used in mortality and morbidity are applied in calculating the numbers of births each year. By a comparison of birth and death rates, demographers can measure the natural increase of a population.[8]

There are crude and specific birth rates. The crude birth rate, which is the most simple to compute, is widely used as a measure of fertility, but the reliability of this index remains questionable. Many births are not registered, particularly those occurring outside of hospitals.[8] Caution should be used when interpreting the overall reliability of the reported rates, especially in rural areas where there is less access to medical care.

Matras discusses three dimensions of childbearing: marriage, intervention, and values of family size.[14] They are closely interrelated, but are yet to be thoroughly assessed. With the advent of the birth control pill and the expansion of family planning education, it is interesting to note that there continues to be significant resistance to the use of such interventions in the control of family size. The question of why some groups are more resistant than others to such interventions may, in some cases, relate to accessibility, availability, and cost. These influences are becoming less of a reality as family planning clinics have expanded and increased their accessibility to more women in the lower socioeconomic groups.

Studies of class value and belief systems as they relate to family size may prove to be fruitful in furthering an understanding of fertility differentials. Investigations in this area have been reported by Blake[27] and Rainwater.[15]

Rainwater found that in working class families successful family planning was inversely related to the level of role segregation between husband/wife. In other words, when there was minimal communication between spouses in areas of domestic affairs, such as the sexual relationship, childbearing, or financial affairs, there tended to be haphazard family planning.[15] A related point of interest concerns working class families. There was a striking lack of knowledge of the physiologic/anatomic processes of conception. Such educational deficits persisted despite the wife's possession of birth control devices. They were available, but rarely used.[15]

The variable of education in family planning is one which is not well investigated. The reported rates reflect that lower educational levels are not necessarily consistent with large families. The rates do indicate that higher levels of education increase the probability that decision making will be shared and that birth control will be used with more reliability. Although some of the families may be considered large, the sizes are desired outcomes and correlate with planned conceptions. Alternatively, large families in the poor and working classes frequently represent undesired outcomes and increased economic strains.[15]

Variables such as occupation, income, and race are often inversely related to fertility rates in the United States. Such differentials are narrowing as birth control information becomes more available and as traditional variations in family size are modified.[8]

Geographic variables reflect differentials, but distinctions between urban and rural areas are sometimes blurred by a lack of uniformity in boundary designations. Differences exist in the meanings of the terms. Suburbs, for example, are considered by some investigators to be within city limits and by others to be outside of the city.[8]

Thomlinson writes that along with social class, geographic area exerts the most influence on variations in fertility. With the accessibility to urban areas increasing, more rural Americans have access to the offerings of city life.[8] This is, however, oversimplified, for the extreme rural areas in the South have serious problems in fertility control because of the isolation and poverty. For example, birth rates in the United States are highest in the southern and Rocky Mountain areas and lowest in the Northeast. These differences relate to the high proportion of rural areas in southern and mountain states, as compared to those in the Northeast.[8]

The influence of religion is another underinvestigated but important area in fertility studies.[8] It is well known that the Catholic religion prohibits many forms of birth control, but variations by age, mixed marriages, geographic location, socioeconomic status, and education need to be investigated to determine 1) correlations within the Catholic population and 2) differentials between the Catholics, Protestants, Jews, and other religious groups.

In summary, the important point to consider in the discussion of fertility is that relationships between birth rates and variables such as class, geographic location, religion, and education have become obscured. Birth control information is widely disseminated and accessible to many women across classes and socioeconomic groups. The accessibility and availability of clinics has increased and cost is now minimal. Questions must be raised as to the validity of the common perspective that socioeconomic status and fertility differentials are directly related.

The relationship between fertility rates and populations may reflect differentials in family socialization patterns within and between classes. It is suggested here that correlations of family socialization patterns and resistance to reliable birth control usage be investigated. Social constructs may, in the long run, be the variables of interest in fertility studies. Interventions might include assisting women and their partners toward decision making which is reflective of personal choices made in mutual best interest.

MIGRATION: A NEW AREA IN POPULATION ANALYSIS

The third determinant in population study is migration. It is an underdeveloped area, primarily because of the difficulies in collecting the demographic data of persons and families who are frequently changing their residences.

Migration and moving are not synonomous. A mover is one who changes his place of residence, while a migrant is a person who changes his place of residence for a lengthy period of time and crosses a political boundary in the process.[8] Not all persons who make a significant move cross political boundaries, but crossing from one boundary to another is an important demographic distinction. It is also true that people who cross political boundaries significantly impact on the composition of social, cultural, and economic characteristics of an area. This is exemplified by three important groups: 1) the blacks migrating from the South to northern cities; 2) the elderly who are migrating to warmer climates such as Florida and Arizona; and 3) young-middle age professionals and semi-professionals, for whom migration represents promotion and a step upward on the ladder of social mobility.

> "Migration disturbs the age-sex composition of the population, thus altering marriage prospects, and perhaps birth and death rates. Often too, it destroys existing social bonds and institutional ties, replacing old allegiances with membership in new churches, schools, factories and cliques."[8]

People migrate for many reasons, among them climate, occupation, education, economic gain, and the quest for adventure. The major incentive for migration for all socioeconomic groups is economic gain. This often has profound implications on population and community composites.

For example, there was a mass movement to the cities during the period of industrialization in the mid-nineteenth century. Large numbers of migrants and their families moved from rural to urban areas, seeking employment in the factories and better lives for their families. The results for many were increased poverty and unemployment. Jobs were limited and, in addition to families suffering from the effects of unemployment, there was the loss of significant social bonds. The migrants were uninformed about urban living and were not prepared for the events that occurred. This phenomenon remains with us today.

A related point of interest is the black migration from the South to northern urban areas. From 1910 to 1940, 1,750,000 blacks moved to northern cities, and from 1950 to 1960, 1,500,000 moved northward.[8]

An important consideration in the rural-urban migration is the community from which one emigrates. When large numbers of young men and women leave a rural area to move to the city for work, the community they leave loses significant numbers of its work force population. This often has serious economic consequences for that community. As mentioned earlier in the discussion on community characteristics, the community composite becomes less heterogeneous, with economic losses leading to a decrease in growth and in the potential for favorable social change.

There are migration differentials as there are mortality and fertility differentials. The twentieth century reflects a significant increase in migration. A high proportion of migrants is characterized by young to middle age adults. Many are students attending school in another part of the country, and there are large numbers of businessmen or salesmen and their families. Migration is often an inherent aspect of occupations, and as middle/upper middle class executives and their families move to urban areas, communities lose their heterogeneity. Community profiles become characterized by large groups of people sharing similar belief systems, economic status, and levels of education. Thomlinson suggests we are becoming a nation of nomads,[8] and to this one might add the concept of the United States as a melting pot is being realized in many communities. The implications have both positive and negative aspects, for uniformity of populations decreases opportunities for cultural exchanges and for the development of understanding between variant groups.

Recently, a counter trend appears to be developing in populations of elderly migrants. Numbers of older people are increasing as are their levels of financial independence. More people are willing to leave their homes for warmer climates.[8] Communities in such areas provide incentives such as modern housing and social activities directed towards the interests of the elderly.

The stereotype of the migrant is generally quite different from the reality of his characteristics. Migrants are traditionally thought of as people moving from place to place for seasonal employment such as apple picking or tobacco picking. They are perceived as being poor and homeless. This may be true for some, but not the majority of migrants. Other differentials exist with regard to age, sex, race, education, and marital status.[8] Demographers are attempting to describe and classify the data to delineate the effects of migration on the characteristics of migrants and on the communities which they enter and leave.

In summary, demographers ask two major questions in their study of migration differentials: "In what manner and to what extent do migrants differ from nonmigrants?" "How much do people making certain types of moves differ from those making other kinds of moves?"[8]

COMMUNITY ACTION FOR HEALTH

In this chapter, discussion has centered on the characteristics of communities and of the populations which comprise them. An acquisition of this knowledge will enable you to assess demographic profiles of communities. Health status of a group is an important part of such a profile. Areas of need will be designated and goals will be established to effect change. The planning and implementation of change is dependent upon a knowledge of health planning and of community resources. Also, persistance when you encounter obstacles to your goals is an important quality. The purpose of this section is to equip you with a basic knowledge of health planning, consumerism, environmental issues, and community resources.

Health Planning

In 1975 President Ford signed into law the National Health Planning and Resources Development Act of 1974.[16] It was a three year program which involved community groups at the local, state, and federal levels in health planning. Established with the act was a National Council on Health Planning and Development. In addition, Health System Agencies (HSA) were set up across the country.

"The HSA will be generally responsible for preparing and implementing plans designed to improve the health of the residents of its health service area; to increase the accessibility, acceptability, continuity, and quality of health services in the area; to restrain increases in the cost of providing health services; and to prevent unnecessary duplication of health resources."[16]

The governing boards of the HSAs consist of consumers and providers, with the consumers constituting a majority.

Health planning and consumerism are two major concerns in the health care delivery crisis. Costs are escalating, services and providers are disproportionately represented, and consumer satisfaction is low. The Planning and Resources Act of 1974 clearly mandates careful health planning to effectively meet the health needs of all communities and their members, and to insure consumer input into this effort. The plan creates problems which fall into three areas: 1) health planning skills and techniques; 2) adequate consumer preparation and participation in health planning; and 3) environmental issues which impact on health planning.

Health planning skills and techniques are critical elements for the effectiveness of this effort. First, a decision has to be made as to whether health care is a right or a privilege. Senator Kennedy's position is that health care is, indeed, a basic right. Included in this right are the availability of a form of comprehensive care, initiation of a national health insurance program, and an emphasis on disease prevention, health care planning, availability of resources, and accessibility to health services.[17] Pickett assists in clarification of the issue by defining the differences between a privilege and a right. A privilege is a "right which is granted as a special favor. Privileges are inherently private matters. A right is a privilege which has been extended to all people and the preservation and protection of that right becomes a public matter."[18] Health care is not yet a right in this country. He adds that health care could be provided as a right through the existing private system by developing a second system of public practice or through a totally public practice.[18] The latter system offers the most widespread availability of services to consumers with reasonable cost.

A knowledge of methodology is critical in health planning. Robinette identifies 12 steps which must be taken to insure adequate planning. Planning helps one plan or initiate controlled change.[19]

STEPS FOR HEALTH PLANNING

1. Form the philosophy.
2. Forecast the future if interventions suggested are not implemented.
3. Establish goals.
4. Gather data.
5. Formulate objectives.
6. Analyze alternatives.
7. Select a strategy.
8. Program—decide what tasks need to be done in what order.
9. Schedule.
10. Budget.
11. Management control.
12. Evaluation and feedback.[19]

These steps can be applied to planning at all levels—local, state, and federal. It is necessary that all steps be taken for the process of planning to be well organized and maximally effective. Planning involves a clear vision of where one is going and of the ultimate goal to be reached. One also needs to have the skills, a willingness to compromise, and the persistance to complete the task.

Consumer Participation

A second issue of critical importance is consumer participation. The primary rationale for having consumer participation in health planning is that consumers are in the optimal position to address their needs. However, the presence of both consumers and providers on health boards leads to conflicts of interests which often impede the effectiveness of the board.

In a discussion of consumer participation on boards of health centers, Paap identified several issues which impact on their effectiveness. First, the sources of information about health needs and related issues come from the providers and other professionals, rather than from the consumers. Second, the time available for decision making is often quite limited, thus decisions are made pending approval (grant applications are a common example). Third, professionals have career investments in their work, whereas the consumer does not. For example, providers such as physicians have personal and professional contact with their colleagues and community members with influence in decision making. Consumers, on the other hand, have much less contact with political and social organizations in the community.[20] They have relatively little influence in decision making and, as a result, become more involved in administrative issues rather than in the areas of community health needs and effectiveness of existing services.

In addressing the issue of consumer participation, Jonas identifies several steps which would provide the consumer with more input and control. Among these are 1) the need to clearly define the objectives for the creation and strengthening of consumer input; 2) the need for consumers to be involved with the evaluation of programs, rather than the administrative processes; 3) the need to realize that conflict is an inherent part of every social organization and that the health care organization shares problems similar to industrial organizations; 4) the need for consumers and providers to see each other as partners with a mutual goal; and 5) the need to realize that a professional degree does not guarantee an ability to produce a program which is effective in meeting the needs of the groups it serves.[21]

Both consumer and provider members of health boards may represent a degree of risk to each other. There may be reluctance on the part of physicians to allow consumer input in decisions which they consider to be the jurisdiction of their professional community. Consumers may be unwilling to compromise on interest issues which are perceived as needs but which do not realistically represent the interests of the overall community.

There are many health problems in communities, and it is logical that change will progress slowly, with an immediate focus on the priority issues. Consumers and providers have a common goal and each group representative brings to the board his values, belief systems, and perspectives on health needs. Majority consumer representation on planning and service boards is a reality which is here to stay. Both groups will have to exercise patience, understanding, and a willingness to compromise for the board to work most effectively.

Environmental Issues

A third area of importance in the Act of 1974 is its impact on environmental issues. In his evaluation, Pond noted its

> "authority to promote activities for the prevention of disease, including studies of nutritional and environmental factors affecting health and the provision of preventive health care services."[22]

Until recently, the quality of our environment and its relation to health has not been given the attention it deserves. Although there are organizations such as the Environmental Protection Agency and the Environmental Defense Fund, their impact has been sporadic and changes have been slow to emerge. Wegman discusses the role of the environmentalist and states that the environmentalist must understand the interdependence of scientific and social or political decisions, as well as the interdependence of all life systems.[23] Decisions made at the political, social, and environmental levels will impact on each other. An example of particular interest is the use of land.[24-25] Careful utilization of available land must be enforced, whether the purpose for use is recreational, industrial, agricultural, or housing. Community health is inextricably linked to the use of available land space. Galanter writes,

> "strategies will vary with local circumstances, but the opportunities to improve the public health by affecting land use decisions do exist—once we recognize that social decision making is a political process—and resolve to engage in that process."[25]

The implementation of the National Health Planning and Resources Development Act will impact on the health of all communities. The quality of change will be significantly influenced by the ways in which consumers and providers compromise on differences and advance common goals.

The importance of knowing community resources has been stressed throughout the chapter. The use of a variety of services is a critical element in community health. Each health service agency should have a resource file, which lists agencies, services they provide, eligibility requirements, and contant persons. It should be the responsibility of all persons employed in an agency to add to the resource file as new services are identified.

Community Resources

Community resources are classified into many categories. They may be institutional, such as hospitals, schools, child protective services, and churches. Others may be social organizations focused on meeting specific community needs. Examples are day care centers, visiting nurses, neighborhood clinics, halfway houses, counseling services, self-help groups, and recreational services for the elderly, the handicapped, and young people. In the local political and civic arena, they may be lobbyist organizations, PTAs, labor unions, women's groups, and the many other special interest groups which have demonstrated considerable effect on elected officials. Such organizations are common to all communities.

The important point is each community has a diversity of available resources at local, state, and federal levels. Social service agencies abound, and it is necessary to select choices in light of their effectiveness in meeting the needs of the groups to which they are directed. Resource files must be updated on an on-going basis, for the community is dynamic and continually undergoing change of a social, political, and economic nature.

Change may be of two basic types: 1) spontaneous change or the movement which is characteristic of all humans and 2) deliberate or planned change. It is planned change which concerns us here. Planned change employs social knowledge to solve problems of man and society. It is a conscious, deliberate, and collaborative effort to enhance the lives of human beings in their respective environments or social systems. [26] It is the application of knowledge for the purpose of creating intelligent action and change. It is the link between theory and practice. A change agent must be concerned with social processes that bear on changing knowledge into action, decision making, and policy formation.

The power structures of the community must be incorporated into the planning of change. Decision makers are generally those persons or groups in a position of power and authority. They can significantly impact on the success or failure of efforts for change.

Despite obstacles, change agents must be willing to take risks, but efforts must be collaborative. It is difficult, if not impossible, to do it alone. As goals and objectives are formulated, incorporate members of target groups who will often generate enthusiasm and time. Change needs grass roots or local involvement. Special interest groups and political activists can given substantial assistance. You need to determine which groups can provide the most support, and then invite their participation.

Public relations are a boon to any change effort. Utilize the media such as radio, television, newspapers, and pamphlets. Community members need information on which to base intelligent decisions. Differences of opinion are constructive inputs to any change effort. Incorporate the expertise of others into your strategies and acknowledge their efforts and assistance.

In summary, planned change requires foresight and skill. Exciting events take place in communities. Everyone belongs to communities, and, as both provider and consumer of community services, one must be knowledgeable of available services, current issues, and the planning for change. Participation is an important element of community health for it enhances the community spirit that is an integral part of social organizations. It follows that social change gives a community movement and life.

THE NURSING ROLE IN COMMUNITY HEALTH

This chapter has given you a basis on which you can build your knowledge of communities and their populations. An understanding of social, cultural, political, and economic structures in communities is a critical element in the delivery of comprehensive nursing care to community members. You have been introduced to community characteristics such as geographic and physical boundaries, to political characteristics such as power bases, to variants in belief systems/norms of groups, and to major determinants in the study of populations. Changes in the structure of health delivery systems have been discussed, with a focus on the areas of law, consumerism, and planned change.

Nursing in the community may assume variant forms which are directed by the goals of the agency by which the nurse is employed. The nursing role incorporates the provision of direct care, casefinding, health promotion, epidemiology, counseling, and political involvements. The nurse is a resource person to many populations, and he or she acts in the roles of change agent and client advocate.

It should be remembered that community health is a multidisciplinary effort. The nurse is a member of a team which includes providers and consumers. Action, innovation, and perserverance are key elements in the attainment of goals which are directed toward improvements in the quality of people's lives.

REFERENCES

1. Smolensky, Jack: *Principles of Community Health,* 4th ed. W. B. Saunders Company, Philadelphia, 1977.
2. Klein, Donald C.: "The Meaning of Community in a Preventive Mental Health Program." *American Journal of Public Health,* 59(11):2008, 1969.
3. Sanders, I.T.: "Public Health in the Community," in Freeman, H., Levine, S., and Reeder, L.G. (eds.): *Handbook of Medical Sociology.* Prentice-Hall, Inc., Englewood Cliffs, N.J., 1965.
4. Hanlon, John J.: *Public Health Administration and Practice,* 6th ed. The C.V. Mosby Co., St. Louis, 1974.
5. *The American Heritage Dictionary of the English Language,* William Morris (ed.). Houghton Mifflin Company, Boston, 1976.
6. Leininger, Madeleine: "Cultural Diversities of Health and Nursing Care." *Nursing Clinics of North America,* 12(1):5, March 1977.
7. Klein, Donald C.: "The Community and Mental Health: An Attempt at a Conceptual Framework." *Community Mental Health Journal,* 1(4):303, 1965.
8. Thomlinson, Ralph: *Population Dynamics.* Random House, New York, 1965.
9. Boulding, K.E.: "Towards a General Theory of Growth." *Canadian Journal of Economics and Political Science,* 19:326, 1953. Reprinted in Spengler, J.J., and Duncan, O.D.: *Demographic Analysis,* Free Press, Glencoe, Ill., 1956.
10. McKinlay, John B.: "A Case for Refocussing Upstream—The Political Economy of Illness," June 1973, in *Proceedings of American Heart Association Conference,* Seattle, Washington, 1973.
11. Jones, Dorothy A. et al.: *Medical Surgical Nursing, A Conceptual Approach.* McGraw-Hill, New York, 1978.
12. Hauser, Philip M. and Duncan, Otis Dudley: *The Study of Populations.* University of Chicago Press, Chicago, 1959.
13. Friedman, Gary D.: *Primer of Epidemiology,* McGraw-Hill, New York, 1974.
14. Matras, Judah: *Populations and Societies.* Prentice-Hall, Inc., Englewood Cliffs, N.J., 1973.
15. Rainwater, Lee: *And The Poor Get Children:* Sex, Contraception, and Family Planning in the Working Class. Quadrangle Books, Chicago, 1960.
16. Health Planning and Resources Development Act of 1974. U.S. Department of Health, Education and Welfare. DHEW Publication No. (HRA) 75-14015, 1975.
17. Kennedy, Edward M.: "The Congress and National Policy," Fifth Annual Matthew B. Rosenhaus Lecture. *American Journal of Public Health,* 68(3):241, March 1978.
18. Pickett, George E.: "The Basics of Health Policy: Rights and Privileges", The 1977 Presidential Address. *American Journal of Public Health,* 68(3):236, March 1978.
19. Robinette, Tasker K.: "What is Health Planning?" *Nursing Outlook,* 18(1):429, Jan. 1970.
20. Paap, Warren R.: "Consumer—Based Boards of Health Centers: Structural Problems in Achieving Effective Control." *American Journal of Public Health,* 68(6):579, June 1978.
21. Jonas, Steven: "Limitations of Community Control of Health Facilities and Services." *American Journal of Public Health,* 68(6):542, June 1978.
22. Pond, M. Allen: "Environmental Quality As An Issue in the Legislative History of the National Health Planning and Resources Development Act of 1974 (PL. 93-641)." *American Journal of Public Health,* 68(6):585, June 1978.
23. Wegman, David: "The Environmental Challenge." *American Journal of Public Health,* 68(5):489, May 1978.
24. Kaplan, O. Benjamin: "Health Input into Land Use Planning: Experiences in a Land Use Program." *American Journal of Public Health,* 68(5):489, May 1978.

25. Galanter, Ruth B.: "Land Use: Public Health is the Bottom Line." *American Journal of Public Health,* 68(5):446, May 1978.
26. Bennis, Warren et al.: *The Planning of Change,* 3rd ed. Holt, Reinhart & Winston, New York, 1973.
27. Blake, Judith: Family Structure in Jamaica, The Social Context of Reproduction. Free Press, New York, 1961.

BIBLIOGRAPHY

Baltzell, E. Digby (ed.): *The Search for Community in Modern America.* Harper & Row, New York, 1968.

Bennis, Warren et al.: *The Planning of Change,* 3rd ed. Holt, Reinhart & Winston, New York, 1975.

Blake, Judith: *Family Structure in Jamaica, The Social Context of Reproduction.* Free Press, New York, 1961.

Bowman, Rosemary Amoson, and Culpepper, Rebecca Clark: "Power: RX for Change." *American Journal of Nursing,* 74(6):1053, June 1974.

Friedman, Gary D.: *Primer of Epidemiology.* McGraw Hill, New York, 1974.

Galanter, Ruth B.: "Land Use: Public Health Is The the Bottom Line." *American Journal of Public Health,* 68(5):446, May 1978.

George, Madelon; Ide, Kazrejaski; and Vamberg, Clara E.: "The Comprehensive Health Team: A Conceptual Model." Reprint from *Journal of Nursing Administration* (1971), Contemporary Publishing Associates, Inc., Mar/April 1971.

Hanlon, John J.: *Public Health—Administration and Practice,* 6th ed. The C.V. Mosby Company, St. Louis, 1974.

Hauser, P.M., and Duncan, O.D. (eds.): *The Study of Population.* University of Chicago Press, Chicago, 1959.

Health Planning and Resources Development Act of 1974. U.S. Department of Health, Education and Welfare. DHEW Publication No. (HRA) 75-14015, 1975.

Jonas, Steven: "Limitations of Community Control of Health Facilities and Services." *American Journal of Public Health,* 68(6):541, June 1978.

Kaplan, O. Benjamin: "Health Input into Land Use Planning: Experiences in a Land Use Program." *American Journal of Public Health,* 68(6): 489, June 1978.

Kennedy, Edward M.: "The Congress and National Health Policy," Fifth Matthew B. Rosenhaus Lecture. *American Journal of Public Health,* 68(3):241, March 1978.

Klein, Donald C.: "The Meaning of Community in a Preventive Mental Health Program." *American Journal of Public Health,* 59(11):2005, Nov. 1969.

Klein, Donald C.: "The Community and Mental Health: An Attempt at a Conceptual Framework." *Community Mental Health Journal,* 1(4):301, 1965.

Leininger, Madeleine: "Cultural Diversities of Health and Nursing Care." *Nursing Clinics of North America,* 12(1):5, March 1977.

Lippitt, Ronald et al.: *Dynamics of Planned Change.* Harcourt Brace World, New York, 1958.

McKinlay, John B.: *A Case for Refocusing Upstream—The Political Economy of Illness, Applying Behavioral Science to Cardiovascular Risk.* Proceedings of American Heart Association Conference, Seattle, Washington, June 1973.

McNeil, Helen Jo: "How to Become Involved in Community Planning." *Nursing Outlook,* 17(2): 44, Feb. 1969.

Matras, Judah: *Populations and Societies.* Prentice-Hall, Inc., Englewood Cliffs, N.J., 1973.

Milio, Nancy: "Dimensions of Consumer Participation and National Health Legislation." *American Journal of Public Health,* 64(4):357, April 1974.

Novella, Dorothy: "People, Power and Politics for Health Care." *National League for Nursing,* 52-1647:1, 1976.

Paap, Warren R.: "Consumer—Based Boards of Health Centers: Structural Problems in Achieving Effective Control." *American Journal of Public Health,* 68(6):578, 1978.

Pickett, George E.: "The Basics of Health Policy: Rights and Privileges," (The 1977 Presidential Address). *American Journal of Public Health,* 68(3):231, March 1978.

Pond, M. Allen: "Environmental Quality As an Issue in the Legislative History of the National Health Planning and Resource Development Act of 1974 (PL93-641)." *American Journal of Public Health,* 68(6):583, June 1978.

Rainwater, Lee: *And The Poor Get Children:* Sex, Contraception, and Family Planning in the Working Class. Quadrangle Books, Chicago, 1960.

Robinette, Tasker: "What Health Planning?" *Nursing Outlook,* 18(1):33, Jan. 1970.

Sanders, I.T.: "Public Health in the Community," in Freeman, H.E., Levine, S.L., and Reeder, L.G. (eds.): *Handbook of Medical Sociology,* Prentice-Hall, Inc., Englewood Cliffs, N.J., 1965.

Smolensky, Jack: *Principles of Community Health,* 4th ed. W.B. Saunders Company, Philadelphia, 1977.

Thomlinson, Ralph: *Population Dynamics.* Random House, New York, 1965.

Wegman, David: "The Environmentalists Challenge." *American Journal of Public Health,* 68(6):540, June 1978.

Werlin, Stanley H., and Schauffer, Helen H.: "Structuring Policy Development for Consumers Health Education." *American Journal of Public Health,* 68(6):596, June 1978.

CHAPTER **3**
HEALTH AND ILLNESS

LINDA L. JARVIS, M.S.N., R.N.

       Man has pursued the search for health since earliest times. The emphasis on health has changed during the years as man has gained new knowledge, increased technical skills, and improved treatment techniques. Initially the stress was on the eradication of disease, then the prevention of disease, and is now turning to the promotion and maintenance of health. It should be noted that this evolution in the approach to health has been both concurrent and separate at various points in time.

As man gained some degree of control over the occurrence and impact of many common communicable diseases, he could begin to investigate the cause and treatment of noncommunicable diseases such as cardiac and respiratory conditions. He was in a position to seek cause and effect relationships in these various conditions, identify risk factors, and begin to identify high risk populations. Likewise, as knowledge about these conditions became commonly known and as lifestyles and health expectations changed, the focus began to grow towards health maintenance and health prevention areas. We are still very much influenced in the health care field by all these components, and the search for disease eradication continues but there is increasing concern and activity in the areas of prevention and health maintenance and promotion. These areas of health focus have a large impact on health care delivery and health care procedures in the present and will for decades to come.

The 1960s and 1970s brought major challenges and some degree of disequilibrium to the health care field. Consumerism reached an all time high. Consumers questioned the health care system, evaluated its services, and found them often lacking and demanded changes.

Legislation in the form of Medicare and Medicaid provided financing for health services for large numbers of people who previously had had little or no health care coverage or benefits. Environmental issues became important topics for concern. Nothing escaped scrutiny—cars, aerosol cans, nuclear energy plants, hair dyes, food colorings, occupational settings, and many others. People became concerned about what was happening to air, water, noise levels, and waste disposal. Our environment was becoming polluted; action was needed. As more leisure time became available to people, there was concern about how it could be spent. What community services in the form of parks, recreation areas, and transportation were available to facilitate use of this time? Indeed, the last two decades have been turbulent and difficult. We have begun to reexamine our priorities and have often found them lacking. Changes are needed in all spheres of our life—social, economic, educational, recreational, and health. As nurses in community health, our concern and attention must be directed to these and other areas of identified need.

Helping people gain, regain, and maintain their optimal level of health functioning has long been a major goal of the community health nurse regardless of the setting in which she worked. As the health crisis of the 1960s and 1970s surfaced, gained momentum, and impacted on health delivery, it has become increasingly important and necessary for community health nurses to examine their basic philosophy about health and health care, to establish a means to provide it to all persons, and search for new ways to implement changes which the consumer public is demanding. We find ourselves working in a wide variety of health settings where innovative health care delivery is necessary. How we accomplish this is the challenge as roles and expectations of community health nurses change in response to identified needs. Health as a concept, a need, and a goal is the focus of both consumers and health care providers.

COMMUNITY HEALTH NURSE AND HEALTH CONCEPTS

This new emphasis on the concept of health is impacting on the role of the community health nurse. Health care in the United States is big business. In 1973, 7.7 percent of the Gross National Product was spent on health care, which meant over $400 was spent per capita.[1] Jesse M. Scott, in 1974, stated that, "Health and accessibility to health care are no longer viewed as privileges but as birthrights."[2] People want and seek quality health care. The nation is faced with a health crisis—how to provide access for all persons to quality health care at reasonable rates. Health care providers are faced with aiding people in their quest for adequate health care and encouraging health promoting choices rather than health damaging ones in all spheres of daily life.

Educational preparation for health care providers has traditionally been conducted in illness settings. Learning about health has been from a curative and restorative view rather than a prevention or health promotion one. This emphasis, however, is beginning to change. Schools of nursing in many areas are teaching students about the concept of health and are providing clinical experiences in areas where students can apply the nursing process to a healthy population. In studying healthy populations, students can begin to appreciate various lifestyle practices and begin to seek knowledge about those practices which tend to maintain or promote healthy states. This data base can aid them in caring for clients regardless of their health state. They will be able to assess the functional level of the client, reinforce those positive steps being taken, and seek to change or eradicate more unhealthy actions.

Take a look around you. Your own health practices as well as those of your peers, your friends, and the general population may leave much to be desired. There are blatant examples of over indulgence ranging from food and drink to tobacco and drugs. People are making efforts, sometimes with little success, to alter many detrimental health habits. Whether they succeed or not will depend on factors such as motivation, perception of dangers of old practices, and perceived value of change efforts. Nancy Milio states ". . . human beings, professional or nonprofessional provider or consumer, make the easiest choice available to them most of the time and not necessarily because of what they know is most healthful."[3] Knowing this, we need to make the health promoting choices easier, more available, and more reinforcing than health damaging choices. As nurses, we should be advocating an approach of preventive care and the maintenance of a healthy state.

The nurse working in community settings with a sound understanding and appreciation of the health concept will be able to provide realistic and attainable nursing care plans for the population with whom she works. Her efforts at preventive care will be directed at primary, secondary, and/or tertiary levels. Primary level prevention refers to preventing the occurrence of a particular condition or disease, secondary level prevention refers to early diagnosis and treatment, while third level prevention focuses on rehabilitation. Whether providing direct care such as medication teaching and administration or dressing changes, casefinding, referral, crisis intervention, health screening, immunizations, or health education, the community health nurse will seek to maintain or improve the health status and functioning of the individual, family, and community.

In order to meet the above goal, it is imperative that nurses carefully examine their philosophy of health and their health care role. We are accountable for our individual health as well as professional practice. We are resource persons with a responsibility to help people evaluate health choices and then make the best one possible. We are expected to be role models. It is very difficult to assist people in healthful habits if we, as nurses, are practicing the same poor health habits we seek to change in others. Particular practices which come to mind are smoking, over indulgence of food and drink, inactivity, and over-work. We need to seek the means to become active change agents for improved health for our clients and ourselves. This involves an evaluation of our personal health philosophy, our professional role philosophy, and an examination of the population with whom we deliver services. Never forget that what we individually believe about health and illness will impact on our expectations of others and the depth and quality of care we provide.

HEALTH AND ILLNESS DEFINITIONS

Health is a dynamic state which is individually perceived. To understand health and illness requires a careful study of both self and the population with whom one works. Factors such as culture, education, economics, geographic location, and health care availability all impact on the health of individuals, families, and communities. Whether or not an individual or family chooses to practice preventive health care will depend in part on the factors cited above. Understanding the health practices and attitudes of the group with whom you work will provide clues to establishing effective health promoting nursing care plans.

There are many definitions of health and illness. The one you choose to embrace for your own reference will depend on your own philosophy, education, and attitudes toward health. It is important to keep in mind that there is no one accepted definition of either term. When examining any definition, the orientation of the author will most certainly be evident. Consider this as you evaluate the following definitions and points of view, representing some current thought on this topic.

HEALTH

1. Health is "a state of an organism with respect to functioning, disease, and abnormality at any given time." (American Heritage Dictionary[4])
2. "Health is a state of complete physical, mental, and social well being and not merely the absence of disease or infirmity." (World Health Organization, 1960[5])
3. "Health is a state of physical, mental, and social well being and the ability to function and not merely the absence of illness or infirmity." (Terris[6])
4. "Health must be defined and measured in terms of adaptive capacity toward environmental circumstances and hazards. When adaptability fails, he is ill." (Sargent[7])
5. "Optimal health is not a condition of an individual but a state of interaction between self and the environment. It is a ceaseless struggle between a basically hostile environment and a series of defenses we are endowed with and which we add to when necessary. The homeostatic balance of forces is our goal and this may be accomplished by decreasing the threat of the environment or raising the capacity of the host to defend himself." (Besson[8])
6. Health is a "dynamic, constantly varying attribute, rather than a complete state of any kind, including disease." (Skrovan[9])

ILLNESS/DISEASE

1. Illness—"sickness of body or mind." Disease is "an abnormal condition of an organism or part, especially as a consequence of infection, inherent weakness, or environmental stress that impairs normal physiological functioning." (American Heritage Dictionary[4])
2. Disease—"A reaction to a stress which extends beyond the bounds of the individual reserve and adaptability." (Francis[10])
3. "Human disease is a dynamic process manifest in diseases, pathologic conditions, impairment of structure and function, psychosomatic disturbances and maladaptive behavior and personality changes. Disease is determined by multiple interacting genetic, environmental, and individual variables, not by single factors acting alone." (Hoyman[11])
4. "Disease is the maladjustment of the existing environment to the host." (Reverley[12])
5. Illness is "failures or disturbances in the growth, development, function and adjustment of the organism as a whole or any of its system." (Engel[13])
6. "Disease is a state in which the individual is no longer in a state of equilibrium with the forces in his external and internal environment." (Beland[14])

It should be clear that there is great diversity of opinion about the meaning of health and illness. However, there seems to be agreement that both terms represent interactive states between social, physical, psychological, and/or environmental factors.

Several points are important to discuss here. Perhaps the most critical one is that health is not only the absence of disease but encompasses all of man's well being including social, psychological, and spiritual dimensions as well as environmental, economic, educational, and recreational factors. It is probable that no one ever reaches a utopian/perfect state of health. Factors such as genetic constitution, stress, and the work-home-leisure environment are constantly impacting on man to variable degrees. A breakdown in any of these areas can impede concentration, task completion, and feelings of well being and produce symptoms such as headaches, gastric disturbances, and generalized pain. This can lead to a state of unhealth even though there is no disease or pathology present.

Another important point is that the health state is dynamic. As stated above, there is a variety of factors which can affect it. However, it is never static but constantly changing in all dimensions as man interacts with his environment. Man's ability to adapt will most likely determine whether he is healthy or ill.

A third point of consideration is that health is an individually perceived state. Attitudes about health are culturally and educationally based. Leininger states "a person's reaction to illness, health maintenance, daily activities, body discomforts, changes in life, food preferences, and various caring and curing treatment practices are all linked with cultural beliefs, values, and experiences."[15] Health attitudes can be changed through the educational process. However, before changes are designed and implemented it is critical to understand the basis of the attitude in question and determine its real impact on the maintenance or promotion of health. Nurse-client conflict about health attitudes/behaviors can impede the nursing process. It is the nurse's responsibility to seek knowledge and understanding concerning cultural practices.

The fourth point to be made is that nurses bring their own cultural beliefs, attitudes, and educational background to any client interaction. These can impact on the quality and quantity of care the nurse is able to provide. It is necessary to be aware of these factors when engaging in client interactions. Often times the cultural and educational differences are not great handicaps and can be resolved with little difficulty. However, in those situations when conflict is impeding therapeutic interaction, it is better to turn the client case over to others, if possible, and take time to examine the conflicts. Ways can then be sought to avoid a similar conflict in the future and to be more understanding of cultural and attitudinal differences.

The health and illness definitions cited earlier should give you some points of references. It is not intended to be an inclusive list. The purpose was to provide you with a selection of viewpoints which you could use in developing your own definition of health and illness. Keep in mind that both are interactive and influenced by a variety of factors.

HEALTH-ILLNESS CONTINUUM

The health-illness continuum is a hypothetical graduated scale for measuring an individual's state of health. Anyone's rank on the scale is dynamic, individualized, and subject to all of the factors mentioned earlier which impact on health. The range of the continuum is from a state of optimal health at one pole to death at the other pole. Terris attempted to diagram the health-illness continuum in Figures 3-1 and 3-2. Figure 3-1 demonstrates that both health and illness states are subject to a variation within that state. Movement along the continuum can be gradual in either direction, static for either condition at a given plateau, or rapid in change in either direction. Changes in any case will be individually determined. Figure 3-2 adds the dimensions of subjective and objective response to a condition as well as the concept of function. Theoretically, as the disease process one experiences progresses, feelings of

HEALTH				ILLNESS			
++++	+++	++	+	+	++	+++	++++

FIGURE 3-1. The health-illness continuum. (From Terris, M.: Approaches to an Epidemology of Health. *Am. J. Public Health* 65(10):1038, 1975, with permission.)

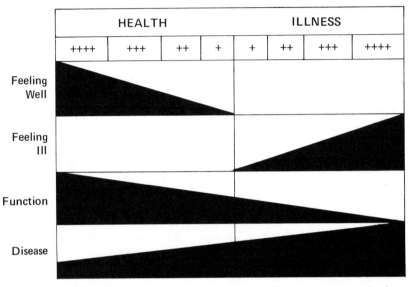

FIGURE 3-2.   The health-illness continuum: subjective and objective aspects and relative disease. (From Terris, M.: Approaches to an Epidemiology of Health. *Am. J. Public Health* 65(10):1038, 1975, with permission.)

wellness decrease, feelings of illness increase, and functional capacity decreases in direct proportion to the unhealthy state. It should be noted that the term disease refers not just to pathophysiologic conditions but also alterations in the social, psychological, and spiritual dimensions of the individual. Terris contends that the subjective aspects of health pertain to how the person feels physically, emotionally, and socially while the functional aspects of health focus on the degree of interference with one's ability to carry out usual activities.[6] "The severity of illness is determined largely by the degree of interference with function."[6]

Dunn views health from a wellness reference point. He contends that wellness is not just a single amorphous condition but rather it is a complex state made up of overlapping levels of wellness which is an everchanging panorama of life itself.[17] It is important to stop considering sickness and wellness as a dichotomy and think of it as a graduated scale.[16]

Because the health-illness continuum considers emotional and social issues as well as physical ones in determining the health status of an individual, it can be less than optimal even though there is no clinical or subclinical disease present. The healthy state is an interrelationship of all three spheres. A breakdown in one will impact on the others. For example, consider a person under stress because of marital difficulties or a student concerned over passing a particular exam. What kinds of things might begin to happen in both of these people? Their ability to concentrate may decrease leading to forgetfulness and wasteful repetition of behaviors, sleep patterns may change requiring more or less sleep than normal but not producing restful sleep, appetite changes may occur leading to anorexia or overindulgence, communication skills may become impaired leading to misunderstandings and unrelayed messages, headaches and gastric symptoms may become evident. There are many other symptoms and changes which could occur. The point, however, is that any individual can experience a health status change from a variety of conditions. Another example involves a bicyclist who fractures his leg in a cycle accident. Assuming he was in optimal health in all three areas, this accident may render him incapacitated and dependent on others for many services. Although the condition is time limited, his ability to carry on activities of daily living, earn a livelihood, and interact socially with others may be greatly impaired causing him many health problems and concerns.

The use of the health-illness continuum will assist the health care provider in gaging the relative level of an individual's health. How well this is done is dependent on the skill, orientation, and philosophy of the practitioner.

MEASUREMENT OF HEALTH AND HEALTH BEHAVIOR

It is interesting and frustrating to note that, as yet, in spite of over two decades of increasing interest and research, there are no reliable tools available for measuring health. In fact, when we attempt to measure health, we resort to negative terms such as morbidity rates, mortality rates, accident rates, and absenteeism. This puts us in a position of identifying what an individual, family, or community does not have rather than its positive attributes.

Dunn suggests that a tool for measuring wellness should be calibrated in biochemical, physiologic, and psychological terms which would enable physicians to recognize low level wellness and develop therapies to raise lower levels to higher ones.[16] The tool should be designed for use by many disciplines. In looking at possible ways to measure levels of wellness in the family one should examine the following:

1. What are the day to day functional and emotional interrelationships of the family members?
2. What activities occupy the family and its members?
3. What values are important to the family and its members?
4: To what degree does the illness or wellness of a family member reflect the health status of the family as a unit?[16]

The nursing process is the tool to use in gathering and analyzing the data suggested above. With a careful analysis of the family members and their interactions, the nurse would be in a strong position to design and implement, with the cooperation of the family, a nursing care plan which would deal with health oriented priorities.

In attempting to measure the health state of individuals, families, and communities, one must seek an understanding of factors affecting health. Beliefs about health and health care of both the consumer and provider impact on the quality of care given and the utilization of care available. Consider the following statements:

1. "The patient's theoretical concept of health, though he may have devoted little conscious time to such beliefs, has a direct bearing upon his health and illness behavior."[17]
2. "The beliefs of the health professional dealing with the patient also extensively influence the care the patient is given during an illness. The professional's beliefs also profoundly influence the development of health care for the broader community."[17]
3. "A person's reaction to illness, health maintenance, daily activities, body discomforts, changes in life, food preferences, and various caring and curing treatment practices are all linked with cultural beliefs, values, and experiences."[15]
4. "To improve the health of the man on the street, you must learn to think like the people in the community."[18]

Health care utilization and delivery is influenced by a multitude of factors. Both the consumer and provider have a responsibility to analyze these factors and then design health programs which will impact favorably on the well being of the population as a whole. People practice health maintenance behavior based on their culture, education, and past experience with health and illness. It is important to keep this in mind whenever noncompliance is an issue in health behavior. There is usually good cause for the action or nonaction and it must be identified if health progress is to be made.

During the 1950s and 1960s a group of social psychologists began to investigate personal health behavior. Rosenstack and others developed what is now known as the Health Belief Model[21] (Fig. 3-3). Use of this model can aid in examining health behaviors, predicting compliance with recommended health regimens. There are three main areas of impact in this model, 1) perceived susceptibility to and seriousness of disease X, 2) modifying factors, and 3) likelihood of action. The perception of susceptibility and seriousness is individualized based on knowledge, emotional factors, and concern about the kind of difficulties the disease can cause.

Modifying factors include prior contact with the disease in family or friends, advice from family, friends, peers, and health professionals, age, sex, and social class.[19] If the perceived benefits of taking a particular preventive action outweigh the perceived barriers to action, the individual will carry through with the desired preventive health behavior.

Critical to this model and the one explaining sick role behavior is the concept of perception. The way an individual, family, and community perceive or detect potential health threats will be instrumental in their eventual health behavior, whether positive or negative. A young mother who has seen her brother suffer the crippling effects of polio will be more likely, theoretically, to comply with preventive immunization programs at the designated time than one who has no intimate knowledge of the disease. Further, efforts at weight control or smoking cessation might be more rigorous for one who has experienced the social stigma of obesity or lived with a family member who has developed emphysema as a direct result of smoking. For these people, the perceived susceptibility is great enough to stimulate action on their part to prevent the condition.

The model for predicting and explaining sick role behavior (Fig. 3-4) also has three components 1) readiness to undertake recommended sick role behavior, 2) modifying and enabling factors, 3) sick role behaviors-likelihood of compliance.[20] While motivation is the key concept in this model, factors such as susceptibility, concern about health matters, and benefits of the treatment regimen also are important. People seem to be questioning the benefit of the treatment more often. For example, if a surgical procedure for cancer is not going to significantly prolong life, some people will decide that quality of life without dealing with the surgical trauma is more important than the recommended surgical treatment. They have weighed the regimen efficacy and found it lacking. Guardians and patients themselves are making decisions about whether or not to utilize heroic life saving measures when cure is not possible and quality of life is low. As consumers become more knowledgable about health and treatment alternatives, they will be challenging the health care provider to take a broader view of these actions and comply with the consumer's wishes, even when these are contradictory to those of the provider. It is a hard lesson to learn.

Utilization of the Health Belief Model to predict both preventive and sick role behavior can be useful to the nurse. It provides a format for data collection and analysis to give clues to behavior from which to design and implement nursing care plans.

Lewis describes the following three areas of health behavior:

1. "An individual's own personal health, the manner in which he manages self maintenance and copes with problems related to his personal well being."
2. "The individual's relationship to his source of health care and the manner in which he

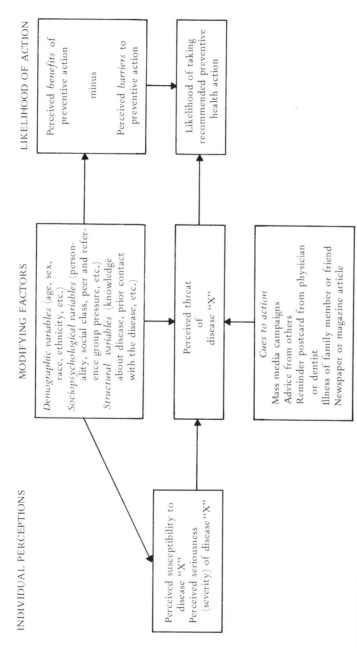

FIGURE 3-3. Health Belief Model. (From Rosenstack, I.: Historical origins of the health belief model, in Becker, M.H. (ed.): *The Health Belief Model and Personal Health Behavior.* Charles B. Slack, Inc., Thorofare, N.J., 1974, with permission.)

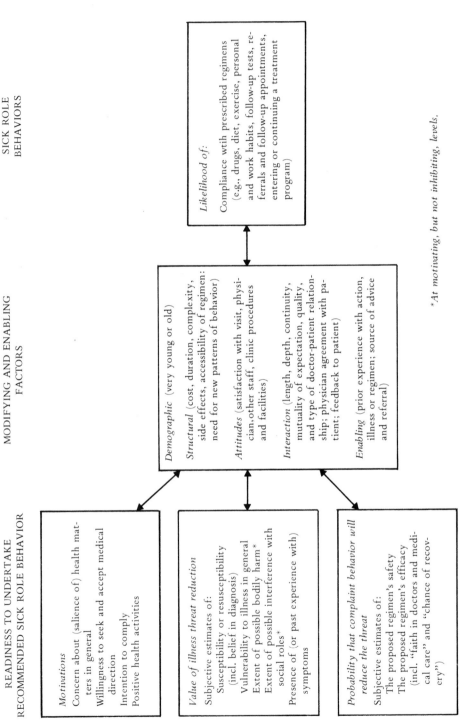

FIGURE 3-4.   Sick Role Model. (From Becker, M.H.: The Health belief model and sick role behavior, in Becker, M.H. (ed.): *The Health Belief Model and Personal Health Behavior.* Charles B. Slack, Inc., Thorofare, N.J., 1974, with permission.)

utilizes the care available, appropriateness of his contact with the health care system, the data he presents to the health care professional, his utilization of the care received."

3. "His relationship to the larger community and the health care system as a whole— active involvement in maintaining or improving community facilities of that community."[17]

The interaction of these three component parts determines the quality and quantity of health care available. Appropriate utilization by the consumer, access to health care through the community, and high quality, respectful, and sensitive care by health care providers can result in desirable health behavior and a higher level of health of the consumer.

In examining factors impacting on the health status of any given population, both individual and public factors must be examined. They will influence the health of the population either positively or negatively. Zubkoff and Dunlop identify three categories of environmental problems:

1. "Those related to the technological process of industrialization such as air and water pollution."
2. "Personal living habits related to such activities as recreation, patterns of leisure that contain little exercise and smoking and other over-indulgences of various kinds."
3. "The syndrome of poverty which has environmental components such as poor housing and sanitation."[21]

In the public domain, they identify two basic types of preventive health services:

1. "Those individually consumed such as immunizations and vaccines, antenatal services, family planning services, multiphasic screening services, child welfare services, health exams and single disease screening services such as tuberculosis and diabetes."
2. "Publically consumed such as water supplies, liquid and solid waste disposal, the control of air and noise pollution, standards of food sanitation, control of substance abuse including drugs, building standards, occupational safety, control of radiologic hazards, transportation safety, control of vectors such as rats and insects and health education."[21]

The interaction of environmental problems plus public efforts to control, prevent, or eliminate them will impact on the health of the population. The nurse has a responsibility to seek data about these factors and utilize this information in the development of nursing care plans. At no time can one assume that health status and behavior is related to a single factor. Physical, social, psychological, and environmental factors all interrelate and thus impact on the health of the individual, family, and community.

From the preceding material, it should be clear that the measurement of health is an inexact science. Our measurement tools are negatively oriented, that is they tell us what is not rather than what is. We do not possess a tool which enables us to reliably define or describe the health state of an individual. We are striving for the development of such a tool. In that pursuit we are examining the beliefs and behaviors of populations regarding health and illness, seeking cause and effect relationships of various factors influencing health, seeking data concerning the behavior of health care providers, and seeking to apply this data to the health behavior of the population in question. It is hoped that these efforts will bring us closer to the development of a health status tool.

RELEVANCE OF THE HEALTH CONCEPT FOR COMMUNITY HEALTH NURSES

Dealing with issues of health and illness is difficult, time consuming, but critically important if we are to have a viable, available health delivery system in this country. Consumers are becoming more knowledgable and sophisticated in their expectations of health care and health care providers. Disease eradication is beginning to take a back seat to prevention and health maintenance and promotion.

Nursing has a role in helping individuals, families, and communities to experience their optimal level of health. Our own attitudes and beliefs about health and health behavior need careful examination. We must never forget that these attitudes and beliefs impact on the quality of care we provide. By a broad understanding of ourselves and the population with whom we work, we can provide effective health maintenance and health promoting care.

Until the time comes that a reliable tool is available for measuring the positive health state of the individual, we can continue to apply the nursing process to collect and validate health data. Our search should be for factors and activities which seem to promote and sustain healthy behaviors. As we collect data on actions which seem to promote healthful living, we can investigate them and, where appropriate, incorporate these suggestions into nursing care plans.

The role nurses play in the quest for improved health levels for all persons should be active, sensitive, and based on scientific knowledge. Because of our close contact in community health with individuals and families, health care providers, and the community at large, we are in an excellent position to influence health behaviors and levels. Knowledge gained about health and illness behaviors should be shared with others. Active participation in the search for ways to promote and maintain health and prevent illness should be sought. This information can then be applied via the nursing process to provide care to the individual, family, and community.

We are on an exciting threshold of health delivery. Social and psychological concerns are gaining as much importance as physiologic ones in understanding the health of populations. Nursing has a large contribution to make to the store of knowledge in the area of health maintenance and promotion.

REFERENCES

1. Compendium of National Health Expenditures. Data compiled by Barbara S. Cooper, Nancy L. Worthington, and Mary F. McGee. U.S. Department of Health, Education, and Welfare. DHEW Publication No. (SSA) 76-11927 (January) 1976, p. 4.
2. Scott, J.M.: "The Changing Health Care Environment, Its Implications for Nursing." *American Journal of Public Health*, 64(4):364, April 1974.
3. Milio, Nancy: "A Framework for Prevention: Changing Health Damaging to Health Generating Life Patterns." *American Journal of Public Health*, 66(5):435, 1976.
4. *The American Heritage Dictionary of the English Language*, William Morris, ed. Houghton Mifflin Company, Boston, 1976.
5. World Health Organization: *Constitution: World Health Organization*. Geneva, 1971.
6. Terris, Milton: "Approaches to an Epidemology of Health." *American Journal of Public Health*, 65(10):1038, Oct. 1975.

7. Sargent, Fredrick: "Man-Environment-Problem for Public Health." *American Journal of Public Health,* 62(5):631, May 1972.
8. Besson, Gerald: "The Health-Illness Spectrum." *American Journal of Public Health,* 57(11):1904, Nov. 1967.
9. Skrovan, Clarence, Anderson, Elizabeth, and Gottschalk, Janet: "Community Nurse Practitioner-An Emerging Role."*American Journal of Public Health,* 64(9):848, Sept. 1974.
10. Francis, Thomas, Jr.: "Research in Preventive Medicine." *Journal of the American Medical Association,* 172(3):994, March 1960.
11. Hoyman, Howard S.: "Rethinking an Ecologic System Model of Man's Health, Disease, Aging, Death." *American Journal of Public Health.* 65(9):516, Sept. 1975.
12. Reverley, Susan: "A Perspective on the Root Causes of Illness." *American Journal of Public Health,* 62(8):1140, Aug. 1972.
13. Engel, G.L. "A Unified Concept of Health and Disease." *Perspectives in Biology and Medicine,* 3:459, Summer 1960.
14. Beland, Irene L., and Passos, Joyce Y.: *Clinical Nursing-Pathophysiological and Psychological Approaches,* 3rd ed. Macmillan Publishing Company, Inc., New York, 1975.
15. Leininger, Madeleine: "Cultural Diversities of Health and Nursing Care." *Nursing Clinics of North America,* 12(1):5, March 1977.
16. Dunn, Halbert L.: "High Level Wellness for Man and Society." *American Journal of Public Health,* 49(6):786, June 1959.
17. Lewis, W.R.: "Health Behavior and Quality Assurance." *Nursing Clinics of North America,* 9(2):359, June 1974.
18. Johnston, Maxene: "Folk Beliefs and Ethnoculture Behavior in Pediatrics." *Nursing Clinics of North America,* 12(1):77, March 1977.
19. Rosenstack, Irwin: "Historical Origins of the Health Belief Model," in Becker, M.H. (ed.): *The Health Belief Model and Personal Health Behavior.* Charles B. Slack, Inc., Thorofare, New Jersey, 1974.
20. Becker, Marshall H.: "The Health Belief Model and Sick Role Behavior," in Becker, M.H. (ed.): *The Health Belief Model and Personal Health Behavior.* Charles B. Slack, Inc., Thorofare, New Jersey, 1974.
21. Zubkoff, Michael, and Dunlop, David: "Consumer Behavior in Preventive Health Services," in Mushkin, S.J. (ed.): *Consumer Incentive for Health Care.* Published for the Milbank Memorial Fund by PRODIST, New York, 1974.

BIBLIOGRAPHY

Becker, Marshall H.: "The Health Belief Model and Sick Role Behavior," in Becker, M.H. (ed.): *The Health Belief Model and Personal Health Behavior.* Charles B. Slack, Inc., Thorofare, New Jersey, 1974.
Becker, Marshall H., Drackman, Robert H., and Kirscht, John P.: "A New Approach to Explaining Sick-Role Behavior in Low Income Populations." *American Journal of Public Health,* 64(3):205, March 1974.
Beland, Irene L., and Passos, Joyce Y.: *Clinical Nursing—Pathophysiological and Psychological Approaches,* 3rd ed. Macmillan Publishing Company, Inc., New York, 1975.
Besson, Gerald: "The Health-Illness Spectrum." *American Journal of Public Health,* 57(11):1904, Nov. 1967.
Compendium of National Health Expenditures. Data Compiled by Barbara S. Cooper, Nancy L. Worthington, and Mary F. McGee. U.S. Department of Health, Education and Welfare, DHEW Pub. No. (SSA) 76-11927, (January 1976) pg. 4.
Dubos, René: *Mirage of Health.* Harper & Row Publishers, New York, 1959.
Dunn, Halbert: "High Level Wellness for Man and Society." *American Journal of Public Health,* 49 (6):786, June 1959.
Engel, G.L.: "A Unified Concept of Health and Disease." *Perspectives in Biology and Medicine* 3:459, Summer 1960.
Francis, Thomas, Jr.: "Research in Preventive Medicine." *Journal of the American Medical Association,* 172(3):994, March 1960.

Hart, S.E.: "An Overview of Health—A Conceptual Model." *National League for Nursing Publication,* No. 52-1472, 1973.

Hoyman, Howard S.: "Rethinking on Ecologic System Model of Man's Health, Disease, Aging, Death." *American Journal of Public Health,* 65(9):516, Sept. 1975.

Johnston, Maxene: "Folk Beliefs and Ethnocultural Behavior in Pedaitrics." *Nursing Clinics of North America,* 12(1):77, March 1977.

Leininger, Madeleine. "Cultural Diversities of Health and Nursing Care." *Nursing Clinics of North America,* 12(1):5, March 1977.

Lewis, W.R.: "Health Behavior and Quality Assurance." *Nursing Clinics of North America,* 9(2):359, June 1974.

Maiman, Lois, and Becker, Marshall H.: "The Health Belief Model: Origins and Correlates in Psychological Theory," in Becker, M.H. (ed.): *The Health Belief Model and Personal Health Behavior.* Charles B. Slack, Inc., Thorofare, N.J., 1974.

Milio, Nancy: "A Framework for Prevention: Changing Health Damaging to Health Generating Life Patterns." *American Journal of Public Health,* 66(5):435, 1976.

Milio, Nancy: "Dimensions of Consumer Participation and National Health Legislation." *American Journal of Public Health,* 64(4):357, April 1974.

Murphy, Michael J.: "The Development of a Community Health Orientation Scale." *American Journal of Public Health,* 65(12):1293, Dec. 1975.

Novella, Dorothy: "People, Power and Politics for Health Care." *National League for Nursing Publications,* No. 52-1647, 1976.

Pender, Nola J.: "A Conceptual Model for Preventive Health Behavior." *Nursing Outlook,* 23(6):385, June 1975.

Reverley, Susan: "A Perspective on the Root Causes of Illness." *American Journal of Public Health,* 62(8):1140, Aug. 1972.

Rosenstack, Irwin: "Historical Origins of the Health Belief Model, "in Becker, M.H. (ed.): *The Health Belief Model and Personal Behavior.* Charles B. Slack, Inc., Thorofare, N.J., 1974.

Sargent, Frederick II: "Man-Environment-Problems for Public Health." *American Journal of Public Health,* 62(5):631, May 1972.

Schweitzer, Stuart: "Incentives and the Consumption of Preventive Health Care Services," in Mushkin, S.J. (ed.): *Consumer Incentives for Health Care.* Published for the Milbank Memorial Fund by PRODIST, New York, 1974.

Scott, J.M.: "The Changing Health Care Environment—Its Implications for Nursing." *American Journal of Public Health,* 64(4):364, April 1974.

Skrovan, Clarence, Anderson, Elizabeth, and Gottschalk, Janet: "Community Nurse Practitioners-An Emerging Role." *American Journal of Public Health,* 64(9):848, Sept. 1974.

Sleeper, Ruth: "Issues in Health Care." The Edna A. Fagan Health Care Lecture Series. *National League for Nursing Publications.* No. 14-1599, 1976.

Terris, Milton: "Approaches to An Epidemology of Health." *American Journal of Public Health,* 65(10):1038, Oct. 1975.

Terris, Milton: "Crisis and Change in America's Health System." *American Journal of Public Health,* 63(4):313, April 1973.

Walsh, Margaret E.: "Health Issues of Today—Perspective For Tomorrow." *National League for Nursing Publications.* No. 14-1613. 1976.

World Health Organization. *Constitution World Health Organization,* 22nd ed. Geneva, April, 1971

Zubkoff, Michael, and Dunlop, David: "Consumer Behavior in Preventive Health Services," in Mushkin, S.J. (ed.): *Consumer Incentives for Health Care.* Published for the Milbank Memorial Fund by PRODIST, New York, 1974.

4
COMMUNITY HEALTH NURSING

LINDA L. JARVIS, M.S.N., R.N.

Nursing is presently in the throes of professional examination and change. Issues are challenging nursing practice and philosophy on all sides. The decisions which are eventually made will impact on the quality and quantity of nursing practice for years to come.

The issues are broad. Perhaps most emotional is that of extended or expanded roles for nurses. Definitions and guidelines for such roles are being developed, implemented, and evaluated in all parts of the country. Also of interest is the issue of independent nursing practice—where is this done, by whom, and under what auspices if any? The need for nursing research to establish a body of nursing knowledge for the legitimization of nursing as a full fledged profession has long been sought. Indeed many nurse-scientists are busily trying to address such issues as what is nursing, what are its unique characteristics, and what is a nurse. When faced with the challenge of new health care providers, answers to these questions have even more impact.

If expanded or extended roles are to be embraced by nurses, there is need for change in state nurse practice acts—a process which was begun in 1971 in Idaho. Distribution of nursing personnel, development of third party payment mechanisms for nursing services, and an increasing need to orient ourselves in a health promotion and maintenance direction rather than in an illness direction are all needs which must be faced directly by nurses and nursing if we are to survive as members of the health team.

The practice of community health nursing has not escaped the impact, confusion, and upheaval of these issues. It is becoming increasingly important for community health nursing to reinforce itself as a specialty with a distinct philosophy, goals, services, and boundaries. As community health principles are integrated increasingly into curricula, there is a real danger that the uniqueness of this specialty will be weakened and perhaps lost forever.

In the pages which follow, we will examine the definition of community health nursing, study some views and theories about nursing and their impact on community health nursing, and examine some current issues in community health nursing practice. It is my opinion that community health nursing is a broad based specialty within the field of nursing which has as its major goal the promotion and maintenance of health and healthful living practices. How this goal is implemented becomes the major challenge for the community health nurse.

VIEWS AND DEFINITIONS OF COMMUNITY HEALTH NURSING

The American Nurses' Association defines community health nursing as:

> "a synthesis of nursing practice and public health practice applied to promoting and preserving the health of populations. The nature of this practice is general and comprehensive. It is not limited to a particular age or diagnostic group. It is continuing, not episodic. The dominate responsibility is to the population as a whole. Therefore, nursing directed to individuals, families or groups contributes to the health of the total population. Health promotion, health maintenance, health education, coordination and continuity of care are utilized in a holistic approach to the family, group and community. The nurse's actions acknowledge the need for comprehensive health planning, recognize the influences of social and ecological issues, give attention to populations at risk and utilize the dynamic forces which influence change."[1]

Tinkham and Voorhies define community health nursing as "the field of nursing in which the family and community are patients. Although it is concerned with the total health-illness spectrum, its primary focus is on the prevention of disease and the promotion and maintenance of the highest level of health and well being."[2]

Freeman describes community health nursing as "a unique blend of nursing and public health practice woven into a human service that, properly developed and applied, could have a tremendous impact on human well being." It is involved in the entire spectrum of health services for the benefit of the community.[3]

Above all else, community health nursing is oriented to the well being of the community at large. Regardless of the definition of the community in which she works, the community health nurse is concerned with the quality of health for all people whatever their age, sex, socioeconomic, or educational characteristics. Although she may deliver direct care to individuals and families and may practice in a wide variety of settings, she must never loose sight of her main focus—the health of the total population.

There are many health settings and target groups with whom she works. Several of these will be discussed in more depth later. For our present purposes, her work settings include schools, occupational sites, official and nonofficial agencies, housing complexes, ambulatory units, hospitals, and theoretically any other setting where health needs can be a major area of focus. As the settings can vary so also can the population target groups— the young, elderly, pregnant, healthy, ill, depressed, rich, poor, educated, uneducated, employed, unemployed, and any others can become the target for community health nursing care.

The focus is health oriented. Positive health practices and attitudes are identified and reinforced and primary, secondary, and tertiary preventive measures are implemented as necessary to prevent illness or modify its impact. This will be discussed in more detail later.

Practitioners in community health nursing come from a variety of nursing backgrounds. The issue of acceptable minimal levels of educational preparation for nursing in general and community health nursing specifically is and will probably continue to be a focus of debate for some time to come. However, according to a 1968 statement by the National League for Nursing, Department of Baccalaureate and Higher Degree Programs, there are two distinct levels of professional nurses practicing in public health.[4] The first is the *public health nurse generalist*[4] who is a graduate of a baccalaureate nursing program which has provided introductory public health content which is needed for professional nursing practice in any setting and is practicing in the field of public health. The second professional level of practitioners is the *public health nurse specialist*[4] who has a master's degree in public health nursing. These practitioners have responsibility for planning, implementing, and evaluating community nursing services.

With the advent of the nurse practitioner movement, many community health nurses are completing programs which will provide them with skills necessary for expanded practice. There are a large variety of programs available including family nurse practitioner, gerontology nurse practitioner, school nurse practitioner, community nurse practitioner, and pediatric nurse practitioner. These nurses are prepared to provide primary care services and long term care of chronic conditions. The exact role, position, and impact they will have on community health nursing is yet to be seen. As decisions about nurse practitioner preparation and job descriptions are evolved in nursing as a whole, they will impact on the practice of community health nursing.

In considering these position descriptions, it is important to keep several issues in mind. One is of the philosophical difference between the so-called technical nurse and the professional nurse. The former is a graduate of an associate degree or diploma program while the latter is a graduate of a baccalaureate program.[5] Since many nursing programs at all three levels provide the student with some degree of community health concepts, this further clouds the distinction between the roles. Also, agencies, due to size, location, and need may hire nurses from any of the three areas which makes for further confusion about the qualifications necessary to practice community health nursing. This is not to say that nurses from nonbaccalaureate programs are not providing quality care, however, I feel that there is a definite limitation in the depth and breadth of nursing care which can be practiced and postpones further the time when the highest of nursing standards can be implemented. This issue of nurse education preparation is still hotly debated and will continue to be in the forefront of nursing issues for some time to come.

NURSING THEORY AND COMMUNITY HEALTH PRACTICE

As stated earlier, community health nursing is a combination of general nursing practice and public health practice applied to a population to maintain or enhance their health and/or prevent illness. The profession of nursing, however, is caught in a search for a scientific body of knowledge to apply to practice, the development of nursing theories, and a definition of nursing. As yet, there is no single theory of nursing to be embraced by students and then applied to practice settings and the clients who seek services. This is a concern of many people. Researchers such as Rogers,[6] Abdellah and coworkers,[7] King,[8] and Nordmark[9] have attempted to address this issue. Their efforts have added much to the understanding of nursing and nursing practice. By the same token, such work also stimulates controversies and ideological conflicts, the very fodder of professional growth and development.

It is not within the scope of this book to provide an extensive discussion of theoretical characteristics and findings, however, a few words are necessary to help the reader understand some of the issues involved.

Professional status designation has been and is sought by large numbers of nurses. One of the critical components of such a designation is a separate body of scientific knowledge. Johnson states: "If nursing is indeed an emerging profession, nurses must be able to identify clearly and develop continually the theoretical body of knowledge upon which practice must rest."[10] She states further, "Nursing stands today as a field of practice without a scientific heritage—an occupation created by society long ago to offer a distinctive service, but one still ill-defined in practical terms, a profession without the theoretical base it seems to require."[10] A similar view was proposed by Brown more than a decade before.[11]

The development of the scientific body of knowledge will clear the way once and for all to call nursing a profession. Among the other characteristics of a profession are the possession af a high degree of skill, control over the kind of people who are admitted to the profession through accrediting bodies that examine and certify the educational institutions, licensure which certifies the practitioner, and a code of ethics.[7] The later qualifications we possess, and we are building, albeit slowly, a body of scientific knowledge.

Research is a mandatory requirement for any profession. The need for prepared, creative nurse-scientists will increase in the years to come. It would be the goal for these nurse-scientists to be prepared in nursing doctoral programs. As it now stands, many of the present nursing researchers have advanced degrees in education, sociology, anthropology, psychology, and other major fields. While this certainly provides for a breadth of knowledge, it also produces researchers who will view nursing from the second perspective of their doctoral major. It seems that this approach can complicate the process of pure nursing research. As more doctoral programs in nursing are developed, it would be hoped that nurse-scientists would come increasingly from this background.

Definitions of nursing are many. The scope of services provided by the nurse and the kind of skills needed by him or her to practice are coming under increasing scrutiny. Decisions made concerning practice, guidelines, licensure, nurse practice acts, educational preparation for practice, and practice limitations will have a momentous impact on nursing. These issues must be squarely faced and clearly dealt with if nursing is to remain a viable member of the health team.

Although not inclusive, the above remarks provide the reader with some of the issues facing nursing and thus community health nursing. Before examining some of community health nursing roles and the scope of practice, a short discussion concerning some theoretical views and concepts and functions of nursing is in order.

Peplau identifies nursing as a

"significant, therapeutic, interpersonal relationship. It functions cooperatively with other human processes that make health possible for individuals in communities. Nursing is an educative instrument, a maturing force, that aims to promote forward movement of personality in the direction of creative, constructive, productive, personal and community living. The nurse functions as a resource person, counsellor, surrogate and technical expert."[12]

Abdellah and coworkers[7] view nursing from a patient-centered perspective with five basic characteristics of nursing practice identified: 1) skills, 2) observation ability, 3) interpretation skills, 4) analysis of nursing problems, and 5) organization of efforts to obtain desired outcomes. A patient-centered approach to nursing attempts to meet the total needs of both acutely and chronically ill patients. Such care is designated as progressive patient care which 1) provides assistance to a patient when, for some reason, he cannot provide for the satisfaction of his own needs, 2) is commensurate with the abilities and skills of the nurse providing the assistance, 3) is derived from a study of the patient's requirements for nursing care, 4) is directed toward making the patient better able to help himself. Such nursing care is carried out in 1) intensive care, 2) intermediate care, 3)self-care, 4) long term care, and 5) home care settings.[7]

Orlando states that learning to understand what is happening between oneself and the patient is the central core of the nurse's practice and comprises the basic framework for the help they give to others. Nursing situations consist of three basic elements: 1) the behavior of the patient, 2) the reaction of the nurse, 3) the nursing actions which are designed for the patient's benefit.[13]

Rogers speaks of man as

"a unified whole possessing his own integrity and manifesting characteristics that are more than and different from the sum of his parts. Man and environment are continuously exchanging matter with one another. The phenomenon central to the nursing conceptual system is the life process of man. Nursing is an empirical science with the aim to assist people in achieving their maximum health potential. Maintenance and promotion of health, prevention of disease, nursing diagnosis, intervention, and rehabilitation encompass the scope of nursing goals. Nursing is concerned with all people where they are— school, home, work, play. The science of nursing aims to provide a body of abstract knowledge growing out of scientific research and logical analysis and capable of being translated into nursing practice. Nursing's body of scientific knowledge is a new product specific to nursing."[5]

King states that generally speaking

"the basic abstraction of nursing is the phenomenon of man and his world. Nursing is a process of action, reaction, interaction, and transaction whereby nurses assist individuals of any age and socioeconomic group to meet their basic needs in performing activities of daily living and to cope with health and illness at some particular point in the life cycle. The moving forces in nursing are imbedded in the dynamics of society in which the process of change alters the environment. Man functions in *social systems* through interpersonal relationships in terms of his perceptions which influence his life and his health."[8]

Helvie and coworkers state

"that every event in health and human behavior is a complex network of multiple factors. No event occurs in isolation but has characteristics of dependency, independency, and/or interdependency. A family consists of a group of individuals interacting and related in a way that maintains the family's homeodynamic balance. Because of changing relationships and forces in his environment, man is continually adjusting and changing in an effort to maintain balance." [14]

Assisting families to develop and maintain health patterns and priorities conducive to good health is imperative for the health of the community.

McKay states that

"nursing is a biopsychosocial process. Open systems are related to and exchange matter with their environment. General systems theory proposes that it is possible to represent all forms of inanimate and animate matter as systems which have common properties though present in different forms. There are universal laws which can be found to describe the structure of these systems and their manner of functioning. The essential components of a system are the *objects* which are the parts of the system, the properties of the objects identified as *attribute,* and the *relationship* among the objects and their attributes which holds the system together. All systems have subsystems, suprasystems, boundaries, and environments." [15]

The preceding statements give some idea of the concepts and theories which are alive and prospering in nursing today. Similarities and overlaps are many. Whenever evaluating theories and conceptual statements, the reader is advised to keep in mind definitions of both terms. Theory is the identification of concepts which, when defined, correspond to observable phenomena and are interrelated.[8] Concepts are abstract ideas that give meaning to our sense perceptions, permit generalizations, and tend to be stored in our memory recall and used at a later time in new and different situations.[8]

The impact these concepts and theories will have on the practice of community health nursing is dependent in part on their utilization and evaluation in the field. Philosophical bents of agencies may well determine the utilization of one approach over another.

ROLES AND FUNCTIONS
OF THE COMMUNITY HEALTH NURSE

Nurses in community health assume many roles, carry out a variety of functions, and provide services through diverse clinical settings. Their work is not considered community health because it is outside the confines of the hospital walls, in fact, many community health nurses work in such settings, nor is it community health because its nursing care is provided in community settings. Since all specialties of nursing now use the nursing process and are family oriented in their approach to patient care, what then makes the care given by community health nurses different?

That is a most challenging and important question to answer. In order to answer we must again examine the definition of community health nursing identified earlier in this chapter by the American Nurses' Association. It included several key statements and words which will help us to clarify this distinction.

The most important statements are contained in the first line. It contains five critical components of community health nursing: the synthesis of 1) nursing practice and 2) public health practice to 3) promote health, to 4) preserve health, and to 5) apply this approach to populations. General nursing care requires the nurse to assess the patient, to establish goals, to implement nursing care plans based on the assessment and established goals, and to evaluate and revise assessments, goals, and nursing care plans as necessary based on obtained data. Public health practice falls into two broad categories of service according to Hanlon. These are: 1) environmental problems sheds and 2) health service marketing.[16] These two areas can be specifically divided into seven categories: 1) activities that must be conducted on a community basis such as supervision of food and water supplies and insect, rodent, and vector control; 2) activities designed for prevention of illness, disability, or premature death from communicable diseases, dietary deficiencies or excesses, behavioral disorders, such as alcohol and drug addiction, mental illness and retardation, allergies, neoplastic diseases, certain hereditary or genetic conditions, occupational diseases, home, vehicular, and industrial accidents, dental disorders, and certain risks of maternity, growth, and development; 3) activities related to provision of comprehensive health care, including promotion of development and equitable distribution of medical and allied health personnel and facilities, assistance in development and maintenance of the quality and quantity of community resources and facilities, including establishment and application of standards for and categorization of hospitals, nursing and convalescent homes, and day care centers, operation of screening programs for early detection of disease, promotion and sometimes operation of emergency medical service systems promotion and sometimes operation of treatment centers, varying from disease speciality clinics to comprehensive health centers, facilitation of and participation in pregraduate and continuing professional and paraprofessional education; 4) activities concerned with collection, preservation, and analysis of vital records; 5) public education in personal and community health; 6) comprehensive health planning and evaluation; 7) research—scientific, technical, and administrative.[16] The application of both the nursing and public health principles gives the nurse great opportunity to provide creative innovative care.

The utilization of either of these components alone would not constitute community health nursing. It is only when they are combined in nursing care delivery, along with the other nursing components, that it can be said that one is practicing community health nursing.

The next two factors critical to the role of a community health nurse are the promoting and preserving of health. This is not to say that all nurses do not see this as a need and a goal. However the nurse in the community has these as her main foci of effort rather than the curative and restoration foci of nurses in other settings. The goal in the community is to prevent illness from ever occurring by promoting healthy living habits and attitudes.

To focus on health rather than illness is critical to the practice of community health nursing. What is critically needed is more knowledge and techniques to help us identify healthy states, practices, and attitudes and then implement measures to maintain, sustain, and promote critical factors necessary to healthful living.

The final characteristic is that the community nurse's efforts are directed toward the total population not just individuals and families. Work with individuals and families is carried out with a view and concern for the health of the larger population. This is done through a holistic approach to nursing care for the larger group. Care is provided on a continuing basis rather than episodically with attention given to health planning, risk factors such as environmental and social conditions, and utilization of interpersonal skills to help initiate and maintain health behavior change where necessary.

The focus of attention on the population as a whole is critical to the concept of community health nursing. Again, it is only when individual and family work is carried out with the welfare of larger populations as the goal that one can be practicing community health nursing. It is the combination of all five components identified above which constitute community health nursing practice.

It is nearly impossible to succinctly characterize the community health nurse; she is a unique health care provider. Williams, in analyzing her role, identifies three barriers to an adequate understanding of the role: 1) a narrow view of defining public health nursing in terms of *where* it takes place and/or whether or not the provider functions in a family oriented fashion, 2) failure to understand the distinction between the foci of clinical nursing and medicine on one hand and public health practice on the other hand, and 3) paucity of service settings in which clinical nursing and medicine and the basic public health strategy of dealing with aggregates or groups are effectively merged and practiced.[17]

The above barriers are very large concerns not only in practice but in nursing education as well. Too often community health concepts are integrated into curricula and then lost. Community health nursing is much more than the application of the nursing process to an individual and/or a family outside a hospital setting. Survival of the specialty will depend on the voices of strong advocates who will insist that both nursing practice and public health practice for the promotion and preservation of health as applied to groups remain the cornerstone of community health nursing practice.

The Standards of Community Health Nursing Practice, as established by the American Nurses' Association, are presented in Table 4-1. These standards provide the guidelines for evaluating the quality of nursing services provided. The consumer, whether individual, family, or a group, is an integral part of the entire process. He participates in the assessment process, the establishment of nursing goals, the implementation of nursing plans, and the evaluation and revision of those plans. Community health nursing then is a collaborative effort between the client and the nurse.

It was stated earlier that community health nursing is concerned with the total population. In order to provide nursing care, individuals, families, and groups become the immediate focus. A family may consist of the nuclear unit, an expanded unit, or a group of individuals who live and interact in a supportive manner for the benefit of the whole. Groups can be defined as any group of unrelated individuals who have one or more characteristics in common. The school or occupational population can be a group. Pregnant women and year old children can constitute separate groups. People having cardiac insufficiency or respiratory impaiment can also form a group. The critical criterion is that they all have in common at least one characteristic which provides a common link between individual members.

As the scope of potential community nursing functions is broad so are the various specialty roles within community health. A later section of this book explores in detail a large variety of specific nursing roles in the field. Roles are developed and carried out in schools, occupational settings, official and nonofficial agencies, hospitals, and other settings. Groups receiving services can be homogeneous or heterogeneous. Regardless of the setting, however, the nurse continues to meet the criteria identified above. She continues to be a competent professional, a counselor, teacher, resource person, and surrogate.[12] Her main interest is always the health and well being of the population at large.

CURRENT ISSUES IN COMMUNITY HEALTH NURSING

As we move into the last quarter of the twentieth century, we find ourselves in the middle of a health care delivery crisis. Not only are the issues mentioned earlier in this chapter impacting on community health nursing practice, but so are such issues as high cost of

TABLE 4-1. American Nurses' Association Standards of Community Health Nursing Practice.*

Nursing practice is a direct service, goal directed and adaptable to the needs of the individual, family and community during health and illness.

Community Health Nursing is a synthesis of nursing practice and public health practice applied to promoting and preserving the health of populations. The nature of this practice is general and comprehensive. It is not limited to a particular age or diagnostic group. It is continuing, not episodic. The dominant responsibility is to the population as a whole. Therefore, nursing directed to individuals, families or groups contributes to the health of the total population. Health promotion, health maintenance, health education, coordination and continuity of care are utilized in a holistic approach to the family, group and community. The nurse's actions acknowledge the need for comprehensive health planning, recognize the influences of social and ecological issues, give attention to populations at risk and utilize the dynamic forces which influence change.

In Community Health Nursing Practice the consumer is the client or patient. Consumers include individuals, groups and the community as a whole. For example, the consumer may be a single individual, family (interpreted in the broadest sense), a school population, an industrial population or selected at-risk segments of the population. Professional practitioners of nursing bear primary responsibility and accountability for the nursing care consumers receive. The purpose of the Standards of Community Health Nursing Practice is to fulfill the profession's obligation to provide and improve this practice.

The Standards focus on practice rather than on the practitioner. They provide a means for determining the quality of nursing which a consumer receives regardless of whether such services are provided solely by a professional nurse or by a professional nurse and nonprofessional assistants.

The Standards are stated according to a systematic approach to nursing practice: assessment, planning, implementation and evaluation. These specific divisions are not intended to imply that practice consists of a series of discrete steps, taken in strict sequence, beginning with assessment and ending with evaluation. The processes described are used concurrently and recurrently. Assessment, for example, frequently continues during implementation; similarly, evaluation dictates reassessment and replanning.

The Standards for Community Health Nursing Practice apply to nursing practice in a variety of settings. In any setting Community Health Nursing Practice must possess the characteristics identified by these Standards if consumers are to receive high quality nursing service. Each Standard is followed by a rationale and assessment factors. Assessment factors are to be used in determining achievement of the Standards.

STANDARD I. The collection of data about the health status of the consumer is systematic and continuous. The data are accessible, communicated, and recorded.

STANDARD II. Nursing diagnoses are derived from health status data.

STANDARD III. Plans for nursing service include goals from nursing diagnoses.

STANDARD IV. Plans for nursing service include priorities and nursing approaches or measures to achieve the goals derived from nursing diagnoses.

STANDARD V. Nursing actions provide for consumer participation in health promotion, maintenance, and restoration.

STANDARD VI. Nursing actions assist consumers to maximize health potential.

STANDARD VII. The consumer's progress toward goal achievement is determined by the consumer and the nurse.

STANDARD VIII. Nursing actions involve ongoing reassessment, reordering of priorities, new goal setting, and revision of the nursing plan.

*(From American Nurses' Association, with permission.)

health services, availability of health care services and providers, educational preparation and criteria for providers, payment plans for health services, consumerism, and professional accountability.

There is much analysis, discussion, and suggestion concerning health care delivery.

Robischon identifies several factors which are influencing practice. Among these are smarter, more sophisticated, and critical consumers, consumer demands that health needs be met, consumer involvement in decisions about health care, a determination to build a better life, a willingness of consumers to group or band together to meet health care needs, a more mobile and larger population, changes in family lifestyles, deteriorating environment, and a changing attitude about health—a positive view that it offers the individual the greatest option for a happy productive life.[18]

Coupled with these population changes are also changes in providers. New types of health care providers are presenting themselves and traditional roles for some are changing. Most blatant among these are the physician assistant and the development of extended roles for nurses such as nurse practitioners or nurse associates. The physician assistant and the nurse associate are both trained by and primarily responsible to the physician, while the nurse practitioner may have preparation in a variety of programs with varying emphasis. Her source of responsibility and employment may be independent, institution/agency based, or physician based. The exact role will be dependent on where and for whom she works—a critical issue for the nursing profession.

Leininger's analysis of the present health care system is that there has been "inadequate identification, utilization and distribution of the health manpower personnel now available and lack of recognition of their full potential and the fact that our present care system is operated and controlled by the medical profession."[19] She proposes that we need to properly utilize present health personnel, allow all health workers direct contact/access to the client, and the establishment of an easily accessible, readily available health system.[19]

What Leininger proposes is an "open, client centered health care system model" (Fig. 4-1). This model offers many exciting and innovative methods of health care delivery. There is care for both healthy and ill populations. The kinds of services are varied and client directed. They range from specialty wellness oriented clinics and centers to settings for curative and restorative efforts. Great emphasis is placed on health maintenance, promotion, and primary care. The services provided can be changed to meet community needs as necessary. What this kind of model could provide for community health nursing practice is an almost pure form of practice. All aspects of community nursing practice could be carried out in established, acceptable facilities/centers and would be oriented to the health needs of the entire population. Since our goal is to have and maintain a healthy population, the model provides for interventions at primary, secondary, and tertiary levels. It is conceivable that dramatic decreases in disease conditions of all types would be realized in a short time with the utilization of this model.

As nurses move more into the primary care independent role and utilize expanded skills, the need for payment reevaluation must be made. At the present time few nurses receive third party payment for their services. If we are to take on an expanded role in health care delivery, private and governmental insurance providers must reexamine the criteria for payment and work with nurses to establish a viable change in the present payment system. Health care quality and quantity could be dramatically improved if there were financial access to the kind of services nurses can provide.

Professional accountability is of concern to all nurses. In the establishment of ourselves as a profession, it is critical that we have a mechanism of professional performance evaluation and an established code of ethics. Peer review and nursing audit are two mechanisms which can help us establish, maintain, and evaluate professional nursing activities. Consumers demand quality nursing care and as a profession it is our prime concern.

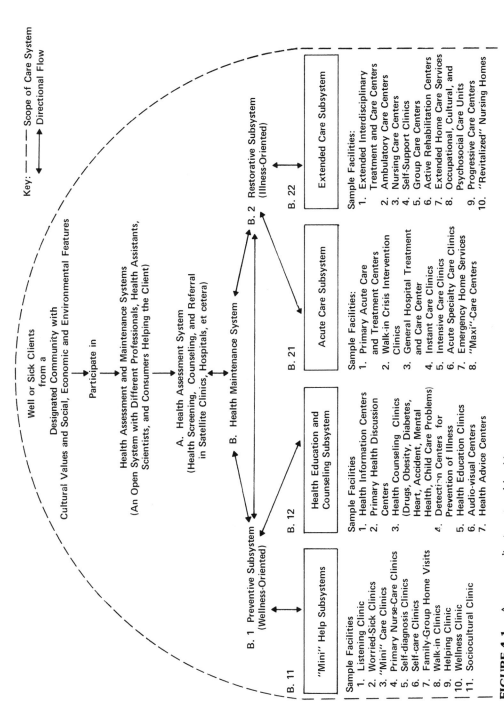

FIGURE 4-1. An open, client-centered health care system model. (From Leininger, M.: An open health care system model. *Nursing Outlook*, 21(3):171, 1973, with permission.)

As the practice of community health nursing evolves and expands, it will be increasingly important to look with a critical eye toward what individuals and groups of community health nurses are doing. Only through evaluation and revisions of nursing care will we be able to provide the kind of care expected by both consumers and the profession.

Community health nursing is in the process of evaluation, evolution, and growth. As our practice horizons expand and population health needs change, we will have an increasing responsibility and opportunity to participate in the planning and implementation of health care services. Our potential for impact on the health of the population has yet to be fully realized.

REFERENCES

1. American Nurses' Association: *Standards of Community Health Nursing Practice,* 1973.
2. Tinkham, Catherine W., and Voorhies, Eleanor F.: *Community Health Nursing: Evaluation and Process.* Appleton-Century-Crofts, New York, 1972.
3. Freeman, Ruth B.: *Community Health Nursing Practice.* W. B. Saunders Company, Philadelphia, 1970.
4. Council on Health Manpower: "Educational Qualifications of Public Health Nurses, in Spradley, B. W. (ed.): *Contemporary Community Nursing.* Little, Brown and Company, Boston, 1975.
5. Rogers, Martha E.: "Nursing is Coming of Age through the Practitioner Movement—Con." *American Journal of Nursing,* 75(10):1841, Oct. 1975.
6. Rogers, Martha E.: *An Introduction to the Theoretical Basis of Nursing.* F. A. Davis Company, Philadelphia, 1970.
7. Abdellah, Faye G., et al.: *Patient-Centered Approaches to Nursing.* The Macmillan Company, New York, 1960.
8. King, Imogene M.: *Toward a Theory of Nursing.* John Wiley and Sons, Inc., New York, 1971.
9. Nordmark, Madelyn T., and Rohweder, Anne W.: *Scientific Foundations of Nursing,* 2nd Ed. J. B. Lippincott Company, Philadelphia, 1967.
10. Johnson, Dorothy E.: "Development of Theory." *Nursing Research,* 23(5):372, Sept/Oct. 1974.
11. Brown, Myrtle Irene: "Research in the Development of Nursing Theory." *Nursing Research,* 13(2):109, Spring 1964.
12. Peplau, Hildegard E.: *Interpersonal Relations in Nursing.* G. P. Putnam's Sons, New York, 1952.
13. Orlando, Ida Jean: *The Dynamic Nurse-Patient Relationship—Function, Process, Principle.* G.P. Putman's Sons, New York, 1961.
14. Helvie, Carl O., Hill, Anne E., and Bambino, Charlotte F.: "The Setting and Nursing Practice." *Nursing Outlook,* 17:35, Sept. 1968.
15. McKay, Rose: "Theories, Models, and Systems for Nursing," in Hardy, M. E. (ed.): *Theoretical Foundations for Nursing.* MSS Information Corporation, New York, 1973.
16. Hanlon, John J.: *Public Health Administration and Practice* 7th ed. The C. V. Mosby Company, St. Louis, 1979.
17. Williams, Carolyn A.: "Community Health Nursing—What Is It?" *Nursing Outlook,* 25(4):250, April 1977.
18. Robischon, Paulette: "Community Nursing in a Changing Climate." *Nursing Outlook,* 19(6):410, June 1971.
19. Leininger, Madeleine: "An Open Health Care System Model." *Nursing Outlook,* 21(3):171, March 1973.

BIBLIOGRAPHY

Abdellah, Faye G.: "Nurse Practitioners and Nursing Practice." *American Journal of Public Health,* 66:245, March 1976.
Abdellah, Faye, et al.: *Patient-Centered Approaches to Nursing.* The Macmillan Company, New York, 1960.

American Nurses' Association: *Standards of Community Health Nursing Practice,* 1973.

Bowman, Rosemary Amoson, and Culpepper, Rebecca Clark: "Power: Rx for Change." *American Journal of Nursing,* 74(6):1053, June 1974.

Brown, Myrtle Irene: "Research in the Development of Nursing Theory." *Nursing Research,* 13(2):109, Spring 1964.

Bullough, Bonnie: "The Law and the Expanding Nursing Role." *American Journal of Public Health,* 16(3):249, March 1976.

Bullough, Bonnie: "Influences on Role Expansion." *American Journal of Nursing,* 26(9):1476, Sept. 1976.

Burton, Lloyd E., and Smith, Hugh H.: *Public Health and Community Medicine,* 2nd. ed. The Williams and Wilkins Company, Baltimore, 1975.

Council on Health Manpower: "Educational Qualifications of Public Health Nurses." *Journal of Public Health,* 61(12):2505, 1971.

Driscoll, Veronica: "Liberating Nursing Practice." *Nursing Outlook,* 20(1):24, Jan 1972.

Hanlon, John H.: *Public Health Administration and Practice,* 7th ed. The C. V. Mosby Company, St. Louis, 1979.

Helvie, Carl O., Hill, Anne E., and Bambino, Charlotte F.: "The Setting and Nursing Practice." *Nursing Outlook,* 16(9):35, Sept. 1968.

Johnson, Dorothy E.: "Development of Theory." *Nursing Research,* 23(5):372, Sept/Oct 1974.

King, Imogene M.: *Toward a Theory of Nursing.* John Wiley and Sons Inc., New York, 1971.

Kinlein, M. Lucille: "Independent Nurse Practitioner." *Nursing Outlook,* 20(1):22, Jan. 1972.

Lambertson, Eleanor, C.: "Perspectives on the Physicians Assistant." *Nursing Outlook,* 20(1):32, Jan. 1972.

Leininger, Madeleine: "An Open Health Care System Model." *Nursing Outlook,* 21(3):171, March 1973.

Lewis, Edith P.: "A Nurse is a Nurse—Or Is She?" *Nursing Outlook,* 20(1):21, Jan. 1972.

McKay, Rose: "Theories, Models and Systems for Nursing." *Nursing Research,* 18:393, 1969.

Mauksch, Inglborg: "Nursing is Coming of Age Through the Practitioner Movement—Pro." *American Journal of Nursing,* 75(1):1834, Oct. 1975.

Nordmark, Madelyn T., and Rohweder, Anne W.: *Scientific Foundations of Nursing,* 2nd ed. · J. B. Lippincott Company, Philadelphia, 1967.

Orlando, Ida Jean: *The Dynamic Nurse-Patient Relationship—Function, Process, Principles.* G. P. Putnam's Sons, New York, 1961.

Peplau, Hildegard: *Interpersonal Relations in Nursing.* G. P. Putnam's Sons, New York, 1952.

A Report of the Secretary's Committee to Study Extended Roles for Nurses: "Extending the Scope of Nursing Practices." U. S. Department of Health Education and Welfare, DHEW Publication NO. (HSM) 73-2037, Nov. 1971, pp. 99-109.

Robischon, Paulette: "Community Nursing in a Changing Climate." *Nursing Outlook,* 19(6):410, June, 1971.

Rogers, Martha E.: "Nursing is Coming of Age Through the Practitioner Movement—Con." *American Journal of Nursing,* 75(10):1830, Oct. 1975.

Rogers, Martha E.: "Nursing: To Be or Not To Be." *Nursing Outlook,* 20(1):42, Jan. 1972.

Rogers, Martha E.: *An Introduction to the Theoretical Basis of Nursing.* F. A. Davis, Co., Philadelphia, 1970.

Schenk, Katherine: "Teaching Distributive Nursing." *Nursing Outlook,* 24(9):574, Sept. 1976.

Shetland, Margaret L.: "An Approach to Role Expansion—the Elaborate Network." *American Journal of Public Health,* 61(10):1959, 1971.

Skrovan, Clarence; Anderson, Elizabeth; and Gottschalk, Janet: "Community Nurse Practitioner— An Emerging Role." *American Journal of Public Health,* 64(9):847, Sept. 1974.

Spradley, Barbara Walton (ed.): *Contemporary Community Nursing.* Little, Brown and Company, Boston, 1975.

Stein, Leonard I.: "The Doctor-Nurse Game." *Archives of General Psychiatry,* 16:699, June 1967.

Tinkham, Catherine W., and Voorhies, Eleanor F.: *Community Health Nursing-Evaluation and Process.* Appleton-Century-Crofts, New York, 1972.

Walker, Elizabeth: "Primary: The Family Nurse Practitioner Program." *Nursing Outlook,* 20(1):28, Jan. 1972.

Williams, Carolyn A.: "Community Health Nursing—What Is It?" *Nursing Outlook,* 25(4):250, April 1977.

CHAPTER 5
HEALTH CARE DELIVERY SYSTEM

LINDA L. JARVIS, M.S.N., R.N.

All states have public and private means of protecting the public health. A clear understanding of the health care delivery system at the local, state, and national levels will aid the community health nurse in providing comprehensive health care.

Our health care system is a complex interrelationship of providers, settings, and consumers. Quality and quantity of services in any given geographic area can vary. In some settings care is fragmented and depersonalized. Long waits for short visits to health providers are common in both public and private settings. Financing of health care is from a variety of sources including taxes, third party payments, contributions, and out of pocket funds. It is often the community health nurse who aids consumers in traveling through the health maze so that comprehensive services are obtained and utilized.

HEALTH CARE ORGANIZATION

The organization of health care in the United States is on three levels—local, state, and national (for purposes of this discussion, the international level of interactions will not be addressed). Each of the three levels consists of public or official agencies, voluntary or nonofficial agencies, and private providers societies.

The public or official agencies are those established by law to provide services for the protection and maintanance of the public's health. Official agencies strive to prevent disease and prolong life for the entire population of any given community. Services are organized through local health departments which are usually designated through local political boundaries such as towns, counties, or townships. Public funds are the primary sources of support for official agencies.

Voluntary agencies on the other hand provide health services to large numbers of people in a variety of settings but are not compelled by law to do so. Many voluntary agencies were started by individuals and groups who recognized a need for a particular service and set about to meet that need. Voluntary services often focus on a single population group, disease entity, or identified need to provide services. Funding for these services may be through contributions, philantrophic gifts, some third party payments, and out of pockets monies.

Private practioners and societies are responsible for the third source of health service at all levels. Private practitioners provide direct service through a variety of modes such as single and group practices. Physicians, dentists, laboratory personnel, and psychologists are some of the providers who render service through the private sector. Professional societies and organizations, while not providing direct care services, do contribute to health care through the establishment and enforcement of professional practice standards, education, and research. Funding for private sector services is primarily from third party and out of pocket funds and membership fees.

Although each of these three provider groups can be defined separately, there is often an overlap of services provided and in some areas there may be great reluctance to combine service efforts or terminate a voluntary agency even though identical services are provided through an official agency. This reluctance may be due to concern over quality and quantity of service which will be provided by one agency if terminated or due to a difficulty in terminating an effort which represents a high degree of individual and group involvement. Whatever the real or assumed reasons, duplication of services is costly and should be avoided whenever possible.

Figure 5-1 shows the basic structure of health services in the United States. In general, these services at the local level tend to be of a direct care nature. State and federal efforts are primarily of a regulatory, support, guidance, educational, and research nature. This tends to be true whether one is viewing governmental agencies, voluntary agencies, or private/professional provider or organizations.

Because of the potential for service duplication, the need for comprehensive health planning is critical. The passage of the Health Planning and Resources Development Act of 1974 which established Health System Agencies responsible for health planning and development takes the broadest possible look at health service. In this manner, it may be possible to strenghten services offered, design new programs to meet identified needs, and cut the overall cost of health services. In order to do this, open and frank discussions and evaluations will need to be carried out by all three sectors to insure quality and quantity of services at a reasonable cost.

Local Health Organization

Although most health services are provided through various private providers, the local health departments provide a variety of services to the community. In general, a health department has three main functions: 1) to determine the health status and health needs of the people within its jurisdiction, 2) to determine the extent to which needs are being met by effective measures currently available, and 3) to take steps to see that the unmet

Federal Level	**Voluntary Agencies** American Cancer Society, American Red Cross, American Heart Assoc., etc.	**Federal Government** Dept. of Health and Human Services, Public Health, Health Services Admin., Health Resources Admin., Food and Drug Admin., Center for Disease Control, N I H, Alcoholism and Drug Abuse and Mental Health Admin., etc.	**Professional Organizations** American Nurses Assoc., American Medical Assoc., American Public Health Assoc., etc.
State Level	**Voluntary Agencies** State Cancer Society, State Lung Assoc., State Red Cross, State Heart Assoc., etc.	**State Government** Department of Health, State Hospitals, Special Schools, etc.	**Professional Organizations** State Nursing Assoc., State Dental Society, State Medical Society, etc.
Local Level	**Voluntary Agencies** Visiting Nurse Assoc., Community Hospitals, Third Party Pay Plans, Civic Organizations, Red Cross, etc.	**Local Government** Health Department, Public Hospitals, etc.	**Private Providers** Medical Society, Dental Society, Nurses, Physicians, Dentists, etc.

FIGURE 5-1. Levels of health organization. (Adapted from Moutin, J.W. and Flook, E.: *Guide to Health Organization in the United States 1951*. Public Health Service Publication No. 196, 1951, Washington, D.C., and Hanlon, J.J.: Public Health Administration and Practices, ed. 6. C.V. Mosby Company, St. Louis, 1974.)

needs are satisfied.[2] These functions are mandated by law and can be met directly or indirectly. Direct intervention would include provision of services while indirect intervention would utilize the services of private, voluntary, or other official agencies. In order to promote healthful living and prevent disease, most health departments will include the following seven categories of service: 1) health education, 2) sanitation, 3) disease control, 4) maternal and child health, 5) vital statistics, 6) laboratory facilities, and 7) mental health.[3]

The local health department is the main link most people have with the state department of public health. The size and local geographic limitations of the health departments are based primarily on political boundaries such as countries, towns, municipalities, and townships.[2] This can lead to some confusion. In an effort to economize and obtain maximum service for health dollars spent, there is a trend toward combining some health departments. Thus we are seeing an increase in city-county and multiple-county health departments.

Just as the location of the health department may vary, so can the staff assignment. In general, however, the following positions will be active: 1) the health officer who usually is a medical doctor with a masters or doctorate in public health, 2) staff physician, 3) public health nurses, 4) public health laboratory technician, 5) dentists, 6) sanitarians, 7) industrial hygienist, 8) statistician, 9) chemist, 10) health educator, 11) social workers, 12) others.[3] The efforts of these professionals are toward the prevention of disease and prolongation of life. They will do this thru many agencies and service organizations. At times their efforts need to be the direct provision of care or service, other times they will serve as educators or consultants.

Voluntary agency efforts at the local level generally provide health care through service, education, and research. Examples of specific organizations and some of their services are the American Red Cross which offers water safety and first aid classes and sponsors blood donor centers; Visiting Nurse Associations which provide bedside nursing care, physical therapy, and support; American Heart Association which supports training and education efforts through cardiopulmonary resuscitation classes, sheltered workshops, and nutritional counseling; and the American Cancer Society which provides bandages for cancer patients, support for patients and families, and education for prevention and identification of cancer and cancer symptoms. The list can go on and on.

In identifying voluntary agencies, Hanlon describes four main types:[2] 1) agencies concerned with specific diseases, for example, the American Lung Association and the American Diabetic Society; 2) agencies concerned with certain organs or structures of the body, for example, the National Society for the Prevention of Blindness, the American Society for the Hard of Hearing, and the National Society for Crippled Children; 3) agencies concerned with the health and welfare of special groups in society, for example, The Maternity Center Association and the National Health Association and; 4) agencies concerned with particular phases of health and welfare, for example, the National Safety Council and the Planned Parenthood Federation of America.

In 1945, Gunn and Platt identified eight basic functions of voluntary health agencies. These functions, listed below, are still relevant and serve as a guide for the existence of such agencies.[4]

1. Pioneering—exploring or surveying to identify new needs not now recognized and new methods for dealing with needs currently identified.
2. Demonstration—carrying out or subsidizing experimental projects to demonstrate practical means of improving public health and for the wider application of proven methods by official and other agencies.

3. Education—the most important single purpose of any agency. These efforts are carried on through workshops, in-service training, and a multitude of other professional and lay education programs.
4. Supplementation of official activities—establishment of new services which official agencies cannot enter due to political, legal restrictions. These are usually time limited until the official agency can provide the service.
5. Guarding citizen interest in health—can guard the public interest by promoting the official health program and by defending it against political and other interference.
6. Promotion of health legislation—support of legislative measures which will improve community health.
7. Group planning and coordination—the need to coordinate activities of various voluntary agencies among themselves and with official agencies so that overlap of service and conflict of interest is minimized.
8. Development of well-balanced community health programs—the cumulative accomplishment of meeting the preceding goals through support and protection of the official health program, voluntary agencies may aid in the establishment of an excellent health program for a community.

Excellent health care services can be provided when there is open, direct, and continuous discussion, planning, and coordination between official and voluntary agencies. Broad health needs can be met by a variety of providers. It behooves us all as citizens, consumers, and health providers to evaluate a given health delivery system critically and participate in efforts to improve or maintain services offered.

Private physicians, dentists, and others provide a large amount of the health services consumed. They may function in single or a variety of group practice modes. The quality of services they provide will depend on considerations such as the extent of educational preparation, specialty orientation, strength of professional standardization and review organizations, the community in which they function, health provider/client ratio, and quality and quantity of health support services available. In selecting a private health provider, individual and family needs should be evaluated, resources for services investigated, and financial expenditures and resources explored. Efforts should then be directed toward finding providers who can best meet the needs of the consumers.

In identifying ways which private physicians can aid in promoting the community's health, Smolensky lists several specific activities.[3] The main sources of support from private practitioners take the form of reporting births; deaths; communicable diseases such as tuberculosis, scarlet fever, mumps, and venereal diseases; infections such as streptococcal and salmonella, and animal bites subject to rabies. All these need to be reported both by telephone and in writing. Explanation to clients about health department services will aid in prompt utilization of such services, availble without cost. Administration of and verification of immunization compliance will combat potential disease outbreaks. Occupational health hazards need to be identified, reported, investigated, and corrected. The last major area of private practice support is in the area of meeting community health needs. This can be done through participation in the planning and implementation of health programs. Cooperation between the private provider and official and voluntary agencies can strengthen the total health program in any given community.

State Health Organization

Services at the state level may be provided through official, voluntary, and private agencies and providers. These services may be direct, indirect, or a combination of the two.

All states have at least one agency which is responsible for the public health of the population.

In general, the state health department provides the following services: 1) seeking the causes of communicable disease in man and domestic animals, 2) investigation of the sources of morbidity and mortality, 3) investigation of the effects of localities, employment conditions, and circumstances on public health, 4) licensing of hospitals and nursing homes, 5) detection and prevention of adulteration of food and drugs, 6) examination for and the prevention of pollution of public water and ice supplies, and 7) preparation and distribution, at cost, of antitoxins, vaccines, and other approved biologic products for the control or prevention of communicable diseases.[3] It is, however, the ability of the state health department to stimulate and assist local health departments in doing the best job possible which really justifies its existence.[2]

Each state develops the internal structures and organization of the health department to meet the various laws, regulations, and needs of its population. This leads to confusion because there may not be direct access from one state to another through a standardized department, bureau, or other designation. It is through this structure that the state provides it services which are primarily supportive, educational, and consultative rather than direct in nature.

Other contributors to the overall health of the public at the state level are the voluntary agencies and professional societies which represent private practices. The primary function of the state voluntary agency is to aid the local units in fulfillment of their missions. Voluntary agencies provide education, service, and research input to health care.[3]

Professional societies aid in educational efforts and in establishing, implementing, and maintaining practice standards. Many professional organizations are also engaged in educational activities through journals and media materials, and through members who make personal appearances as speakers or consultants. These efforts are directed toward improving and/or maintaining health.

Federal Health Organization

The most complex level of our health system is at the federal level. Prior to 1980, the Department of Health, Education and Welfare was the agency responsible for the national health through the work of its major branches—the Public Health Service, the Social and Rehabilitative Services, Social Security Administration, and the Office of Education. Under Public Law 96-88 signed October 17, 1979, effective April 2, 1980, HEW was separated into two independent agencies—the Department of Health and Human Services, Patricia Roberts Harris, Secretary, and the Department of Education, Shirley N. Hufstedler, Secretary. Educational activities are conducted through the new Department of Education. The Public Health Service, the Social and Rehabilitative Services, and the Social Security Administration are within the Department of Health and Human Services. The Public Health Service will continue to consist of six major agencies: 1) National Institute for Health, 2) Food and Drug Administration, 3) Health Service Administration, 4) Center for Disease Control, 5) Health Resources Administration and, 6) Alcohol, Drug Abuse and Mental Health Administration. Hanlon identifies the functions of the Public Health Service to "take the form of research, demonstrations, interstate and international quarantine, advise on technical matters and loan of officers to state and local health departments and other federal agencies with particular health interests. Probably its most significant contribution is made through financial grants-in-aid to state and territorial health agencies for the expansion and improvement of their programs and those of local jurisdictions they include."[2] There are ten regional HHS offices across the country in such major cities as Boston, Atlanta, Chicago, Seattle, and San Francisco.

The original purpose for establishing the Department of Health, Education and Welfare was to pull together, under one agency, the many agencies which provide services affecting the health and productivity of the population. Critics and admirers of the agency are vocal in their evaluation of the relative merit of the Department. Those in favor or supportive of HEW cite such accomplishments as three Nobel prize winners, the great strides made in cancer research, the development of rubella vaccine, and synthesis of the first laboratory gene.[3] Detractors claim the Department has become an uncoordinated, wasteful, ineffective bureaucratic nightmare with rigid and unflexible regulations, dissemination of inaccurate information through regional offices, and duplication of programs with inadequate planning and follow-up.[3] The reorganization of this agency into two separate departments is an effort to provide more adequate services to the population and deal with some of the issues which have surfaced during the last few years.

Because states are free to develop their own programs to meet the needs of its population and because the federal government guidelines tend to be minimal, there has been a great variety of programs developed. Coordination of programs and funds has often been lacking. Delays in delivery of federal monies to states has sometimes been slow. As a result, the quality and quantity of services has been erratic and often times inadequate. In an effort to better coordinate federal funds to states, many states are reorganizing their bureaucratic structure so that health, social, and welfare funds are centrally channeled and can meet total needs of clients and families rather than isolated needs.

The fair and equitable allocation and utilization of funds to states for the needs of its citizens is a dynamic process which will need constant scrutiny, evaluation, and implementation. Although the Health Planning and Resources Development Act of 1974 is designed to help better distribute and utilize funds, it will not provide a total answer to health needs and costs. That quality can only be met through the combined efforts of consumers, providers, and governmental and voluntary agencies striving for the common goal of effective, available, high quality health care and services.

The voluntary health agencies at the federal level are "responsible for supervising and guiding the activities, functions, responsibilities, programs and projects of its state officers."[3] National level agencies promote education, research, and service through their local and state offices. Private providers, associations, societies, and organizations provide leadership, guidance, and support for the local and state membership. They contribute to health care through education, lobbying, research, and standards of practice activities. Direct services are rarely, if ever, provided.

In summary, the basic organization of health care in the United States is carried out at the local, state, and federal levels. Services are of a direct and indirect nature provided by official agencies, voluntary agencies, and private providers. There can be no denying that the system is complex, overwhelming, and supports duplication of effort and time. The merits or lack thereof of the system can and have been debated by many. There will be no easy or swift solution to the problem we encounter.

HEALTH CARE PROVIDERS

Community health nurses have always worked as a team with other health care providers. The original health team consisted of a physician, sanitarian, and a nurse. As time passed and the scope and practice of public health expanded, additional health providers were added. Today the community health nurse often finds herself being asked by consumers to clarify the title, function, and preparation of various team members and those members of the expanded team in the many referral resources utilized. Although the potential list of direct and indirect health providers is enormous, the following pages describe some whom the nurse is most likely to contact and utilize in providing nursing services to clients.

Ironically, there is much confusion about the role of the nurse professional and her level of preparation. Many lay persons see a nurse as a nurse as a nurse. The title "nurse" is often given to anyone who wears a white uniform and works in a hospital or for a physician. As more and more professional nurses shed the traditional white uniform for street clothes and various other types of apparel, the once fool-proof means of identifying a nurse will be lost. As professional nurses gain more knowledge and skill, their many functions also change. This can be confusing to the consumer. It is of major importance to the survival of nursing that both professionals and consumers understand the various levels of preparation for nurses and the multitude of roles they assume. Nurses, too, need to understand the differences and likenesses among their professional peers.

Nursing care is delivered through three separate levels of nursing preparation. The registered nurse is one who has completed an approved program of study in an associate degree, diploma, or baccalaureate program and has successfully written and passed the standard National League for Nursing examination. Once a nurse has passed the N.L.N. boards he or she is a registered nurse. During the time from graduation until successful completion of the boards, the nurse is appropriately titled a "graduate nurse." Advanced educational preparation through masters and doctoral programs and various practitioner programs equips nurses to carry on a variety of advanced roles including independent practice, leadership, and research.

The second level of nursing is provided by practical or vocational nurses. Programs for practical nurses are 8 to 15 months in length. In all states the practical nurses are licensed.

Third level nursing care is provided by nurses' aides or nursing assistants. Training for this role is done on the job by individual institutions and agencies. They provide for personal care of clients. Their primary sites of employment are hospitals, nursing homes, and home health agencies. A license is not necessary and the quality and duration of preparation programs varies greatly between settings.

There is also confusion about who a doctor is. This title is applied to a variety of persons among them medical doctors, osteopaths, chiropractors, psychologists, and educators. When one is talking about "Dr. X," it is imperative that one establish the kind of doctoral preparation one has. The most commonly known doctor is the medical doctor (M.D.). This is a person who has completed a prescribed and approved program of premedical and medical school preparation. Completion of medical school allows one to earn the title M.D. National Board examinations are taken in three parts; during the second and final years of medical school and during the internship year. After completion of medical school, doctors take a one year internship which is hospital based. This may be either a straight (in one specialty area) or rotating (two or more specialties) experience. Following the internship most physicians take a residency of two to five years depending on the chosen specialty. Physicians can be board certified or a diplomate of that board by completing an approved internship and residency, a written plus oral examination, and varying years of practice. There are 20 specialties and they include such areas as family practice, surgery, anesthesiology, obstetrics/gynecology, pediatrics, psychiatry, and neurology. All physicians must pass examinations in order to be licensed to practice medicine.[5]

Osteopathic physicians constitute another category of doctors. Their education is like that of medical doctors but includes extra hours of osteopathic manipulation. It is defined as "a system of medical practice based on the theory that disease is due chiefly to mechanical derangement in tissues, placing emphasis on structure integrity by manipulation of the part. The uses of medicine, surgery, proper diet, psychotherapy, and other measures are included in osteopathy."[5] An internship year is usual as well as advanced preparation in a specialty area with licensure included as a practice requirement.

Chiropractors also assume the title of doctor. Their practice involves external, physical manipulations of the spine in order to treat illness. They are licensed to practice. Formal medicine has little if any contact with these practitioners.

Dentists comprise a large segment of the total health team. They too are called doctors and must complete a prescribed program of study, usually a minimum two years of predental and then four years of dental school. Unlike physicians, dentists do not have to engage in an internship or residency in order to practice, although this is required if they intend to become board certified. There are eight dental specialties which include orthodontics, endodontics, periodontology, and public health dentistry.[5] Both a written and practical examination are required for practice. The major focus of dental practice is in the private sector (the degree one obtains is either a D.M.D. (Doctor of Dental Medicine) or D.D.S. (Doctor of Dental Surgery). According to Wilson and Neuhauser there is essentially no practice difference between the two degrees.[5]

Podiatrists or chiropodists are specially trained doctors who diagnose and treat various conditions of the feet. The degrees offered are either the D.S.C. (Doctor of Surgical Chiropody) or Pod.D. (Doctor of Podiatry). Both require a minimum of two years of college prior to entering a four year podiatry school. All podiatrists are state licensed.

Veterinarians serve an important role in the health knowledge and practice for humans. They receive the doctor of veterinary medicine degree (D.V.M.) and provide care to pets and other animals. They are engaged in research to help determine and understand the interrelationship of animal and human health. This is important because diseases can be transmitted from animal to man by a variety of means and because animals such as hogs, cattle, and sheep are used for human food consumption.

Psychologists who are prepared at the doctoral level are able to administer and interpret various psychological tests of intelligence, aptitude, and so forth and to conduct different kinds of therapy programs under the supervision of a psychiatrist. Educators, prepared at the doctoral level, are also participating in the evaluation and planning for children with learning disabilities and various other handicaps. As community health nurses are becoming more involved in the evaluation of children for learning disabilities and behavioral difficulties, contact with the psychologist is increasing. They practice in a variety of settings including schools, hospitals, and outpatient departments.

Additional professional health team members include social workers, nutritionists and dietitians, physical therapists and occupational therapists. Social workers function in a variety of settings and usually specialize in individual, group, or community work.[5] Social welfare policy and services are a main area of focus. To qualify as a professional social worker a Master of Social Work (MSW) degree is required, which is usually a two year graduate program.

Nutritionists are concerned with "carrying out nutritional programs for the promotion of health and prevention of disease."[5] Dietitians focus on the feeding of individuals and groups based on knowledge and management skills in nutrition. Dietitians tend to be hospital based while nutritionists are generally community health based such as in outpatient departments or community clinics. Both roles require preparation at the college level and masters and doctoral programs are available.

Work with physical and occupational therapists is common in the community. Clients may travel to a center for service or may receive the therapist in the home. Occupational therapists complete four years of college leading to a Bachelor of Science in Occupational Therapy with additional preparation available. Much of their work includes assistance in environmental modification for the handicapped client. Also important is the provision of alternate activities to maintain interest and utilize time in a satisfying, constructive manner. Physical therapists focus primarily on restoration or improvement in musculoskeletal function. Preparation comprises completion of a four year bachelors program, a 12 month certificate course for an individual with a bachelors degree, or masters degree training. In order to practice, physical therapists must be licensed. [5]

Pharmacists provide a vital service to the health of the population by preparing, prescribing, and dispensing drugs and medicine. [5] Their education is five years in length leading to a Bachelor of Science in Pharmacy. The first two years are preprofessional and the latter three years are professional. Pharmacists engage in a 6 month to 12 month apprenticeship or internship under the supervision of a licensed pharmacist. They must pass a state board examination before they are eligible to practice as licensed pharmacists. Most pharmacists practice in the retail or community pharmacy which may offer a wide variety of health, health related, and miscellaneous items. Masters and doctoral programs in pharmacy are also available.

The last health team member to be mentioned is the sanitarian. The kind of contact consumers and community health nurses have with this member may be limited. Sanitarians are responsible for "helping people understand the laws that protect their health; providing technical advice and assistance so as to bring about voluntary compliance or, if necessary, enforcement of the laws." [3] Among the specific areas of concern are safety of well water and public water supplies, rabies cases, food poisonings, sewage disposal systems, epidemiology of typhoid fever and dysentery, and education of professional and consumer groups. Educational preparation is via one of three routes: 1) college degree with a major in sanitation or sanitary engineering; 2) college degree and 16 semester units in public health courses; and 3) college degree including at least 30 semester hours of basic science and one year of full time experience in a health department. [3] A license or Certificate of Registration is required before one can practice in any state. Graduate preparation is also available in this field.

In addition to the professional health care provider one will encounter, there are also many para- and nonprofessionals who participate in the total health care program. Although space has not allowed for extensive elaboration on such positions, one should be aware that many of the professions employ persons with and without formal training to extend the service they are able to provide. For example, nursing may employ nursing assistants and nurses' aides, physicians may employ physician assistants, dentists may employ dental hygenists and assistants, and psychology and social services may employ persons at various educational levels to assist in providing care. In order to avoid giving misinformation, one should actively clarify the title, preparation, and limitations of allied workers.

In summary, the number and variety of health care providers is staggering. There are questions being raised on all sides as to the need for so many roles. As the number of providers increases, so do costs to the consumer. All professions must take a hard look at the services they provide and at the qualifications needed to carry out the expected services. Where possible a moratorium should be placed on new role development until it has been determined that the task cannot be adequately handled by a provider already established in the system.

HEALTH CARE SETTING

Just as there are a variety of health care team members, there are also many health settings in which the community health nurse may work. An understanding of the various sites and kinds of services provided in different health settings is necessary in order to utilize such facilities to their fullest. For a detailed outline of health care services in the United States, the reader is referred to Wilson and Neuhauser. [5]

In this section we will discuss a sampling of these settings and examine some of the services they provide. Because the hospital is the first health care setting most people think of in terms of service areas, this will be our beginning point. The hospital represents a service available to clients on the total community health care continuum. It often centralizes many diagnostic and treatment modalities such as x-ray, laboratory, and counseling. As community needs, research data, and financial resources have changed, so have the foci, services, and direction of many hospitals.

Hospitals fall into various categories based on such factors as 1) ownership, 2) type of patient treated and services provided, 3) average length of patient stay, 4) medical and osteopathic facilities, 5) teaching and non-teaching orientation. [5] Hospital ownership may be at the federal, state, or local level. Federal hospitals include those providing services for current military personnel and their families (Army, Navy, Air Force), the Veterans Administration which services discharged military personnel with and without service connected disabilities, and the Public Health Service hospital whose recipients of service include merchant seamen, personnel and dependents of the U.S. Coast Guard and Coast and Geodetic Survey, American Indians and Eskimos, federal employees injured on duty, persons addicted to narcotic drugs, and others. [5] State hospitals provide long term care for mentally ill, mentally retarded, and tubercular clients. Local hospitals may come under district, county, city/county, or city control. The type of client seen, the type of services provided, and the revenue sources available will depend on its organizational structure. Many of these hospitals provide care for both indigent and private patients.

In addition to the large number of governmental hospitals mentioned above, there are also many nonprofit or voluntary hospitals. These may be operated by churches, community corporations or associations, or industrial or union groups. Their services may be open or restricted. Open care would mean universal eligibility while restricted services would require membership in a group such as a particular industry (railroads) or a union. One other type of voluntary hospital is the cooperative hospital. The Kaiser Foundation is an example of this model in which comprehensive care is provided through group practice, paid for through prepayment by members and controlled by users of the institution.

The last major type of hospital is the proprietary or profit kind. These may be owned by individuals, partners, or investors. In any event, the purpose is to make money.

The term *teaching hospital* refers to one which has an approved internship and residency program and may offer clinical facilities for medical students. Medical schools may own these hospitals or may provide operating services without ownership.

As hospital stays have shortened, the need for home care and followup has increased. To meet this need, many hospitals have established continuing care services, usually under the auspices of the nursing department, but sometimes located in the social service department. The community health nurse working in such a setting would aid in discharge planning with the client and family, floor staff, and community resources. She would assist in or make necessary referrals for home care and followup. In such a role she must be familiar with community resources and serve as liason between the hospital, client, and community.

Health care in the home may be provided by a variety of organizations. With the establishment of Medicare and Medicaid programs which are federally funded, the term *Home Health Agency* was established to refer to an agency which was eligible for receiving federal funds. This term includes visiting nurse associations, home care programs, and combined agencies. A home care program is defined by Wilson and Neuhauser as "an organized program, hospital or community based, for the provision of a spectrum of medical services, equipment and supplies to patients in their homes, generally patients with chronic illness."[5] Visiting nurse associations provide nursing services in the home through the direct efforts of a registered nurse or by home health aids under the supervision of a registered nurse. Nurses provide direct and indirect nursing care, education, and counseling. Additional services through this voluntary agency might be physical and occupational therapy.

A combined agency is one which offers the services of both voluntary and official agencies such as visiting nurse associations and local health departments. By joining efforts, the scope of services can be expanded and resources utilized in a more effective manner. Administration structures can vary and should be clarified to provide for adequate understanding of the organization. Funds coming into the combined agency are primarily from taxes, contributions, and third party payers. The nursing roles from the two agencies in this type of setting usually merge. In health departments the nurses usually direct their efforts toward health promotion and preventative measures. Nurses from visiting nurse associations traditionally provide bedside care. In the combined agency there may not be this sharp demarcation of role. In fact, this orientation might well broaden the scope of nursing service the registered nurse is able to provide.

Ambulatory settings are either hospital or community based. Hospital based services are carried out in ambulatory care units or clinics. The population served may be indigent, private, or both. Teaching hospitals often provide service to both population groups. Service is provided through the house staff consisting of interns, residents, and attending physicians or by private physicians with offices located in the clinic area. The services provided vary depending on the size and expertise of the unit but include such specialties as medicine and surgery.

Community based settings include neighborhood health centers, mental health centers, and drug treatment centers. Neighborhood health centers provide comprehensive health services to a population in a geographic area. Efforts are of a health maintenance and disease prevention orientation. Comprehensive mental health services including crisis intervention, counseling, and education are provided to a geographic area through the services of a mental health center. The kind and location of services will depend on the needs and facilities of the community. Both professional and lay personnel are employed in such settings.

Drug treatment centers function as primarily self-help or methadone programs. The methadone programs are generally hospital based whereas the self-help program is community based. Methadone is used as a long term heroin substitute for heroin addicts. The self-help program is a drug free group approach to dealing with drug addicts. Both approaches may include counseling, short term residential facilities, and hot line services.

Private practitioners provide their services in office settings located in a variety of locations. Some may be residential, hospital, clinic, or office suite based. These physicians and nurses may work in solo, group, or partner practices. Supplemental services such as laboratory and x-ray are done through referral or contract means. Payment for service is usually out of pocket or from third party sources.

Nursing homes provide a variety of health care services ranging from minimal to constant professional nursing services. There are basically three types of nursing homes: 1) skilled nursing facility; 2) intermediate care facility; and 3) residential facility. The skilled nursing facility (SNF) provides 24 hour service and professional nursing care. Medicare and Medicaid may pay for services if certain guidelines are met. Services in an intermediate care facility (ICF) may be covered by state Medicaid but not by Medicare. The ICF is considered a less expensive alternative to a skilled nursing facility. The residential facility is generally considered to be a rest home and neither Medicare nor Medicaid funds are available for such placements. There are generally four levels of care provided in nursing homes. The higher the level designation the more skilled nursing care is needed. Many nursing homes provide more than one level of care. Wilson and Neuhauser identify three types of services offered in nursing homes as: 1) nursing care provided by R.N.s and L. P.N.s as well as support services like physical and occupational therapy; 2) personal care such as help in walking, bathing, dressing, etc.; and 3) residential care which provides room and board in a protected environment. [5]

The last service to be mentioned is that provided by hospices. Hospices provide care and support to dying patients and their families through spiritual, emotional, and medical interventions. "Hospice is a medieval term, used because it signifies that the doors are open to the troubled on a journey from one life to the next; it also emphasizes that spiritual and emotional care are as important as medical care." [6] Hospice facilities may be part of a hospital unit or a separate entity altogether. The movement, which originally started in England, is making progress in the United States. The approach is interdisciplinary in nature and includes nurses, clergy, psychiatrists, and physicians. Help efforts are directed toward relief of pain, support and understanding of the dying patient, and support of the family members who will survive. "The goal of hospice care is to help a patient continue life as usual—work, being with a family, doing what is especially significant before life comes to a close, and feeling a part of on going life." [6] The hospice offers help and support as the patient and family need it. It is a facility which one moves in and out of as necessary. As the population, lay and professional alike, come to grips with the reality of mortality and the very real need to face it squarely, greater use of such facilities will be carried out. People need to actively participate in their rites of dying for it is a part of living.

The above identified health care facilities represent some of the major ones which a community health nurse may work with or utilize as referral sources. It is the responsibility of the nurse to investigate each facility directly to determine scope of services provided, eligibility requirements, and payment options. With this information she will be in a position to make recommendations in order to meet client needs.

HEALTH RESOURCES

The identification and investigation of potential resources is a constant task of the community health nurse. It is knowledge of services available in the community which allows the nurse to provide comprehensive care. A file of some kind, perhaps a Rolladex or card file, should be compiled which will include such information as name of agency, service or person, address, phone number, type of service provided, cost and eligibility requirements. As changes are made, cards can be updated or removed.

The kinds of agencies/services to be compiled are limitless. Since the focus of the nurse is to consider all aspects of the client's life, information on emotional, social, religious, recreational, health, educational, and vocational services is helpful. This will allow the nurse to plan and carry out a nursing intervention for almost any identified need even though she does not directly provide the service.

One seeks information from a variety of sources. Local and state governmental offices can provide information about programs to meet a myriad of needs ranging from vocational and special education to welfare services, housing, and health services. By traveling the governmental maze in search of information, the nurse can be sensitized to the many frustrations encountered in trying to obtain exact information. This effort can save clients much time and aggravation as they seek services.

Voluntary agencies provide direct and indirect services. Some communities publish directories of voluntary agencies. United Fund also can supply a list of agencies which provide services. The telephone book, both white and yellow pages, is another source for agency contact. The police and fire departments can provide information about their services. Both of these departments may offer educational or direct care programs such as cardiopulmonary resuscitation.

The scope of services a nurse is able to provide both directly and indirectly is broad. She will best be able to do this when a thorough knowledge of the health care delivery system in the area is gained. In addition, she will need to seek names and services provided by private providers and the large number of official and voluntary agencies providing health and health related services. In most instances there will be no single available source book for this information. It will be obtained through much documentation work and plain old footwork. All information obtained, however, should be completely recorded so that a resource file can become a permanent on going part of the service. Comprehensive health services will only be provided when a thorough understanding of the community and its resources is possessed.

REFERENCES

1. Health Planning and Resources Development Act of 1974, pp. 4, 7-9.
2. Hanlon, John J.: *Public Health Administration and Practice*, ed. 6. The C.V. Mosby Company, St. Louis, 1974.
3. Smolensky, Jack: *Principles of Community Health*, 4th ed. W.B. Saunders Company, Philadelphia, 1977.
4. Gunn, S.M., and Platt, P.S.: *Voluntary Health Agencies: An Interpretative Study*. The Ronald Press Co., New York, 1945.
5. Wilson, Florence, and Neuhauser, Duncan: *Health Services in the United States*. Ballenger Publishing Company, Cambridge, Mass., 1974.
6. Craven, Joan, and Wald, Florence S.: "Hospice care for Dying Patients." *American Journal of Nursing*, 75(10):1816, Oct. 1975.

BIBLIOGRAPHY

Althouse, Harold L.: How OSHA Affects Hospitals and Nursing Homes." *American Journal of Nursing*, 75(3):450, March 1975.

Callender, Marie: "National Approach to Long Term Care." *Nursing Outlook*, 21(1):22, Jan. 1973.

Craven, Joan, and Wald, Florence S.: "Hospice Care for Dying Patients." *American Journal of Nursing*, 75(10):1816, Oct. 1975.

Education for Allied Health Professions and Services. Department of Health, Education and Welfare, Public Health Service, Bureau of Health Manpower, Washington, D.C., 1967.

Gunn, S.M., and Platt, P.S.: *Voluntary Health Agencies: an Interpretive Study.* The Ronald Press, Co. New York, 1945.

Hanlon, John J.: *Public Health: Administration and Practice,* 6th ed. The C.V. Mosby Company, St. Louis, 1974.

Health Planning and Resources Development Act of 1974. U.S. Department of Health, Education and Welfare, DHEW Publication No. (HRA) 75-14015.

Ingles, Thelma: "St. Christopher's Hospice." *Nursing Outlook*, 22(12):759, Dec. 1974.

Keith, Pat M.: "A Preliminary Investigation of the Role of the Public Health Nurse in Evaluation of Services for the Aged." *American Journal of Public Health*, 66(4):379, April 1976.

Kobrzycki, Paula: "Dying with Dignity at Home." *American Journal of Nursing*, 75(8):1312, Aug. 1975.

Linn, Margaret; Guret, Lee; and Linn, Bernard S.: "Patient Outcome as a Measure of Quality Nursing Home Care." *American Journal of Public Health*, 67(4):337, April 1977.

Martinson, Ida M., et al.: "When the Patient Is Dying—Home Care for the Child." *American Journal of Nursing*, 77(11):1815, Nov. 1977.

Moutin, Joseph W., and Flook, Evelyn: *Guide to Health Organizations in the United States 1951.* Federal Security Agency, Public Health Service, Bureau of State Services. Public Health Service Publication No. 196, 1951, Washington, D.C.

Paige, Roberta, and Looney, Jane Kinkbiner: "When the Patient is Dying—Hospice Care for the Adult." *American Journal of Nursing*, 77(11):1812, Nov. 1977.

Shetland, Margaret L.: "An Approach to Role Expansion, the Elaborate Network." *American Journal of Public Health*, 67(10):1959, Oct. 1977.

Smolensky, Jack: *Principles of Community Health.*, 4th ed. W.B. Saunders Company, Philadelphia, 1977.

Wilson, Florence, and Neuhauser, Duncan: *Health Services in the United States.* Ballinger Publishing Company, Cambridge, Mass. 1974.

CHAPTER 6
POLITICS AND PRACTITIONERS

MAXENE JOHNSTON, M.A., R.N.

When we begin our health careers as students, we are taught and we are questioned. We soon begin to develop our own questions. Eventually, we become practitioners, and the questioning continues: What contributes to the kind and quality of care patients receive? What changes can we expect in health care? Where do the changes occur? Who and at what level is the best person to effect change? Why has health become so "political?" How much government is involved? And where do patients fit in the overall picture of health politics?

These are the types of questions that nurses ponder in an attempt to cope with the puzzling qualities of health care practices in our country. These are also the types of issues that need attention if we are to sort out and understand the sociocultural and political environments in which nursing is practiced.

The purpose of this chapter is fourfold:

1. To provide some general information on historical and contemporary factors affecting community health and nursing practice.
2. To identify current trends, mandates, and folk influences on health, and their impact on patients and practitioners. By trends I mean the particular directions health beliefs and practices take over time. Mandates, on the other hand, are definite orders or charges for action. These either come from those in positions of authority or can take the form of instruction given by a constituency to an elected legislative body. Mandates involve the patient, practitioner, and politician in a dynamic set of

interrelationships that has a profound effect on health care. Folk influences add yet another dimension to the quality of life we see in our communities. These influences are indigenous to our society and reflect our customs, traditions, and beliefs, as well as modify our behavior.

3. To discuss the relationships between health groups and the people they serve. One aspect of these relationships involves the realization that patient care is now provided through a vast and complex health industry. Providing health services has become an industry made up of a myriad of businesses. It is only natural then that the role of health "broker" would evolve to bring consumers, providers, and manufacturers together to exchange goods. The health broker concept reflects the realities of the business relationships in today's health care practices while other aspects include the sociocultural components of patient-practitioner relationships.

4. To describe the political nature of the agencies and settings in which nurses work and provide some guidelines to assist nurses in their ongoing interactions in these settings.

You might wonder at this point what, if any, help or relevance this has to community health nursing. How will this information affect your practice? This is a most likely question and one that carries with it an air of uncertainty and eagerness for meaning. Perhaps the best way to approach an answer to such a multilevel question is to recall the story of Michael Farraday being asked of what good were his studies in electricity. Farraday allegedly replied, "What good is a baby?"

Needless to say, none of us is naive enough to believe that an awareness of the enormous sociocultural and political nature of our health practices and institutions will provide us with any immediate gains such as a new remedy or method for relief of trauma. To understand the relevance of these issues to community health, we must take the long point of view. We must develop a sense of history about medicine to really comprehend the uneven political nature of today's challenges in health.

COMMUNITY HEALTH: AN ADAPTIVE HISTORY AND A CHANGING PRESENT

In studying health historically, a commonly unnoticed fact is the radical difference between ancient and modern science. Ancient science was known to be observational and descriptive. On the other hand, modern science is manipulative. The difference is drastic and carries with it considerable consequences.

If modern science is manipulative, it is by the same token ecologically disruptive. With ancient science, like ancient medicine, man was able to understand his environment. It directed and supported his adaptive efforts. It enabled him to live within his world. What it did not do, however, was to encourage or empower him to change his world. But this change did eventually come about.

With the advent of modern science, with the rise of the modern city, with the development of industry and electronic inventions, and with the clustering of large numbers of people in new work and living networks, a new array of diseases was born. But the tuberculosis, typhoid, typhus, diphtheria, scarlet fever, infantile diarrheas, and others were not really new diseases. They were new only in their epidemic dimensions and reflected the ecologic disruption that was occurring in the adaptive nature of the population. Naturally, community health nursing practice during this time was strongly influenced by such pressing health needs. Our concerns were focused on the obvious—the diseases, the illnesses. Keeping citizens well did not have the appeal that treating the sick enjoyed.

Now the infectious diseases have been controlled for the most part. This brings us to the medicine of today and perhaps the near future. In his book *The People Shapers* Vance Packard explains today's science as a series of manipulative techniques focused on our current biologic revolution.[1] In essence, he is suggesting that yesterday's science fiction has become today's modern medicine.

It is a well known fact that many of the diseases and disorders we see today do not stem from specific pathogens but rather from economic, iatrogenic, social, political, and cultural factors. These are the pathogenic agents of today's world. These are modern microbians. They are also the conditions influencing the nature of contemporary community nursing practice.

Today nurses are well prepared to deal with individual and family problems and health needs, but this is not enough. In order for nurses to successfully use their skills and abilities, we need to have an awareness of the sociocultural and political nature of our practice as well as the settings and the communities in which we work.

As nurses we have come to recognize that we are not autonomous but are part of a health care delivery system that is politically based. We have seen a growing interest by nurses in developing a greater understanding of the sociocultural and political context in which nursing has developed and in which nurses now have to function as professional health care workers.[2] This is the result of several changes in society in general and in nursing in particular.

Nursing in the United States is practiced in a society experiencing a variety of value and role changes. Traditional jobs and roles for males and females are being challenged as no longer functional, appropriate, or desirable. As a result, more men are becoming nurses while at the same time more traditional expectations and values continue to influence the patterns by which status and rewards are distributed among male and female nurses. The fact that male nurses are promoted to leadership positions more readily and command higher salaries when compared to their female counterparts seems indicative of the lingering traditional notion that most often men are heads of households and therefore should command more status and more pay.

Changing values have also brought about the proliferation of new nursing roles; nursing care specialists, liason nurses, nurse practitioners, midwives, epidemiologists, and a cadre of nursing specialities directed to expanding services to specific patient populations. Such role changes have brought nurses into direct confrontation with other professionals, generated new legal definitions of practice, and created ambiguities in the expectations of patients and practitioners. These role changes, however, are a direct result of the change in the nurse.

Generally, nurses no longer find it acceptable to cope with inequities and inadequacies found in community practice. We have found that all communities have their share of such problems, ranging from barriers that prevent handicapped people from being fully independent to nursing homes that are unsafe and unhealthy. However, because today we know more about assertiveness and the rights of individuals, more nurses are acting and developing skills to deal with problems encountered in providing what we know people need and want. Community health nurses are now initiating legislation, testifying in response to legislation, defining underserved populations, and developing competent practitioners to meet those needs. They are not only found in visiting nurse and home health agencies but are working in schools, hospitals, and ambulatory settings to provide a level of care that reflects a health rather than illness model as well as continuity and coordination to the chaotic and episodic nature of patient care. Nurses are changing the inequities in community care and speaking out on the inadequacies. They have become, in essence, more political.

HEALTH POLITICS: TRENDS, MANDATES AND POLICIES

It would be reassuring to learn that most health issues and their solutions arise from professional and humanitarian commitments and beliefs. Yet over the years we have seen the divisive nature of professional, political, and consumer approaches to a number of causes such as the welfare of elderly people, the care of the mentally ill and handicapped, the struggle for equal rights of minority groups, the demands for family planning provisions, the issue of abortions for poor women, as well as the dilemma of the self-care movement.

Understanding these conflicts calls for a degree of insight into our own ideals, beliefs, and assumptions about the commitments and intentions of these various groups. Until we can do this and can adjust our expectations to the realities of the times, we risk increasing the sense of confusion, disappointment, and frustration we experience when confronted by the trends, mandates, and priorities in health care. They are often difficult at best to understand but predictable when anticipated. Therefore, a discussion of trends, mandates and folk politicians and their impact on health practices and programs is warranted.

Trends

There have been many trends in this country which have affected the way people live as well as affecting those in future generations. One only needs to trace our technologic advances to find the social and behavioral changes they bring along. Since new technology and inventions do not necessarily interrupt the established rules, values, or morals of a society, many of the behavioral and attitudinal changes that result from such discoveries are often considered trends, phases, or the current "in-thing." This fosters disbelief by some and a display of countertrends and worried rhetoric by others. Several examples may serve to illustrate this point.

The care of children is one area in which we continue to see many trends or shifts in the direction of established practice. What is considered to be the proper method of feeding an infant, either by breast or bottle, has certainly fluctuated over the years. It is also interesting to note that, as in the instance of breast feeding, trends vary among different socioeconomic groups. Currently, breast feeding is seen primarily as the method of choice by many women in the middle and upper socioeconomic levels of society while bottle feeding is found more frequently as the choice of lower income women. As Margaret Mead has said, such trends usually are either coming in at the top of society and going out at the bottom or vice-versa.[3]

This phenomenon can also be observed at national and international levels. We see many countries giving up what other countries now want. In the United States we are currently experiencing a trend toward developing more humanistic hospital facilities by providing rooming-in or alternative birthing centers, while other countries attempt to build bigger and more sterile nurseries and delivery rooms.

Other approaches to solving health problems have led to trends in almost every area of practice. We have seen movement in the direction of hospice and home-care programs for terminally ill patients, day-care treatment instead of nursing home placement for geriatric patients, increased acute care specialization in hospital services, regionalization of maternal-child health services, "free clinics," neighborhood health centers with comprehensive services and women's health care clinics, community based psychiatric care, and independent living programs for those people with handicapping conditions. These and other trends in health care often result from the mood and preferences of the consumer or the economic gains behind the approach rather than from simply the inherent therapeutic value of practice. In some instances, however, the high cost of care has forced some trends that have actually enhanced patient care rather than having the opposite effect.

For example, over the past several years we have seen increasing numbers of women wanting to have their babies at home. There are many reasons for this. First of all, it costs a lot of money to have a baby in the hospital. Second, more and more women are questioning their relationships with professionals and are fleeing from patronizing, paternalistic physicians to secure the relationships and environments that allow them to experience a more liberated labor and delivery. There is also an increased desire on the part of fathers to participate in this event. This patient or consumer trend provided the impetus for a contemporary movement by professionals to establish alternative birthing and maternity centers in hospitals in order to promote these desired components of care.

On the other hand we also have seen many revenue producing patient care programs set a trend of care in one direction that may be difficult to redirect to other, perhaps more reasonable practices. What this means is that we are still more likely to see patients admitted to the hospital for evaluations, work-ups, and treatments than to see them treated as outpatients or in the community since much of the cost of hospital based care is reimbursed and therefore reinforced through existing medical and health insurance programs.

This is not to say that hospitalization is not reasonable nor therapeutic but rather to suggest that trends and movements redirecting how and where people are cared for are more likely to result from various economic realities rather than from an accounting of the social, cultural, and psychological disadvantages of our current system and the human costs involved over time.

Changing the nature of care from, for example, acute to preventive becomes difficult given these realities. This makes sense when you consider that overall, most health services and programs have been and will probably continue to be perceived in one way by the patient group, another by the practitioner group, and still another by the politicians who are responsible for observing trends in health care and identifying national priorities and legislative mandates.

Mandates

Early in the 1960s, this country saw a thrust toward mandating health planning and regulation setting. It was an attempt by the federal government to decentralize the control of health planning from the federal-national locus in Washington to the state, and more specifically, to the regions of this country. Many people responded to the promises of the Regional Medical Programs (RMP), later tried to become involved in Comprehensive Health Planning (CHP), and now are helping to build Health Systems Agencies (HSA).[4] The focus, however, has now come around to increasing the amount of consumer participation in planning and regulating local health resources.

Participation has become a key to respectability in the health arena. High demands for the consumer's voice to be represented run parallel to the frustration and concern of educators and practitioners that they too have a vehicle of influence in the health programs and priorities in their communities. HSAs may provide a unique opportunity for many of the health professions to enter into direct communication in regional health affairs. But, as we have already seen in some states, the interactions between the politicians, consumers, and professionals are still a matter of ethnocentric notions of who should be in control and who is more qualified to make decisions. The sad result is often more hard feelings rather than better health planning.

Political decisions will continue to be made that affect the health of the patients we care for and the nature of our practice. Political decisions will be made, whether it be on fluoridation of water, pasteurization of milk, or the number of health clinics for a given area, but they should be informed political decisions. In recent years, however, this has been difficult to achieve since relations between medicine, the public, and government at all levels have become increasingly adversarial. As we enter the era in which we need decisions on a type of national health insurance and a national policy on health for this country, the people and the bureaucracy will be meeting in a never ending merry-go-round of more demands for services, fewer dollars for delivery, and heightened skepticism that neither group offers any hope to make any competent decisions.

It just might be, however, that in the final analysis what the government needs to do and what the public sector needs to do will not be compatible. There are often unrealistic expectations of what the other party should be accomplishing and contributing. But once the goals of mandated program or policy are identified, other questions then need to be addressed. First, will there be enough time to make the goals workable? Second, will there be enough cooperation between state and federal governments and health professionals to make the goals achievable?

There are of course considerable problems with mandating or legislating desirable outcomes. Having the law state that consumers and professionals must participate in health planning will not necessarily be enough to create the social equity and quality controls that were intended. Such orders or mandates are vulnerable to the influence of the multi-tier social and bureaucratic structures on to which they are grafted. A good example of this is the Professional Standards Review Organization (PSRO).

PSROs were mandated by the government to develop quality assurance programs and were designated to review the cost and quality of health care provided by Medicare, Medicaid, and maternal/child health programs in hospitals and skilled nursing facilities.[5] But, early in their development, PSROs were actively fought off by many medical practitioners who perceived such government regulations as increased control and interference in the private practice and use of health services. In time, however, more and more PSROs have been established and are beginning to influence issues of cost control and quality medical care.

The desire for more and more participation in government and for more "home-rule" over health issues by professionals and consumers has not subsided but instead has become more vocal. There appears to be more lobbying for decisions to be made on local levels. Those who support this approach believe that decisions should be made close to the area where they will have the greatest impact. Warde's comments that follow support this observation:

"Health care providers operating hospitals, clinics and centers have long been indisposed to countenance and interference from the outside, either in terms of consumer participation or governmental control. Health professionals have been particularly resistent to local government controls and prefer to live with the border regulations of a more remote national government. The arguments against local government of professional incompetence and of being too political are well known but not well founded. Certainly no level of government has a monopoly on wisdom.

In fact, efforts at the local level where government officials and citizen groups combine can have a powerful impact on services and there are some significant successes to date. The establishment of new federal and state structure interrupts and dilutes this process. There may be an immediate effect of a diminution in the collective capacity of government to provide health care. Nor is the possibility too remote that the presence of state and federal agencies at the local level will be viewed as a true alternative which may lead to further tests of 'mandated services' and a reduction in local government appropriations for health and mental health."[6]

Overall, a stronger relationship between consumers and professions other than medicine and government has indeed been mandated both by law and by the public, and offers a potential center for change in the utilization and development of community health resources.

Folk Politicians

When someone refers to the concept of folk beliefs, there is a frequent association in the minds of most individuals with nonscientific, unproven bizarre notions, customs, and habits. What this is in fact is a demonstration that a distinction exists between the legitimate, formal, and acceptable systems in our culture and those that are seen as informal and not openly sanctioned by the majority of the culture.

Most people would agree that in Western Society we have many informal, nontraditional sources that influence our behavior and ultimately the health of individuals and communities. These sources should be considered to be our folk politicians. They often bring about changes without being hampered by a professional point of view. This also allows them to have a limitless ability to absorb and assimilate new ideas and new perspectives.

Examples of this folk politician concept can be found in all communities. Organized consumer-patient groups are one example. They have become active, self-appointed representatives of various health issues and diseases. Other examples include the many novels and movies that depict health problems and community concerns. The proliferation of these types of folk politicians has had a major impact on the attitudes and knowledge of the public. Today's public knows more than they ever did about the frustrations and successes of the handicapped; the pressures and conflicts of doctors, nurses, and administrators; the joys and sorrows of the retarded; and the health problems and diseases of the poor.

Books, films, and newspapers continue to have a great impact on areas affecting health and illness. But, the greatest politician we have today is our television. No other vehicle has had the profound impact on the living and health patterns of the American public as we have seen from the messianic quality of television. It has become by far the most precise example of a highly industrialized culture in which communication and information exchange about society and human conditions takes place collectively and electrically at a highly technical, unilateral level.

Television, for the most part, has become a contemporary politician most influential in instilling social and moral values, changing levels of public awareness, and stimulating social action. However, the people in television as well as in radio and movies are not publicly elected representatives subject to the same scrutiny and a surveillance of other public leaders. They have a responsibility for the quality of our lives but in fact do not have the dramatic social influence provided by folk politicians of the media.

As our technology advances and our communication resources become more sophisticated, it will become increasingly important to be aware of the variety of scientific, professional, and folk influences affecting the health of individuals. Recognizing the types of formal and informal politicians in a community can assist the nurse in understanding and planning appropriate approaches to contemporary health issues.

THE PEOPLE AND POLITICS OF CURING AND CARING CULTS

Health organizations, such as those that provide community health services, are clearly the caring and curing cults in our culture. They are devoted to producing an intangible commodity called "health."

As practitioners in these health organizations or systems, we religiously worship good health and normalcy and are intellectually committed to these ideals. But the commodity, health, is dependent not only on various practitioner groups (physicians, administrators, technicians, various support staff) but interdependent with housing, education, environmental policies, and the distribution of wealth.[7] Therefore, it is not likely that the mass promotion of the well being of people could take place in the absence of engaging in some political activity whether by default or design.

The People

The individuals concerned with health matters are mainly found in three main social groups in our society. There are the politicians who legislate the health priorities, the patients who consume the health services, and the practitioners who provide the health knowledge and know-how. There are of course a myriad of other extended networks involved in health such as the commercial brokers for health medicines, equipment, health housing (hospitals, clinics, offices), as well as the professionals involved in selling health care treatments and standards.

These groups have many common problems and similar concerns, but each group retains its own special organization, patterns of behavior, values, economic base, and language which distinguishes them from the other groups and provides the interactive qualities for the politics of health care in this country.

Much of the literature on the relationships between health groups and those they serve has emphasized the importance of having a working knowledge of social organization. This is invaluable to one's understanding of his relationship to effective or ineffective health programs. These relationships have a particular significance in community health practice. Freedman explains that for the health professional this requires gaining both a "clear picture of the structure of the community in which he has to carry out his duties and the study of health workers and institutions in relation to the public they set out to serve."[8]

We know that the effects on medical behavior of social relationships within groups being served by health and medical programs are found in many factors. These factors include patterns of power and authority which permit those in dominant positions to facilitate or impede acceptance of medical changes by others; class and caste differences which affect access to and utilization of health and medical facilities; factionalism, which can have a differentiating effect on responses of antagonists to health and medical programs; and family, kinship, and other social factors which in themselves can influence or link people in medical decisions.[9]

The politics that exist between the practitioners and patients in a given community are important to assess. However, it is equally as important to understand that nurses are faced with politics in their own work setting as well.

The Politics

The notion that politics and practitioners have anything to do with one another has formerly been considered to be unpleasant and as compatible as oil and water. The fact of the matter is that this is no longer the case. Not only is politics being mentioned more frequently in patient care settings but the art of influencing policy is essential if the nurse is to carry out responsibilities that result in the improved health and well being of patients.

Traditionally nurses have preferred to think of health care as something outside of politics. Schrock has suggested that the concept of politics conveys ideas of partisanship to nurses, of fighting for power, of inequality, and of many other things which people often translate into the notion of dirty politics.[2] Care, on the other hand, is thought of as being clean. It follows then that caring agencies are usually idealized as places where people are not discriminated against, where everybody gets his fair share, and where there are not two levels of care, one for the privileged and one for the others.

There are those who also argue that there is little or no room for politics in nursing. Their frame of reference has politics associated with corruptness, self-serving, counter-productive behavior, and therefore has no place in the day-to-day care of those who are ill and in matters of life and death. Such "Rip Van Winkle" thinking is just that—years behind. It ignores today's reality that medical decisions at all levels involve, or have an impact on, groups of individuals who are organizationally based in facilities dictated by policy. Rarely do people, particularly in life and death matters, act alone, autonomous and independent of the input, inspiration, and interests of others.

Politics in its purest form is merely the art of influencing thinking and action in the decision-making process. It is the art of influencing policy. In this regard, politics is power, the power to bring about change.[10] Simply stated, the politician can be and often is a change agent, a role well known to the nursing profession. The term politics need not have a negative connotation. In fact, to be "political" should be viewed as a respectable means of working in any organization that develops as a result of the human need for cooperation.

The New Game in Town

Much has been written about the political behavior of nurses as a whole, or rather the lack of it. The socialization of nurses and women into general caring, tendering, and nuturing roles has, in the past, often limited the simultaneous development of the skills necessary to influence policy and shape decisions affecting their practice and/or patient care. But this has changed dramatically in the last few years.

An increasing number of nurses are joining and participating in local and national governmental affairs. They are serving on numerous committees which affect the standards and quality of care in our country. We now see nurses making the time, using their energy, finding the available resources, developing the self-direction, confidence, and assertiveness to enable them to move into active roles in the agencies, schools, industries, and communities in which they work and live.

Agency work settings have perhaps become the most active political arenas for nurses. Most nurses recognized the importance of political wisdom in their jobs long before it became fashionable to take stands, unite around causes, or fight government interference in health care. There is a lot of evidence to support the increased competition between administrators, physicians, and nurses for effective influence on agency policy and operations. Mullane suggests that the nature of the competition between physicians and nurses over nursing care policy is changing, since today more nurses are less willing to direct and influence patient care through the slow, circuitous, self-negating route of the doctor-nurse game.[11]

Nurses are now becoming comfortable and knowledgeable about playing institutional politics and have incorporated a different set of strategies into their problem-solving approaches. Although the name of the game may be different, many of the doctor-nurse rules remain the same. The key, however, to playing institutional politics seems to be in understanding the basics of the informal organization as it affects the formal authority relationships inherent in the agency's formal organizational pattern. The difference here is that the formal organization will emphasize positions in terms of authority and functions whereas the secret of the informal organization is knowing the people and their relationships.[12]

A Guide to Political Action for Nurses

When dealing with institutional politics such as planning strategies for change or mounting a campaign to influence policy, there are a few basic areas that you should assess.

First, collect *who really decides* data. It is extremely important to know who the real decision makers are and who needs to be influenced. Many a disappointed person has left a committee meeting being turned down while a proposal for the ultimate good "thing," program, or action was thrown out. They may have written a convincing project but somehow they had not convinced the people. It just is not enough to do the paperwork—the peoplework is "where it's at."

I experienced an apt example of this principle several years ago when planning some proposed changes for the environment and design of a pediatric clinic setting. Fortunately, before it became necessary to approach the administrative layers of the agency with this request, I learned that no changes of this type have ever occurred without the "blessings" of the master mechanic. Consequently, I pursued an informal link between the master mechanic and myself and was able to get his advice and perceptions of the proposal. All major difficulties were compromised privately and the project, therefore, presented little concern and was supported publically. Essentially, it is important to identify and consult with the person in any organization who perceives he has the responsibility, expertise, and authority in a given area, no matter if real or imagined, in order for you to have any influence over the decisions or policies that affect that area.

The next piece of information you need is *where is he or where are they coming from* data. A prerequisite to influencing any change is to understand the facts of a situation and the points of view of others involved. Whether you want to think of it as their frame of reference or their world's view is not as important as the fact that you think of it. In other words, until you can get into someone else's shoes, you may not know when you step on their toes.

Knowing how you will be perceived by others can also help you prepare for the concerns and anxieties inherent in change. In a more global sense on the subject of perception, Hsu has commented that "The common man in China will accept science if it is disguised as magic, whereas the common man in America will accept magic if it is disguised as science."[13]

Whether you alone set about to introduce change, influence policy, or bring about new decisions, or are invited and asked to do this, understanding the perceptions of others is vital to any successful intervention. Oscar Lewis presents us with a fine example of the undesirable outcome that can result from not understanding the perceptions of a community nor recognizing that any "outsider," as are most health workers with the people they serve, will be seen as potentially disruptive.[14]

Many years ago the residents of the Mexican village of Tepoztlan asked to be helped with their lack of medical resources, pointing out that they lacked a doctor among other things. This request was honored and a medical cooperative was established which included a doctor. But, despite the initial success, the clinic suddenly lost patients and was soon abandoned. Some of the major obstacles were thought to be due to a generalized lack of interest in changing local ways of doing things, lack of rapport between doctor and patients based on the doctor's ignorance of native illness concepts and an attitude of superiority, continued faith of the villagers in their local curanderos, and the local interest groups headed by the leading curandero viewing the medical cooperative as a threat to their power. Outsiders, no matter how many positive measures they provide, will be perceived by some people as a threat to their own status and interests.

The role of an outsider can of course be assigned to anyone. For example, the community health nurse is often perceived as an outsider by the hospital nurse. These categories are arbitrary and have no foundation in reality since nursing practice is based on a philosophy of care that is not limited or bound to a particular work environment. However, since such ethnocentric notions exist between people in various speciality and occupational areas, the relationship between practitioners often reflects attitudes in which one group is seen as incorrect, inferior, or perhaps immoral.[15]

Finally, to be successful with institutional politics you need to know *what is the best timing* data. Knowing when to approach someone, when to give an overview of an issue or to supply detail, and when to approach the right person at the right time—all adds to one's political skill and potential success.

Another point needs to be made about the notion of timing. Perhaps this is nothing more than common sense, but nonetheless it is important to realize that one's boss or the person to whom you report should always be aware of any statements or reports you plan to make to a group in which he or she is present. In other words, never surprise the boss with anything that is not already seen or known about. This qualifies for the category of poor timing and puts the boss in an uncomfortable spot, having to respond publically to this new information while displaying a degree of reassurance that he or she is knowledgeable and in control of the activities of the employees.

SUMMARY

To summarize briefly then, I have tried to discuss some of the sociocultural and political realities in our Western medical system, examine the interactive nature of these realities, and describe their impact on health programs and policies at the various levels of our society. I have indicated that nursing practice is not autonomous but is part of a health system that is politically based. In order to practice successfully in such a system, it is important to have an understanding of several areas affecting community health:

1. The organizational politics of a health setting or agency.
2. Current national and local trends and mandates affecting community health practice.
3. The folk politicians of a community and their influence on health matters.
4. The relationships between health groups and the people they serve.

In the final analysis, there can be no real comprehension of community health without a thorough understanding of its politics and practitioners. This, indeed, presents a challenge and a dedication to inquiry for us all.

REFERENCES

1. Packard, V.: *The People Shapers.* Little Brown and Co., Boston, 1977.
2. Schrock, R.A.: "On Political Consciousness in Nurses." *Journal of Advanced Nursing,* 2:41, 1977.
3. Mead, M.: Lecture: World Congress of Mental Health. Vancouver, B.C., Canada, 1977.
4. Perry, J.W.: "The Next Decade: Issues and Challenges." *Journal of Allied Health,* 7(1):19, 1978.
5. Powell, D.J.: "The Struggles Outside Nursing's Body Politic." *Nursing Forum,* 15(4):349, 1976.
6. Warde, J.J.: "The Role of Local Government in Health Planning." *Journal of Health Politics, Policy and Law,* 1(4):387, Winter 1977.
7. Schrock, R.A.: "Politics and Professionalism." *Nursing Times,* May 5, 1977.
8. Freedman, M.: "Health Education: How It Strikes an Anthropologist." *Health Education Journal,* 14:18, 1956.
9. Lieban, R.W.: "The Field of Medical Anthropology," in Landy, D. (ed.): *Culture, Disease, and Healing.* Macmillan Publishing Co., New York, 1977.
10. Mullane, M.K.: "Politics Begins at Work." *R.N.,* 39:45, July 1976.
11. Mullane, M.K.: "Nursing Care and the Political Arena." *Nursing Outlook,* 23(11):699, 1975.
12. Longest, B.B., Jr.: "Institutional Politics." *Nursing Digest,* 5(3):14, 1977.
13. Hsu, F.L.K.: "A Cholera Epidemic in a Chinese Town," in Paul, B.D. (ed.): *Health, Culture, and Community.* Russell Sage Foundation, New York, 1955.
14. Lewis, O.: "Medicine and Politics in a Mexican Village," in Paul, B.D. (ed.): *Health, Culture, and Community.* Russell Sage Foundation, New York, 1955.
15. LeVine, R., and Campbell, D.T.: *Ethnocentrism: Theories of Conflict, Ethnic Attitudes, and Group Behavior.* John Wiley and Sons, New York, 1972.

BIBLIOGRAPHY

Ashley, J.: "This I Believe About Power in Nursing." *Nursing Outlook,* 21(10):637, Oct. 1973.
Beauchamp, D.E.: "Exploring New Ethics for Public Health: Developing a Fair Alcohol Policy." *Journal of Health Politics, Policy and Law,* 1(3):338, 1976.
Bowman, R.A., and Culpepper, R.C.: "Power: Rx for Change." *American Journal of Nursing,* 74(6):1054, June 1974.
Brandon, W.: "Politics, Administration, and Conflict in Neighborhood Health Centers." *Journal of Health Politics, Policy and Law,* 2(1):79, 1977.

Bush, P.: "The Male Nurse: A Challenge to Traditional Role Identities." *Nursing Forum*, 15(4):390, 1976.

Butler, R.N.: *Why Survive? Being Old in America.* Harper & Row, New York, 1975.

Clapp, L.: *The Congressman: His Work as He Sees It.* Doubleday and Co., New York, 1963.

Davis, K.: *National Health Insurance—Benefits, Costs, and Consequences.* The Brookings Institution, Washington, D.C., 1975.

Ellis, J.H.: "The New Orleans Yellow Fever Epidemic in 1878: A Note on the Affective History of Societies and Communities." *Clio Medica*, 12(2):189, 1977.

Falkson, J.: "We Need a National Health Policy." *Journal of Health Politics, Policy and Law*, 2(3): 310, 1977.

Green, M.J.: *Who Runs Congress?* Bantam Press, New York, 1972.

Griffith, S.: *Congress: Its Contemporary Role.* New York University Press, New York, 1975.

Grissum, M., and Spengler, C.: *Woman Power and Health Care.* Little, Brown and Co., Boston, 1976.

Heilbroner, R.: "Middle Class Myths, Middle Class Realities." *The Atlantic Monthly*, 37:42, Oct. 1976.

Hopping, B.: "Professionalism and Unionism: Conflicting Ideologies." *Nursing Forum*, 15(4):373, 1976.

Hott, J.R.: "The Struggles Inside Nursing's Body Politic." *Nursing Forum*, 15(4):325, 1976.

Isaacs, M.: "Toward a National Health Policy: A Realist's View." *American Journal of Nursing*, 78:848, May 1978.

Kalisch, B., and Kalisch, P.: "A Discourse on the Politics of Nursing." *Journal of Nursing Administration*, 6:29, March-April 1976.

Kemp, K., Carp, R.A., and Brady, D.: "Abortion and the Law: The Impact of Hospital Policy of the Roe and Doe Decisions." *Journal of Health Politics, Policy and Law*, 1(3):319, 1976.

Lawrence, J.C.: "Confronting Nurses' Political Apathy."*Nursing Forum*, 15(4):363, 1976.

Lipsky, M., and Lounds, M.: "Citizen Participation and Health Care: Problems of Government Induced Participation." *Journal of Health Politics, Policy and Law*, 1(3):285, 1976.

Moscovice, I., et al.: "Health Services Research for Decision-Makers: The Use of the Delphi Technique to Determine Health Priorities." *Journal of Health Politics, Policy and Law*, 2(3):388, 1977.

Moss, F.E., and Halamandaris, V.J.: *Too Old, Too Sick, Too Bad: Nursing Homes in America.* Aspen Systems, Germantown, Maryland, 1977.

Navarro, V.: "The Crisis of the Western System of Medicine in Contemporary Capitalism." *International Journal of Health Services*, 8(2):179, 1978.

Navarro, V.: "Social Class, Political Power, and the State." *Journal of Health Politics, Policy and Law*, 2(1):499, 1977.

Powell, D.J.: "The Struggles Outside Nursing's Body Politic." *Nursing Forum*, 15(4):341, 1976.

Raheja, K.: "Nursing in Transition." *Nursing Forum*, 15(4):413, 1976.

Schoenmaker, A.: "Male versus Female Admissions Choice." *Nursing Forum*, 15(4):406, 1976.

Schrock, R.: "Politics and Professionalism." *Nursing Times*, 73:671, May 1977.

Smith, D.: "The Hospital Support Game Revisited." *Journal of Health Politics, Policy and Law*, 2(2):257, 1977.

Smith, J.G. (ed.): *Political Brokers: People, Organizations, Money, Power.* Liveright/National Journal, New York, 1972.

Steiner, G.: *The Children's Cause.* Brookings Institution, Washington, D.C., 1976.

Stevens, R.: *American Medicine and the Public Interest.* Yale University Press, New Haven, 1971.

Strickland, S.P.: Politics, Science, and Dread Disease: *A Short History of United States Medical Research Policy.* Harvard University Press, Cambridge, Massachusetts, 1972.

Tolchin, S., and Tolchin, M.: *Clout, Woman Power and Politics.* Putnam and Sons, New York, 1976.

CHAPTER **7**

HEALTH CARE LEGISLATION AND FINANCING

SISTER ROSEMARY DONLEY, Ph.D., R.N.

Contemporary discussions about health quickly evolve into talk about federal regulations and the cost of health care. It seems that the interrelationships among health care costs, federal legislation, and care patterns cannot be denied or overlooked. The health care system has not always been so complex and interdependent. In the not too distant past public discussions about health care, or medical care as it was then called, centered around the treatment of illness, hospitalization, surgery, and nursing care of the person and his disease.

In the early 1960s when health professionals spoke about medical care, their discussions were also confined to care delivery and professional practice. Students in schools of the health professions heard passing reference to the Hill-Burton Act. In schools of nursing, courses in professional adjustments or trends in nursing underlined the importance of medical, pharmacy, and nurse practice acts. There was little attempt, however, to integrate legislation with practice or to measure legislative impact within the hospital. The cost of illness and hospitalization was given more attention. There were frequent admonitions about the careful use of supplies. Nursing students were asked to calculate the cost to the patient if he continued to follow a special diet or drug regimen. Physicians would consult with patients about their ability to pay for certain tests or treatments. The resultant medical decision was often influenced by what the patient could afford. Most hospitals had charity wards. Practicing physicians and nurses were expected to do a certain amount of free work each year. However, as is evident from this description, cost analyses were simple. Responsibility for the cost of hospitalization and illness was considered within the domain of hospital administration or Blue Cross, the universal synonym for hospital insurance.

Today the public addresses health care within the framework of federal legislation and regulation. Health care costs are a national concern. [1] Nurses have been slower than other health care professionals in acknowledging the impact health legislation has had upon their practices and finances. It is, therefore, imperative that any modern text about nursing examine the interrelationship of cost, legislation, and care delivery practices. There are several ways to accomplish this goal. This chapter will help you identify and trace some interrelationships between health care systems, federal regulation, and cost of health care.

A logical way to begin the analysis of the health care system is to study each of its component parts: health programs, health legislation, and health care costs. Health programs can be identified, defined, and then compared and contrasted with older or more established health or medical care models. An interesting way to look at programs is to locate them within the community. You can begin your list with the hospital and its acute care programs. You will soon discover that hospitals have highly specialized functions and well defined units of care (intensive care units, coronary care units, step-down units, for example). Patients who are not acutely ill are transferred to extended care facilities or skilled nursing homes. Some people seek care in ambulatory care settings. Some hospitals have primary care centers. Others operate home care programs, day hospitals, hospices, or health maintenance organizations.

Hospitals have developed brochures which describe and define their services. These may be helpful to you as you refine your list of health programs. As you conduct your survey be certain to examine the visiting nursing or home health agencies in your area. Clients of home care agencies receive health services within their homes. A major focus of these programs is client and family education.

The work place is another area worthy of investigation. Industry based health programs offer health services to the majority of adults in the United States. These programs, like the school health programs, are often overlooked in examinations of the health system because of the historical emphasis on illness and treatment in hospitals. Most communities also have a variety of clinics or professional offices where physical and mental health services are provided. Some of these follow the traditional practice arrangement of a solo practitioner—usually a physician—rendering medical care on a fee for service basis. Other ambulatory settings house interdisciplinary teams of health practitioners who offer a spectrum of services to children as well as adults. When you have generated a list of health programs, you will be ready to compare present services with practices in the 1950s or 1960s.

Health legislation can be understood most easily if it is related to the organizational structure of the United States Congress. Every two years when a new session of Congress convenes, jurisdictional patterns and responsibilities are confirmed or rearranged. Some committees, for example, the Human Resources Committee in the Senate and the Interstate and Foreign Commerce Committee in the House, have the power to authorize or establish legislative activity within their domains of jurisdiction, that is, human resources and commerce. Health legislation falls within the purview of these committees. Acting through subcommittees (Health and the Environment in the House and Health and Scientific Research in the Senate), members of congress draft bills which establish new health programs or extend, modify, or expand existing health laws. The Health Services Bill and the 1978 amendments to the Health Maintenance Organization Act of 1974 are examples of authorizing legislation passed by the 95th Congress before its adjournment. The other side of the legislative coin is the appropriations process. Just as committees are organized to write laws, other committees are formed to examine proposed or existing legislation and decide on appropriate levels of funding. Appropriations Committees with health subcommittees exist in both the House and Senate. Real power rests within appropriations committees. For even if a law is passed by Congress, its implementation may be postponed or seriously threatened if adequate funding is not legislatively mandated. The Labor-HEW appropriations bill for 1979 contains the compendium of the appropriation legislation in health. Compare for any existing or new law the dollar figure recommended by the authorizing committee with the money designated by the appropriations committee. This will give you a sense of the double-edged process of health legislation. There is another set of committees with which you should be familiar. The Senate Finance and House Ways and Means Committees play unique legislative roles in health. Because they have jurisdiction over tax matters, they can use this structure to authorize and finance health bills. The Medicare Act of 1965, which these committees authored, is an example of a law which defines health programs that will be reimbursed or paid for through the Social Security system. No separate authorization is needed.

When you study health legislation in this manner, you are examining it within a jurisdictional framework. This is the orientation that is necessary if you wish to influence or lobby for any bill. Health legislation can also be considered from an issue or topical perspective. Categories can be derived from existing laws, for example, manpower, health services, health finance, research, and regulation. Other classification systems could follow from the subject, for example, children, adolescent health, and older Americans. This approach cuts across committee jurisdictions and sessions of congress. Analysts concerned with policy research often use this methodology to demonstrate the need for legislative coordination. For example, the 96th Congress will examine several bills designed to support training programs for physicians, nurses, and allied health professionals with the goal of developing a national policy on the education of health manpower. Viewing legislation against criteria of comprehensiveness, scope, and policy direction provides a different assessment than considering each bill against its legislative predecessor.

Another way of studying health legislation is to look at the passage of a law as a political and historical event. This direction is similar to a case analysis. Redman illustrates this method in his narrative about the legislative enactment of a plan to develop a national health service corps.[2] An educational advantage of this approach is that it will acquaint you with a variety of federal documents and enable you to establish or strengthen a relationship with your congressman or senator and the staffs of his district and Washington offices. As has been intimated, the documents you will need to conduct your research are available in Federal Repositories which are located in designated public or university libraries in your region and/or through the offices of your congressman or senator. These documents flow from and record the process by which a bill becomes a law.[3] Among the documents you will need are:

1. *Congressional Records* for the days when the bill is introduced, referred to committee, initially debated and voted on in each House, and acted upon after the conference committee report is filed.
2. Reports on hearings on the bill before the House and Senate subcommittees.
3. Committee reports from the House and Senate.
4. Conference report.
5. *Federal Register* which records the development of regulations and program implementation.

If you become intrigued with the political process, you may wish to spend some time in Washington as an intern or fellow. The National League for Nursing and the American Nurses Association offer summer fellowship experiences for nursing students. [4,5]

Perhaps the most puzzling area to investigate is the cost of illness and treatment. Because this country is considering national health insurance, there is much conflicting dialogue and a developing literature on the subject of costs. The usual starting point is a study of the present health care system and how it is financed. Most Americans have some insurance against the risk of illness. Usually this is a work related fringe benefit over which the policy holder and his family have little real control. For those age 65 and over, individuals with specified disabilities, government workers and their dependents, veterans, and those who need kidney dialysis or transplantation, the federal government provides a health insurance program, Medicare. [6] Medicaid, a federally aided, state administered system, offers a medical assistance program to people with low income. [6] In some states medicaid extends coverage to the medically indigent. Medicare and Medicaid are authorized under titles XVIII and XIX of the Social Security Act as amended.

Other groups of people are self-insured or purchase insurance to augment their work related programs. Still others have no health insurance. When Senator Ted Kennedy announced his plan for National Health Insurance to the 95th Congress in August of 1978, he said of this group:

> "The nation as a whole will spend $252 billion in 1981 on health care and that money will pour into a system without cost controls, without quality controls, with uneven access to care, and without any prospects for improvement.
>
> In fact 26 million Americans still have no insurance coverage whatsoever, 19 million more have minimal, and totally inadequate coverage, and 51 million Americans live in areas without sufficient access to health care." [7]

As you begin to look at the present insurance system, you will discover that benefits vary from policy to policy and from region to region. Medicare offers the only uniform benefit package. When analysts relate insurance systems to costs, they conclude that reimbursement policies encourage the use of the most costly services—hospitals. [8] They also note that the person who needs/demands care and the provider who controls access to the health system are separated from the third party who pays the bills. [9] In discussing the impact of the reimbursement system on nursing, the American Nurses' Association emphasizes that present mechanisms effectively limit public access to nursing service. [10] In supporting coverage of nursing service as a health benefit, ANA argues that paying the nurse when she is the actual provider of care will lower health care costs. [11]

The insurance system is not the only factor associated with spiraling hospital costs. Excess hospital beds, the use of expensive technology and diagnostic aids, and the over-supply of physicians are also indicted as causal agents. [12,13]

The preceding paragraphs have provided a study outline of the health care system. The central thesis of this chapter, however, is that health care delivery, health costs, and the legislative process are linked together. The key to this interaction is health legislation. Since the enactment of Health Insurance for the Aged and Disabled, the official name for the Medicare act, federal initiatives have had major impact on care programs and costs. What are some of the factors which have stimulated health legislation?

FACTORS INFLUENCING HEALTH CARE LEGISLATION

Political Factors

It is difficult to isolate any single factor as an explanatory trigger for the growing federal involvement in health care. However, explanations which trace political, bureaucratic, and public interest are worth examining. Earlier in this chapter an allusion was made to the Hill-Burton program. Advanced in 1946 as a method for establishing health care facilities in rural areas, Hill-Burton became a vehicle for congressmen and senators to bring federal money back home to build hospitals. The Hill-Burton Act illustrates political influence on health care legislation. The outcomes are evident. Hill-Burton money increased or diversified the industry in a region, provided jobs for local people, and rendered health services more accessible. The institutions built with Hill-Burton funds demonstrated in a very concrete manner the power of the congressman or senator. Grant programs to finance health services or construction became political devices. Over time there developed political health constituencies created to insure the flow of federal health dollars back to the districts.

During the Johnson administration and the era of the Great Society, major federal investments were made in a variety of social, health, welfare, and educational programs. Some congressmen and senators came to be known nationally because of their interest in and advocacy for health.[14] Even today it is possible to bestow upon several national figures the title of "Mr. Health." The use of health issues to create a political image is not confined to the Congress. President Carter, for example, recognized that health was of popular interest when he promised national health insurance during the 1976 campaign.

In addition to creating health monuments, political figures have also created health images. Consequently any discussion of the dramatic growth in federally mandated health programs must consider the political dimensions of health legislation and the impact of health bills and programs on the careers of health politicians.

Bureaucratic Factors

Once health programs are legislated, their existence triggers an administrative or bureaucratic response. Cursury evaluation of the growth of the Department of Health and Human Services supports the conclusion that bureaus and departments have developed around various legislative programs. Certainly the Health Care Financing Administration (HCFA), the major agency in the Department of Health and Human Services constructed to manage Medicare and Medicaid, was spawned by the Title XVIII (Medicare) and Title XIX (Medicaid) of the Social Security Act.[15] Over time, bureaucracies created by federal mandate have become powerful and informed advocates for expanded or new health legislation.

The Provider Community

Health care providers also play unique roles in the health legislative arena. The historical involvement of health experts in legislation makes interesting reading. It can be said that federal legislation has encouraged the development of new health providers and has stimulated new organizations of various professional groups who have joined the establishment in lobbying for their self-interests.[16] In the formulation of health legislation, committees hold public hearings on proposed bills. Various health experts and representatives of professional health organizations give testimony about the issues raised by the bill under consideration as well as the predicted effects of the proposed legislation. These statements are part of the public record and are compiled in hearing reports. If you were to study a major piece of health legislation, the Medicare Amendments for example, it would be possible to trace the position of the American Medical Association and the American Nurses' Association from the early days when Medicare was first considered until present times. A study of the records would document distinctly divergent approaches by two large professional groups. Although organized medicine opposed Medicare, physicians have been major financial beneficiaries of the program. Professional nurses, early supporters of Medicare legislation, have experienced no significant financial benefits from Medicare.

While the ANA and AMA may not represent the practicing nurses or physicians, the structure and access of these organized lobbies have enabled both groups to quickly mobilize campaigns, provide data, and inform the media about their view-points. Individual nurses are often uninformed about the position of the ANA and may be generally naive about the impact of health legislation upon their professional practice. Physicians, because of their historical role as direct providers, quickly experience the financial consequences of health legislation. Because of their financial and social positions, doctors are powerful advocates with congressmen and senators.

The recent impact of individual and organized health care providers on health legislation can be examined within the more contemporary context of national health insurance.[17] The preceding discussion conveys the impression that organized medicine and individual doctors are more actively involved in major health legislation than nurses. If you wish to test this thesis, the following interview schedule could be used with physicians and nurses. Analyses of the responses of doctors and nurses in your survey will enable you to assess the level of knowledge, concern, and involvement within each profession.

A timely set of questions would be:
1. What is your stand on national health insurance?
2. What impact would a national health insurance program have on your practice?
3. What is the position of your professional association on national health insurance?
4. Do you agree with this position?
5. What have you done to advance your views?

Diagnosis and treatment of illness, the hallmark of the hospital, medical advances, and the growth of the hospital industry had been dependent on the skill and dedication of doctors and nurses. What has happened to this simple vision? The growth in technology and computerized diagnostic techniques has revolutized medicine. Physicians, trained in highly complex procedures, leave their residencies and establish a practice base in community hospitals. Regional Medical Programs (RMP) (PL89-239), a federally funded effort designed to bring the expertise of the academic health centers to the people through advanced training for nurses and doctors, also contributed to the development of specialized care units (intensive care, coronary care, infant referral center).[18] These identifiable results of health laws (manpower training and RMP) have spawned entirely new federal initiatives. The Congress is now concerned with the growing number of physician-specialists and their influence on the cost of health care. Amendments to manpower legislation which will come before the 96th Congress will offer financial support for doctors who choose primary care rather than specialist training. The Health Planning Act of 1974 created a major effort to control the duplication of services, equipment, and specialized care units. The Medicare law possesses the ability to generate countless companion bills. The Professional Standards Review Organizations Act of 1972 (PSRO) and the Medicare and Medicaid Fraud and Abuse Act of 1977 illustrate this principle. Within the provider category, health legislation stimulates health legislation.

The Consumer Movement

Consumers also have become influential in health care legislation. The patient and his family are now discussed in the literature as partners or health care consumers. The National Health Planning and Resources Act of 1974 (PL 93-641) dramatically underlines the emerging role of the citizenry. Given by legislative mandate a majority vote on health planning boards, the consumer member is in a position not only to make personal health decisions but to engage in policy decisions about the placement of health care facilities and services.

Citizen groups have also become vigilant supporters of patient rights, procedures to guarantee informed consent, food product labeling, and patient package inserts in prescription drugs. Often consumers and providers are pitted against each other in health debates. On issues such as teenage pregnancy and federal funding for abortion, consumer groups oppose each other. Perhaps the most significant initiative by consumers has occurred in the interest of federal support for research and treatment of disease entities. The National Cancer Institute stands as a monument to public belief that a war on cancer could irradicate the disease.

Relation of Health Care Legislation to Other National Issues

In considering factors which stimulate or retard the development of health legislation, health questions must be examined within the gamut of issues which face the American public. The 95th Congress found many of its health bills undermined by growing public concern about inflation and government spending. In fact "Proposition 13" became a watch word in the closing days of the 95th Congress. A decade before, Lyndon Johnson found that public reaction to the Vietnam War eroded into his efforts to build a great society. [19]

In discussing the administrative position on national health insurance, President Carter cited inflation and concern over the economic health of the country as the reason to support his incremental approach to national health insurance. [20] The escalating cost of health services has become an obsessive concern both within Congress and the health care community. The complex problems operative in a highly technologic society are reflected in health care. The debates which have developed around the need to contain hospital costs emphasize that the health care delivery system does not exist or operate within a vacuum.

A brief review of one action of the 95th Congress in its closing days indicates the impact federal legislation has on program development and expansion. In October 1978, Congress passed the Health Services Bill which extended fiscal support for community health centers, migrant health services, veneral disease programs, genetic disease and hemophilia programs, home health services, hypertension programs, immunizations, lead-based paint programs, and grants to states for comprehensive health programs. This single bill also established three year demonstration projects for hospital based primary care centers and a new program directed toward teenage pregnancy prevention and health care services. The Health Services Bill is an obvious example. However, health maintenance organizations (HMO) became more visable and available because of federal legislative initiatives in support of HMOs. An alphabet of programs can be traced to federal health laws. PSROs came to monitor appropriateness of care and bed utilization (PL-92:603); HSAs were constituted to plan for and evaluate the need for health facilities and equipment (PL93-641); OSHA was developed to monitor the health and safety of the work place (PL91-596). The regulatory process formulated to implement the Medicare Act has achieved in itself the stature of a major health program. The Medicaid packages designed by each state offer yet another illustration of the legislative stimuli to the development of health programs.[6] This programmatic thrust is not confined to the federal sector. Hospitals and health care agencies have created departments and programs to capture federal funds through grants or contracts. They have also established internal control operations to aid in meeting federal guidelines especially in the area of reimbursement.

What impact has government spending via health legislation had on health? Today this question is usually expressed rhetorically by raising another question about federal spending: "Can we afford national health insurance?" In considering the implications of federal government involvement in health, some indirect costs can be traced to manpower legislation, regulatory controls, and seed money for demonstration projects. The major influence, however, has been experienced through direct government spending via Medicare and Medicaid. Commenting on the costs of health care, the Office of Budget Management concludes in its special analyses of the 1978 budget of the United States Government:

"Total national expenditures for health rose from $12 billion in 1950 to $139 billion in 1976—more than an eleven-fold increase. Per capita expenditures grew from $78 to $638 over the same period. The percentage of the U.S. gross national product (GNP) spent on health has almost doubled in the last quarter century, from 4.6% in 1950 to 8.6% in 1976. If the rate of increase in recent years continues, the proportion of GNP spent on health will double again to 17% by the year 2000. The amount spent on health by the private sector and Federal, State, and local governments has risen substantially since 1950. However, the Federal Government's share of total health spending has more than doubled since 1965. The share of state and local government expenditures has remained about the same, while the share of private health spending has declined by 17%. The Federal Government now pays almost one-third of all health expenditures in the country. That includes more than 60% of the costs for medical research, 45% for health facilities, 40% for medical education, and 30% for health services."[21]

In defending its program to control hospital costs, the Department of Health, Education, and Welfare* noted that Medicare and Medicaid payments to hospitals have increased at a rate of 19 percent a year since 1967 and that one quarter of the Social Security tax now is used to support Medicare. In fiscal year 1976, the federal government spent $139.3 billion for health. Forty percent of this money paid hospital bills.[22]

It is hard to resolve or untangle the impact of the federal health standards or dollars on health programs or costs. The voluntary health care system seems almost dependent

---

*HEW became two independent agencies under Public Law 96-88, signed October 17, 1979, effective April 2, 1980: the Dept. of Health and Human Services, Patricia Roberts Harris, Secretary; the Dept. of Education, Shirley N. Hufstedler, Secretary.

on federal spending. It is difficult to believe that the federal initiatives in health will lessen. Inflation will cause legislation to be more regulatory than authorizing. The focus in the eighties will be directed more toward outcome evaluation and detection of fraud and abuse than toward program development. From the financing side, current proposals outline payment on the basis of charge, reimbursement for costs, reimbursement for average costs, prospective budgeting, and capitation payments. Another reimbursement model being proposed recommends that hospitals be considered as public utilities.[23] Perhaps analyses developed around all sides of the national health insurance question will yield a system of reimbursement that is more rational.

Although Americans have come to believe that health care is a right, responsibility for exercising and protecting this right is yet to be developed. As students of nursing you will come to define more clearly your professional practice. Historically nursing has considered man within a holistic frame of reference. Man has been described as the study and subject of nursing. You are fortunate to be entering practice at a period when the health care system is being reshaped. Certainly a time of challenge, one responsibility of professional nursing is to participate in the development of a health care system that is oriented to maintaining health and engaging the active, informed involvement of the public.

REFERENCES

1. Inglehart, J.K.: "A Private Sector Answer." *National Journal,* 50:1935, 1977.
2. Redman, E.: *The Dance of Legislation.* Simon and Schuster, New York, 1973.
3. Zinn, H.: *How Our Laws Are Made.* U.S. Government Printing Office, Washington, D.C., 1974.
4. "Interns Share Observations on Washington Experience." *The American Nurse,* 10:12, 1978.
5. "Top Health Officials Welcome NLN's 1978 Public Policy Fellows." *NLN News,* 26:3, 1978.
6. Markus, G., and O'Sullivan, J.: *Medicare—Medicaid.* Congressional Research Service, Library of Congress, 77-216 Ed., Washington, D.C., 1977.
7. Kennedy, Senator Ted: "A New National Health Insurance Program." Congressional Record, October 2, 1978, S16814.
8. Institute of Medicine: *Medicare and Medicaid Reimbursement Policies: Summary and Conclusions of a Final Report.* U.S. Department of Health, Education and Welfare, SSA-PMB-74-250: March, 1976.
9. Jeffers, J.R., Bognanno, M.F., and Barlett, J.C.: "On the Demand Versus the Need for Medical Services and the Concept of 'Shortage'." *American Journal of Public Health,* 61:57, 1971.
10. American Nurses' Association: *Summary Proceedings, American Nurses' Association 50th Convention.* The American Nurses' Association, Kansas City, Missouri, 1977.
11. American Nurses' Association: *Reimbursement for Nursing Services: A Position Statement of the Commission on Economic and General Welfare.* The American Nurses' Association, Kansas City, Missouri, 1977.
12. Inglehart, J.K.: "Controlling the MD Spiral." *National Journal,* 23:866, 1977.
13. Institute of Medicine: *Controlling the Supply of Hospital Beds.* No. 2-04602, 1976.
14. Cohen, R.: "The Kennedy Staff—Putting the Senator Ahead." *National Journal,* 49:1883, 1977.
15. Conley, J., and Havemann, J.: "Reorganization—Two Plans, One Department Down, Much More to Come." *National Journal* 49:1876, 1977.
16. Inglehart, J.K.: "HMO's—An Idea Whose Time Has Come?" *National Journal,* 8:311, 1978.
17. Gehrig, L., and Lesparre, M.: "NHI: Forecasting the Political Climate." *Hospitals,* 50:45, 1976.
18. *National Health Planning and Development and Health Facilities Assistance Act of 1974.* Committee Report of Labor and Public Welfare to accompany S2994. 93-1285: 13-19, 1974.
19. Kearns, D.: *Lyndon Johnson and the American Dream.* Harper & Row, New York, 1976.

20. Carter, Jimmy.: Presidential Directive/DPS-3, *National Health Insurance*. The White House, July 29, 1978.
21. *Federal Health Programs, Special Analysis K, Budget of the United States Government, 1978.* Office of Management and Budget, Washington, 203-204, January, 1977.
22. *Hospital Cost Containment, A Summary of Legislation Pending before the House of Representatives.* U.S. Department of Health, Education and Welfare, Washington, March, 1978.
23. *Reimbursement of the Providers of Health Services.* Staff Study for the Subcommittee on Health and the Environment, of the Committee of Interstate & Foreign Commerce, House of Representatives, U.S. Government Printing Office, Washington, D.C., 1976.

8

HEALTH EDUCATION IN COMMUNITY HEALTH NURSING

LINDA L. JARVIS, M.S.N., R.N.

Throughout one's lifetime there are multiple choices to be made about health, both individually and collectively. Healthful living is influenced by such forces as religious practice, occupational choices, recreational choices, one's culture, social mores, and the environment. We learn to make healthful choices, sometimes through trial and error, other times through didactic input. In all instances, learning leads to some kind of a behavior change. A behavior change which will lead to healthful, happy, and productive living is the goal of health education.

This chapter will identify a definition of health education, the scope and impact of health education, and the community health nurse and health education.

DEFINITION

The need for sound health education permeates the activities of health providers, educators, and agencies in all sectors of our lives. The need to develop and implement effective health education programs has never been greater. The definition for health education as established by the Joint Committee on Health Education Terminology is: "A process with intellectual, psychological, and social dimensions relating to activities which increase the abilities of people to make informed decisions affecting their personal, family, and community well being. This process, based on scientific principles, facilitates learning and behavioral change in both health personnel and consumers, including children and youth." [1]

Inherent in this definition is the responsibility the individual has for his own health status. Health choices made by the individual impact on the family unit and the community. It also points to the fact that individuals, families, and communities have choices concerning health—some will have a positive effect, others are detrimental. Health education both influences and considers psychological, intellectual, and social dimensions of the target population and the health provider. In the end, once exposed to a health education program, the desired outcome is a change in health behavior or attitude. It is never sufficient, therefore, to merely give information, instead the presentation of information must result in a desired behavior or attitude change. To this point Hanlon states "skillfully developed and properly used, health education can become a powerful force in social improvement and change. Its ultimate goal, of course, should be to encourage and assist the public in taking individual and group actions to protect and improve its own health."[2]

SCOPE OF HEALTH EDUCATION

Perhaps more than any single topic, health education should be a constant part of people's lives from cradle to grave. It has become particularly important for people to understand the impact such factors as stress, smoking, exercise, chronic disease, air pollution, recreational choices, occupational choices, and a myriad of other options have on individual and group health.

If health education is to aid people in making choices which will maintain and promote healthful practices, prevent disease, promote long life, avoid accidents, and aid in living and enjoying life to the fullest, educational efforts must be planned and implemented for all kinds of populations.

The term *target populations* is commonly used to designate a group of people sharing one or more characteristics who are identified as needing special attention, education, or other health intervention to increase their perception of an issue/problem, enhance their health practices, or intervene in some manner in order to prevent disease or accidents. If one accepts that persons use health education to live to the fullest, then target populations can be identified for reinforcing efforts as well as corrective activities. People do not have to be a health risk to receive health education. For some people this may come in the form of reinforcement for present healthful behavior, for others it means seeking ways to share information which will encourage the individual to change his "health damaging" behavior to "health generating"[3] behavior.

With the above in mind, school age children, adolescents, the elderly, mothers and fathers, geographic neighbors, a city, unimmunized children, smokers, joggers, the overweight, the underweight, a fifth grade class, a group of junior high school teachers—all of these people can become the goal of the health educator.

Historically, health education as a course of study in the United States has been offered in schools since 1787.[4] Course work was directed primarily toward "physical training, anatomy, physiology and hygiene."[4] In the intervening decades to the present, prompted by many social reforms, educational research, and advanced scientific and social knowledge and technology, health education has become a means of maintaining and improving health in many of life's arenas.

Who, then, are the health educators? Hanlon states that "everyone involved in or concerned with health in any way is a health educator."[2] The list of such educators would include nurses, doctors, dentists, physical and occupational therapists, teachers at all school levels, voluntary health agency and governmental personnel, parents and health educators. The complexity of educational material will depend on one's level of preparation.

There are many universities and colleges in the United States which offer baccalaureate, masters, and doctoral level programs in health education. Some of these educators will work in schools, others will work in a variety of voluntary or official agencies or community organizations, and some will provide services in direct health care settings such as hospitals and neighborhood health centers.

As the various components of the Health Planning and Resources Development Act of 1974 are implemented, it will be interesting to note the educational direction which is taken, for one of the Act's charges is for the development "of effective methods of educating the general public concerning proper personal health care and effective use of available health services."[5] In the end, all of us, professionals and lay persons alike, are health educators, for we all have information to share which will, hopefully, lead to a healthier, enriched life.

IMPACT OF HEALTH EDUCATION

As stated earlier, all of us are potential recipients of health education programs and those of us in the health field, at whatever level, will participate in the planning and implementation of many such programs. What then are some of the factors or issues one must consider when planning such programs?

To be most effective, health education efforts must involve the target population in identification of health and learning needs and planning and implementation of the program. The health educator must keep in mind that there is no one way to do this nor is there a single health education methodology which one can identify and use as the framework for all educational programs. Principles of teaching and learning, however, can be used. These include identification of learner(s), identification of learning need(s), establishment of learning goals, organization of content and selection of teaching methodologies, implementation of the content, evaluation of the learning, and revision of goals, content, and methodology where necessary.

Learners represent all ages and stages of life. They will be affected, to some degree, by their cultural background, their age, educational level, socioeconomic level, and health attitudes. In identifying any learner group, it is useful to determine their health belief frame of reference. In doing such an assessment, utilization of the health belief model as described by Rosenstock will aid the health educator in identifying the degree of perceived threat, personal susceptibility to the threat, and activities directed toward threat reduction.[6] In terms of health promotion/disease prevention, this information can be used to establish appropriate learning goals and teaching content and methodology. Of course the health belief model can also be used in education efforts directed at illness behavior and sick role behavior.[7,8]

In health promotion/disease prevention, the educational task becomes one of identifying motivational factors which will either reinforce present health promoting behavior or will stimulate a behavior change to health promoting activities. Ardell states, "A fundamental principle of health promotion is that each person has the capacity to determine his own health potentials and is the only one who can assume the basic responsibilities for his own well-being."[9] Our task becomes one of identifying cues which will stimulate positive health action and identifying barriers which can be modified or eliminated so they don't interfere with beneficial health behaviors. Health education, then, is always a two-way street between the learner and educator. Educational efforts can be successful only if this is the guiding beacon for the health educator.

Some additional specific factors about the learner which must be considered are his age (it will influence directly his attention span), interest in subject matter, time of learning sessions, language comprehension, location of meetings, availability of child care, and direct and indirect cost. As stated earlier, in order to be most successful, any educational effort should include the learners in planning and implementation.

Since a major goal is to stimulate a positive behavior change and not just the provision of information, such involvement can represent a greater learner committment. Educational programs on a topic such as dental care for a group of second graders will be much different from one planned for a group of fifth graders. The time involved, complexity of learning activities, and attention spans for learning activity will be much greater for the fifth graders than for the second graders. Likewise a program planned for mothers will have a higher probability of being attended and thus utilized if their child care needs, convenience of time, and central location are taken into account during planning efforts. The elderly, when they become learners, need to have available transportation, easy access to and from the meeting place, and consideration given to possible visual and auditory impairments.

Identification of learning needs can originate from a variety of sources, among them are individuals, schools, boards of health, civic organizations, local, state and national governmental agencies, and voluntary agencies. The identified needs can be directly health related as in the need for childhood immunizations, safety oriented such as proper ways to cross streets or poison prevention in the home, recreation directed such as the need for regular exercise or ways to organize a community recreation program, occupation oriented such as safety education, environmentally oriented such as controlling air pollution (smoking, cars, etc.) or solid waste control oriented such as trash disposal and recycling units. All of these areas—health, safety, recreation, occupation, and environment affect the quality of life of the individual, family, and community. Educational efforts are directed toward supporting behavior change to enhance the quality of life in all of these spheres.

Once needs have been identified it will be necessary to determine which ones can and should be approached first. It should be clear from the list above that the identified needs operate across several levels. It is assumed that more than one need would be addressed at a time. For example, among the most common culprits of environmental pollution are car exhausts, industrial exhausts and smoking. Each requires careful study and participation on several levels to begin to realize a change. Smoking cessation at the individual level can be a starting point. Restricted use of cars and/or increased public transportation utilization can be explored at the individual and local level and fuel modification and filter utilization can be explored by the industries at the local level with encouragement of local, state and national anti-pollution law enforcement and Environmental Protection Agency participation. Schools can conduct anti-smoking and physical fitness programs to reach young people in an effort to sway their health choice making.

Once the learner and learning needs have been identified, the health educator is ready to establish learning goals. Learning objectives should be learner oriented. For guidance in the preparation of learning objectives, the reader is referred to the books *Preparing Instructional Objectives* by Robert F. Mager, *The Process of Patient Teaching in Nursing* by Barbara King Redman, and *The Teaching Function of the Nursing Practitioner* by

Margaret L. Pohl. To quote Dr. Mager, "An objective is an *intent* communicated by a statement describing a proposed change in a learner—a statement of what the learner is to be like when he has successfully completed a learning experience. It is a description of a pattern of behavior (performance) we want the learner to be able to demonstrate."[10] Clearly, the learner is the cog in the educational wheel. He must know what he is to learn and what behaviors on his part will demonstrate that learning has taken place.

The development of clear, concise, usable, behavioral objectives takes time and practice. The objectives serve as a guide to developing content and learner evaluation tools. Since a behavior or attitude change is the major goal of health education, objectives need to be written so that behavioral changes are observable and measurable. Examples of observable, measurable behavior include the number of times teeth are brushed per day, use of dental floss, participation in an exercise program, participation in a weight control program, participation in a health education program, and so forth. A word of caution is necessary at this point. One must be careful not to equate, necessarily, a behavior change with an attitude change. For example, one may stop smoking because it is too expensive or jeopardizes the health of a family member rather than because cigarette smoking is hazardous to one's personal health. To determine the motive behind the smoking cessation requires more careful intervention and observation technique. So, although the smoking behavior has ceased (a desirable outcome), motivation for such behavior may be nonhealth related (not a desirable outcome). One is then faced with the choice of accepting the behavior as it now stands or seeking ways of focusing on the health impact of smoking and helping the learner internalize these attitudes. Whether or not such an effort should be explored would depend on the learner needs, educator priorities and time, and overall health priorities, time, and fund availability.

Once objectives have been established one is ready to design the content and select educational resources. The use of the media can enhance the educational presentation if it is utilized judiciously. Media may include posters, slides, movies, transparencies, or video tapes. Teacher demonstrations with the opportunity of learner demonstrations can be useful in determining if a skill has been learned. Media can be commercially prepared or hand done. Whatever mode is chosen, one should take into account the age of the learner, attention span, cultural characteristics, and length of presentation. Never show a film, slides, videotape, or other media without first previewing it yourself. Many teaching programs have been based on a poor choice of media material.

Sources for media are many. They include schools, libraries, governmental agencies, voluntary agencies, commercial organizations, and industries. Some materials are available free of charge while others are available for a small rental fee or purchase charge. Keep in mind that money spent must be paid by someone. If a charge is to be made for health education materials make sure the learner is aware of this before committing himself.

Informing the public of health education programs can be done through such media as radio, television, newspapers, flyers, and posters. Many local radio and television stations have free time available for such public service announcements and are cooperative in providing guidelines for utilization of the service. Other methods include word of mouth, door-to-door informing, and announcements made through schools, clubs, and other organizations. Whatever mode is chosen should be compatible with the community target group and be planned and implemented with their full support and participation.

The evaluation and revision of educational programs and learning must be an integral part of the entire educational plan. Evaluation should focus on the learner to determine if he has met the objectives and also on the educator to determine his or her effectiveness.

Evaluation of both will use the learning objectives to determine acquisition of learning. Because programs may cover different lengths of time and the behavior change may have to be viewed longitudinally, smoking cessation is an example, evaluation may have to be done more than once. Evaluation may be done with paper and pencil tests, return demonstrations, direct behavior observation, completion of questionnaires, or telephone interviews. Whatever method is chosen should be geared to obtain desired information, completed in a short period of time by the learner, and be economically sound in terms of time and money for learner and educator. Students should receive feedback on their evaluations.

Educators need input concerning the impact of the overall program and their perceived effectiveness as teachers. Evaluations may be written or verbally solicited. Hopefully, the atmosphere will be such that criticisms can be made without concern of repercussions. The purpose of education is to share knowledge and information with the learner who takes this material and engages in behavioral and/or attitudinal changes. If he does not perceive the encounter as educationally beneficial, then education has not taken place.

Specific information should be sought about such points as reasonableness of the objectives, style of presentation, suitability of media materials, student input and feedback, and time factors. Information on these points, as well as evaluation by the students, can aid the educator in making necessary revisions. Revision should be implemented, where possible, in succeeding programs.

Health education programs can be planned for all sectors of a given population and/or community. The educator responsible for the planning of the program, regardless of the length, will go through the basic steps for the teaching-learning model. These include identification of the learner, identification of the learning need(s) and establishment of learning goals, organization of content and selection of teaching methodologies, implementation of the content, evaluation of the learning, and revision of goals, content, and methodologies where necessary.

COMMUNITY HEALTH NURSE AND HEALTH EDUCATION

It is accepted that the community health nurse is a health educator by virtue of her professional preparation. Because of the contact with large numbers of people representing many strata of society, the nurse is often in an excellent position to assess health education needs and make recommendations for such programs to the appropriate professionals.

Whether teaching the individual, family, or community, the community health nurse has a constant goal—the improvement or maintenance of health and healthful practices. It is not necessary that the nurse take responsibility for teaching all learners, rather, she may be most effective as a catalyst to identify both learners and learning needs. Her exact educational role will depend on such variables as scope of need, her interests and educational skills, resources in the community for teaching activities, and the priority of the learning need. Efforts should always be directed toward community involvement and direct participation in planning and meeting educational objectives.

Since nurses working in community health are familiar with local, regional, and other resources, they are in a strong position to correlate need and resource. Sharing with peers and consumers the need for recreational programs or facilities, mothers' groups, play groups for children, day care services, drug and alcohol hot lines, death and mourning programs, and other identified needs can sensitize community leaders to concerns and means of resolving them. Keeping people free of disease is not enough. Nurses must become active in meeting other needs which will improve the quality of lives—whether the needs are recreational, occupational, social, or environmental.

People will seek health knowledge and interventions based on their individual and group health beliefs. The identification of these beliefs is a major step nurses will take in providing health education programs. Their efforts will be directed to the individual, family, and community with the hope and intent that the learners will share with others what they have learned.

In short, the title of health educator can be conferred on all persons who provide educational input for the purpose of improving or maintaining the highest quality of life possible. As nurses, our opportunities for such education have always been many. In these times, however, our educational horizons have expanded.

REFERENCES

1. *"New Definitions: Report of the 1972-73 Joint Committee on Health Education Terminology."* Health Education Monographs 33:63, 1973.
2. Hanlon, John J.: *Public Health Administration and Practice,* 6th ed. The C. V. Mosby Company, St. Louis, 1974.
3. Milio, Nancy: "A Framework for Prevention: Changing Health Damaging to Health Generating Life Patterns." *American Journal of Public Health,* 66(5):435, May 1976.
4. Means, Richard K.: *A History of Health Education in the United States.* Lea and Febiger, Philadelphia, 1962.
5. *Health Planning and Resources Development Act of 1974.* U.S. Department of Health, Education, and Welfare, DHEW Publication No. (HRA) 75-14015, 1975, p. 16.
6. Rosenstock, Irwin: "Historical Origins of the Health Belief Model," in Becker, M.H. (ed.): *The Health Belief Model and Personal Health Behavior.* Charles B. Slack, Thorofare, N.J., 1974.
7. Kirscht, John P.: "The Health Illness Model and Illness Behavior," in Becker, M.H. (ed.): *The Health Belief Model and Personal Health Behavior.* Charles B. Slack, Thorofare, N.J., 1974.
8. Becker, Marshall H.: "The Health Belief Model and Sick Role Behavior," in Becker, M.H. (ed.): *The Health Belief Model and Personal Health Behavior.* Charles B. Slack, Thorofare, N.J., 1974.
9. Ardell, Donald B.: "High Level Wellness Strategies." *Health Education,* July/Aug. 1977, p. 2.
10. Mager, Robert F.: *Preparing Instructional Objectives.* Fearon Publishers, Palo Alto, 1962.

BIBLIOGRAPHY

Ardell, Donald B.: "High Level Wellness Strategies." *Health Education,* July/Aug. 1977, p. 2.

Becker, Marshall H. (ed.): *The Health Belief Model and Personal Health Behavior.* Charles B. Slack, Inc., Thorofare, N.J., 1974.

Burton, Lloyd E., and Smith, Hugh H.: *Public Health and Community Medicine,* 2nd ed. The Williams and Wilkins Company, Baltimore, 1975.

Bureau of Health Education: *Focal Points.* U.S. Department of Health, Education and Welfare (October 1978) p. 1-7.

Bureau of Health Education: *Focal Points.* U.S. Department of Health, Education and Welfare (January 1978) p. 1-7.

Corry, James M., and Gray, Bryan J.: "Ending the Constant Crises in Health Education." *Health Education,* July/Aug. 1977, p. 26.

Corry, James M.; Munson, Howard E.; and Read, Donald A.: "A Dedication to Positive Change." *Health Education,* Jan./Feb. 1977, p. 9.

Hanlon, John J.: *Public Health Administration and Practice,* 6th ed. The C. V. Mosby Company, St. Louis, 1974.

Health Planning and Resources Development Act of 1974. U.S. Department of Health, Education and Welfare, DHEW Publication No. (HRA) 75-14015, 1975, pp. 1-20.

Huskey, Dorothy A.: "Community Health Education: The Past, The Present, The Future." *Health Education* Nov./Dec. 1976, p. 2.

Mager, Robert F.: *Preparing Instructional Objectives.* Fearon Publishers. Palo Alto, 1962.

Means, Richard K.: *A History of Health Education in the United States.* Lea and Febiger, Philadelphia, 1962.

Milio, Nancy: "A Framework for Prevention; Changing Health Damaging to Health Generating Life Patterns." *American Journal of Public Health,* 66(5):435, May 1976.

Pohl, Margaret L.: *The Teaching Function of the Nursing Practitioner,* 2nd ed. Wm. C. Brown Company Publishers, Dubuque, Iowa, 1973.

Redman, Barbara King: *The Process of Patient Teaching in Nursing,* 3rd ed. The C. V. Mosby Company, St. Louis, 1976.

Simmons, Jeanette (ed.): "Making Health Education Work." *American Journal of Public Health,* (Supplement) 65(10):1-49, 1975.

Smolensky, Jack: *Principles of Community Health,* 4th ed. W.B. Saunders Company, Philadelphia, 1977.

Werlin, Stanley H., and Schauffer, Helen N.: "Structuring Policy Development for Consumer Health Education." *American Journal of Public Health,* 68(6):596, June 1978.

Willgoose, Carl E.: *Health Education in the Elementary School,* 4th ed. W.B. Saunders Company, Philadelphia, 1974.

CHAPTER 9

TOOLS AND RESOURCES FOR THE COMMUNITY HEALTH NURSE

LINDA L. JARVIS, M.S.N., R.N.

Nurses working in community health settings bring with them the knowledge base gained through their educational program as well as experiences and insights gained through a variety of patient care activities. It is hoped that their educational program provided an opportunity to study wholistic man and to develop some sensitivity toward the role of such factors as culture, art, religion, politics, psychology, sociology, ethics, and economics in the belief and value systems of different groups. Acquisition of such knowledge is an on-going process and requires active pursuit by the nurse. It is through this understanding of man—his beliefs, values, and needs—that we are able to provide a level of nursing care which addresses the uniqueness of man in his particular culture and environment.

The depth of nursing care which can be provided will depend on the variety of skills and knowledge possessed by the nurse. Each nurse will bring to her position her own perceptions of health, illness, and nursing. As she provides nursing care, interacts with her peers, and seeks to expand her knowledge base, she will be able to provide increasingly complex nursing care. Nursing in the community is dynamic and can be exceptionally rewarding.

CLIENT SERVICES

Community health nurses work in a variety of settings as will be seen in later chapters. However, regardless of the setting in which the nurse works or the target population receiving services, there are common tools and resources which will be useful in providing nursing care. Prevention of illness and maintenance of health are common goals in all areas of community health nursing.

The cornerstone of nursing practice is the *nursing process* which consists of five components. Through assessment, planning, implementing, evaluation, and revision the nurse is able to provide skilled, informed nursing care to the individual, family, and/or community. The process provides the framework for obtaining data about health status, for setting goals, for designing and implementing a nursing care plan to meet those goals, and for evaluating the effectiveness of the nursing care plan and making revisions where needed. The nursing process is equally applicable in wellness and illness situations.

The assessment allows one to collect data about the present status of the client as well as pertinent past history. The collection of such data should be initiated at the first client contact and completed in as much depth as possible. Sufficient time, at least 45 to 60 minutes, should be allowed for this initial assessment. While trying to be as complete as possible, keep in mind that data may be added to the history sheet as they become available. Assessment, as are all other components of the nursing process, is an on going activity.

The assessment includes a client history, a physical examination, analysis of data collected, and based on this information, the establishment of nursing diagnoses. Yura and Walsh, in discussing the role of the nurse in client assessment, emphasize the importance of viewing the client in a wholistic manner in order to determine his state of wellness or illness.[1]

The form which one uses for this assessment will depend on the format favored by the institution in which one works. However, regardless of the setting the following areas should be addressed: 1) biographical data such as name, birth date, sex, marital status, education level, type of employment, religious preference, language spoken, telephone numbers and addresses of home and employment site, and emergency contacts; 2) past health/illness history; 3) family history of health/illness status; 4) growth and development status; 5) lifestyle preferences; 6) coping patterns; 7) client's perception of health/illness; 8) occupational data; 9) socioeconomic status including insurance coverage; 10) physical examination including evaluation of mental/emotional status; 11) nutrition history, and 12) environmental assessment.

With this data and the knowledge base of what constitutes wellness for specific age/stage groups, the nurse will be able to determine the health status of the individual and define nursing diagnoses. If there are no identified health problems or needs, then the nursing actions might be to reinforce or support healthy behavior patterns and maintain intermittant health care contact. The identification of a health need or problem, however, will prompt the nurse to vigorously specify each one and establish specific steps to be taken to meet or resolve the problem/need. More frequent contact may be needed and referrals to other health care providers or agencies might be necessary.

Once the nursing diagnoses have been made, the nurse will work with the client and/or family in an effort to resolve or reduce the impact of the identified problem or need. Planning has little chance of success if it does not include the client/family. Decisions made for people rather than with them have little influence or longevity. Nursing actions should take into account the variety of characteristics which influence the client/family such as culture, lifestyle, religion, socioeconomic level and others. Nursing interventions may focus on a single diagnosis or deal with several at the same time. The decision of which approach to use will depend on such variables as degree of severity of various problems/needs, priority designation of the client/family, and time factors.

Having completed the nursing assessment and plans, nursing interventions are then implemented. The nursing care plan becomes the guide for the nurse as she participates in the resolving of client/family problems/needs. Communication channels need to be kept open between the nurse, client/family, and other health care providers. It may be that the nurse enlists the assistance of many people in providing care for the client/family. As the plans are implemented, careful observation and data collection continues. It is an ongoing process throughout the implementation phase. Revision may need to be made to meet changes in client/family needs as the plans are implemented. The nurse will utilize her communication skills to provide designated nursing care. Evaluation and revision will take place as the nursing care plan is implemented. Client/family response to such intervention may range from complete recovery to stabilization at some point along the wellness continuum. As client/family responses are identified, they can be evaluated in terms of desired outcomes and revisions then made. One always looks at how goals were met in determining effectiveness of nursing interventions. The responses of the client/family to interventions is of paramount importance. Revisions may or may not be made depending on level of client/family response to interventions, unexpected changes in behavior, and priority of the nursing goal being evaluated.

The five components of the nursing process, although discussed as separate entities, are interrelated. One can do no part of the nursing process without addressing all parts. It is an ongoing, dynamic process which requires that the nurse use her entire nursing skills and knowledge arsenal to fully utilize it. It is a tool of great power which allows nurses to determine where they are going in terms of nursing care, evaluate where they have been, and forge new directions as client/family responses indicate.

Assessment of the community provides the nurse with information about demography which includes statistics about the people, residence information, educational levels, physical size and characteristics, medical services and facilities, health status, and economic status. In doing a community assessment, the nurse will be able to identify various cultural/ethnic characteristics, religious persuasions, and lifestyle patterns. Such information will provide direction to the nurse as she seeks to better understand the community in which she works. Knowledge about beliefs, values, and practices in various social, cultural, ethnic, and religious groups can increase sensitivity to their unique characteristics. This should help to hasten trust bonds and improve communication with various groups.

When one does a community assessment, the purpose is generally to understand the community and to identify assets and liabilities. A good place to start is by reviewing demographic data which will provide an overview of the community. The nurse can then devise a plan to systematically explore the community. Perhaps a first step might be to travel by car and foot the major sections of the community. This provides a visual picture of the scope and diversity of the community. Another action might be to seek in depth data about a variety of services, facilities, and conditions in the community. For example, one might look at housing, educational facilities, health care services and facilities, transportation services and facilities, special needs services and facilities such as for the aged, the disabled, or preschool children, recreational facilities, and occupational opportunities and sites. Collection of information on such topic areas will provide the opportunity to visit governmental offices as well as community sites. These activities may provide insights into the various needs of the community which the nurse can then participate in meeting.

Community assessments take time. It is time which is well spent as it provides the nurse with a global view of the community and its characteristics, allows her to identify strengths and weaknesses, and provides an opportunity for her to introduce herself to a number of people in the community. It should be kept in mind that community assessments are on-going projects which need frequent updating to deep abreast of changes. The forms which are used to record community data, again, will vary from agency to agency. Regardless of the format, however, every effort should be made to make the assessment as complete and permanent as possible.

As a result of the community assessment, the nurse will begin to identify a variety of agencies and community services which may be tapped when designing client care plans. The development of a *community resource file* can be of invaluable service when one is trying to find resources to meet client needs. A useful way to file such information is on file cards or in a large loose leaf notebook which can be kept in alphabetical order. Information should include: 1) name, address, and phone number of agency, service, or individual; 2) specific type of service provided; 3) eligibility requirements; 4) cost, acceptance of third party payment; 5) transportation options/availability; 6) special notes such as facilities for the disabled, availability of interpretors, etc.; 7) date and time of site visit with comments about suitability as a referral source.

With the above information, all nurses in the agency will have access to the resource data and can make additional comments as necessary. All resource files should be reviewed and updated every 6 to 12 months so that information is current. Between such updating, new information can be added, dated, and signed by the nurse as it becomes available. Resource files are invaluable time savers when maintained properly.

Record keeping will be done on the forms in the particular setting. Every client should have some form of record kept on him which will provide assessment data with nursing diagnoses, the nursing care plan and evaluation, and revisions which have been instituted. The record may be narrative or problem oriented in design. It does not matter so much which design is used, so long as every client has a record which is current. All nurses who interact with or for the client should enter such data in the record which provides an ongoing account of client/family progress and activities. It is a legal record which should be carefully and completely maintained. Nurses are responsible for fully documenting all client/family nursing care activities.

Nursing audits should be carried out through a recognized structure within each agency. Nursing audits will evaluate the quality of nursing care given and determine if it was satisfactory or in need of improvements. Careful recording of nursing activities in client records, therefore, becomes the source for determining quality and quantity of nursing care given. Such nursing audits should be sought as a means of strengthening or improving nursing care. Nursing audits should never be punitive in nature. It is, in its purest form, a means of determining if adequate nursing care has been provided. Areas of weakness can be identified and ways then explored to assist nurses in improving deficit areas.

Client and nurse contacts take place in a variety of ways. Some meet through agency visits, home visits, educational programs, health screening programs, and telephone calls. The initial client/family contact is important as it sets the stage for all future contacts.

The *telephone* is a common source of client/family contact for the nurse. It is also an invaluable tool in seeking community resource information and in making referrals. Through use of the telephone, the nurse makes contact with the entire community. Telephone usage should be thoughtfully carried out. When speaking with anyone by phone, enuciation is imperative. Always identify yourself by name, title, and the agency for which you work. State the purpose of your call concisely. Repeat any information which was not clearly understood. If you are seeking specific information, repeat it to the informant to be certain you have recorded it properly. If you are conversing with a client and are making an appointment for a visit, be sure to repeat the date, time, and place at least twice to determine that you were heard correctly. Once the conversation has been completed, thank the callee for their time if appropriate. Good public relations by phone can be invaluable as you seek information and assistance in providing client care.

For those nurses who make home visits, the use of the *black bag* may be necessary. The black bag contains equipment needed to assess, treat, and teach the client/family. The exact contents of black bags will vary but in general they should contain: 1) a sphygmomanometer, 2) stethoscope, 3) oral and rectal thermometers and cases, 4) scissors, 5) hemostat, 6) forceps, 7) instrument basin, 8) tape measure, 9) alcohol, 10) soap solution, 11) apron, 12) paper towels, 13) hand soap, 14) cotton balls, and 15) lubricant. Additional equipment can include rubber gloves, Band-Aids, dressing materials, syringes, needles, and medications. The exact contents will depend on the needs of client/families during the home visit. Remember that the inside of the bag is clean and should remain so. The exact technique for handling the contents of the bag should be reviewed by the nurse during her orientation to the agency.

In doing the assessment and designing and implementing the nursing care plan, it may be necessary to include a variety of people in the plan to meet client/family needs. The process used is that of *referral*. Referrals can be to other health persons in the agency such as physical and occupational therapists, nutritionists, social workers, physicians, or home health aids, to community agencies of various kinds, to medical centers, and others. All referrals should be made with the understanding and consent of the client/family. Know the referral source either directly through personal contact or indirectly through information contained in the resource file. Open communication should be maintained between the nurse, client/family, and the referral agent. Appropriatness of referral, satisfaction with service, and meeting of established goals should be used in evaluating the referral.

Any referral should be made with thought. The goal is, in general, to promote the highest level of independent functioning in the client/family. Close supervision is needed to determine when the client/family can take on more care responsibilites. Such activity should be encouraged. A physical therapist, for example, may teach the nurse and home health aide to do a set of exercises. As the family is ready to take over such actions, they may be taught the exercises and the nurse or physical therapist will be there for instruction, support, and encouragement.

Health screenings under the auspices of a health department, community agency, or hospital are carried on to identify persons with or at risk of developing a certain disease. Screenings are done for such conditions as hypertension, diabetes, glaucoma, and sickle cell anemia. It should be emphasized that such screenings are not diagnostic but rather identify persons who need additional work up for a specific diagnosis.

Screenings are useless unless some plan has been made for follow up on those with positive findings. Referral may be made to a private physician, clinic, or health center. The need for referral for further examination is necessary as it gets high risk clients into the health care system for treatment if needed. It is always possible that a client with positive findings will refuse a referral. Educational efforts should be directed toward factual information about the disease, diagnostic measures, treatment programs, and general anticipated effects of early diagnosis and treatment. An open, honest approach to clients which allows for discussion and questioning will provide information and support for the decision. Health screenings can be valuable aids in identifying high risk groups but only if a total plan for referral and followup has been made.

In addition to the community resources which the nurse uses for referrals and services, there are additional sources which assist the nurse in performing her nursing role. A prime source of information, exchange of ideas, and support are her *nursing peers and nursing supervisors in the agency*. Client/family care approaches can be discussed with the group to find effective ways of meeting and resolving client needs and problems. In most cases nursing peers are eager to share successful nursing care approaches and will discuss plans they have tried which have been less than successful. This kind of open, honest sharing can aid in the growth and development of all nurses as client/family care successes and failures are shared. Other team members such as social workers, physicians, psychologists, and physical and occupational therapists can also provide important input as you try to design and implement appropriate nursing care plans.

Information about third party payments, social security benefits, veterans benefits, and other problems can be obtained by contacting the appropriate *private or governmental agency*. Pharmacies, drug companies, and local hospital pharmacists can provide information about various medications. Agencies should have some kind of resource materials section available which would contain various textbooks, drug books and information sources, telephone books, and various commercial catalogues. Depending on how sparce community facilities are, telephone books and catalogues can be lifesavers when trying to obtain information and problem solve for and with clients/families.

Once one becomes sensitized to the resources in the community, it is just short of amazing how much support is available. A systematic search of the community for people, agencies, and organizations which are interested in public and health services can uncover a vast array of resources available for tapping. If, by chance, the nurse finds a dirth of existant resources, she can begin a campaign to stimulate such services if they are needed in the community. People, in general, are desirous of being needed and helping one another; often all that is needed is a little direction.

STATISTICS

Statistics are useful in providing data for the establishment of various public health programs. Two terms which are used to describe these statistics are *vital statistics* and *biostatistics*. Vital statistics refer to "statistics dealing with births, deaths, marriages, etc."[2] Biostatistics is the "application of statistical processes and methods to the analysis of biological data."[2] Although time consuming to gather and process, statistics aid in describing the population. A census, done every 10 years, provides information about such population characteristics as enumeration, age, sex, marital status, educational level, residence characteristics, and so forth. Because of our very mobile society, the 10 year census reports seldom fully describe the population for a very long period of time, at least in many urban areas. Census tracts describe small geogrpahic areas and they are stored in libraries and governmental offices for review and other uses.

Vital statistics are usable only if there is some comparison with a given population parameter. For example, morbidity or incidence of a given disease may be expressed in number of cases per 1,000, 10,000, or 100,000 population. A rate of 10 cases of any disease per 1,000 would have much greater significance then 10 cases in 10,000. Since communicable diseases are reportable to the department of public health, an estimate of disease incidence can be made. However, there is so much paper work as well as various social pressures on physicians that reporting is not as complete as it could be. This lack of accuracy, of course, makes statistics and projections made from them more difficult. Also a factor in nondisease reporting is the fact that many childhood communicable diseases do not get reported because these children are not seen by physicians but are treated at home. This is particularly true during epidemics of diseases.

Birth and death rates are primarily determined by birth and death certificates. Of course it is necessary to evaluate such birth and death rates within the limits of some population parameter as stated above. Since most babies are born in hospitals, their birth certificates are easily available. Babies born in other settings, however, are harder to count as birth certificates may not be sought or delayed in acquisition. A partial source of birth data can be attained at the time of school entry. However, such information still is an estimate of actual births. Whether or not the designation of illegitimate is entered on a birth certificate varies from state to state. Some states place it on the original certificate and it goes with the individual for life. Others place it on the certificate but not on subsequent copies. Although failure to identify one as illegitimate may interfere with accurate statistics on the incidence of such births, it is questionable if anything is gained for the individual to have to face the social stigma which is still prevalent in our society as a result of the label.

Death certificates are a little easier to account for. However, the problem here is in terms of cause of death, not that the death occurred. It is a particular problem when several conditions exist simultaneously. Hanlon cites use of the *International Classification of Diseases, Injuries and Causes of Death* from the World Health Organization as being useful in determining the actual cause of death.[3] Information about cause of death is valuable in analyzing statistics about any disease. Deliberate misrepresentation of the cause of death is more common in deaths due to suicide and syphilis than many other conditions. The social stigma of a particular cause of death influences reporting accuracy.

All vital statistics are useful in determining target public health programs. Immunization programs, health screening programs, and various educational efforts can all be traced to needs identified through vital statistics. They are time consuming to collect, but provide a very real base for public health decision making.

DISEASE CONTROL

Epidemiology is "concerned with defining and explaining the interrelationships of the host, agent and environment in causing disease."[4] Epidemiologic investigations are carried out for communicable and non-communicable diseases and various health and safety conditions. These include, but are not limited to, cardiac disease, hypertension, smoking, safety, alcoholism, and environmental pollution. Epidemiology involves a search for cause and effect relationships. Also sought, particularly in instances of communicable diseases, are sources of infection and contacts.

In attempting to investigate, control, and eliminate communicable/infectious diseases, *Vector control* becomes important. The primary vectors of concern are rodents and arthropods.[6] Rodents include rats, skunks, raccoons, squirrels, and others; while the list of arthropods includes flies, roaches, lice, ticks, and mosquitos. Any current attempts at rodent and insect control are generally a cooperative venture between public and environmental health programs. Various rodenticides and insecticides, if used unwisely, can be very damaging to our increasingly fragile environment.

Another means of disease control is through *immunization programs*. Efforts are underway to raise the level of immunizations among children 14 years old and younger to 90 percent. Standard immunizations are given for diphtheria, pertussis, measles, rubella, mumps, tetanus, and polio. Additional immunologic agents are available but are not routinely given. In some areas, children are barred from school attendance until their immunization program is initiated or completed. Even with 45 states having compulsory immunization plans, millions of children are not protected. Nurses participate in both emergency and regularly scheduled immunization programs.

Education concerning agent-host-environment interrelationships is needed by both health care providers and consumers. Large scale campaigns are conducted to inform people of cause and effect relationships, potential hazards and remediation steps. The control of any disease or condition requires a cooperative effort between the public and health care providers. The more people are aware of hazards and potential solutions the greater the possibility for informed decisions. Nurses provide a vital link between the source of information and the public. The methods of disseminating information are varied but include formal and informal input sessions and use of media such as radio, television, and newspapers. Evaluation of effectiveness must be ongoing and changes made where appropriate. It should be remembered that change through education can be slow and persistence is imperative.

Once a disease or condition has been diagnosed, *treatment plans* must be implemented. These may be personally or environmentally directed depending on disease etiology. Specific treatment may involve medication administration, home or hospital confinement, search for contacts, environmental action as in the use of rodenticides or insecticides. Treatment will be directed toward cure of the disease/condition and elimination of the causative agent whatever it is. To do this most effectively, research is ongoing to determine the most effective treatment approaches, seek cures to disease, and improve environmental conditions.

Nurses play a key role in the entire disease control picture. Activities include case finding, treatment, evaluation, education, research activities, and prevention measures. It is an ongoing process which requires constant deligence and involvement.

RESEARCH

Nursing research, generally, is carried on to provide answers to effective approaches to patient care. Community health nurses can involve themselves in research to determine the most effective ways to teach the client/family/community, treat disease and health conditions, and provide preventive services. Research need not be elaborately designed in order to be effective.

In general, research involves the following components: 1) statement of the problem, 2) review of the literature, 3) identification of dependent and independent variables, 4) research design, 5) definitions of terms, 6) statement of hypotheses, 7) data collections, 8) data findings and analysis, and 9) conclusions.[3] This outline provides a framework in which the nurse can begin to seek answers to patient care questions and issues. Although research may be pure in nature, applied research is most likely to be the type pursued by most nurses in the field.

Funding for research activities may come from local agency funds or a variety of local, state, and federal governmental sources. Requests for research funds usually require some kind of proposal which states the problem, proposed methodology to explore the problem, personnel to be involved, subjects to be used, and estimated costs. Rights of subjects are to be protected and various regulations may have to be met in order to obtain funds.

The term research often puts people off to the point that efforts to systematically seek answers to questions are delayed or avoided. This is unfortunate as much time is wasted and nursing care innovations are postponed or never identified. Simple questions can serve to start beginning research studies. Support from supervisors, local health department personnel, nearby schools of nursing, and regional offices of the Department of Health and Human Services may be sought and utilized. In any event, efforts at small research projects can be successful, reinforcing to the nurse, and stimulate the pursuit of knowledge about other issues.

The community health nurse has a large number of resources at her disposal. These resources can expand the scope of practice and effectiveness if used in a professional manner. It behooves the nurse to seek them out and utilize them to their fullest. Such efforts will pay dividends in personal satisfaction and the delivery of high quality client/family care.

REFERENCES

1. Yura, Helen, and Walsh, Mary B.: *The Nursing Process: Assessing, Planning, Implementing and Evaluating.* Appleton-Centruy-Crofts, New York, 1978.
2. *Taber's Cyclopedic Medical Dictionary,* 13th ed. F.A. Davis Company, Philadelphia, 1977.
3. Hanlon, John J.: *Public Health Administration and Practice,* 6th ed. The C.V. Mosby Company, St. Louis, 1974.
4. Rinehart, Joan M.: "One Way to Learn the Research Process." *Nursing Outlook,* 24(1):39, Jan. 1976.

BIBLIOGRAPHY

Benaliel, Jeanne Quint: "The Interaction Between Theory and Research." *Nursing Outlook,* 25(2): 108, Feb. 1977.

Chavigny, Katherine: "Self-Esteem for the Alcoholic: An Epidemiologic Approach." *Nursing Outlook,* 24(10):636, Oct. 1976.

Gulbrandsen, Mary Wachter: "Guide to Health Assessment." *American Journal of Nursing,* 76(8): 1276, Aug. 1976.

Hanlon, John J.: *Public Health Administration and Practice,* 6th ed. The C.V. Mosby Company, St. Louis, 1974.

Houer, Julie, and Zummier, Marie J.: "Nursing Quality Assurance, The Wisconsin System." *Nursing Outlook,* 26(4):242, April 1978.

Hubbard, Susan, and Devita, Vincent.: "Chemotherapy Research Nurse." *American Journal of Nursing,* 76(4):560, April 1976.

Jarvis, Linda L.: "Childhood Immunizations." *Issues in Comprehensive Pediatric Nursing,* 3(3):36, Sept. 1978.

Lambertson, Martha; Keen, Margaret; and Adomanic, Ann: "Peer Review in a Family Nurse Clinician Program." *Nursing Outlook,* 25(1):47, Jan. 1977.

Mayers, Marlew Glover: *A Systematic Appraoch to the Nursing Care Plan,* 2nd ed. Appleton-Century-Crofts, New York, 1978.

Morris, Williams (ed.): *The American Heritage Dictionary of the English Language.* Houghton-Mifflin Company, Boston, 1976.

Nordburg, Beatrice, and King, Lynette: "Third Party Payment for Patient Education." *American Journal of Nursing,* 76(8):1269, Aug. 1975.

Norris, Catherine M.: "Restlessness: A Nursing Phenomenon in Search of Meaning." *Nursing Outlook,* 23(2):103, Feb. 1975.

Rinehart, Joan M.: "One Way to Learn the Research Process." *Nursing Outlook,* 24(1):38, Jan. 1976.

Rosenau, Ann M.: "Helping Practioner Students Put Concepts into Action." *Nursing Outlook,* 25(7): 446, July 1977.

Schare, Barbara L.: "An Undergraduate Research Experience." *Nursing Outlook,* 25(3):178, March 1977.

Talahere, Laurel, and Graves, Patricia: "A Tool for Assessing Families of Burned Children." *American Journal of Nursing,* 76(2):225, Feb. 1976.

Terris, Milton: "The Epidemiologic Revolution, National Health Insurance and the Role of Health Departments." *American Journal of Public Health,* 66(12):1155, Dec. 1976.

Taber's Cyclopedic Medical Dictionary, 13th ed. F.A. Davis Company, Philadelphia, 1977.

Wandelt, Mohal A.: *Guide for the Beginning Researcher.* Appleton-Century Crofts, New York, 1970.

Wolff, Helen, and Erickson, Roberta: "The Assessment Man." *Nursing Outlook,* 25(2):103, Feb. 1977.

Yura, Helen, and Walsh, Mary B.: *Human Needs and the Nursing Process.* Appleton-Century-Crofts, New York, 1978.

Yura, Helen, and Walsh, Mary B.: *The Nursing Process: Assessing, Planning, Implementing, Evaluating.* Appleton-Century-Crofts, New York, 1978.

UNIT **II**
COMMUNITY HEALTH NURSING ROLES

In the early development of community health nursing roles, the primary role was that of visiting nurses from either official or nonofficial or voluntary agencies. The major designations were visiting nurses from voluntary agencies such as Visiting Nurse Associations and public health nurses from official agencies such as Public Health Departments. As the roles of community health nurses have expanded, we find the nurse working in a variety of settings with many population groups.

There is some confusion, debate, and disagreement over the terminology to be used in commonly identifying this specialty of nursing. Although nursing through the auspices of the American Nurses' Association has adapted the term *community health nurse* to identify this specialty role, this terminology is not necessarily used throughout the country. The federal, state, and local governments often refer to this role as *public health nursing*.

This discrepancy in terminology is acknowledged in Chapters 13 and 14. Chapter 13 employs the more traditional terminology of *public health nursing* and addresses the nursing role in official and combination agencies. The term *community health nurse* is used in Chapter 14 which focuses primarily on the home care nursing role in voluntary, combination, and proprietary agencies. This should not be taken as acceptance of these designations but rather an attempt to recognize that terminology differences do exist, even though there is similar role function. Students may well encounter both terms which can lead to confusion.

Other nursing roles are identified to show the breadth of community health nursing activities. As nursing specialties have developed in general, roles within the community health nursing rubric have become broad based and diversified. The chapters within this unit look at some of these roles.

10

NURSING ROLE
IN AMBULATORY CARE

LOUISE G. DAUGHERTY, M.S.N., R.N., AND GWENDOLYN J. BUCHANAN, M.S.N., R.N.

Acceptance of the inevitability of rapid and continuous change in the delivery of health care services challenges all nurses as never before to identify their role in the development and maintenance of quality client care. Relentless questioning of the old, rigidly structured bureaucratic systems in which nurses usually find themselves must continue if new, innovative, and humanistic approaches in the delivery of nursing care are to become a reality. Bureaucratic health care systems focus on organizational structure and maintenance whereas the focus for nursing is individualizing the system to meet the client's needs. The nurse in individualizing the health care system requires a knowledge base for meaningful interventions, an understanding and acceptance of the client, and authority to make the system flexible. Philosophically these requirements are widely accepted today but operationally they provoke controversy and system upheaval.

Unfortunately it is the vertical client who is caught in the philosophical-organizational conflict. Before continuing, let us identify the vertical client as an individual who receives his health care from a system while remaining in a nonhospitalized status. Holistic, comprehensive, quality care for the vertical client is the goal of the professional ambulatory care nurse, but historically the system as a provider of care has dealt with these clients by forcing them into a structured organization with little or no attention paid to their personal needs, feelings, dignity, or privacy. This structured approach has had a dehumanizing effect on both clients and ambulatory care nurses. The client's unresponsiveness to his care and the nurse's irritation with the system has led both to receive little or no satisfaction from the interaction.

Conflict, dissatisfaction, and increased consumerism have created changes in areas of our health care system. One of these areas is the ambulatory care setting and, in most instances, the change emitted from nursing. Nursing implemented ambulatory care nursing as a humanistic, holistic interaction where the vertical client became an individual and the system became less dehumanizing. From a task oriented functional nurse role, ambulatory care nursing has become an accepted speciality with established priorities and authority to insure quality health care delivery.

DEFINING THE ROLE

The concept of ambulatory care nursing within structured systems is developmentally in its infancy and definitions of nursing roles are still vague. However, as specialists in ambulatory care nursing, we know what the roles are, what can be accomplished, and we are continuing to define the dynamic, generalized role as we in the specialty believe it to be. The nucleus of our role is self-directedness. This basic stance includes a systemic assessment (nursing process) and the formulation of different approaches to holistic nursing. The different approaches are responses to the changing needs of the vertical client, family, and significant others in their therapeutic as well as preventive care. This philosophic stance demands that the basic values which emphasize the dignity, privacy, and individuality of each client and his family be integrated into these approaches. These are not new approaches. Their freshness comes from the reformulation and the application of approaches in response to new knowledge, new humanistic problem solving, and more opportunities for the ambulatory care nurse to function independently and freely. Given the opportunity and the support, the creativity of ambulatory care nurses can be and is phenomenal!

The diversity in practice as the ambulatory care nurse grows within a specialized generalist role is, in itself, a professional challenge which predominates in this area of health care delivery. The terminology *specialized generalist* is meant to denote specialization in the setting and type of clients, i.e., vertical. The term generalist denotes a nursing approach to clients with differing problems and their own control over their care. A spirit of pioneering and exploring within constructive assertiveness becomes an essential characteristic of the nurse. Flexibility, honesty, and the ability to accept both success and failure must be preserved. Our ultimate objective is excellence in care with the client as our reason for being.

SCOPE OF SERVICE

Nursing is responding to increased consumer demand for health services with the development of new and innovative programs in institution and community ambulatory care. In these programs, nursing has assumed the responsibility of independent practice and collaborative roles by working with other health professionals to deliver primary health care for clients in their homes, in clinics, and in hospitals. The nurse's clinical practice encompasses client education, health counseling, health maintenance, and preventive and primary care. Though some of these functions can overlap with other members of the ambulatory care health team, e.g., physician, clinical pharmacist, dietitian, and social worker, it is the congruous interrelation of all that can increase the successful delivery of comprehensive care.

Consumer satisfaction and responses to these services have increased recognition and acceptance of the nurse as a provider of primary care in ambulatory settings. Quality services have been demonstrated in ambulatory care by nurses in health care delivery systems throughout the United States and Canada.

Dr. John W. Runyan, Jr., writes,

"It is becoming increasingly apparent that continuing care for the mounting population of chronic disease patients by the physician on a one-to-one basis is impossible and that the attempt may be a misdirection of the physician's time and talents. The care of most chronic disease patients is patient education, counseling and empathy, with adjustments in a simple therapeutic program from time to time. One only has to look about in a teaching institution to see that the interest of the medical students and house staff wanes as soon as the diagnosis is made and treatment is stabilized."[1]

Dr. Runyan wrote for his colleagues in medicine to introduce the nurse clinician program in Memphis and Shelby County of Tennessee. Faced by overwhelming demands for continuing care of the chronic disease client, Dr. Runyan turned to "our traditional partner in patient care, the nurse, for assistance in this problem."[1]

Nurse conducted diabetic clinics, for example, are well established in health care delivery systems throughout our nation. The nurse is responsible for assessing the client's capacity to engage in and accomplish therapeutic self-care and for providing and managing the amount and quality of care required.[2] These nurses are successfully providing on-going continued care and supervision of the client. There has been rapid growth of continuity programs where each client has his own doctor or nurse whom he can contact at any time of need. The nurse's client load is assigned just as the physician's. One recognized outcome of these programs is that the client's visits to the emergency department is greatly reduced.[3] The reward for nursing practice is the increased trust and confidence of the client in "his" nurse.

Pioneering in nursing practice in ambulatory care continues to forge new frontiers in health care delivery. Nursing in oncology, cardiology, neurology, rehabilitation, and emergency care, as well as other subspecialty areas in health care delivery, is dynamically evolving. Programs which reflect the caring philosophy and deep concern of the nurse for the client continue to develop in ambulatory care settings. Nursing roles remain to be discussed or evolved in the health care delivery for the vertical client.

HISTORICAL DEVELOPMENT OF ROLE

As in any great endeavor, the beginnings of ambulatory care nursing were small, the results of personal vision and dedication. Excerpts from nursing history serve as reminders, however, that recent professional progress may not be claimed solely by the ambulatory care nurses of today. They are the fruit of seeds planted by pioneer nurses with a commitment to humane rather than human services. Without this intense commitment to this goal, treatment of the vertical client could have remained at a relatively undeveloped stage.

From the time of Christ, as the Apostles began to organize churches, we hear of deaconesses. They were at first assistants to the clergy, probably preached, gave advice, and visited the sick and poor. This contact with the sick inevitably involved doing some actual nursing. [4] Around the year 400 (in Rome), Paula, considered to have been the first person to systematically train nurses, is described in old English prose: "She was marvelous, debonair, and piteous to them that were sick, and comforted them and served them right humbly, and gave them largely of such food as they asked. They laid their pillows aright and in point; and she rubbed their feet and boiled water to wash them." [4] This fourth century description of a nurse so well states the humane rather than the human service described earlier. In the seventeenth century, the Hospitaller Sisters of the Mercy of Jesus had for their life's work visiting the sick, health visiting (equivalent to district nursing), some care of lepers, and the custody of the insane.

The military has been equally as strong a stimulus as religious movements for innovative action by nurses to improve or initiate care for the vertical client. History describes nurses who went into the battlefield to care for the wounded and staff the emergency "lean-to" clinics to render immediate first-aid for those who bore the battle.

History repeatedly reminds us that the concept of ambulatory care is neither new nor original. Responses to major crises in health care were patterned after what we now define as ambulatory care. Soon after the colonies declared their independence, health care services for the vertical client were developed. America's first dispensary, in 1786, was established in Philadelphia. [5] In 1893, New York City opened milk stations, patterned after charitable clinics in France, to assist and teach mothers about infant feedings. [6] Nursing practice in American school clinics has continued since they were first organized in the early 1900s. Industrial nursing has been a very specialized area of practice for preventive as well as therapeutic health care delivery since industrial clinics were first organized at the turn of the twentieth century.

Public clinics and health centers, modeled after the "settlement house" movement, were organized in urban slums. Jane Adams, 1880, in Trynbu Hall of Chicago (her home), provided a day nursery, a kindergarten, and a library for her neighbors. These neighbors represented over 30 nationalities, were people who clung to their own customs, and, at the same time, wanted for their children the education and the opportunity that they felt America had to offer. Community services were provided by nurses in health department clinics by the antituberculosis society and the Milk and Baby Hygiene Association. In 1893, nurses with a vision, Lillian Wald and her friend Mary Brewster, ventured into New York's slums. What they heard and saw, while nursing the sick or sharing the family troubles, helped them to recognize social causes which complicated the health problems of their clients. They provided preventive teaching, health counseling, and consultative social services. [5] Ambulatory care nurses today continue to expand their services while continuing with the same services offered by Wald and Brewster.

There are many types of organized ambulatory care services in the health care delivery system in the United States today. These are found in public health agencies; industrial health units; elementary through high school health services; university student health centers; medical and nursing practice; independent nurse clinics; hospice programs; satellite clinics; mental health centers; health maintenance organizations; special government programs such as neighborhood health centers, Indian centers, and geriatric centers; special voluntary programs such as crisis intervention centers; alcoholic and drug dependency centers; and hospital ambulatory care clinics and emergency departments. We can now recognize that within the single identity of the ambulatory care nurse is a diversity and multiplicity of roles. Some are prescribed by the daily demands of the area of practice and others surface as a sensitive response of the nurse seeking new and improved services to meet the client's needs.

The entry of the nurse practitioner into health care services can be identified as a response to meet such needs. Communities without any health care service, clinics with inadequate medical staff coverage, emergency rooms and admission services with long, exhausting waits brought justified consumer complaints and demands for improved services. Nursing rallied to these deficiencies in service and nurse practitioners assumed roles which were, in the past, medically oriented. Their advanced assessment and interpretative skills promote independent and interdependent functioning in the delivery of holistic and quality health care to the client and family. However, their role must be considered and remain an extension of nursing rather than an extension of delegated tasks by physicians. Nurse practitioners who use their assessment skills to strengthen this knowledgable care of clients are moving ambulatory care into the twentieth century. Consumer acceptance has been positive and support from consumer groups to expanded nurse services has begun.

As change continues to follow quickly on the heels of previous change in the ambulatory nursing role, plateaus become fewer and fewer. No longer can we coast and rest on the new plateau until the change becomes traditional. Some researchers are noting that in the next five years health will be redefined to mean not merely the absence of illness, but the opposite of illness—a positive condition of well-being.[7] Too few individuals recognize the relationship between personal behavior and health. The same will be true for mental health: we will talk about emotional wellness. Our concern will be with the normal problems of normal people—problems of everyday life. This job cannot be left primarily to other health professionals. Ambulatory care nurses will be the therapeutic resource to the vertical client and family. The nursing role in ambulatory care will be yours and ours to develop, refine, and change. How well the challenge is met will be dependent on our ability to observe, interpret, and respond as only nurses can: as the health care provider focusing on holistic, humanistic care who facilitates the client in his responses to this condition or situation.

EDUCATIONAL PREPARATION

The educational preparation of ambulatory care nurses covers the entire spectrum: associate degree programs, diploma programs, baccalaureate degree programs, and masters programs. Nurses prepared at the graduate level are expected to serve as role models in the delivery of holistic care and be identifiable change agents within the ambulatory care systems.

Presently, nursing licensure does not reflect differences in the standards of nursing practice. However, renewal of licensure in many states requires continuing education credits for active registered nurses, and ambulatory care nurses must involve themselves enthusiastically in the profession and professional organizations.

Nurse practitioners/clinicians receive their additional education for the expanded role from several formal program sources: specific programs developed by individual hospitals; continuing education programs; health maintenance organizations; and university programs, usually at the graduate level. A current trend is developing toward incorporating nurse practitioner programs into the baccalaureate degree curriculum with specific tracks of specialty. From the first formal program for expanded role nurse midwives at the

State University of New York in 1931, there has been a growth spurt of extended nurse programs during the past decade. This surge of programs coincides with the beginning of federal support in 1972. [8]

As the ambulatory care nurse's role continues to expand there is little room today for the nurse who brings to the setting only a collection of rote techniques of the past or who views continuing education useful only for job advancement. Nor is there room for the nurse who views holistic nursing for something-to-do-if-we-have time. Only nurses with the confidence that extended skills can be used in assertive nursing practice and who have a commitment to the care of clients on a continuum are needed in ambulatory care.

EMERGING TRENDS

The rigidity which marked earlier decades of nursing education is less apparent today. We are beginning to see more nursing programs relate what is taught in the classroom to the ambulatory area of practice. Concomitantly, the opportunity to have clinical experience in the ambulatory setting gives the student greater understanding of and opportunity for personalizing a technique (its progression and application) and evaluating advantages and disadvantages as well as impact on the vertical client. It is also in the ambulatory environment that the student nourishes not only nursing skills but also capacities for awareness, empathy, and communication with the client and family. Ambulatory care settings are increasingly available for the student's leadership experiences.

That so many ambulatory care nurses have survived as learners and continue to grow personally and professionally is more often a tribute to their individual initiative and perserverance rather than to any particular design of hospital inservice programs. Too often these inservice programs were and are organized by groups that made decisions about learning activities without any knowledge of what is needed or wanted by the nursing personnel in this area. In other hospitals, nurses have not had the opportunity or been encouraged to enhance their enthusiasm for professional development. Inservice program orientation frequently focuses only on institutional maintenance and procedure updates. A few examples may illustrate how a collaborative inservice program can enhance the growth of the ambulatory nursing role.

As the dynamic advances of cancer research affects the modality of treatment, there are new concepts in the philosophy of care of clients with cancer. Memorial Sloan-Kettering Cancer Center has established ambulatory care facilities for followup care of clients who have completed a prescribed course of chemotherapy and for care of new undiagnosed clients. [9] The unit opened in 1973 and is designed to deliver rapid, thorough treatment and provide comfort for the client during his visit to the clinic. The oncology nurses coordinate the client's care throughout his stay in the ambulatory care system. Nursing practice includes administration of intravenous chemotherapy, identification of priorities of care and supervision of care, the completion of an interim history, and coordination and planning of care with the client and his family. Each nurse maintains a case load of clients. With increasing numbers of clients and changes in the complexity of treatment, flexibility and knowledge updating are essential to meet the changing methods in the delivery of care. This program, as others, enjoys the support of the consumer and provides care that permits the client to remain at home while continuing to receive treatment.

Another example is in the diabetic clinic. New possibilities in the treatment of the diabetic client suggest that the nurse remain current in knowledge to assist the individual client reach his maximum health potential. There is increased emphasis on dietary limitations as regulation and not deprivation. The total client must be considered: culturally, socially, and intellectually to help him to continually adjust to the disease, accept responsibility for his actions, and utilize teaching efforts of the nurse to better his situation. Practitioners of these clinics emphasize that with the development of clinical standards they have successfully provided on-going continued care and supervision of the clients with diabetes.

Time spent educating the client and family is recognized as important because how well the family copes with the problem directly affects the individual and his continued status as a vertical client. The client has a right and responsibility to participate in his care; he is a part of the ambulatory care team!

The emergency departments have become the most readily available resource for clients desiring entrance into the health care delivery system. Allegheny General Hospital in Pittsburgh is one of many hospitals to utilize the nurse practitioner to make decisions and perform tasks normally undertaken by the physicians in the emergency department. The nurse takes complete histories, does physical examinations, and identifies resources for care.[10] An illustration of this concept is the rape victim in the emergency area for treatment. The ambulatory care nurse performs the pelvic examination and gathers legal evidence, following the prescribed method of collecting documentation. She also knows the resources, that is, support groups, available to the victim and assertively initiates contact.

The Beth Israel Ambulatory Center, in Boston, has established an entry into the health care delivery system for the nonemergency client, by-passing the emergency department. In this setting the nursing staff frequently is the provider of primary care and assumes complete responsibility for client management. The director, Dr. Delbanco, states, "The person who can perform a task most effectively, most appropriately, and with the greatest cost effectiveness is the person who should do it."[11]

To clarify our point, we do not suggest that the inservice departments have the sole responsibility for providing the knowledge leading to role expansion. Growth, after all, is a personal process that occurs only with personal involvement. Nurses must also rely on their own personal resources, discuss problems, ideas, and creative thinking with their peers, and actively identify their learning needs as related to quality care of the vertical client.

Dr. Martha Rogers very clearly outlined the need of continuing education. We cannot rely solely on our initial program of nursing as our role changes. New knowledge must be laid on this foundation, or we can find ourselves replaced with other health care providers in the ambulatory care setting.[12]

While limited nursing research has been done in ambulatory care, there is clearly the need for studies directed toward outcome of care, as well as process. We must deal with the necessity of long range followup evaluation of the effect of ambulatory care nursing role expansion rather than relying solely or even primarily on immediate effects.

As the focus of care continues to shift to the ambulatory setting there are surely more questions that will require answers. Some could be: What skills does the nurse in an expanded role need in the future? Are the educational programs appropriate to accomplish these anticipated changes? Is there an improvement in outcomes of client care when a nurse functions in an expanded role? Only nursing research can provide these answers!

LEGAL CONSIDERATIONS

An ambulatory care nurse must be currently licensed to practice professional nursing in the United States. However, as the nursing role in ambulatory care continues to expand, there has been increased concern over the legal definition of nursing practice and this is still being debated by both the health and legal professions in many areas. Almost every state today has been or is in the process of studying, introducing, effecting, and/or revising changes in the nurse practice acts to legitimize current practices. Each nurse must be familiar with her state's practice act since each state individually writes its nurse practice act.

A further step in elevating the standard of nursing practice is certification by the American Nurses' Association. Certification is based on the assessment of knowledge through a nationally administered written examination and by peer review, an objective performance evaluation of the applicant in a specific area of nursing practice. [13] Reevaluation for certified nurses will be every five years to determine whether or not the individual's practice reflects the changes in the client's needs and advances in technology, nursing, and learning. [13] The American Nurses' Association has made the commitment to defining standards of nursing practice and to the development of precise methods for monitoring the care given. [14,15]

Actually there is no certification for ambulatory care specifically. However, the diversity of ambulatory care nursing makes many of the nurses functioning in this role eligible for certification under one of the five ANA's standards for certification.

Ambulatory care nurses, as all nurses, are liable for their actions. This is not the result of the role expansion: liability exists in even the most limited and traditional role. Liability is more public today and stresses acts of omission as well as commission.

Malpractice insurance is not a prerequisite for functioning in the ambulatory nurse's role. However, as more legal action involving nurses is appearing in the judicial system, the nurse should not assume that she is adequately insured for malpractice by her employer. It is worth her time to thoroughly investigate what, if any, coverage is provided. Ambulatory nurses staffing nurse administered clinics and nurse practitioners are especially open to legal action because of the absence of a physician. Unfortunately there are clients/consumers who still adhere to a belief in the mystical powers of the M.D. title and therefore can and do challenge the nurse's care.

LEGISLATIVE IMPACT ON ROLE

The ambulatory care nurse must concern herself with the rising cost of health services and justify her services in monetary terms as well as her effectiveness in relation to results. It is the legislators and administrators, our main source of funding, that emphasize business methodology with us. Accountability has become a major emphasis in terms of both cost and effectiveness.

As pressures on health care services increase, it becomes essential that programs to maintain high quality health care become implemented as quickly as possible. It is important that nursing be prepared and be a leader in evaluating our own quality and cost effectiveness. Criteria of care must be developed and utilized essentially in the same way for inpatient and outpatient nursing services. With increasing emphasis on hospital and community based ambulatory care programs, it is essential to develop mechanisms to assess the efficiency of services provided in such settings. Quality control constitutes evaluating outcomes and modifying practice to ensure reaching desired outcomes. Quality control must be perceived by practitioners as an integral part of all nursing care. Nurses in ambulatory care, as in other areas of health care delivery, must assume the responsibility for the maintenance and improvement of the quality of patient care and the development of a systematic methodology for monitoring the quality of nursing care.

If primary care nursing practice is to remain viable, it must have third party reimbursement. Presently the most likely form of payment for nurse's service is that made to a clinic or institution, designated as a payment for services rendered by a nurse.

States have the option, in accordance with their own laws, to reimburse the nurse practitioner for services under Medicaid. [16] The Rural Health Services Act mandates coverage of nurse practitioner services for health clinic services only in rural areas. [16]

The impending passage of national health insurance legislation suggests a substantial increase in ambulatory care client load. Many believe that recognition of the nurse as a health care provider under this legislation would mean significantly greater access to health services for some consumers. Other nursing concerns are questions as to whether national health insurance will allow the consumer to choose ambulatory care service instead of hospitalization or to receive health teaching to prevent illness. Once again the American Nurses' Association has expressed its concern related to reimbursement for nursing services and also urged that the preventive approach to health care be supported by national health insurance legislation.

CONCLUSION

In the past few years ambulatory nursing has had the satisfaction of seeing many of its cherished ideas take hold in even the most conservative institutions. No longer are we peripheral to the planning and decision making that will directly affect our nursing practice for holistic client care. We have demonstrated a willingness to take risks, to assume newer responsibilities, and to be accountable for our performance. At long last we are actively involved in restructuring the health care delivery system for the vertical client and family. In this period of role definition and reevaluation, we must keep in mind that there will be changes and more changes. Nevertheless, it is certain that ambulatory care nursing will be in tune with the consumer's needs and promises to be an even more dynamic and self-fulfilling role in the decades ahead.

REFERENCES

1. Runyan, John W.: "Nurse Clinicians in Diabetic Care." *Metabolic Therapy,* 4(3):3, Fall 1975.
2. Brady, Rodney: "M.B.O. Goes to Work in the Public Sector." *Journal of Nursing Administration,* 4:45, July-Aug. 1973.
3. Sirota Adair L.: "Private Care in a Public Clinic." *American Journal of Nursing,* 74(9):1643, Sept. 1974.
4. Goodnow, Minnie: *Nursing History in Brief.* W.B. Saunders, Philadelphia, 1938.
5. Jamieson, Elizabeth, and Sewall, Mary: *Trends in Nursing History.* W.B. Saunders Comapany, Philadelphia, 1944.
6. Roemer, Melton I.: "From Poor Beginnings, The Growth of Primary Care." *Hospitals,* 49:38, March 1975.
7. Farson, Ricard E.: "Human Potentialities," in *Crossroads: Quality of Life Through Rhetorical Modes.* D. C. Heath and Company, Lexington, Mass., 1972.
8. Levine, E.: "What Do We Know About Nurse Practitioners?" *American Journal of Nursing,* 77:1799, March 1977.

9. Wollnech, Lorraine: "Management of the Child With Cancer On an Outpatient Basis." *Nursing Clinics of North America,* 11(1):36, March 1976.

10. Walker, Lynn L.: "The Emergency Department as Entry Point Into the Health Care System." *Hospital Topics,* 53(2):47, March-April 1974.

11. Downey, Gregg W.: "Outpatient Center Improves Care." *Modern Hospital,* 120(6):77, June 1973.

12. Driscoll, Joan, and Reeser, Frances E.: "Today's Nursing Choice: Involvement or Obsolescence?" *Hospital Care,* 4(2): March 1973.

13. *Certification for the Adult and Family Nurse Practitioner.* Fact Sheet, American Nurses' Association, Kansas City, 1977.

14. American Nurses' Association: *Standards of Nursing Practice.* ANA, New York, 1974.

15. Cornell, S.A.: "Development of an Instrument for Measuring the Quality of Nursing Care." *Nursing Research,* 23:108, March-April 1975.

16. U.S. Department of Health, Education and Welfare: "Medicaid and Medicare Programs: Rural Health Clinic Services." *Federal Register,* 7, 14 July 1978.

CHAPTER 11
NURSING ROLE IN OCCUPATIONAL HEALTH

CAROL A. SILBERSTEIN, M.Ed., R.N.

CAUSE FOR CONCERN

In this era of preventive health care, the providers of that care would be remiss if they ignored the work place as one area of potential health problems both in terms of illness and injury. The injury rates in industries have increased nearly 29 percent from 1960 to 1970. The National Safety Council estimates 14,000 annual deaths due to on-the-job accidents and 2.2 million disabling injuries. [1]

Occupational disease is a subject much debated by management, labor, government, and health professionals. Examples of known occupational diseases include coal workers' pneumoconiosis, asbestosis, berylliosis, and silicosis. Several toxins used in various manufacturing processes are known to be cancer causing agents, including asbestos, benzene, and vinyl chloride. These problems have far reaching consequences as we examine the statistics of morbidity and mortality due to the epidemics of cancers. The concern for the economic impact of health care must include an evaluation of the incidence of disease and disability which results directly from occupational exposures. The Department of Health and Human Services estimates 390,000 new cases of occupational diseases each year and approximately 100,000 annual deaths resulting from occupational disease. [2]

These estimates are based on our present knowledge concerning occupational health hazards. In a rapidly changing technologic society, manufacturing processes introduce increasing numbers of new chemicals, new production methods, and new stresses, both physical and psychological. There is a vital need for health professionals, including nurses, to document the impact of these physical and chemical stresses on the human organism. Only when these data are available will we be able to provide the worker with a safe and healthful work environment.

Physiologic responses to occupational toxins occur from absorption through the skin, inhalation, or ingestion. Exposure to these chemicals can result in respiratory or cardiac disease, cancer, neurologic dysfunction, systemic poisoning, or a decrease in life span. Of increasing concern are the effects of the exposure on the developing fetus. These diseases produce acute and/or chronic effects and may result in permanent disability or death. One major problem is the identification of latent periods, that is, that period of time between exposure to a toxin and the appearance of symptoms. Many toxic exposures produce no immediate symptoms but in 7, 10, or 20 years after the exposure the worker becomes disabled. Coal workers' pneumoconiosis and byssinosis (from exposure to cotton dust) are examples of occupational diseases with a long latency period.

Individuals in the workplace are usually not exposed to a single hazard, but rather there are multiple factors involved. Chemicals, heat, noise, vibration, as well as the individual's particular response to physical and chemical stress are important factors. In addition to the workplace exposures, the employee's personal habits may affect the response to hazards. Medications alter the chemistry of the body, and the effect may be not only additive but also synergistic, as in the case of alcohol and barbituates. Smoking is a habit of many workers. Those employees who smoke and are exposed to carbon monoxide increase their chances of developing physical symptoms. Asbestos workers who smoke have a significantly increased incidence of cancer over those asbestos workers who do not smoke.

Occupational diseases are not restricted to blue collar workers or to the heavy industries. Job illness and injury rates among agricultural workers are exceeded only by those in mining and construction. Dentists are being studied for the effects of x-rays and mercury exposures. Cosmetologists display excess cancer rates, respiratory diseases, and cardiac disease. Finally, operating room personnel, including nurses, have an increased incidence of spontaneous abortions, birth defects, and hepatic and renal disease.[3] It must be remembered that executives are subject to occupationally induced diseases also. They may not have direct exposure to dust, fumes, or chemicals but the physical and psychological stress frequently results in increased incidence of gastrointestinal disorders and/or cardiovascular disease.

HISTORY AND LEGISLATION

Concern for the hazards of occupations is not a new idea. Mining, probably the oldest industry known to man, has always been known as a hazardous occupation. The miner of antiquity was a slave, criminal, or prisoner. Therefore, there was no reason to improve his working conditions. One of the earliest references to the control of such hazards is a second century A.D. document in which miners were encouraged to cover their heads with cloths and sacks, and their noses and mouths with fish bladders in order to decrease the inhalation of dust. Galen recognized the problems of acid mists and the subsequent development of pulmonary edema. In 1500 Agricola identified not only the problem of silica and tuberculosis but also lung cancer. Agricola did not realize it at the time, but the cancers were due to the mining of a radioactive ore in siliceous rock.[4] Ramazzini in 1700 published the first systematic study of trade diseases. He discussed occupational disease as related to corpse bearers, midwives, stone cutters, wet nurses, weavers, runners, farmers, groomers, and a variety of other common occupational problems.[5] Because of this treatise Ramazzini is frequently referred to as "the father of occupational medicine" and his famous question, "What occupation does he follow?" is a familiar if unpracticed one.

Although Ramazzini's work influenced the worker's health and safety and increased interest in the worker's environment, legislation was slow to follow. Percival Pott, a physician in England, noted in 1775 an increased incidence in scrotal cancer among chimney workers. He found that young boys who were used as chimney sweeps because of their small physical size, were exposed to large amounts of soot, and he identified this as the causative agent of the scrotal cancers. Literature frequently points out a variety of political, economic, and social problems, and indeed this has been a vehicle for identification of disorders related to occupational exposures. Probably the most famous person identified in this respect is the Mad Hatter in Louis Carroll's *Alice in Wonderland*. Although this is a children's fantasy, Carroll was making a very active political point concerning the well known hazard of felt hat makers exposed to mercury. Although mercury was a known neurotoxin, and workers exposed to mercury developed various behavioral disorders, manufacturing processes were not changed. Carroll attempted to create enough social turmoil to force industry to develop safety measures to avoid exposures.

As the Industrial Revolution spread across Europe, the United States was just beginning to become an industrial country. The problems that had confronted the health professions in Europe now confronted the Americans. The first steps in solving the problems were legislative. In 1836 Massachusetts passed the first Child Labor Law and 30 years later appointed a special police officer to enforce the law that prohibited the employment of children under 10. Legislation was slow in coming because again, as in years past, there was an expendable work force. People from Europe were immigrating to the United States in droves, and if they were injured or became ill on the job they were easily replaced. Since the individual states have the power under the Constitution to govern themselves, the Federal Government could only deal with control of working conditions for persons employed in federal jobs. In 1884 the Bureau of Labor was created, and in 1914, as part of the Public Health Service, an Office of Industrial Hygiene was formed. Through this office research, training, and consultation became available to industry. During this time an outstanding physician, Dr. Alice Hamilton, began to speak out concerning the hazards of the workplace. Her investigations led to improved working conditions for people exposed to lead, silica in mines, carbon disulfide in the viscose rayon industry (for making tires), and mercury poisoning in the quicksilver mines of California.

In recent years concern has increased about the safety of the working environment. In 1970, the Occupational Safety and Health Act was enacted by the Congress of the United States. This Act covers all workers engaged in activities related to Commerce. The state agencies are designated to implement standards and programs as approved by the Department of Labor, and therefore can, by agreement with the Federal Government, undertake the enforcement of the Federal Act. The coverage of the Act is comprehensive and involves all workers employed in places of work engaged in a business affecting commerce. Two major departments were identified and developed under the Occupational Safety and Health Act. First is the Occupational Safety and Health Administration (OSHA) which falls under the Department of Labor. The responsibilities of OSHA include the promulgation, modification, and enforcement of occupational safety and health standards, the investigation and inspection of industry, the issuance of citations and penalties for health violation, the implementation of programs for education and training, the development of records, and the reporting of deaths, injuries, and illnesses. The second organization founded under the Occupational Safety and Health Act is the National Institute for Occupational Safety and Health (NIOSH). This Institute, under the Department of Health and Human Services, has the primary responsibility of developing research facilities. Included in its activities are planning, directing, and coordinating efforts to develop and establish criteria documents and the development of research, training, and related activities to assure a safe and healthful work environment. NIOSH personnel are responsible for administering these research activities, developing innovative methods and approaches for dealing with occupational safety and health, and supporting training programs. This agency also provides consultation services to educational institutions and occupational sites who request their services.

The establishment of these two federal agencies has had an immediate effect on problems relating to occupational safety and health. In the political arena discussions center on such aspects of occupational health as the funding for increased research. NIOSH has recently funded several Educational Resources Centers for Occupational Safety and Health. These centers have specific responsibility for the education and training of health manpower in the area of occupational health. The place of occupational health within the health care delivery system is another issue of national concern. Priorities must be set for health care action. The economic impact of occupational disease is of national concern. The cost of health care is rising at an alarming rate. It is therefore beneficial to eliminate those illnesses which can be eliminated. Control devices, screening programs, and educational programs can be developed which will help to decrease the incidence of disease directly related to occupational exposures.

The Occupational Safety and Health Act has created increased research into the development of alternative production of technology which will decrease the workers' exposure to hazardous chemicals. Industry has been encouraged to share data concerning physical responses to individual physical or chemical stressors in the work environment.

With the increased data being collected via the OSHA mandates, health professionals are being recognized as having invaluable skills essential to the health care of workers. Nurses are assuming increased responsibilities within the occupational setting. Nurses are no longer being seen as the person to put on bandages or give out pills but rather are involved in data collection, assessment processes, program planning, implementation of health programs, and decision making regarding the worker health programs. Data collection is a vital part of the nursing responsibilities. A recent study conducted for NIOSH by the University of Washington reported that 31 percent of over 1100 medical conditions found among 908 participants were diseases which were probably of occupational origin with an additional 10 percent of participants giving a medical history which was suggestive of occupational disease origin. Only 2 percent of these illnesses were reported on the employer's log required by OSHA, and only 3 percent were found in the Workmen's Compensation records. [3]

Academia has also responded to the legislation related to occupational safety and health. Increased numbers of universities and colleges are sponsoring programs for education and training. Full time academic study is now available in most of the areas of occupational health including occupational medicine, occupational health nursing, industrial hygiene, safety, toxicology, epidemiology, and biostatistics. Many of these programs offer interdisciplinary courses which help individual disciplines recognize the scope and expertise of members of the occupational health team. Continuing education programs are offered by government agencies, private industry, and universities to further disseminate vital information concerning occupational safety and health. National conferences sponsored by such organizations as the American Academy of Occupational Medicine, the American Association of Occupational Health Nurses, the American Association of Industrial Hygienists, and the National Safety Council add further opportunities for sharing and disseminating new knowledge which is rapidly becoming available as research in occupational diseases is expanded.

The public has also become more aware of the effects of chemicals on the environment. More emphasis must be placed on facilitating cooperation between those people concerned with problems in the general environment and those people concerned with the work environment. The general environmentalists were quite active and did succeed in eliminating the use of DDT as a pesticide because of its effects on wildlife. The banning of DDT resulted in the widespread use of parathion, another pesticide which has less harmful effects on wildlife, but parathion is far more hazardous to those involved in its production than was DDT. This is an example of the necessity for the careful documentation of health effects of specific chemicals, the need for widespread dissemination of that information to government, academia, and the public, and the need for a careful decision making policy, taking into consideration the total picture rather than a fragmentary view.

The Environmental Protection Agency is responsible for administering the Toxic Substance Control Act passed in 1976. Enacted to regulate commerce and to protect human health and the environment, this act requires toxicity testing on all new chemical substances before they are used in a production process. The act places the responsibility for obtaining and supplying these data on the manufacturers and processors of these agents. The purpose of this act is to protect the workers, the public, and the environment from potential hazardous exposures. Tragedies, such as the exposure of Japanese villages to alkyl mercury in seafood which resulted in neurologic disease in adults and birth defects in children, may be avoided in the future here in the United States. The act also provides for adequate authority to regulate and take action concerning those new chemicals and/or mixtures which present an unreasonable risk to health or the environment. The economic impact of this act is yet to be realistically evaluated. It seems evident that the cost of this testing will be added to the production costs.

RESPONSE OF THE NURSING PROFESSION

Occupational health nursing is a new and rapidly growing area of specialization within the nursing profession. The occupational health nurse's primary consideration is the health care of the working population. Occupational health nursing was recognized as a clinical specialty after the American Industrial Revolution. In 1888, Betty Moulder was employed by a group of coal mining companies to care for the sick and injured miners and their families. Shortly thereafter in 1895, Fletcher Proctor, a former governor of the State of Vermont, introduced district nursing to several villages in Vermont. The nurses' responsibilities were to care for the residents of the village who were employees of the Vermont Marble Company. Ada Mayo Stewart was selected to be the first nurse to implement this program. As the specialty grew it seemed timely that New England, the birthplace of American industry, should also become the birthplace of the first organized American industrial nursing movement, and in 1915 the Boston Industrial Nurses Club was formed. Recognition came slowly, but in 1917 the first special education course for industrial nurses was offered through the College of Business Administration at Boston University. Meanwhile industrial nurses recognizing the need to attain increased knowledge in their chosen speciality began to organize in local, state, and regional groups. Finally in 1941 the American Association of Industrial Nurses was founded. Catherine R. Dempsey, an industrial nurse working in Massachusetts, was selected the first president. In 1977 the organization formally changed its name to the American Association of Occupational Health Nurses, Inc. During these years the organization was constantly striving to improve the health care provided to workers in the workplace. There was constant communication between management representatives, labor unions, governmental consultants, and health professionals in an effort to control and prevent occupational diseases. In keeping with its stated purpose of "maintaining the honor and character of the nursing profession; improving community health by improving nursing service to employees; and developing and promoting standards for occupational health nurses and occupational health nursing," the American Association of Industrial Nurses, in conjunction with the American Board for Occupational Health Nurses (ABOHN), and the American Nurses' Association (ANA) endorses and supports certification programs for occupational health nurses.[6]

The American Nurses' Association certification program is in the area of community health nursing and incorporates all areas of community health including occupational health. The nurse, upon successful completion of the program, is certified as a generalist in community health nursing.

The ABOHN certification program is designed for the registered nurse practicing in the occupational health setting, whether she is a diploma graduate, a baccalaureate graduate, or a graduate with a master's degree. Upon completion of the required number of continuing education courses and verification of the nurse's expertise in occupational health nursing, the nurse may sit for the board examination. Upon successful completion of the exam she becomes a certified occupational health nurse. The completion of this program identifies the nurse as having met specific criteria to be recognized as a qualified and competent occupational health nurse. Both of these certification programs are endorsed and supported by the American Association of Occupational Health Nurses and the American Nurses' Association.

As we look at the field of occupational health nursing, we see an area of nursing practice that is just being recognized as a separate area of expertise for nurses. Occupational health nursing as such has not been identified and taught as an integral part of nursing in most educational programs, whether they are diploma programs, associated degree programs, or baccalaureate programs. The nurses practicing in the industrial setting had to develop their own "on the job" training programs, identify their roles, develop their job descriptions, increase their assessment skills, and learn new skills never taught in their basic nursing programs. The trend is changing. Educators responsible for nursing programs are beginning to integrate concepts of occupational health into the basic nursing program. In the nursing assessment tool developed by Faye McCain, she includes questions concerning the patient's occupation.[7] Patients admitted to the hospital with cancer may have developed the disease because of occupational exposure to asbestos (mesothelioma of the lung), benezene (leukemia), or vinyl chloride (angiosarcoma of the liver); and a patient with kidney disease may have been exposed to lead or cadmium. Tables 11-1 through 11-4 present more detailed lists of hazards and agents and the occupational settings in which they occur. Knowledge of the patient's occupation is vital in planning his nursing care and subsequent return to his home and job.

The graduate nurse who chooses to enter the specialty of occupational health nursing

TABLE 11-1. Selected biologic hazards and their sites of action in occupational settings*

Hazards	Site of Action	Occupation Exposure
Rabies	Nervous System	Veterinarians Zoologists Farmers Ranchers
Viral hepatitis	Liver	Hospital workers Oral surgeons
Q fever	Systemic, particularly respiratory system	Stockyard workers Wool handlers Laboratory workers
Tuberculosis	Respiratory system	Health professionals
Tetanus	Nervous system	Construction workers Farmers Any job involving the likelihood of traumatic injury

*For further information see *Occupational Diseases: A Guide to Their Recognition.* U.S. Department of Health, Education and Welfare, Public Health Service, Center for Disease Control, National Institute for Occupational Safety and Health, June 1977. 1-607.

brings with her skills from her basic educational program. These may include communication, beginning physical assessment skills, counseling techniques, basic knowledge of pathophysiology, health education, health screening, rehabilitation, and nursing principles. These are a good beginning, but, if the nurse desires a career as a clinical specialist in occupational health nursing, she must develop increased skills and knowledge in the areas of physical assessment, epidemiology, biostatistics, environmental control, safety, toxicology, and, of course, occupational health. Additional courses in administration, management, budgeting, personnel relations, and labor relations would be helpful. Such a program requires graduate education on the master's level. Indeed the accreditation document, Standard Interpretation and Audit Criteria for Performance of Occupational Health Programs, recommends that those nurses holding supervisory positions or nurses in one nurse units in industry have earned a master's degree in occupational health nursing or in public health nursing.[8]

THE OCCUPATIONAL HEALTH TEAM

The industrial setting is very different from the hospital environment. The goals and objectives vary considerably. The nurse who works in a hospital sees the patient as the focus for her work. The goal is to help the individual regain his highest level of wellness. In industry, increased production and increased profits are the priorities. Health enters the picture only as it interferes with production, as in increased rates of absenteeism, or with profit, as in high workmen's compensation claims or increased health insurance costs. The nurse, then, must sell her product, a healthy worker, in terms of the cost effectiveness of said worker. In order to do this she must be aware of the products and processes of the industry in which she is practicing. The work setting involves a multitude of different specialties working in many different situations. Many of these specialties are unfamiliar to

TABLE 11-2. Selected occupations and agents causing occupational dermatoses*

Occupation	Agent	Occupation	Agent
Aircraft workers	Resins Bichromates Chromic acid Solvents	Florists	Bacteria Fertilizers Fungi Herbicides Pesticides
Automobile workers	Asbestos Oils Rubber Lead	Insecticide makers	Aldrin Arsenic trioxide Chlordane Dieldrin
Bakery workers	Dusts Flour Heat Species Fungi	Laundry workers	Malathion Methosychlor Bleaches Chemical dusts Enzymes Fiberglass
Clerks	Ink removers Solvents Copy paper Duplicating materials	Painters	Acetone Benzine Chlorinated hydrocarbons Chromates
Dry cleaners	Acetic acid Ammonia Benzine Carbon tetrachloride Waterproofing chemicals	Road workers	Asphalt Cement Epoxy resins Herbicides Ultraviolet radiation
Embalmers	Bacteria Formaldehyde Fungi Ionizing radiation	Wood workers	Amino resin glues Formaldehyde Phenolic resin glue Varnishes

*For further information see *Occupational Diseases: A Guide to Their Recognition.* U.S. Department of Health, Education and Welfare, Public Health Service, Center for Disease Control, National Institute for Occupational Safety and Health, June 1977. 1-607.

the nurse. Therefore, it is essential that an interdisciplinary team approach be utilized in planning and implementing the health care of the worker. Members of this health team include the nurse, the physician, the industrial hygienist, safety officer, management, labor representatives, and other health professionals that may be needed for consultative purposes (Fig. 11-1). The occupational health nurse should communicate with the physician to establish the scope of the occupational health program. Together with the other members of the occupational health team an overall plan for the health and safety program should be constructed. Vital to this interaction is the acceptance of each member of the team as a peer with specialized skills essential to the success of the overall program. It is essential that each member of the team be familiar with the expertise of the others. For example the nurse should be aware that the industrial hygienist has expertise in the areas of air analysis, environmental study, monitoring techniques, and the interpretation of the results of these tests as they relate to guidelines and standards set by the Occupational Safety and Health Administration. If the nurse, in surveying her workplace, sees

TABLE 11-3. Selected chemical hazards, their sites of action and occupational settings*

Hazard	Site of Action	Occupation
Ethylene chlorohydrin	Respiratory and neurologic	Drug makers Dye workers Potato growers
Dicholoroethyl ether	Respiratory	Dry cleaners Oil processors Soap makers Textile workers Furniture workers
Acetic acid	Respiratory	Drug workers Dye makers Food preservers Laundry workers Rubber workers
Ketones	Skin Nervous system	Adhesive makers Dye workers Garage mechanics Shoe makers
Carbon tetrachloride	Skin Central nervous system	Chemists Firemen Ink makers Insecticide makers Refrigerant workers
Calcium cyanamide	Mucous membranes	Cotton workers Fertilizer workers Herbicide workers Steel workers
Isocyanates	Respiratory	Insulation workers Toy makers Paint sprayers Rubber workers
Arsine	Hematopoietic	Bronzers Etchers Jewelers Lead burners Paper makers
Beryllium	Respiratory	Beryllium workers Ceramic workers Electronic workers Nuclear reactor workers
Cadmium	Respiratory Kidney	Alloy makers Battery makers Engravers Welders Pesticide workers
Lead	Hematopoietic	Battery workers Ceramic workers Painters Plumbers

TABLE 11-3. *(Cont.)*

Hazard	Site of Action	Occupation
Phosphorus	Skin Respiratory tract Mucous membrane	Fireworks makers Incendiary makers Metal refiners Munitions workers
Ozone	Eyes Mucous membrane	Arc welders Food preservers Sewage treators Wood agers
Sulfur dioxide	Mucous membranes Respiratory tract Eyes	Brewery workers Firemen Glassmakers Ice workers Paper workers Tannery workers

*For further information see *Occupational Diseases: A Guide to Their Recognition.* U.S. Department of Health, Education and Welfare, Public Health Service, Center for Disease Control, National Institute for Occupational Safety and Health, June 1977. 1-607.

TABLE 11-4. Occupational carcinogens and their target organs*

Carcinogen	Target Organ	Carcinogen	Target Organ
Vinyl chloride	Brain Lung Liver	Chloromethyl methyl ether	Lung
		Chromates	Lung
Asbestos	Larynx Lung Gastrointestinal tract Pleural cavity	Mustard gas	Lung
		Nickel	Lung Nasal cavity
Benzene	Hematopoietic (blood cells)	Soots and tars	Lung Scrotum Skin
Coke oven emissions	Kidney Lung Skin	Uranium	Lung
		4-Aminobiphenyl	Bladder
Chromium	Larynx Nasal cavity	Benzidine	Bladder
		B-Naphthylamine	Bladder
Arsenic	Lung Skin	Ionizing radiation	Hematopoietic (blood cells) Lung Gastrointestinal
Bis(chloromethyl) ether	Lung		

*For further information see *Occupational Diseases: A Guide to Their Recognition.* U.S. Department of Health, Education and Welfare, Public Health Service, Center for Disease Control, National Institute for Occupational Safety and Health, June 1977. 1-607.

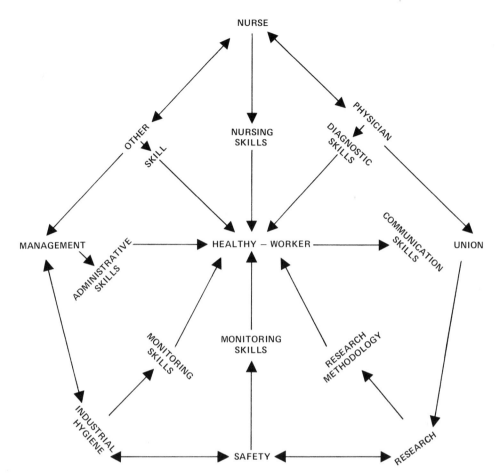

FIGURE 11-1. Working model of an interdisciplinary team. (From Silberstein, Carol: Implementing and Evaluating the Nursing Process. *Occupational Health Nursing,* Nov. 1976, pp. 10–12, with permission.)

dust or vapors or smells unusual odors from a particular chemical process, she should communicate this to the industrial hygienist so that he can evaluate the situation and take appropriate action. Similarly, if she notices poor housekeeping, cluttered workbenches, barriers or stairs, or broken guardrails on machines, she should communicate this to the safety officer.

Representatives of both management and labor are essential members of the health team. No matter how well an occupational health program is planned, if one does not have the cooperation of the administrative decision makers and the consumers, the program will fail. Although several members of the health team have been identified, in reality the nurse usually works alone in a health unit for which she has the primary responsibility, with the periodic consultation of a physician. In these instances the nurse must be even more aware of the occupational environment and have a firm knowledge of community resources available to her for appropriate evaluation of that work environment.

Industries themselves vary in size, scope, hazards, and processes. The nurse may choose a large chemical company which produces a variety of chemicals. She may have a complete medical unit with full time medical and nursing staff or she may be alone in a one nurse unit of a small chemical company. Her only resource of additional manpower may be a foreman or security people trained in first aid. Other options for work settings include industries which manufacture heavy equipment, foundries, rubber and related industries, industries producing household products, drug companies, insurance companies, food processing companies, or hospital personnel health programs. It must be remembered that the hospital employs workers who need health care. The nurse may function as a director of a health unit, a nursing supervisor, a staff nurse, or she may be a consultant for a variety of small companies which are not large enough or are nonhazardous and therefore do not require the presence of a full time health professional. Infinite opportunities are available for the nurse to identify the specific setting in which she feels she has the most to offer and feels most comfortable.

ROLES AND FUNCTIONS OF THE OCCUPATIONAL HEALTH NURSE

The nurse who chooses occupational health as her area of expertise is entering a challenging and rapidly growing area of nursing care. Her main concerns are health maintenance, health promotion, and health education. She brings with her all the skills and knowledge obtained in her basic program and will practice these daily. In the daily activities of the occupational health unit, the nurse may deal with minor lacerations, broken bones, and major trauma such as amputations, burns, or multiple injuries. She will deal with minor complaints such as colds, headaches, and splinters. The knowledge gained in medical-surgical nursing will be applied in her care of the worker with respiratory disease or the individual returning to work after a myocardial infarction. She will use the skills learned in psychiatric nursing to help individuals recognize problems and seek appropriate counseling. Nursing care of expectant women is also an active part of her day as more and more women remain on the job during their pregnancies. In addition to maintaining and practicing these familiar nursing interventions, the nurse must develop new skills in toxicology, epidemiology, and environmental control. This knowledge is gained through on the job training and in continuing education courses. Frequently these courses are taught by experts in fields other than nursing, and it becomes the nurse's responsibility to integrate these concepts into her nursing care. For example, environmental control of hazardous dust and vapors is the responsibility of the industrial hygienist or the safety officer, but the nurse needs to know the physiologic effects of these hazards so she can initiate proper health screening, health monitoring, and health education programs.

Occupational health nursing provides for the implementation of the nursing process in the health care of workers in the occupational setting. Nursing responsibilities in the area of occupational health are many and complex. Since the responsibility is to work with a healthy population, the focus of nursing care becomes one of primary prevention.

The management of the industry provides the physical set-up for the health unit. It is up to the nurse to design, implement and evaluate the nursing section of the occupational health program. In order to do this effectively, the occupational health nurse must clearly delineate in writing the philosophy, objectives, administrative structure, responsibilities, and activities of the nursing section of the occupational health program. Interrelationships and lines of communication with all members of the occupational health team should be clearly stated in policy statements. The nurse must have the authority to communicate directly with all members of the team where a worker's health and safety are concerned. The occupational health nurse acts as an independent practitioner of nursing. It is essential that she have skills in professional judgment, decision making, problem solving, nursing assessment, nursing care, counseling skills, and evaluation techniques.

The occupational health nurse is responsible for the immediate nursing assessment and nursing care of individual employees who present themselves in the clinic with health complaints. In addition to these responsibilities the nurse must develop educational programs for the employees. These programs include health information about major health problems such as cancer, obesity, or alcoholism, as well as health information about specific health problems related to that industry, such as ultraviolet radiation, noise, or dust. By keeping accurate and current health data on all the employees, past and present, the nurse has a valuable source of information concerning the prevalence and incidence of specific diseases within the working population. From these data can be determined specific patterns of symptoms and signs and how these relate to specific industrial products or processes. These data then help management decide if a process is hazardous to the health of the work force and what measures to take to make it safe. It has been demonstrated in many cases that industry has had to stop a particular process because it was causing disease among the workers. If accurate health records are maintained, this information becomes readily available, and vital decisions can be made on hard data. These records also allow the nurse to recognize a potential problem in the work area, for if she sees a number of workers from one area in the plant there may be an unrecognized exposure. She can then consult with the industrial hygienist who will monitor the area and make the necessary technical alterations to avoid undue exposure of the worker.

Retirement planning is another area of important health care. Many companies have excellent benefit programs for the retiring employee. These programs are usually explained in detail to the individual several months before retirement. It is equally important for the nurse to provide health information to these individuals and their families. Programs on the physiology of aging, sexuality and aging, and the psychological impact of retirement are vital to a good retirement program. The occupational health nurse has available to her the information concerning employees who will be retiring. She should contact these people and invite them and their spouses to participate in a retirement planning program. These classes should be arranged several months in advance of retirement so that the retirees will have ample time to ask questions and have discussions with others who are retiring. Some means of communication should be available after retirement so that the employee has some referral agencies available if needed.

The nurse is interested not only in developing screening programs for recognized major health problems such as hypertension, cardiovascular disease, or diabetes, but also in developing preventive programs for recognition of potential health hazards within the work setting which may result in respiratory disease, dermatologic problems, musculoskeletal disorders, or mental health problems. The nurse actively participates in the program of preplacement examination, periodic medical assessments, and in the treatment of occupational illness or injuries. Treatment of nonoccupationally related disease, such as common respiratory infections or injuries incurred off the job, is determined by the company policy. In a medical emergency the nurse will intervene until further specialized care is available. As a result of the nursing assessment, individual nursing care plans are developed. The care plans are directed toward therapeutic and preventive nursing care, including assessment of the health status, plan of nursing care, methods of implementing that care, results of the therapeutic interventions, and evaluation of the quality, the effectiveness, and the efficiency of the nursing care. Included in these nursing practices are the tasks of case finding and medical referrals. Employees who return to work after serious illnesses are screened by the nurse and evaluated for future job placement. When a job description is provided to the nurse, it is easier to decide if the employee is physically capable of returning to that work situation. The job description will tell the nurse the specific requirements of the job. Is it a sedentary job? Does it require heavy lifting? Does the process require rapid hand movements? All of this information will help the nurse properly assess the returning employee.

It is the responsibility of the occupational health nurse to develop an adequate record keeping system not only to meet the federal and state requirements but also for her information, so that potential health problems can be recognized and corrective measures taken before major illnesses ensue. Adequate record keeping, including nursing care plans, will help identify health hazards and allow for the initiation of epidemiologic studies.

The nursing process is an effective tool in the evaluation of the particular occupational health setting in which the nurse is practicing. The first step in any process becomes a complete assessment of the work situation. This includes the age, sex, and race of the employees. This information will help to identify specific workers who may have potential health problems due to sensitivity to particular chemicals or other hazards in the work place. Next she should evaluate the plant itself using a problem solving approach. Management should provide a tour of the plant, identifying any physical hazards such as guardrails, ventilation problems, slippery floors, heat stress, or noisy areas. Although the nurse is not expected to be an expert engineer, she can tell quickly whether or not problems exist. Merely by using one's senses one can see if there are mists, dusts, or smoke. Odors can be detected which may indicate increased exposure to particular chemicals.

After becoming familiar with the plant environment, the nurse must then communicate with the industrial hygienist, safety officer, or other individual who is responsible for knowing precisely what chemical or physical hazards exist within that plant. She should become familiar with all of the potentially toxic materials used in the manufacturing process. She must have knowledge of the routes of exposure (inhalation, absorption, or ingestion) and of the signs and symptoms of excessive exposures.

The nurse should then review the records in the occupational health unit, looking for such problems as neuropathology, dermatologic problems, and pulmonary or other systemic diseases. Once these data have been obtained, they must be organized. Now a profile of the work force and the occupational settings has been obtained. The physical hazards should be noted, identified, and education programs developed. The chemical hazards should be listed, identified by specific chemical names, routes of exposure, the number of workers potentially exposed, in what area of the plant, as well as the signs and symptoms of a toxic exposure both in the acute and chronic states. Emergency nursing measures to be taken for acute exposure, as well as those involved in caring for patients over a long period of time, should be recorded. This information should be kept in a readily available, easily obtained record system (Fig. 11-2).

Once this information has been appropriately organized, planning the occupational health program appropriate for the plant and the employees may be started. In the planning phase, as in the assessment phase, it is essential to involve all members of the health team. This may include simply the nurse and the manager, or it may include the nurse, physician, management, labor, industrial hygienist, and safety officers. During this planning, essential components of the program can be identified, and all health team members can agree on the philosophy and objectives of the health unit. Medical surveillance must be initiated, and

WORK AREA	NUMBER OF WORKERS IN AREA	NUMBER OF CLINIC VISITS FROM AREA/MONTH
EXPOSURE	RECOMMENDED TLV	LAST MEASUREMENT
SIGNS AND SYMPTOMS PROTECTIVE EQUIPMENT CONTROL MEASURES EDUCATIONAL PROGRAM NURSING ACTION		DATE: VALUE: LAST WALK—THROUGH SURVEY BY MEDICAL DEPARTMENT

FIGURE 11-2. The industrial hazard reference file. (From Silberstein, Carol: Implementing and Evaluating the Nursing Process. *Occupational Health Nursing,* Nov. 1976, pp. 10-12, with permission.)

specific activities, including preemployment physicals, identification of sensitive individuals, screening, health care, and educational programs can all be developed at this time. The appropriate protection mechanisms can be instituted. For example, if there is an area of the plant that is particularly noisy, the industrial hygienist will measure the levels. The nurse, the industrial hygienist, and the safety officer will then meet and decide on the type of program to initiate. Can the noise be eliminated or decreased by engineering changes? Do the workers need to wear hearing protection? If so, the nurse will then participate in planning an education program for workers, explaining to them that elevated noise levels can cause permanent hearing loss. The safety officer or the nurse then will explain how to use the hearing protection.

After an appropriate time interval the program evaluation process should be implemented. Criteria should be developed in the planning phase of the process so that objective and subjective data can be obtained for appropriate evaluation. The evaluation criteria should include information that will tell the occupational health team the number of problems identified, number of problems acted upon, the results of these actions, the frequency of a specific diagnosis in occupational health hazards, and the number of visits to the health unit. Once these data are accumulated, the occupational health team members will be able to identify whether or not special services or special education programs need to be developed for these workers.

THE OCCUPATIONAL HEALTH NURSE AND THE COMMUNITY

The occupational health nurse functions in an industry within a community, therefore there are many interactions which are appropriate. The nurse should be aware of the community services which are available to the employees. When employees visit the health clinic, the nurse is the most knowledgeable in treating problems directly related to the job. Nonoccupational illness should be treated by the worker's private physician, or referral should be made to the appropriate community agency. The worker identifies the nurses as an immediate source of health information. In this sense all of the health problems, both personal and family, are brought to the nurse. The nurse must be aware of the employee's family as a support system. The worker may come to the clinic to discuss problems of drug addiction in a teenager, terminal cancer in an aging parent, or sexual problems within the marriage. In most industrial plants the nurse is not responsible for the health care of the family, although when occupational health nursing was first established the nurse did have the responsibility of caring for the workers and their families.

It is well known that workers who have family problems may be affected on the job. Therefore the nurse must provide the opportunity for the employee to talk with a health professional in order to make an appropriate referral.

Employees must also be provided with appropriated instructions in terms of personal hygiene on the job. Cases have been reported where family members have developed berylliosis or cancer not from an occupational exposure but from exposure to the toxin via the contaminated clothes of the worker.

The occupational health nurse should be totally familiar with health activities provided by the community. These include mental health programs, home health care agencies, screening programs, Red Cross programs, or Family Service Agencies. Community based health services frequently provide mobile units which will come to local industry for hearing testing, immunization programs, vision screening or blood donor programs. This list is by no means all inclusive but is intended to demonstrate the need for knowledge of the community services available to the workers.

If the industry is an extremely hazardous one, plans should be made with local civil defense authorities, hospitals, the Red Cross, and local law enforcement agencies to handle any disaster situation which might arise at the plant resulting in injuries to the employees or the surrounding population.

Throughout this chapter emphasis has been placed on the need for communication between members of the health team, with workers, and with local community agencies. A very real need for communication, and one which is seldom recognized, exists between the community health nurse and the occupational health nurse. When the community health nurse visits a patient for the first time, an initial health assessment is made. This, with the information received from the referral source, is used to plan the nursing care of that individual. The occupation of the patient is usually noted with no further data. This information is essential to the nursing care of that patient. If, for example, the community health nurse is visiting a patient with chronic obstructive pulmonary disease who is expected to be able to return to work, the nurse should have knowledge of the specific job. If he works in a parking garage, a relatively sedentary job which a patient with chronic obstruction lung disease should be able to handle, he is exposed to increased levels of carbon monoxide. This individual already has an increased red cell mass (to compensate for the decreased pulmonary oxygenation) and exposure to carbon monoxide further compromises his ability to oxygenate his tissue. If this patient is returning to an industrial setting where his job involves wearing a face mask respirator, it is imperative that the occupational health nurse know his specific disease and his condition. If the worker has chronic bronchitis, then the respiratory mask would further hamper his breathing capacities. On the other hand if the worker has emphysema, the respirator may actually be helpful, since the filter acts in the same way as pursed lip breathing.

A frequent problem in community health nursing is lead poisoning in children. Once the diagnosis is made it is usually the nurse who is asked to assess the home for sources of lead. One frequently ignored source is the occupation of the family members. Employees frequently do not change clothes at their place of employment. When the family member comes home after work he may bring a significant amount of lead home on his work clothes. This becomes the source of exposure to the children in the household. Some occupations resulting in lead exposure include battery makers, book binders, printers, painters, demolition workers, foundry molders, jewelers, metal workers, roofers, ship workers, and welders. Lead is not the only health hazard that may be found on work clothes. Asbestos and beryllium have been reported as causative factors of diseases.

The community health nurse should also be aware of the manufacturing processes within her specific area. Effluents from smoke stacks and individual waste disposal methods may provide a source of exposure to a variety of chemicals for the community at large. The contamination of the James River, Hopewell, Virginia, by kepone, a pesticide which produces neurologic disorders, is an example of a community health problem resulting from improper waste disposal. The community health nurse would only become aware of such a problem after appropriate agencies such as the Environmental Protection Agency had done the necessary sampling and verified the problem. The nurse would then be intensely involved in the screening process which would identify those members of the community who were affected by the contamination.

SUMMARY

The occupational health nurse provides nursing care for a healthy working population. The focus of that care is primary prevention. An interdisciplinary approach within the industrial setting is essential to the functioning of an occupational health program.

Knowledge of the principles of safety and industrial hygiene are essential. The toxicology of those chemicals to which the workers are exposed must be identified, and the nursing care must be delineated in writing. The nurse has administrative authority to design, implement, and evaluate the occupational health nursing program.

She functions as an independent practitioner, a provider of care, a consultant, a teacher, and a researcher. Close contact must be maintained with community agencies not only for the individual and his family but also for the community as a whole.

REFERENCES

1. Hearings on Small Business and the Occupational Safety and Health Act of 1970 Before the Subcommittee on Environmental Problems Affecting Small Business of the H. R. Select Committee on Small Business, 92 Congress, 2nd Session, June 22, 1972.
2. The President's Report of Occupational Safety and Health, 6.P.O. Document No. 2915-0011, May 1972.
3. Ashford, N.A.: *Crisis in the Workplace: Occupational Disease and Injury. A Report to the Ford Foundation.* The MIT Press, Cambridge, Mass., 1977.
4. Agricola, G.G.: *De Re Metallica*, 1556. Translated by Hoover, H.C., and Hoover, L.H. in Min. Mag., London, 1912.
5. Ramazzini, B.: *De Morbis Artificum*, 1713. Translated by Wright, W.C. University Press, Chicago, 1940.
6. Lee, Jane A.: *The New Nurse in Industry, A Guide for the Newly Employed Occupational Health Nurse.* U.S. Dept. of Health, Education and Welfare, Public Health Service, NIOSH, Cincinnati, Ohio—January 1978.
7. McCain, F.: "Nursing by Assessment—not Institution." *American Journal of Nursing,* 65:82, 1965.
8. *Standards, Interpretation and Audit Criteria for Performance of Occupational Health Programs.* Report to the National Institute for Occupational Safety and Health. Occupational Health Institute, Chicago, 1975.

BIBLIOGRAPHY

Brown, M.L.: *Occupational Health Nursing.* Springer Publishing Company, Inc., New York, 1956.
Cahall, J.: "The Use of the Nursing Process in the Industrial Setting." *Occupational Health Nursing,* Nov. 1976, pp. 7-9.
Copplestone, J.F.: *Preventive Aspects of Occupational Health Nursing.* Edward Arnold, London, 1967.

Sarason, Seymour: *Work, Aging, and Social Change.* The Free Press, New York, 1977.

Schilling, R.S.F.: *Occupational Health Practice.* Butterworths, London, 1973.

Silberstein, C.: "Implementing and Evaluating the Nursing Process in the Occupational Health Unit." *Occupational Health Nursing,* Nov. 1976, pp. 10-12.

"Symposium on Occupational Health Nursing." *Nursing Clinics of North America,* Vol. 7, No. 1, 1972.

Zenz, Carl: *Occupational Medicine, Principles and Practical Applications.* Year Book Medical Publishers, Chicago, 1975.

12
NURSING ROLE
IN SCHOOL HEALTH

MARILYN L. STEMBER, Ph.D., R.N.

School nurses have experienced an increasing role in the delivery of health care services since their inception at the turn of the century. While the roles and functions of all health professionals have evolved over time, school nurses have experienced even more dramatic changes. This chapter examines the general perspective of school health nursing, identifies skills and knowledge that are basic to practice, and suggests guidelines for school health programs.

HISTORICAL VIEW

In the early 1900s Lillian Wald and Lina Rogers of the Henry Street Nurse Association demonstrated in a one month project the worth of a nurse in the school.[1] Wald was able to show that through nursing followup, children could be readmitted to school following a communicable disease, reducing the incidence of absenteeism.[2] Increasing knowledge about pathogenic organisms during the first decades of the century permitted school nurses to be concerned with three variables in the disease process: 1) characteristics of pupil (host); 2) characteristics of the pathogen (agent); and 3) characteristics of the environment contributing to the host-agent interaction. For example, the tubercle bacillus was known to thrive among those who were sick, malnourished, and lived in poor housing. Programs designed to improve the nutrition of school aged children were undertaken. Detection programs in high risk areas with accompanying steps to improve conditions in slum areas resulted in dramatic reductions in tuberculosis.

It is interesting to note that by 1910 medical examinations in schools were required in 337 cities in the United States with 1194 physicians, 371 nurses, and 48 dentists employed by school systems. The primary focus of these early services was to serve children by protecting the common health of all children. With the high incidence of infectious diseases and the increasing knowledge of their control, it was natural that much of the effort was waged against smallpox, tuberculosis, and diphtheria.

As control of contagious diseases became more successful, school nurses found their role shifting to an emphasis on health education. The development of health educational programs was guided by the philosophy that every child should be taught early in life to preserve his own life and health as well as that of others. Assisted by the efforts of the Women's Christian Temperance Union (WCTU), laws were passed mandating that specific health instruction, particularly related to the use of narcotics and alcohol, be a part of a broad program of instruction in hygiene. From the time of the WCTU crusade to World War I, the recognition increased for the interrelated aspects of healthful school environment, health services, and health instruction.

As school nurses joined forces in health education with the educators, they also began to be hired by boards of education. Increasing numbers of nurses were employed by the educational system rather than by the health care system. This major change in the authoritative and supervisory structure for school nursing has systematically contributed to some of the role ambiguity and conflicts experienced by many school nurses today.[3] Concomitant with employment by educational systems was an increase in tasks delegated by the educational system. Rather than nurses defining their major contributions in a school health program, many of the tasks and responsibilities of the school nurse were promulgated by school administrators.

The Children's Charter of 1930 was the prominent policy for child health programs following World War I. A major national conference of federal health and educational professionals was held in 1945 to consider the health needs of school children and identify strategies for meeting those needs. While legislation prior to this date had been directed at ameliorating preventable physical and mental health conditions noted in the World War I servicemen, it was disconcerting to participants that the same problems were noted again among the World War II inductees. One result of the 1945 conference was the creation of the Committee on the School Age Child. This committee drafted a report released in 1951, "Better Health for School-Age Children," that assisted in shaping school health programs.

Federal grants in the 1960s and the 1963 and 1965 ammendments to Title V of the Social Security Act expanded programs in prevention and treatment of childhood diseases and handicapping conditions and provided comprehensive health services to more than a half million children and teenagers.[1] During the 1950s and 1960s, the specification of school nurse responsibilities became more precise. However, the priority of tasks continued to be defined by the school principal, the primary administrative authority. School principals, in general, wanted school nurses to provide immediate first aid when anything happened, to be in charge of admitting students back into school, to be available when students got sick during the school day, and so forth. Thus, health care delivery to children in the school setting, rather than being broad based and derived from an underlying philosophy of community health nursing practice, was determined by the expectations of their nonhealth professional supervisors.

An early effort by school nurses to define their role in school health programs and to promote standards for care was begun under the leadership of Gertrude Cromwell.

Cromwell headed the Committee on School Nurse Policies and Practices of the American School Health Association, a group that began work on guidelines for school nurses and standards of practice. In 1955, the Committee issued a statement entitled "Recommended Policies and Practices for School Nursing," a report published in the January 1956 issue of the *Journal of School Health*.

Another example of nursing's attempt to define and clarify the areas of responsibilities of the school nurse is the 1967 *Guidelines for School Nursing*[4] prepared by the School Nursing Committee of the American School Health Association. The report was based on an evaluation of current nursing practices and on trends which appeared to be guiding the future course of school nursing. Functions and activities were identified for achieving objectives established by the school district. The responsibilities of the nurse in the school program were derived from several major areas: 1) the organization and implementation of school health services, 2) responsibilities related to pupil health, 3) coordination of the school health program, 4) teaching and educational evaluation, 5) the health of school personnel, and 6) the professional responsibilities of the school nurse. In the latter category recognition was made that the school nurse had a dual professional role as a member of the nursing profession as well as the teaching profession.

SCOPE OF SERVICE

A number of publications specifying the responsibilities of school nursing have appeared in the literature. Identified responsibilities included health appraisals to assess the health status of students, counseling students and their parents to secure medical, dental, or other treatment, assisting teachers in adapting health programs to meet needs of students, serving as a consultant and resource person in the educational program, being a liason with the school and the community agencies, protecting student health by attention to environmental health factors, providing emergency care for illness and injury incurred in the school, serving as a team member in identifying, evaluating, and providing for handicapped children, and cooperating in community health planning.

These kinds of responsibilities have been included in statements by professional organizations[5,6] about the role of the school nurse. Included in the school nurse role are assisting in the establishment and enforcement of school policies, implementing programs for the protection and promotion of the health of the pupils, maintaining a school environment that is conducive to health living, building components of the curriculum that have significance for health, managing health services, handling special health programs, and relating school health programs to those of the community.

Furthermore, job descriptions of school nurses identify a variety of other responsibilities: implementing state laws, making home visits, supervising vision and hearing tests, readmitting students who have been absent, planning and implementing immunization programs, and ordering first-aid supplies. Added to that are such activities as counseling of students with special health problems, health teaching, emergency care, and so forth, usually providing a very encompassing job description for the school nurse.

ROLE AMBIGUITY AND CONFLICT

The major problem is not the narrowness of scope of health care services or restriction in the parameters for providing health care, but rather what the school nurses actually are doing, what they think they should be doing, and what others expect them to do.

These questions are paramount today. Several studies, such as one by Blauvelt,[7] address these concerns. Blauvelt conducted a survey to determine what the agreement was between what school nurses were doing, what they thought they should do, what supervisors thought they should do, and what principals wanted them to do. The purpose of the study conducted in 1974 was to determine what functions were actually being performed and those that respondents would like to see performed.

Blauvelt reported returns from over 200 health room personnel, 194 principals, 28 supervisors, and a panel of national leaders. The following findings were confirmed. There was no significant level of agreement on the relative appropriateness of 16 selected school nurse functions between nonnurses and nurses, between principals and nurses, between principals and nonnurses, between supervisors and nurses, between supervisors and nonnurses, and between the national panel and nonnurses. There was a significant level of agreement between nurses and the national leaders on what functions should be performed in the school health setting.

Another major finding was that nurses were not performing the functions they thought they should be performing. It was also found that neither nurses nor nonnurses were performing the functions that supervisors felt to be most important. Finally, there was not a significant level of agreement between what principals thought should be done in school health rooms and what nurses and nonnurses assigned to those rooms were actually doing. The results of this study highlight the major problems of low clarity and role disagreement. Nurses in this study were functioning in a situation in which they not only were unable to enact roles they desired, but their activities were not in agreement with what the supervisor expected of them nor with what the principal expected of them.

School nurses often dispair over the fact that colleagues in the school setting are quick to describe the role of the school nurse.[3] A systematic study was conducted by Forbes[8] to identify teachers' expectations of the nurses' roles and functions in the school. A study sample of 115 randomly selected teachers identified various activities in an open-ended questionnaire. Responses were categorized as relating to 1) administration of the school health program, 2) the nurse's role as a faculty member, 3) functions in the community, 4) health appraisals, 5) counseling and guidance, 6) health education, and 7) health protection and safety. The variety of responses led the author to conclude there was not a consistent pattern of activities that was associated with the professional school nurse. These findings suggest that teachers have not developed a consistent concept of the professional role of the nurse.

A 1973 issue of *Journal of School Health* reported a study[9] undertaken by the School Nurses Professional Improvement Committee in the state of Washington to determine the appropriateness of selected nursing tasks, to determine the most frequently performed tasks, and to determine the tasks that nurses most frequently share with others. Included in the questionnaire were 149 health related tasks drawn from *Standards for School Nurse Services* prepared in 1970 by the Department of School Nurses, National Educational Association.

This survey of nurses serving 42 schools revealed that nurses were involved to a great extent in nearly all of the health related tasks, but a majority of the tasks were also being performed by students, parents, and teachers in the school setting. The fact that these health related tasks were also performed by others in the school setting contributed to difficulties in defining the school nurse's role; respondents perceived that their work lacked "unity and structure."[9]

Two primary program changes were recommended as a result of this study. One was to give priority and nursing time to those tasks recognized as most appropriate, e.g., promoting health, education resources, prevention of injuries, provision of emergency care, health counseling, and referrals. Second, the study disclosed certain tasks were performed exclusively by nurses in the school setting. For example, the nurse alone had responsibility for vision rescreening and referrals. The nurse was also central in interpreting medical recommendations. Exclusive tasks were assigned a high priority. It is interesting to note that routine screening of vision, dental health, and physical well being received low priority ranking. Again, this study described the overlapping of responsibilities and roles of the nurses in the school setting.

In a recent report, Crowley and Johnson[10] described multiprofessional perceptions of school health that were ascertained using the Delphi technique. In order to arrive at consensus about a definition for a national school health conference to be held in 1977, the 495 respondents of the first Delphi questionnaire reacted to a question about the nature of school health. The contrasting responses by professional groups are quite enlightening in understanding the role ambiguity in school health. Respondents who were employed in state government offices were proponents of the view that school health is a problem oriented service activity program. The educational participants who were invited to the conference concurred with this view. However, primary practitioners were generally supportive of the preventive service activities concept, while members of academic communities and professional organizations were backers of the comprehensive service, education, and environmental definition. On the second round of the Delphi survey, the 142 respondents, when presented with the data from the first round, moved toward preferring a more comprehensive view of school health comprised of services, health education, and a healthful environment.

The image of nursing and the nurse's role is generally derived from the white uniformed hospital nurse. In an attempt to help school administrators to understand the practice of nursing as it is administered in schools vs. the practice of nursing in hospitals, Macdonough[11] compared the role of the nurse in the two settings. She contrasted the fact that the in-hospital patient has accepted nursing care, while in school health programs the agreement for care is not established so that the major responsibility of the school nurse is to counsel parents about the need for medical attention and/or the acceptance of the nurse recommendations. Second, in the hospital a patient knows he is ill and wants to get well. In the school situation the family and the student often do not recognize the problem, and not only do they not seek help, but they may resent and resist efforts on the part of the school nurse to assist them. In another comparison, responsibility for health was contrasted. She stressed that hospital nursing service is provided around the clock with the nurse responsible for the health status of patients. In a school health program the student and his family must assume major responsibility for health care. This means in schools an increased emphasis on teaching and demonstrating good health practices is required.

Another contrast made by Macdonough was that in the hospital the main goal of nursing care is cure. In school nursing, the goal is generally prevention and health promotion. This perspective, rather than stressing what the nurse will do to make the patient well, stresses prevention of illness and disability and promotion of optimal health for the student. The difference in independence and isolation also was compared. There are large numbers of nurses in hospitals and the work in a hospital situation is assigned to the nurse by others. School nurses not only work in isolation from other professional nurses, the kind of work load and priorities in the school system are self-assigned. Therefore, broad based assessment skills, epidemiologic knowledge, and program planning skills are also necessary. The common expectations of principals that the school nurse should be there to take care of any first-aid injuries and to deal with any illness oriented problems may be a carryover of the image from the hospital setting to the school setting.[11,12]

A major change that has influenced the role of the school nurse is the increase in interdisciplinary members that are concerned with the school health program. In earlier decades, the classroom teacher, the parent, the principal, and sometimes a school physician, were the primary individuals with whom the nurse worked. Particularly in the larger school systems, the school nurse is now expected to share professional decisions with guidance counselors, psychologists, speech and reading consultants, and specialized teaching personnel who instruct the emotionally disturbed, the retarded child, and the auditorial and neurologically handicapped child. Multidisciplinary team functioning involves clarification and redefinition about the tasks and responsibilities belonging to the individual team members.

Another factor that is contributing to the changing role of the school nurse is changing child health needs that now demand new and different approaches.[13] Societal changes have resulted in increased sexual activity among school aged children, sometimes resulting in teenage pregnancy or venereal disease.[14,15] The misuse of drugs and alcohol, smoking, and many other problems that were formerly problems of the adult generation are now reaching younger populations and are having implications for the school health program.[16,17] Schools are playing a major role in identifying abused children and protecting them from further abuse.[18]

Oda[19] suggested that the school nurse role is undergoing change in divergent directions. She suggested that in some areas school nursing is moving toward role definitions stressing health education, counseling, and consultation. Others are projecting that nurses will be utilizing increased technologic health assessment skills in school settings. At the same time that some school nurses have moved away from the medical or pathology model into health education and consultation, other nurses have created emerging roles that are designed to provide primary care by quality in-depth assessment of physical, psychosocial, psychoeducational, behavioral, and learning problems, as well as providing comprehensive well-child care. She further suggested that regardless of the nurse's focus—whether it is more pathologic or prevention oriented—expanded or altered roles may not be understood or accepted by colleagues in the school setting, by students and families who utilize health services, and by communities at large. Role expectations of others may or may not be congruent with the nurse's. It is obvious then that this role discrepancy can profoundly affect the practice of school health nursing.

Another reason for the lack of role clarity was highlighted historically. Nurses employed in school settings are often responsible to at least two or more supervisors.[20] Traditionally, in the organizational structure of a school, the site administrator or principal is responsible for all activities that go on in the school. In addition, school nurses often have nursing supervisors outside the school setting to whom they are also directly responsible. It may be that school nurses are also responsible to the director of special services which adds an additional layer of administrative accountability. It would appear that the conflicting expectations of these various administrators may contribute to role ambiguity.

The purpose of the remaining sections of this chapter are to clarify educational and certification requirements of the position and to identify appropriate knowledges and skills required for current role definition. While it is clearly understood that the role of the school nurse is dynamic and is dependent in part on the individual situation, in general, role parameters can be specified that are helpful for school nurse practice.

REQUIREMENTS OF THE POSITION

Educational Preparation

The minimum educational requirement for school nurses varies from state to state and from setting to setting. Henderson and Nite[1] noted that this variation was in part due to employment arrangements. Since school nurses may be employees of state, county, or municipal school systems, health departments, visiting nurses services, or other private health care institutions, there is no standardization of educational requirements. Bryan[21] observed the following:

"School nurses have the most varied requirements and titles of any group within the nursing profession. Some states have no certification requirements; others require a year of study beyond the baccalaureate degree."

The leadership for establishing educational standards has primarily come from professional organizations. As early as 1938, the Education Committee of the National Organization for Public Health Nursing published minimum qualifications for nurses in school nursing positions.[1] The rising expectations in school nurse preparation can be seen by examining some major reports. For example, the Committee on School Nurse Policies and Practices in its 1959 report to members of the American School Health Association made recommendations regarding the school nurse's professional preparation. This report stated graduation from an accredited school of nursing was the minimum, and the possession of a bachelor's degree was strongly recommended. Areas delineated for special preparation were in school health, prevention and control of disease, nutrition, psychology and child development, organization and administration, practices of public health nursing, health counseling, health education, and mental health.[22]

The American Nurses' Association presented a document, *Functions and Qualifications of School Nurses*[6] in 1966, that grew from the concern that Boards of Education employed nurses with a variety of professional preparation ranging from the attainment of a diploma in a hospital school of nursing to completion of a master's degree. Two recommendations were made: 1) preservice preparation in nursing evidenced by graduation from a school of nursing with state accreditation at the time of graduation and 2) preparation for school nursing as evidenced by possession of a baccalaureate degree. Field experience in school nursing was cited as a component of the baccalaureate degree.

In the early sixties, the National League for Nursing undertook a study to determine what the nurse needs to know to carry out the functions of a school health program. The study concluded that while much of what the nurse needs to know can be attained in a baccalaureate program in nursing, some work beyond the first degree is necessary to give the nurse an orientation to the school system.

Following the ANA position paper of 1965 recommending the baccalaureate degree as the minimum preparation for beginning professional nurse practice, the School Nurse Committee of the American School Health Association concurred in a 1967 report.[4] Nursing education at the baccalaureate level was recommended as a first step because it provides preparation in basic and nursing sciences and a background in liberal education comparable to that of other professions. Graduate education in school nursing would prepare for specialist practice. A master's program curriculum would focus on general areas of man and his environment, the educational system, the field of specialization, and responsibility to society.

Given that the basic requirement for nursing practice was to be the baccalaureate degree, Stobo[23] in a 1969 report suggested that the nurse in the school system should probably be prepared at the master's level. She argued that because nurses work collaboratively with numerous personnel in the school system, they are expected to make judgments and professional decisions with guidance counselors, psychologists, social workers, speech and reading consultants, specialized training personnel, as well as those who are teaching in general and special programs. In an increasing number of schools, the master's degree is becoming the preferred degree to be held by teaching and specialized staff members.

Stobo's recommendations were also based on the findings of a national conference entitled "Educational Preparation of the Nurse for School Health Work," which was held in March, 1967 with the sponsorship of the United States Children's Bureau. The Conference attendees represented boards of education, departments of health, state departments of education and health, educational divisions within universities, and national professional associations for nursing. Two general recommendations emerged from this conference. First, preparation for school nurse professionals should be at the graduate level, with commonalities of preparation in maternal child health nursing, public health nursing, and mental health. Second, interdisciplinary courses were suggested to be developed and included in the preparation of all school professional staff members. Common core courses would be the result of interprofessional collaboration among representatives from the fields of medicine, ecology, guidance, social work, nursing, and other related disciplines.[21,23]

It was clear in Stobo's report that nursing educators should develop master's programs in school nursing. She noted with concern that numbers of school nurses had attended graduate programs in other academic fields such as health education, guidance, and home and family life. She argued that the attainment of a degree in another area forces a professional hybrid, a sacrifice to the goal of nurses being highly competent in their own field.[23]

Another major trend is the development of school nurse practitioner programs for the preparation of a primary care specialist in the school setting. This development has paralleled the expanded role of nursing in all specialty areas. School nurse practitioner programs have been described in some detail in the last decade.[24-28]

"Guidelines on Educational Preparation and Competencies of the School Nurse Practitioner," a joint statement of the American Nurses' Association, the American School Health Association, and the Department of School Nurses/National Education Association, was issued in 1977 and appeared in the May, 1978 Journal of School Health.[29] This document identified the functions and responsibilities of school nurses, provided a definition of school nurse practitioners and described the major components of the school nurse practitioner program.

The Guidelines describe the competencies that should be demonstrated at the completion of the formal course of study. It suggested that although planning for programs should be carried out by representatives of nursing, medicine, school systems, other professional disciplines, and the community at large, educational programs for school nurse practitioners should be carried out in health centers under the auspices of an accredited baccalaureate nursing program.

It was recommended that faculty for these programs be composed of nursing, medicine, and school systems as members of the curricular team. Course content was identified and included growth and development, interviewing and counseling, family dynamics, positive health maintenance and health education, childhood illnesses, exceptional child, mental health, community resources and delivery of child health care service, family/nurse/physician/school relationships, and clinical experience.[29]

The statement also said that nurses prepared at the baccalaureate level should be selected for admission to school nurse practitioner programs, however the sponsoring institution should have flexibility for developing student admission policies for the program. The recommended length of this continuing education program was the equivalent of one academic semester of intensive preparation followed by a preceptorship period of six to eight months under the direction of medical instructors and nurse practitioners. The report suggested that concepts and skills of the school nurse practitioner should be available in baccalaureate nursing curricula as soon as possible.

A 1973 survey[30] of educational requirements for school nurses included responses from all 50 states. Twenty-six states identified the B.A., B.S., or the B.S.N. degree as basic educational requirement for regular, permanent, or life certification. Twenty-four states identified specific academic areas of course work that were required for permanent certification. Frels[30] noted that among the courses identified were school nursing, education, psychology, foundations of education, curriculum and teaching methodology, adult and adolescent psychology, guidance and counseling, exceptional children, principles and practice of community health nursing with a supervised field practice, and principles of organization and administration of public health. Eight states identified additional academic preparation for the school nurse supervisor. This included course work in administration, supervision, and curriculum. Several states indicated an M.A. degree or 30 hours of additional education was required.

In spite of the survey showing that over half of the states require a bachelor's degree as a minimum, the nursing profession's recommended standards are for a bachelor's degree with school nurse practitioner preparation. Continuing education programs such as the one described at the University of Colorado[12,26-28] will offer professional nurses the opportunity to develop skills and competencies not included in their basic preparation. The desirability of master's degree preparation appears to be on the horizon.

Certification

Many state boards of education have mandatory certification requirements for nurses employed by school boards. Under these requirements, preparation for nurses resembles the preparation required of teachers. Certification is a legal procedure which authorizes an individual who has completed specific requirements to perform certain services in the schools. In the teaching profession, certification and licensure are sometimes used interchangeably. However, as the ANA document entitled *A Rationale for School Nurse Certification*[5] suggests, certification in the nursing profession must be distinguished from licensure. While licensure to practice indicates that the nurse has met certain minimum legal requirements established by the state and is registered to practice therein, certification is the process by which state officials assure the public that licensed professional nurses have completed additional requirements for practice in the school.

The history of the American Nurses' Association involvement in certification of school nurses began as early as 1959 when the ANA published "Essential Consideration for Certification of School Nurses Employed by Boards of Education." The guide was developed for the purpose of acquainting school nurses and state nurses' associations with the purposes of certification, certification patterns, and methods for securing certification.

Between 1959 and 1964, the number of boards of education employing school nurses and number of nurses employed by schools increased approximately 80 percent. Only about half of the states had certification requirements and there was little standardization among states who required certification. It appeared to ANA leaders that a more comprehensive statement on certification was needed. Addressed to both the profession of education and nursing, *A Rationale for School Nurse Certification* was published in 1966.[5] It clearly stated that the nursing profession has the responsibility for establishing professional standards to assure a high quality of nursing performance in school health programs. Nursing was charged with the obligation to devise and enforce professional standards, to recruit and select students for programs, to prepare practitioners, to accredit programs, to evaluate nursing practice, and to promote continuous growth in professional competence.

This document suggested that education and nursing alike share a mutual interest in the standards which are established for any one of the disciplines involved. The nurse as a member of the educational system works with members of teaching and administrative staff of the school. Therefore, professional colleagues represent not only nurses but a variety of disciplines in both health and education who are concerned about the professional preparation of the school nurse. A number of states have reported that cooperative action by both professions has been facilitated by an interdisciplinary advisory counsel.

School nurses who are interested in certification should become familiar with pertinent legal regulations in their states. Current certification is reflecting increased academic preparation in general education and more extensive student teaching, practicum, or internship experience. The survey on certification reported by Frels[30] noted an increasing number of states certifying school nurses. As of January 1973, 28 states had a school nurse certification requirement. Nineteen of the states had a mandatory requirement and 9 had a permissive requirement. Most states used the credential "School Nurse Certificate." However, a variety of other titles are used, such as "Special Service Certificate," "School Nurse Endorsement", and "Nurse Teacher Certificate."

Another finding of the survey was that regular or permanent certificates were valid from three years to life. Twenty-two states indicated that they issue a provisional or limited certificate. States varied on the length of time that the limited certificate was valid and this ranged from one to five years. Additional educational preparation was generally required for renewal ranging from four credit hours per year to the acquisition of a master's degree.

In addition to certification and licensure, another concept often discussed is credentialing. Bryan[21] reported that school nurses who have obtained the basic education in nursing by completing the baccalaureate degree may be eligible for credentialing in nursing. In several states nurses now take up to a year of special graduate studies before being eligible for a school nurse credential. Courses usually include work in child growth and development, mental health, curriculum development, advanced pediatrics, and health education methods and media.

In summary, educational requirements, certification, and standards for practice have contributed to improving the quality of health services for the nation's young people. Regulatory procedures such as those established by state certifying authorities and professional standards contribute to a uniformly high quality of nursing personnel for all children and youth.

DETERMINING ROLES AND ACTIVITIES: AN AGGREGATE FOCUS

The school health program is concerned with the health of the aggregate of school children. Rather than focusing on nursing care given to individual children, the health of all school age children is central. This view of school nursing 1) implies the need for skill in assessment of a population and identification of high risk populations; 2) requires program planning skills in order to set goals and priorities; 3) involves implementation strategies at the individual, group, and the environmental levels; and 4) requires evaluation at the program level. This approach enhances the likelihood that nursing's role and activities are based on population needs, are clearly planned with multidisciplinary and consumer input, are implemented on a rational basis, and are evaluated in light of the health status of the school age population.

Assessment

A systematic assessment includes the characteristics of the students and their community, their status of health, and the services available in the community. Assessment is needed in order to effectively plan, implement, and evaluate the school health program. The first step is to broadly describe the characteristics of the student group. What are the age ranges of the population? Other attributes to assess are the sex distribution, race or ethnic group identification, family characteristics, and marital status of the parents. What are the housing conditions and employment status of the area? Demographic data, secured from school records and from census reports, provide a backdrop from which to assess other characteristics.

A second type of data necessary for obtaining a systematic data base is information about the health status of the population. Hogue in Hall and Weaver[31] has provided a list of health indicators that may be utilized for assessing the general level of health status in a population.

1. Level of social functioning was cited. In the school age child, ability to attend school is an indicator of the general functioning. Absenteeism has been used by a number of investigators[33,39] who have noted that absence records are a measure of health for a school population that remains fairly consistent over time.

2. Symptoms and complaints may be utilized as health indicators. Reasons for the child's absences or complaints and symptoms observed in the health room are examples.

3. Disabilities and impairments may be indicators. The proportion of children with visual impairments or hearing loss can be examined. The number of children with learning disabilities or other impairments and the number of children with handicaps, physical and mental, provide other data about the health status of a school population.

4. Biologic indicators of disease were cited as a possibility. Elevated blood pressure, for example, is associated with certain disease processes. The incidence of streptococci in throat culture examinations may be used as another health status indicator.

5. Disease categories may be used, for example, the number of cases of acute diseases such as measles, heart disease, and dental disease.

6. Mortality rate may be used. Although mortality rate may be used as an indirect assessment about health status, it is likely not to be a helpful measure in a given school population.

7. Measures of population growth and population pressures can be used. Indicators that might be appropriately used are rates of drug and alcohol usage, rates of juvenile delinquency, proportion of children living in substandard housing, proportions of families living at poverty level, as well as divorce rates and employment rates in the community. Another set of indicators is measure of growth and nutritional status, such as height and weight of children or degree of iron deficiency anemia.

8. Health indicators might include measures of health care utilization such as rate of dental care, number of children seen by family physicians each year, and the number of hospital admissions.

Hogue suggested that a principal criterion for determining which indicators of health status should be used is the availability of data and the feasibility of collecting additional data. In the school system, it is apparent that much of this data is already recorded on school records. However, the status of most records in school systems is that they are simply cards in a file; the information has not been summarized and tabulated in the way that might be most beneficial for utilizing them.

Promising advances for assessment are the information systems that have been developed for school systems. Johansen and Orthoefer[34] reported on the development of a school health information system in Rockford, Illinois. The computerized school nursing record provides a complete system for obtaining baseline data on each child, as well as a baseline data about the school health program. In a second article, Smiley[35] reported on the use of computers for assisting school health programs in Ontario. This information system is designed to record history, screening, and followup data. It records all health problems, need for services, health conditions, and services provided. It will provide summaries at any time about the current assessment of any parameter of the data recorded.

Although computerized systems will provide an excellent mechanism for providing summary data on the health of the school's population, considerable data are readily available in most schools. For example, one estimate of health status is the absentee rates. School systems are required to record attendance rates. By summarizing these reports, the school nurse may get baseline data about absentee rates in the school system. Fricke[13] reminded nurses that school records are the basis for epidemiologic studies:

> "School nurse records provide a rich source from which to obtain data for the purpose of identifying factors which influence the status of health. Causes of accidents, reasons for absenteeism and reasons for visits to the nurse's office are but a few which when accurately assessed provide a valid basis for action and direction."

Other data sources are the census reports for the district's population, planning commission surveys, information from hospital records, and statistics from local health agencies. This information contributes to the assessment of the school and community's needs.

One source of data at the county and state levels is the record of reportable diseases. Infectious diseases are reported to central locations in all states and there are additional registries for certain other diseases or conditions such as rheumatic fever and congenital anomalies. These are kept by state health departments and medical centers. National surveys might be important for national trends. Types of information that may be useful are the national family growth studies, the health and nutrition examination survey, and the health interview survey. These documents are published by the National Center for Health Statistics.

Data that are unavailable from secondary sources might be obtained by several methods. Survey techniques such as interviews or questionnaires may be used. For example, in a recent needs assessment of teenage mothers, a group of graduate students and I obtained and organized secondary data, but it was necessary to interview a sample of teenage mothers to identify needs and services desired. This information could not be readily obtained by other methods.

Another way to obtain assessment data is by direct observation. Observing pupils, families, and teachers in the school and community can yield much information about community and school needs. Teachers can be helpful in recognizing students appearing to have hearing or sight problems. Other observations might be made in the cafeteria, playground, and hallways. For example, one option for observing nutritional patterns is to observe the foods students select in school cafeterias when choices are available. In order to determine the nutritional patterns of the community, observations might be made in supermarkets to get a perspective on the kinds of foods that are served in the home.

Discussion with parents or school children or community members is another way to derive information about what the needs are in the school or the community served by the school. Discussions with students will often provide insightful information about the needs that are perceived by them. Discussion groups through Parent-Teacher Associations may be another way to incorporate parental concerns and desires for school program activities.

Neuman and Mayshark[36] reported a similar methodology in asking the community to provide information about what residents perceived were the needs and what schools might do. In a statewide study in South Carolina, respondents were asked to identify the major health problems seen by the community, and then to determine what community agencies might be most beneficial in solving their problems. Among rural respondents, the school was ranked second to all other agencies for four of the six major health problems. Specifically, the school was thought to be an important agency in meeting the community needs of illegitimacy, accidents, unemployment, and alcoholism. From the urban respondents, the same problems emerged, but with the addition of drug abuse and venereal disease. Again the school was seen as a predominate community resource for prevention of drug abuse, venereal disease, illegitimacy, alcoholism, and accidents.

All respondents, regardless of rural or urban residence, agreed on areas in which the school presents the greatest potential for possible solutions for currently perceived health problems.[36] The interesting implications for program development is that while the urban respondents saw drugs and venereal disease as important health needs, the rural areas did not see these as problems. Thus, if programs can be developed which correspond with the need for drug and venereal disease counseling in the schools in urban settings, they are likely to be well accepted. However, if drug programs and venereal disease programs were to be offered in rural areas, it is likely that the community would not be receptive to the programs; they did not see these as major problems and did not identify the school as a logical and important source of information in these areas.

Surveys of students may be particularly important in assessing various areas where there are few other ways to get at an accurate assessment. For example, student surveys of sexual activity may be the basis for programs on sex education. More importantly, parents and principals may be more supportive of controversial programs when a need has been clearly identified and communicated. Teacher surveys have also been suggested[37] for systematically assessing current health related instruction and perceived need for additional instruction or consultation.

One of the reasons for describing the sociodemographic characteristics of any group is that often those characteristics are associated with known differences in health parameters. For example, we know there are certain risk elements associated with various age levels. There are differences in death rates by age, race, and sex. The leading cause of death in children is accidents and safety programs clearly might be a priority. Other causes of death are congenital malformations, cancer, influenza, and diseases of the heart. While deaths from congenital malformations decline after the preschool years, suicide and homicide are increased risks as adolescence approaches.

In a study of Headstart children, Stone and Kudla[38] found that among 100 randomly selected children, allergies were more prominent in the white sample (13 percent) than in the black sample (1 percent). Similarly, speech abnormalities were more prominent in the white sample—17 percent—as compared to 7 percent in the black sample. Relating to differences in sex, they found in their survey that females had a higher percentage of enuresis (bed wetting) than the males, 17 percent and 3 percent respectively.

Few studies in school health have specifically identified the types of students and families who are at risk for poor health. An example of one study in this area, however, is the Basco, Eyres, Glasser, and Roberts study[39] designed to identify high risk children and families. The purpose of that study was to delineate child and family characteristics associated with illness and absentee behavior in school populations. In the first phase of their study, 2,000 school records of 1st, 4th, 7th and 10th grade students were analyzed. The results showed that of 23 student, family, and social variables studied, grade point average, age/grade relationship, social class, parent's marital status, school location, grade level, and racial identification were found to be associated with total episodes of absences from school.

In the second phase of their study, they looked at an absent subsample of 384 pupils, interviewing family members of these students. They found three factors, school location, grade level, and social class, were associated with episodes of absences at a statistically significant level. They found that children whose parents were divorced or separated had more absences than children from intact homes, but that this difference was not statistically significant as it was in phase 1. Another correlation of interest in this study was that the child's attitude towards school showed a strong association with total absences; children reporting that they enjoyed school had fewer absences than children who disliked or were afraid of school.

Additional findings from the study by Basco and her colleagues are that children from families in which a member has a chronic disease with functional limitations had a mean of 8.4 episodes of absence, almost 4 episodes more than children who came from a family without chronic illness. A comparison was made of absenteeism in children from families in which a death occurred in the past year and those in which no death occurred; it was found that when a death occurred there was a mean of one episode more in those families.

In examining the relationship of income and absenteeism, the researchers noted a consistent pattern. Approximately 4.4 absences were noted in families with an income of more than $7,000. Less income, however, was associated with higher absentee rate. For example, the rate for the income range $3,000 to $5,000 was 9.0, while the mean was 9.9 for families who had income of less than $3,000. Similarly, when social class was related with absences during the 1969-70 school year for 351 pupils, it was found that the lower the class the higher the rate of absences. When the adequacy of diet was related to absenteeism it was found that the mean absences for an adequate diet was 4.3, for a fair diet it was 5.4, and for a poor diet it was 6.0. The definition of an adequate diet was that there was adequate provision for all four food groups. Fair diets provided three of the four groups and poor diets provided only one or two groups.[39]

Ferinden[40] has presented evidence that certain characteristics of children are associated with learning difficulties. Research findings suggest that symptoms such as clumsiness, coordination difficulties, the tendency for children to use both right and left hands, delayed speech and articulation disorders, and family history of learning disorders are indicators for identifying students as high risk for later learning difficulties. Since these delayed motor developments can be screened with perceptual motor instruments, the identification and size of this high risk population can be estimated.

Factors associated with health status of particular populations or groups within the population are vital knowledge in overall assessment. Thus, the school nurse needs to be aware of the epidemiologic findings and associated risks for particular subgroups of the school population. This kind of information may assist the nurse in planning and implementation activities. If high risk groups can be identified, special programs can be developed to meet their needs. Thus, when limited resources are available, selected students can receive special services from the school health program. Ford[41] has aptly summarized this importance of need assessment and suggested that nurses

"can through epidemiological and demographic methodologies identify the health needs of target populations found in the school and in school neighborhoods, determine the nursing needs within these health needs, establish priorities, identify strengths and form patterns of delivery of service."

Finding the sources of data and conceptualizing the types of data required to make an accurate inventory of the health status of the school population is only one part of the health assessment procedure. Another vital component is the assessment of services currently available. School health services should not be planned in isolation from the context. If other community agencies offer services that cover particular areas, it is not expeditious for school health programs to duplicate those when other areas have not been well covered by any agency in the community. It has been suggested[37] that coordination of community agencies is often overlooked. Services can be organized to complement existing ones, gaps in service can be recognized and assigned for coverage, and access to adequate planned resources can be determined. Given the limited resources and finite amount of time that a school nurse has in a school health program, the assessment of the needs and services of the community must be determined with a broader view than simply assessing the children that are present in the school system.

Data gathered from a variety of sources must be assimilated. One problem encountered in this task is that the data may not be available for similar years. For example, the census data may be up to 10 years old, while the school health program data may be based on last year's screening program. National data is often one to five years old.

Trending and extrapolating data may be required. Furthermore in some situations, data may not be available and some synthetic estimates must be made in order to complete the data requirements for assessment.

Program Planning

Information generated by a school population assessment is the basis for program planning. Planning begins with the identification of goals and objectives. Alternative approaches for goal achievement must be specified, priorities must be set, and a formal plan developed. It cannot be overemphasized that planning must occur in cooperation with many other people. School personnel, including teachers, principals, and other special services in the school, must be involved in the planning process. The community with its many resources is another important component of the planning linkage system. Broad based involvement in planning will result in a school health program that is not only acceptable, but reflects the professional as well as the client's perspective on the priorities of needs and services.

Another important benefit from the involvement of numerous people within the school and community is that if there is agreement on the goals, the objectives, and the plan for doing them, there will be greater clarity about the role of the school nurse. Furthermore, involvement of administrators, teachers, parents, and community resources in the plan for the school health program will serve to educate them about the types of needs in the school population, as well as the kinds of nursing services that might be appropriately chosen for meeting those needs.

It is obvious that prior to the program planning process activities involving others, the preparation of a systematic data base, the identification of cost benefit ratios of various strategies, and an estimation about the time involved per student in certain activities are essential pieces of information. These data will assist the planning group in setting priorities and achieving agreement about the plan for services. To illustrate, in planning for vision screening, the nurse may present data which show that while a number of students were evaluated and discovered to have defects, the number of corrections achieved through their referrals was very low. A question might be raised here about whether or not it would be a better practice to screen less often and expend more effort in followup.

Another program planning activity relates to the appropriate use of manpower. The usefulness of the traditional nurse-to-student population ratio for manpower estimates is questionable. Apparent from the earlier discussion on assessment of needs, some school populations have far greater needs than other school populations. Thus, the use of the standard nurse-to-school population ratio may not be the best plan for determining the manpower requirements.

A second consideration relates to auxilliary personnel. Many school systems have adapted the use of volunteers, clerical assistants, trained aides, and technicians to assist with the school health program.[42-43] The use of these assistants has been shown to be highly effective in screening programs, managing first aid stations, and in triaging certain complaints. When assistants were first in the school health programs, their functions were primarily clerical in nature (e.g., recording, filing, checking transfer). In recent years, they have been more involved with the health care of pupils. They have assisted in screening programs and in managing certain health problems.

McFadden and O'Brien[44] reported the use of assistants in assuming a major responsibility for a particular category of students. In a nursing audit of school health records, categories were determined for students: category 1 was for students with no apparent health or social problems and who were under the supervision of a doctor; category 2, which was tabbed by a different color, included students with health and social problems that were currently under the supervision of the family physician or the staff nurse; and category 3 included children with severe health and social problems to be carried by the public health nurse covering the school with the doctor as necessary. In this report, the authors described the increased responsibility of the assistants for the followup on children in category 1. They reported use of the paraprofessional reduced the amount of nursing time spent on nonnursing activities. Nurses in the experimental schools spent 68 percent of their time on professional activities compared with 58 percent in the control group.

Program planning allows for a perspective on the entire year. When planning occurs on a day-by-day basis or a week-by-week basis, all priority components of the school health program may not be addressed, resulting in failure to achieve the goals. In practice, full weeks of a school health program may be devoted to one activity, while other weeks may represent more balanced program priorities. It is only with a program perspective and scheduling that includes the entire academic year that the implementation will occur in all of the goal areas determined to be important.

It should be noted that even when the goals and objectives have been identified and prioritized, there is still a fair degree of planning at the program level. For example, given that a high priority is safety in the school, planning must be done in order to determine the best mechanism for achievement. The intervention may be on an individual level with safety as a topic in student interacation whenever the timing is appropriate. On the other hand, intervention could be at the group level in terms of providing classroom instruction on safety or involving the teacher in designing units on safety in the curriculum. Thirdly, the intervention may be at an environmental level. The monitoring of the safety hazards in the school system may be one way in which the nurse may intervene at an environmental level (e.g., safety in relation to playground equipment and rules that are in operation). While it is sometimes apparent that intervention needs to be geared at all three levels, it may be that one level is more cost effective than another.

Implementation

It was noted in the previous section that implementation may occur on the individual level, may involve group strategies, and may involve environmental manipulation. The kinds of activities that are generally implemented were discussed under the scope of practice. Major areas include screening and early detection, the management of acute and chronic illness, emergency care, group and family counseling, health education programs, environmental control, and working with the community.

While flexibility must always be an important parameter, the plan provides the blueprint for implementation of the school health program. Tasks and functions by themselves are open for role ambiguities and lack of role agreement. When the tasks and functions are clearly linked to an overall plan that is based on appropriate and identified comn unity needs, there is greater clarity and greater consensus about the functions in implementation.

Competency in the skills identified in the plan is of crucial concern in discussing implementation. Because many functions are similar to nursing practice in other settings (i.e., developmental assessment, pediatrics, patient teaching and counseling in generalized nursing practice), only those activities which are more unique to the nursing role in school settings are discussed here. Screening tests, counseling, primary care, and health education are discussed in the following sections.

SCREENING TESTS

Screening tests are preliminary health evaluations used to assess a particular aspect of the health status of the pupil. They include procedures such as testing for vision and hearing, assessing growth and development, screening for scoliosis, dental or cardiac findings, and identifying the incidence of conditions such as strep throat and anemia. The nurse practicing school nursing must understand the scientific bases and be proficient in the technique of various school health screening tests and examinations. Furthermore the nurse must know the general provision of the law and regulations concerning the types and frequency of certain mandatory examinations.

When choosing a screening test to use for a given condition, Eisner and Oglesby[45] have provided some criteria to consider when selecting screening devices. They suggest the major consideration is the sensitivity and specifity of the competing test. Sensitivity relates to whether or not the test may result in too many over-referrals or too many under-referrals. The test is insensitive if it results in too many under-referrals and is overly sensitive if it results in too many over-referrals.

A second criterion is cost. Cost becomes a major consideration in relation to the benefit to be derived. While costs are fairly easy to ascertain, it is often difficult to estimate benefits. Although we may want to consider the economic benefits of preventing disability over a long period of time, Eisner and Oglesby suggested it is more useful in school programs to consider the immediate benefits of obtaining health defect correction. Thus, the benefit of a screening program is dependent on the number of children who receive treatment. Another consideration in the cost/benefit ratio is the level of effectiveness of a given treatment; when the treatment for a given condition is somewhat variable, fewer children will benefit in the long run than when treatment is fairly effective.[45]

Another criterion for deciding which screening test should be included in a school health program is the acceptability of the test. Vision and hearing programs have long been established in the school system and most parents welcome the opportunity to have their children tested to determine if vision or hearing is less than normal. However, procedures which break the child's skin and other intrusive procedures such as urine tests may need to be carefully considered before they are implemented in a school health program. Laboratory tests that may be important in screening in some situations are: 1) blood tests for anemia, 2) urine testing for detecting asymptomatic urinary tract infections, and 3) tuberculin tests for tuberculosis case finding program, depending on the prevalence of TB in the community. For legal protection, signed parental permission is advised for procedures that are more intrusive, such as those which penetrate the child's skin.

Vision Screening

The basic intent of vision screening is to discover children who have some type of visual impairment. The frequency of vision testing is often determined by state regulations. Routine vision screening of all children in schools is sometimes required on an annual basis. In other cases, it is required to be done at certain grade intervals. If there are no state regulations, some general guidelines might be followed. All children entering kindergarten should be screened if they have not had an eye test during the preschool year. All new pupils to a school district without vision testing are good candidates for the vision screening program.

Pupils may be referred with signs and symptoms of visual difficulty. Teacher/nurse observations suggestive of possible eye problems include excessive rubbing of the eyes, head tilted forward, difficulty in reading or in performing other close work, eye irritation, holding the book close to eyes, squinting and stumbling over small objects. All of these are signs that may be correlated with difficulty in vision.

There are a number of tests for vision screening, including the Snellin "E" chart that is often used in younger children. Additional tests that might be used are the Titmus screener, the cover test, the near-vision test, and the tracer vision screener. Color vision screening often uses the Ishihra test.

Screening programs often use trained technicians, aides, and volunteers (e.g., local sororities, clubs, or homeroom mothers) to administer the initial screening of large numbers of students. Advance screening arrangements are made through the principal and teachers involved. When nonprofessionals are used, pupils who do not satisfactorily pass the initial screening test should be evaluated by the school nurse prior to the referral for care. If defects are noted, the school nurse confers with the students and parents, either at school or in the home, and assists in arrangements for satisfactory professional care. Families may be referred to their usual source of eye care or it may be necessary to acquaint them with resources in the community. Because many resources have certain eligibility requirements, the school nurse needs to be acutely aware of community resources.

Defects in color vision occur more prominently in boys than in girls. One average that is often cited is a 3 percent rate for boys and a 0.1 percent rate among girls. Since the defect is more rare among girls, in some cases only boys may be selected for routine testing. Students with color deficiency are generally not referred, but counseled regarding vocational choices. New technology in color lens however, may provide some alternatives in the future.

Although most of the findings of the vision screening program will be related to refractory problems and are generally correctable with eye glasses, it should not be overlooked that vision screening should also determine problems in muscle balance, problems related to inflammation from infections in the eye, and developmental anomalies.

Hearing Screening

Byrd[46] suggested that a careful analysis of any screening program for the detection of hearing losses should be made if it does not identify from three to five pupils per 100 children. He noted that seldom does the number of children with hearing loss in any school district fall below that figure. The obvious importance of hearing for the learning process is well known.[47] It may also affect the child's speech and personality. Many children with hearing handicaps may be improperly labeled as disobedient, uncooperative, or slow learners because they cannot respond properly to instructions of classroom teachers. Thus, the child with the hearing loss may be handicapped in numerous ways.

Similar to vision screening, hearing screening procedures may be mandated by state regulations. In other situations, students in selected age groups, such as kindergarten, first, third, fifth, and eighth grades, may be examined, as well as others with known or suspected hearing impairments. Pupils with a history of speech defects should have a complete hearing and speech evaluation.

In recognition of the fact that the audiometer is the only satisfactory method for detection of hearing losses in school children, many states require by law that schools employ an audiometrist for periodic screening of pupils or require audiometric certification by school nurses or teachers or persons employed to assist in screening. The audiometer is designed to test hearing from low to high pitch sounds in varying ranges of intensity. In hearing screening tests, losses of over 20 decibels need to be retested. In retesting if a 20 decibel loss in noted in only one ear, it is not generally judged to be a significant loss. A loss of 20 decibels or more in both ears, however, is often noted as a significant hearing loss. A loss of 30 decibels or more in one ear is judged to be significant. Thus, a loss of 20 to 30 decibels or more demands careful attention and further appraisal of the child's hearing status.

A model program for the identification of hearing losses in school children and the results are presented in an article by Stephens, Rounthwaite and Hutchison.[47] These authors delineated the testing technique, the equipment used, and the regrouping and retesting of the initial screening test. Prevalence rates are reported, as well as the false/positive findings on the initial screening test. They noted that in many cases failure on the screening test with subsequent normal responses led to the discovery of problems which in themselves required further investigation. Students whose hearing losses were not sufficient to warrant further evaluation were marked for repeat testing annually to detect possible deterioration in hearing.

The importance of early detection and medical attention for the child with hearing loss is illustrated in data provided by the Palo Alto School District in California.[48] In a given year, 186 children received medical attention following the hearing screening program. Of the cases that received attention at the elementary school level, 46 percent recovered normal hearing. The recovery rate fell to approximately 13 percent at the junior high school level and to slightly less than 5 percent at the high school level. Thus, the need for early detection is apparent.

Nurses who are proficient in examination of the ear with an otoscope can detect ear infections and are able to prevent hearing loss through prompt treatment. Educating the parents and children about the relationship of ear infection and loss of hearing is an important aspect in followup. However, if hearing loss has already occurred, strategies can be employed to assist in compensation. Preferential seating near the front and center make it easier to listen and watch other children as they speak. A child with a marked loss in one ear should be seated with the better ear toward the class.

Scoliosis Screening

Another screening program that has been advocated in many school systems in recent years is the scoliosis screening program. Early detection and treatment of scoliosis can often prevent major, expensive, and sometimes hazardous surgery. Benson, Wade, and Benson[49] noted that spinal curves often develop during early adolescence and may progress during the time of rapid growth. If the back is braced during this rapid growth period, deformity can be minimized and surgery may be prevented.

Routine scoliosis examinations have been conducted in schools in many areas of the United States. Minnesota and Delaware have been cited for their leadership in the development of these screening programs. Major phases of the program have been identified. First, boys and girls are screened by the school nurses and physical education teachers who have had instruction in scoliosis screening. In the second phase, the students who are noted to have a possible scoliosis deformity are screened by an orthopaedic physician. In phase three, if the orthopaedic physician concurs, referral for treatment is made to the parents.

The report[49] of the school screening for scoliosis in the Sacramento area noted that of the 7,815 students screened by the school nurse and physical education teacher, 17 percent were reexamined by the orthopaedist. Of those, 221 (2.82 percent of the total seen) were referred to their private medical doctor for x-ray and further evaluation. Followup showed that 139 were evaluated by a physician. Of that 139, 87 percent were diagnosed as having a spinal deformity that required treatment.

Communities around the country have demonstrated that school screening for scoliosis can be accomplished in a very short time. A rapid, effective method, taking no more than 30 seconds per child, has been utilized to detect spinal curvatures.[49] As with most screening programs, the followup of the school nurse is a most important component. The general grades that are routinely screened in many areas are 5th, 6th, 7th, and 8th grades.

The most common methods of treatment are the Milwaukee bracing with exercise, exercises alone, and interval observations by the physician. It has been noted that the parents and community have a very limited understanding of scoliosis. The result of this lack of knowledge in the community is that parents may not respond to the referrals sent by the school for followup. Secondly, the lack of community knowledge and understanding is not supportive to students who are wearing the sometimes cumbersome Milwaukee brace; an educated school community would provide a more understanding atmosphere for students who are currently in treatment.

Cardiac Screening

Another program that has been implemented in some school systems in recent years is a cardiac screening program. With the demise of the routine physical examination and health assessment programs, programs have been implemented to detect cardiac abnormalities. One simple screening program is blood pressure readings to determine hypertension.

Heart sound screening is a further screening device that has been used in some school programs to detect cardiac irregularities. Eisner and Oglesby[50] reported on a heart sound screening program in which a microphone is placed on the child's chest to pick up heart sounds. Frequency, duration, and other characteristics are analyzed by a portable analog digital computer. Results are displayed as being within normal limits, outside normal limits, or technically unsatisfactory. When compared with the results of examinations by cardiologists, this method has proven to be sensitive and specific. It can be used with both preschool children and school age children. These authors argue that although the prevalence of heart disease is low among children, it is still high enough to merit a screening program. Early detection is important in many cases, as several of the predominant cardiac conditions are progressive in nature. Secondary changes may be avoided if abnormal heart sounds can be detected in early phases of the disease.

Strep Throat Screening

Related to the prevention of rheumatic fever in school children is the screening for hemolytic streptococcus. It has been estimated that for children from 5 to 19 years of age in the United States, the incidence of rheumatic heart disease is 1.7 per 1000 individuals.

Feeney[51] reported that each year approximately 60,000 children in the United States are victims of rheumatic fever. Generally accepted is the fact that the precurser of the disease is an infection with group A hemolytic streptococcus.

In a three year demonstration project in New Jersey,[52] nurses in 16 schools tested every child known to have a sore throat. This project showed that a school centered program to detect and control strep infection is feasible, efficient, and low in cost. While some schools provide the opportinity for children with sore throats to come to the school nurse for a throat culture, other schools routinely screen in specific grades (1st and 7th, for example) to detect asymptomatic streptococcal infections.

Many school systems use an outside lab to culture and interpret the findings. Feeney[51] reported the use of a foil-lined envelope that contained silica gel crystals. After the sterile swab is used in the pharynx and tonsillar areas, it is inserted into the foil-lined envelope using aseptic technique. The envelopes are placed in another protective envelope and mailed to the state health department laboratories.

The experiences reported in the literature show that parental acceptance of strep screening and physician confidence in the program generally were very high. Chobin, Kangos and Miller,[52] for example, reported 87 percent of the permission cards were signed by parents by the end of the first year of the program, and 95 percent rate by the end of the second year. The isolation rate of group A hemolytic strep from asymptomatic school children during the first year was 7.7 percent, 4.4 percent during the second year, and 4.1 percent during the third year. Of children referred to physicians, 98.6 percent returned forms indicating they had received treatment.

COUNSELING

School children's reliance on the school nurse or the nurse's office as an escape from the stresses of the classroom, playground, or home is a familiar phenomenon. The nurse has the opportunity to assess the complaint in the broad context. Stamler and Palmer[53] noted that many children make frequent contacts with the nurse with vague requests or complaints. After a brief encounter it can be noted that the child recovers.

Counseling is a method for assisting others to identify feelings and real or imagined problems and to problem solve and arrive at decisions which assist in better adjustment. The goal is to increase the ability to function effectively so that experiences are satisfying and responsibilities are fulfilled. Counseling requires directive and nondirective interviewing skills. It also requires empathetic listening, focus on feelings, attention to physical complaints when indicated, and helping the child, parent, or teacher to develop insight and greater control of the situation.

The school nurse is a key person in building sound mental health. This may be achieved by working with an individual student or group of pupils, through family counseling, and through teacher and staff education and counseling. The nurse may be involved in a team effort, sharing this responsibility with the psychologist and sometimes principals and teachers. For example, when an individual student requires counseling over a period of time, the case conference method might be effective. The teacher, nurse, and mental health professional can discuss the dynamics and plan for management. One member may take the primary responsibility for implementing the plan, but all must stay involved and informed to jointly support the required changes.

In addition to students presenting themselves with complaints or being referred for such behaviors as disruption or depression, the school assessment will have identified target groups for health counseling such as: pregnant teenagers, children with alcohol or drug dependence, students who want to quit smoking, children with high absenteeism, children with speech problems, children with a death in family, or overweight children.

Counseling can occur on a one-to-one basis, but small groups have been shown to be very effective. Student groups may be established for special problem areas. Using a nonthreatening atmosphere, a peer exchange can be provided. Students can assist each other with problem identification and problem solving with the nurse assuming a consultive role. The nurse as the group leader facilitates group process and draws out the shy members while controlling the dominate and disruptive members.

A number of mental health problems are likely to be related to family relationships. In dysfunctional families, children may develop and accept an unhealthy role for survival. A child may accept a label which may perpetuate negative expectations. "Dumb," "lazy," and "clumsy" are examples of these labels. Another problem in families is communication. Messages are often mixed and inconsistent, and clarification may not be permitted. Mental health consultation with families, then, is likely to examine expectations, individual needs, communication patterns, and openness of expression. Depending on the nature of the problem and the resources of the school and the community, referral may be appropriate.

Divorce is a crisis that an increasing number of children and families face. Children must adapt to the loss of a parent with its accompanying changes. Other family relationship problems might be less severe and more transient. When a child comes to the health room with a stomach ache, the nurse might ask such questions as whether there was trouble at the breakfast table that morning. The nurse can then help the child gain insight and determine how such incidents might be handled.

The nature of mental health problems may be different by age groups. Child abuse is more common in the younger age groups.[18] In the 5- and 6-year-old group, separation anxiety, student-teacher relationships, peer interaction, and shyness are frequently noted. Problems related to learning, developmental problems, acceptance by peers, and family problems are commonly noted in the elementary schools. A new baby in the home, illness or death in the family, and divorce have been cited as common family problems.

In junior high and high school, many of the same problems are seen. There is increased concern over self-image and peer acceptance. Acting out, withdrawal, drug and alcohol abuse, and absenteeism may be indicators of mental health status. Suicide, homicide, delinquency, and anxiety are increasing mental health problems in the adolescent population.

The emotional health of children is dependent on a healthy environment. The mental health of teachers and their understanding of this area are major components. Drake[54] reported teacher groups have selected such areas as understanding the adolescent, developing and reinforcing self-concept in the classroom, detecting drug abuse, reinforcement and extinguishing behavior, and dealing with attention-getters in the classroom as areas they would like to pursue. Monthly sessions in these areas were found to be supportive to problem solving for teachers and this is likely to create a healthier environment for students. The nurse must also be available to counsel with teachers and staff individually so that they can be supported while they make decisions to reduce their own tensions.

The potential for development in mental health and counseling programs is unlimited. The school can be an effective locus for preventing emotional illness, promoting positive mental health, and treating emotional problems.

Primary Care

Seven million of the more than 55 million children of school age in the United States have never visited a physician's office, clinic, or hospital except when prompted by an extreme illness or emergency.[24] In many settings, school health programs have been redesigned to provide primary care to these children. Complete and continuing care is provide by school nurse practitioners who identify physical, nutritional, emotional, and developmental problems that may interfere with the health of students and their ability to learn.

On an appointment basis, routine examinations of well children are made. A health history, a complete physical exam (including inspection, palpation, percussion, and auscultation) and a neurologic evaluation are components of the examination. Teaching and counseling are important aspects of the encounter. Parents are invited to attend, and parental attitudes and participation have been noted to be favorable.[24]

The medical management of primary care requires collaboration with local physicians. Consultation provides medical backup and a referral system. Although practices vary from school district to school district, nurses commonly manage anemia, constipation, allergic and dermatologic conditions, upper respiratory infections, and bacterial infections. They also manage emotional problems such as school phobia and poor self-concept. In the psychosocial area, they may consult with, refer to, or jointly manage with other school or community professionals.

Children are also seen as they present themselves with signs or symptoms of illness. Again nurses obtain histories and use appropriate examination and laboratory tests to determine the nursing diagnosis and plan for care. Decisions are made about exclusion from school, treatment if necessary, or counseling for the child and sometimes the parents.

Practitioner preparation is recommended as a basis for primary care activities. In a study with a small sample size, eight school nurse practitioners were compared with a matched sample of school nurses. Nurses with primary care preparation were shown to be more specific in management of health problems, to exclude only about half as many pupils, to refer only about half as many pupils for care, consultation, or further evaluation, to be more specific in advice to parents, and to have more parents agree with and follow their advice.[55]

Various primary care delivery systems have been described. Nader[56] discussed a school based community health primary care model in Cambridge, Massachusetts. Health centers in the schools are designed so that a child can be followed in a single integrative service from birth through adolescence. Staffed primarily by nurse practitioners, they offer primary care services to preschool and school aged children.

The extent of effort in primary care activities will depend on the preparation of the nurse and the students in the school. If 90 percent of the children utilize family physicians on a regular basis, the Cambridge model would be inappropriate. In other schools, the nurse may provide comprehensive health care appraisal and services to many school age children.

HEALTH EDUCATION

Although patient or client education is an important part of the professional nursing practice in all settings, health education is a major opportunity and responsibility in the schools. In few other situations is the climate so favorable for learning. Not only is education a major goal, but the opportunity is present for repeated and sequential educational experience over all the years that children are enrolled in schools.

The contribution of the nurse in health education is made in a variety of ways. Nurses must take advantage of informal or incidental teaching opportunities. A vital contribution can also be made to formal health instruction. These activities include development of the health curriculum, planning and consultation with teachers, and formal teaching in the classroom.

A sequentially planned curriculum in health education is as important as such a plan for every other subject. Curriculum planning needs strong administrative leadership and the school nurse as a health specialist should have an active and continuous role in health curriculum activities. Although state and local curriculum guides may be available, they are often inadequate or out of date.[57] Nurses have knowledge about the age-specific appropriateness of many topics. They also bring the results of the school assessment and can assist in planning and implementing educational experiences consistent with that school's and community's needs. In this way health education should be relevant and meaningful to the students.

The curriculum should identify the health topics and specify the grade or grades in which each will be taught. Failure to coordinate health education in this manner results in omission and neglect of some areas and unnecessary repetition in others. Grade level appropriateness is another major issue to be resolved. A number of topics for health curriculum have been published. Byrd[46] for example, listed 20 broad areas in health with 500 health topics for curriculum construction and learning experiences.

The lack of interest in health and inadequate preparation of teachers for teaching health have been cited as major problems.[57] The nurse can be a valuable resource for the classroom teacher as well as assisting in teaching some microunits of the content. The enthusiasm and commitment of the nurse can be contagious.

Consultation with teachers about the materials and activities for health education can be a valuable contribution. Brainstorming sessions and sharing health textbooks, other literature, and audiovisual materials can provide ideas and increase the knowledge and skills of teachers. An audiovisual file on health might be maintained by the nurse. As materials are used, teachers could contribute their review of films available from the school district, health department, local university, or other organizations. The availability of other teaching aides such as models of the ear, eye, or heart might be noted in the file. Information about speakers and exhibits could stimulate their use. With familiarity of community resources, information about personnel and materials to enrich the instructional program could also be shared with teachers.

In some areas of health education, the nurse may formally teach some of the content. This requires that in addition to the specific information on health, attention be given to teaching methods and techniques. Creative and appropriate learning experiences are essential to effective learning. Team teaching might also be implemented. Health content can be combined with an art expression, literature, or mathematics class.

Health education has been primarily directed at providing information to students, rather than adopting good health practices. For example in nutrition education there is little evidence to support that information alone leads to better eating habits. Since food behavior is dependent on family patterns, parent-teaching should be included. Homework involving parents might be assigned. Other mechanisms might be constructed for active involvement of the student. Compositions on foods they dislike or meals they like best might be shared with the class. A vegetable tasting party might be a way to see if students might change their minds about some dislikes in vegetables. Other ways are to have students involved in meal planning games—for a class picnic, a slumberparty supper, or a Saturday evening supper after the soccer event. Students might develop contracts about what they would like to change about what or the way they eat. How well they have met their commitment would be reinforcement at a later time. Students might also select special topics such as sugar, salt, food additives, or organically grown foods. Involvement in activities will help develop an awareness and sensitivity to good eating and will translate into the start of a lifelong eating pattern.

Igoe[24] has discussed two other important health education focuses: 1) to increase pupil's responsibility and independence for their own health care and 2) to enable pupils to develop confidence in their right to expect a collaborative relationship with health personnel. What does it mean to be healthy or sick? How can one be more responsible for one's health? How can symptoms be evaluated and decisions made about whether or not to seek care? What does one need to know to be a better consumer of health care services?

This affective and cognitive learning and participatory behavior can begin as early as kindergarten. All through the school years, appropriate consumer behavior can be reinforced in the school nurse's office. The child can be helped to communicate his needs and to ask appropriate questions. Igoe[24] provided other examples. In the fourth grade, when students learn about immunizations, they learn how to maintain their own immunization records. With a sound basis for decision making, many students call their parents' attention to the need for booster injections.

As the developmental level increases, more complex consumer health can be introduced. Fifth and sixth graders can learn to evaluate the severity of such symptoms as headache or abdominal pain so that they can decide when further evaluation by a nurse or physician is needed. In high school, students should learn to manage common minor illnesses as well as manage their life style so that they prevent illness and promote health. Health education directed at self-care and health promotion may have long range implications for preventing illness, disability, and chronic diseases in adult life.

The nurse is even more likely to be directly involved with health education developed for specific target populations. For example, children with asthma were a selected group in the Galveston, Texas school system. The overall goals of the program were to increase the children's understanding about their asthmatic condition and to assist them in assuming greater responsibility and involvement in managing their condition. Identified as more specific goals were: 1) to reduce the number of asthmatic attacks requiring emergency care, 2) to decrease the number of school days missed, 3) to improve attitude toward self, 4) to improve perception of self-control for health behavior, and 5) to increase the children's and parents' knowledge of asthma and its management.[56]

Using a cooperative model, this asthma project used both school and community professionals to conduct weekly sessions. Structured lessons and an affective educational program were used. Meetings were conducted for parents, but attendance was poor. An exception was noted—when children showed their parents a tape of their classes and examples of their learning, almost all of the mothers and one father attended and participated in teaching breathing exercises to the children. Because of the low parent involvement, a patient education book "Teaching My Parents About Asthma" was designed for both parents and children during a second phase of the program.[56]

The teaching activities of the nurse are interwoven with many other activities. Informal teaching can occur whenever opportunities or problems present an opening. The school setting provides an ideal setting for coordinated continuous health education. Through participation in the health curriculum planning, providing encouragement and resources for teachers, and direct teaching in the classroom or with groups with special needs, the school nurse implements a significant part of any health program.

Program Evaluation

The evaluation of a program is based on the objectives and goals identified in the planning phase. One aspect of program evaluation is simply a reporting of whether or not the activities that were planned were indeed carried out. While a report presenting the number of students surveyed with the number of defects found and corrected is useful, this type of program evaluation is far too commonplace. A major question is what difference does that service make in terms of the health of the group.

Discussions on the evaluation of health care have been predominate in the literature in the past decade. It has been suggested that evaluation should be in the areas of structure, process, and outcome. Structure describes the personnel, equipment, records, facilities, and so forth. Process refers to what the providers do and can range from the assessment process, to the intervention itself, to the evaluation. In nursing, process is often evaluated in performance ratings. Thus, if the nurse is good at counseling strategies, process would be rated high. Likewise, if health appraisal or screening programs were conducted in an appropriate manner, process would be rated high. Outcome, on the other hand, refers to the effect of the health care or the process on clients. While the health status of the student, the satisfaction of the student, or the level of disease in the population may be used as outcome measures, there is still considerable difficulty in determining what are suitable outcome measures.

Recent evaluation models focus on both process and outcome in an attempt to link the kinds of processes that are conducted by nursing personnel with the outcome it has for clients. Is the manner in which services are provided related to outcome? While it will take considerable research to establish these kinds of process-outcome linkages, it should be recalled that we are not alone in school health practice with this dilemma.

An example highlights the important issue of selecting outcome criteria. In health education programs, measuring the level of knowledge before and after may be a useful indicator of whether or not the content was learned, but if the intent of the educational program was to change behavior, then a paper-and-pencil test measuring knowledge may not be the appropriate outcome criterion to select. Cosper, Hayslip and Foree[58] reported a teaching project on overweight students. The 23 students in the experimental group were offered a nutrition counseling and education experience. Although the level of knowledge was significantly higher ($p < 0.001$) in the experimental group than the control group, there was no difference in dietary intakes as measured by a 24-hour recall in the two groups.

A useful strategy for evaluation in school nursing was presented by Dickinson.[59] This educator suggested that nursing could become accountable in education through the use of behavioral objectives. He suggests that nurses must use the same techniques as those employed by the classroom teachers if they are to demonstrate their accountability in an educational institution. He suggests that behavioral objectives must be written in a way that can be evaluated in terms of goal achievement. A requirement for a behavioral objective is that it is written clearly in student behaviors that can be seen or heard. Behavioral objectives include what must be accomplished by the student. Thus, rather than being nurse directed in focus, they are student directed. An example provided in the Dickinson article is the following:

"Upon graduation, each learner will be able to: upon being asked what he should do daily for health and appearance, list the following: 1) brush teeth at least 2 times per day; 2) take a shower or bath; 3) comb hair; 4) elimination with cleaning; 5) brush clothes; 6) change stockings and underwear; 7) check for signs of physical defects or deficiencies; 8) exercise to keep muscle tone; 9) eat balanced diet."

This example demonstrates how achievement of the objective can be determined from the students. A program with behavioral objectives for students tells nurses and administrators exactly what the school health nurses are accomplishing instead of what nurses are doing.

A variety of designs can be used to evaluate a school health program. A systems framework and design is highly appropriate. Herberg[37] presented a model for analyzing a school's health program using a systems approach. It identifies structural properties as well as relationships between the school and the community in which the program is embedded, the school itself and its health program, the instructional and service units, and the kinds of services rendered and outcomes achieved.

Surveys might be quite informative. Cauffman and her colleagues[60] reported the findings from a survey of parents who had received at least one notification from the school about a defect. With 92.5 percent of the 495 parents interviewed, it was found that notification factors were more potently related to success of referral than either attitudinal or socioeconomic factors. More than one notification, notification by more than one professional, and use of more than one method of contact were significantly related. Although both telephone calls and visitations were more effective than written notices, a telephone call, less costly, was equally as effective as a home visit. Thus evaluation and cost-effective analysis of survey studies provide a good basis for decision. In other cases, a classic experimental or quasiexperimental design may be followed. Tuthill and his colleagues,[33] for example, used experimental and control schools. In the Cosper and colleagues' study[58] cited earlier, experimental and control groups were structured to determine the influence of a special dietary program.

Weber[61] noted that research is an almost untouched function of the nurse in school health services. There are many areas that need further research. What is the mixture of skills that is most effective in attaining objectives? What is the economic soundness of employing nurses? What would happen if we changed some elements of the existing structure? What kind of professional process behaviors are related to successful outcomes? What types of clues are associated with future problems? What resources best meet certain needs? What kind of parental involvement is more successful? Answers to some of these questions are becoming known through some isolated research studies. Much more needs to be done.

Evaluation, the last step of the nursing process, is the most neglected area of all. Reports most often are an account of services provided: the number of children seen for counseling, the number of children screened for various entities, the number of conferences with parents and teachers, the number of classes taught. How can we measure the extent or impact of our services? Did the educational program have any effect on health behavior? Does visual or hearing correction have an impact on learning? Evaluation strategies must be determined in the program planning phase. After implementation, data must be obtained and examined to assist in evaluation.

Evaluation and accountability are even more important in a time of impending budget cuts in many school districts. Chinn[62] noted that unless it can be demonstrated that nursing skills in the educational setting enhances or promotes learning, justification for retaining the school nurse is certainly questionable.

STRATEGIES FOR ROLE CLARITY

Children are learners who are regularly and readily available in school systems throughout the country. What better place for highly skilled nurses to provide preventive, problem oriented, or therapeutic health care through dynamic, relevant programs. Successful programs require clarity about the role of the school nurse. Since expectations of others in the school and community vary widely, nurses must be certain about the general nature and practice of school nursing and must be willing to negotiate from that position.

One critical element for role clarity is the nurse's competence in defining school health practice. Hawkins[20] stressed that the vagueness in nursing roles may often be due to the fact that the nurses do not have a clear notion about what their roles are to be.

"If she waits for her role to be made clear to her, it may develop inconsistently and unsatisfactorily. But, if she insists on being the expert who knows what is proper to her role, her judgment will sway others. There was some evidence that if nurses could agree among themselves, misunderstandings, inconsistencies, and uncertainties on the part of others could be substantially reduced."

The purpose and scope of professional practice must be well articulated. Members of a profession often assume that consumers and other professionals know what they do and how their skills can be utilized. This unjustified assumption precipitates misunderstandings which prevent real cooperation. Language is important. In communicating with others, words must be chosen carefully since specialty groups frequently derive unique meaning for many commonly used terms.

Knowing the students, school, and the community is another prerequisite for role specification. If practice is epidemiologically based on a complete and accurate school population and community profile, the likelihood of different expectations is reduced. If planning and priorities are accomplished in conjunction with school and community persons, goals and strategies will be shared, understood, and supported.

One trap to avoid is the *task trap*. Practice is not a list of tasks apart from situation specific objectives. When the tasks undertaken are not accomplishing goals, readjustments are required. Ongoing evaluation in addition to summative evaluation provides general parameters for the scope and focus of school nursing.

Nursing in schools offers an innovative, flexible practice site. With clarity about the everchanging practice of school health accompanied by knowledge and sensitivity about the target population and the appropriate skills necessary for accomplishing aspects of practice, school nurses will meet the challenge of influencing the health status of the adults of tomorrow.

REFERENCES

1. Henderson, Virginia, and Nite, Gladys: *Principles and Practice of Nursing.* Macmillan, New York, 1978.
2. Macdonough, Georgia P.: "School Health—1977." *Journal of School Health,* 47:425, Sept. 1977.
3. Humes, Charles W., Jr.: "Who Should Administer School Nursing Services?" *American Journal of Public Health,* 65:395, April 1975.
4. School Nursing Committee of American School Health Association: "The Nurse in the School Health Program: Guidelines for School Nursing." *Journal of School Health,* 37:1, April 1967.
5. American Nurses' Association: *A Rationale for School Nurse Certification.* American Nurses Association, New York, 1966.
6. American Nurses' Association: *Functions and Qualifications of School Nurses.* American Nurses Association, New York, 1966.
7. Blauvelt, Louise: "Closing the Gaps in School Health Services." *Journal of School Health,* 47:422, Sept. 1977.
8. Forbes, Orcilia: "The Role and Functions of the School Nurse as Perceived by 115 Public School Teachers from Three Selected Counties." *Journal of School Health,* 37:101, Feb. 1967.
9. Berg, Beryl: "In Health-Related Tasks, Where Does the School Nurse Function?" *Journal of School Health,* 43:316, May 1973.
10. Crowley, Eileen A., and Johnson, Judith L. "Multiprofessional Perceptions of School Health: Definition and Scope." *Journal of School Health,* 47:398, Sept. 1977.
11. Macdonough, Georgia P.: "Comparison of Nursing Roles." *Journal of School Health,* 42:481, Oct. 1972.
12. Igoe, Judith Bellaire: "Bridging the Communication Gap Between Health Professionals and Educators." *Journal of School Health,* 47:405, Sept. 1977.
13. Fricke, Irma B.: "School Nursing for the 70s" *Journal of School Health,* 42:203, April 1972.
14. Kappelman, M., Khan, M., Washington, Vivian et al.: "A Unique School Health Program for Pregnant Teenagers." *Journal of School Health,* 44:303, June 1974.
15. Veerhusen, Pamela, Cooksey, Phyllis, and Fredlund, Delphine: "Pregnancy: A Crisis in Health Education." *American Journal of Public Health,* 62:821, June 1972.
16. Caskey, Kathryn K., and Blaylock, Enid V.: "The School Nurse and Drug Abuse." *Nursing Outlook,* 18:27, Dec. 1970.
17. Wake, F. R., Thomas, Eleanor, and Bergin, Jane: "Nurses, Smoking, and School Children." *The Canadian Nurse,* 69:19, July 1973.
18. Murdock, C. George: "The Abused Child and the School System." *American Journal of Public Health,* 60:105, Jan. 1970.
19. Oda, Dorothy S.: "Increasing Role Effectiveness of School Nurses." *American Journal of Public Health,* 64:591, June 1974.
20. Hawkins, Norman G.: "Is There a School Nurse Role?" *American Journal of Nursing,* 71:744, April 1971.
21. Bryan, Doris S.: *School Nursing in Transition.* The C. V. Mosby Co., St. Louis, 1973.
22. Mayshark, Cyrus, and Shaw, Donald D.: *Administration of School Health Programs: Its Theory and Pracitce.* The C. V. Mosby Co., St. Louis, 1967.
23. Stobo, Elizabeth C.: "Trends in the Preparation and Qualifications of the School Nurse." *American Journal of Public Health,* 50:669, April 1969.
24. Igoe, Judith Bellaire: "The School Nurse Practitioner." *Nursing Outlook,* 23:381, June 1975.
25. Joint Statement of the American Nurses' Association and the American School Health Association: "Recommendations of the Educational Preparation and Definitions of the Expanded Role and Functions of the School Nurse Practitioner." *Journal of School Health,* 43:594, Nov. 1973.
26. Silver, Henry, K.: "The School Nurse Practitioner Program: A New and Expanded Role for the School Nurse." *Journal of American Medical Association,* 216:1332, May 24, 1971.
27. Silver, Henry K., Igoe Judith B., and McAtee, Patricia R.: "School Nurse Practitioners: A Concise Description of Their Functions and Activities." *Journal of School Health,* 47:598, Dec. 1977.
28. Silver, Henry K., and Nelson, Nancy: "The School Nurse Practitioner Program: A New Concept in Providing Health Care." *Journal of Nursing Administration,* 1:4, May-June 1971.

29. A Joint Statement of the American Nurses' Association, the American School Health Association, the Department of School Nurses/National Education Association: "Guidelines on Educational Preparation and Competencies of the School Nurse Practitioner." *Journal of School Health*, 48:265, May 1978.
30. Frels, Lois: "National Survery—School Nurse Certification." *Journal of School Health*, 44:340, June 1974.
31. Hall, Joanne E., and Weaver, Barbara R.: *Distributive Nursing Practive: A Systems Approach to Community Health*. J. B. Lippincott Co., Philadelphia, 1977.
32. Ball, B.: "School Nurses Have Expanded Roles, Too." *Nursing 73*, 3:61, Sept. 1973.
33. Tuthill, Robert W.; Williams, Carolyn; Long, Gene; et al.: "Evaluating a School Health Program Focused on High Absence Pupils: A Research Design," *American Journal of Public Health*, 62:40, Jan. 1972.
34. Johansen, Sonja, and Orthoefer, Joseph E.: "Development of a School Health Information System." *American Journal of Public Health*, 65:1203, Nov. 1975.
35. Smiley, J.R., Allin, R.W., Best, E.W.R., et al.: "The Use of Computers in Assisting School Health Programs in Ontario." *Canadian Journal of Public Health*, 64:141, March-April 1973.
36. Newman, Ian M., and Mayshark, Cyrus: "The Community Health Problems and the School's Unrecognized Mandate." *Journal of School Health*, 43:562, Nov. 1973.
37. Herberg, Edward N.: "Sociological Perspectives on School Health Programs." *Journal of School Health*, 42:10, Jan. 1972.
38. Stone, Donald B., and Kudla, Kenneth J.: "An Analysis of Health Needs and Problems as Revealed by a Selected Sample of Project Head Start Children." *Journal of School Health*, 37:470, Nov. 1967.
39. Basco, Dolores, Eyres, Sandra, Glasser, Jay H., et al.: "Epidemiological Analysis of School Populations As A Basis For Change in School Nursing Practice." *American Journal of Public Health*, 62:491, April 1972.
40. Ferinden, William E.: "The Role of the School Nurse in the Early Identification of Potential Learning Disabilities." *Journal of School Health*, 42:86, Feb. 1972.
41. Ford, Loretta C.: "The School Nurse Role—A Changing Concept in Preparation and Practice." *Journal of School Health*, 40:21, Jan. 1970.
42. Lum, Margaret C.: "Current Concepts in the Use of Non-Professional Assistants in School Health Services—A Selected Review." *Journal of School Health*, 43:357, June 1973.
43. Moir, Berta H.: "A School Health Program is a Community Enterprise." *Nursing Outlook*, 3:342, June 1955.
44. McFadden, Grace M., and O'Brien, Margaret J.: "Increasing the Effectiveness of School-Community Health Programs—A Nursing Viewpoint." *American Journal of Public Health*, 60:335, Feb. 1970.
45. Eisner, Victor et al.: "Health Assessment of School Children: Selecting a Screening Test." *Journal of School Health*, 42:21, Jan. 1972.
46. Byrd, Oliver Erasmus: *School Health Administration*. W.B. Saunders Co., Philadelphia, 1964.
47. Stephens, M.M., Rounthwaite, F. J., and Hutchison, D.A.: "Identification of Hearing Loss in School Children: A Model Program and Results." *Canadian Journal of Public Health*, 61:297, July-Aug. 1970.
48. Callan, L.B.: "The Growing Influence of Health Problems of School Health Education." *Journal of School Health*, 41:137, March 1971.
49. Benson, Karen D., Wade, Betty, and Benson, Daniel: "Results of School Screening for Scoliosis in the San Juan Unified School District, Sacramento, California." *Journal of School Health*, 47:483, Oct. 1977.
50. Eisner, Victor, and Oglesby, Allan: "Health Assessment of School Children: Heart Sound Screening." *Journal of School Health*, 42:270, May 1972.
51. Feeney, Rita: "Preventing Rheumatic Fever in School Children." *American Journal of Nursing*, 73:265, Feb. 1973.
52. Chobin, Nancy, Kangos, John, and Miller, Joseph: "From Project to Ongoing Program." *American Journal of Nursing*, 75:1489, Sept. 1975.
53. Stamler, Carolyn, and Palmer, James O.: "Dependency and Repetitive Visits to the Nurses Office in Elementary School Children." *Nursing Research*, 20:254, May-June 1971.
54. Drake, Richard E.: "The School as a Focus of Community Mental Health Services." *Nursing Clinics of North America*, 5:657, Dec. 1970.

55. Hilmar, Norman H., and McAtee, Patricia A.: "The School Nurse Practitioner and Her Practice: A Study of Traditional and Expanded Health Care Responsibilities for Nurses in Elementary Schools." *Journal of School Health*, 43:431, Sept. 1973.
56. Nader, Phillip R.: *Options for School Health: Meeting Community Needs.* Aspen Systems Corporation, Germantown, Md., 1978.
57. Editorial: "The Role of the School Nurse in Health Education." *American Journal of Public Health*, 61:2155, Nov. 1971.
58. Cosper, Barbara Anne, Hayslip, Donna Elaine, and Foree, Sherrell Bell: "The Effect of Nutrition Education on Dietary Habits of Fifth-Graders." *Journal of School Health*, 47:475, Oct. 1977.
59. Dickinson, Donald J.: "School Nursing Becomes Accountable in Education Through Behavioral Objectives." *Journal of School Health*, 41:333, Dec. 1971.
60. Cauffman, Joy G., Warburton, Edward A., and Schultz, Carl: "Health Care of School Children: Effective Referral Patterns." *American Journal of Public Health*, 59:86, Jan. 1979.
61. Weber, Kirsten: "Current Concepts in Community Health Nursing and Their Implications for Secondary School Health Services in British Columbia." *Canadian Journal of Public Health*, 63:137, March-April 1972.
62. Chinn, Peggy: "A Relationship Between Health and School Problems: A Nursing Assessment." *Journal of School Health*, 43:85, Feb. 1973.

BIBLIOGRAPHY

Abdellah, Kaye G.: "School Nurse Practitioner—An Expanded Role for Nurses." *Journal American College Health Association*, 21:423, June 1973.

Archer, Sara Ellen, and Fleshman, Ruth: *Community Health Nursing.* Duxbury Press, North Scituate, Mass., 1975.

Ball, B.: "School Nurses Have Expanded Roles, Too." *Nursing 73*, 3:61, Sept. 1973.

Beitz, D.E.: "Health Appraisal in Secondary Schools." *Journal of School Health*, 46:322, June, 1976.

Bellaire, Judith M.: "School Nurse Practitioner Program." *American Journal of Nursing*, 74:2192, Nov. 1971.

Benson, Evelyn Rose, and McDevitt, Joan Quinn: *Community Health and Nursing Practice.* Prentice-Hall, Inc., Englewood Cliffs, 1976.

Bivins, Emma C., and Lucye, Helen S. "A Case for New Directions in School Dental Health Education." *American Journal of Public Health*, 59:509, March 1969.

Brewer, K.: "The School Nurse: A Lesson in Diversified Care." *American Nurse*, 10:3, Jan. 15, 1978.

Brown, M.: "Secondary School Nursing: A Changing Focus . . . Eastern Ontario." *Canadian Nurse*, 73:42, Oct. 1977.

Cady, Ruth: "Oh Where, Oh Where Should Health Educators Be?" *American Journal of Public Health*, 62:79, Jan. 1972.

Cahn, Lorynne, and Petersen, Robert: "Education and Mental Health: A Need for Inter-disciplinary Involvement." *Journal of School Health*, 43:218, April 1973.

Cahn, Lorynne, and Petersen, Robert: "In Health-Related Tasks, Where Does the School Nurse Function?" *Journal of School Health*, 43:316, May 1973.

Califano, Joseph A., Jr.: "School Health Message." *Journal of School Health*, 47:334, June 1977.

Campbell, Marie, T., Garside, Alma H., and Drey, Marie E.C.: "Community Needs and How They Relate to the School Health Program: S.H.A.R.P.—the Needed Ingredient." *Journal of School Health*, 60:507, March 1970.

Chen, Shu-Pi C.: "Role Relationships in a School Health Interdisciplinary Team." *Journal of School Health*, 45:172, March 1975.

Coleman, Jane, and Hawkins, Wilber: "The Changing Role of the Nurse: An Alternative to Elimination." *Journal of School Health*, 40:121, March 1970.

Cowen, David L.: "Denver's Preventive Health Program for School Aged Children." *American Journal of Public Health*, 60:515, March 1970.

Creighton, Helen, and Squaires, G. Marjorie: "School Nurses: Legal Aspects of Their Work." *Nursing Clinics of North America*, 9:467, Sept. 1974.

Cromwell, Gertrude E.: *The Nurse in the School Health Program.* W. B. Saunders Co., Philadelphia, 1963.

Crosby, Marian H., and Connelly, Mary Grace: "The Study of Mental Health and the School Nurse." *Journal of School Health,* 40:373, Sept. 1970.

Densen, P.M. et al.: Childhood Characteristics as Indicators of Adult Health Status." *Public Health Reports,* 85:981, Nov. 1970.

Dougherty, S.E.: "A School Health Program for the Children of Migrant and Seasonal Agricultural Workers Progress Report." *Journal of School Health,* 41:115, March 1971.

Haggerty, Robert J., Roghmann, Klaus J., and Pless, Ivan B.: *Child Health and the Community.* John Wiley and Sons, Inc., New York, 1975.

Hamburg, Morris, and Hamburg, Marian V.: *Health and Social Problems in the School: Case Studies for School Personnel.* Lea and Febiger, Philadelphia, 1968.

Hammond, E.: "A Nurse's Concern Regarding Factual Knowledge of V.D.: A Regional High School." *Journal of School Health,* 42:599, Dec. 1972.

Hopp, J. W.: "Values Clarification and the School Nurse." *Journal of School Health,* 46:60, Sept.-Oct. 1976.

Hurster, Madeline: "The Identification of Value Orientations of Sixth Graders, With Specific Reference to Health Concepts in the School Health Education Study Curriculum." *American Journal of Public Health,* 62:82, Jan. 1972.

Hyman, Herbert Harvey: *Health Planning: A Systematic Approach.* Aspen Systems Corp., Germantown, Md., 1975.

Johansen, S. et al.: "The School Nurse and Health Education." *Health Visitor,* 49:283, Sept. 1976.

Julifs, B.L.: "Kaleidoscope of Community Health: Can Health Be Taught? The Role of the School Nurse in Health Education." *American Nurses' Association Clinical Sessions,* Appleton-Century-Crofts, New York, 1974, p. 289.

Kanfer, Frederick H., and Goldstein, Arnold P.: *Helping People Change.* Pergamon Press Inc., New York, 1975.

Kark, Sidney L.: *Epidemiology and Community Medicine.* Appleton-Century-Crofts, New York, 1974.

Lampe, J.M.: "A New Approach to Delivery of Health Care to School Children as Instituted by Denver, Colorado, Public Schools." *Journal of School Health,* 42:272, May 1972.

Levey, Samuel, and Loomba, N. Paul: *Health Care Administration: A Managerial Perspective.* J. B. Lippincott Co., Philadelphia, 1973.

Lynch, Annette: "There is Health in School Health." *Journal of School Health,* 47:410, Sept. 1977.

McAtee, Patricia A.: "Nurse Practitioners in Our Public Schools: An Assessment of Their Expanded Role as Compared with School Nurses." *Clinical Pediatrics,* 13:360, April 1974.

MacMahon, Brian, and Pugh, Thomas F.: *Epidemiology Principles and Methods.* Little, Brown and Co., Boston, 1970

Nader, Phillip, Conrad, Jane, Williamson, Mildred, et al.: "The High School Nurse Practitioner." *Journal of School Helath,* 48:649, Jan. 1978.

Oda, Dorothy S. (ed.): "Will the Real School Nurse Please Stand Up?" *American Nurse,* 10:4, Jan. 15, 1978.

Pan American Health Organization: *The Role of the Nurse in Primary Health Care.* World Health Organization, Washington, D.C., 1977.

Reinhardt, Adina M., and Quinn, Mildred D.: *Current Practice in Family-Centered Community Nursing,* Vol. I. The C. V. Mosby Co., St. Louis, 1977.

Reinke, William A., and Williams, Kathleen N.: *Health Planning: Qualitative Aspects and Quantitative Techniques.* The Johns Hopkins University School of Hygiene and Public Health, Baltimore, 1972.

Ross, Donald C., Meinster, Martha O., and Gingrich, Lois J.: "A Program for Expanding the Mental Health Functions of the School Nurse." *Journal of School Health,* 48:157, March 1978.

Somers, Anne R.: *Promoting Health: Consumer Education and National Policy.* Aspen Systems Corp., Germantown, Md., 1976.

Spradley, Barbara Walton: *Contemporary Community Nursing.* Little, Brown and Co., Boston, 1975.

Susser, Mervyn: *Causal Thinking in the Health Sciences: Concepts and Strategies in Epidemiology.* Oxford University Press, New York, 1973.

Thompson, Virgina M.: "Role of the School Nurse." *Journal of School Health*, 47:358, June 1977.

Wilson, Charles C., and Wilson, Elizabeth Avery (eds.): *Healthful School Environment*. National Education Association, Washington, D.C., 1969.

Wold, Susan J.: "School Nursing: A Framework for Practice." *Journal of School Health*, 48:111, Feb. 1978.

CHAPTER 13
NURSING ROLE IN PUBLIC HEALTH

MARILYN B. MAJOR, M.P.H., R.N.

Public health nursing is an exciting and stimulating field. The nurse's individual caseload of families represents a range of ages and conditions along the health-illness continuum, and therefore a wide variety of health services is provided in the home, schools, and community clinics. Regardless of the setting, the objectives of public health nursing are health maintenance and personal independence. These goals challenge the professional to draw upon a wide range of nursing skills as well as upon his or her knowledge of the community and its institutions. The nurse must deal not only with immediate health needs but directly with the individual person, the individual's family, and the institutions concerned with health care delivery.

The majority of public health nurses operate within the context of an official health department or a combination agency. Thus the structure and functions of these agencies must be understood in order to fully perceive the scope and responsibilities of this branch of nursing. The major financial support for an official health department comes primarily from local taxation supplemented by state support. Many professional activities of these departments are mandated by state law. Generally the official health department is directed by a health officer who must be a physician. Under his authority there may be several divisions which are responsible for implementing various programs and activities. Typical divisions include dental, environmental health, laboratory, public health nursing, health education, and clinical services (Fig. 13-1). Because the health department is supported by tax monies, services are provided either free of charge or at a nominal fee.

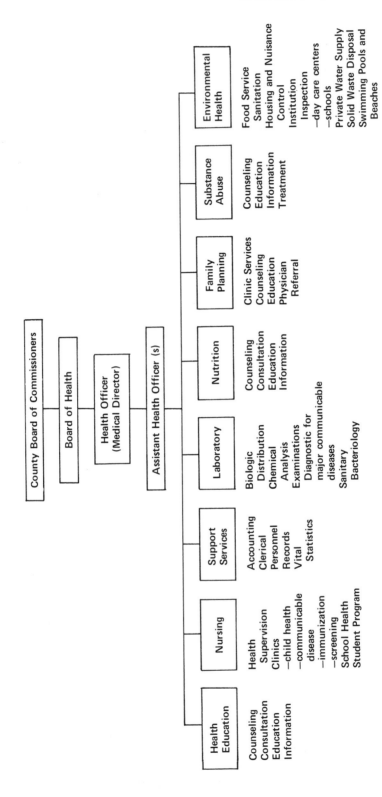

FIGURE 13-1 Organizational chart of an official health department

A combination health agency is partially supported by tax funds but additional monies come from third party payment such as patient fees and community contributions. A combination agency provides bedside nursing services in addition to the community health maintenance services typical of an official health agency. This additional function may be either similar to that provided by the Visiting Nurse Association or the VNA itself may be included in the same organizational structure (Fig. 13-2).

HISTORICAL DEVELOPMENT

The present role of the nurse must be seen in its historical context. The evolution of public health nursing in the United States came out of a restricted view of both its purpose and service group. In the nineteenth century, the main responsibility of official health agencies was control of communicable diseases and sanitation. Between 1875 and 1900, district nursing services were developed in various cities. Such services were frequently affiliated with religious organizations or private agencies, such as the Visiting Nurse Society.

In 1893, Lillian Wald and Mary Brewster established the Nurses' Settlement on the east side of New York City. This enterprise was later called the Henry Street District Nursing Service. The guiding principle of the Henry Street Settlement was the "determination to bring the best of everything to the service of all."[1] Five years later on the west coast, the Los Angeles Health Department employed a nurse to provide nursing care to the sick poor in their homes. In New York in 1902, a nurse from the Henry Street Settlement was loaned to the city health department on an experimental basis to work in the schools. Her responsibility centered on working with the families of children who were excluded from school because of a communicable disease and determining when a child could return to school. This program effectively reduced the numerous and lengthy school absences resulting from communicable diseases. Its success led to the employment of a group of nurses to provide similar services for other city schools. Eventually the scope of their responsibilities was extended.

During the same period, another Henry Street nurse was assigned to the Division of Infant Hygiene of the New York City Health Department; her work resulted in the regular employment of a nurse for infant hygiene. Expanding the scope of nursing involvement, the New York City Health Department then appointed three public health nurses to visit tuberculosis patients at home in order to instruct them on personal hygiene and their disease process. In 1907, Alabama became the first state to legally approve the employment of public health nurses by local boards of health.

The concept of the guardianship of public health as one of the chief functions of the municipality, the community, the state, and the federal government arose out of the Henry Street philosophy that the nurse and the physician must be available without exception to the poor as well as the rich. After the initial employment of public health nurses, the movement grew rapidly. In the 30 year period from 1920 to 1950 the number of public health nurses increased from 11,000 to 25,461.[2] By 1968 there were 50,492 professionals employed in public health.[3] Although public health nursing arose from the private sector and originally was geared to providing home nursing services to the poor, it is now firmly established in the public domain and serves persons from every socioeconomic level.

Originally, the public health nurse was considered to be a generalist, providing all types of services. One of her more important functions was bedside nursing, and according to one scholar, "she endeavors to discover and remedy physical defects and habits as well

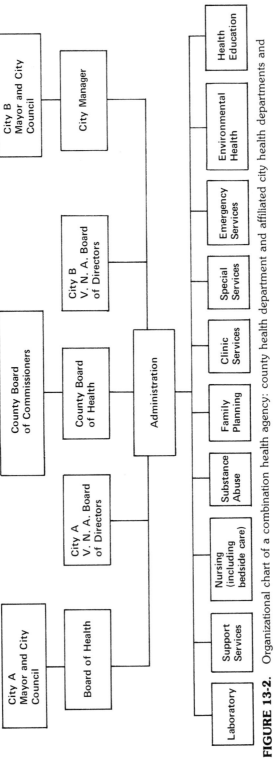

FIGURE 13-2. Organizational chart of a combination health agency: county health department and affiliated city health departments and visiting nurse associations.

as unsanitary conditions. She gives various members of the family definite instruction regarding the prevention of disease and the development of sound health."[4] As public health nursing became institutionalized and bureaus emerged, the concept of a specialized public health nurse evolved. The progress of medical science and the increased knowledge of prevention, diagnosis, and treatment of disease conditions also contributed to the emergence of the public health nurse specialist.

As early as 60 years ago, some professionals saw the specialist as a leader whose successors could utilize her pathfinding methods in broader types of service. In the 1920s, Lavina Dock observed that "the trend is steadily toward general service of staff nurses, adequately supported by highly trained and experienced experts as consultants or supervisors."[2] This trend has continued. Today the concept of public health nursing embracing a broad range of services is widely accepted, and there is a growing specialist role for those who receive training in newly developed practitioner programs.

EDUCATIONAL PREPARATION

The educational qualifications of public health nurses exhibit a great deal of variety. The nursing divisions of many official health departments require the nurse to have baccalaureate preparation in nursing with public health nursing experience as part of the educational preparation. In some cases, agencies prefer that their employees also have previous experience. Although the baccalaureate prepared public health nurse is the ideal, sometimes the realities of the employment situation demand modifications. Many official agencies have difficulty recruiting qualified personnel. Generally, the employment situation revolves around the principle of supply and demand: if an agency has a large number of qualified applicants from which to choose, the nursing director can increase the entry level qualifications of those hired. On the other hand, if there are no baccalaureate prepared nurses available, an agency may be forced to hire less qualified individuals.

Licensure as a registered nurse in the state where one plans to practice is a basic requirement for public health nursing service. Those who have additional educational preparation and training for expanded roles, such as nurse midwives and family nurse practitioners, often find that some state legislation on nursing practice is confining and restrictive. These laws often prevent effective functioning of nurses attempting to meet community needs.

SCOPE OF SERVICE

When comparing public health nursing to other branches of nursing, both similarities and differences become readily apparent. Public health nursing integrates many theories and practices from other branches of nursing. For example, professional competence is dependent on sound knowledge of anatomy and physiology. Every professional nurse needs to be proficient in technical nursing skills and knowledgeable about the etiology of various disease processes. Interviewing and communication skills are essential for exchanging information with patients, families, and other professionals. The principles and practice of the teaching-learning process are utilized by all nurses. One of the goals in teaching a patient or family new skills is that there will be a change in behavior. The nurse must be aware of the steps in the change process and how to use them with both individuals and groups. Although the extent of utilization varies, all professional nurses must be cognizant of the purposes and procedures for making an effecive referral and the resources available in a given community.

There are, however, many unique aspects of public health nursing. It is essential that the public health nurse be knowledgeable about the principles of family dynamics and understand how cultural values affect decision-making and health practice. Thus, concern is directed at all aspects of health: physical, emotional, and social well being.

This definition views health as a multifaceted, interactional entity. Health is not just the absence of illness or disease. There is a positive focus to public health nursing which includes all aspects of one's total being. The concern is with individual members of a community but not just the individuals alone. The public health nurse is also involved with how the health of these individuals influences families and the community. The converse situation is also important, that is, how the community and its families influence individual members. Health is, indeed, an interactional process and this is the underlying precept for public health nursing.

While there is a great deal of emphasis on health promotion or primary prevention, there are actually three levels of prevention within which many of the services provided by the public health nurse can be categorized. Primary prevention deals with those activities which are specifically directed at maintaining health and preventing illness. Discussing the nutritional or immunization needs of a newborn infant with the child's parents is an example of this type of health promotion.

Secondary prevention focuses on the diagnosis and treatment of a disease condition. For example, if the public health nurse discovers during her newborn assessment that the infant has unequal skin folds on his left and right buttocks and upon flexion and external rotation of the hips there is a clicking sound, she may suspect the child has a congenital anomaly. She will advise the parents of her observations and suggest that they contact a physician for further evaluation. The public health nurse may share her findings with the physician either verbally or in writing. Regardless, she will contact the family again to determine if there was followup and the results. The nurse will need to assess the family's understanding, ability, and willingness to accept the physician's diagnosis and recommended treatment. This includes a determination of the family's financial resources for providing treatment.

Tertiary prevention deals with the rehabilitative process. In the example of an infant with congenital dislocation of the hips, the public health nurse should monitor the progress of the treatment program. She will assess the residual effects of the condition on the infant's growth and development, i.e., how it affects the child at home, with playmates, and at school. During the entire process, support and encouragement must be continually provided to the family.

Given the focus of public health nursing, the nurse often functions independently and frequently is the sole health professional in a given situation. Effective and efficient utilization of the referral process on behalf of the families being served is an essential professional skill. In many cases, she may suggest that a family seek medical care for a member who is ill. This requires knowledge about the resources available in the community, eligibility requirements, and the types of services various agencies provide. If many members of a family have health needs or if one member has multiple health needs, the public health nurse may become the coordinator of the health services for that family. When many agencies are providing services to a family, there is frequently a need for such coordination and maintenance of open channels of communication.

Community resources that are potential referral agencies are part of two larger systems, health and welfare (social services). Knowledge of these systems is imperative if comprehensive service is to be provided. This awareness fosters the establishment and maintenance of good communication between the nurse and other health professionals as well as between the nurse and professionals from the welfare system, such as social workers. The strength of the referral process often rests on the liason that is established between health and non-health professionals. The public health nurse may also act as an advocate on behalf of a family she serves. Occasionally, for one reason or another, an agency does not fulfill its obligations to an individual or family. Sometimes there are so many agencies involved and communication between them becomes so confused that the public health nurse needs to reopen communication on the family's behalf. The quality of the nurse's ability to work with community agencies can affect the quality of service that is provided.

Understanding of the principles and practice of health planning and administration of health services is important for the public health nurse and supervisor as they plan, implement, evaluate, and administer the various programs offered by an agency. If the service is truly flexible and responsive to the needs and age distribution of the community, it should naturally vary from agency to agency.

Knowledge of standard public health practice is of paramount importance for the public health nurse. The principles of epidemiology and the processes of communicable and chronic diseases are inherent. In the past, public health nurses spent a great deal of time working with persons who contracted communicable diseases. Although the common communicable diseases are much less prevalent today, the occurrence of Legionnaire's disease in the mid-1970s highlights the continuing importance of epidemiology. As the incidence of communicable disease has diminished, however, the focus of public health nursing service has shifted. Service throughout the life cycle and at all stages in the health-illness continuum has become the goal of any responsive professional public health nursing service (Table 13-1).

In many agencies, maternal and child health services continue to receive high priority. These services include expectant parent classes and visits to high risk antepartum patients, especially those women under 18 and those over 35 years of age. Home visits to families with new infants are important in order to assess the infant and the family's adjustment to the new infant. This provides an ideal time to discuss the need for continued health care and immunizations, the growth and development of an infant, and its stimulation and nutritional needs. The nurse can assess the postpartum status of the mother, the plans for a postpartum checkup, and the need for family planning information. Additonal needs (financial, nutritional, transportation, and housing) should be determined by the public health nurse. All of these functions are significant because many young families are not aware of the community resources available, such as immunization, child health, and family planning services.

As the percentage of the elderly in the population of the United States increases, the needs of our older citizens are becoming more apparent. The public health nurse must be aware of these needs. Many senior citizens suffer from chronic diseases, isolation, limited income, and lack of knowledge about community resources.

To a certain extent, staffing arrangements affect the quality and type of services provided. In official agencies, two patterns of staffing have emerged. In many agencies, the public health nurse is assigned a geographic area which may be determined by using census tract or elementary school district boundaries. One public health nurse becomes responsible for providing all of the services needed in her district or geographic area. In turn, several nurses are assigned to a nursing supervisor who oversees the group's work in the broader

TABLE 13-1.   Public health nursing service through the life cycle. (Key * = continuous; # = if present; & = PRN)

Services	Infancy	Preschool years	Early school years	Adolescent years	Young adult years	Middle adult years	Later adult years
Accident prevention	*	*	*	*	*	*	*
Chronic diseases	#	#	#	#	#	*	*
Communicable diseases	0	0	0	0	0	0	0
Exercise patterns	*	*	*	*	*	*	*
Family planning				*	*	*	
Genetics	#			#	#	#	
Growth/development	*	*	*	*	*	*	*
Intellectual stimulation	*	*	*	*	*	*	*
Learning	*	*	*	*	*	*	*
Mental health	*	*	*	*	*	*	*
Nutrition	*	*	*	*	*	*	*
Physical health	*	*	*	*	*	*	*
Protection from environmental hazards	*	*	*	*	*	*	*
Safety	*	*	*	*	*	*	*
Social health	*	*	*	*	*	*	*
Use of leisure time	*	*	*	*	*	*	*

geographic area. A set of standing orders to cover medical procedures is needed for professional guidance and legal purposes. These are usually developed by the nursing division in cooperation with the health officer.

The second staffing pattern is the formation of a nursing team. This team serves a large geographic area and all of the nurses work in the entire area. In this team approach, several public health nurses are responsible for providing services in any given community. The team approach requires effective communication among team members to prevent duplication of service. It also permits the individual public health nurse to be a specialist in a specific professional competence rather than a generalist. This team will also have a supervisory nurse. The team staff pattern is widely used in combination agencies where bedside nursing services are provided in addition to those concerning health supervision, communicable diseases, maternal and child health, and school services.

In a combination agency the team will usually be augmented by the services of licensed practical nurses, a physical therapist, and home health aides. In such an agency, the public health nurse will have specific medical orders for each patient receiving bedside nursing services in addition to the standing orders for medical procedures. This calls for knowledge of the techniques and skills required for the provision of bedside nursing services as well as the generalized public health nursing service. Individual patient orders must be renewed on a regular basis. The time period varies and is dependent upon the source of payment. Because of the requirements of third party payers such as Medicaid, Medicare, or private insurance companies, considerable time must be spent by agency personnel just to meet the requirements for payment. The resultant difficulty is that the emphasis on compliance with the rules for third party payment can overwhelm the public health nurses attempting to provide service. The elaborate procedures for obtaining payment are one of the contributors to the high cost of health care in this country.

Over the last several decades, there has been extensive discussion and concern over the scope of federal legislation for national health care. National health insurance will surely affect the role of public health nurses to some degree, and it is unclear whether any third party program can reduce the number of forms to be completed. Yet, the nursing profession has to convince both the general public and legislators at all levels of the value of nursing services so that it will be included in any reimbursement program.

Paperwork is an inevitable part of public health, and there is a wide variation in the type of recordkeeping in nursing divisions. The narrative format record is probably the most common type. Each visit a nurse makes is reported in a narrative style and, while the record tends to become rather voluminous, at least all of the data are included.

Some agencies combine the narrative format within nursing process categories: data collection, nursing diagnosis, nursing goals, nursing action, implementation, and evaluation. This approach provides the public health nurse with a framework in which to organize the information. It also provides data regarding the progress which the family and the nurse are making.

A third record style is the Problem Oriented Record (POR). The actual record format is much more compact than other styles. This form lists the problems of each family member and the solutions to be attempted. The time required to set up the original problem list and initial assessment is considerable, but once the problem list is completed, recording of individual visits takes a short period of time. One of the weaknesses in the POR is that only the problems of individual family members are identified in the record while their strengths and coping mechanisms are omitted.

The public health nursing record is a legal document which is the only complete written record of the services provided by a public health nurse. Therefore, it is important to remember that if information is omitted from the record, the legal interpretation is that the public health nurse did not provide the service. Thus, the nursing record serves as documentation of the service provided, its quality, and professional accountability.

To further evaluate the quality of service and determine accountability the nursing audit was developed. Maria Phenauf was an early leader in the development of the nursing audit for use in public health nursing agencies. The Phenauf audit tool is directed toward those records where bedside nursing service is provided. Because of its particular focus, it is difficult to utilize on the health supervision records which are found in most official agencies. To meet this need, the public health nursing staff of the Oakland County Division of Health, Pontiac, Michigan developed an innovative nursing audit tool for use with the health supervision records.

The Oakland County Public Health Nurse Family Record Audit was created to help analyze caseloads and answer several questions. How much difference does the nursing input make in a family? Is the family making progress? Are the goals and objectives being met? The purpose of the audit is to look objectively at the agency's work by identifying and assessing both strengths and weaknesses in the services rendered.

The five public health nursing functions identified in the Oakland County Division of Health audit are an adaptation of Maria Phenauf's tool which in turn is based on the seven functions of professional nursing developed by Lesnik and Anderson. The Oakland County functions are: 1) observation of the situation, 2) evaluation of the total situation and plans for nursing action, 3) implementation of the nursing plans, 4) coordination of other services, intra-agency and interagency, and 5) organization of the family folder.

The audit tool is used in Oakland County to assess the quality of service as reflected in closed family folders. It may also serve as an appraisal tool in two additional manners: by the supervisor and nurse together and by the individual nurse. Given sufficient data the nursing audit may be used to modify nursing service. Strengths and weaknesses in the nursing service can be identified and modified for efficiency in quality, cost, and accountability (see Appendix at end of this chapter).

Clearly, the scope and purpose of public health nursing in an agency setting has changed since its inception more than 150 years ago. The focus shifted from simple, single goals to complex multipurpose services. Accompanying this development was the evolution of professional procedures and guidelines to improve service. While public health nursing may appear to be a complicated field, it offers an opportunity and challenge to the creative, innovative individual to utilize the full range of nursing skills in a variety of settings.

REFERENCES

1. Dock, Lavina L.: *A Half Century of Public Health: Jubilee Historical Volume of the American Public Health Association.* Mazÿck P. Ravenel, ed. American Public Health Association, New York, 1921, p. 441.
2. George Rosen: *A History of Public Health,* New York, 1958, p. 381.
3. Roberts, D.E., Saba, V.K., and Allen, H.K.: "Census of Nurses in Public Health." *American Journal of Nursing,* 70:2394, Nov. 1970.
4. Moore, Henry H.: *Public Health in the United States.* Harper and Brothers, Publishers, New York, 1923.

BIBLIOGRAPHY

Ceglarek, Joan E., and Rife, Joyce K.: "Developing a Public Health Nursing Audit." *Journal of Nursing Administration,* 7:37, Dec. 1977.

Futrell, May DiPietro, and Kelleher, Marie J.: *The Nurse's Guide to Health Services for Patients.* Little, Brown and Company, Boston, 1973.

Hanlon, John J.: *Public Health: Administration and Practice.* The C.V. Mosby Company, St. Louis, 1974.

Leavell, Hugh Rodman, and Clark, E. Gurney: *Preventive Medicine for the Doctor in his Community.* McGraw-Hill Book Company, New York, 1965.

Lesnik, Milton Jack, and Anderson, Bernice E.: *Nursing Practice and the Law,* 2nd ed. J.B. Lippincott, Philadelphia, 1955.

Moore, Harry H.: *Public Health in the United States.* Harper and Brothers Publishers, New York, 1923.

Phaneuf, Maria C.: *The Nursing Audit: Profile for Excellence.* Appleton-Century-Croft, New York, 1972.

Ravenel, Mazÿch P.(ed.): *A Half Century of Public Health.* American Public Health Association, New York, 1921.

Rosen, George: *A History of Public Health.* MD Publications, Inc., New York, 1958.

Smillie, Wilson G.: *Public Health: Its Promise for the Future.* The Macmillian Company, New York, 1955.

Smolensky, Jack: *Principles of Community Health.* W.B. Saunders, Philadelphia, 1977.

Will, Marilyn B.: "Referral: A Process Not A Form," *Nursing 77,* 7(12):44, Dec. 1977.

APPENDIX. OAKLAND COUNTY PUBLIC HEALTH NURSING AUDIT TOOL*

INTRODUCTION TO AUDIT TOOL

Definition of scoring terms are as follows:
Yes—Clearly stated in the record.
No—Not stated in the record.
Partial—Stated some of the time.

I. OBSERVATION OF SITUATION

1. *Physical Environment:* Description and location of where visit occurs, and noted changes.
2. *Social Environment:* Description of family constellation and living pattern, which may include religious and ethnic influences.
3. *Economic Environment:* Identified source of income, which may include how it is used.
4. *Educational Environment:* Description of formally and informally acquired knowledge.
5. *Emotional Environment:* Description of demonstrated feelings, verbal and/or nonverbal, such as hostility, joy, sorrow, apathy, hate, love, and reverence.
6. *Problems and Needs as Seen by the Family:* Family members will have different viewpoints; therefore, we should be specific about informant.
7. *Problems and Needs as Seen by the PHN:* PHN evaluates needs of entire family.
8. *Resources:* Existing or previous individual, family, or community sources of support, supply, and assistance. Examples of such sources of support are occupation, and/or source of income, agency, medical, or other resources such as friends, relatives, neighbors.

II. EVALUATE TOTAL SITUATION AND DRAW UP PLANS FOR NURSING ACTION

1. *Available Information Is Reviewed:* Information gathered from such sources as referral source, other family records, other PHNs, physicians, school records, dentists, and other agencies servicing the family. The key word in definition is *available.*
2. *Assessment of Needs:* PHN evaluates needs and assigns priorities to problems.
3. *Family and Patient Coping Abilities:* Statement of how family deals with situations or meets difficulties.
4. *Acceptability of Nursing Service:* Statement of family response to PHN service.
5. *Barriers to Action:* Restraints or obstructions restricting PHN intervention or family movement. These may be as diverse as mental or physical handicaps,

---

Audit and nursing record material used with permission of the Oakland County Division of Public Health, Pontiac, Michigan.

individual PHN limitations, social and economic factors, language barriers, or improper timing of PHN action. Absence of barriers to action is implied unless barriers are specified in dictation.

6. *Nursing Diagnosis:* A labeled, concise conclusion derived from observation and evaluation and upon which nursing action is based.

7. *Written Nursing Goals:* Goals are the desired end result. Goals must be written, i.e., appear as heading in dictation.

8. *Written Nursing Plans:* Written activities designed to reach a stated nursing goal.

III. IMPLEMENTATION OF NURSING PLANS

1. *Evidence of Planning with Family:* PHN and family establish tasks or activities to achieve a written goal. "Evidence" is obvious data, not implied data.

2. *Evidence of PHN Action:* Written evidence of direct care, demonstrations, instruction, counseling, listening, supportive action, planning with family.

3. *Evidence of Followup:* Followup is an act to carry out plans. (Example: Family might make appointment and PHN would followup.) Intent of followup can be implied, e.g., NAHFS (not at home for service)—MOVED.

4. *Evidence of Flexibility:* Nursing action changes to respond to family's situation and needs. Flexibility is present unless nursing action obviously not responsive to changing family needs.

5. *Assessment of Goals:* Reevaluation of written goals during service.

6. *Legal Practice:* Use of agency policy as mandated by law and current administrative directives.

IV. COORDINATION OF OTHER SERVICES—INTRA- AND INTER-AGENCY

1. *Referral to Other Services:* Family is directed toward specific services, if need indicated. May include communication with services before family is seen. If no need indicated, score as YES.

2. *Followup of Referrals Made by PHN:* PHN obtained information from family or services that family acted on referrals. When no referral made, score a YES.

3. *Feedback to Source of Referral:* Feedback is verbal or written communication to source of referral. Verbal or written communication is necessary on all professional referrals, except birth certificates. PHN's judgement is accepted regarding feedback to nonprofessionals, e.g., indiscreet neighbor or hostile relative. If referral not received as written form, then feedback information should appear in dictation. Score a self-referral as YES.

4. *Clarification of Agency Roles:* PHN explained Health Department services and/or other agencies' services to family.

5. *Conferences on Behalf of Family:* A communication to facilitate provision of health services to individual and family as need indicated. This includes PHN's

supervisor, other professionals, or nonprofessionals. If no need indicated, score as YES.

V. RECORDING FORMAT

1. *Referral Source:* Statement of origin and nature of referral.
2. *Family Record Forms Complete:* Admission, family data sheet, (front and back of sheet), medical data, T.B. and C.D. forms, and referral forms.
3. *Agency Dictation Guide Used:* Definition: Implies only that guide format, individual items (i.e., Diagnosis, Goals, Plans, etc.) are audited.
4. *Summaries—Periodic, Transfer, Closing:*
   Periodic summaries are to be done every 12 direct service visits or 18 months, whichever comes first. Summaries may be done more often if evaluation of services is needed.
   Transfer and closing summaries are to be written when record is transferred or closed. Anytime service is reinitiated there must be an update of summary at the time of closure.
5. *Family Record in Sequential Order:* Family data sheet, continuation sheets, and summaries in chronologic order. Reports should be grouped by department and person in reverse chronologic order (current date on top). All reports, letters, or miscellaneous should be taped, stapled, or otherwise secured to the record.
6. *Evidence of Supervisor Review:* Initial of supervisor at the farthest point she has reviewed and signature at the closing or transfer.
7. *Evidence of PHN Review:* Dictation corrected and signed in ink by PHN.

COMMENTS

To apply only to the mechanics of the audit.

AUDIT TOOL

I. OBSERVATION OF SITUATION	Yes (8)	No (0)	Partial (4)
1. Physical Environment.	_____	_____	_____
2. Social Environment.	_____	_____	_____
3. Economic Environment.	_____	_____	_____
4. Education Environment.	_____	_____	_____
5. Emotional Environment.	_____	_____	_____
6. Problems and Needs as Seen by Family.	_____	_____	_____
7. Problems and Needs as Seen by PHN.	_____	_____	_____
8. Resources.	_____	_____	_____

II. EVALUATE TOTAL SITUATION AND DRAW UP PLANS FOR NURSING ACTION

	Yes (8)	No (0)	Partial (4)
1. Available Information Is Reviewed.	_____	_____	_____
2. Assessment of Needs.	_____	_____	_____
3. Family and Patient Coping Abilities.	_____	_____	_____
4. Acceptability of Nursing Service.	_____	_____	_____
5. Barriers to Action.	_____	_____	_____
6. Nursing Diagnosis.	_____	_____	_____
7. Written Nursing Goals.	_____	_____	_____
8. Written Nursing Plans.	_____	_____	_____

III. IMPLEMENTATION OF NURSING PLANS

	Yes (6)	No (0)	Partial (3)
1. Evidence of Planning with Family.	_____	_____	_____
2. Evidence of PHN Action.	_____	_____	_____
3. Evidence of Followup.	_____	_____	_____
4. Evidence of Flexibility.	_____	_____	_____
5. Assessment of Goals.	_____	_____	_____
6. Legal Practice.	_____	_____	_____

IV. COORDINATION OF OTHER SERVICES – INTRA- AND INTERAGENCY

	Yes (4)	No (0)	Partial (2)
1. Referral to Other Services.	_____	_____	_____
2. Followup of Referrals made by PHN.	_____	_____	_____
3. Feedback to Source of Referral.	_____	_____	_____
4. Clarification of Agency Roles.	_____	_____	_____
5. Conferences on Behalf of Family.	_____	_____	_____

V. RECORDING FORMAT

	Yes (2)	No (0)	Partial (1)
1. Referral Source.	_____	_____	_____
2. Family Record Forms Complete.	_____	_____	_____
3. Agency Dictation Guide Used.	_____	_____	_____
4. Summaries—Periodic, Transfer, Closing.	_____	_____	_____
5. Family Record in Sequential Order.	_____	_____	_____
6. Evidence of Supervisor Review.	_____	_____	_____
7. Evidence of PHN Review.	_____	_____	_____

COMMENTS

Please complete on back of this page.

PROCEDURES AND GUIDELINES FOR AUDIT COMMITTEE

I. PURPOSE:

Nurses in this agency are accountable for the quality of service delivered.

II. PHILOSOPHY:

Public Health Nurses are professionals and are self-directing as well as self-evaluating.

III. OBJECTIVES:

A. A.N.A. standards for quality assurance have been accepted as an agency standard. According to these standards, the purposes for peer review which includes record audit are:
   1. To evaluate the quality and quantity of nursing care.
   2. To identify the strengths and weaknesses of nursing care.
   3. To provide evidence to be utilized as the basis of recommendations for new or altered policies and procedures to improve nursing care.
   4. To identify those areas where practice patterns indicate that more knowledge is needed by the practitioners.
B. The record audit will evaluate, on a monthly basis, the quality of service of PH field nursing section as reflected in the family records.
C. Field staff will utilize the audit tool on an individual basis to identify strengths and weaknesses of nursing care, as reflected in recording, on a regular basis.
D. Use of record audit will be included as part of staff expectations in orientation and reinforced periodically by nursing supervisors.

IV. FUNCTIONS OF AUDIT STANDING COMMITTEE:

A. Perform audit on a monthly basis, using developed definitions and tools on a designated sample number of records.
B. Measure quality as reflected in the audited records; compute and analyze averages of results.
C. Report to administration on a quarterly basis a summary of audit results including evidence of strengths and weaknesses identified, with recommendations for new or altered policies and procedures to improve nursing service, if indicated.
D. Participate in orientation session for new staff on the use of record audit.

V. MEMBERSHIP:

A. Ten members, one representing each field nursing supervisor group.

B. One of the ten members shall be a nursing supervisor.

C. Each supervisor will be responsible for appointing a replacement if a member of her group leaves the committee with more than six months remaining of a term. The replacement member will complete that term and have the option to be replaced or to be appointed for a complete term.

D. Staff should have completed or be completing minimum of one year employment as field staff before being recommended for audit committee membership. At the discretion of the supervisor, appointment can occur before the completion of one year of employment.

E. Before completion of a term a retiring audit committee member must be responsible for notifying supervisor of the replacement need.

VI. TERM:

A. 18 months beginning in March or September according to the supervisor rotation schedule.

B. Any extension in the term of an individual will be up to the audit committee and supervisor. Six months extension limit.

VII. ORIENTATION OF NEW COMMITTEE MEMBERS:

A. One retiring member and the co-chairperson will be responsible for orienting new members. Orientation will take place within one month before the new members' first audit committee meeting. (Orientation will not be included in term.)

B. A week before the planned orientation meeting, the prospective members will be given a packet containing:
   1. The numbered reference packet which belonged to retiring member.
   2. Definitions.

C. The videotape of audit committee may be shown prior to the orientation meeting.

D. Each member being oriented will audit the sample record to provide a basis for comparison and discussion. Discussion should cover similarities and differences in scores and why these occur, as well as variance in auditing decisions of individuals and the averaging that occurs.

E. An overview of audit committee activities shall be included in the orientation: history of the audit, philosophy of the audit concept, current activities such as special projects and subcommittees, place of audit in quality assurance, different criteria (structure, process, outcomes) used to judge quality of nursing care (our audit uses process). Also remind new members that the audit is based on the use of the nursing process in a field visit as recorded by the nurse.

VIII. AUDIT PROCEDURE:

A. Selection of records.
   1. Only closed records will be audited.
   2. The clerk will pull every third closed record during the current month, minimum of 25, from each office. If there are less than 25 closed in the current month, pull from closed file.
   3. Submit all closed records to audit committee recorder according to the schedule by each month.
   4. Recorder for current month will review and select records. An average of 20 records shall be audited each month. An attempt will be made to select records that have been opened in the last three years.
   5. The following records will be excluded from audit.
      a. Hearing
      b. One visit
      c. No field service visits recorded in the last three years
      d. Child health conference only
      e. Student dictation only
      f. Auxiliary health worker only
B. Recording dated prior to guide for recording PHN visits (1972) need not be audited.
C. Use audit tool and audit tool definitions.

IX. QUARTERLY REPORT:

A. Quarterly report to be prepared by subgroup appointed by the chairperson after March, June, September, and December meetings.
B. Report to be discussed by total membership in April, July, October, and January for evaluation of results and recommendations if any.
C. Report to administration will include analysis of variables, hypothesis as to changes noted, and recommendations.

X. FREQUENCY OF MEETINGS:

Meetings will be held monthly on the first Friday A.M. of the month, alternating between north and south health offices.

XI. CHAIRPERSON DUTIES:

A. To serve for six months.
B. Establish agenda.
C. Coordinate and lead meeting.
D. Receive communications for the committee.
E. Keep audit book updated.
F. Appoint subcommittee for preparing quarterly report.
G. Maintain a log of procedural changes suggested by the committee. The log will be submitted to administration annually for review and incorporation as necessary into guidelines and definition.

XII. CO-CHAIRPERSON:

A. To serve as co-chairperson for six months and become chairperson for six months.
B. To serve as chairperson in the absence of the chairperson.
C. To participate in orientation of new committee members.

XIII. RECORDER:

A. Rotate on monthly basis according to seniority to alternate between north and south health offices. The chairperson is not included in the rotation.
B. Reserve room for meeting.
C. Review records for auditing according to guidelines under selection of records (VIII-5).
D. Prepare monthly report with recorder from previous month.
E. Write minutes of meetings, have typed and distributed to members of committee with one copy for book.

FAMILY DATA SHEET

9999	999
DIST. /	CVT

NAME: (Family)   **BROWN, ERNEST III**   **CROSSFILE/**

STREET	POST OFFICE	ZIP CODE	DIRECTIONS	TELEPHONE NO.
100 N. Main Street	Everytown	41000		777—2435
STREET	POST OFFICE	ZIP CODE	DIRECTIONS	TELEPHONE NO.
STREET	POST OFFICE	ZIP CODE	DIRECTIONS	TELEPHONE NO.
STREET	POST OFFICE	ZIP CODE	DIRECTIONS	TELEPHONE NO.

HOUSEHOLD ROSTER

NAME (Individual)	ADM	Sex	Mar.	Rel.	B' date	Immunization Needed	SIGNIFICANT NOTES
Ernest III		M	M	H	3/5/50		
Gail		F	M	W	3/26/51		
Ernest IV		M	S	S	8/14/73		

OCCUPATION and/or SOURCE OF INCOME

8/73	Ernest III	Laborer

AGENCY, MEDICAL or OTHER RESOURCES

	Ernest III	Blue Cross
	Gail	Dr. A. OB
	Ernest IV	Dr. C. Ped.

FAMILY DATA CONTINUATION SHEET

FAMILY
NAME: <u>BROWN</u>

Date	
9/5/73	**HOME VISIT MADE**

9/5/73

HOME VISIT MADE

SOURCE OF REFERRAL:

Nursery at Pontiac General Hospital on first born infant discharged with thrush, mother borderline toxemia.

PURPOSE OF VISIT:

Followup receipt of referral and assess how mother is doing.

ENVIRONMENT:

Bilevel, older home. Clean & attractive.

SITUATION:

ERNEST IV: Birthdate, 8-14-73; birthweight, 6 lbs. 4 oz.; discharge weight, 6 lbs. 2 oz.; present weight, 6 lbs. 12 oz. On Enfamil, 4 oz. each feeding on demand (every 3-1/2 to 4-1/2 hours). Cereal will be started at 5-6 weeks.

Has pediatrician's appointment on 9-6-73. The physical assessment revealed good color, skin turgor and muscle tone, small spot of thrush still on tongue (medication continues to be taken), normal bowel movements, circumcision healed, cord off and healed, very small amount of cradle cap and no clear evidence of jaundice, genitalia in good condition, stools are normal. The soft spot was slightly puffy and is larger than normal for newborn baby. During the home visit, mother gave the baby his bath and discussed with PHN thermometer technique.

GAIL: Asked questions quite freely of PHN. She has to make an appointment for her six-week check-up. Had been borderline toxemic during pregnancy. Is supposed to be taking medication now but doesn't because it makes her sleepy and she doesn't want to feel that way during the day when she wants to be taking care of the baby. PHN to bring blood pressure cuff at next home visit. Discusses with PHN calling the doctor for either an order change or dosage change. Her flow has begun to stop. Will plan to discuss birth control with her doctor at her six week check-up.

NURSING ACTION:

1. Observed bath and discussed with mother different techniques. Noted

Date	
9/5/73 cont.	

that mother was very comfortable in handling the baby and used good technique when giving the baby his bath.

2. Explained physical assessment findings to the mother.
3. Left information on growth, Poison Control Center, and bottle feeding.
4. Noted the baby still has some thrush on his tongue and is still on medication.
5. Discussed blood pressure problem with mother and strongly encouraged her to call doctor for medication or dosage change.
6. Allowed mother to ventilate and provided supportive counseling.

NURSING DIAGNOSIS:

Young mother with apparent good adjustment. Normal newborn is gaining weight and needs to continue medical followup.

PLANS:

1. Revisit within one week to go over growth and development of baby.
2. Check mother's blood pressure and see if she has followed up by calling her doctor for any changes.
3. Check results of doctor's visit for the baby.

RESOURCES:

1. Dr. A., Ob-Gyn.
2. Dr. C., Pediatrician.

Family and neighbors have proven very helpful to this mother and frequently dropped in during the visit.

Jane Doe, PHN

9-11-73

Home Visit cancelled—PHN ill.
Rescheduled for 9-19-73.

Jane Doe, PHN

9-19-73

HOME VISIT MADE:

PURPOSE:

1. To take mother's blood pressure and discuss present status of medication treatment.
2. Discuss postpartum checkup.
3. Check the results of the baby's visit to the pediatrician.
4. Instruct and teach the growth and development and encourage questions.
5. Write mutual goals and set time limit to reevaluate these.

Date	
9/5/73 cont.	

ERNEST IV: SITUATION:

Next pediatrician appointment is 10-12-73. Pediatrician stated that he was doing fine and he now weighs 7 lbs. 3-1/2 oz. He is on cereals and will be starting fruits tomorrow. He had a rash on the inner thigh —air drying and different ways of healing this were discussed with the mother.

GAIL: Blood pressure taken during home visit—it was 117/80. She is off medication. She has her postpartum checkup this week. Birth control was discussed. Gail has questions ready for her obstetrician. Plans to return to work on 11-5-73. She works the afternoon shift at Pontiac Motors in the same building as her husband. Gail's mother will baby-sit for them.

ERNEST III: (Father). Mother stated his health is good. They do have an internist they could go to for his medical supervision.

NURSING ACTION:

1. Discuss growth and development of 1-1/2 month old with mother.
2. Together decided on the following goals to be evaluated in 11/73.

NURSING GOALS:

1. Evaluate blood pressure problem and supervise within the home.
2. Establish an effective birth control method that is safe for her.
3. Answer questions about growth and development.

PLANS: Gail:

1. Evaluate health status—medical supervision.

Ernest IV:

1. Follow for normal growth and development.
2. Teach regarding physical growth and development.
3. Start on an immunization routine.
4. Teach mother about creating a safe environment for him at home.

Jane Doe, PHN

10-10-73   HOME VISIT MADE:

PURPOSE OF VISIT:

1. Follow for normal growth and development.
2. Teach regarding physical growth and development.

Date	
9/5/73 cont.	
	3. Start on immunization routine.
	4. Teach about safety.
	5. Evaluate for transfer due to team realignment.
	SITUATION:
GAIL:	Was very interested in safety material and asked some questions about this during discussion with PHN.
	Discussed with PHN growth and development of two-to-three month old baby. Did not have many questions about this. In discussion about continuing PHN visit, stated she really didn't need the PHN visiting. This PHN concurs.
PLANS:	1. Write summary note.
	2. Close and reopen upon referral.
	Jane Doe, PHN
10-25-73	Record review. Concur with closing.
	B. Smith, Nursing Supervisor

FAMILY FOLDER SUMMARY SHEET

FAMILY
NAME: <u>BROWN, ERNEST III</u>

SUMMARY

10/16/73

REFERRAL:

Normal infant with thrush, mother borderline toxemia, thrush resolved, and mother exhibited good knowledge in infant care. Mother and baby doing well. Mother to return to work 11/73.

Jane Doe, PHN

PLANS: 1. Close
2. Reopen upon referral

CHAPTER 14

NURSING ROLE IN HOME HEALTH CARE

BEVERLY MEDEIROS GALLAGHER, M.S.N., R.N.

       The primary purpose of visiting persons in need of nursing care in the home is to provide skilled nursing care, which may be supplemented with other health services, to clients in their place of usual residence on an intermittent, or visiting, basis. The public, the health professions, and in particular those who require health services are increasingly recognizing the value of providing or receiving nursing care in the home. It is frequently less expensive, often preferable to institutional care, and more comfortable, both physically and psychologically, because care is provided to clients in familiar surroundings. Health and illness teaching has the potential for being far more effective when patients and families are instructed and evaluated in their usual home environment. This chapter will primarily consider nursing care provided by home health agencies, which the National League for Nursing defines as agencies which provide multidisciplinary health care to the sick, the disabled, and the injured in their place of residence.[1]

Some of the common types of home health agencies are visiting nursing associations, home care units of hospitals, private home health agencies, and home health units of official health departments or combination agencies. The agency may be of the nonofficial, nonprofit type, governed by a board of directors and financially supported by third party payments, fees, and donations, such as a visiting nurse association. Official health departments and combination agencies, which have characteristics of both official and nonofficial agencies, also provide home health care. Proprietary agencies, which are profit making, are another source of home health services. Regardless of the type of agency which provides the service, nurses involved in home health care primarily care for individuals and families who have diseases or disabilities. This type of care is known as morbidity care. Some clients may have terminal illnesses and thus require support in their wishes to die at home. Families and individuals are helped through the grieving process and are assisted by the nurse to die as comfortably as possible. The role of the home health nurse, however, is also one of case finding, health promotion, and preventive health care for the family, as well as the usual nursing functions of referral and collaboration. Community health nurses who primarily provide morbidity care may also care for well individuals, depending on the needs of the community.

Clients who receive nursing care in the home are usually either homebound or have nursing needs which can best be met in this setting. A common misconception is that nursing services in the home are restricted to low income groups. The majority of the nurse's caseload may well consist of low income individuals, but this is partly because low income groups have proportionately more frequent and more severe episodes of illness than do higher income groups.[2] Also, visiting nursing began as a service primarily for the sick, poor population. Unfortunately, this image has prevailed and may cause higher income groups to be reluctant to accept or refer themselves for home health services. If the nursing service is not restricted to a certain group, such as those affiliated with a certain hospital, charity, or outpatient department, then the service should be available to all members of the community, regardless of income.

Thus the nursing care of persons in the home involves a variety of services and is provided under the auspices of a number of different types of agencies. Regardless of the type of service provided, the community health nurse involved with home care functions as a coordinator, a teacher, and a provider of direct patient care. Nursing care in the home does not just involve helping persons to get well again; many times home care means helping persons to die. Unquestionably, the popularity of caring for persons in the home is rapidly increasing, as many have come to realize that it is often preferable, more economical, and more effective than institutional care.

HISTORICAL DEVELOPMENT

EUROPE

In one manner or another, people have always cared for the sick. This practice can be traced back to primitive man by the deciphering of carvings and cave paintings. One can assume that the most knowledgeable people cared for or advised the sick in other households, but whether this care was provided in a manner which even resembled visiting nursing is unknown.

The Jewish people felt a strong personal and social responsibility for the care of the sick and the less fortunate. Visiting the sick was considered a duty, and the care of the sick was a service extended to both Jews and Gentiles alike.

The care of the sick by those of different households is known to have been practiced extensively during the time of Christ and for many years thereafter under the auspices of the Christian church. The neighbors of the sick are known to have visited and sought assistance for the sick. Early in the Christian era, human sympathy influenced a number of groups to visit the sick and the less fortunate. The first known organized home visitation of the sick began when the Christian church established orders of deaconesses who had specific responsibility for the care of the needy poor. To these first nurses, it was a pleasure to be able to execute the duties of the church and to demonstrate publicly their support for the teachings of Christ. These orders were active until the fifth and sixth centuries when monasteries assumed the major responsibility for the care of the sick. Visiting nursing was an integral part of the monastery services and special funds were appropriated for the visitation of the sick. The nurses felt a holy calling for their work. Their care was of a purely palliative nature, to relieve suffering, not to cure or prevent disease. Since there was not yet a profession of nursing, no standardized training was required for nursing practice. It was based on love, sympathy, and religious enthusiasm. Throughout the Christian era, nursing care in the home remained an important activity.

After the fall of the Roman Empire, Europe became a barbaric land, with war the usual state of affairs. From 600 to 1600 A.D. there was little organization in the care of the sick. Religious and military nursing orders were established which were exclusive, primarily attracting women of noble birth. To many of these women, the care of the sick was not the most important reason to engage in nursing practice; such an activity was also a means of atonement for one's sins. Although the care of the sick in the home was an unscientific and disorganized practice for which nurses were not properly educated, these early attempts should not be criticized. Brainard,[3] instead, suggests that we admire the great self sacrifice of these women who attempted to provide a nursing service under the worst conditions.

In the beginning of the 17th century, there was an awakened consciousness concerning the suffering of the unfortunate. Those with more resources felt a responsibility toward helping the poor and the sick. The prevailing attitude toward the underprivileged changed to one of attempting to understand the causes of such indigence and illness. Many women who lacked the necessary preparation for nursing responded to this concern by attempting to provide nursing care to needy individuals in the community.

St. Vincent de Paul significantly improved the quality of home nursing care by insisting that educational preparation was necessary and by discouraging the indiscriminate giving of material goods. He believed that such indiscriminate giving could even be deleterious. St. Vincent established the Sisters of Charity in 1633. This was a nursing order which devoted much effort to the care of the sick in the home and one which remains active today.

By the 18th century in Europe, many endeavors had demonstrated the benefit and necessity of having nurses in the community who cared for the sick in the home. According to Brainard,[3] the following factors influenced the growth of home nursing care during this period:

1. The new social consciousness to the appalling conditions in which mankind lived and the realization that those who were more fortunate had a responsibility to help the sick and the poor.
2. The growth of medicine from a purely palliative and curative service to one which had preventive aspects to it. The concepts of sanitation, hygiene, and inoculation helped to foster this change.
3. Nursing care had changed from a service which involved the uneducated and inexpert care of the sick into a profession with rules and regulations governing its practice.

Florence Nightingale, born in 1820, did much to improve nursing care in the home by proving the necessity and benefit of education for nursing practice. Ms. Nightingale was the first person to insist that nursing, and especially visiting nursing, was not amateur work. Her students were taught about preventive health and health maintenance, as well as about the cure and care of diseases. She had some ideas about community health nursing which were quite profound for the time, as she stressed that the health of individuals depended upon the health of the community and vice versa. Instead of giving her students some rather vague ideas about the care of the sick, she taught by a clear framework based on scientific principles which demonstrated that there was a process to nursing practice.

In 1859 nursing care in the home expanded further when Mr. William Rathbone of England founded a nursing service much like the present day visiting nurse associations. Previous attempts of organizations had included visiting nursing as part of their activities, but this visiting was not the sole purpose of the organization, as was Rathbone's. The nurses were taught some quite modern principles based on Ms. Nightingales's philosophy of nursing. With the development of this service, nursing care in the home grew from a few charitable endeavors by philanthropists or religious organizations to a well recognized community service. Increasingly, more communities were recognizing the necessity of having a home nursing service.

When the Pilgrims left for America in 1620, nursing care in Europe was provided primarily by Catholic sisters. The care of individuals in the home was just beginning to be recognized as a valuable service. Thus, the Pilgrims came to America with little knowledge of nursing care, although the need for health services was great. In some colonies a large majority of the residents died from illnesses during their first year. During the 17th, 18th, and early 19th centuries, kind but untrained women cared for the ill, and few efforts were made to establish services to provide care in the home. One of the earliest organized home visiting services was the Ladies Benevolent Society of Charleston, South Carolina, established in 1813. Development of this service was stimulated by the health needs resulting from the War of 1812 and a yellow fever epidemic in 1813. These care providers were not trained nurses but were kind, charitable women. Much effort was directed to seeking employment for their clients instead of the continual distribution of material relief. This service was the first one known in America by which the sick and the poor were visited on an intermittent basis in their homes, as all clients are today.

The alarming social and health conditions of the 19th century certainly exemplified the need for health services in the home. Epidemics were severe and frequent. Industrialization, urbanization, and immigration increased the morbidity and mortality rates. Yellow fever, typhus, and cholera were common diseases. During this period, Americans continued to be concerned about the atrocious social and health problems. Winslow, a prominent public health historian, noted that the emphasis had finally turned to helping people rather than things.[4]

The Women's Board of the New York City Mission in 1877 established a home nursing service, based on the principle that a nurse could minister to the sick person's bodily ills, just as the missionaries did to one's spiritual ills. These efforts were so successful that other services were soon organized.

Two of the earliest autonomous associations which provided nursing care in the home were the Boston Instructive District Visiting Nurse Association (1886) and the Visiting Nurse Service of Philadelphia (1886).[5] These associations were established by the efforts of nurses and private citizens to provide skilled nursing services to the sick poor in the home. Interested, well-to-do citizens recognized the needs of the less fortunate citizens and assumed a major role in donating and securing the monies necessary to establish and maintain such services, similar to the manner in which some voluntary agencies are supported today.

By the end of the 19th century, a number of communities had established home nursing services. Some services were under the auspices of the Church, others were autonomous, and some were managed by charitable agencies. Visiting nurses often became specialists in tuberculosis control, infant welfare, school nursing, or rural health. The public and the medical profession strongly supported home nursing care. Winslow believed that the nurse in the home was the most important figure in the public health movement, since half of the infant deaths were preventable by the services of a nurse in the home.[4] By 1910 there were over 1902 agencies which provided home nursing services.[6] This increase was not without concern, however, since there were not yet mechanisms for quality assurance of these services. A national organization was needed to help establish and enforce standards of care. In June 1912, the National Organization for Public Health Nursing was thus established to stimulate and to standardize public health nursing practice.

Following World War I, nursing care services in the home expanded rapidly and enthusiastically. With such growth, the need to determine what the educational preparation should be for this group of nurses became even more apparent. Some agencies provided inservice education programs. The Instructive District Visiting Nurse Association of Boston in 1906 was one of the first agencies to offer a postgraduate course specifically for nurses who practiced home care.[7] Soon after, many universities established similar programs for the postgraduate education of public health nurses. By 1925 the recommended preparation for public health nursing practice was a high school education and a nursing education which included both theory and practice in public health nursing.

The Depression came in 1929 when community health nursing agencies were at their height. Unemployment rates increased; ill families presented the visiting nurses with numerous social problems in addition to the usual nursing problems. Voluntary agencies had to be more selective about the type of services they offered and to whom they offered them. Health promotion and health education, always a priority in the past, had to be ignored. The standards of community health nursing which took so long to develop were indeed in jeopardy. Gardner states that by well meaning ignorance most of the underlying principles of visiting were violated. An example of this is that on occasion, nurses were engaged in relief giving without the usual thorough investigation of the financial needs of the family. Before the Depression, relief was only offered by public health nurses after its necessity was confirmed.

The Social Security Act was passed in 1935. Among its benefits was the allocation of funds for the financial support of the education of nurses employed in community health practice. This funding helped to strengthen the educational status of community health nurses by financing their education.

Nursing care in the home was affected by World War II just as were other types of nursing practice. Nurses were needed by the thousands each month to serve in the military. Many volunteered. Communities recognized the value of having a home nursing service and believed that it was just as important to keep nurses in their community as it was out in the field with the military. Voluntary agencies continued to struggle financially to survive. This group became involved in morbidity type care, while the official agencies became active primarily in preventive care and health promotion. This pattern remains in many communities today.

During the 1950s and 1960s, home health agencies began to expand the scope of their services. The health team grew in numbers and in types of professionals and nonprofessionals. Medical knowledge was greater. Multidisciplinary teams were used in home health agencies. There were changes in the recommended educational preparation of community health nurses during this period. Baccalaureate programs began to include both theoretical and clinical content of community health nursing. By 1964 the American Nurses' Association defined a public health nurse as a graduate of at least a baccalaureate nursing program.

Another significant force which has had a profound effect on nursing care in the home is the institution of Medicare and Medicaid in 1965. It seems likely that the issue of who will pay for whom and what will continue to be a strong determinant of the quality, scope, and delivery of home health services.

Undoubtedly, the provision of nursing care in the home is not a new type of service at all. Visiting the sick, the unfortunate, and those in need of nursing care at home is practiced with many of the same motives and often a similar philosophy as it was nearly two millennia ago. According to Fitzpatrick, caring for the sick in the home was the first type of nursing service—the very origin of nursing—and perhaps even the oldest human service known to mankind.

PREPARATION FOR PRACTICE

The educational preparation of a group of nurses significantly influences the type and the quality of the nursing care that the group is able to provide. As a group, nurses undoubtedly have much closer personal contact with more of the public than do other members of the health team; thus, it is critical that community health nurses are adequately prepared for their roles.

Home health nursing, like other areas of community health nursing practice, involves the prevention of illness and the promotion and maintenance of health.[8] Because nursing care is provided in the home, the home health nurse is regularly involved in providing nursing care to families and significant others as well as to individual clients. The nature of home health care puts nurses in situations where they must be able to make independent judgments and act interdependently in the home. The home health nurse may have much less support for her judgments by other health professionals than the nurse employed in an institutional setting. The community health nurse caring for persons at home implements the nursing process without the continual presence and assistance of other health professionals.

To fulfill these functions, home health community nursing practice requires that the nurse apply knowledge from the natural sciences, the social sciences, and the humanities, as well as from nursing education. A baccalaureate nursing education, which includes community health nursing theory and practice, is the appropriate educational preparation for home health nursing practice at the staff level.[9] One of the primary purposes of baccalaureate education, to prepare a beginning nurse to provide health care to persons, families, and groups in a variety of settings by use of the nursing process with humanistic and scientific concepts,[10] is a statement similar to the role description of community health nursing practice according to the American Nurses' Association. This statement describes community health nursing as a practice which is general and comprehensive, including all ages and diagnostic groups, and directed to individuals in families and groups. The nurse integrates the biologic, psychological, and social sciences, and knowledge of nursing, community, and ecology.[8]

Another issue which affects nursing education according to Ozimek is the current emphasis on prevention of illness, the maintenance and restoration of health, and the education of people to live more healthful lives. She further believes that one of the greatest challenges of health professionals is caring for an affluent, educated society who is informed and sophisticated about its health problems.[11] Because community health nurses who care for clients in the home continually relate to persons of many different ages, socioeconomic groups, and cultural groups, they need to have extensive preparation in the social sciences. A baccalaureate education, with its emphasis on problem solving and self-direction as well as its strong behavioral science content, best helps the nurse to prepare for this type of role.

Instead of specifically emphasizing the number of years of basic education or the actual degree that the community health nurse should have, the World Health Organization Expert Committee on Community Health Nursing emphasizes the *type of orientation* of the program from which the nurse has graduated. The Committee believes that community health nurses are best educated by a people oriented, not institution oriented curriculum, which emphasizes health, not disease. The Committee recommends that the entire program be community and health oriented, with disease and institutional care regarded as mere episodes in an individual's life span. [12] Although a number of nursing curricula have changed to have a health focus, the majority of nurses who are now considered prepared for community health practice since they hold a baccalaureate degree in nursing may well have been educated in a disease oriented curriculum. The fact that perhaps the majority of nursing graduates have been educated in this manner has implications for the type of inservice education programs that community home health agencies may wish to offer. Many staff may benefit from additional knowledge of concepts of health promotion and preventive health care.

Since 1937, the United States Public Health Service and the Department of Public Health in each state have cooperatively compiled periodic data regarding the educational preparation, along with a number of other characteristics, of public health nurses. The study has increased in depth and scope and is currently undertaken biennially. The fact that this costly and time consuming study continues to be executed in such depth reflects the importance of the service of community health nurses to the nation. The most recent educational survey was in 1972 in which the educational level of a projected number of 57,000 registered community health nurses was surveyed. The author considered statistics which pertain to groups of nurses for whom home health care is a primary function. These groups include nurses employed in combination, voluntary, and organized home health agencies.

By comparing the results of the Public Health Survey of 1972 with the recommended standards for professional nursing practice according to the National League for Nursing, [13] it is clear that the majority (66 percent) of the nurses under consideration did not at this time meet these standards. [14] The amount of preparation varies among agencies; combination and voluntary agencies have the highest percentages of staff meeting the recommended educational standards. Regarding regional differences, the western part of the country had the highest percentage of completely prepared nurses; the southern states had the lowest. [14] Although the majority of nurses who engage in home health care do not meet the recommended standards for their role, one must recognize that educational preparation is only one of many factors which determines the quality of nursing care rendered. One should not infer that the nursing care that these nurses provide is inferior. Many of these nurses and administrators may have broadened their understanding of community health nursing by other means, such as by participation in continuing education programs, workshops, or management courses. They may have learned a second language, necessary for their work with clients, and perhaps they have had many years of experience. One's life experiences, such as exposure to other cultures or experience with child rearing, similarly enrich community health nursing practice.

Recognizing the need for assisting community health nurses to prepare themselves for their role, the Public Health Service offers Public Health Special Purpose Traineeships to enable registered nurses to complete a baccalaureate program. The program awards money to nursing students who agree to pursue a career in community health.

There also are a number of innovative home health care programs that demand that home health community nurses be completely prepared for their roles. One example is the use of community health nurses with extended assessment skills, often called nurse practitioners. Such a nurse who worked in a rural area in Iowa was of much value to the entire community. [15] For a number of her elderly clients, the process of making a clinic appointment, getting to the clinic, sitting in the waiting room, and then returning home several hours later was too difficult to manage on their own. The persons who have the most difficulty may well be those who most need health care. A primary care provider, such as a visiting nurse practitioner, also can be of much value to the nursing staff of the home health agency by functioning as a consultant and a staff educator, as well as a provider of direct patient care. The employment of the nurse practitioner is also another manner by which home health agencies can help better prepare the nursing staff for their roles.

Thus, although the educational preparation of the group of community health nurses surveyed by the Public Health Service differs from the standards for professional nursing practice recommended by the National League for Nursing [13] and by the Council on Health Manpower, [9] one must recognize that the educational preparation of a group is only one measure of its preparedness. Moreover, there are a number of alternatives available which can help nurses to prepare themselves for home health nursing practice.

SCOPE OF HOME HEALTH SERVICES

During the past 10 years, there has been a steady increase in the number of agencies which offer nursing services in the home. Geographically, more individuals now have these services available. In 1963, only 56 percent of the American population had access to these services, with 1163 agencies providing home health care. By 1972, the comparable figures were 92 percent of the population, with 3151 agencies. [14] A number of agencies were established after the Medicare and Medicaid programs were instituted in 1965 since these programs authorized reimbursement of fees to the agencies. When reviewing these figures, it is important to note that the availability of home health services varies greatly among different geographic areas. In some communities, 100 percent of the population has access to these services; in others, only 7 percent. [14] For example, urban residents may have a variety of options as to the agency from which they receive home health care: the visiting nurse association; the home care department of the local hospital; or a private agency. In contrast, the rural resident may have no home health services available. Since 1962, however, the trend has been to establish home health services in less developed rural areas where there previously have been none. The availability of home health services also varies considerably with the extent of urbanization. As the size of the community and the extent of development increase, so does the likelihood of the community's having the services of a home health agency. [14]

Where Home Health Services Are Provided

The primary purpose of a home health agency is to provide nursing care to individuals and families in their place of residence on a visiting basis. However, many agencies offer services in settings other than in the home, such as in senior citizen centers, social service agencies, schools, well child clinics, and industrial sites. Some nurses primarily involved in home care are employed part-time in institutions to coordinate the discharges of prospective clients. The extent to which nurses engage in nursing practices in addition to home care depends on the availability of other nursing services in the community. Urban communities tend to have a number of different agencies to meet their health needs and thus may not need the services of the home health nurse in settings other than the home. In rural areas, the nurse may have to assume a number of roles. Thus, although nurses primarily concerned with home health care are seen most in that setting, they also may provide other types of community health nursing care.

Types of Services Provided

The 1972 survey by the Public Health Service indicated that a great majority of home visits by community health nurses were made to care for sick patients, and that these clients required a greater number of both services and visits by nurses and other health team members than the care of essentially healthy clients. [14]

In 1973, the National League for Nursing surveyed urban home health agencies regarding the type, length, and cost of care which clients required over a period of three months. Sixty-three percent of the clients were 65 years of age or older; one quarter lived alone. Most clients had been referred to the home health agencies by institutions. Half received care primarily from private physicians, and half used clinics or group health organizations. Circulatory disorders were the most common diagnosis, with neoplasms second. Allergic, endocrine, metabolic, and nutritional disorders were the next most frequent problems for which clients needed home health care. [16] On the basis of these surveys, one can infer that much of home health care involves the care of an ill client who is over 65 years of age. Because these clients receive these services, they are able to remain living in their own homes or may be able to return home from the hospital at an earlier date.

Health professionals employed in home health agencies work closely with professionals employed in institutions which refer clients to the home health agencies. The primary health provider determines the client's medical needs, and ideally the hospital staff, home health agency staff, client, and family jointly determine what types of services will be needed from the community. In some agencies, nurses of the home health agency spend several hours weekly coordinating the discharge of the client from the hospital to the community. After the client's health needs have been determined, the client is instructed regarding care. Typical activities of the home health agency nurse in the home are instructing clients in their physical care, helping them to cope with the difficulties they suffer as a result of illness, obtaining necessary supplies and equipment, and referring clients to other appropriate resources in the community. If the client has a family, they, too, are included, as appropriate. The community health nurse is legally responsible for reporting any changes in the condition of the client to the primary health provider. In addition to the above, the nurse also acts as advisor to the client and family concerning health maintenance. Frequently, many serious health problems of family members are unknown until the community health nurse, working in the home, identifies them. The community health nurse who provides nursing care in the home, regardless of the type of care given, serves as coordinator, teacher, counselor, and sometimes as direct care provider, although her focus varies according to the health needs of the family.

Types of Agencies Which Provide Home Health Services

Agencies which provide nursing care in the home are of many types. Among the more common of these are the voluntary (nonofficial, nonprofit); the official (tax supported, nonprofit); the combination (supported by taxes and fees, nonprofit); and the proprietary (private, for profit). The structure of the agency significantly determines the types of services and programs it offers and thus is an important consideration for the community health nurse.

THE VOLUNTARY AGENCY

The voluntary agency is supported by nontax funds such as fees, third party payments, income from investments, and charities such as the United Fund. Third party payments may be from official sources such as Medicare and Medicaid, private insurance companies, or other voluntary agencies such as cancer societies and heart associations. The type of financial support received varies among agencies and is significantly determined by the population served. For example an agency in a higher income community may be supported mostly by private insurance payments, whereas it is not unusual for the voluntary home health agencies in lower income communities to be supported primarily by Medicare and Medicaid funds.

Because voluntary agencies are governed by a board of directors instead of by legislation (as official and in part combination agencies are), they have considerably more freedom than do official agencies in determining their programs, providing that they keep within the requirements for licensure, certification, and accreditation. Voluntary agencies began in this country for the purpose of responding to the needs of the community, and many continue to enjoy this flexibility. The voluntary home health agency may have responsibility for a city, town, or perhaps a county. In sparsely populated rural communities, the home health agency may be responsible for a number of towns. In recent years, many small voluntary agencies have been forced to merge with each other to meet the needs of the consumer and the standards of quality imposed upon them. The voluntary agency is privately governed by a board of directors composed of interested community citizens.

Community health nurses employed in voluntary agencies can expect their services will be paid for by clients, third party payers, and charities, unless the services are free. Clients who have no insurance benefits nor sufficient financial means to pay for home health care are eligible for free services in many agencies.

THE OFFICIAL AGENCY

Home health services which are under the auspices of official agencies are provided at the local level. These agencies are financially supported by tax funds and official monies which may be granted for a specific purpose, such as for a program to increase the number of immunized persons in the community. Official home health services are administered by the local board of health or health officer in the community. Like voluntary agencies, official agencies may be responsible for more than one town or city. There has been a trend toward the merger of small official agencies to better meet the needs of communities. The activities of the community health nurse employed by an official agency are under the control of the local or county government. Some of the services that this nurse provides in addition to home health care may be of the type mandated by law, such as communicable disease control. For example, the nurse may spend her mornings caring for clients in the home and her afternoons assisting with an immunization program.

THE COMBINATION AGENCY

The combination agency is jointly administered by a board of directors as well as by local governmental authorities who are involved in the health care of that community. Financial support is by taxes, fees, endowments, third party payments, and perhaps federal grants. This type of agency is a combination of the voluntary and the official agency which have combined to provide more effective health care. The community health nurse employed in a combination agency will be providing some services for which clients or third party payers may be billed. Other services, of the type mandated by law, will be free. The community health nurse who is employed in a combination agency may have the opportunity to practice a variety of types of nursing care in addition to home health care, such as well child care, tuberculosis case finding and control, or teaching nutrition to senior citizens. The nurse's role may consist of caring for both sick and well clients.

THE PROPRIETARY AGENCY

The proprietary agency is profit making as opposed to the three types of nonprofit agencies which have been described. Proprietary agencies are owned by an individual or a group which directly receives the profits from the income of the agency. (A nonprofit agency must return excess income for agency use after expenses are met.) A proprietary agency can be reimbursed by Medicare funds if it is established in a state with a licensure law and if it has been licensed. A proprietary agency is reimbursed with Medicaid funds according to state regulations. Although proprietary agencies have been under scrutiny to ensure that they deliver services of adequate quality since all of them may not be under regulations, there is no valid evidence that one type of agency provides higher or lower quality care than another.[17] In fact, because proprietary agencies may not be under regulation by Medicare and Medicaid, they may be able to be even more accommodating to their consumers.

Home Health Team Members

Home health care often requires the services of a number of disciplines. As greater numbers of more seriously ill and disabled individuals are discharged earlier from the hospital, one can expect to see increased demands upon home health agencies. In a National League for Nursing survey,[16] nearly one quarter of the cases reviewed regarding the care of the sick in urban communities required the services of health care providers in addition to nursing. Physical therapy and home health aide services were needed by nearly 12 percent of the sample. The sample consisted of mostly elderly, ill individuals and thus the need for physical therapy and home health services is partially explained. However, since the majority of home health care does involve this population, this survey does provide a valid view of home health services. If the population had been younger, healthier, and in need of preventive or promotive care, nutritionists and social workers would probably be the more active disciplines.

The value of the services of a homemaker-home health aide is particularly important to recognize because it is often this care which really enables the individual to remain at home, outside of an institution.

Homemaker-home health aides are nonprofessionals who have been trained both to care for the home and to provide personal care. Homemakers are nonprofessionals who only care for the home and do not give personal care. This distinction between roles is frequently confused by consumers and providers of health care, but it is an important one to understand.

Undoubtedly, all of the many services of the health care team contribute to an individual's well being, but it is the home health aide who, under the supervision of a community health nurse, provides for most of the individual's basic needs. Typical activities of the aide are:

promoting the client's personal hygiene; encouraging compliance with medical and nursing orders; doing light housework; shopping; preparing meals; and reporting changes in the client's condition to the nurse. Homemaker-home health aides may also work with healthy families when a parent is ill or absent.

Health team members who often are needed to care for persons in the home in addition to nurses, physical therapists, and home health aides are nutritionists, occupational therapists, speech therapists, physicians, and social workers. Services may be arranged for by contractual agreement with other agencies. The number of services an agency offers has been found to increase as the size of the nursing staff of the agency increases.[14] In some cases, nursing may be the only service required, but some clients may require all services. Frequently, the professionals employed in a home health agency act only as consultants to each other and thus do not provide direct patient care.

Services which supplement professional services, in addition to those of the home health aide, are meals-on-wheels programs, the home delivery of medications and supplies, patient transportation services, chore services, homemaking services, and dental and podiatry care.

The following case history is known to the author and serves to demonstrate the use and integration of health services in the home:

Mrs. Mary Smith was a 28-year-old woman who was hospitalized for evaluation of more frequent and severe exacerbations of rheumatoid arthritis. She and her husband had three young children. Mr. Smith was employed and received an adequate income. Mrs. Smith was to be discharged on a new treatment program of chemotherapy, physical therapy, and occupational therapy. Although she felt symptomatically better as she approached discharge, she was considered to be an appropriate candidate for home health care since her disease was a chronic one with remissions and exacerbations. The coordinated services of many health team members were necessary.

Discharge planning began when a nurse who spent several hours weekly coordinating hospital discharges with home health services arranged a conference with the Smiths, their physician, a social worker, a physical therapist, hospital staff nurses, and the community health nurse who would care for the family after discharge.

The following activities resulted from this conference and the subsequent care the family received:

1. The community health nurse, the physical therapist, and the occupational therapist visited the home prior to Mrs. Smith's discharge to adapt her surroundings to her needs. A raised toilet seat and safety bars around the toilet were installed. The height of the bed was changed, a bedboard added, and furniture rearranged to promote energy conservation.
2. With the family's agreement, the services of a homemaker-home health aide were instituted upon discharge to help with child care, personal care, and the care of the home. The frequency of the visits was adjusted according to the family's needs.
3. The community health nurse, who served as coordinator of her care, believed that a priority of her nursing care was to ascertain that the family thoroughly understood the disease process and that their expectations were realistic. The nurse helped the Smiths to adjust their daily schedules so as to conserve Mrs. Smith's energy. The nurse also emphasized the importance of the family's preserving their close relationship despite the stress of a chronic illness. She was equally concerned that the health needs of other family members not be forgotten.

4. A social worker from the home health agency visited the family to suggest a number of alternatives for coping with the financial and emotional problems which this illness imposed. The social worker alerted the family to the types of difficulties that they might encounter during this crisis, and she was able to suggest some realistic means of coping with them. The social worker helped the family to identify and build upon their strengths. A conference was arranged with the Smiths, the social worker, and the children's school teachers so that the teachers would be aware of the stress the children were experiencing.

5. The occupational therapist and physical therapist visited as needed to reassess Mrs. Smith's needs.

After these many services were begun and were well established, the professionals adjusted the frequency of their visits as needed. The services of the homemaker-home health aide remained most important to the family. The Smiths were most satisfied with the home health services that they received and agreed that Mr. Smith would not have been able to remain employed and that the family would not have had the opportunity to remain together as a family without these services.

LEGAL AND QUALITY CONTROL CONSIDERATIONS

There are three processes of importance to home health agencies which affect the characteristics of their services by regulating the type and quality of services that the agency offers. They are licensure, certification, and accreditation. All three activities are concerned with the promotion of quality home health care, regarding either the agency as a whole or the individual practitioner. In a time when both consumers and providers of health services are demanding higher quality and more accessible health care, it is important that community health nurses understand these processes and their respective implications.

Licensure

Licensure is a legal requirement which each individual state has the option of requiring for the home health agencies in that state. (Registered nurses must be licensed to practice nursing in that state according to state licensure laws and nurse practice acts.) An agency in a state which requires licensure must meet specific standards of licensure and be licensed. When statistics regarding licensure were compiled by the Department of Health, Education, and Welfare in July 1977, 18 states had licensure laws. Seven other states were considering licensure.[18] Agencies which provide health care in the home and licensure are licensed by each state's department of health or board of licensure. The actual standards for licensure are established by each state but consider many of the same types of factors as do the federal Medicare regulations. The opportunity to be licensed is particularly important to proprietary agencies since they cannot be reimbursed for services by Medicare funds without being licensed.

Although the licensing of agencies is one means of quality assurance, less than half of the states have such laws. Perhaps there will be an increase in the number of states with this law as the number of home health agencies increases. A consistent means of monitoring the types and quality of services available may become necessary, since home health services are not always so visible as institutional care. The uniform licensure of agencies is one means of standardizing the quality of care.

Certification

The second activity which affects home health nursing services is certification. There are two types of certification processes which are of importance. The first type refers to the American Nurses' Association certification program which awards certificates to individual nurses who have voluntarily demonstrated excellence in their specific area of practice. The second type of certification to be considered is the federal certification program by which agencies must be certified if they wish to receive reimbursement from Medicare.

CERTIFICATION OF THE INDIVIDUAL PRACTITIONER

The American Nurses' Association certification program is a voluntary process by which nurses are recognized for their demonstration of high standards of nursing practice. The nurse who qualifies is issued a certificate which indicates that she has met the necessary criteria regarding both achievement and performance in a specific area of nursing practice. (Licensure as a registered nurse signifies that the nurse has met the minimum standards of safe, effective practice. Certification further indicates that the individual is both knowledgeable and able to properly apply that knowledge.) Nurses are certified for five years if they meet the criteria and may be recertified thereafter if the standards continue to be met. As home health care expands, the quality of these services needs to be assured. Certification for excellence in community health nursing practice helps to raise the quality of care rendered by stimulating growth in professional knowledge and by fostering the application of this expertise.

CERTIFICATION OF THE AGENCY

Requiring certification of agencies that wish to receive Medicare funds is another means of promoting high quality care. In 1966 the 89th Congress of the United States passed Title XVIII, the Medicare amendment to the Social Security Act of 1935, which provides federal medical and hospital insurance for the aged and disabled. Some home health agencies, particularly voluntary agencies, may well receive the majority of their financial support by official third party payers such as Medicare and Medicaid. In order to be eligible to receive reimbursement from Medicare, an agency must meet the federally determined Medicare requirements and thus be *Medicare certified*. The latest requirements for Medicare certification of home health agencies have been written by the Department of Health and Human Services and consider the following factors:

1. The structure of the agency. As mentioned previously, profit-making agencies receive Medicare funds only if licensed.
2. The agency's requirements for the education and experience of the employees.
3. The government of the agency. The agency must have a professional advisory committee to determine the activities, functions, and organization of the agency.
4. The specific provisions for supervision of agency staff.
5. The existence of a means for determining and evaluating the budget, the capital expenditures, and the financial structure of the agency.
6. The existence of a clear, specific plan of treatment for clients. Some of the factors that the plan must include are the diagnoses, mental status, types of services involved, equipment requirements, frequency of visits, rehabilitation potential, prognoses, nutritional status, medications, and necessary therapies for the client.

7. A clear statement of the expectations and practices of each member of the health team.
8. A plan regarding supervision and functions of home health aides.
9. A protocol for the conformance of the health team with the physician's orders and provisions for the periodic review of this plan. [19]

The states of Massachusetts, Connecticut, New Jersey, Rhode Island, and Oregon have additional standards for some of these items which are higher than those stated above. Certification is another process which helps to monitor the quality of home health services of the agencies which participate in the Medicare program.

Accreditation

Another means of promoting high quality home health care is by accreditation, a voluntary evaluation program initiated in 1966. The program is jointly executed by the American Public Health Association and the National League for Nursing. It is available to organizations which offer nursing care and related services to individuals outside of institutions. The agency seeking accreditation is evaluated against its own stated purposes and its efforts to meet the health needs of the community which it serves. Some of the major purposes of accreditation are the following:

1. To promote improvement in community health services, with coordination and integration of health care.
2. To promote experimentation and innovation in providing services and in the optimum use of manpower.
3. To help consumers, potential staff, and educational programs in identifying agencies which are concerned with high quality health services.
4. To encourage self-study and self-evaluation in community health agencies. [1]

The criteria for accreditation have been established by a number of health professionals who are experts in home health care and community health nursing services. The criteria are revised as necessary by representatives from a number of health disciplines. The accreditation process begins with an extensive self-study period by the agency and the writing of a self-study report. Thereafter, a site visit is made by representatives of the program to confirm or expand upon the data of the report. A decision is then made about the granting of accreditation. If accredited, an agency must submit interim reports every three years; the entire process is repeated every five years. As of May 1977, there were nationally 81 home health agencies accredited by this program. [20]

In summary, licensure, certification, and accreditation are three processes which promote the monitoring and regulation of home health services. It is important to recognize, however, that since there is not a licensure law in every state and since not every agency has to meet Medicare certification standards unless it wishes to participate in the Medicare program, there is no uniform means for controlling the quality of home health care. This issue should be of concern to community health nurses, since there may be a number of agencies for whom there is no means of quality control.

LEGISLATION AFFECTING NURSING CARE IN THE HOME

There are several major pieces of legislation which significantly influence the delivery of home health care. This legislation helps to improve and expand services, monitor the quality of services, finance programs, and prepare staff to provide health care in the home. The following are among the major pieces of legislation.

Medicare

Medicare, Title XVIII of the Social Security Act of 1935, provides up to 200 yearly home visits to a client who has been certified by a physician as needing professional home health services. Part A of Medicare is hospitalization insurance which pays for 100 home health visits within a 12 month period *after* a hospitalization in a hospital or skilled nursing facility for at least three days. Part B is supplementary medical insurance which pays for 100 additional home health visits within the calendar year. The client is not billed for the covered home health services and thus does not have to make cash payments to the agency. In order to receive Medicare benefits for home health services, the client has to meet the following criteria:

1. The services must be ordered by a physician and the client must be under the care of a physician.
2. The services must involve care which is of a skilled nature. The client's health problems must require skilled professional care.
3. The client must be homebound.
4. The client must satisfy the three day institutionalization requirement if he uses Part A of Medicare.
5. The client's condition must be unstable. There must be a health problem that requires continual reassessment, treatment, and evaluation.
6. The agency from which the client receives care must be certified by Medicare. [19]

For many older and disabled Americans, Medicare is inadequate for coverage of their home health needs. An individual who has only Part A coverage and who has not been institutionalized cannot receive benefits. An individual who requires home health care but who can be somewhat self-sufficient in leaving home cannot receive benefits. For elderly or disabled persons who can just barely do their own marketing and whose ability to still do so is of great importance, there are no home health benefits. There is also a restriction on the number of visits an individual can receive by a home health agency; an individual who suffered from a chronic illness could use all of his benefits and still require services. Medicare will also not pay for the services of a home health aide unless the client also requires nursing care, physical therapy, or speech therapy.

However, to many individuals Medicare benefits have been a tremendous help. Although the benefits are restricted to individuals and to agencies which meet specific criteria, the program is excellent for eligible consumers and providers. The benefits include payment for certain supplies, equipment, and a variety of professional health services such as physical therapy, occupational therapy, speech therapy, and the services of a nutritionist and social worker. For many home health agencies, the guaranteed payment by Medicare has allowed expansion in the size and scope of agencies and services. Medicare representatives periodically monitor participating agencies to ascertain that they meet the criteria for participation.

Since Medicare was instituted in 1965, there has been a steady increase in the numbers of all types of its participating agencies. The greatest increase has been in proprietary agencies. [21]

In summary, Medicare has significantly affected home health agencies since its establishment. As well as an increase in the numbers of agencies participating in the program, it is likely that the program has stimulated an improvement in the quality of services rendered by participating agencies. Home health care has received much attention recently by legislators, providers, and consumers of health care, and it is likely that some of this interest is the result of the expansion of services resulting from the Medicare program. Home health care also has been received by many individuals who may not have been willing to receive it without Medicare benefits. Medicare has undoubtedly meant increased paperwork for providers, which considerably increases the amount of desk work for community health nurses. For agencies which did not meet the certification requirements prior to joining the program, Medicare may well have changed patterns of staffing and organization which often increases operation costs. Thus the Medicare program, although of much benefit to a number of providers and consumers of home health care, has not been without legitimate concern in many areas.

Medicaid

Medicaid is Title XIX of the Social Security Act. It is a federal (but state administered) program for eligible low income families and individuals. The client does not have to make direct payments for the health services received—the government pays the bill. Home health benefits are one of the benefits of the Medicaid program, and the coverage is comprehensive. An agency which participates in the Medicare program, or meets the same criteria if it does not participate, is eligible for receiving reimbursement from Medicaid. Proprietary agencies currently are not reimbursed by Medicaid funds. The Medicaid regulations define home health services similarly to Medicare, but there is no limitation on the number of home visits that a client can receive. There are no homebound restrictions for Medicaid recipients, and home health care can be provided after a client's condition has stabilized. In general, Medicaid requirements are much less restrictive than those of Medicare, which enables greater numbers of clients to receive more comprehensive home health services.

Title XX

Title XX is an amendment to the Social Security Act which was instituted in 1975 to provide social services in the home to the aged and disabled. Funds are forwarded to each state by the federal government; the allocation of money is at the state's discretion. The purpose of Title XX benefits is to foster self-sufficiency and self-support while helping to prevent inappropriate institutionalization. The services sponsored by Title XX are the type which can be effectively coordinated with professional home health care to provide the client with comprehensive home health services. Some of these are the following:

1. Homemaker services, to be provided by a trained homemaker.
2. Chore services, which are provided by an untrained person and includes repairs, heavy house cleaning, yard work, and shopping.
3. Home management, which includes meal preparation, consumer education, and assistance with home maintenance.
4. Homemaker-home health aide services. [22]

These services are vital to many individuals who are able to remain in their homes but who need help with the care of the home and with daily activities. For the elderly and disabled, Title XX is of much value.

The Health Revenue Sharing and Health Services Act of 1975

The Health Revenue Sharing and Health Services Act of 1975 (PL 94-63) awarded $3 million in grant money to support the development and expansion of home health services. The purposes of the grant are to: 1) meet initial costs of establishing home health agencies where none are available; 2) expand the services available in existing agencies; and 3) compensate personnel during their participation in the above two activities. [22]

The money is available to either public or nonprofit agencies, but an agency must meet the requirements for Medicare certification. (The reason for this provision is that the purpose of the financial support which this program awards is to help agencies become financially viable and stable.) Preference in awarding the money is given to areas that serve large proportions of elderly or indigent persons. Thus, the law attempts to help communities that lack home health services and whose residents are primarily elderly or poor. Of the 56 grants made in 1976, 46 were to agencies in these areas. The total amount of these grants also has increased from $3 million in fiscal years 1976 and 1977 [23] to $6 million in fiscal year 1978. [22] Unquestionably, this program is one effective solution to the problem of the maldistribution of home health services in the United States.

Title III Grants for State and Community Programs on Aging

This program was developed in 1974 as a division of the Older American's Act to develop a coordinated system of social services for the elderly. One purpose of the program is to prevent unnecessary institutionalization by providing support services which enable persons to live at home. All work is at the state and local levels, with each state divided into a number of service areas. Within each service area, agencies regarding elderly affairs must be established to coordinate the services. Each state must also have one central agency to coordinate all of these activities. Four services of the Title III Grants are the provision of transportation, home services, legal counseling, and home repairs and renovations.

The Rural Health Clinics Bill

The Rural Health Clinics Bill (PL 95-210) was passed in December 1977 to provide for the coverage of services by nurse practitioners and physician's assistants, without the presence of a physician, by Medicare and Medicaid funds. The Bill also states that the rural clinic can be reimbursed for home nursing services if there is no home health agency in the community. The nursing care can be provided by registered and licensed practical nurses. This bill helps to enable residents who live in rural communities without home health services to receive the services of a nurse in the home.

The Medicare-Medicaid Anti-Fraud and Abuse Amendments (PL 95-142)

In October 1977, Congress passed the Medicare-Medicaid Anti-Fraud and Abuse Amendments. The purpose of this law is to increase the power of the government in identifying, prosecuting, and punishing persons involved in fraudulent activities concerning Medicare and Medicaid programs. The law considers a number of different types of unlawful behavior, such as the provision of health services to clients to a greater extent than necessary and the practice of illegal remunerations. Congress inserted into this amendment a mandate which stated that the Secretary of Health, Education, and Welfare must evaluate and recommend revisions in current laws pertaining to home health care by January 1979. The purpose of this insertion was to improve the distribution, coordination, and financial support of home health services.

SUMMARY

Caring for the sick and the less fortunate in the home was one of the first kinds of nursing care and is one whose benefit and necessity continues to be appreciated by both consumers and providers of health care. The question of the cost effectiveness of this type of care recently has become an important issue as the costs of institutional care continue to rise. Emphasis on the quality of life for the elderly has lent support to the provision of comprehensive services for the elderly who wish to remain living in their own homes. Society's criticism of the inappropriate institutionalization of the elderly and the ill has influenced many to see home care as an attractive, suitable alternative to the institution. Many persons, both young and old, enjoy earlier hospital discharges, when they are appropriate candidates for home health care.

Recognizing the benefits of home health care, the federal government has enacted a number of programs. Some help to solve maldistribution problems of home health services by financially supporting the establishment and activities of new home health agencies. Others educate both professional and nonprofessional home health providers, establish support services in the community, and monitor the quality of the home health services delivered. The community health nurse who provides care in the home acts as the coordinator of the services the client receives. These services may be of many kinds such as physical therapy for a hemiplegic adult, nursing care for a terminally ill child, or counseling by a psychiatric social worker for a family whose children are neglected. The community health nurse also is primarily responsible for supervising the activities of home health aides who provide nonprofessional personal and homemaking services to clients of all ages in the home.

Inevitably, home health care will continue to be recognized as a necessary community health service as both providers and consumers of health care confirm its benefits and as the costs of institutional care remain prohibitively high.

REFERENCES

1. National League for Nursing, Council of Home Health Agencies and Community Health Services: *Accreditation of Home Health Agencies and Community Nursing Services.* Pubn. No. 21-1622, National League for Nursing, New York, 1976.
2. Milio, Nancy: *The Care of Health in Communities: Access for Outcasts.* Macmillan Publishing Co., New York, 1975.
3. Brainard, Annie M.: *The Evolution of Public Health Nursing.* W. B. Saunders, Philadelphia, 1922.
4. Winslow, C. E. A.: "The Role of the Visiting Nurse in the Campaign for Public Health." *American Journal of Nursing,* 11:909, August 1911.
5. Fitzpatrick, M. Louise: *The National Organization for Public Health Nursing; 1912-1952: Development of A Practice Field.* National League for Nursing, New York, 1975.
6. Dock, Lavinia L.: "The History of Public Health Nursing." *Public Health Nurse,* 14:524, Oct. 1922.
7. Tinkham, Catherine W. and Voorhees, Eleanor F.: *Community Health Nursing: Evolution and Process.* Appleton-Century-Crofts, New York, 1972.

8. American Nurses' Association Division on Community Health Nursing Practice: *Concepts of Community Health Nursing Practice.* American Nurses' Association, Kansas City, 1975.

9. Council on Health Manpower: "Educational Qualifications of Public Health Nurses." *American Journal of Public Health,* 61:2506, Dec. 1971.

10. Ozimek, Dorothy: *The Baccalaureate Graduate in Nursing: What Does Society Expect?* Pubn. No. 15-1520, National League for Nursing, New York, 1974.

11. Ozimek, Dorothy: The Future of Nursing Education. Pubn. No. 15-1581, National League for Nursing, New York, 1975.

12. Report of the World Health Organization Expert Committee: *Community Health Nursing.* WHO Technical Report Series #558, World Health Organization, Geneva, 1974.

13. National League for Nursing-Division of Baccalaureate and Higher Degree Programs: *Baccalaureate Education in Nursing: Key to a Professional Career in Nursing.* 1977-78 Pubn. No. 15-1311, National League for Nursing, New York, 1977.

14. Saba, Virginia K.: *Surveys of Public Health Nursing 1968-1972.* DHEW Pubn. No. (HRA) 76-8, U.S. Government Printing Office, Washington, D.C., 1975.

15. Williams, Glenys O.: "The Elderly in Family Practice: An Evaluation of the Geriatric Visiting Nurse." *The Journal of Family Practice,* 5:369, March 1977.

16. Levenson, Goldie: *Type, Length, and Cost of Care for Home Health Patients.* Pubn. No. 21-1589, National League for Nursing, New York, 1975.

17. *Home Health Line,* 1(13):88, 1976.

18. U.S. Department of Health, Education, and Welfare: *Survey of Regional Offices to Determine Number of States as of July, 1977 Licensing Home Health Agencies, Those in the Process of Legislation, and Those Actively Discussing Legislation.* 1977, Unpublished data.

19. U.S. Department of Health, Education, and Welfare, Health Care Financing Administration: *Conditions of Participation of Home Health Agencies in Federal Health Insurance for the Aged and the Disabled—Code of Federal Regulations.* Title 20. Chapter III, Part 405.

20. National League for Nursing, Council of Home Health Agencies and Community Nursing Services: *Home Health Agencies and Community Nursing Services Accredited by NLN/APHA, May 1977.* Pubn. No. 21-1645, National League for Nursing, New York, 1977.

21. U.S. Department of Health, Education, and Welfare, Health Resources Statistics: *Health Manpower and Health Facilities.* 1975, p. 449.

22. Proskauer, Martha (Congressional Research Service): *Federal Programs That Finance Home Health Care Services.* Library of Congress: October 21, 1977, p. 12.

23. U.S. Department of Health, Education, and Welfare, Health Services Administration, Office of Planning, Evaluation and Legislation: *Home Health Grant Program Evaluation Methodology.* Report No. OPEL 77-11, July, 1977, p. 6.

15
NURSING ROLE
IN EDUCATION

LINDA L. JARVIS, M.S.N., R.N.

Education is defined as "The act or process of imparting knowledge or skill; systematic instruction; teaching, the obtaining of knowledge or skill through such a process."[1] It is an interactive process between teacher and learner. Nursing education involves the imparting of and acquisition of nursing knowledge and skills. Community health nursing education includes learning of both nursing and community health theory and skills.

Nursing education is carried on at various levels. Many models for nursing education have been suggested. We began as an apprentice vocation and have struggled, against sometimes almost insurmountable odds, to establish nursing as a profession with the privileges of such a designation.

Community health nursing has, since early times, enjoyed a special position in nursing. Although early nurses had all of their basic preparation in hospitals, special instruction was available for nurses who were working in community settings. Early community nursing work, especially among the poor, was begun as people became aware that private nursing in the home was beneficial to the health of the client and family. Nursing care to the client and family included illness care and teaching, health teaching, and community resource utilization. Lillian Wald, a pioneer in community health nursing at the Henry Street Settlement House in New York City, became the first to use the term *public health nurse* as an appropriate description of the nursing activities carried out with clients in community settings.[2]

The focus of this chapter is on community health nursing education. Because the history of general nursing education has characterized progress made in community health nursing education, both will be reviewed to give the reader some idea of the struggles encountered and the progress made. In order to provide the highest possible level of community health nursing care, excellence in education is needed. Knowledge about nursing and public health theory is necessary to effective practice so that the health of target populations can be improved and/or maintained.

HISTORICAL DEVELOPMENT OF NURSING EDUCATION

Modern nursing education can be traced to Pastor Theodore Fliedner and his wife Friederika of Kaiserwerth, Germany in 1836 when they established a training school for deaconesses. It was this training school which Florence Nightingale attended. The experience at the Fliedner's training school and the work done during the Crimean War guided Miss Nightingale toward the nursing education program she was to develop at St. Thomas' Hospital in London, England. Her writings included *Notes on Hospitals* and *Notes on Nursing* which were instrumental in improving hospital care and preparing women to deliver high quality nursing care based on theory and not instinct.

In the United States, the Civil War prompted the entry of women into formal nursing roles, often to the disapproval of physicians and families. Dorothea Dix was appointed by Secretary of War Simon Cameron to organize women nurses for the war effort.[3] Prior to this appointment, she had been instrumental in initiating mental health care and treatment reforms. She faced and met the tasks of recruiting, training, and placing young women in nursing positions for the Union Army.

The Confederate Army had nursing services provided primarily through the auspices of men who were recovering from wounds or were not strong enough to go into combat. It was not unitl the middle of the war that southern women began to provide nursing care to a large extent. The attitude had been that women of "good" background should not be exposed to caring for strange men. Few nurses for the Confederacy had had any formal nursing training.

For both the North and South many untrained nurses provided valuable nursing care to the wounded and dying. In all, approximately 10,000 women served as nurses during the Civil War.[3] Kalisch and Kalisch identify seven separate groups of women who provided nursing services during the war: 1) the nurses recruited by Dorothea Dix for the Union Army, 2) Sisters of Charity or other religious groups, 3) short term "nurses" employed to do menial hospital chores, 4) black women employed through the War Department, 5) uncompensated volunteers, 6) women camp followers, and 7) women employed by various relief organizations.[3] For most of these women there had been little if any formal training or hospital experience prior to serving. What they did posess was a desire to help the wounded and dying and a strong determination to do a job which needed doing. In spite of nonsupport from many families and physicians, these women were able to perservere and provide a humane service needed by the wounded and dying soldiers. This was happening at a time when women were expected to stay in the home and rear children and were considered as subordinate to men.

In the United States the experience of the Civil War emphasized the need for prepared nurses. Late in the 1800s there developed special apprentice training programs for the preparation of nurses. Even then there was concern that nurses might be over educated through such training programs. In general there were no uniform standards for admissions, study advancement, or graduation requirements. Nursing recruitment and education was hospital based with service to the hospital as the major goal and quality education secondary.

In July 1872 the New England Hospital for Women and Children in Boston established the first nurses training school in the United States.[3] In 1873, Linda Richards became the first professionally trained nurse when she completed the one year program offered at the New England Hospital. Three other schools soon opened in New York, New Haven, and Boston for the training of nurses. The first school in the U.S. to be patterned after Florence Nightingale's St. Thomas Hospital program in London was the New York Training School at Bellevue Hospital. The Connecticut Training School for Nurses at New Haven State Hospital and the Boston Training School for Nurses at the Massachusetts General Hospital were also modeled after the Nightingale plan. Students were admitted, generally, between the ages of 25 and 35, represented the entire range of educational background, and were often members of the middle and upper classes. They were subjected to long hours of hard physical work which included scrubbing and polishing as well as patient care. Once finished with the basic nursing program, these nurses usually worked in private homes since hospitals used students to provide patient care.

Schools of nursing continued to proliferate during the next decades. As they were part of the personnel structure of the hospitals with which they were affiliated, the quality of student varied as did the educational curriculum. In all instances, however, student nurses were exposed to rigid rules and regulations regarding their private as well as professional lives.

The increase in nursing theory provided to nurses evolved slowly with general lack of support from physicians. Although physicians had begun to see the need for skilled nurses, there was a common attitude that theoretical instruction should be strictly limited. There was, and continues to be in many quarters, the concern that nurses might become overeducated. As nursing theory improved, so did the quality of nursing care and thus the overall health of the client also improved.

In the early part of the 20th century, nursing education continued to be provided through hospital schools under very authoritarian conditions with students providing patient care. Because many students were being graduated without adequate preparation and standards concerning curriculum requirements were unequal, it became evident that a standardized licensure procedure of some type was needed. In 1903, North Carolina became the first state having a state nursing licensure law. Other states soon followed with similar laws which varied much with regard to requirements for registration. Today all nurses are required to pass the standardized National League for Nursing written examination in order to become registered. Each state still establishes its own nurse practice acts and there is variation between states.

It was after World War I that much attention was given to university based education for nurses. In 1923 the first major evaluation of nursing education supported by the Rockefeller Foundation was reported by Josephine Goldmark in a study entitled *Nursing and Nursing Education in the United States.*[4] The study, commonly known as the "Goldmark Report," spoke of the need to establish university schools of nursing to prepare nurse leaders, to establish a common basis of education, not apprenticeship, and to take nurse education out of the hospital framework in order to better prepare nurses for public health nursing. Nursing education properly belonged to those who were dedicated to a liberal educational approach.

Although nursing programs were offered in universities as early as 1906, it was not unitl 1924, following the release of the Goldmark Report, that the Yale School of Nursing was opened as an autonomous collegiate school.[5] Both community and hospital work were included in the curriculum plan. Other collegiate nursing programs soon opened at Western Reserve University, Vanderbilt University, and the University of Chicago, but there were many concerns voiced about such nurses being overtrained and too costly in providing service.[3] Even as collegiate programs were being established, there were some schools which added two years of liberal arts education to a basic hospital training program which lead to a baccalaureate degree. The general evoluation has been from a five year program, often divided two and three years as described above, to the common two-two year program of today. The contemporary collegiate nursing programs are divided into a lower division of basic sciences and an upper division of nursing science courses.

As the collegiate programs continued to develop, hospital training programs also pro-liferated, but there was growing concern about the quality of the programs and the students they graduated. In 1926 the Committee on the Grading of Nursing Schools began a study of nursing schools. In 1934 the Committee's published findings recommended 1) reducation in the nurse supply and improvement of the quality of training, 2) replacement of students with graduates for routine ward duty, 3) assistance to hospitals to help meet costs of graduate services, and 4) public support for nursing education.[3]

It was during this time that efforts were also being made to grade schools of nursing. As a result of grading of schools of nursing, the poorer ones were forced to cease operation. The direction in many hospital and all collegiate schools of nursing was toward quality educa-tional programs for students rather than utilization of students for staffing and service for the hospitals.

Early community health nursing efforts were directed toward bedside care. In 1891 there were approximately 130 nurses working in community health; by 1919 the number had in-creased to nearly 9000.[3] These nurses were aware very early that preventive and health promotion efforts were important if bedside care was going to be effective and the health status improved. Nurses needed special preparation in order to meet these health needs.

In addition to having formal training in hospitals, public health nurses also received addi-tional public health preparation through a variety of collegiate postgraduate programs, on the job training in district nursing associations, or through special fieldwork connected with hospital training.[3] Schools developed which provided programs of varying lengths of time to prepare nurses to work in public health. Public health nurses carried case loads, did health teaching and promotion, informed clients of community resources and services, and pro-vided various welfare services. From the beginning, nurses charged for their nursing ser-vices. In the early part of the 20th century, public health nurses were becoming an accepted part of the city, county, and state health departments. Gradually their practice was becom-ing more of an advisory and teaching nature. Areas of work also began to expand as public health nurses worked in schools, maternal child clinics, and industries. Much work was done with the poor and uneducated.

In 1925, Mary Breckenridge started the Frontier Nursing Service in Kentucky to bring health care to a remote rural area. Through her efforts nurses brought improved maternity care to the area served as well as general public health and nursing services. The program is still functioning today.

During this period much effort was directed, nationally and individually, to the improve-ment of the nation's health. Public health nurses played a major role in the movement as the scope of their work increased. The passage of the Sheppard-Towner Act (1921) provided matching federal money to deal with the problems of maternal and infant health. Much of this effort was directed toward education of both lay persons and professional nurses. Family planning education was initiated by Margaret Sanger, a public health nurse in New York City. Communicable disease control was increased. Health promotion was empha-sized. The public health nurse was involved in community and professional efforts to im-prove and expand health services and was seeking and demanding academic education for all public health nurses.[6]

Public health nursing efforts were extended during the depression as federal monies were utilized to put unemployed nurses into service. Among the programs developed were Federal Emergency Relief Administration (F.E.R.A.) grants for care of the ill in their homes, the Works Progress Administration (W.P.A.), Civil Works Administration (C.W.A.), and the Social Security Act of 1935. These various programs extended the work of public health nurses, expanded local health departments, and provided educational monies to prepare nurses to work in public health.

As we moved from WW II and into the 1950s, the country was faced with nurse shortages. Many of the military nurses had returned to families rather than staying in nursing. In 1948, Dr. Esther Lucille Brown published a report entitled *Nursing for the Future* which recommended that nursing education be university based and schools of nursing be accredited and identified as such.[7] During this period, prompted by the war, the number of licensed practical nurses was increasing and standards for educational preparation were meager and unstandardized. The popularity of practical nurses and aides for the delivery of nursing care spread due to continuing conflict over economic issues, nursing education criteria, and perceived need for highly trained nurses to provide care in the home and hospital. As nursing struggled to become a profession, set backs were encountered at each step.

In 1952 an associate degree program project was established at Teachers College, Columbia University with Mildred L. Montag as the project director.[3] The purpose of these two year community and junior college nursing programs was to prepare nurses in a shorter period of time in order to ease the nurse shortage. They were prepared for bedside service. There were seven two year programs which initially tested this idea and they were shown to be effective, based on state board results and peer review. It has been over two decades since the first associate degree programs were initiated and we had, in 1977, 656 associate degree programs.[8]

As nursing moved into the 1960s and 1970s, education was moving more into the collegiate and community college areas with a decrease in the number of diploma programs which operated. Diploma programs decreased from 494 in 1973 to 367 in 1977.[8] The health care crisis had surfaced in the 1960s and great concern was voiced about access to and availability of health care. Monies were made available for the education of nurses such as the Nurse Training Act of 1964. Nursing research was being emphasized. Expanded roles in nursing began to emerge and the term "nurse practitioner" became vogue. Technology was advancing at a rapid rate and nurses were being called on to function in highly technical areas such as Coronary Care Units. Continuing education for registered nurses began to take on increased importance and significance. Minoritites, including men, were seeking nursing education as were increasing numbers of college graduates coming into nursing after completing prior degrees. Graduate preparation in public health nursing was becoming more available. The late 1970s, however, were marked by great reductions in nursing education monies, and at this point there is real danger that money for nursing education will be nonexistant. Many special studies and people have been instrumental in the development of nursing education as known today.

Public health nurses have long enjoyed a special status in the nursing profession. Traditionally, their education has required special theory and practice above the basic nursing program in order to function at an optimal level. Collegiate preparation has been the desired level of education. Both women and men have been actively involved in expanding the role of the nurse and eagerly sought opportunities to expand and improve health services for the individual, family, and community. Effectiveness has been achieved because early in the specialty the importance of health teaching and promotion had been realized. Support in both educational and practice efforts has come from the American Nurses' Association, the National League for Nursing, and the National Organization for Public Health Nursing (now part of N.L.N.)

As nursing struggles to be recognized as a profession, there is confusion within the ranks as to the need for some specialties. The integration of community health concepts into general nursing curricula is commendable. However, it is imperative that the uniqueness of community health nursing principles not be lost in such a move. The making of home visits to individuals and families is not community health nursing. As Carolyn Williams has pointed out, community health nursing must never lose sight of the fact that our focus is the promotion of health related behavior and the provision of personal health services to many aggregates.[9] We must not lose sight of the importance of the aggregate approach from both a clinical and planning view. We must strive to maintain our unique identity so that the focus of community health nursing will not be lost.

The people, educational programs, organizations, legislation, and studies instrumental to the development of nursing and community health nursing are many. The appendix to this chapter contains an outline highlighting some of these important people and events.

COMMUNITY HEALTH NURSING EDUCATOR PREPARATION AND ROLE

Community health nurses are both recipients of and providers of educational experiences. Their preparation includes content from both nursing and public health. Ideally, there are two levels of nursing practitioner in the field. The scope of services and role played will depend on the position they fill and the needs of the community and agency. Although it is desirable and is my bias that all community health nurses should possess a baccalaureate degree in nursing, this is not the case nationwide due to the insufficient number of baccalaureate prepared nurses in many parts of the country and the ever increasing demand for nurses to work in the community. This is one of many problems facing community health nursing.

The public health nurse generalist is prepared at the baccalaureate level to provide general nursing care in the community.[10] Her educational preparation includes lower and upper levels of instruction with a solid base in the social, physical, behavioral, and biologic sciences. Upper level courses provide nursing theory and clinical practice built on the foundation of lower level courses in public health, child, maternal, medical, surgical, and psychiatric areas. Care emphasis is directed toward the individual, family, and community. Carolyn Williams makes a strong plea for all community health nursing educators to focus on group or aggregate level care rather than individual, clinically oriented care.[9] Community health nurses, regardless of the site in which they work, must keep in mind that the target group is the focus, not the individual, although attainment of the group goal may be through one to one contact.

The public health nurse specialist is prepared at the master's level with a degree in public health nursing from a school of public health accredited by the American Public Health Association or from a graduate school of nursing accredited by the National League of Nursing.[21] There is, at the present time, much debate concerning nursing education in community health at the graduate level including site of the educational program and specific content.[10-13]

The specific skills needed by nurses in community health include utilization of the nursing process as a tool for the delivery of nursing care, various assessment skills including physical assessment and community assessment, community health planning and financing, legislative process, and epidemiology as applied to nursing in the community. The sophistication with which the nurse is able to utilize these skills will depend on her level of preparation and understanding and the support and needs of the agency with which she works.

Baccalaureate prepared nurses will provide community health nursing skills in a variety of settings. These settings may include city and county health departments, visiting nurse associations, schools, industries, and other such settings. The master's prepared community health nurses will provide direct care requiring a high degree of skill and serve as role models in appropriate settings, administrators, supervisors, consultants, expert practioners, or researchers in family and community health.[10]

Community health nurses who choose to work primarily as educators may do so in baccalaureate and graduate nursing programs, in various direct service organizations, in continuing education projects such as the work done by nurses in the Area Health Education Centers, or in housing projects discussed later in this book. Regardless of the population with whom the educator works, she will seek to identify learning needs and learners, establish objectives, design content, select teaching methodologies, implement the program, and evaluate its effectiveness. Whether the nurse educator teaches lay persons, peers, student nurses, or allied professionals, the teaching steps she follows will be the same.

All nurses in community health nursing education must be registered in the state in which they practice. Each state has its own Nurse Practice Act which defines the limits of nursing practice. Some nurses have completed various practitioner programs and are certified for that specific practitioner focus. Examples include family nurse practitioners, school nurse practitioners, and gerontology nurse practitioners. In all cases, nurses are responsible for their professional actions regardless of their chosen area of work. This accountability is an integral part of the quest for professionalism.

Funding to prepare nurses to become educators has been variable. During the 1960s and early 1970s monies were more readily available than is presently the case. Nurse Training Act monies are available through legislation and appropriations by Congress in varying yearly amounts. During the 1980s money from this source will fluctuate and probably correspond directly to the national economic picture. There are various sources of financing available for nurses from a variety of public and private funds. Guaranteed student loans are available for some educational expenses. For the most current listing of available funds for nursing education, students should contact the student financial aid office at the school they wish to attend, local banks, local, city, and county governments for special nursing grants and scholarships, and the local ANA chapter for financial assistance information. Money for educational efforts has definitely dwindled in the past eight to ten years. Whether it will ease in face of the present economic/inflation crisis is not known. Financing one's nursing education will be more difficult in the future.

LEGISLATION

The appendix to this chapter identifies several important pieces of legislation which have been instrumental in the development of community health nursing. As comprehensive health care, consumer participation, funding, peer review, and nursing role clarification become more prevalent, further legislation may greatly influence the extend to which nurses may practice. Legislation being considered in such areas as family planning, health maintenance organizations, health services for youth, and home health care will impact directly on the scope of services community health nurses are able to provide.

The reader is referred to N-CAP, the Nurses Coalition for Action in Politics, for current information on federal legislation. Congressmen and Senators can also be contacted at both the state and federal levels to determine the status of pertinent health legislation. Only as we become more involved in the political process and health planning will we be able to have a favorable impact for the improvement of health care.

Community health nursing has a long history of involvement for the improved health status of various groups through improved educational preparation of nurses. We serve as educators to individuals, groups, communities, students, and peers. Education is the basis of quality community nursing care through increased understanding and sensitivity concerning health needs. Even in these times of economic stress, it is hoped that nurses will continue to strive for excellence in community health nursing education. It is only through the enforcement of the highest standards of nursing education that the health of the community can be insured.

REFERENCES

1. *The American Heritage Dictionary of the English Language,* William Morris (ed.). Houghton Mifflin Company, Boston, 1976.
2. Wales, M.: *The Public Health Nurse in Action.* The Macmillan Company, New York, 1941.
3. Kalisch, Philip A., and Kalisch, Beatrice J.: *The Advance of American Nursing.* Little Brown and Company, Boston, 1978.
4. Goldmark, Josephine: *Nursing and Nursing Education in the United States.* Macmillan Company, New York, 1923.
5. Diers, Donna: "A Combined Basic Graduate Program for College Graduates." *Nursing Outlook,* 24(2):92, Feb. 1976.
6. Tinkham, Catherine W., and Voorhies, Eleanor F.: *Community Health Nursing-Evolution and Process.* Appleton-Century-Crofts, New York, 1972.
7. Brown, Esther Lucille: *Nursing for the Future.* Russell Sage Foundation, New York, 1948.
8. Educational Preparation for Nursing—1977. *Nursing Outlook,* 26(9):568, Sept. 1978.
9. Williams, Carolyn A.: "Community Health—What Is It?" *Nursing Outlook,* 25(4):252, April 1977.
10. Council on Health Manpower: "Educational Qualifications of Public Health Nurses," Spradley, B.W. (ed.): in *Contemporary Community Nursing.* Little, Brown and Company, Boston, 1975.
11. Ruth, M. Virginia, and Partridge, Kay B.: "Differences in Perception of Education and Practice." *Nursing Outlook,* 26(10):622, Oct. 1978.
12. Flynn, Beverly C.; Gottschalh, Janet; Ray, Dixie; et al.: "One Master's Curriculum in Community Health Nursing." *Nursing Outlook,* 26(10):633, Oct. 1978.
13. Ulin, Priscilla: "What Master's Students Want to Know." *Nursing Outlook,* 26(10):629, Oct. 1978.

BIBLIOGRAPHY

Archer, Sarah Ellen, and Flishman, Ruth P.: "Community Health Nursing—A Topology of Practice." *Nursing Outlook,* 23(6):358, June 1975.
Brown, Esther Lucille: *Nursing for the Future.* Russell Sage Foundation, New York, 1948.
Bullough, Bonnie, and Bullough, Vern L.: *The Emergence of Modern Nursing.* The Macmillan Company, New York, 1964.
Cady, Louise: "Extending the Role of Public Health Nurses." *Nursing Outlook,* 22(10):636, Oct. 1974.
Diers, Donna: "A Continued Basic Graduate Program for College Graduates." *Nursing Outlook,* 24(2):92, Feb. 1976.
Dietz, Lena Dixon, and Lehozky, Aurelia R.: *History and Modern Nursing,* 2nd ed. F.A. Davis Company, Philadelphia, 1967.
Educational Preparation for Nursing—1977. *Nursing Outlook,* 26(9):568, Sept. 1978.

Flynn, Beverly C., Gottschalh, Janet, Ray, Dixie, et al.: "One Master's Curriculum in Community Health Nursing." *Nursing Outlook*, 26(10):641, Oct. 1978.

Goldmark, Josephine: *Nursing and Nursing Education in the U.S.* Macmillan Co., New York, 1923.

Kalisch, Philip A., and Kalisch, Beatrice J.: *The Advance of American Nursing*. Little Brown and Company, Boston, 1978.

McNeil, Jo: "An Administrator's View of Staff Educational Needs." *Nursing Outlook*, 26(10):641, Oct. 1978.

Nursing Organization Curriculum Conference: *Curriculum Bulletin No. 1*. National League of Nursing Education, New York, Department of Services to Schools of Nursing, 1950.

Nutting, M. Adelaide, and Dock, Lavina L.: *A History of Nursing*, vol. 2. G.P. Putnam's Son, New York, 1935.

Ostrand, Lillian, and Willis, Winnie: "Faculty Preparation—An MPH or MSN Degree." *Nursing Outlook*, 26(10):637, Oct. 1978.

Ruth, M. Virginia, and Partridge, Kay B.: "Differences in Perception of Education and Practice." *Nursing Outlook*, 26(10):622, Oct. 1978.

Spradley, Barbara Walton (ed.): *Contemporary Community Nursing*. Little, Brown and Company, Boston, 1975.

Standards of Community Health Nursing Practice. The American Nurses' Association, 1974.

Tinkham, Catherine W., and Voorhies, Eleanor F.: *Community Health Nursing—Evolution and Process*. Appleton-Century-Crofts, New York, 1972.

Ulin, Priscilla R.: "What Master's Students Want to Know." *Nursing Outlook*, 26(10):629, Oct. 1978.

U.S. Department of Health, Education and Welfare: *Health Planning and Resources Development Act of 1974*. DHEW Publication No. (HRA) 75-14015, 1975.

Wales, Marquerite: *The Public Health Nurse in Action*. The Macmillan Company, New York, 1941.

Warner, Anne (ed.): *Innovations in Community Health Nursing*. The C.V. Mosby Company, St. Louis, 1978.

Williams, Carolyn A.: "Community Health Nursing—What Is It?." *Nursing Outlook*, 25(4):250, April, 1977.

Wilson, Florence A., and Neuhauser, Duncan: *Health Services in the United States*. Ballinger Publisher Company, Cambridge, 1974.

APPENDIX. PEOPLE AND EVENTS IN NURSING EDUCATION AND COMMUNITY HEALTH NURSING

People

Date	Name	Contribution to Nursing Education and Community Health Nursing
1836	Pastor Theodor Fliednor and Friederike Fliednor	Established first modern nursing deaconess order in Kaisersworth, Germany. Initiated modern nursing.
1850–1910	Florence Nightingale	Symbol of modern nursing. Trained at Kaisersworth, Germany. Organized nursing services during Crimean War, Established St. Thomas School of Nursing in London. Emphasized the need for trained nurses to improve health. Established framework for early schools of nursing through writings and experiences of Crimean War.
1861–1865	Dorothea Dix	School teacher in Boston, humanitarian for mental health reforms, organized nurses for Union Army during Civil War.
1861–1865	Walt Whitman	Writer, poet, untrained male nurse during Civil War in military hospitals of both Union and Confederate Armies.
1861–1865	Louisa May Alcott	Writer, *Hospital Sketches*. Untrained nurse during Civil War.
1861–1865	Mother Mary Bickerdyke (Mary Ann Ball)	Untrained nurse from Galesburg, Ill. Assigned to Cairo, Ill. to care for wounded, stressed cleanliness, good food, organized nursing care. Politically powerful.
1861–1865	Ella King Newsom	Trained by Sisters of Mercy at Memphis Hospital. Organized hospitals for the Confederate Army. Emphasized cleanliness and good treatment.
1861–1865	Kate Cumming	Volunteer nurse during Civil War with the Confederate Army.
1873	Linda Richards	First trained nurse in the U.S. Graduated from New England Training School, Boston, Mass.
1879	Mary E. P. Mahoney	First black graduate nurse, attended New England Hospital for Women & Children.

People

Date	Name	Contribution to Nursing Education and Community Health Nursing
1881	Clara Barton	Former school teacher, during Civil War had organized War Relief efforts, organized American Red Cross.
1886-1956	Lavinia Dock	Author of nursing textbooks, reform nurse, charter member of Society of Nurse Superintendents which became the American Nurses' Association.
1891-1940s	M. Adelaide Nutting	Author, educator, nurse leader, first nurse to hold a professorship in a university at Teacher's College, Columbia University, pushed for educational research in nursing to improve nursing education standards, leader in preparing nurses for the war effort (WW II), stressed the need for improved education for public health nurses. Member of the Committee for the Study of Nursing Education with Isabel Stewart. Directed the NLNE's evaluation of nursing school standards entitled *A Standard Curriculum for Schools of Nursing.* Director of the Department of Nursing and Health at Teacher's College, Columbia University which offered excellent special public health courses for nurses.
1893	Mary Brewster	Trained nurse, established Henry Street Settlement House in New York City with Lillian Wald to provide home nursing services.
1983-1940s	Lillian Wald	Author, nurse leader in public health nursing and nursing education. First to use the term "Public Health Nurse," established school nursing in 1902, instrumental in expanding the practice and scope of services of public health nurses—school nursing, urban public health nursing, rural public health nursing, industrial public health nursing, leading organizer of the national organization for Public Health Nursing and its first president, pushed for establishment of a federal bureau for the pro-

People

Date	Name	Contribution to Nursing Education and Community Health Nursing
		motion of children's health—later known as the U.S. Children's Bureau. Member of the Committee for the Study of Nursing Education.
1898	Sophia Palmer	Editor of American Journal of Nursing, made first public statement about nurse's licensure to the Federation of Women's Clubs of New York State.
1916	Margaret Sanger	Public health nurse in New York City established first birth control center in America, pioneer in contraception education.
1925	Mary Breckenridge	Established the Kentucky Frontier Nursing Service to promote health in a rural area of Kentucky. All nurses in the Service were trained midwives. Still in operation today.
1918-1940s	Annie Goodrich	President of A.N.A. Member of the Committee for the Study of Nursing Education." Educator, Chief Inspecting Nurse of the Army Hospitals at home and abroad. Recommended establishment of the Army School of Nursing. The first Dean of Yale School of Nursing.
1921-1941	Isabel Stewart	Educator, pushed for financial aid for nurse education, spoke for quality in nursing education.
1923	Josephine Goldmark	Social worker, author, secretary for the "Committee for the Study of Nursing Education." Wrote the report for the committee, focus on education for public health nurses. The report, entitled *Nursing & Nursing Education in the United States,* emphasized desirability of collegiate preparation for nurses.
1941	Lucille Petry	Educator at University of Minnesota. Member of nurse education staff of the Public Health Service, Director of the U.S. Cadet Nurse Corps.
1948	E. Lucille Brown	Nurse educator, research staff member of Russell Sage Foundation, wrote *Nursing for the Future* which recom-

People

Date	Name	Contribution to Nursing Education and Community Health Nursing
		mended changes in nursing practice and education.
1951	Mildred Montag	Nursing educator. Project Coordinator for the initial development of nursing programs in junior and community colleges. Her dissertation in 1951 has been used as the model for the two year nursing programs. Used the term "technical nurse."
1970	Jessie Scott	Nursing educator; Assistant Surgeon General; Director, Division of Nursing of the United States Public Health Service.

Educational Programs

Date	Program	Contribution to Nursing Education and Community Health Nursing
1872	New England Hospital for Women and Children, Boston	First general training school for nurses in America.
1873	New York Training School Bellvue Hospital, New York City	First American nurse training school modeled after Florence Nightingale's St. Thomas School of Nursing in London.
1873	The Connecticut Training School for Nurses at New Haven State Hospital, New Haven, Conn.	Second American school of nursing based on Nightingale plan.
1873	Boston Training School for Nurses at Massachusetts General Hospital, Boston	Third school of nursing in United States based on Nightingale plan.
1891	Provident Hospital School of Nursing, Chicago	First school for black nurses in the United States.
1899	Teacher's College Columbia University, New York City	Established a course in hospital economics as a postgraduate course to prepare nurse educators and supervisors.

Educational Programs

Date	Program	Contribution to Nursing Education and Community Health Nursing
1909	Nurse Training School, University of Minnesota, Minneapolis	Due to the efforts of Richard Olding Beard, the Nurse Training School was organized as an integral part of that institution. It was a three year diploma program under the college of medicine.
1918	Army School of Nursing	Established by the Committee on Nursing of the Council of National Defense to ease nurse shortages, especially for war effort. Annie Goodrich was the Dean of the school which lead to a diploma.
1923	Western Reserve University, Cleveland, Ohio (now Case-Western Reserve University)	Collegiate program endowed by Frances Payne Bolton, initially offered a B.S. in nursing and later a M.N.
1924	Yale School of Nursing New Haven, Conn.	First autonomous collegiate school, established following the Goldmark Report through funds from the Rockefeller Foundation, the first separate university department with its own dean and budget. Annie Goodrich was the first dean. Twenty eight month course which included public health. Initially students were required to have at least two years of college work to be admitted, later, only baccalaureate graduates were accepted.
1924	Census of Public Health Nurses in the United States	Census supported by the National Organization for Public Health Nursing to determine number of PHNs and scope of service.
1930	Sage Memorial Hospital School of Nursing, Ganada, Arizona	Nursing program for Indian Women.
1943	Cadet Nurse Corps	Provided nursing education supervised by the U.S. Public Health Service under the Bolton Act. Nursing students had to provide essential military or civilian nursing service for the duration of the war. Lucille Petry was the Director of the U.S. Cadet Nurse Corps.
1940s	Practical Nursing Programs	Established to provide nursing services to the health system in response to WW II.

Educational Programs

Date	Program	Contribution to Nursing Education and Community Health Nursing
		The term "practical nurse" was approved by the American Nurses' Association, the National League of Nursing, and the National Organization for Public Health Nursing. Standards were few and duties were varied depending on the site of employment and perceived need.
1952	Associate Degree Nursing Programs established	Mildred Montag was first project director for these two year programs in junior and community colleges, designed to relieve the nurse shortages. Graduates termed "technical nurses."
1960s	Extended role for nurses and nursing, "nurse practitioner"	Various research and educational programs conducted to show nurses could do such tasks as take health history, do physical exams, and treat certain conditions. Standards and licensure are issues still being debated as well as the appropriate level of education preparation.
1970	National Health Service Corps	Designed to recruit nurses with strong public health backgrounds and nurse practitioners to provide health care in underserved areas.

Special Nursing Reports and Studies

Date	Committee, Report and/or Study	Contribution to Nursing Education and Community Health Nursing
1917	The Standard Curriculum for Schools of Nursing	M. Adelaide Nutting was chairperson and Isabel Stewart was committee secretary. Committee was designed to establish curricula standards.
1919	Committee for the Study of Nursing Education (Goldmark Report),	Committee established to determine the type of preparation needed by the public health nurse. Report published

Special Nursing Reports and Studies

Date	Committee, Report and/or Study	Contribution to Nursing Education and Community Health Nursing
	Nursing and Nursing Education in the United States	in 1923. Main recommendation for the establishment of collegiate schools of nursing to prepare nurse leaders.
1925	Committee on the Grading of Nursing Schools, *Nurses, Patients and Pockets*	Composed of representatives from ANA, NLNE, NOPHN, AMA, American College of Surgeons, AHA, and APHA. Report published in 1928. Purpose was to study supply and demand for nursing services, examination of nurses' jobs, and the grading of nursing schools.
1927	A Curriculum for Schools of Nursing	A Revision of the 1917 report "The Standard Curriculum for Schools of Nursing." Provided updated recommendations, including emphasis on public health nursing.
1948	The Brown Report, *Nursing for the Future*	Published by E. Lucille Brown, on the research staff of Russell Sage Foundation, included recommendations for the examination and accredidation of all schools of nursing and the open publication of the accredited schools. Supported public responsibility for assuming part of the financing of nursing education.
1948	National League for Nursing, *Nurses for a Growing Nation*	Projected needs for nurses and education into the 1970s, spoke of need to increase baccalaureate degree graduates and to increase/expand the facilities for such educational increases.
1961	The Surgeon General's Consultant Group on Nursing, *Toward Quality in Nursing*	Identified need for more nurses, more money to educate nurses, need for federal aid. Examined the types of programs offered and recommended that a program plan be developed which would allow for the professional advancement of the nurse.
1962	*Collegiate Education for Nursing*	Completed by Margaret Bredgman, recommended that nursing programs in colleges be on a par with other programs in the college. Adequately prepared faculty and facilities were

Special Nursing Reports and Studies

Date	Committee, Report and/or Study	Contribution to Nursing Education and Community Health Nursing
1965	American Nurses' Association, *Position Paper on Education for Nursing*	necessary for quality educational programs. Prepared by the ANA Committee on Education. Recommended that preparation for beginning professional nurses should be baccalaureate degree and for beginning technical nurses should be associate degree. All education for licensed nurses should be in institutions of higher education.
1967	National Commission for the Study of Nursing Education, *An Abstract for Action* (Lysaught Report)	Jointly supported by ANA and NLN, direct outgrowth of the Surgeon General's Consultant Group on Nursing, purposes were to conduct increased research into nursing service and education, improve and expand nursing education programs, increase financial support for nursing education, insure that quality nursing service would be more accessible.
1971	*Extending the Scope of Nursing Practice*	Supported by H.E.W. it concluded that an expansion of the nurse's role was necessary if quality health care was to be available to all persons.

Nursing Organizations

Date	Name of Organization	Contribution to Nursing Education and Community Health Nursing
1893	American Society of Superintendents of Training Schools for Nursing (became the N.L.N.E., then the N.L.N.)	Purpose was to promote fellowship among its members and establish a universal standard of training. Established at the Columbia Exposition held in Chicago.

Nursing Organizations

Date	Name of Organization	Contribution to Nursing Education and Community Health Nursing
1896	Nurses' Associated Alumnae of the United States and Canada (became the A.N.A.)	An organization of nurses to insure quality nursing care for all people and secure the welfare of nurses. Isabel Hampton Robb, first president.
1900	International Council of Nurses	Idea for an international fellowship germinated at the Columbia Exposition in Chicago, 1893. Formed from the national nursing association of each member country. To further the interests of nursing and nurses.
1908	National Association of Colored Graduate Nurses (later joined A.N.A.)	Association of Black Nurses formed in large part because they were not allowed membership in some state nursing associations.
1911	American Nurse's Association	Originally the Nurse's Associated Alumnae of the United States and Canada. The purposes remained the same as the original organization.
1912	National Organization for Public Health Nursing (later joined N.L.N.)	Composed of nurses and nonnurses who were interested in furthering and stimulating interest in public health nursing.
1912	National League of Nursing Education (became N.L.N.)	Originally the America Society of Superintendents of Training Schools for Nurses, with name change still held to earlier purposes.
1933	Association of Collegiate Schools of Nursing (became N.L.N.)	Purposes included the professional and collegiate development of nursing education, support between collegiate schools of nursing, and the promotion of nursing research in the service and education realm.
1946	World Health Organization	Purpose is the attainment of the highest possible health standards for all people.
1952	National League for Nursing (N.L.N.)	Formed with the merger of NLNE, the National Organization for Public Health Nursing, and Association of Collegiate Schools of Nursing. Both nurses and nonnurses can be members.
1952	National Student Nurse Association	Formed under the leadership of both the ANA and NLN. Purposes included preparation for participation in professional nursing organizations and nurse recruitment.

Legislation

Date	Legislative Action	Contribution to Nursing Education and Community Health Nursing
1903	State Nurse Licensure	North Carolina first state to enact a state-wide nurse registration law.
1931	Student Nurse Work Hours, California	Only state at that time to limit student nurse work to eight hours per day.
1921	Sheppard-Towner Act	For the improvement of maternal and infant welfare, included home visits, health education and health screening, expanded public health services.
1933	Federal Emergency Relief Administration Grant, Civil Works Administration, The Works Progress Association	All provided increased community nursing services, thus providing health care to those in need and employment for nurses.
1935	Social Security Act of 1935	Provided training for nurses in health departments, and a variety of health services to different population groups.
1941	Fair Employment Practices Committee (F.E.P.C.)	Established to investigate discrimination complaints and attempt to redress grievances, a step forward for black nurses.
1943	Bolten Act	Established the Cadet Nurse Corp. The U.S. Public Health Service subsidized the education of nursing students who would agree to provide military or civilian services.
1943	National Health Insurance	A comprehensive national health insurance program was proposed by President Harry Truman and which was opposed by the AMA, AHA, and other groups.
1944	The Public Health Service Act	Consolidated and revised the laws pertaining to the Public Health Service. Included areas such as administration, research, federal-state corporations, hospitals, medical examinations and medical care, leper care, narcotics addicts, biological products, quarantine and inspections, and the National Cancer Institute.
1946	The Hospital Survey and Construction Amendments of 1946 (Hill-Burton Act)	Established funds for nursing home and hospital construction, amended many times since enactment.

Legislation

Date	Legislative Action	Contribution to Nursing Education and Community Health Nursing
1954	Brown vs. Board of Education of Topeka	Outlawed racial segregation in public schools.
1962	Health Service for Agricultural Migratory Workers	Provided grants to establish health clinics and family services for migrant workers and their families.
1964	Social Security Amendments of 1965, Title XVIII, Health Insurance for the Aged (Medicare)	National health insurance program for the aged providing basic hospital and post-hospital care. Revisions have been made in 1966, 1967, 1971, and 1972.
1965	Social Security Amendments of 1965 Title XIX, grants to the states for Medical Assistance Programs (Medicaid)	A medical assistance program for people receiving federally aided public assistance and medically indigent persons. Revisions made in 1966, 1967, 1971, and 1972.
1966	Comprehensive Health Planning and Public Health Service Amendments of 1966	Act to extend and improve health planning and public health service.
1970	Communicable Disease Control Amendments of 1970	Reestablished grants of communicable disease control. Amended 1972.
1970	Family Planning Services and Population Research Act of 1970	Established an office of population affairs, authorized grants for family planning services and research but not abortions.
1970	Occupational Safety and Health Administration Act of 1970	Designed to promote occupational safety and health and to enforce laws and regulations for the health and safety of employees.
1973	Health Maintenance Organization Act of 1973	Assistance in the development and expansion of H.M.O.s.
1974	Health Planning and Resource Development Act of 1974	Provides for the planning and reorganization of the health care system on a local, state, and national bases to increase availability and accessability to the nation's citizens.
1974	Supplemental Security Income for the Aged, Blind and Disabled Title III (S.S.I.)	A federal minimum income program for people previously covered by adult public assistance programs which were federally supplemented.

16
NURSING ROLE
IN MIDWIFERY

JOAN E. MULLIGAN, Ph.D., C.N.M.

The purpose of this chapter is to provide an overview of the development of American nurse-midwifery, to describe present requirements for education and practice, and to comment on the place of nurse-midwives in the spectrum of providers of care to childbearing and birthing women.

DEFINITIONS

It is always helpful to know what a writer means when certain terms or phrases are used. The following are definitions of terms used in this chapter. The sequence of definitions roughly approximates the change over time in the who, what, when, where, and how these words pertain to childbearing and birthing experiences.

Midwifery. The work of a midwife.

Midwife. Woman with woman assisting; a woman whose work is helping women with childbirth; mid as with, wife as woman, rather than married woman.

Lay midwife. A twentieth century American term, a woman who assists women during the childbearing and birthing experience and who has generally acquired the knowledge and skills necessary to so assist by personal study and experience with other lay midwives; a term used to differentiate from the nurse and physician midwife.

Man midwife/male midwife. A seventeenth century European term, introduced to describe birth attendants skilled in the use of obstetric instruments and knowledgeable about the birth process. [1]

Granny midwife. A twentieth century American term that came to represent the stereotypic ignorant, unsafe, generally rural midwife; closely equivalent to the eighteenth century British term Sairey Gamp, the stereotype of the ignorant nurse.

Barber-surgeon. A thirteenth century European term used to describe members of the Guild of Barber-Surgeons. The right to use surgical instruments belonged officially to surgeons. Earlier, the term was used to describe the barber who performed surgical procedures. [1]

Obstetric. Of or pertaining to pregnancy and childbirth; of or pertaining to obstetrics.

Obstetrics. The branch of medicine concerning the care of women during pregnancy, labor, and the puerperium.

Obstetrician. Nineteenth century British term derived from the Latin *obstetrix* to designate physicians trained in midwifery and to differentiate from man/male midwife; one who practices obstetrics. [1,2]

Diploma mills. A twentieth century American term used to describe mail order and other unaccredited ways to obtain a medical or nursing diploma.

Nurse-midwife. "A registered nurse who by virtue of added knowledge and skills gained through an organized program of study and clinical experience has extended the limits of her (his) practice into the area of management of mothers and babies throughout the maternity cycle so long as progress meets criteria accepted as normal." [3]

Certified nurse-midwife (CNM). "An individual educated in the two disciplines of nursing and midwifery, who possesses evidence of certification according to the requirements of the American College of Nurse-Midwives." [3]

Nurse-midwifery practice. "The independent management of care of essentially normal newborns and women, antepartally, intrapartally, postpartally, and/or gynecologically occurring within a health care system which provides medical consultation, collaborative management, or referral and is in accord with the functions, standards and qualifications for nurse-midwifery practice as defined by the American College of Nurse-Midwives." [3]

The phrases *childbearing* and *birthing* will be used in this chapter in preference to the medical phrases pregnancy, labor and delivery, and puerperium. *Prebirth, birthing,* and *postbirth* will be used in preference to the medical terms prenatal (antepartum), intrapartum, and postpartum.

The term *childbearing woman* will be used in preference to the medical term pregnant woman or the social term *mother* to describe the prebirth state. The term *mother* will refer to the social status acquired by a woman postbirth.

The use of nonmedical terms to describe the physiologic states of women is deliberate. Readers should engage in an exercise of free association around the words "childbearing," "birthing," "pregnant," "antepartal," and so forth as a means to understanding the way words guide our approaches to people, and as a means to a beginning appreciation of the differences underlying the practice of midwifery by present day practitioners.

HISTORICAL DEVELOPMENT AND CONTINUING ISSUES IN NURSE-MIDWIFERY

The tradition of women helping women with "women's business" [1] began with women. To learn about nurse-midwives and nurse-midwifery is to learn about changing beliefs underlying the practices governing the care and management of childbearing women and their birthing experiences. The care and management practices reflect the sanctions over time governing who does what to whom, how, when, and where. Management practices and practitioners were and are influenced by the state of knowledge at any given time, by the social-cultural beliefs underlying behavior expected of both men and women, and by beliefs about childbearing. Without some sense of these changes, it is most difficult to appreciate the emergence of the nurse-midwife.

Nurse-midwifery, like other choices open to nurses, must be viewed as an occupational outgrowth of the social, scientific, demographic, organizational, economic, and political beliefs underlying the influences surrounding childbearing and childbirth. In short, as more couples become aware of the personal satisfaction to be obtained through full participation in childbearing and birth, and as these couples become informed about and disenchanted with modern technologic management of birth, they seek alternatives to medical management. The search for alternatives leads to alternative providers. Presently, middle and upper income couples are seeking the assistance of both lay and nurse-midwives. Additionally, the expertise of perinatal specialists is needed by those couples who are truly at risk of pregnancy related mortality and/or morbidity. The presence of nurse-midwives frees such specialists for attention to the at-risk population while at the same time providing the not-at-risk populations with safe care.

The declining birthrate, the high income of specialists, and the moderate income of general and family practice physicians increases the competition for childbearing clients; this is an economic fact of medical practice. The presence of nurse-midwives intrudes into this market. However, nurses seeking spheres of economic reward and social influence can find nurse-midwifery a challenging career choice, despite the past and present obstacles to practice.

The resurgence of popular interest in midwifery in the late twentieth century is paralleled by the early twentieth century struggle to establish obstetrics as a proper medical specialty and to eliminate the granny midwife. These late twentieth century efforts to expand and extend nurse-midwifery practice must be viewed in the context of the history of lay midwifery and the development of obstetrics as a proper medical specialty.

To historians, one of the most puzzling phenomena to explain is why women, who for centuries had been the traditional attendants at birth, were displaced by mostly male physicians. [1,4,5] It is a fact that in 1677, 99 percent of all American births were attended in the home by midwives. It is a fact that by 1977, 99 percent of all American births were attended in the hospital by physicians, who were mostly male. How and why had this change occurred?

Wertz and Wertz,[4] writing about birth from colonial times to the present, offer an explanation derived from the change in belief in magic to belief in science. Birth was demystified by science which meant that the natural process was amenable to some forms of human interventions. Physicians, mostly men, possessed the knowledge and technical equipment for intervention, thus women could seek, and were more open, to physician intervention in the case of birth difficulty. Additional explanation is needed to account for this change in America. Similar changes in belief occurred in Great Britain and Europe, yet midwifery remained an option there.

Donegan,[5] writing on the period 1760 to 1860, argues that demise of midwifery came as a result of an entanglement of social and economic factors geared to open opportunity for women to enter medical education, determined to preserve women's modesty, and in response to upper and middle income women wanting access to medical skills generally possessed by men.

Litoff,[2] analyzing the state of midwifery and midwives in the period 1860 to the present, attributes the decline of midwifery to a combination of several factors; improved obstetric practice desired by upper income women; the growth of safe, hospital based birth; lack of organization by lay midwives in contrast to the organization of male midwives and later proponents of the new medical specialty of obstetrics; lack of financial support for education of lay midwives; and finally poor supervision and regulation.

Donnison's[1] extensive historical research on British midwifery, covering the period of the seventeenth century to the present, offers an explanation based on the development of obstetric instruments, the exclusion of women from learning opportunities, poor regulation of practice, poor compensation for services, and the fact that upper class women chose to employ the skills of the man/male midwives.

Midwifery was women's business as long as there was limited understanding of the childbearing state and birthing, and as long as there were few effective means to change the outcome. As knowledge of the anatomy and physiology of childbearing and birth accumulated from the studies by male physicians, and as knowledge about these processes became available to barber-surgeons to apply to the difficult childbearing cases attended by midwives, there emerged the man midwife. The instruments used to crush skulls in order to extract the dead fetus had always been the instruments of the barber-surgeon.[1] Midwives generally called the barber-surgeon to assist in difficult births. With the invention of the forceps and their possession by male midwives, another era of birth management began. The education of eighteenth and nineteenth century American physicians in Britain brought to America a similar era.

The tradition of calling upon the man midwife in time of difficulty continues to the present. The lay midwife of today, as in times past, and the nurse-midwife of today leave to the physicians the management of difficult childbearing and birthing states. Whatever explanation for the past decline of midwifery one selects, it is important to see the influence of the past on the present.

Figure 16-1 attempts to summarize this history.* It is especially worth noting that at the time the twentieth century American midwifery controversy began and when the first suggestion for nurse-midwives appeared, American maternal and infant mortality rates were notoriously high. The term *midwife* became synonomous with the term *granny midwife* which was in turn associated with high mortality rates.[6] Attention directed to midwifery practice and its association with mortality rates deflected for a time attention to equally dismal medical practice.[7] Table 16-1 is a simple representation of three options presently open to childbearing women.

Very clearly, the emergence of nurse-midwifery in Britain and America is related directly to organized efforts to reform and/or exclude lay midwifery. There had been short lived efforts in the eighteenth century to establish education for American midwives. There were educational programs in nineteenth century America, but unlike Britain, formal programs in America did not develop and endure until the twentieth century. In 1861, Florence Nightingale opened a school for midwives with the intention of certifying the graduates as midwifery nurses, since she held the opinion that a proper midwife should be

---

Donnison,[1] Donegan[5] and Litoff[2] provide extensive documented descriptions of the process of acquisition of knowledge and skills for the management of childbearing by male midwives and the exclusion of lay midwives from access to this knowledge. Wertz and Wertz[4] provide detailed discussion of the social/cultural influences on birthing.

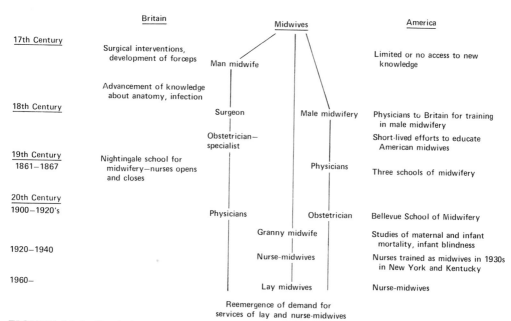

FIGURE 16-1. Brief chronology of events leading to emergence of American nurse-midwifery. (Derived from Donnison,[1] Litoff,[2] and Donegan.[5])

capable of dealing with all cases of childbearing and birth. Graduates of the school were intended to serve the rural poor. The school closed in 1867 following persistent outbreaks of puerperal fever in the wards of the school. Nightingale's dream of government support for another school was not to be fulfilled in her time.[1]

As early as 1911, visiting nurses trained as midwives were proposed as a solution to the American midwifery problem. In 1914, Fred J. Taussig, a St. Louis physician, in an address delivered to the National Organization of Public Health Nursing, introduced the term nurse-midwife when proposing the establishment of midwifery schools, to which only graduate nurses would be admitted.[2] It was more than a decade before such a school was established.

The first American nurse practitioners, as that term is now understood, were the 1931-32 nurse-midwife graduates of the New York Lobenstine School. The school was named to honor Ralph W. Lobenstine, physician and chairman of the medical board of the Maternity Center Association. These graduates, like current nurse practitioners, were to bridge the gap between the less advantaged and the medical care system. They were to attend to the childbearing needs of normal women, leaving the pathology to medical management.[2]

However, any discussion of nurse-midwifery must start with lay midwifery. A brief history derived principally from the work of Litoff[2] and Wertz[4] follows.

Childbearing women in the American colonies were attended by midwives. As early as 1716, the New York Common Council established rules to govern the midwifery practice of both males and females. In 1765 a course in midwifery for women and men was offered in Philadelphia. The first American midwifery text was published in 1807. In 1848 a formal training program was established at the Boston Female Medical College which awarded certificates in midwifery to those successfully completing the program. By the

TABLE 16-1. American midwifery in the 1970s: A summary of three childbearing/birthing options*

Characteristics	Lay midwives	Nurse midwives	Physicians
Pre-education	General	Nursing	Medicine, osteopathy
Education for practice	Apprenticeship	In institutions accredited by certifying boards and boards of parent disciplines (ACNM/NLN; ACOG/AMA; AOA)	
Registration and licensure	Varies with states and territories	Registered and licensed to practice parent discipline, nursing, or midwifery; RN may or may not require separate license to practice midwifery.	Registered and licensed to practice parent discipline, nursing, or medicine. MD/DO do not require separate license to practice midwifery.
Certification	None at present	American College of Nurse-Midwives (ACNM)	American College of Obstetricians and Gynecologists (ACOG)
Organization of practice	Solo, group	Solo, groups for profit, nonprofit groups	Solo, groups for profit, nonprofit groups
Practice site	Home	Home, hospital	Generally hospital. Not all physicians oppose home birth; many who support the option belong to the American College of Homebirth Physicians.
Reimbursement	Negotiated	Negotiated, third party payers, salary, fee for service	Negotiated, third party payers, salary, fee for service
Management style as a reflection of belief system	Natural methods; birth as a spiritual as well as physiologic experience	Natural with some dependence on technology; birth as a spiritual as well as physiologic experience	Highly dependent on technology; birth as a physiologic process
Knowledge Base: Anatomy & physiology of childbearing & birth	Required	Required	Required
Recognition of deviations	Required	Required	Required
Interventions	Natural	Natural, some analgesics, some local anesthetics, episiotomy, low forceps (rare)	Whole panoply of technology

Permission to use obtained from J.E. Mulligan, School of Nursing, University of Wisconsin-Madison.

end of the nineteenth century, male midwives had become established as the acceptable managers of birth for most upper and mid-income women. Women were considered too physically frail and lacking in intellectual capacity to learn the skills of the new midwifery. Further, such study might affect their later ability to bear children. [8]

The transition of lay midwifery from the realm of women's work to the realm of men's work, that is, the emergence of male midwives, led to the establishment of midwifery as required learning in nineteenth century American medical schools. Rarely was midwifery taught as a clinical subject; content in midwifery as with other medical subjects, was of a didactic nature.

A century earlier American physicians studying in Britain imported to the United States the science of obstetrics developed in London and Edinburgh. These returning physicians imported also their learnings about the British midwifery controversy. In time the male midwife disappeared from the American scene, his domain to become the domain of the physician. The establishment in 1888 of the American Association of Obstetricians and Gynecologists signaled the formal recognition and incorporation of the management of childbearing and birth in the domain of medical practice. Midwives were effectively excluded from the conduct of women's business for all but the lower income women. Upper income women believed physicians superior to midwives, and, besides, they could afford to pay for the services of the physician. Low income women, however, could neither afford the physician, nor could they as easily overcome their modesty which prohibited male attendance during birth. Immigrant women and low income urban and rural women continued to be served by midwives.

Contrary to popular opinion, not all midwives were unskilled. Immigrant midwives had been trained in Europe and midwives were being trained in America. The spectre of the stereotypic shuffling, untrained, ignorant granny midwife that emerged from the early twentieth century studies of maternal and infant mortality, continues to haunt the house of midwifery to this day, despite the fact that some midwives were conscientious about their work.

The stereotype, a convenient mechanism for avoiding thought, enabled traditional historians, educators, and policy makers to ignore the fact that prior to 1900 three schools of midwifery existed: the College of Midwifery of New York City, empowered in 1883 by the New York Supreme Court to issue certificates; the Playfair School of Midwifery in Chicago, established in 1896; and the St. Louis College of Midwifery. The municipally supported New York Bellevue School of Midwifery was founded in 1911; that school closed its doors in 1935.

The stereotype obscures also the fact that Connecticut, New York, and New Jersey had established regulatory, supervisory, and training programs for midwives. The populations served by the midwives had markedly lower maternal and infant mortality rates than those not so served. The plans of those states could have served as models for the rest of the country. They never did.

At the same time, diploma mills for physicians, nurses, and midwives flourished in the last decades of the nineteenth century and the first two decades of this century. Neither the physician, nurse, nor midwife diplomates were very competent. The 1910 Flexner Report[6] and the 1923 Goldmark Report[9] recommended sweeping changes in medical and nursing education. In 1912 Abraham Jacobi, president of the AMA, advocated the training and registration of midwives so they could attend normal births in order to free doctors to learn more about abnormal pregnancies. [2] The New York Committee for the Prevention of Blindness and many public health officials in New York, Georgia, and

elsewhere agitated for improved midwifery training and regulation. The midwifery controversy would continue until the late 1930s.

In the meantime, the idea of a nurse-midwife grew slowly. A recommendation to
establish maternity centers throughout the city of New York was made, following a 1915
study on maternity care conducted by the New York City Health Department. The purpose of establishing the centers was to reduce the high maternal and infant mortality
rates. The Maternity Center Association (MCA), a voluntary organization, was established
in 1918 to locate these maternity centers throughout the city. When established, nurses
in the centers provided many services including prenatal instruction, the selection of
candidates for hospital birth, and helping others prepare for birth at home.[2]

The expansion of MCA activities led to the decision to employ nurses trained as midwives. The Bellevue School for Midwives agreed in 1923 to admit the nurses employed
by MCA for midwifery training. The Commissioner of Welfare did not support the plan.
Another decade would pass before the first American trained nurse-midwives would begin
to practice.

In the meantime, another organization came to be in the early 1920s. Mary Breckenridge,
a nurse with American public health nursing education and British midwifery training,
went to Leslie County in the hills of Kentucky to begin a service that continues today.
Before leaving Britain, Mary Breckenridge went to study maternal and nursing care delivery
in the highlands of Scotland, a fit model for the Kentucky plan. Litoff states that Breckenridge believed that if "a successful nurse-midwifery program could be established . . . (in)
Kentucky, . . . similar work could be performed anywhere in the United States."[2]

The Kentucky Committee for Mothers and Babies chose Heyden, Leslie County as the
site for the first nursing center. When the center opened in 1925, American nurses trained
as midwives in Britain and British nurse-midwives staffed the center. In 1928 the name was
changed to the Frontier Nursing Service. In 1939, when Britain declared war against
Germany, the British nurse-midwives began to return to Britain. To ensure trained nurse-
midwives, the Frontier Graduate School of Midwifery came into being in 1939.

Both the Maternity Center Association and the Frontier Nursing Service received wide
publicity and support for their services which resulted in improved health status and survival
for childbearing women. The establishment in 1931 of the Association for the Promotion
and Standardization of Midwifery gave additional visibility to nurse-midwifery. The Association wanted, among other things, to establish a school for nurse-midwives in New
York.[2] In 1931, the Lobenstine Midwifery Clinic and School opened in Harlem. Graduates
of accredited nursing schools were the only nurse admitted. In 1934, the clinic and school
joined with the Maternity Center under the name of MCA.[2]

Despite the wide publicity and demonstrated effects on the health of childbearing
women which resulted from the services of these two organizations, the United States was
generally not ready for the widespread implementation of nurse-midwifery services. There
is no one adequate explanation for this fact. Clearly, the efforts of medical educators to
improve obstetrical education and the high status ascribed to the practitioners of medicine
were contributing factors. Concerted efforts to persuade couples of the benefits of medical
care, combined with the change of birth site from home to hospital and the preference
for physician service held by middle and upper income women also helped to postpone
the development of nurse-midwifery in this country.

Further, neither the American Nurses' Association (ANA) nor the National League for
Nursing (NLN) seemed able to find a place for the nurse-midwives in their organizations.
Perhaps the best explanation for the lack of space for nurse-midwives in these organizations

rests in the fact that they did not fit the organizational structures of that time period nor the ideologies of the organizations.

The nurse-midwives in Kentucky had formed the American Association of Nurse-Midwives in 1929. In 1954 nurse-midwives attending the annual ANA convention planned the formation of their own organization; in 1955 the American College of Nurse-Midwifery came to be.[43] The American College of Nurse-Midwives (ACNM), established in 1969, brought the membership of the New York based American College of Nurse-Midwifery and the Kentucky based American Association of Nurse-Midwives together. One of the goals of this new group was to further the legal recognition of nurse-midwives. Another goal was to evaluate and accredit nurse-midwifery educational programs. Nurse-midwives, unlike the lay midwife, now had an organization. Nurse-midwives could now begin to establish the requirements for the education and practice of American nurse-midwifery.

The exclusion of nurse-midwives from incorporation into both the ANA and NLN is a historical fact. In the forefront, as the first providers of primary health care (before any of us had ever heard of the phrase) and as the first nurse practitioners (as we now understand the meaning of that term), the early nurse-midwives deprived the ANA and the NLN of their knowledge of the conduct of women's business and were themselves deprived of the resources of the larger organizations. There is no way of knowing what nurse-midwifery might have contributed to both, nor what both would have contributed to the promotion of nurse-midwifery and thus to the wellbeing of childbearing women.

The fact remains, that in 1976 the Center for Health Statistics discussed nurse-midwives in the narrative of its report on midwifery but omitted reporting either the geographic location of nurse-midwives or the ratio of nurse-midwives to population, while reporting both the geographic location and the ratio of lay midwives.[11] As late as 1977, despite the presence of 18 accredited nurse-midwifery programs, the Center could only report an estimated 4300 persons active in the field of midwifery, with no differentiation made between nurse and lay midwife.[12] As of 1980, there is yet no American nurse-midwifery textbook by a nurse-midwife; American nurse-midwifery students rely on obstetrics and pediatric texts similar to those used by medical students and practicing physicians and on a classic English midwifery text now in its eighth edition.[13] One final piece of evidence that suggests that nurse-midwifery continues to struggle for recognition rests on the fact that in the recently passed and funded Rural Health Services legislation,[14] its rules and regulations for implementation omit specific reference to either the nurse-midwife or the American College of Nurse-Midwives. In view of these facts, one must conclude that the historic struggle to establish nurse-midwifery as a visible, widely available, accountable, and safe alternative to a medically managed, technologic childbearing and birthing experience continues.

This section concludes where it began, with lay midwives. Recent demands for home birthing away from the technology of the hospital, coming primarily from middle and upper class women and men, has led to the reemergence of the lay midwife.[15,16] This trend is opposed by the American College of Obstetricians and Gynecologists.[17] The ACNM[18] has taken a somewhat cautious stance on the subject of home birth.

NURSE MIDWIFERY: PREPARATION FOR EXTENDED AND EXPANDED NURSING PRACTICE

Despite the evidence presented above of low nurse-midwifery visibility, nurses seeking greater participation in the health provider market through advanced education, especially as that market pertains to the childbearing, birth, and the postbirth period, cannot be accommodated by existing, accredited nurse-midwifery programs. In the 1930s there were two nurse-midwifery programs; in 1980 there are 18 accredited programs. A discussion of the educational and clinical preparation of American nurse-midwives and their scope of services follows.

Educational and Clinical Preparation

Admission to a nurse-midwifery educational program requires the applicant to be a registered nurse currently licensed to practice nursing, or to be eligible to become registered and licensed as a nurse.

It is an education that derives from selected aspects of medicine built upon the bases of nursing and in preparation for the conduct of women's business. Since that business sometimes requires relief from pain and surgical procedures, nurse-midwife students, unlike most other nurse practitioners, learn to use selected local anesthetics such as a pudendal block; to do and repair an episiotomy and to repair vaginal tears should these occur; and learn the immediate resuscitation of the newborn. Programs in nurse-midwifery differ somewhat from each other due to, among other factors, their medical settings—the client population may be very large and predominantly low income or moderately large and of mixed income. Whatever the setting and client population, however, each program must meet the requirements established for accreditation by the American College of Nurse-Midwives.

Since its beginning in 1955, the ACNM has pioneered the accreditation process for nurse-midwifery and thus nurse practitioner education. The work of that organization is described below in some detail as it is a model for other practitioner programs. When the American College of Nurse-Midwifery began in 1955, one of its concerns was the "evaluating and rating of nurse-midwifery programs."[2] By 1978, the American College of Nurse-Midwives could be credited with the following accomplishments: the adoption of a philosophy[19] from which derives the bases for educational programs and the preparation of a statement outlining the functions, standards, and qualifications for the practice of nurse-midwifery[20] intended to implement the philosophy and which provides goals for the education programs. Additionally, by 1977 the College had revised procedures for approving educational programs in nurse-midwifery[21] in order to ensure that the 1972 standards for evaluating procedural functions for practice,[22] the statement of functions, standards and qualifications, and the statement of purpose of nurse-midwifery education[23] would be accomplished.

To meet ACNM requirements for accreditation, basic nurse-midwifery educational programs are usually located in or affiliated with institutions of higher learning.[23] Two present exceptions are: The Nurse-Midwifery Program, United States Air Force, Andrews Air Force Base, Washington, D.C. and the Frontier School of Midwifery and Family Nursing, Wendover, Kentucky. Programs are established where there is already a nurse-midwifery service within the institution, or where contracts for appropriate clinical experience can be negotiated.[24] Faculty of the programs must meet requirements for academic appointment, must have at least one year's experience in clinical nurse-midwifery, and must be current in clinical practice.[24] Educational programs are located in areas where there is a large enough patient population to provide each student with "15 new antepartum visits, 70 return antepartum visits, 20 labor management experiences, 20 deliveries, 40 immediate postpartum visits, 20 newborn assessments, and 40 postpartum/family planning gynecological visits."[24]

Finally, programs are located in states where legislation is not prohibitive.[25] That is, the medical and nursing practice acts and the pharmacy acts of the state are not deterrents to the practice of nurse-midwifery. It can be, however, that although state laws do not hinder practice, the by-laws and administrative and medical staff policies of institutions within the state can act as restraints on practice. Thus, where nurse-midwifery services and educational programs do exist, they are the outcome of considerable negotiation within the states and institutions, between those who have developed birthing services on a medical model and those who wish a birthing service on a nurse-midwife or health model.

Students entering an accredited midwifery program take a core of courses which carry academic credit determined by the level of the program.[23] In other words, depending on whether a student enters a certificate program or a program leading to a master's degree, the assigned credit value of the course work varies. Certificate programs admit registered nurse students with academic credentials ranging from diploma to doctorate. Credit value of certificate nurse-midwifery course work is determined by the institution offering the program. The value of credits so earned, when applied toward meeting baccalaureate degree requirements, is determined by the admitting institution. In other words, a registered nondegree nurse may be able to apply the nurse-midwifery certificate credits toward a baccalaureate degree, depending upon the policies of the particular university. Students in both programs must acquire knowledge of the medical management aspects of all phases of normal childbearing and of the newborn period. Depending on the program, students augment and supplement their nursing knowledge and the special knowledge of nurse-midwifery necessary to "labor sit" (a vernacular phrase for nurse-midwifery care rendered during birthing). The core curriculum includes the "theory and practice of nurse-midwifery . . . history taking, physical and pelvic assessment, nurse-midwifery management, process of antepartum, intrapartum, postpartum, family planning/gynecology, neonatology, parent education and professional aspects of nurse-midwifery."[24] Nurse-midwives learn skills derived from surgery, anesthesiology, pharmacology, nutrition, and internal medicine.

Educational programs are located in a variety of academic administrative units such as schools of public health, nursing, medicine, or colleges of allied health professions. One exception is the Frontier Nursing Service School of Midwifery and Family Nursing which continues as an autonomous institution. Admission to a nurse-midwifery program requires that the student first meet the academic admission requirement and then the nurse-midwifery program requirement. Satisfactory completion of graduation requirements is represented by a certificate of completion or a master's degree in public health or nursing. The variety of educational settings is such that readers are advised to obtain information about accredited programs from the American College of Nurse-Midwives, 1012 14th Street, N.W., Washington, D.C. 20005. Specific content of each program varies with each setting. All nurse-midwives are expected, however, to have knowledge about all the skills to manage the normal progression of pre- and post-childbearing and birthing. Some of these skills are the ability to assess fetal growth and position by palpation, assess the adequacy of the bony pelvis, and, like other nurse practitioners, obtain a history, perform a physical examination, and know when to ask for consultation and when to refer.

Upon recommendation of faculty, students of nurse-midwifery programs apply for admission to the certification examination set by the American College of Nurse-Midwives. Satisfactory completion of the examination entitles the use of the initials CNM (Certified Nurse-Midwife).

The site of practice for nurse-midwives is similar to other providers, that is, hospital, clinics, offices, and, in some cases, the home. Brennan and Heilman[26] describe their practice based in Roosevelt Hospital, New York. Others practice in childbearing centers such as the Maternity Center Association-New York or the Childbearing-Childrearing Center at the University of Minnesota-Minneapolis. A few nurse-midwives have organized to provide home-birth services.[27] However, the majority of nurse-midwives assist birthing in the hospital setting and the pre-post childbearing process in offices or clinic settings. In all settings, nurse-midwives have associations and agreements with medical and hospital back-up and clearly stated protocols for accepting couples who seek out the nurse-midwife or are referred for management of all aspects of the childbearing and birthing experience. *Nurse-Midwifery in the United States, 1976-1977*[28] provides a well documented and carefully analyzed report on this population of nurse practitioners.

Despite the fact that the majority of American childbearing women continue to obtain their care from mostly male physicians and most continue to experience a medically/technologically managed hospital based birth, "childbirth in the last analysis is women's business."[1] The education of nurse-midwives is an education for the conduct of women's business. That education is likely to enhance the possibility for nurse-midwifery accommodation to the increasing search for a more human childbearing and birthing experience. Nurse-midwife education can and does dramatize the differences between bith experiences derived from the medical model and those derived from a health/nursing model. The personal rewards of nurse-midwifery and the satisfaction of women and men following their experience with a nurse-midwife assisted birth are many. Readers interested in the movement toward a less technologically managed birth experience are referred to NAPSAC,[29] Arms,[30] and Haire.[31]

Scope of Services

Like other nurse practitioners, nurse-midwives are concerned with the maintenance and promotion of health of their specific client population, the early identification and control of deviations from normal, the use of medical consultation, referral and the provision of supportive nursing services in the event of major deviation from normal, and continuity of care.

Nurse-midwifery practice exists in the environment of generally receptive and supportive medical, nursing, and hospital administrative practices. Like others in an extended and expanded role, the medical management aspect of nurse-midwifery practice is guided by protocols jointly agreed upon by nurse-midwives, other nurses, physicians, and hospital, clinic, or office administrators.

The nurse midwife, like other nurse practitioners, works with nurses, physicians (especially obstetricians and pediatricians), pharmacists, family members, clerks, nutritionists, social workers—in other words, the whole range of client support personnel. One major difference is that the client population is in some phase of childbearing.

Nurse-midwifery practice differs from that of other nurse practitioners in respect to surgery and anesthesia, so that the client population served by nurse-midwives receives a range of services beginning with the diagnosis of conception; care and instruction required during the prebirth period; close attention and support during birthing; conduct of the birth itself which may include the use of local anesthesia and/or the performance and repair of an episiotomy; assessment and care of the newborn immediately at birth; attention to the mother and father immediately and in the postbirth period; and, finally, assistance to the couple in choosing a conception control method.

Nurse-midwifery service is open to any childbearing woman whose medical and/or childbearing history places her in the range of normal. It is conjecture that perhaps because low income women are frequently classified as high risk they may, in fact, not have as easy access to nurse-midwifery services as do higher income women whose nutritional state, general health status, and other factors are less likely to place them in the high risk category. Thus, in the 1970s we may be seeing a reversal of history; that is, urban higher income women may want, seek, and be able to obtain nurse-midwifery services in preference to physician services, while urban low income women receive their care from physicians.

Persons seeking nurse-midwifery services generally learn about the service through friends, reading, or telephoning local hospitals and clinics.

Depending on the geographic location and practice setting, salaries for nurse-midwives are comparable to salaries paid other nurse practitioners. The 1978 ACNM reported the mean 1976 income of certified nurse-midwives at $16,171.[31] Annual income was affected by such factors as the management of birth, whether the basis of income was a fixed salary or fee-for-services, and education.[31]

In general, nurse-midwives are enthusiastic about their work and the personal satisfaction that comes at the time of birth, when parents view their newborn for the first time. However, the maze of laws, rules, and regulations to regulate health care providers, in particular midwives, promulgated by state legislatures and regulatory agencies over the past 50 years continues to impede the full participation of nurse-midwives in the health care system in the 1970s.

Legal Considerations in the United States

Nurse-midwives are perhaps the victims of their history. Like other nurse practitioners, their right to practice under the laws of various states is mixed. While it is a fact that a nurse or a physician licensed to practice in one state and wishing to move to practice in another state must meet the requirements for licensure in the new state, this is possible only because each state has laws governing the practice of nursing and medicine. This is not so in the case of nurse-midwives. Their certification of competency by the board of the American College of Nurse-Midwive is not a guarantee of the right to practice.

The most current and complete report on the status of licensure to practice nurse-midwifery is found in the special issue, Summer 1976, of *Journal of Nurse-Midwifery*.[32] In 1970, the Legislation Committee of the ACNM began plans to conduct a nation wide survey to determine how state laws affected nurse-midwifery practice, which states had laws that interfered with nurse-midwifery practice, and ways to establish sound guidelines for the legal base of practice.[32]

Forman and Cooper describe the legal situation succinctly: "Old laws are not suited to new situations."[32] It is not sufficient to seek laws governing nurse-midwifery practice, it is necessary to examine also laws governing the practice of medicine and nursing and lay midwifery. The practice of nurse-midwifery may be governed by actual legislation or by rules and regulations promulgated by various state administrative boards or by the interpretation of the existing laws by states' attorneys-general. Of major interest, of course, is the control of practice where it is not prohibited. For example, are the controls vested in a board of medicine, a board of nursing, or some other administrative board responsible for licensing, or is there a separate board to license nurse-midwives?

The survey found that 49 of the 50 states, including four federal jurisdictions,[32] had permissive laws, that is, laws that neither supported nor prohibited practice.[32] Five states had laws interpreted by states' attorneys-general—laws restrictive in that they conflicted with other state laws. No states had laws that were clearly prohibitive.

Further survey results revealed that 25 states had either statutes or rules of a regulatory agency or joint statements between professional groups in which specific reference was made to nurse-midwifery, nurse-midwives, or ACNM certification.[32] Thirty states had a variety of legal arrangements whereby practice was enabled.[32] Arrangements to enable nurse-midwifery practice vary from nursing practice statutes (16 states), lay midwife statutes (7 states), physician assistant statutes (4 states), or general health statutes (3 states).[32]

Certification of qualification to practice is the business of the American College of Nurse-Midwives; permission to practice nurse-midwifery, as evidenced by licensure or other administrative means, is the business of states. Although the laws of 49 states and jurisdictions permit practice, actual practice occurs in only 38 of the 49. In 17 of these states only nurse-midwives engage in full practice; 15 states permit full practice by both lay and nurse-midwives; and in 6 states, with some exceptions, full practice by lay midwives is possible.[32]

Certainly, the problems of certification to practice are relatively simple in comparison to the complex arrangements to make that practice a reality. Readers interested in pursuing the topic further are advised to address their requests to the Legislative Committee, c/o ACNM, Washington, D.C., 20005. Readers residing in states where nurse-midwifery is not a reality are urged to become involved in the process of legislative change; those residing in states permitting nurse-midwifery practice but where this service is lacking are encouraged to explore the policies and guidelines of local hospitals which may act as obstacles to nurse-midwifery services.

There can be very little doubt that the historic roots of American nurse-midwifery continue to be hazards on the pathways to a gentler birthing experience.

Once upon a time it was fashionable for middle and upper income women to experience medically managed hospital based birth and for low income women to experience a midwife managed home birth or perhaps a rather bungled medically managed hospital based birth. The time is now upon us when middle and upper income women in some states can choose between the nurse-midwife choreographed birth or the technologically synchronized birth. Low income women, by virtue of their physical state, may still not have this choice in many states. As so often in the past, the wishes and choices of middle and upper income women later become the reality for the low income women. Now the choice of a woman (since most nurse-midwives are women) to help in "women's business" is open to higher income women, as many of their lower income sisters continue to engage in "women's business" under the management of mostly male physicians.

LEGISLATION AND NURSE MIDWIVES

Certainly it must soon be recognized by health planners and policy makers that nurse-midwives have a major place in reducing costs and improving the quality and availability of health care services in regionalization plans for childbearing and birthing services. PL93-641[33] mandates a restructuring of services, including those of childbearing and birthing. The law and its rules and regulations[34] is based on a medical, technologic model: no provisions are made for the establishment of birth centers nor the utilization of nonphysician childbearing-birthing providers. Similarly, in the rules and regulations of PL95-210[35] establishing rural health services, no reference was made to the nurse-midwife, nor did the legislation for Maternal Infant Care[36] acknowledge the existence of nurse-midwives.

It is difficult to imagine how planners and policy makers, faced with infant and maternal mortality rates higher than most industrialized nations[37] and faced with evidence from numerous sources that in the presence of nurse-midwives infant and maternal rates drop,[38,39] can continue to propose and pass legislation ignoring a population of providers who have demonstrated their value in American and in all industrialized societies. But they do!

The position of nurse-midwives in Europe, Africa, and Asia is long established. The European Common Market provisions attend to exchange of health providers.[1] Nurse-midwives and midwifery in Europe and Britain will undoubtedly undergo changes in requirements for practice. While the importation of American medicine may pose a threat to their position eventually, their contribution to the well being of women and children is longstanding. Readers interested in pursuing this topic further should contact the International Confederation of Midwives, 57 Lower Belgrave Street, London, SWIW, ORL, England.

SUMMARY

Midwives have been the attendants at birth since the beginning of our history. They have been women helping women. As medical knowledge advanced, the business of birthing entered the domain of medicine and men. In the 1920s the American midwifery controversy peaked, leading to, among other changes, the establishment of nurse-midwifery in the Harlem section of New York and in Kentucky. The intervening years brought major changes in the medical management of birthing and reducing maternal and perinatal death rates, resulting in an American population convinced that childbearing and birthing are in the domain of medical practice. Medicine was not excluded when all institutions became suspect in the 1960s. Now in 1980 as nurse-midwives continue the struggle for recognition, a new breed of lay midwife practices in every state of the union. Some women and their partners are rejecting the medical model of birth; birth attended by a lay midwife is an emerging alternative for many.[29,40]

Nurse-midwives can provide a third alternative, the compassion and essence of the lay midwife combined with the knowledges and skills derived from nursing and medicine. Public awareness of this alternative is growing.

ACKNOWLEDGEMENTS

I wish to thank Susan Kiley, Nancy Ropel, and Linda Runstrum, students, Baccalaureate Program, and Sarah L. Turner, R.N., Ph.D., Assistant Professor, University of Wisconsin-Madison School of Nursing, for their suggestions and assistance in the preparation of this chapter. The criticisms and suggestions of historian Patricia Spain Ward, Humanistic Studies Program, College of Medicine, University of Illinois at Chicago are gratefully acknowledged.

REFERENCES

1. Donnison, Jean: *Midwives and Medical Men.* Schocken Books, New York, 1977.
2. Litoff, Judy Barrett: *American Midwives.* Greenwood Press, Westport, Ct., 1978.
3. American College of Nurse-Midwives: *What is a Nurse-Midwife?* Washington, D.C.
4. Wertz, Richard, and Wertz, Dorothy: *Lying-In.* Free Press, New York, 1977.
5. Donegan, Jane: "Midwifery in America, 1760-1860." Unpublished Dissertation, Syracuse University, 1972.
6. Flexner, Abraham: *Medical Education in the United States and Canada: A Report to the Carnegie Foundation for the Advancement of Teaching.* Carnegie Foundation, New York, 1910.
7. Meigs, Grace L.: *Maternal Mortality From All Conditions Connected With Childbirth in the United States and Other Countries.* Department of Labor, Childrens Bureau, Washington, D.C., Misc. Series #6, Publication #19, 1917.
8. Haller, J., and Haller, R.: *The Physician and Sexuality in Victorian America.* W.W. Norton, New York, 1974. See also Walsh, Mary R.: *Doctors Wanted: No Women Need Apply.* Yale University Press, New Haven, 1977.
9. Goldmark, Josephine: *Report of the Committee for the Study of Nursing Education and Report of a Survey.* Macmillan Company, New York, 1923.
10. Breckenridge, Mary: *Wide Neighborhoods: A Story of Frontier Nursing Service.* Harper & Row, New York, 1952.
11. U.S. Department of HEW, PHS, HRA: *Health Resources Statistics.* U.S. Superintendent of Documents, Washington, D.C., HRA Publication #76-1509, 1976.
12. U.S. Department of HEW, PHS, HRA: *Health United States 1976-1977.* Superintendent of Documents, Washington, D.C., HRA Publication #177-1232, 1977.
13. Myles, Margaret F.: *A Textbook for Midwives,* 8th ed. Longman, Inc., New York, 1974.
14. PL95-210 Rural Health Clinic Services Act: *Federal Register* (February 8, 1978), Vol. 43, #27, [4110-35], 5373. Final Rules and Regulations published in 1978 now includes nurse-midwives. *Medicare and Medicaid Guide,* Reg. 405.2401, #20, 868, 1978.
15. The Fremont Health Collective: *Women and Health.* 2(3):19, Nov./Dec. 1977.
16. Exchange: *Women and Health.* 3(1):17, Jan./Feb. 1978. Reports the formation of the National Midwives Association with headquarters at P.O. Box 163, Princeton, NJ.
17. American College of Obstetricians and Gynecologists, District II: *Position Paper on Out-of-Hospital Maternity Care.* New York, adopted January, 1976. See also *Network News,* National Women's Health Network, June Edition, 1977, p. 1.
18. American College of Nurse-Midwives: *Statement on Homebirths.* October 1973. *Annual Report 1975,* p. 20, *Annual Report 1977,* p. 11, Washington, D.C.
19. American College of Nurse-Midwives: *Statement of Philosophies.* Washington, D.C., 1972.
20. American College of Nurse-Midwives: *Functions, Standards, & Qualifications.* Washington, D.C., 1975.
21. American College of Nurse-Midwives: *Policies & Procedures of Approval for Programs in Nurse-Midwifery Education.* Washington, D.C., 1975.
22. American College of Nurse-Midwives: *Standards for Evaluation of Nurse-Midwife Procedural Functions.* Washington, D.C., 1972. Retitled *Guidelines for Evaluation . . . ,* 1977.
23. American College of Nurse-Midwives: *Statement of Nurse-Midwifery Education.* Washington, D.C., May, 1977.
24. American College of Nurse-Midwives: *Criteria for Evaluation of Educational Programs in Nurse-Midwifery.* Washington, D.C., 1977.
25. American College of Nurse-Midwives: *Guidelines for Establishing New Basic Education Programs for Nurse-Midwives.* Washington, D.C., 1973.
26. Brennan, Barbara, and Heilman, Joan R.: *Complete Book of Midwifery.* E.P. Dutton, New York, 1977.
27. Epstein, Janet F., and McCartney, Marian: "A Home Delivery Service That Works." *Women and Health* 3(1):10, Jan./Feb. 1978.
28. American College of Nurse-Midwives Research & Statistics Committee (eds.): *Nurse-Midwifery in the United States, 1976-1977.* Washington, D.C., 1978.
29. Stewart, David and Stewart, Lee (eds.): *21st Century Obstetrics Now.* NAPSAC Publications, Chapel Hill, N.C., 1977.

30. Arms, Suzanne: *The Immaculate Deception*. Houghton Mifflin Company, Boston, 1975.
31. Haire, Doris: *The Cultural Warping of Childbirth*. International Childbirth Education Association, Seattle, 1972. Reprinted in *Environmental Child Health*. Special Issue, Vol. 19, June 1973.
32. *Journal of Nurse-Midwifery*. Special Issue, Vol. 21, #2, Summer 1976.
33. PL93-641 National Health Planning and Resources Development Act of 1974.
34. *Federal Register*. Part II, p. 48504, September 1977.
35. PL95-210 Rural Health Services Act.
36. PL88-156 Ammendments to Title V, SSA, Maternal and Infant Care Project Ammendments, 1964.
37. U.S. Department HEW, PHS, HSA: *Improvement in Infant and Perinatal Mortality in the United States 1965-1973*. U.S. Government Printing Office, Washington, D.C., Publication No. (HSA) 78-5743, 1978.
38. State of California Department of Public Health, Bureau of Maternal and Child Health: *The Use of Nurse Obstetric Assistants in a Rural County Hospital Maternity and Newborn Program*. Berkeley, Ca., 1978.
39. *Frontier School of Midwifery & Nursing*. Frontier Nursing Service, Wendover, Ky., Annual Reports.
40. "New Interest in Home Deliveries." Maternal and Child Health Information, MCH Service, HSMHS, DHEW Publication No. 29, January, 1973, p. 1.

BIBLIOGRAPHY

"Alternative Patterns of Nurse-Midwifery Care." *Journal of Nurse-Midwifery*, 21(3), Fall 1976.

American College of Nurse-Midwives: *Nurse-Midwifery in the United States 1976-1977*. Washington, D.C., 1968.

Ashley, Jo Ann: *Hospitals, Paternalism and the Role of the Nurse*. Teachers College Press, New York, 1977.

Barker-Benfield, G.T.: *The Horrors of the Half-Known Life: Male Attitudes Toward Women and Sexuality in 19th Century America*. Harper & Row, New York, 1976.

Beebe, Joyce: "The Future of Nurse-Midwifery Education." *Journal of Nurse-Midwifery*, 22(3):16, Fall, 1977.

Bureau of Maternal and Child Health, Department of Public Health, State of California: *The Use of Nurse Obstetric Assistants in a Rural County Hospital Maternity and Newborn Program*. Berkeley, Ca., 1967.

Chafe, William H.: *The American Woman: Her Changing Social, Economic and Political Role, 1920-1970*. Oxford University Press, New York, 1972.

Chepaites, Joseph B.: "The First Federal Social Welfare Measure: The Sheppard-Towner Maternity and Infancy Act, 1918-1932." Unpublished dissertation, Georgetown University, 1968.

Cherner, Anne: "Midwives and the Medical Profession." Unpublished thesis, Radcliffe College, 1976.

Danziger, Sandra Klein: "The Use of Expertise in Doctor-Patient Encounters During Pregnancy." Unpublished dissertation, Boston University, 1977.

Donegan, Jane Bauer: "Midwifery in America, 1760-1860: A Study in Medicine and Morality." Unpublished dissertation, Syracuse University, 1972.

Donnison, Jean: *Midwives and Medical Men: A History of Inter-Professional Rivalries and Women's Rights*. Schocken Books, New York, 1977.

Ehrenreich, Barbara, and English, Dierdre: *Witches, Midwives and Nurses: A History of Women Healers*. The Feminist Press, Old Westbury, N.Y., 1973.

Ehrenreich, Barbara and English, Dierdre: *For Her Own Good*. Anchor Press, Doubleday, New York, 1978.

Flack, H.I.: *Eternal Eve: The History of Gynaecology and Obstetrics*. Doubleday, New York, 1951.

Fremont Women's Birth Collective: "Lay Midwifery—Still an 'Illegal' Profession." *Women and Health*, 2(3):19, Nov./Dec. 1977.

Haller, John S., and Haller, Robin M.: *The Physician and Sexuality in Victorian America*. W.W. Norton, New York, 1977.

"Ina May and the Farm Midwives." *Spiritual Midwifery*, The Book Publishing Company, Summertown, Tenn., 1975.

"Legislation and Nurse-Midwifery Practice in the U.S.A." *Journal of Nurse-Midwifery,* 21(2), Summer 1976.

Lemons, J. Stanley: *The Woman Citizen: Social Feminism in the 1920's.* University of Illinois Press, Chicago, 1975.

Levy, Barry S., Wilkinson, Frederich S., and Marine, William M.: "Reducing Neonate Mortality Rate With Nurse-Midwives." *American Journal of Obstetrics and Gynecology,* 109(1):50 Jan. 1971.

Litoff, Judy Barrett: *American Midwives 1860 to the Present.* Greenwood Press, Westport, Conn., 1978.

Montgomery, Theordore A.: "A Case for Nurse-Midwives." *American Journal of Obstetrics and Gynecology,* 105(2):309, Oct. 1969.

Mulligan, Joan E.: "Three Federal Interventions on Behalf of Childbearing Women . . . ." Unpublished dissertation, University of Michigan, 1976.

Mulligan, Joan E.: "Professional Transition: Nurse to Nurse-Midwife." *Nursing Outlook,* 24(4):228, April 1976.

Oakley, Ann: *The Sociology of Housework.* Pantheon Books, New York, 1974.

Oakley, Ann: *Woman's Work.* Vintage Books, New York, 1976.

Shaw, Nancy S.: *Forced Labor: Maternity Care in the United States.* Pergamon Press, New York, 1974.

Stewart, David, and Stewart, Lee (eds.): *21st Century Obstetrics Now.* NAPSAC Publications, Chapel Hill, N.C., 1977.

"The Future of Nurse-Midwifery Education." *Journal of Nurse-Midwifery,* 22(3), Fall 1977.

Wertz, Richard W., and Wertz, Dorothy C.: *Lying-in: A History of Childbirth in America.* The Free Press, New York, 1977.

17
NURSING ROLE IN DEVELOPMENTAL DISABILITIES

MARGARET REGISTER BEAN, M.N., M.S., R.N.

The assumption underlying the nursing care of children with developmental disabilities is that the nursing process is directed toward helping each person to attain and maintain his maximum level of health. Clark and McMahan cite the World Health Organization's definition of health as "a state of complete physical, mental, and social well-being and not merely the absence of disease or infirmity."[1] The nursing process involves helping the developmentally disabled to reach and maintain optimum health in each of these areas. The developmentally disabled includes any child who has a delay in development or has specific disorders, such as cerebral palsy or blindness, which interfere with achieving a complete level of physical, mental, and social well-being.* The nurse's background knowledge and clinical skills in the areas of psychology, nursing (including allied health fields), and sociology enable her to solve some problems through direct intervention and to identify when expertise and consultation are needed from other professionals. Nursing intervention offers a total approach in the provision and coordination of services for the child with developmental disabilities. To practice in this specialty area two conditions are necessary. The nurse must first accept the premise that it is the right of each individual to develop to his maximum capacity, be it great or small. Second, the nurse must acknowledge a personal commitment to the achievement of that goal.

---

* The terms developmentally disabled and handicapped are used interchangeably in this chapter.

HISTORICAL DEVELOPMENT

Formerly, nursing care of the developmentally disabled was largely conducted either in acute care hospitals, residential institutional settings, or health department clinics. The predominate focus was in institutional settings where the majority of these children were referred. Robinson and Robinson[2] relate this trend which began in the 1920s and 1930s to the eugenics movement. In these institutional settings, the nurse performed traditional roles geared toward meeting physical needs through functions such as giving medications, caring for basic hygiene, and maintaining a healthy physical environment. For those children who remained at home, public health nurses counseled parents in techniques of home management. The public health nurse was required to provide a multiplicity of services and was considered to be a one person team. State crippled children's programs were available to provide diagnostic and treatment services. With the advent of new techniques and knowledge, public health nurses became more involved with prevention and case finding through clinics such as those for well-child care and family planning. School nurses also assumed increasing responsibility for identifying children with handicaps.

In the 1960s, nursing leaders began to arrive at conceptual frameworks for focusing on the nurse's role and to isolate specific components of function in the care of the developmentally disabled. Coyner cites the work of several nurses who made significant literature contributions during this period:

"Barnard (1968) advocated a family-community health nurse approach to care of the mentally retarded child; LeLouis (1967) demonstrated the benefits of a limited motor stimulation program to promote early sitting behavior in 10 normal infants. In her work with severely retarded young children Pothier (1968) successfully implemented a home-based sensory-motor training program. A significant contribution directed to the advancement of nursing skills in early identification of developmental disorders was the publication of Una Haynes' 'A Developmental Approach to Casefinding' by the U.S. Public Health Service in 1969. One nurse author who titled an article 'Nursing's Concern in the Mentally Retarded is Long Overdue' expressed the feeling of the few practitioners actively serving this population in various community settings."[3]

Other nurses cited by Coyner who made significant contributions to the literature include Eugenia Waechter, Martha Adams, Ilse Wolff, Shirley Steele, and Marcene Powell.

In the 1960's there was also the advent of diagnostic and evaluation clinics and university affiliated centers. The former were set up to provide diagnostic and referral services for multiply handicapped children. The university affiliated center offered diagnostic services secondary to the primary roles of professional training and research. Coyner discusses the development of early intervention programs during the same period as a result of " . . . advancements in diagnosis, remediation, and special techniques of management for many handicapping conditions."[3] The staffs of many of the aforementioned programs serving the developmentally disabled were composed of multidisciplinary teams. The nurse found herself working with professionals such as physical therapists and occupational therapists who performed specialized functions for which nurses had formerly been responsible. Identifying the unique components of the nurse's role became a concern of many nurses working on these teams. The nurse's dilemma in terms of her unique contributions in working with the developmentally disabled was typical of that depicted by Hans Mauksch in relation to the nursing profession as a whole. He describes the nurse's earlier role as being similar to a sheet of cookie dough where she was responsible for everything. As new disciplines developed, they represented cookies cut from the original dough. The nurse's role consisted of the remaining fragments.[4] Nurses who pioneered in these multidisciplinary settings had the responsibility for analyzing the remaining framework and identifying the nurse's unique contributions. The final product as established by these nursing pioneers was to see nursing as providing a total approach to the provision and coordination of services to the developmentally disabled individual and his/her family.

In the 1970s, these pioneers made even greater advancements in the area. Sally O'Neil[5] helped nurses to apply a scientific approach in the application of principles of behavior modification. Betty Bell[6] developed a preschool type setting for severely physically handicapped children. This program was used by other disciplines as a clinical placement for students. Patterson advocated that nurses could be the greatest contributors in the field of developmental disabilities. She based this belief on the nurse's "relating abilities," "common sense approach," and "presence" in nearly every setting beginning with the nursery.[7] Kleeschulte[8] developed a consultant service for public health nurses throughout the state of Alabama to guide them in casefinding and facilitating development in the developmentally disabled child. In the June 1975 edition of *Nursing Clinics of North America*, one of the topics was "Symposium on the Child with Developmental Disabilities." Issues discussed centered around national concerns; classes for parents; coping in physically handicapped children; deaf-blind children; the physically handicapped, severely retarded child; sociosexual development of the handicapped; behavior modification; minimal brain dysfunction; and the institutional setting.[9]

A comprehensive description of the nurse's role in working with the mentally retarded child was published in a book by Kathryn Barnard and Marcene Powell (1972).[10] Kathryn Barnard and Helen Douglas edited a publication (1974) which was a literature review to evaluate " . . . pertinent areas of knowledge and their potential contribution to assessing child health." This publication represented the initial stage of the final goal which was " . . . to develop methods to identify children in adverse situations so that preventive services can be offered at a time when habilitation or remediation is most influential in promoting optimal health."[11]

These are a few of the many works which could be cited as these pioneers continue to make great strides in developing the nurse's role in the care of the developmentally disabled. These nurses are acquiring national strength and are continuously contributing to nursing knowledge through practice, research, and publications. Being scattered throughout the country, nurses need a support system and professional sharing. Through membership in the American Association of Mental Deficiency, many nurses find an opportunity to exchange ideas and to gain professional support. Maternal Child Health Nursing Consultants are available through the Department of Health and Human Services. They offer much needed consultation in areas such as funding for special projects, recruiting new personnel, and providing continued educational opportunities. Maternal Child Health Nursing Consultants in state health departments are also becoming very supportive and interested in enhancing the nurse's role in the care of the developmentally disabled. Nursing leaders in this area are currently seeking recognition through the American Nurses' Association as a special interest group.

EDUCATIONAL PREPARATION AND CLINICAL EXPERIENCE

Nurses with educational preparation at all levels become involved in nursing care of the developmentally disabled. Most find that their entire basic educational preparation is helpful since a multiplicity of problems is usually present. However, severe gaps in knowledge and skills are also felt. For some, the only educational experience available in the undergraduate program is a visit to a residential setting for the retarded. Many nurses feel so inadequately prepared that they consider pursuing other professions such as physical therapy. However, those who seek this solution report a preference for the nursing role. Some nurses supplement their basic preparation by attending workshops in other professional fields and specialized programs in nursing care of the handicapped. Thus, the basic educational needs of the nurse working with the developmentally disabled are not clearly established.

I propose that theory and clinical experience in developmental disabilities be provided at the baccalaureate level. Baccalaureate graduates who practice in this particular area of nursing would need both to complete a specialized training program and take certifying exams. For nurses seeking higher level positions such as in research and teaching, master's and post-master's positions are available to them.

To assist in the enrichment of baccalaureate preparation in the care of the developmentally disabled, practitioners are helping to identify basic theory and clinical experiences which should be included. Nursing educators are aligning themselves with practitioners to learn more about special educational needs. Core content necessary for an understanding of the developmentally disabled includes knowledge in the areas of 1) child health (including pediatric nutritional needs), growth, and development; 2) anatomy and physiology; 3) neurophysiology; 4) disease conditions which produce handicaps and mental retardation; 5) child psychology; 6) the parenting process, including influencing factors; 7) introductory genetics; 8) the psychological and sociologic dynamics of family life; 9) the coping process resulting from birth of a developmentally disabled child; and 10) techniques for facilitating development. Instruction and clinical experience should be provided in the assessment of growth and development, the bonding process, mother-child interaction, and techniques of child management. Students need the opportunity to apply basic principles and knowledge by working directly with developmentally disabled children and their families in a variety of supervised settings such as nurseries, kindergartens, day care programs, specialized preschool programs, schools, institutions, diagnostic and evaluation clinics, and university affiliated facilities.

Additional content which should be included in the basic educational preparation was identified by nurses at a conference entitled, "The Nursing Role in Early Intervention Programs for Developmentally Disabled Children," which was held in Salt Lake City, Utah, in 1976. They advocated that:

" . . . a base of knowledge for this special area of nursing practice includes learning experiences regarding role identification, assertiveness training, promoting the ability to find and utilize all resources available in a given service area, develop decision-making ability, and initiate political awareness, i.e., how to 'work' and work within 'the system'."[3]

Undergraduate Specialization

Nurses who specialize in the care of the developmentally disabled need further preparation and certification beyond the baccalaureate level. More in depth knowledge is needed in pediatric neurology, orthopaedics, cardiology, hematology, and nutrition. Greater expertise should be developed in assessing and interpreting the child's growth and development, parental interaction, the bonding process, and techniques of child management. More in-depth knowledge and clinical experience in counseling parents as they work through the grief process are necessary. Nurses who specialize at the baccalaureate level also need theory and clinical experience in techniques to facilitate the child's movement processes, speech and language development, and independence in self-help skills. Coyner supports my view that nurses can be taught to apply principles developed by specialists such as the Bobaths, Rood, and Mueller. The Bobaths and Rood have completed much work in identifying techniques for facilitating physical development in the child with cerebral palsy. Mueller developed techniques for stimulating normal feeding behaviors in children with cerebral palsy.[3] Techniques identified by Ayers[12] are useful in working with the child who has delays in sensory motor development which frequently result in learning disabilities. Ayers's techniques are useful for both the preschooler and the school age child. Knowledge and expertise in these areas contribute to the nurse's teaching role and supplement her background for assessing the child's problems and planning nursing intervention. One physical therapist, Joan Mohr,* who trained with the Bobaths and Mueller, offers special workshops to help nurses apply this information. Nurses at the baccalaureate level who have specialized preparation in developmental disabilities function in a variety of settings. Nurseries, preschool programs, headstart centers, kindergartens, and schools represent educational programs where the nurse offers a total, coordinated approach to the care of the child and his family. High risk newborn nurseries, intensive care centers, follow-up programs for high risk infants, health department clinics, and pediatricians' offices represent areas in the health care system where the nurse who specializes at the baccalaureate level functions. The baccalaureate level practitioner provides direct services to the child and his family through functions such as assessment, teaching, supporting, counseling, coordinating, and advocating.

Master's and Post-Master's Levels

Programs are available which offer in-depth preparation at the master's and post-master's levels. The Child Development and Mental Retardation Center in Seattle offers a post-master's program in "Nursing of Children with Handicaps." It is offered as a master's program which requires the student to attend four consecutive quarters. The program is also available in a four-summer sequence which the student attends for five weeks each year. It is set up to enable the nurse with a master's degree in another area of nursing to become a specialist in the area of developmental disabilities. A certificate rather than an additional master's degree is given for this summer program. Clinical experiences are provided at the Child Development and Mental Retardation Center and in nearby hospitals, schools, and preschool programs. Theory and course content are provided through lectures, seminars, and independent study.

"This program is planned for the nurse who wants to—

Apply and expand her knowledge from the physical, social, and related sciences to the problems of the handicapped child and his family.

Adapt clinical nursing skills in observations, developmental assessments, and therapeutic relationships to children and their families.

---

*One workshop entitled "Introduction to Neuro-Developmental Treatment Approach for Cerebral Palsy" was conducted by Joan Mohr in February 1978 in Chattanooga, Tennessee. Nurses from seven states who work with the developmentally disabled attended the workshop.

Develop and integrate clinical nursing practice within the framework of the community.

Utilize findings and contribute to research in the care of the handicapped child."[13]

Nurses who specialize at the post-master's level frequently work in programs such as the university affiliated facility or the diagnostic and referral clinic. Increasingly, nurses in developmental disabilities are going into private practice. Those at the post-master's level also work in high risk intensive care units, nurseries, followup programs, schools, preschool programs, health department clinics, and pediatricians' offices. The post-master's level practitioner is more involved in research, professional training, and publishing than the baccalaureate level person.

Types of Service

With specialized educational preparation and an overall background from fields such as the behavioral sciences, the nurse is well prepared to provide services to the developmentally disabled. The nurse's primary goal is to help the child to reach and maintain a maximum level of health. Defining the specific functions of the nursing role is an evolving process. The basic components can be identified but may have to be redefined in the particular setting where the nurse is functioning. The basic components of the nurse's role in the care of the developmentally disabled include: 1) assessing; 2) planning and implementing nursing interventions such as teaching, supporting, coordinating, counseling, and advocating; and 3) evaluating and revising nursing interventions.

ASSESSMENT

As a part of the basic nursing process, the nurse must first identify the problem. Assessment is a continuous process and covers many areas including: 1) the background history, 2) the parenting process, 3) the physical assessment, 4) the developmental assessment, 5) the child's acquisition of independence in self-help skills, and 6) the physical environment.

Background History

Much important assessment information is gained from an interview with the parents. Events that occurred prenatally and postnatally may have influenced parental response to the child. If the child had to be hospitalized for extended periods due to prematurity or an illness, the separation may have had a negative effect on the attachment process as described by Klaus and Kennell.[14] If the child's appearance and reactions conflicted with prenatal expectations, these factors may have interfered with parent-child interactions as presented by Klaus and Kennell in relation to the work of Solnit and Stark (1961).[14] For example, I worked with a family whose infant screamed and threw herself backwards when cuddled. The baby was content to be left alone on her back in the crib. The parents became quite frustrated in their attempts to relate to the child. I used this assessment information in planning a program to gradually decrease the child's negative response to cuddling.

Information should also be carefully recorded regarding the child's history of injuries and illnesses. Parents sometimes only allude to very significant symptoms. In one situation when I was completing a history, the mother mentioned sleepwalking as a problem with her child. A neurologic evaluation revealed that the walking episodes were manifestations of a seizure disorder. After the child was placed on an appropriate medication, the problem disappeared.

In addition, clues relevant to the parental coping ability may be gained during the history taking. Parents may manifest denial by stating that they see no problems with the child but that the doctor felt the child should be evaluated. Other parents emphasize only one problem when the child may have multiple handicaps. For example, parents of retarded children frequently refer only to the child's speech delay. Other parents indicate an acceptance of the problem when they ask for services to enable their child to develop to maximum capacity. The accepting parent is also interested in learning more about the child's condition.

The background history can also reveal significant information about the reaction of other siblings to the handicapped child. Sometimes they are ashamed and refuse to participate in the care of the disabled child. The child may also be prohibited from interacting with siblings' friends. Other children, however, demonstrate an accepting attitude with respect to a disabled brother or sister. These siblings want the handicapped child to be included in all family activities.

In addition to siblings' reactions, it is important to see if parents spend time with their normal child as well as with the developmentally disabled child. It is so easy to become engrossed in meeting the multiple needs of the disabled child and to ignore the other children. Robinson and Robinson relate this reaction to one of nonacceptance.[2] I recall an incident where the parents never found time to followup on their son's abnormal vision screening because all their time was devoted to meeting the needs of the severely physically and mentally handicapped sister. Later, when the son was being tested for the Army, he was turned down because of poor vision. The mother said she remembered the school sending home a note requesting that the child's vision be checked, however, the parents were so tied up with the daughter's care that they did not have time to follow through on the recommendation.

The Parenting Process

Bean and Ritchie define parenting as " . . . a process through which a child's physical, emotional, social, and mental development is nurtured."[15] Assessing the parenting process is crucial in working with the developmentally disabled child and the family because extra adjustments are added to the parenting role. The parents have to work through the process of adjusting to the child's being different from the one which they anticipated. They have to face friends and relatives with the facts that the child will not develop normally. Parents often find that relationships with old friends are not the same after the birth of a developmentally disabled child. Public reactions frequently are upsetting to the parents. I have heard parents comment that the stares and questions such as "What is wrong with him?" make it difficult to take the developmentally disabled child shopping or out to a restaurant.

The nurse needs to set up special periods where she can observe the interaction between parent and child. Some important factors to consider in any observation of parent-child interaction include: 1) eye contact, 2) touch, 3) methods of child management, 4) efforts to teach the child, 5) verbal communication, and 6) attempts to play with the child. Betty Caldwell's "Home Inventory for Infants"[16] and the "Fels Parent Behavior Rating Scales" as described by Baldwin and others[17] provide guides for the nurse to use in observing similar types of behaviors. The "Home Inventory for Infants" is helpful in observing mother-child interaction and other factors within the home setting on children primarily from birth to three years of age. It is broken down into six basic categories including:

1. Emotional and verbal responsiveness of mother.
2. Avoidance of restriction and punishment.

3. Organization of physical and temporal environment.
4. Provision of appropriate play materials.
5. Maternal involvement with child.
6. Opportunities for variety in daily stimulation.[16]

Each of these categories is subdivided into specific component parts. Caldwell now has a home inventory tool to be used with children between the ages of three and six years.

"The Fels Behavior Rating Scales" " . . . cover thirty variables of parent behavior which are designed to include the most important aspects of the parent-child relationships." The eight major areas covered are:

1. Home atmosphere.
2. Contact of child and mother.
3. Control influence of parent and child.
4. Babying and protectiveness.
5. Criticism and evaluation of the child.
6. Readiness of explanation.
7. Emotional relationships between parent and child.
8. Miscellaneous. [17]

Each of these areas is further broken down into more specific parts.

Floyd developed a tool for observing maternal and infant interaction during feeding time. One observation is the mother's cuddling behavior.[18] Observing for the reciprocation of responses between parent and child is an essential component of this assessment. Another means of assessing maternal-child interaction is use of a one way mirror. At this time the nurse uses a parent-child interaction tool to systematically record behaviors occurring during a particular activity. A home visit is also a good place for studying parent-child interaction.

In addition to assessing interaction, it is important to identify the parent's stage of acceptance that the child is developmentally disabled. This assessment is crucial if intervention is to be successful. Young discusses three stages which the parents go through "from the time of conception to the resolution of chronic grief." [19]

The first of these is "denial" and occurs because the family cannot believe their child is handicapped. The second stage is "awareness" and is characterized by the parents' beginning realization of what has happened and their responding possibly with anger. The third state is "restitution" and lasts until either the child or parents die(s). During this period, the parents may develop either an adaptive or a maladaptive response. The former is characterized by a reorganization of relationships and coping with the child's treatment and defect. The maladaptive response is seen in parents who either spend all their time with the child or ignore him completely. [19]

Chinn, Drew, and Logan list five stages described by Rosen as being typical of those which parents go through in accepting the retarded child. These include:

1. Awareness of a problem.
2. Recognition of a basic problem.
3. Search for a cause.
4. Search for a cure.
5. Acceptance of the problem. [20]

Robinson and Robinson discuss each of these in detail. They mention that other authors have developed categorizations for identifying stages which parents go through in accepting the retarded child. Robinson and Robinson also related that:

" . . . two indices of acceptance are the degree to which the mother functions in her usual manner, continuing her association with her friends, and the degree to which both parents meet the needs of their normal children as well as those of the retarded child. (Wortis, 1966)"[2]

Even after the parents adjust to the initial impact of having a handicapped child, Robinson and Robinson support the idea that they will continue to experience crises which require intervention. For example, 20-year-old Jim had a severe seizure disorder that was diagnosed in the preschool years. During this time, the parents went through the initial adjustment process in accepting their child's handicap. As the parents sought services and tried to maintain some organization in their lives, there were continuous crises which required readjustment. After a few years in school, Jim had to be placed on a homebound program. This was discontinued due to poor responsiveness resulting from tremendous doses of medication. By the time Jim was 17 years of age, a left cortical resection was done to remove the part of the brain where the seizure activity was localized. Without the operation, doctors said Jim would gradually become totally dependent. The surgery was successful and the seizures decreased, however, Jim had a resultant right hemiparesis.

At age 20, when he was seen at the clinic, Jim scored at a fourth grade level on educational tests. He was placed in a special program for occupational training and assistance in separation from his parents. For about two years Jim remained in the program and was making good progress. Then one day I ran into him and his mother on the elevator. After a happy greeting, the mother said, "Call me sometime." As Jim walked on ahead, the mother whispered, "The seizures have started again." The writer could see the hurt in the mother's face as once again the family approached still another crisis.

Thus, with good assessment information about the child and his parents, the nurse is ready to identify areas where nursing intervention will be appropriate and those where a referral is necessary. Continuous reassessment is needed throughout the intervention process.

The Physical Assessment

In conjunction with the developmental evaluation, it is important to do a physical assessment to identify problems that might require treatment or consultation, and determine growth and development. Both Haynes's publication *Developmental Approach to Case Finding*[21] and Alexander and Brown's book *Pediatric Physical Diagnosis for Nurses*[22] are excellent resources to use when doing a physical examination. An important component of this part of the evaluation is to look for the presence or absence of reflexes. Fiorentino[23] explicitly illustrates how the child reacts when reflex development is either normal or abnormal. In terms of developmental programming, it is particularly important that the nurse know whether the child is fixated in abnormal patterns. For example, the child who has residual components of the assymetric tonic neck reflex should not be left lying in a position facilitating flexion toward the side where reflex flexion has already occurred. The nurse also needs to determine if protective extension, righting reactions, and equilibrium responses occur at an appropriate age, otherwise, the child will have difficulty with walking. Since the physical therapist has expertise in these areas and in reflexology, consultation and sharing of information is necessary.

The Developmental Assessment

Assessing the developmental level of the child is of major importance in identifying what services are needed and in counseling with the parents. There are several tools available to guide the nurse's observations in determining the child's functioning in relation to the norms of children the same age. This information provides a frame of reference for further teaching and counseling. For example, if the child is functioning below his chronologic age, he will demonstrate behavior more typical of a younger child. The four-year-old who is functioning at a two-year level will act more like a child in the latter age category. Delays in development may result from such things as a lack of stimulation, a disorder in learning, a medical problem, or a combination of these. A diagnosis cannot be made on the basis of results from screening tools; consultation with other professionals is needed to explore identified problem areas. Including parents in the developmental testing appointments increases their awareness of the child's problems and provides a better understanding of techniques used in testing.

The Denver Developmental Screening Test (DDST)[24] is one tool which is helpful in assessing children from birth until six years. It is adaptable to both well-child clinics and preschool programs and takes approximately 20 minutes to administer to each child, yet some items can be completed in a group setting. The DDST provides a time range rather than definite ages during which most children develop a particular skill. This approach allows for variations in the specific time at which a milestone must be achieved to be considered within normal limits. The areas included in the DDST are personal-social development, fine motor-adaptive skills, language development, and gross motor skills. If a speech articulation handicap is suspected, administration of the Denver Articulation Screening Test[25] may be necessary since the DDST concentrates more on language comprehension.

Another test often used in conjunction with the DDST is a Developmental Screening Inventory.[26] It includes the same areas as the DDST except that adaptive behavior is a separate component. According to Knobloch and Pasamanick, adaptive behavior " . . . is concerned with the organization of stimuli, the perception of relationships, the dissection of wholes into their component parts, and the reintegration of these parts in a meaningful fashion."[27]

A third screening tool is the Developmental Profile by Alpern and Boll.[28] From this test the nurse can determine specific age levels of the child, including physical age, self-help age, social age, academic age, and communication age. The Developmental Profile is designed to test children from birth through preadolescence.

The Acquisition of Independence in Self-Help Skills

Self-help skills are those activities which enable the child to care for his own needs. Feeding, dressing, and toileting are the major areas included. A good assessment of the child's level of functioning in these areas is necessary. Developmental screening tests do not sufficiently itemize the component parts of self-help skills. Bensberg[29] presents check lists which are helpful in this area. Once the nurse has established a base line showing where the child is functioning in each area of self-help skills, she then looks for signs of the child's readiness to develop new skills. One important factor to consider is whether the child can attend and make eye contact. If not, this area would require intervention before the child could progress to higher level skills. In terms of feeding, if the child is not eating with his fingers, he is not ready for spoon feeding. Finger feeding requires hand to mouth movements which depict readiness for learning to use utensils. In evaluating readiness for new achievements in dressing, the nurse checks to see if the child assists with dressing by pushing his arms and legs through garments and whether he can remove articles of clothing. Two questions relating to readiness for bowel training include: 1) Does the child withhold bowel functioning for even a limited period? and 2) Is the child bothered by soiled pants? A question to identify readiness for bladder training would be: Can the child remain dry for two hours?[30] Once an identification of a baseline representing the child's specific achievements in self-help skills and assessment of his readiness for developing new skills is completed, the nurse has sufficient data to plan a program with the parents for facilitating further independence in self-help skills.

The Physical Environment

There is no substitute for a good assessment of the home situation. Major factors to observe include the availability of materials for stimulation (toys, books, homemade playthings, and housekeeping articles, e.g., pots and pans), safety features, the accessibility of the home for the child and his care, and the proper utilization of special devices and adaptive equipment. The Caldwell "Home Inventory for Infants"[16] and "Home Observation for Measurement of the Environment, Preschool Version,"[31] referred to earlier, are quite helpful in evaluating the home. The nature of the developmentally disabled child's problems may cause him to be more prone to accidents, consequently, environmental safety precautions are necessary. It is not unusual to find homes that are physically inaccessible to the child. For example, I made a home visit to see a child, Robert, who had Prader-Labhart-Willi-Fanconi Syndrome. Gellis and Feingold present the major diagnostic features of the syndrome as including: "Obesity, hypogonadism, short stature, hypotonia, and mental retardation, [with] frequent diabetes mellitus or abnormal glucose tolerance test."[32] Robert was slow in developing speech, was obese, and had hypotonia and hypogonadism. His obesity was demonstrated by the fact that at five years of age he weighed 147 pounds and was 47 inches in height. The excess weight made it difficult for Robert to ambulate. The steps leading into his home were steep and unsteady. When Robert entered the house, an older sibling stood behind to provide support, while the mother remained inside the door and held Robert's hands. It is unlikely that this type information would have been revealed in an office interview.

In the home setting, the nurse is in a better position to assess whether special equipment is adaptable. Parents are frequently given patterns for making special devices, however, no one checks to see if they meet the child's needs.

PLANNING AND IMPLEMENTING NURSING INTERVENTIONS

Teaching

A second component of the nurse's role is teaching. There are many areas in which the nurse can instruct parents in the care of developmentally disabled children. Some important topics include: 1) techniques to facilitate development, 2) child management, 3) self-help skills, and 4) basic health needs.

Techniques to Facilitate Development

One essential component of teaching is guiding parents in methods to facilitate development when the child is functioning below her chronologic age. An important principle is to start at the child's level and to guide her through a normal sequence. This approach is necessary regardless of the child's chronologic age. Curricula that are geared to normal developmental progression offer the nurse many ideas for providing or suggesting methods of stimulation. One that is useful with children from birth through six years of age is the "Portage Guide to Early Education."[33] The kit includes a manual, checklists, and a card file. The latter is filed according to five developmental areas, including infant stimulation, socialization, language, self-help, cognitive, and motor. Each of these sections is broken down into activities for each year of development until age six. For example, there is a series of cards on providing developmental stimulation in the area of language for the child who is in the one-to-two-year age group.

In working with a child who has a specific disability such as Down's syndrome or cerebral palsy, the nurse will need to work with other specialists in developing a program for parents. Finnie[34] gives many helpful suggestions for working with the child who has cerebral palsy.

The following case history gives examples of how the nurse might teach a parent when the child is delayed in development. This child was seen by an orthopaedist and a physical therapist who gave suggestions which were incorporated into the teaching plan. Twenty-one-month-old Jean had a mild left hemiparesis which apparently resulted from damage to the central nervous system as a result of prolonged labor and a difficult delivery. She tended to externally rotate her hips and had some tightness in that area. Jean had difficulty in supinating the left arm and in using the fingers on that hand. Instead of crawling, Jean scooted and used very little hip rotation. She also slumped when sitting. In teaching the mother how to facilitate Jean's development, I concentrated on eight specific areas:

1. To improve hip rotation and to decrease tightness the mother was encouraged to let Jean lie prone over a large bolster. In this position, her arms and hands were free for reaching and grasping. While in this position, the mother could rotate Jean's hips from side to side. Reaching for bubbles and playing with a favorite toy were activities which helped sustain the length of time she would remain over the bolster. Another method of encouraging hip rotation was to let Jean straddle the bolster and perform activities such as working puzzles. While one parent was helping with the activity, the other could passively rotate Jean's hips from behind.
2. To improve back extension and sitting balance, lying prone over a bolster as described above was encouraged. The mother was also instructed to rock Jean back and forth as she lay prone over a large plastic wheel. When pushed toward the floor, Jean would throw her hands out and pull her head up while extending her back.
3. To encourage use of the left hand and the development of a pincer grasp, two-handed activities and toys with small parts were suggested. Pushing a large wheel in free play was an excellent way to get two-handed involvement. Toys mentioned included a hammer, a peg board, and a small pole with removable rings. Working puzzles with knobs and putting small pellets into a container were activities suggested to facilitate the acquisition of a pincer grasp in the left hand.

4. To promote the further development of equilibrium reactions, tilting Jean on a tilt board in both the sitting and standing positions was demonstrated. The mother was also instructed in making this device.
5. To encourage reciprocal creeping, a tunnel through which Jean could crawl during play activities was recommended. Knee walking was also suggested.
6. To decrease drooling, blowing bubbles and sucking through a straw were encouraged.
7. To promote the development of language, the mother was instructed in making a speech book in which objects and people were cut out of magazines and pasted in with Jean's assistance. The pictures were categorized into sections such as clothes, people, vegetables, and so forth. Jean was encouraged to label the objects. Praise was used as a reinforcement for all attempts to speak. In addition, Jean was encouraged to follow simple directions.
8. To provide external stimulation for Jean's left arm and hand, rubbing different textures over the skin was recommended.

Child Management

A second area of concern in teaching parents is in relation to techniques of child management. Many parents feel that because the child is developmentally disabled he should not be disciplined. The nurse can help parents to understand that limit setting is as important for these children as for the nonhandicapped. Parents are taught that consistency and firmness are important in dealing with their child. Lewis emphasizes the importance of teaching the process of parenting rather than giving parents specific behaviors to perform. He emphasizes the significance of interpreting " . . . why parents should do something rather than just telling them what to do. This method helps them to become a 'generator of ideas'; otherwise, they stop when the situation changes."[35] Lewis identifies six principles which the professional can teach in relation to the process of parenting.

"The first one involves modeling and stresses the idea that the child will repeat behaviors which are demonstrated by his parent. For example, the parent who slaps his child while saying 'I told you not to hit,' is being inconsistent between his behavior and what he expects of the child. The second principle is centered on reciprocity and requires that parents treat children as people and not as property. A parent who applies this principle will not yell at his child because he himself does not like to be yelled at. The third principle states that each age of the child has certain rules and developmental milestones which in turn should affect what we expect of a child. For instance, the five-year-old dislikes certain foods or will refuse a broken cookie. These dislikes are irrational and will disappear by themselves. The parent must accept in his contract that he will live with certain things until the child grows out of that stage. The fourth principle is concerned with negotiation. The child gets his way part of the time, and the parent gets his way part of the time. The fifth principle relates to 'whose problem is it, the parent's or the child's?' Children frequently eat when they are hungry rather than at meal times. It is the parent's problem that they expect everyone to eat at meal times whether they are hungry or not. The sixth and final principle is one of weight which states that the parent's reaction to negative behavior should be in line with the severity of the misconduct. Severe retribution through punishment is more in line with criminal activity. A parent's goal in relation to transgressions should be to educate the child. This approach may involve: (1) repeating the rule, (2) explaining the consequences of a violation, and (3) if the child continues to violate the rule, he should be removed from the situation."[35]

Along with teaching these basic principles relevant to the process of parenting, the nurse can guide parents in techniques of behavior modification as described by Whaley and Malott.[36] The first important consideration in using this approach is to get a baseline representing how often the child is already performing the desired behavior. One approach to increasing this response is to provide tangible reinforcement immediately after the child responds appropriately. For example, if a child makes eye contact only one or two times out of 25 times that his name is called, this information provides baseline data indicating a need for increasing this behavior. The nurse would then select something tangible, such as orange juice, that the child likes and use it to reinforce the desired behavior. Each time the child makes eye contact following his name being called, the nurse immediately gives the child a sip of orange juice or another tangible substance. Social reinforcement (e.g., verbal praise) is paired with tangible rewards so the child eventually performs the behavior for a more sophisticated reinforcement. Giving the rewards, such as juice and social praise, every time immediately after the child responds is called continuous reinforcement.[36] This schedule of continuous reinforcement must gradually be changed to one of intermittent reinforcement, otherwise, the desired behavior is soon extinguished after the continuous rewards are terminated. Extinction behavior represents the stopping of a behavior when the reward is no longer paired with the behavior. To prevent extinction, the schedule of continuous reinforcement must be changed to one of either fixed-ratio or variable-ratio. On a fixed-ratio schedule, the child now has to perform the behavior a specific number of times before a reward is given. When the reward is given after an unspecified number of responses, the process represents a variable-ratio schedule. The latter is more effective in behavior management since it produces consistent responses from the individual because he is uncertain when the next reinforcement will occur. With the fixed-ratio, it only comes after a certain number of responses and may promote pauses in the desired behavior after the reinforcement.[36] In applying reinforcement techniques in behavior management, negative behaviors are ignored, provided the child's safety is not at risk.

Self-Help Skills

These principles of behavior modification can also be applied in teaching self-help skills. As mentioned previously, when self-help skills are broken down into small steps, part of the task is already accomplished. I used principles of behavior modification in teaching self-feeding to Tina. The mother was instructed to stand behind Tina and to place her hand over the child's hand. This position enabled the mother to guide Tina's hand in scooping food as well as taking it to her mouth. When she could grasp the spoon and scoop the food independently, the mother was instructed to decrease assistance by moving her hand to the child's elbow. The mother eventually was able to eliminate her assistance completely. Another child was toilet trained by rewarding her with orange slices when her behaviors approximated those outlined for that skill. The child was first given orange slices for going to the potty. The second step involved giving orange slices only when the child sat on the potty. The third step required the child to void in the potty following which an orange slice was given.

Basic Health Needs

Additional areas for teaching include the components of basic health care. Parents frequently have trouble providing an adequate diet for the physically handicapped child.

Through basic nutritional counseling, the nurse can assist parents in getting essential amounts of the basic four food groups into the child's diet. Establishing good sleeping habits is another basic health need which may be difficult to develop. Some of the most common concerns include the child's desire to sleep with his parents, refusal to stay in bed, and frequent demands made around bedtime. Through basic health teaching, the nurse can help the parents to solve many of these problems. Inglis[37] describes techniques and presents excellent case histories of nursing interventions to help parents in managing sleep problems. According to Inglis, "The approach is solidly based on both the principles of behavior modification and those of changing the home environment." A unique component of this program is " . . . the telephone support for parents. Through this the nurse is, in effect, applying behavior modification strategies to the parents by reinforcing their efforts."[37]

Instructing parents in the need to seek early treatment for conditions such as middle ear infections prevents the development of further handicapping conditions. Parents should be taught to avoid using cotton swabs to clean the child's ears since the wax is merely pushed further into the ear canal. Basic teaching in environmental control of allergens helps to prevent allergic conditions. For example, frequent vacuuming and dusting helps to eliminate dust which causes allergic respiratory problems for many children.

Supporting

A third major component of the nursing role is providing support. Throughout the continuous process of adjustment which families face as the result of having a developmentally disabled child, the nurse has many opportunities to offer support. In defining support, Barnhart and Stein include such descriptions as:

> " . . . to undergo or endure, esp. with patience or submission; tolerate. . . . to sustain (a person, the mind, spirits, courage, etc.) under trial or affliction. . . . to maintain (a person, family, establishment, institution, etc.) by supplying with things necessary to existence; provide for. . . . to uphold (a person, cause, policy, etc.) by aid or countenance; . . . to hold up or add strength to, . . ."[38]

The nurse may have to tolerate many things from families of the developmentally disabled, including the parents' using her as a scapegoat for their anger. Explanations by the nurse may actually be misinterpreted to enable the parents to deny realities. They occasionally report to other agencies actions and responses by the nurse which never occurred. By having a good relationship with other agency personnel, the nurse can clarify misconceptions as being a part of the adjustment process. I have learned that it is wise to hear both sides of the story before reprimanding paraprofessionals on the basis of a negative parental report. To provide support, the nurse must develop broad shoulders and be accepting rather than retaliating.

Barnhart and Stein's definition of to sustain is " . . . to keep (a person, the mind, the spirits, etc.) from giving way, as under trial or affliction."[38] With the periodic crises which families encounter as a result of having a developmentally disabled child, they become vulnerable to periods of becoming immobilized. Frequently, all that may be needed is someone to clarify the situation, a nonjudgmental person to listen, the provision of needed items, the confirmation of an issue, or a referral to an appropriate resource. The mother who is suddenly overwhelmed with the child's care and needs to get out of the house for some fresh air may simply require assistance in finding a babysitter. Frequently, just being there and letting the family know she cares is all that is required of the nurse. There are times when the family just needs someone to listen.

Financial burdens are not uncommon in families who have a developmentally disabled child. The child frequently requires such things as the care of several specialists, adaptive equipment, medications, and special diets. All of these can be expensive items. By being familiar with special services, e.g., crippled children's clinics, and monetary assistance, e.g., Social Security Income (SSI), the nurse can support the family in meeting financial needs. I recall an incident where a mother frantically called to report that her hyperactive daughter, Annette had set the closet on fire and burned all her school clothes. I sent one of the child development workers* to take the mother to a secondhand clothing store, where she replaced the items at minimal cost. In helping with these maintenance needs, the nurse must remember that families have pride and this may prevent their discussing financial difficulties. In a situation involving a child, Lois, who was partially deaf, the clinic staff was amazed that the mother did not follow up on recommendations for service. Both mother and child were always attractively dressed and the home setting was very adequate and comfortable. At the time the child development worker staff was added to the clinic, the mother had already delayed getting services for over a year. The mother was accepting of the worker's visit to the home to guide her in techniques to facilitate Lois's language development. During her visits, Lois was fascinated with the activities and started making progress. The mother was amazed at how much the child learned. As she developed awareness of Lois's capabilities, the mother expressed concern about getting continued services for her daughter. Further discussion revealed that the mother had wanted to get these earlier but did not have the money. Her parents were providing financial support and the mother did not feel she could ask them to pay additionally for special treatment services. The family's level of living had sidetracked professionals from exploring this avenue and the mother was too proud to ask for help. The worker assisted her in applying to crippled children's services for financial assistance. The mother mentioned in a post-service followup interview that she did not know what she would have done without the worker.

Sometimes the nurse provides support to the parents by upholding decisions they have made. For example, grandparents and friends occasionally react negatively to the parents' setting limits on the child. They may make such comments as "poor little Johnny should not be punished." The nurse upholds parental interpretations to others that the developmentally disabled child needs limit setting. A second example is seen in the parents who are told "He is just immature," or "He is just like his father was and he did all right." The nurse must uphold the parents as they begin to accept the realities with respect to the child's problem.

In addition, a pat on the back is a valuable means of providing support. Parents need to be told they are doing a good job. It is also important to the parents for the nurse to share their excitement when the child shows improvement.

Coordinating

A fourth function which comprises an important aspect of the nursing role is coordinating. A developmentally disabled child usually has more than one problem. Common occurrences

---

*The child development worker is a paraprofessional who makes home visits to observe the child in the home environment and to guide the parents in techniques to facilitate the child's development. The workers also provide support and counseling for parents. The child development workers are under the nurse's supervision.

are orthopaedic handicaps; ear, nose, and throat disorders including hearing losses; visual handicaps; speech and language problems; socialization maladjustments; emotional disorders; and disturbances in learning. The development of multidisciplinary diagnostic teams has been a valuable contribution in helping parents to identify what their child's problems are and in recommending appropriate services. Prior to this time, parents went from one specialist to another with no central person to pull the material together for them.

As a part of the team, the nurse has a key function in coordinating the process for the family. It is helpful to explain the role of other professionals and to interpret the components of their evaluation and/or treatment. When parents are confused by results and suggestions interpreted to them by another team member, the nurse can clarify misconceptions and explain recommendations. When she has questions about the situation, the nurse can either consult with the other professionals or ask them to clarify the information for the parents.

In seeking services, families again encounter difficulties such as problems in contacting the specific agency, getting accepted for service, working out financial arrangements, and planning for transportation. Feelings of uncertainty about the program itself are not uncommon. Familiarity with the agency and personnel enables the nurse to answer many of the parents' questions, thereby alleviating their fears. For the parent who is afraid her child will regress, the nurse can explain that children are grouped according to their abilities. Other parents are apprehensive that the child will pick up bad habits. For instance, one child with Down's syndrome developed a limp when placed in a preschool program for multiply handicapped children. A little investigation revealed that another child in the same class had a similar problem. The parents were advised to simply ignore the behavior and the limp soon disappeared. Minor misunderstandings between the parent and agency personnel may result in the child's being withdrawn from the program. Letting the parents discuss the situation and identifying possible alternatives help them to decide on the best course of action. There are times when the total family is unable to adapt to the infant's or toddler's attending a special program. In these cases, a homebound program with a paraprofessional supervised by the nurse is an alternative. Periodic consultation with the physical therapist might be indicated. The nurse coordinates her services with the professional, the paraprofessional, and the family.

Counseling

A fifth aspect of the nursing role is counseling. Barnhart and Stein's definitions of counseling include ". . . advice; opinion or instruction given in directing the judgement or conduct of another . . . to urge the doing or adoption of; recommend (a plan, etc.)."[38] The counseling role encompasses the performance of the functions of assessment, teaching, supporting, and coordinating—all of which are performed through a systematic model which is founded on certain specific features and is geared toward providing advice and directing parental behavior. Robinson and Robinson[2] also include some of these basic functions in their description of the counseling role. Ourth identifies the three significant features of the nurse's role in counseling: 1) The first involves an awareness by the nurse as to how she is perceived by the family. 2) The second feature is to identify the parents' needs and to meet them before discussing the child. 3) The third aspect of the nurse's role is to listen to the parents discuss concerns which they have about their child. I identify these three features of the nurse's role in counseling as important approaches to be used in performing other functions, such as teaching. One could say that the three features identified by Ourth form a model for the nurse to follow as a part of the counseling role in all nursing interventions.[39]

In looking at these three features more specifically, I find the first consideration is the nurse's professional appearance. Does she appear to be a threatening force who sets out to evaluate others? The nurse must project a nonjudgmental, accepting attitude. It is best accomplished when the nurse acknowledges that families' patterns of living may differ from what she perceives as appropriate. Gans[40] presents some interesting data which demonstrate the necessity of understanding and respecting the traditions and patterns of living of other cultural groups before successful intervention can be achieved. The nurse must view the parents' approach to situations as being meaningful to them and representative of their values. Accepting different values and patterns of living is essential to a nonjudgmental approach. The nurse must also develop awareness in terms of who the parents identify her with. I have frequently encountered parents who felt inadequate in their ability to care for the child. Consequently, the nurse was viewed as a threat and an agent who might remove the child from the home. Such misconceptions must be clarified.

The second part of the framework is to identify the parents' needs and to help meet them before discussing the child. For instance, on a home visit to see a developmentally delayed two-year-old child, I discovered the family had lost their furniture due to inability to meet payments. There were no facilities for refrigeration and cooking. The mother was wondering how she would prepare the evening meal and keep milk chilled for the baby. At that moment, the mother was more concerned about meeting basic physical needs than hearing about her son's developmental delay. A second example depicting parental need to discuss issues other than the child which are of concern to them is seen in final conferences where diagnostic findings are shared. I frequently find the entire session is spent in discussing family problems other than those of the child. One mother talked for one and a half hours about her health problems and the recent death of a family member. Near the end of the session, she commented, "Oh my goodness, I came here to talk about my child and I spent the entire time discussing other problems." I assured the mother that it was also important to discuss other things that were bothering her.

The third aspect of the framework is to listen to the parents discuss concerns which they have about their child. When they are ready to discuss the child's problems, the nurse can more effectively intervene.[39] For example, when Mr. and Mrs. Thomas brought their nine-month-old son, who they suspected had cerebral palsy, to the clinic, they anxiously observed the assessment process and asked questions concerning methods for stimulating his development. They also wanted to know about materials to read on cerebral palsy. These parents were ready to listen and to take advantage of the nurse's teaching.

The assumption underlying these three features of the framework is that the nurse cannot convince the family of anything. The secret, according to Ourth,[41] is in developing an involvement which helps the family to understand that they have a child with a problem. I feel it is most important for the nurse to listen to the parents in a supportive manner as they express feelings and discuss problem situations. When decisions have to be made, the nurse provides sufficient information to enable the parents to decide for themselves. Many times they have already reached a decision but need someone to confirm that it is the best course of action. It may be helpful to mention actions taken by other parents. If the nurse lacks sufficient information or expertise to perform the counseling role, she should refer the family to a specialist.

Advocating.

The sixth function which is a part of the nursing role is advocating. The nurse is in a strategic position to serve as an advocate within the community for the total family. Working with the developmentally disabled requires a commitment from the nurse to become involved with committees and activities at the local, state, and national levels which are geared toward promoting the establishment of services for this population. Serving on local boards of agencies who offer programs to the developmentally disabled opens doors to improving service quality. Political involvement is important especially in relation to getting special legislation passed. Supporting national associations such as the National Association of Mental Deficiency and the National Association for Retarded Citizens Advocacy is imperative. Just helping to create an awareness of the needs of the developmentally disabled is of major importance.

Another method through which the nurse can advocate better services is by assuring professional and public accountability not only for her services but for those of other nurses working in agencies serving the developmentally disabled. Encouraging the hiring of qualified nurses is a beginning point. Sharing information about educational opportunities that are available can help to improve the qualifications of nurses already employed. Additionally, special grants may be obtained to sponsor workshops for preparing nurses to work with the developmentally disabled. The nurse should also become involved in education programs for the general public to assist them in identifying, seeking, and evaluating needed services.

EVALUATING AND REVISING NURSING INTERVENTIONS

In the process of assimilating assessment information into intervention programs, the nurse must identify techniques for evaluating the success of interventions. Some approaches that might be used include parental response questionnaires to determine if the services met the parents' expectations. Measuring changes in the child's functional performance and increases in parental effectiveness are other useful sources for obtaining evaluative information. Obtaining this data will require the nurse to continually reassess the child and the family. Evaluative information is then used in changing nursing intervention to achieve other desired outcomes.

An additional method of evaluation which is especially important to funders is cost effectiveness. The nurse must identify the cost of the intervention and compare it with similar services rendered by other agencies. If the value of the service is not in relation to the cost, it is doubtful that anyone will be willing to pay for it.

Case History Representing the Nurse's Role

The following case history summarizes the roles of the nurse in working with the developmentally disabled. The Jones triplets were nine months of age when they were first brought to the clinic. The mother was unaware that she would have a multiple birth until a few months prior to the delivery. The babies were delivered at 32 weeks gestation. James was the first born and weighed two pounds and thirteen ounces. Having fewer problems at birth, he was discharged after five weeks in the premature nursery. James was rehospitalized at ten weeks with bacterial meningitis and seizures. A shunt was performed to relieve intracranial pressure. The illness caused severe brain damage and the resultant seizure disorder.

John was the second born and weighed two pounds and two ounces at birth. He was on a respirator for two and a half months due to respiratory distress. After discharge, John continued to have respiratory problems and was hospitalized at one point with pneumonia.

The third triplet was Jerry, who weighed two pounds and twelve ounces. He had respiratory distress in the neonatal period and was kept on a respirator for three weeks. At two months, Jerry was discharged from the nursery. He tended to progress without further complications.

DEVELOPMENTAL AND PHYSICAL ASSESSMENT

When the family first came to the center, I completed a developmental assessment on each child. The tests initially used included a Denver Developmental Screening Test and a Developmental Screening Inventory. On the original assessment, James completed tasks below a one-month level. Preliminary reflex testing revealed the presence of the tonic labyrinthine supine and the asymetrical tonic neck reflex. The mother was present during the testing and expressed concerns about James's low functioning. On the basis of the assessment information, he was referred for a physical examination, an ophthalmologic evaluation, and a physical therapy assessment. Summary reports were requested from the neurologist. Generally, the physical therapist felt James's functioning was at a brain stem level with no response to light, touch, sound, or movement. The ophthalmologist described James as having very poor vision as a result of brain damage.

On the initial developmental assessment with John, gross motor skills were found to be within normal limits for his chronologic age. Fine motor, language, and personal social skills were within normal limits when John was given credit for prematurity. An important observation, however, was that John would remain preoccupied with one toy or activity for unusual lengths of time. This behavior was identified as one for continual observation. On the basis of assessment information, John was also referred for a physical examination, a physical therapy assessment, and an ophthalmologic evaluation. The physical therapist felt John showed some residual components of the tonic labyrinthine supine reflex which should have become integrated earlier. He also had a diminishing palmar grasp and a plantar grasp. The presence of the latter was not unusual for John's age. The ophthalmologist felt John had a resolving right lateral rectus paresis resulting from the prematurity. Continued followup for muscle imbalance problems was recommended.

Jerry's developmental screening revealed that he was functioning within normal limits for his chronologic age in gross motor and personal social skills. Fine motor and language skills were within normal limits when Jerry was given credit for prematurity. Referrals to a pediatrician and a physical therapist were recommended. They, too, found Jerry to be within normal limits.

ASSESSMENT OF SELF-HELP SKILLS

Both John and Jerry showed normal development in this area. They were eating from a spoon and finger feeding. James was still taking baby food from a special feeder with a nipple. Even with this device it was very difficult to feed him because he arched his back and refused the food. James also had a loud suck which the mother was concerned about.

ASSESSMENT OF BACKGROUND HISTORY

After completing a developmental assessment on each child, I held an intake interview with Mrs. Jones to gather background history and to begin to assess the mother's coping ability. Prenatal complications included unusual weight gain, especially in the early months of the pregnancy, and premature delivery. The pregnancy had come at an inconvenient time, as it interfered with the mother's plans for finishing college. Her religious background, which emphasized the family unit, helped Mrs. Jones more readily accept the mothering role. After she first went home from the hospital, many people offered assistance. Mrs. Jones mentioned that it was very helpful at first; however, she felt a gradual loss of control of her family. Eventually, the mother was able to arrange for 12-year-old twins who lived next door to assist in the afternoons. Mrs. Jones said this arrangement worked much better since she could direct their activities.

In terms of reactions to service from hospitals and clinics, Mrs. Jones had a good experience in the hospital where the triplets were delivered and treated for early complications. Procedures were explained and the parents were made to feel a part of the children's care. Problems came later when clinic services were sought.

Along with discussing past history, Mrs. Jones talked about other problems with the triplets. James had always had a tendency to throw himself backward, making it difficult to carry him. John was slow to gain weight. Jerry seemed normal in development, but the mother worried that he had been overlooked since she had so little time for him.

ASSESSMENT OF THE PHYSICAL ENVIRONMENT

The family lived in an adequately furnished home. The environment was clean and not cluttered. It was safe for the babies to crawl on a blanket on the floor. Each baby had a crib and there were toys available. The church had purchased a washer and dryer for the family.

ASSESSMENT OF THE PARENTING PROCESS

Interaction between the mother and babies was observed. She seemed to spend an equal amount of time with each triplet and showed no preference for which one she carried. The mother demonstrated a lot of touch, eye contact, and verbal communication.

In terms of parental acceptance, the mother had already gone through the stages of accepting that James was severely handicapped. She asked for suggestions on what to do for him and followed up on activities which I demonstrated. The mother did express concern as to whether the stimulation would really make any difference. At the same time, she happily reported any change in his behavior. I felt Mrs. Jones was overwhelmed by the tremendous responsibilities which had suddenly fallen upon her.

From the assessment information, I realized that the parents would need continued counseling throughout the evaluation process. Both Mrs. Jones and the triplets were enrolled in a six-week diagnostic demonstration session. I met with the mother and triplets at the clinic one time per week for one and a half hours. The twins who assisted the mother at home attended part of each session to learn how to work with the babies. The activities performed during each meeting included continuous assessment, teaching, supporting, coordinating, and counseling.

TEACHING

In performing the teaching role, I guided the mother in techniques to facilitate each child's development.* Some approaches demonstrated in the six-week session are described below.

---

* I would like to express appreciation to Sharon Vanderbilt, R.P.T., Director of Physical Therapy Department at T. C. Thompson Children's Hospital, and Imogene Konvalinka, M.A., speech pathologist at Team Evaluation Center, Inc., for assistance in planning the triplets' stimulation program.

James

1. Holding James prone over my knees with his head turned in a position opposite from the side he usually held it due to the asymetrical tonic neck reflex. James was gently rocked in this position to provide vestibular stimulation.
2. Having James prone in the position described above but with myself sitting on a large bolster (12 inches in diameter by 6 feet in length) and gently bouncing him.
3. Positioning in a prone position over a small wedge to encourage integration of the tonic labyrinthine supine reflex and to promote the development of head control. James's head was kept in midline as much as possible.
4. Swinging back and forth in a hammock swing to provide vestibular stimulation.
5. Carrying James over the shoulders to decrease his tendency to arch backwards. It was suggested that Mrs. Jones carry James with his head and shoulders tilted backwards over her shoulder. This position required Mrs. Jones to hold James by his hips and legs rather than around the shoulders.
6. Placing James down in a side lying position and rolling him to the supine position for diaper changes. Placing James down on his back would promote the continuation of the tonic labyrinthine supine reflex.
7. Touching James's arms, face, and legs with various textures and exposing him to lights and sounds for sensory input.
8. Positioning in a sitting position with the head forward to facilitate James's taking food. Later, a homebound program was set up to assist Mrs. Jones in using a spoon to feed James. The speech pathologist and physical therapist related the loud suck to neurologic damage which enhanced the feeding problems.

John

1. Encouraging segmental rolling (moving hips and shoulders separately) as occurs in normal development. John was placed on his back and his leg was passively flexed to facilitate rolling. John was also passively encouraged to roll from a prone position. Favorite toys were placed on each side to encourage voluntary rolling.
2. Encouraging the development of body rotation (in addition to that encouraged through rolling) as in an activity described by Freeman and associates.[42] John was placed on a small beach ball and rocked from side to side but was allowed time to right himself before being tipped to the other side. Freeman and associates also suggest placing a toy at midline so the child will come back to that position to get the toy.
3. Encouraging the development of activities requiring John to bring both hands together in the middle of his body. Some of these included putting rings on a stand, banging blocks, and reaching for suspended objects.
4. Rocking in an all-fours position to encourage weight bearing and weight shift. John was placed in a creeping position on his hands and knees and rocked from side to side and forwards.
5. Encouraging eye tracking. Bright objects were slowly moved from side to side to encourage this response. John tended to fixate on me rather than follow the object.

Jerry

1. Encouraging Jerry to imitate sounds.

2. Providing activities to encourage the development of receptive language such as labeling the body parts on a doll.
3. Getting him to turn small knobs, to pick up pellets, and to play with blocks to promote the development of fine motor skills.
4. Rocking Jerry on a balance board to encourage the development of protective extension, righting, and equilibrium reactions.

SUPPORTING

During the teaching sessions and even after the completion of the evaluation, I had many opportunities to provide support for the mother. I would patiently listen as Mrs. Jones discussed the constant frustrations encountered in trying to obtain services for the triplets. Many of the obstacles, such as getting immediate service, just could not be overcome through the current system. I reassured the mother that she was doing everything possible for her children. Mrs. Jones frequently needed someone to sustain her during these difficult periods.

Frustration with existing programs became so great at times that the mother would decide to investigate private services. Knowing that this solution was financially impossible, I helped the mother to see that trying to get private services was not the most realistic approach. Sometimes support through meeting maintenance needs is best accomplished by helping the family to take advantage of existing resources.

Still another manner in which I provided support to Mrs. Jones was to uphold her in the decision that stimulation was necessary for James. When she was feeling low because of the skeptical attitudes of other professionals, I would reassure Mrs. Jones that stimulation would help to prevent contractures which would interfere with normal body functioning and make James's care more difficult. He also needed as much stimulation as possible to allow him to develop to his maximum capacity. Some of the mother's negative feelings could have resulted from the need to "blame" someone, however, I felt she was justified. I acknowledged that the mother should neither spend all her time with James nor feel guilty about the limited time available for him. Emphasis was also placed on achievements which James made and the mother was praised for working so patiently.

COORDINATING

In performing the coordinating role, I frequently had to set up new appointments and clarify situations for the mother. An orthopaedic consultation was obtained because of her concern about John's feet turning out when he was placed in a standing position. After the initial orthopaedic evaluation, I referred the mother to the Crippled Children's Clinic where she could get follow up orthopaedic care. I also talked to the director of the specialized preschool center about the possibility of allowing all three children to attend the program even though only James and John needed the services. It was difficult for the mother to get someone to baby-sit with Jerry while she attended the program with the other two children. The director agreed to make arrangements for keeping Jerry at the school while his brothers were in the stimulation program. Even after the children's evaluations were completed, the mother called me for assistance with coordinating appointments.

COUNSELING

The activities performed in the areas of assessment, teaching, supporting, and coordinating were integrated into the counseling function. The assessment of Mrs. Jones's coping process showed that she had accepted James's handicap and was ready to start seeking services and planning for the future. Teaching techniques to facilitate his development were integrated throughout the counseling process. The mother brought up the subject of how they would care for him in the future. Mrs. Jones explained that because of her religious beliefs, she could never put James into an institution. The parents believed that the family would be re-joined in Heaven, where James would have a perfect body. Mrs. Jones said she could never face her son in eternity if she resorted to institutionalization. Mrs. Jones also discussed how her husband seemed to not accept the fact that James would never develop pro-gressively. Each day when the father came to get his family, I discussed some of the things the children were doing. She also acknowledged the added strain placed on him by having to use his lunch time to transport the family. Due to the father's work schedule, there was not sufficient time to get him involved in the sessions where he could observe the problems encountered with James. Near the end of the evaluation process, however, the father was able to discuss in an interpretive conference the severity of his son's handicap. He also ex-pressed appreciation that someone had finally looked at the "total child."

Many times Mrs. Jones expressed frustration at having to wait in clinics and being unable to get professionals to explain things to her. I encouraged her to be assertive and to let others know that she expected explanations. Mrs. Jones was also advised to remind person-nel of her appointments and the problems encountered by running into a feeding time in the clinic.

Throughout the counseling process, I worked through the framework of considering how the parents perceived me, meeting their needs first and discussing the children when the parents were ready. They identified me as a support person and relied on me to help them through crises. On some group days, the mother came in overwhelmed with situations that had occurred prior to the session (e.g., a bad clinic appointment). I let her talk about these problems and helped to work out solutions when possible. Clues from Mrs. Jones would in-dicate when she was ready to continue group activities.

ADVOCATING

As an advocate, I am involved in improving the quality of care available for the triplets. For example, I was instrumental in getting the director of the preschool program to hire a nurse to coordinate the program for infants. I encouraged the director to send the nurse to a specialized workshop to improve her skills in working with the developmentally delayed child.

Service Providers

TEAM MEMBERS

A large variety of professionals participate on teams serving the developmentally disabled. Pediatricians, nurses, social workers, physical therapists, occupational therapists, speech therapists, nutritionists, psychometrists, psychologists, audiologists, and educators are the most common members of multidisciplinary teams. Other professionals such as geneticists, neurologists, orthopaedists, and ophthalmologists provide consultation but are not usually permanent members of the team. Service agencies such as in institutional and school settings may also include recreation and music therapists in addition to the above team members. No one program would be likely to have all these disciplines. School systems are more likely to initially employ nurses, physical therapists, speech therapists, social workers, educational diagnosticians, and psychometrists. Preschool programs do not usually include the last two groups.

Each professional performs many functions on the team, but each has a unique contribution to make. Pediatricians do in-depth pediatric surveys and offer consultation in genetics and neurology. The physical therapist specializes in facilitating the child's gross motor development. Occupational therapists concentrate on fine motor skills, eye-hand coordination, and sensory motor development. Speech therapists are concerned with the child's speech and language development. The latter three therapists frequently work as a special team in meeting the needs of the severely physically handicapped child. Psychologists are concerned with the child's social, behavioral, and emotional adjustment. Some are behaviorally oriented while others are analytical. Psychometrists are licensed to administer and interpret I.Q. tests. Educational diagnosticians use this information in analyzing the child's pattern of learning and determining his/her academic achievement. These diagnosticians are particularly helpful in identifying the most appropriate methods through which to teach the child. Nutritionists analyze the child's diet for appropriate nutrients and advise on a therapeutic nutritional program. Recreational therapists use play in a developmental manner to entertain and relax the child. Music therapists apply sound and movement in developing coordination skills and promoting relaxation. Each of these professionals counsels parents and performs many other activities, however, these functions distinguish them from other professionals. On an effective team, interfacing of roles makes it difficult for the observer to identify a particular professional.

SUPPORT PERSONNEL

The late sixties and early seventies witnessed a real interest in the use of paraprofessional personnel which is continuing. One type program in which they are involved is the early intervention program which uses paraprofessionals as home visitors to teach the mother how to provide a stimulating environment. They carry toys into the home and demonstrate games that can be played with the child. Suggestions for homemade toys are also given to the mother. Preparation for this role is frequently accomplished through completion of a training program that varies in length from several weeks to as much as six months. Some of these programs require the paraprofessional to go to another area for the training.

A second group, health professionals, extends their services through use of the paraprofessional. I have four who are referred to as child development workers. They go into the home of developmentally disabled children and guide parents in techniques to facilitate the child's development. They also provide support and counseling for parents and help them to coordinate services. These workers receive a 12 week training program. It includes spending 9 weeks as a participant observer in three different agencies which serve developmentally disabled children. Special lectures and assignments are also part of the training program. Another professional group that relies on paraprofessionals is physical therapists. Their assistants perform routine tasks as directed by the therapist. For example, the assistant might be assigned to roll a child over a beach ball to improve his protective extension. This paraprofessional group frequently is required to complete a two-year program in a university setting.

Institutions, preschools, schools, and other agencies also employ these workers. Sometimes they perform routine duties like helping to serve meals in a preschool program. In some of these settings, the paraprofessional functions much like the child development worker. Training varies tremendously and usually consists of some type of on-the-job program with continuing education provided.

Volunteer groups are effectively utilized in some programs. These groups need to be well organized and supervised in order to offer a continuous service. Senior citizens are also used to provide special services to the developmentally disabled. In some institutions, they come in at mealtimes and feed patients. In the center where I work, a senior citizen supervises the playroom. The children love the enchanting elderly people who play games and read stories to them.

Where Services Are Provided

INFANT AND PRESCHOOL PROGRAMS

An increasing number of infant preschool programs are available to serve the developmentally disabled child. Some of these are under the direction of the United Cerebral Palsy Association, Inc. Others are supported by a combination of funds which include private money, endowments, and federal grants. These programs frequently include the services of nurses, physical therapists, occupational therapists, and social workers.

State and private kindergartens also accept developmentally disabled children, but they may not have special services available. Some contract for these from local agencies (e.g., speech and hearing centers) and assume responsibility for transporting the child for therapy. Headstart programs accept developmentally disabled children. Specialized multidisciplinary professional teams are sometimes hired, as part of the Headstart system, to provide consultation and treatment.

Parent-Child Centers serve children up to age three. King describes this type program as using a family-centered approach.[43] Mothers and children come into the center for special activities. The program includes teaching in relation to good health practices, growth and development, and home life. Outside consultation is sought when the children have special needs. Nurses in these programs assume an increased responsibility in case finding and referral.

SCHOOL AGE PROGRAMS

At school age, developmentally disabled children may attend public schools where they are either integrated into the regular program or assigned to separate classes. Others are enrolled in special schools. The current trend is to integrate developmentally disabled children into the regular classrooms, thereby eliminating the stigma of "special" classes or "special" schools. Nurses have traditionally functioned within the school system. Other disciplines such as physical therapy, speech therapy, and occupational therapy are being added to provide total care for developmentally disabled children.

The program curricula vary according to the needs of the child. Children who have normal intelligence but severe delays in speech and motor development are taught to communicate their knowledge through methods other than speech and writing. For instance, special head devices are available with lights that the child uses in pointing to a particular picture on a board in front of him. If the child wanted ice cream, he could direct the light to the picture of an ice cream cone.* Children who are not retarded but have been diagnosed as having learning disabilities or learning problems attend regular classes with special resource assistance. Special schools and classes are also set up to serve children whose problems are primarily either visual or auditory. Other programs are available to serve the child with emotional and behavioral problems.

Educable mentally retarded children are taught academic subjects at a level which they can comprehend. During high school, emphasis is placed on vocational training in preparation for employment. When the educable retarded child becomes an adult, she works on public jobs, usually maintains a nuclear family unit, and may or may not have children. In the adult world, these individuals are not considered retarded, since they assume a place in society just like anyone else but with less complex jobs.

With moderately retarded children, emphasis is placed on caring for personal needs and solving problems of daily living. Academics are incorporated into the curriculum as the individual shows readiness for these. During high school years, the focus is on vocational training in preparation for work in sheltered workshops or special job placements. Some of these are set up as a part of special school systems. Sheltered apartments may also be a part of these programs.

For the profoundly retarded child, there are day care type programs available either in public or special schools. The program is directed toward facilitating normal physical functioning and preventing the development of further handicapping conditions, such as contractures. These children will never achieve independent functioning, consequently, they continue to require custodial care. Some profoundly retarded children continue to reside with the natural parents as long as they can care for them. "Foster, adoptive, and family boarding placements" are other alternatives as suggested by Wolfensberger.[44]

INSTITUTIONAL CARE

A large number of services for the developmentally disabled are still provided in institutional settings. The services rendered in these have improved with the introduction of specialized personnel. The trend is to return these residents either to their own homes or to special programs within the community. This change in approach is based on the normalization principle. Wolfensberger refines the definition of this principle to mean: "Utilization of means which are as culturally normative as possible, in order to establish and/or maintain personal behaviors and characteristics which are as culturally normative as possible.[44]

Institutions in conjunction with a number of community programs help to facilitate the normalization principle. Special schools and institutional programs offer short-term services where moderately, severely, and profoundly retarded children reside for extended periods, usually six months. During this time, an intense program is implemented to evaluate the developmental potential of the child. Respite care units are also set up within special facilities to give parents temporary relief from the care of the severely disabled child. The length of time which a child may stay ranges from 24 hours to several months. The child with severe physical and mental handicaps is difficult to care for and puts extra strain on the parents.

---

* This type equipment has been developed and is available for purchase from Dr. Sam Sparks, Director; Sensory Engineering Laboratory; 17505 68th St. N.E.; Bothell, Washington 98011.

The respite care unit provides them with an opportunity to leave the child in a protective environment during periods of unusual stress or when the parent just needs to get away.

Sheltered apartments provide an opportunity for older teenagers and adults to live with some degree of independence. More of this type program are needed. Wolfensberger speaks of the need for various types of sheltered apartments. He comments that:

> "Particularly in large population centers, sheltered living residences could be graded rather easily from those with minimal supervision to those with more intensive supervision. These graduations must be much more extensive than the frequently encountered institution/halfway house/independence trichotomy."[44]

These approaches which are directed toward maintaining the developmentally disabled person within the community will expand the need for nurses, especially in providing support to families and coordinating services.

UNIVERSITY AFFILIATED CENTERS

The major goal of the university affiliated center is to promote better service delivery through professional training, in-depth diagnostic workups, and research. The latter service is frequently directed towards developing improved diagnostic techniques and identifying effective treatment approaches. The staffs include a variety of professionals.

DIAGNOSTIC AND EVALUATION CLINICS

A smaller multidisciplinary unit is found in diagnostic and referral clinics. The major goal of these clinics is to identify the child's problem and to refer him/her to another agency for service. The diagnostic and referral clinics are also scattered throughout the country.

CRIPPLED CHILDREN'S CLINICS

State crippled children's programs are known for long-term service to the developmentally disabled. According to Norris,[45] these are a part of the office of Maternal and Child Health with each program set up as an independent unit under a state department. Special clinics treat conditions such as seizure disorders, orthopaedic handicaps, speech and hearing problems, and allergies. Special programs are now being included for developmentally delayed infants. Norris also mentions that:

> "The provision of quality services has been a central concept to the crippled children's program. When standards for care can be met, existing community facilities for ongoing diagnosis, treatment, and follow-up are used. When this is not possible, large pediatric services are utilized with follow-up services provided by traveling teams or field clinics. When necessary, crippled children's programs may fund primary care services, support specialized diagnostic services, and supplement the cost of treatment when parental need is indicated."[45]

HEALTH DEPARTMENT CLINICS

Health department clinics offer a tremendous service in terms of early case finding, continuous counseling, and ongoing health supervision. The health department also focuses on the prevention of handicapping conditions through prenatal care and family planning.

As a part of the health department staff, I advocate the hiring of nurses who have a clinical specialty in developmental disabilities either at the master's or post-master's level. In addition to working directly with families, they would be great consultants for the entire staff since this area of nursing incorporates many fields of knowledge and clinical expertise.

NATIONAL ASSOCIATIONS AND FOUNDATIONS

A large number of national associations and foundations are available, including the Association for the Blind, the Easter Seal Society for Crippled Children and Adults, the Muscular Dystrophy Association of America, the National Foundation-March of Dimes, the National Cystic Fibrosis Research Foundation, the National Association for Retarded Citizens Advocacy, the National Cerebral Palsy Association, Inc., and the Epilepsy Foundation of America. Each national association or foundation is represented throughout the country by local chapters in many cities and towns. If one is not close by, the national association should be contacted for assistance. Programs offered vary with the particular association or foundation. Some of the more common services include public education through lectures and free literature, purchase or loan of special equipment, funding for special programs (e.g., school programs and camps), transportation, research, parent groups, information and referral services, special clinics, and purchase of medical services. [46]

LEGAL CONSIDERATIONS IN THE UNITED STATES

Licensure

To practice nursing in the area of developmental disabilities the practitioner must be licensed as a registered nurse in the state within which she functions. I feel that an application for licensure should be rejected if the applicant's baccalaureate curriculum did not include core content and clinical experience in the nursing care of the developmentally disabled child and his family. This approach would prevent nurses from practicing in the area without exposure to fundamental theories and principles. This policy was suggested by consumers and professionals at the White House Conference on Handicapped Individuals. They expressed concern that many professionals are working in the area of developmental disabilities who have had no basic preparation. Including core content in the basic baccalaureate curriculum would serve both to insure a higher level of practice and to make the nurse more aware of the needs of the developmentally disabled.

Certification

Special certification should also be required for all nurses who work with the developmentally disabled and their families. To become certified, a nurse would complete a program including theory and clinical experience previously identified under the section on educational preparation required to specialize at the undergraduate level in care of the developmentally disabled. A higher level of certification should be available for practitioners at the master's and post-master's levels. At the present time, nurses are not required to be certified to function in the area of developmental disabilities. The need has been identified as a result of the specialization which is necessary for the practitioner. In addition, the consumer needs to be protected from those individuals who are not adequately prepared. Certification as opposed to a separate license would be sufficient to guarantee a level of professional expertise. The American Nurses' Association should be responsible for implementing the certifying process.[47]

Nurses also have a responsibility to work toward certification of those paraprofessionals whom they supervise. At the White House Conference on Handicapped Individuals, the handicapped strongly urged that both professionals and paraprofessionals be certified to insure quality service.

Accountability

To insure efficient and effective services, the nurse needs to build a system to document her work and to demonstrate quality of services. Identification of the criteria which constitute each nursing function provides a means for numerical coding of specific services to which a cost factor can be applied. It is then possible to determine whether the service rendered is justifiable in terms of cost. For example, for the nursing function of completing a developmental assessment on a child, criteria would be identified to define the specific activities involved. These might include 1) to administer and score a Denver Developmental Screening Test, a Developmental Profile, and a Developmental Screening Inventory and 2) to summarize findings in a functional profile. This service would be given a computer code such as 04. A specific cost would be determined for the services by identifying how much of the nurse's time was spent on this function in relation to her total salary. This cost is then compared to that of other agencies who render the same service and evaluated in terms of total agency output to determine whether it is cost effective. Along with efficiency, having each function defined in terms of specific criteria also helps to assure a more accurate level of practice. The nurse is cognizant of what activities constitute a particular function.

To insure quality, the planning process must include a method of evaluation. For example, in teaching the nurse would assess parental knowledge prior to and at the end of the session. If a significant increase occurred, this information could be an indication of successful nursing intervention provided certain variables had been controlled. Consumers also have a contribution in terms of what constitutes effective services and they must be included in planning. At the diagnostic and evaluation clinic where I am employed, parents are called several weeks following the evaluation to get their reaction to the services and to see if they followed up on recommendations. Changes in the program are made on the basis of parental suggestions. If parents did not follow up on recommendations, an evaluation is made to determine the cause. If they were unrealistic, other suggestions might be given. Failure to complete recommendations frequently indicates that the family needs further supportive services, such as help to work out transportation problems. All parental input is used to reassess services and to plan new strategies.

An additional approach to assuring quality service is through the Professional Standards Review Organizations (PSROs). Norris notes that this organization was:

" . . . designed to involve local practicing physicians and other health care professionals in the ongoing review and evaluation of health care services covered under Medicare, Medicaid, and Maternal and Child Health Programs."[45]

According to Norris, the PSROs would be concerned with "the necessity for care, . . . the quality of care," and how "economical" services were that met the patient's needs.[45] Since many programs serving the developmentally disabled receive financial assistance from these sources, they will eventually come under the peer review system. The PSROs employees use techniques such as questionnaires and interviews to gather information about the quality and economic feasibility of the service. The nurse who reviews my agency is hired by the state health department and is housed in the regional health office.

McClure refers to barriers which nurses often encounter in relation to accountability. [48] The first barrier is "misguided egalitarianism." This trend toward going overboard in making all levels of nursing practitioners feel equal must be substituted by the practice of acknowledging differences in nurses and reinforcing them for individual contributions. I feel that levels of certification in developmental disabilities would help to alleviate this problem. The second barrier discussed by McClure is "professional passivity." Nurses exhibit a "psychological inertia" which causes them to "respond to others rather than to initiate action." McClure further comments that "to be accountable means to be willing to seize responsibility, not to wait until it is thrust upon us." This problem emphasizes the need for the assertiveness training identified earlier as a component of basic baccalaureate education in the area of developmental disabilities. The third barrier identified by McClure is "meaningful peer review." This process of reviewing peers becomes a "laissez-faire system" with professionals refusing to criticize each other. [48] Nurses in developmental disabilities must assume a consultative, supportive, and evaluative approach to reviewing services of their peers.

Financial Structure/Funding

Multiple sources of funding for service to the developmentally disabled are available at the local, state, and national levels. At the local level, federal and state monies are supplemented by county funds, special drives, endowments, and special foundations. The fund-raising drive is a successful technique used to gather money either for health and welfare in general or a specific purpose. Most large towns have an organization whose functions are to conduct an annual drive for collecting operating funds and to allocate and distribute the money to health and welfare agencies. The name of the organization tends to vary in each town. In the Chattanooga area it is referred to as the United Fund of Greater Chattanooga, Inc. Drives for specific purposes are conducted by special groups. For example, the Shriners sponsor annual circuses to raise money for crippled children. The Blind Association holds annual candy sales to raise money. The particular approach used, whether sale of articles or special events, varies with the particular community.

At the state level, money is available through departments such as the Department of Public Health, the Department of Mental Health, the Department of Education, and the Department of Human Services. Each of these departments receives appropriations from the federal government to supplement state funds. The specific names of these offices may vary with individual states. For example, the Department of Human Services (formerly known as the Department of Public Welfare) as it is called in Tennessee, is referred to as the Department of Family and Children's Services in Georgia.

Nationally, the Department of Health and Human Services offers continuous financial support and short-term grants to many programs. Norris (1975) mentions that:

"The Department of Health, Education, and Welfare administers more than 300 categorical programs authorized by Congress. In order to carry out this mission, a wide variety of partnerships are required at the national, state, and local levels involving public and private agencies and organizations." [45]

LEGISLATION AFFECTING THE ROLE OF THE NURSE IN THE CARE OF THE DEVELOPMENTALLY DISABLED CHILD

Much legislation has been passed which directly and indirectly affects the role of the nurse in the care of the developmentally disabled. Some acts and amendments have resulted in the development of new programs which have created job opportunities for nurses. Other legislation has resulted in control measures. Norris in Table 17-1 cites examples which summarize how nursing practice has changed since 1912 in relation to legislative actions affecting care of the handicapped.

Some legislation has both directly and indirectly affected nursing practice. Norris refers to the signing into law of the Children's Bureau (1912) which made a study (1925) of rural and urban crippled children's programs in 14 states that " . . . provided the facts necessary to recommend future federal legislation to benefit children with handicaps."[45] Norris also mentions that:

> "These early Bureau efforts and the Sheppard-Towner Act (1921-1929) provided the knowledge and experience upon which the Social Security Act was based. Since its inception in 1935, the original purposes of the Maternal and Child Health programs that came into being at that time have been fostered, improved, and expanded."[45]

Robinson and Robinson cite developments between 1955 and 1960 "which led to the rapid growth of the National Institute on Health and special appropriations for research in mental retardation."[2] These same editors mention the President's Panel on Mental Retardation which was appointed by John F. Kennedy in 1961. It "presented the problem of mental retardation as a matter of grave national concern and federal responsibility."[2] A

TABLE 17-1. Legislative actions affecting the handicapped and changes in nursing practice since 1912[*]

From	To
Treatment	Prevention and early case finding
Treatment of most obvious single conditions	Treatment of less obvious and multiple conditions
Focus on individual	Focus on individual in the context of his family and other social institutions
Services for special population groups such as poor or rural	Services for all on a statewide or regionalized basis
Reduction of mortality	Reduction of mortality as well as reduction of morbidity and improved quality of life[†]
Crisis or episodic care	Ongoing services for health maintenance
Physically oriented medical care	Multidisciplinary comprehensive health care
Inpatient hospital care	Ambulatory and increased emphasis on primary care
Professional accountability	Public accountability

[*] Reprinted with permission from Norris.[45]
[†] The original publication was "Reduction of morbidity and improved quality of life." This was changed in personal communication with Geraldine Norris on January 30, 1980 to read as stated above.

similar President's Panel continues to meet annually to discuss issues and to make recommendations.

Other legislation has related directly to the nurse's functions. Norris comments that "in 1967 Title XIX of the Social Security Act was amended to require early and periodic screening, diagnosis, and treatment (EPSDT) of children eligible for Medicaid."[45] Nurses were to provide many of these services. Norris also discusses "the 1972 amendment to Title XI of the Social Security Act (P.L. 92-603) (which) provides for the creation of Professional Standards Review Organizations (PSROs)"[45] which was discussed earlier. The provision of effective and efficient services is now a professional mandate.

The Rehabilitation Act of 1973[49] and the accompanying amendments represented federal action to help the physically and mentally handicapped to realize their full potential. Norris[45] mentions that this act authorized the 1974 establishment of the Office for the Handicapped in the Office of the Assistant Secretary for Human Development. In 1974, as part of the Rehabilitation Act Amendments, the White House Conference on Handicapped Individuals Act was passed.

"It spoke to the quality of life available in the United States for many; however, the rights and benefits are frequently denied the handicapped. Seven million children and at least twenty-eight million adults were identified with mental and physical handicaps. The Act also emphasized the need to grant equal rights to those individuals. Previously the handicapped individual or his family had assumed all responsibility for care; however, it was time for all levels of government to accept this challenge."[49]

The White House Conference on Handicapped Individuals Act further authorized the president to call the White House Conference on Handicapped Individuals which was held in May of 1977. The mission of the conference was:

"to stimulate a national assessment of those problems faced by individuals with mental and physical handicaps; to generate a national awareness of those problems; and to develop recommendations for legislative and administrative actions to allow individuals with handicaps to live their lives independently, with dignity, and with integration into community life."[49]

Participants at the conference emphasized the need for nurses to have educational preparation in the area of developmental disabilities. They also identified levels of certification and consumer involvement in planning as methods for improving nursing service.

Other legislation passed during the 1970s included laws requiring schools to provide special services to the developmentally disabled. In 1975, a federal education law (94-142) mandated educational opportunities to the handicapped. Ballard and Zettel identify the four major purposes of the law as to:

Guarantee the availability of special education programming to handicapped children and youth who require it.

Assure fairness and appropriateness in decision making with regard to providing special education to handicapped children and youth.

Establish clear management and auditory requirements and procedures regarding special education at all levels of government.

Financially, assist the efforts of state and local government through the use of federal funds.[50]

These educational laws are having a tremendous impact on the roles of school nurses; they must assume responsibility for providing health care services to the developmentally disabled. Coordinating services of other disciplines and serving as a liaison with the family are important components of this role. Assessment of the home setting is a necessity.

Thus, historically and presently, legislative actions have had a tremendous impact on the nurse's role in developmental disabilities. These acts and amendments affect the nurse in terms of the place of employment, the specific job functions, and the level of accountability.

CONCLUSION

The nurse has many direct services to offer in meeting the total needs of developmentally disabled children and their families. In all her activities, the nurse's primary goal is to help the child to reach and to maintain a maximum level of health. Since health is a multifactored condition, nursing must encompass the many component parts. This goal is accomplished through the functions of assessing, teaching, supporting, coordinating, and counseling. With her orientation to the total child, the nurse has less opportunity to specialize with respect to a particular problem area, consequently, she must coordinate services with those professionals who concentrate on one aspect of the child's care. By focusing on the total family, the nurse can best advocate their needs and desires to the community.

In performing these services, the nurse must ascertain that she is accountable in terms of efficiency and effectiveness. Meeting this requirement necessitates that the nurse will acquire and maintain a level of professional expertise. She must also be knowledgeable about sources of funding and current legislation since these affect the boundaries of her practice.

ACKNOWLEDGMENTS

I wish to acknowledge the children and parents who are represented in the chapter and the staff on the Team Evaluation Center, Inc. I would also like to express appreciation to Paula Millen, P.N.P., M.S., R.N., for proofing and consultation; Polly Pullen and Madelyn Williams for typing; Beckie Baker, B.S., Marcia Jenison, M.Ed., C.C.C., David Thompson, M.A., Betsy Brown, M.Ed., and Susan Brewer, Ph.D. for consultation; Hattie Ballard, Lee Clinton, Betty Sparks, and Pat White, Child Development Workers, for support and excellent patient service. Eugenia Henry, M.A., Fran Maurer, B.S.N., R.N., Camille Cook, M.P.H., R.N., Marian Langley, M.P.H., R.N., Hazel Fowler, M.P.H., R.N., Ann Peterson, M.P.H., R.N., and Conrad Shackleford, M.D., for professional support and consultation.

REFERENCES

1. Clark, D.W., and MacMahon, B. (eds.): *Preventive Medicine*. Little, Brown and Company, Boston, 1967.
2. Robinson, N.M., and Robinson, H.B.: *The Mentally Retarded Child: A Psychological Approach*, ed. 2. McGraw-Hill Book Company, New York, 1976.
3. Coyner, A., and Lloyd, L.: "Nursing Role in Early Intervention Programs for Developmentally Disabled Children." Proceedings of Conference, University of Utah College of Nursing, Division of Continuing Education and Utah State Division of Health, U.S. Department of Health, Education, and Welfare, 1976.
4. Mauksch, H.O.: "The Organizational Context of Nursing Practice," in Davis, F. (ed.): *The Nursing Profession: Five Sociological Essays*. John Wiley & Sons, Inc., New York, 1966.

5. O'Neil, S.: Child Development and Mental Retardation Center. University of Washington, Seattle, Washington, 1970.
6. Bell, B.J.: Center for Developmental and Learning Disorders. University of Alabama, Birmingham, Alabama, 1970.
7. Patterson, N.: Notes taken by Susan Ritchie, M.P.H., at "Workshop on Developmental Disabilities." Child Development Center, Memphis, Tennessee, March 1976.
8. Kleeschulte, S.: Center for Developmental and Learning Disorders. University of Alabama. Birmingham, Alabama, 1970.
9. Worthy, E.J. (eds.): "The Symposium on Child with Developmental Disabilities," in Sharp, E.S., and Worthy, E.J. (eds.): *The Nursing Clinics of North America,* 10:2:307, June 1975.
10. Barnard, K.E., and Powell, M.L.: *Teaching the Mentally Retarded Child—A Family Care Approach.* The C. V. Mosby Company, St. Louis, 1972.
11. Barnard, K.E., and Douglas, H.B. (eds.): *Child Health Assessment Part 1: A Literature Review.* DHEW Publication No. (HRA) 75-30, 1974.
12. Ayers, A.J.: *Sensory Integration and Learning Disorders,* ed. 3. Western Psychological Services, Los Angeles, 1974.
13. "Post-Master's Program in Nursing of Children with Handicaps." Brochure, University of Washington School of Nursing, Seattle, Washington, 1970.
14. Klaus, M.H., and Kennell, J.H.: *Maternal Infant Bonding.* The C. V. Mosby Company, St. Louis, 1976.
15. Bean, M.R., and Ritchie, S.K.: "Parenting Without Neglect," in Bean, M., and Ritchie, S. (eds.): *Understanding and Enhancing the Normal Process of Growth and Development in the Infant and Preschool Child—Preventing Neglect.* Unpublished Monograph of the Proceedings of Regional Workshop for Community Health Nurses, Team Evaluation Center, Inc., Chattanooga, Tenn., 1976.
16. Caldwell, B.M.: "Home Inventory For Infants." Unpublished Copyright Copy of a Description of the Inventory, Center for Early Child Development and Education, University of Arkansas at Little Rock, Little Rock, Arkansas, 1970.
17. Baldwin, A.L., Kalhorn, J., and Breese, F.H.: "Patterns of Parent Behavior," *Psychological Monographs,* 58:3, 1945.
18. Floyd, L.: "Parenting in the Seventies," in Bean, M.R. (ed.): *The Nurse as a Facilitator of Parenting.* Unpublished Monograph of the Proceedings of Workshop for Public Health Nurses, Team Evaluation Center, Inc., Chattanooga, Tenn., 1977.
19. Young, K.Y.: "Chronic Sorrow: Parents' Response to the Birth of a Child with a Defect." *Maternal Child Nursing,* 2(1):38, 1977.
20. Chinn, P.C., Drew, C.J., and Logan, D.R.: *Mental Retardation, a Life Cycle Approach.* The C. V. Mosby Company, St. Louis, 1975.
21. Haynes, U.: *A Developmental Approach to Casefinding.* Children's Bureau Publication No. 449, Washington, 1967.
22. Alexander, M.M., and Brown, M.S.: *Pediatric Physical Diagnosis for Nurses.* McGraw-Hill Book Company, New York, 1974.
23. Fiorentino, M.R.: *Reflex Testing Methods for Evaluating CNS Development.* Charles C Thomas, Springfield, Ill., 1973.
24. Frankenberg, W.K., Dodds, J.B., and Fandal, A.W.: *Denver Developmental Screening Test Manual/Workbook for Nursing and Paramedical Personnel.* Manpower Development and Training Act, University of Colorado Medical Center, 1973.
25. Drumwright, A.F.: Denver Articulation Screening Test, University of Colorado Medical Center, Lit. 17, 1971.
26. Knobloch, H., Pasamanick, B., and Sherard, E.S.: "A Developmental Screening Inventory." Division of Child Development of the Department of Pediatrics, and the Department of Psychiatry, The Ohio State University College of Medicine, and The Children's Hospital, Columbus, Ohio.
27. Knobloch, H., and Pasamanick, B.: *Gesell and Armatrudas' Developmental Diagnosis,* ed. 3. Harper & Row, Publishers, New York, 1974.
28. Alpern, G.D., and Boll, T.: *Developmental Profile.* Psychological Development Publications, Indianapolis, 1972.
29. Bensberg, G.J. (ed.): *Teaching the Mentally Retarded—A Handbook for Ward Personnel.* Southern Regional Educational Board, Atlanta, 1965.

30. "Diapers Away." Pamphlet on Toilet Training the Mentally Retarded Child at Home, U.S. Department of Health, Education, and Welfare, Social and Rehabilitation Service, Division of Mental Retardation, Arlington, Va.

31. Caldwell, B.M.: "Home Observation for Measurement of the Environment, Preschool Version." Unpublished Instruction Manual, Center for Early Child Development and Evaluation, Little Rock, Arkansas.

32. Gellis, S.S., and Feingold, M.: *Atlas of Mental Retardation Syndromes.* Superintendent of Documents, U.S. Government Printing Office, Washington, 1968.

33. Bluma, S.M., Shearer, M.S., Frohman, A.H., et al.: *Portage Guide to Early Education.* The Portage Project, Cooperative Educational Service Agency #12, Portage, Wis., 1976.

34. Finnie, N.R.: *Handling the Young Cerebral Palsied Child at Home,* ed. 2. E.P. Dutton and Company, Inc., New York, 1975.

35. Lewis, M.: "Parenting with the Infant and Young Child," in Bean, M.R. (ed.): *The Nurse as a Facilitator of Parenting.* Unpublished Monograph of the Proceedings of Workshop for Public Health Nurses, Team Evaluation Center, Inc., Chattanooga, Tenn., 1977.

36. Whaley, D.L., and Malott, R.W.: *Elementary Principles of Behavior.* Appleton-Century-Crofts, New York, 1971.

37. Inglis, S.: "The Nocturnal Frustration of Sleep Disturbance." *Maternal Child Nursing,* 1(5):280, 1976.

38. Barnhart, C.L., and Stein, J. (eds.): *The American College Dictionary.* Random House, New York, 1963.

39. Ourth, L.: "Techniques of Behavior Management," in Bean, M.R. (ed.): *The Nurse as a Facilitator of Parenting.* Unpublished Monograph of the Proceedings of Workshop for Public Health Nurses, Team Evaluation Center, Inc., Chattanooga, Tenn., 1977.

40. Gans, J.G.: *The Urban Villagers.* The Free Press, New York, 1962.

41. Ourth, L.: "Techniques of Behavior Management." Notes from paper presented to a public health nursing workshop, Chattanooga, Tenn., Oct. 15, 1977.

42. Freeman, J., Gould, V., Merkley, F., et al.: *A Developmental Curriculum for Infants Exhibiting Developmental Delay.* Project Atypical Development Ameliorated through Prescriptive Techniques, Developmental Disabilities Projects Fund, Health and Welfare Agency, California, 1975.

43. King, J.B.: "Teenage Parents," in Bean, M.R. (ed.): *The Nurse as a Facilitator of Parenting.* Unpublished Monograph of the Proceedings of Workshop for Public Health Nurses, Team Evaluation Center, Inc., Chattanooga, Tenn., 1977.

44. Wolfensberger, W.: *The Principle of Normalization in Human Services.* National Institute on Mental Retardation, Toronto, 1972.

45. Norris, G.J.: "National Concerns for Children with Handicaps," in Sharp, E.S., and Worthy, E.J. (eds.): *The Nursing Clinics of North America,* 10:2:313, June 1975.

46. *Directory of Community Services.* Metropolitan Council for Community Services, Inc., United Fund of Greater Chattanooga, 1978.

47. "ANA" Certification: Recognition of Excellence." Article based on a speech presented by Joan Olden, R.N.: *AORN Journal* 19(3):676, 1974.

48. McClure, M.L.: "The Long Road to Accountability." *Nursing Outlook,* 26(1):47, 1978.

49. *The White House Conference on Handicapped Individuals—Final Report.* Vol. 2, Part A, U.S. Government Printing Office, Washington, 1977.

50. Ballard, J., and Zettel, J.: "Public Law 94-142 and Section 504: What They Say About Rights and Protections." *Exceptional Children,* 44:177, Nov. 1977.

51. Bean, M.R., and Boll, B.J.: "Nursing Intervention in the Care of the Physically Handicapped, Severely Retarded Child," in Sharp, E.S., and Worthy, E.J. (eds): *The Nursing Clinics of North America* 10:2:353, 1975.

BIBLIOGRAPHY

Braley, W.T., Konicki, G., and Leedy, C.: *Daily Sensorimotor Training Activities.* Educational Activities, Inc., Freeport, New York, 1968.

Buscaglia, L.: *The Disabled and Their Parents.* Charles B. Slack, Inc., Thorofare, N.J., 1975.

Campbell, D.R.: *How to Really Love Your Child.* Victor Books, Wheaton, 1977.

DeAngelis, C.: *Basic Pediatrics for the Primary Health Care Provider.* Little, Brown and Company, Boston, 1975.

McDiarmid, N.J.,Peterson, M.A., and Sutherland, J.R.: *Loving and Learning Interacting with Your Child from Birth to Three.* Harcourt Brace Jovanovich, New York, 1975.

Dodson, F.: *How to Father.* Nash Publishing, Los Angeles, 1974.

Gelfand, D.M., (ed.): *Social Learning in Childhood.* Wadsworth Publishing Company, Belmont, Cal., 1969.

Gellis, S.S., and Feingold, M.: *Atlas of Mental Retardation Syndromes.* U.S. Department of Health, Education and Welfare, Washington, 1968.

Ginott, H.G.: *Between Parent and Child.* Avon Books, New York, 1971.

Johnson, T.R., Moore, W.M., and Jeffries, J.E. (eds.) *Children are Different,* ed. 2. Ross Laboratories, Columbus, Ohio, 1978.

Johnson, V.M., and Werner, R.A.: *A Step-by-Step Learning Guide for Retarded Infants and Children.* Syracuse University Press, Syracuse, 1975.

Koch, R., and Dobson, J.D. (eds.): *The Mentally Retarded Child and His Family.* Brunner/Mazel, Publishers, New York, 1971.

Korones, S.B., Lancaster, J., and Roberts, F.B.: *High-Risk Newborn Infants.* The C. V. Mosby Company, St. Louis, 1972.

Mercer, R.T.: *Nursing Care for Parents at Risk.* Charles B. Slack, Inc., Thorofare, N.J., 1977.

Miller, M.M.: *Sunday's Child.* Holt, Rhinehart, and Winston, New York, 1968.

O'Neil, S.M., McLaughlin, B.N., and Knapp, M.B.: *Behavioral Approaches to Children with Developmental Delays.* The C. V. Mosby Company, St. Louis, 1977.

Smith, D.W., and Wilson, A. A.: *The Child with Down's Syndrome.* W. B. Saunders Company, Philadelphia, 1973.

Vaughan, V.C., McKay, R.J., and Nelson, W.E.: *Nelson Textbook of Pediatrics,* ed. 10. W. B. Saunders Company, Philadelphia, 1975.

Walters, C.E., (ed.): *Mother-Infant Interaction.* Human Sciences Press, New York, 1976.

Williams, S.R.: *Nutrition and Diet Therapy.* The C. V. Mosby Company, St. Louis, 1969.

CHAPTER 18

NURSING ROLE IN GERONTOLOGY

MARIAN G. SPENCER, M.S., C.A.G.S., R.N.

Aging is a universal phenomenon, yet, when is a person old? This is difficult to answer, although the tendency is to cite a chronologic figure of age, usually 65. The retort of some elders would be, "As old as I look and young as I feel." Undeniably, aging is relative and multidimensional. The biopsychosocial clock ticks from birth to the terminal event of death. All the years in between these two points in time represent aging. Once the human organism reaches biologic maturity, at about 16 years, time-dependent changes set in. Aging is a gradual slowing down process and is normal for all living organisms.

Biologic aging varies among individuals. The role of aging differs for each person within organs and organ systems. Moreover, individuals do not change as they grow older, they become more what they always have been. There is a gradual slowing down of intellectual functioning, memory deficits, and decreased speed in performance of those tasks requiring speed. However, there are those persons at age 40 who have lost mental flexibility and interest in new experiences, in contrast with persons aged 80 who possess flexibility of thought and interests as well as intellectual acuity.

Alteration or loss of social functions performed within the family/community network can change the person's self-concept and feelings of personal worth. The physical-social environment has impacts on the biopsychosocial aspects of aging for each individual. The inner strengths and resourcefulness of older people enable them to adapt and adjust to life changes.

Current societal values have placed severe curtailment on older people's freedom to maintain control over their life situations. The worship of youth and productivity limits their ability to function in the mainstream of the economy which responds to rapid technologic advances. While independence is a highly valued trait in this society, the society does little to help aging persons maintain their independence. We have a system of human waste and obsolescence. We operate within a system of laws, programs, and services which increasingly forces old people into dependent roles. An attitudinal change from that of patronizing older people to accepting older people as having the same human needs as the dominant society throughout their life cycle is needed.

DEMOGRAPHIC FACTORS: FUTURE PREDICTIONS[1]

Old people as a group are not static. In the United States there are approximately 33 million persons aged 65 plus. The projected population growth for the U.S. up to year 2035 is 40 percent, or from 217 million to 304 million persons. The elderly population is expected to more than double in size by 2035, from 33 million to 71 million. The population projections increase the average age of our population from the current figure of 29.9 years to 38 years by 2035.

The rapidity of growth of our aging population will undoubtedly have a sizeable impact upon the need for health and support services. While aging is not synonymous with illness, the incidence of chronic disabling conditions increases with advancing age.

The elderly population has increased nearly 7 times since 1900, that is, from 4.9 million in 1900 to 32.8 million in 1977. Moreover, the elderly population has grown older. The population aged 75 and over has grown about 17 times. About one-fourth of the elderly population is aged 75 plus. This proportion is expected to increase to over one-third by the year 2035. Currently, the 85 plus group members 1 of every 16 elderly persons; by the year 2035, they will number 1 of every 10.

Future predictions are that the elderly will continue to grow numerically at a more rapid rate than the population as a whole. Even more dramatic is the growth of elderly persons who live alone. Between 1960 and 1976 the number has increased from 3.8 million to 7.9 million. Single person households among the 75 plus group outnumber the rates for the younger aged elderly. Contributing factors are 1) longer female life span; 2) improvement in financial security through the added benefits of Supplemental Security Income, Medicare, Social Security with incremental benefits, and broader coverage under private pension plans. Other influential factors include geographic mobility of families resulting from better educational and job opportunities, ease of accessibility of transportation and communication systems, and smaller family size (depression era cohorts lower birth rates).

While it is difficult to predict trends in income levels given the current state of the economy with uncontrolled inflation, it is likely that future elderly persons will enjoy better financial resources. Future elderly will be better educated and will have worked at higher salaried occupations.

IMPLICATIONS FOR NEEDS AND SERVICES

Human service requirements will escalate to meet the myriad needs of older people. Need will be the determinant for care. Currently, 95 percent of the elderly are community based. The other 5 percent, or approximately 1 million, are in nursing homes or related facilities. In view of projected increases in the aging population, maintaining the aforementioned percentages will present a major challenge for the health delivery system.

The maxim that "man does not live by bread alone" is not a simplistic truism. Old people have the same needs as people of all age groups. The aging process alters their roles and functions. The struggle for adaptation and survival is heightened. Aging individuals sustain multiple losses. According to Havighurst:

> "The suggested developmental tasks of old age more specifically imply adjustment to losses. They include: adjusting to decreasing physical strength and health, adjustment to retirement and reduced income, adjusting to death of spouse, establishing explicit affiliation with one's age group, meeting social and civic obligations, and establishing satisfactory living arrangements". [2]

How the individual adjusts to these age related changes is dependent upon previous patterns of coping acquired throughout his or her lifetime. Self-image, health, and economic status play significant parts in one's personal pattern of adjustment. Professionals working with older people should be sensitive to the subtleties and nuances age decrements impose upon the adaptive capacities of old persons. Rolelessness is the hallmark of the aged today.

Senescence is a phase of human development. It is a winding down process. The human clockworks tick more slowly. The biologic clock signals decreased energy and vitality as well as time related changes in organs and organ systems. The psychological clock chimes the warning of decrease in mental acuity, that is, decline in speed of intake and the process of information, decline in speed of performance of tasks, and ego constriction in the interpersonal realm of family and friends. The sociologic clock slows to an occasional tick, meaning, time has run out for the individual to acquire or maintain status or prestige. The basic anchorages (Cath) which give form and substance to life and living are gradually lost,

FUNCTIONAL – STRUCTURAL CHANGES IN NORMAL AGING

While the effects of aging are cumulative, the role of aging differs for each individual. Major theories of aging may be classified under two groups, the first "programmed" and the second "wear and tear." In programmed aging each developmental stage of the body is switched on and off accordingly due to some mechanism in the individual's genetic endowment. In DNA replication there are possible errors occurring in the template messenger RNA which affect cell metabolism and gradually impair organ function and eventually the whole organism. [3]

Aging is associated with depletion of cellular and functional reserve. This renders the older adult more susceptible to chronic disabling conditions. Health maintenance and disability prevention have had great psychosocial attributes. When possible these afford aging persons the opportunity to live with a sense of dignity and worth. However, 80 percent of the elderly population is plagued with chronic health problems, such as cardiovascular disease, cancer, arthritis, chronic pulmonary disease, diabetes, and glaucoma. Chronic illness may occur at any age, but with advancing years the vulnerability increases more rapidly. The need for acute care among the healthy aged is undifferentiated when compared with the general population.

Health care professionals are inadequately prepared to assess the health needs of older people. A basic understanding of normal aging processes is essential to understanding the altered manifestation and response in patterns of illness behavior. HEW publication, *The*

Practitioner and the Elderly, Working with Older People: A Guide to Practice, provides descriptive information on changes in aging. A detailed narrative follows.[4]

Skin and Subcutaneous Tissues

The obvious and outward signs of these changes represent the image an individual presents in his social relationships and also are factors in his concept of self. Gray hair, wrinkles, warts, and other manifestations, therefore, represent clearly a deteriorating or less attractive image for the individual himself and for others. Emotionally, they are one more stress or strain which the ego must grapple with in adapting to the aging process.

CHANGES IN APPEARANCE

Functional Changes

The sterotyped picture of an aged person is that he or she is small and lean; however, the range of variation in external appearance is probably as great as for younger groups. The changes that occur with aging in the skin and subcutaneous tissues are largely responsible for the alterations in external appearance:

    a. General skin appearance. The skin becomes progressively lax, inelastic, dry, wrinkled, and also becomes thinner (atrophic). Focal pigmentary discolorations (yellow and brown) occur.

    b. Ecchymoses (minute hemorrhages resulting in the familiar black and blue spots and markings). Because of an increased fragility of the dermal and subcutaneous vessels, ecchymoses result from relatively trivial trauma.

    c. Angiomas and keratoses (types of warts). Other frequent skin changes are senile angiomas and warts on the face, scalp, and trunk.

    d. Fissures. Fissures often develop about the mouth.

    e. Hair. The graying and whitening of hair is an almost universal change. Aside from inherited baldness, there is a progressive loss of hair from the frontal and vertical areas of the scalp in men and a general thinning of the hair in women.

    f. Sweating. Old people also sweat less than younger ones.

Structural Changes

The structural changes consist of an atrophy of the epidermal layer except for the focal areas of hyperkeratosis (excessive deposit of callus). The latter can be considered premalignant lesions in the sense that malignant tumors, most often basal cell carcinomas, develop at such sites. The dermis undergoes basophilic degeneration which involves degenerative changes in both collagen and elastic fibers. The skin adnexal structures, i.e., the sweat and sebaceous glands and the hair follicles, undergo atrophy, and there is atrophy of the subcutaneous tissues.

    It is not difficult to match structural changes with changes in the appearance of the skin:

    a. The fissuring is due to atrophy of the epidermal layer.

    b. The wrinkling and loss of resiliency can be related to the changes in collagen and elastic fiber and the drying to loss of sweat glands.

    c. The secretion of the sebaceous glands contains a factor which protects against hyperkerotic changes, and loss of this substance permits the development of these tumors.

d. Atrophy of the hair follicles accounts for the balding.

e. The loss of subcutaneous tissue is particularly important since this layer affords both an insulating layer and a cushioning against trauma. The former may be responsible, in part, for the inability of old people to regulate body temperature, and the latter to the development of decubitus ulcers (skin sores) at points of pressure.

ENVIRONMENTAL FACTORS VERSUS INTRINSIC AGING EFFECTS

It should be emphasized that many of these changes in skin are most marked in the exposed portions of the skin because prolonged exposure to actinic rays can result in changes similar in many ways to those seen in aging. This constitutes an example of the difficulty often encountered in distinguishing between intrinsic aging effects and environmental factors.

Musculoskeletal System

The stooped posture, stiffened joints, and porous bone structure represent not only a less attractive physical image but also a limitation in mobility and independent activities of daily living, both at home and in the community.

Functional Changes

Changes include bent appearance, slow movements.

a. Height. Some reduction in height.

b. Posture. Typical posture partially bent hips and knees, stooping back, and flexed neck.

c. Muscle power. Loss of muscle evident. Rapid, voluntary movements less easy to perform due to a combination of changes involving both muscle and nervous system. Inactivity accelerates the process.

Structural Changes

a. Muscle. Changes are thinning of the individual fibers, loss of cross striation—hyaline appearance—disappearance of muscle fibers replaced with scar tissue which does not expand or contract at will.

b. Posture. Changes in ligaments, joints and bones. Ligaments and joints become stiffened.

1. Ligaments calcify and ossify.
2. Stiffening of the joints results from erosion of cartilaginous joint surfaces, their ossification, as well as degenerative changes in soft tissues which line joint cavities (synovium osteoarthritis).
3. Calcification and ossification of the ligaments of the vertebrae, lipping of the vertebrae.
4. Intervertebral discs become thinner—curvature of the spine.
5. Cartilages and ligaments and joints which join rib cage to sternum and vertebrae impair movement of rib cage and affect respiration.
6. Bones become porous and lighter, losing elasticity (osteoporosis). Some bones change

shape. The angle between the neck of the femur and the shaft changes from obtuse to right angle. This altered structural change increases stress and predisposes to fractures. Changes in bone structure of the vertebrae, intervertebral discs, and ligaments all combine to produce kyphoscoliosis (hunched back) of the elderly.

RELATION TO ORGAN SYSTEMS AND BODY ACTIVITIES

These changes in muscle have an important influence on a number of other organ systems and many activities.

a. Daily tasks. Create difficulty in carrying out ordinary daily tasks.

b. Respiratory system. Impair the efficiency of the respiratory system because of impairment of muscles of respiration.

c. Excretory functions. Involvement of the muscles of the abdomen and pelvis creates problems of defecation and urination.

d. Energy stores. Muscles store glycogen, and loss of glycogen stores leads to loss of reserve sugar, the energy requirement for emergency activity.

Nervous System

Functional Changes

Deficits referrable to the nervous system include the loss of some tendon reflexes and loss of efficiency of sensory organs, for example, a raised threshold for taste and smell.

a. Tactile discrimination and appreciation of vibrations are diminished.

b. Increased threshold for pain.

c. Reflexes generally slow and adjustment to stimuli becomes slower and less efficient.

d. Recovery of balance from changes in position is retarded.

e. Susceptibility to shock is increased due to loss of neural control of circulation.

f. Decrease in speed and accuracy of a variety of cognitive and psychomotor functions. There is decline in some intellectual abilities especially in the very old. Impairment in short term memory, but long term memory may be intact well into old age. There is an increase in factual knowledge with age (experience) and in its coordination and ordering, and this may offset some of the other mental decrements.

Structural Changes

There are both gross and microscopic changes which occur with advancing age which may be, to some degree, associated with identifiable personality changes. Opinions differ as to whether the structural changes represent intrinsic aging effects or are the consequences of vascular impairment.

a. With advancing age there is progressive atrophy of the convolutions (gyri) of the brain surface and widening and deepening of the spaces (sulci) between the convolutions.

b. There is some loss of bulk of brain substances and some dilation of the canals (ventricles) which contain cerebrospinal fluid.

c. Microscopically, a progressive loss of brain cells (neurons) can be detected and the remaining neurons acquire a brown pigment (lipofuscin). Corpora amylacea, small, sandlike bodies, progressively increase in number within the brain substance.

d. Some of these changes are believed to be intensified in senile dementia and are intensified, at least in focal areas, following occlusion of cerebral vessels. It is not unusual to see old people who exhibit very few of the identified behavioral changes noted until they have suffered one or more strokes. Following this there is a sudden and rapid deterioration in the direction of senile dementia.

PERSONALITY CHANGES

Many behavioral problems observed in the elderly may be related to cerebrovascular system changes as well as changes in the nervous system. Many symptoms may mimic those of mental illness and may present severe management problems for institutions or other caretakers caring for the patient. Families and/or significant others may find these changes distressful and may need counseling and help with their feelings.

a. Old people have been described as developing a narrowing of interest and a failure to accept new ideas.

b. They are often melancholy and pessimistic.

c. They are labeled as having a loss of intensity of emotional response and a loss of adaptibility.

d. Old people may exhibit abnormal possessiveness.

e. In advanced senility, there is mental confusion with intervening lucid periods.

Some observers believe that many of these characteristics represent only an exaggeration of earlier traits. Professionals must be aware of and sensitive to the shades of gray in personality assessment.

THE SPECIAL SENSES

Less attention has been paid to age related impairment of the special senses. Total loss of function of one or more is still compatible with life. It is self-evident that loss of some of these functions can have profound personality effects and create serious problems in coping with the environment.

Vision

There is a high rate of retention of good vision throughout advancing years. Visual efficiency may decline.

PRESBYOPIA (FARSIGHTEDNESS)

This is a condition of decreased near vision resulting from progressive rigidity of the lens and reduced ability to accomodate. Clinical manifestation is usually about age 40. It is correctable with eye glasses.

SENILE CATARACT

Senile cataract is usually present to some degree in all old people, but it is possible to live beyond 80 without significant handicap from a cataract. Increasing opacity of the lens may gradually reduce visual efficiency. Rapidity of development is highly variable. There is no need to delay removing the opacifying lens. This can be done whenever the visual needs of the patient require.

GLAUCOMA

This condition is associated with increased intraocular pressure. Persistent increased intraocular pressure can cause asymptomatic destruction of optic nerve tissue leading to gradual loss of visual fields and ultimately to blindness. The tonometer test to measure intraocular pressure in people over age 35 should be routine in health assessment. The test should be done at regular intervals to detect glaucoma at a treatable stage before visual loss.

Older adults should have a complete eye exam annually for detection screening of visual deficits. Visual changes may limit activities, passive and active. Many vision problems prevent enjoyment of travel, shopping, reading, television, and other forms of diversion and may be the most difficult physical handicap to which the older person must adapt.

Hearing

PRESBYCUSIS (HEARING LOSS WITH AGE)

This generally begins about age 30, but usually does not cause difficulty until the middle years of life or later. Hearing loss begins in the higher frequencies and progresses to lower frequencies. The condition can result from a combination of many factors, such as aging of the brain and the total auditory system, effects of disease, trauma, and noise.

Decreased hearing acuity in elderly persons often causes limitations of social relationships and enjoyment of activities such as church attendance, radio, concerts, television, and social visiting. Social participation is important to the mental health of the elderly. A hearing disability can have serious implications when it leads to isolation, which in turn may result in withdrawal, frustration, and concomitant personality changes.

Speech

Changes in pronunciation, voice, and language usage are common in the aged. Aphasia (or dysphasia) is less common and refers to various impairments in the ability to use or understand words as a result of brain lesions. Factors which may be responsible for changes in pronunciation and vocal usage include lesions involving motor nerves controlling muscles used in respiration and articulation, lessened resilience of tissues and cartilages used to produce voice, and a lessening of finer muscular control in the oral structures used in speech.

Smell and Taste

Progressive loss of sense of smell is common, also a loss of the sense of taste as the taste buds diminish in number. These changes may be partly responsible for loss of appetite and other pleasureable sensations. Loss of sense of smell can create a hazardous situation since it may involve inability to detect odors of dangerous gases or something burning.

Tactile

With advancing age there is progressive loss of ability to experience heat, cold, and touch sensations. Vibration sense of the extremities is also often lost, although it may remain in some nonagenerians.

CARDIOVASCULAR SYSTEM

A problem in assessing aging phenomena in humans involves differentiation between various degenerative phenomena within the specific organ due to intrinsic causes. An example of degeneration changes due to intrinsic causes would be heart function affected by diseases of the coronary arteries, valves, or primary diseases of the myocardium; extrinsic causes may be hypertension, arteriovenous fistula, chronic anemias, generalized arteriosclerosis, or chronic pulmonary disease. In addition, other intrinsic causes may be due to so-called mechanical wear and tear phenomena.

Functional Changes

There is a decline in cardiac output at rest. The heart becomes less capable of responding to extra work which in young persons is characterized by an increase in rate and stroke volume. The heart does not enlarge with age unless there are underlying intrinsic and/or extrinsic causes such as previously mentioned. In the absence of these conditions, the heart is usually normal or small in size in old people. There is progressive increase in peripheral resistance to the flow of blood and also a tendency for increased systolic blood pressure.

Structural Changes

There is some increase in the interstitial fibrous tissue. Atrophy in voluntary muscle fibers does not occur here. The muscle cells progressively accumulate brown pigment (lipofuscin) in a manner similar to nerve cells. Senile amyloidosis (excessive deposit of starchlike material) of the heart is quite common. These changes may occur even in the absence of significant narrowing of the coronary trunk arteries. These alterations are probably responsible for the diminishing cardiac output.

The arteries elongate with advancing age, become tortuous, and calcify. There is fibrosis of the lumen (inner channel) which becomes narrower. These changes cause the pulse wave to be propagated more rapidly in older people and may be responsible for the tendency toward higher systolic blood pressures.

Basement (supporting) membrane thickening advances progressively with age in vessels of all sizes, even down to capillaries. In small vessels the muscle fibers hyalinize and perivascular fibrous tissues increase. These changes cause an impairment of diffusion of nutrients into the tissues as well as the removal of waste substances. Aging changes may occur secondary to these vascular alterations.

RESPIRATORY SYSTEM

Changes within the respiratory system may lead to a limiting of mobility and activities of all kinds. Shortness of breath and other breathing difficulties produce varying degrees of fear and anxiety in older persons similiar to the apprehensions which accompany heart conditions.

There are three components of this system which may show age related impairment: *ventilation* (breathing), *diffusion* (exchange of oxygen and carbon dioxide between lungs and blood), and *pulmonary circulation*.

Functional Changes

Total lung capacity declines, while there is an increase in residual volume. There is a reduction in vital capacity and its subdivisions. Maximum voluntary ventilation and other tests that require effort decline with age because of an age related decrease in maximum pulmonary ventilation and maximum oxygen consumption.

Structural Changes

Aged related factors which interfere with ventilation are weakness of the muscles of respiration, marked obesity, and skeletal abnormalities of the rib cage. There is also diminished resiliency of the lungs, probably due to changes in elastic fibers. Reduction in diffusing capacity is probably due to a reduction in alveolar capillaries plus mild maldistribution of inspired gas.

Pulmonary arteriosclerosis occurs at a much slower rate than systemic arteriosclerosis, primarily because of the lower operating pressures in pulmonary circulation.

EMPHYSEMA

Old people may experience dyspnea (shortness of breath) without manifest evidence of obstruction to exhalation common in other forms of emphysema. Pulmonary function in older persons should be followed periodically to promptly identify changes which may be due to developing clinical disease.

GASTROINTESTINAL TRACT

Food and enjoyment of it is a primary satisfaction available to many older persons, so that digestive difficulties, modified diets, and intestinal upsets are often major problems to the elderly, representing one or more areas of deprivation for them. There is great preoccupation with food intake and excretion. Food fads are not uncommon, and these are often difficult to resolve by those supplying food regularly to the aged. Bowel incontinence represents a major nursing management problem to those caring for the aged.

Functional Changes

Complaints referrable to the gastrointestinal track are common among aged persons. Loss of sense of smell and its effect on appetite has been mentioned, as has loss of taste buds in the oral cavity. The latter may be further impaired by glossitis. The intake of food may be further reduced because of ill-fitting dentures.

The stomach shows a reduction in gastric motility, but this is not sufficient to delay gastric emptying. There is diminished peristalsis throughout the gastrointestinal track due to the generalized weakening of muscle activity, which also involves the smooth muscle of this system. This may be responsible for constipation which is common in old people. Other factors contributing to constipation are dehydration and changes in pH of the feces. There is a rise in fecal pH with age which results in killing of the lactobacilli.

Hemorrhoids, when present, further complicate processes of elimination, and bleeding from these hemorrhoids may be responsible, in part, for anemia in the aged. Anemia in the aged may be due to impaired iron absorption.

Ordinarily, there is no impairment of liver and pancreatic function in the healthy aged. Generally, there is no evidence of impaired function of the gall bladder or bile ducts, although the frequency of calculi (stones) increases with advancing age.

Structural Changes

There is atrophy of the mucosal lining of all segments of the gastrointestinal track with advancing age. There is thickening of the basement membrane and submucosal connective tissue which may account for impairment of absorption. Age related vascular changes also occur in this system and further contribute to impaired absorption. Liver biopsies obtained from aged persons may show abnormalities suggestive of non-specific hepatitis in the liver or gastrointestinal tract. There is some increase in fibrosis (scarring) in the pancreas.

URINARY TRACT

Urinary incontinence is a major management problem for nursing in long-term care facilities and hospitals. It also causes shame to patients and difficulty in understanding and acceptance among relatives and friends. However, bladder retraining programs have a measure of success in many facilities, adding to morale improvement for both patient and staff.

Functional Changes

The *filtration rate* in the kidneys of persons in their 80s is about 50 percent of that of individuals in their 20s. *Renal blood flow* is also about 50 percent of that of the young group. *Tubular function* is comparably diminished.

Polyuria (excessive urination) and *nocturia* (nighttime urination) are common among the aged. In the male this is most often due to prostatic enlargement, which occurs in about 75 percent of males over age 55. This is often accompanied by *infections of the bladder* due to urinary stasis. In the female *infections of the urethra with extension into the bladder* are common and usually account for these symptoms.

Structural Changes

The structural changes in the kidneys which alter renal function consist of *hyalinization* (obsolescence) of *glomeruli (kidney filters)*, *interstitial fibrosis* with some loss of tubules in the cortex, a peculiar soft hyaline which compresses and produces atrophy of collecting tubules, and vascular changes already noted. Contributing to this decrement in renal function are the age related diminution in cardiac output, dehydration, and anemia.

REPRODUCTIVE ORGANS

Female

The most consistent aging phenomenon is *menopause*. There is variation in the age of onset. There are concomitant behavioral problems which will not be detailed here. There is a period of time during which low grade estrogenic activity continues; this appears to be due to the takeover of secretion of estrogenic substances by the adrenal glands. Gonadotropic (pituitary) activity continues at a high level for some years following the onset of menopause. Eventually, there is atrophy of all the genitals.

Male

In the male, climacteric occurs considerably later in life and is accompanied by a cessation of spermatogenesis, with less marked atrophy of the genitalia. Depression, irritability, and impotence may occur.

ENDOCRINE SYSTEM

Functional Changes

No significant pituitary changes have been demonstrated and, in fact, certain hormones such as gonadotrophins actually are secreted in increased amounts for a period of time following menopause. Despite a decrease in oxygen consumption with advancing age, it appears that there is no perceptible thyroid deficit. There is a fall in the secretion of adrenal 17 ketosteroids but not of other adrenal hormones. There is a deficit in anabolic steroids, particularly those secreted by the gonads which are important in that they are probably responsible for the loss of muscle protein.

There are knowledge gaps about the influence of aging on hormone production and utilization. It appears unaffected. Endocrine function appears normal, but under stress conditions abnormalities can be detected. There is a decline in glucose tolerance with age which presents a problem in making a diagnosis of diabetes mellitus.

Structural Changes

Structural changes occur in the endocrine glands in aging and reflect age related adaptive processes.

HEMOPOIETIC SYSTEM

Bone Marrow

Information about aging changes in bone marrow is limited. There is evidence of a diminution of functional and reserve capacity which becomes evident only under conditions of stress. There is diminished leukocytic response to infection and a retardation of recovery from anemia due to hemorrhage.

Lymphoid System

Responses of the lymphoid system, including the spleen, appear to diminish with age; there is a reduction in volume of lymphoid tissues and the response to external antigens is diminished. For example, the regional lymphadenopathy (enlargement of lymph nodes) associated with infections of the skin is often absent in old people.

Blood Volume

Blood volume may diminish with age. This may be due to indirect effects since blood volume is related to height, weight, surface area, muscle mass, protein content, and other variables, some of which diminish with age.

Blood Chemistry

Anemia is not a characteristic of aging; the hemoglobin level is normal in healthy old people. However, nutritional state and dehydration may affect the level of hemoglobin. The total and differential white cell counts also do not change significantly with advancing age. Serum proteins do change with age. There is diminution in the proportion of albumin and a proportionate rise in globulin, primarily the beta globulins; these changes may be most impressive in the unwell elderly.

NUTRITION AND METABOLISM

The social aspects of eating are lacking for many elderly who live alone. Lacking motivation for adequate meal planning and preparation, these aged fall into a vicious cycle of poor nutritional intake to lowered energy to further poor food intake. Home delivered meal programs and/or group nutrition programs for the elderly have boosted their psychic and physical energy through improved nutritional intake. Diabetes is often most difficult for the elderly to manage in view of strong preference for sugar and starchy foods which are quick and easy to prepare and consume.

Nutritional Deficiencies

Many changes seen in senesence resemble nutritional deficiencies. The capillary fragility responsible for ecchymoses, even following trivial trauma, suggest vitamin C and vitamin K deficiencies. The hyperkeratotic changes in the skin resemble those seen in vitamin A deficiency, and the fissuring around the mouth, the glossitis, the angular stomatitis suggest a deficiency in various vitamin B components. Other changes suggesting nutritional deficiency are the loss of lean body mass, water depletion, and sometimes even fat depletion. Obesity in some aged persons may actually mask a protein loss. The process of demineralization of bone suggests a deficiency in mineral intake. Regarding the water content changes with aging, it is noteworthy that intracellular water falls off by about 15 percent between age 40 and age 80.

Indirect Factors

Indirect factors also point to a nutritional deficiency. The usual changes in eating habits of old people can be listed as follows:

1. They have reduced water intake as a rule.
2. Characteristically, they develop a preference for sugars.
3. The motivation for preparing and eating an adequate diet is often lost along with other motivations.
4. The decreased appeal of food may be related to loss of taste buds and reduced sense of smell, as already noted. The loss of teeth or ill-fitting dentures may also be a factor.
5. There is reduction in the quantity of enzymes and gastric acidity, which may impair absorption.

On the other hand, as has been noted, the basal metabolic rate decreases with age, indicating that the nutritional requirements of the aged are reduced.

Table 18-1 is an outline for "Levels of Nutritional Assessment for the Elderly."[5] This should prove helpful to the community nurse or primary care nurse working with older clients.

BLOOD LEVELS

A common method of assessing the normalcy of a metabolic process is the measurement of blood levels of the biochemical components of the process. It is to be remembered that such measurements have only limited value since changes in the blood represent the combination of the level of synthesis and discharge into the blood stream, the uptake by the tissues utilizing the particular component, and the efficiency of the excretory mechanism. Some of these measures rise with age, others fall, and still others remain constant.

RATIO OF ORGAN-BODY WEIGHT

Varying patterns of change in relation to age occur in respect to the ratio of organ weight to body weight. This ratio can also be considered as dependent on changes in nutrition and metabolism. This ratio for such organs as the spleen and liver shows a rise to a peak during middle age, followed by a decline. A similar curve obtains for dilatation of the large arterial trunks. The ratio for the heart reaches a peak at about 40 and remains constant thereafter. The ratios for kidney, brain, pancreas, and testes remain essentially constant after adult growth; the ratios for the lungs and prostate increase throughout the life span; and the ratios for the thyroid and some endocrine glands diminish progressively after adult growth has been reached.

TEMPERATURE MAINTENANCE

Temperature maintenance can also be considered to reflect alterations in nutrition and metabolism—proper nutrition being essential for maintaining the insulating qualities of the subcutaneous tissue and metabolism for providing energy for the production of heat. It has been observed that adjustment to adverse environmental temperatures is less rapid and complete as persons become older. The rectal temperature can fall as low as 70 to 90°F, and mortality from hypothermia in old people is about 85 percent. This constitutes a real

TABLE 18-1. Levels of nutritional assessment for the elderly*

Levels of Approach	History		Clinical Evaluation	Laboratory Evaluation
	Dietary	Medical and Socioeconomic		
Minimal	1. Meals eaten per day, week; regularity 2. Frequency of ingestion of protective foods (four food groups) 3. Supplemental vitamins, protein concentrates, mineral mixes 4. General knowledge of nutrition, sources of information	1. Chronic illness and/or disability; occupational hazard exposure; use of tobacco, alcohol, drugs. 2. Symptoms such as bleeding, fainting, loss of memory, dyspnea, headache, pain, changed bowel and/or bladder habits, altered sight and/or hearing, condition of teeth, and/or dentures 3. Therapy (prescribed or self-administered) such as drugs, alcohol, vitamins, food fads, prescription items, eyeglasses, hearing aids 4. Names, addresses, and phone numbers of persons providing medical or health care; close family or friends 5. Lives alone, with spouse, or companion 6. Sources of income	1. Height and weight; cachexia; obesity 2. Blood pressure, pulse rate and rhythm 3. Pallor, skin color and texture 4. Condition of teeth and/or dentures and oral hygiene 5. Affect during interview and examination 6. Vision and hearing appraised subjectively and objectively by examiner 7. Any gross evidence of neglect	1. Hemoglobin 2. Blood and/or urine sugar 3. Urinalysis (color, odor, bile and sediment by gross inspection; pH, glucose, albumin blood, and ketones by stick test) 4. Feces (color, texture, gross blood; occult blood by guaiac test)
Mid-level†	In addition to the above: 1. Food preferences and rejections 2. Overt food fads 3. Meal preparation facili-	In addition to the above: 1. Family history of spouse, parents and siblings, other relatives, persons living in same household	In addition include: 1. Head and neck examinations (otoscopic, ophthalmoscopic, dental and oral cavity, nose and throat)	In addition include: 1. Serum lipids (including B-lipoproteins) 2. Serum iron and iron binding capacity

TABLE 18-1. Continued

Levels of Approach	History		Clinical Evaluation	Laboratory Evaluation
	Dietary	Medical and Socioeconomic		
	...ties and knowledge 4. Food budget 5. Usual daily diet: Protective foods (meats, dairy products, fruits and vegetables, cereals); Nutrients (protein, fat, carbohydrates, iron, water and fat-soluble vitamins, minerals, trace elements, and water); Empty calorie food (alcohol, candy, sucrose)	2. Pain: location, frequency, character, duration 3. Mental hygiene: attitudes, fears, prejudices, symptoms of psychoses, possible psychosomatic symptoms and signs 4. Income: amount and adequacy for nutrition, housing, health, utilities, clothing, transportation, etc.	2. Chest (inspection, palpation, auscultation and percussion, bi-manual examination of breast tissue) 3. Abdomen (inspection, auscultation, percussion, and palpation) 4. Rectal and pelvic 5. Inspection and palpation of extremities (evaluation for temperature, edema, pulse, discoloration, ulcers) 6. Gross neurological evaluation; motor and sensory	3. Urinalysis 4. Electrocardiogram 5. Peripheral blood smear for differential white blood cell count and red cell morphology 6. Chest film 7. Post-voiding residual urine by catheterization (if indicated)
In-depth†	In addition include: 1. 24-hour dietary recall, preferably for each of several widely separated days; analysis of nutrient intake; evaluation of adequacy, e.g., relate to activity, body weight, laboratory data, affect, etc. 2. History of past and present food preparation and practices 3. History of dining practices and facilities, including companionship	In addition include: 1. System review 2. Social history 3. Economic history including specifics on sources and amounts of income 4. Mental evaluation (attitudes toward aging)	If indicated, include: 1. Complete sensory and motor neurologic examination 2. Sigmoidoscopy 3. Ophthalmologic examination (ophthalmoscopic examination with pupils dilated, refraction, dark adaptation, color perception, visual field examination) 4. Audiometry	If indicated, include: 1. Serum total protein and albumin; serum creatinine and/or blood urea nitrogen (BUN) 2. Roentgenographic evaluation of bones and joints suspected of being fractured, harboring infection and affected by rheumatic and/or metabolic bone disease and/or metastatic or primary neoplastic disease 3. Glucose tolerance tests

4. Blood and/or urine vitamin assays for water-soluble and fat-soluble vitamins
5. Trace element assays of blood, urine, and/or tissue
6. Kidney-ureter-bladder (KUB) film for stones in urinary tract or gall bladder.
7. Bacteriologic cultures of any chronic infections
8. Barium enema, upper gastro-intestinal series, gall bladder series and intravenous pyelography
9. Fluoroscopy of chest
10. Angiography for coronary arteries, aorta, peripheral vessels
11. Bone marrow for unexplained anemia
12. Renal clearance studies
13. Histologic evaluation of biopsies of tissue suspected of being neoplastic

*With permission from Christakis.[5]
†The aged, quite unlike children and youth, are the end result of lifetimes of physiologic aging, disease, and disabilities and cannot be evaluated as if they belonged to younger cohorts. In the above table, it is assumed that mid-level evaluation procedures may be carried out in ambulatory care settings and that in-depth level procedures may be conducted as hospital or research procedures. The placement of these in actual practice will depend on availability of facilities and personnel.

danger to the aged living alone without sufficient food and heating facilities. (This is a very important consideration for the elderly residing in parts of the country where winter weather can be harsh, in light of the current expense of heating fuel and their inability to get out of the place of residence due to travel problems. There may be harmful shortages of both home heating and food supplies).

HEALTH MAINTENANCE-DISABILITY PREVENTION

Health is a major concern of older persons. The findings of numerous research studies identify health status as a prediction of morale among the elderly. A common perception of health among older people is in terms of their ability to be active. In other words, health is important to older adults only as it becomes poor health and interferes with their independence and daily functioning. Many old people are preoccupied with body functions and justifiably so, as they may experience many unpleasant symptoms. As has been stated previously, to be old is not to be ill. There are important considerations which make illness in the aged complex. First, it is common for old people to have more than one disease at a time; second, symptoms of disease in the elderly are not as noticeable or easily delineated or may manifest in different forms than in younger people.

The aforementioned description of age changes which limit body functioning provides the professional nurse with an armamentarium for assessment with the cognizance that if persons live long enough, they are bound to experience age related afflictions. These age related afflictions may be further complicated by the accumulation of chronic disabling conditions of a lifetime. This builds the case for health maintenance which emphasizes health rather than illness. Health maintenance programs should offer those services related to disease prevention and promotion and maintenance of the maximum level of personal independence. The more positive aspects of the older individual's capabilities or potential should be reinforced instead of magnifying disabilities. Health maintenance, in this instance, utilizes periodic health examinations, immunizations, accident prevention, mental health programs, health education, and health counseling.

Never underestimate the importance of functional assessment of the elderly client as a key factor in matching needs and services. Functional assessment in this context[6] means any systematic attempt to measure objectively the level at which a person is functioning in any of a variety of areas such as physical health, quality of self-maintenance, quality of role activity, intellectual status, social activity, attitude toward the world and toward self, and emotional status. Once these data are collected, the nurse should make a nursing diagnosis as a basis for planning intervention strategies with the elderly client and for significant others, including other health team members, as deemed appropriate. Realistic goals should be set with some predictable, measurable outcomes. This presupposes that the nurse is knowledgeable about community resources and collaborates to establish appropriate linkages to obtain a full spectrum of services for her clients.

There is a range of possibilities for decision making in examining need indicators for long term health care management. In Table 18-2, Williams[7] has described services and facilities according to the functional status of the older client. The findings about the individual client are matched with the descriptions in the first column, *Health and/or Functional Status*, which are arranged in ascending order of disability. The second column, *Health and/or Support Services Required*, matches the types of services needed for the varying degrees of disability. The third column, *Alternative Settings or Levels of Care*, describes the possible

TABLE 18-2. Services and facilities according to functional status of older client*

Health and/or Functional Status	Health and/or Support Services Required	Alternative Settings or Levels of Care
1. Medically stable; mentally alert; *able to care for self fully in an independent living setting* (i.e., alone if necessary).	*Medical:* No more than regular preventive and maintenance ambulatory care. *Nursing:* None *Social:* No special needs except socialization. †	At home, alone or with family or friends. Persons at home alone require occasional visits or telephone calls to make sure they are still able to function.
2. Medically stable; mentally alert; ambulatory with or without mechanical assistance; *in need of some, but less than daily help with personal care (e.g., bathing, preparation of reimbursement), and/or help with meal preparation, shopping, cleaning, laundry, finances.*	*Medical:* No more than regular preventive and maintenance ambulatory care. *Nursing:* If needed, periodic visits by public health or visiting nurse, home health aide, or equivalent. *Social:* Help with meal preparation or shopping, cleaning, laundry, finances or other nonpersonal care; and socialization. †	At home with assistance of family or friends; OR housekeeper or homemaker (full time assistance is not necessary); OR if only in need of meal preparation, provision of meals (e.g., Meals-on-Wheels); OR semi-independent apartment; OR unsupervised boarding home or housing for handicapped persons (all with assistance of public health or visiting nurse, or home health aide, or equivalent).
3. Medically stable but possibly in need of limited rehabilitational services; ambulatory with or without mechanical assistance; not more than minimally confused; not requiring constant supervision and able to manage own medications; *in need of minimal daily assistance with bathing, dressing, or toileting.*	*Medical:* No more than regular preventive and maintenance ambulatory care. *Nursing-Personal:* Limited, but daily assistance with activites of daily living. *Rehabilitation:* Services available on an ambulatory basis or from visiting therapists. *Social:* Probably needs recreational planning, assistance and socialization. †	At home with regular assistance of family or friends at least periodically throughout the day (i.e., not in need of constant supervision); OR at home with a day care program plus family or friends evenings and weekends; ‡ OR at home with daily home health aide and provision of meals; OR supervised boarding home.
4. Medically stable, but possibly in need of rehabilitational services; not more than minimally confused, not requiring constant supervision; able to ambulate at least within a dwelling with or without mechanical assistance, AND	*Medical:* No more than regular preventive and maintenance ambulatory care. *Nursing:* Nursing plan plus supervision with limited assistance with activities of daily living or medications. *Rehabilitation:* Should be available on an ambulatory, visiting therapist, or inpatient	At home with family or friends capable of providing needed assistance including managing medications; OR at home with home health aide (1-2 hours a day) plus frequent visits by public health or visiting nurse; OR

TABLE 18-2. Continued

Health and/or Functional Status	Health and/or Support Services Required	Alternative Settings or Levels of Care
in need of assistance with bathing, dressing, or toileting once or twice daily, OR unable to manage own medications. OR Special therapeutic diet.	basis. Social: Probably needs recreational planning, assistance and socialization. †	intermediate care facility (health related facility).
5. Medically stable or changing in predictable ways, (e.g., improving, declining or terminal); not more than moderately confused (needs some supervision), AND needs help with ambulation; OR needs complete help with bathing, dressing, or toileting; OR frequently (e.g., daily) incontinent.	Medical: Regular visits and other visits as required. Nursing: Nursing plan plus supervision and assistance in activities of daily living, medications or incontinence with the aim of at least maintaining person at current level of function. Rehabilitation: Periodic but not daily services as needed, available either by a visiting therapist or an inpatient basis. Social: Probably needs recreational planning, assistance and socialization. †	At home with continual assistance by family; OR At home with home health aide during day (6-8 hours) and family evenings and weekends; OR intermediate care facility with more than usual staff; OR nursing home.
6. Medically stable or changing in predictable ways (e.g., improving, declining or terminal), AND needs administration of medications with skilled observation of their effects; OR confused, requiring 24 hour /day supervision, but not dangerous nor abusive; OR in need of regular rehabilitational services; OR always incontinent; OR needs total assistance with activities of daily living (including eating).	Medical: Regular visits, and extra, but usually not daily, attention as needed. Nursing: Up to 24-hour-a-day assistance with ambulation, toileting, bathing, dressing, feeding, care for incontinence; administration of medications; supervision for confusion Rehabilitation: Periodic services as needed, available either by staff members or visiting therapists. Social: Probably needs recreational planning, assistance and socialization. †	At home with family available 24 hours a day with help from home health services; OR skilled nursing facility.
7. Medically unstable with sustained exacerbations or complications of chronic illness; OR in need of extensive reha-	Medical: Availability of physician daily and for emergencies; availability of consultants. Nursing: 24 hours a day care and supervision.	Chronic hospital.

TABLE 18-2. Continued

Health and/or Functional Status	Health and/or Support Services Required	Alternative Settings or Levels of Care
bilitation requiring frequent physician attention; OR requires daily specialized care such as tracheostomy care, inhalation therapy, intravenous fluids and similar therapy.	*Rehabilitation:* Planned and supervised daily PT, OT and regular speech therapy. *Social:* Recreational planning services and socialization.†	
8. Acutely ill or disabled or able to benefit from diagnostic or therapeutic services beyond those possible on an ambulatory basis. (This includes acute psychiatric disorders and persons abusive or dangerous to themselves or others, not controlled by regular medications.)	Full range of physician and other hospital services 24 hours a day.	Acute general hospital: OR as appropriate, psychiatric unit of a general hospital or a psychiatric hospital.

*With permission from Williams.[7]
†Persons of every functional status may need efforts to stimulate and maintain personal involvement with others, and assistance in coping with their present situation and in preparing for institutional care, if that becomes necessary.
‡Day care provides meals, supervision, nursing, and recreation and may include physical therapy, occupational therapy, and speech therapy.

settings in which the necessary services might be provided for the various degrees of disability. The guide succinctly identifies options and levels of health care/service needs.

HEALTH SERVICES SYSTEM

The range of health related needs of older people is great. Moreover, the range of health related services must be equally great to meet their needs. Inflation and the spiraling costs of health care add to the plight of the aged in need of such care/services. Although Medicare and Medicaid benefits accrue to those older persons needing acute care and nursing home care respectively, the coverage for total health care needs remains grossly inadequate. Home health care services suffer from inadequate funding and lack of accessibility. Nursing home care is overutilized due to lack of availability of viable alternative community resources. Costs continue to escalate without improvement in the quality of care or services provided. The summation of this is that the current system for health care/services is in disarray. Older people are victimized by the continued inflationary cost spiral nationally as well as the less than humane modus operandi of the health delivery system.

GERONTOLOGY NURSING

The nursing process provides a framework for delivery of nursing services. When the basic knowledge of normal human aging is added, this more systematic approach facilitates the understanding and management of the multidimensional aspects of health care needs of the aging client. The nursing process interfaces with all the standards of nursing practice, but important in this context are standards of community health nursing and standards of gerontologic nursing.

Nurses prepared at the baccalaureate level are at the entry level of practice for community health (public health) nursing. This is an important consideration in the education of nurses for professional practice, the underlying assumption being that the selected aspects of the biologic and behavioral sciences in combination with scientific theories of gerontology and nursing theories allow for a more accurate and intelligent problem solving approach in the use of the nursing process to meet health and nursing needs of community based older adults.

The baccalaureate prepared nurse should be competent to provide comprehensive nursing care for older adults. Each person ages differently. The unique response of the individual to aging must be determined in order to properly place him or her along the wellness-illness continuum. Nursing diagnoses must reflect the differential diagnoses of disease entities due to the atypical pattern of disease manifestation in the aged, as well as differences in disease diagnoses and clinical case management for improving health status.

The baccalaureate nurse functions in a primary nursing role in delivering health care to the aging population. She has an interdependent team role and uses the nursing process to design and implement nursing care. The sites in which she might work include nursing homes, long term care facilities, and acute care facilities. The exact role she carries out will be somewhat dependent on the work site.

The master's prepared nurse in gerontology provides primary health care as a gerontologist specialist or nurse practitioner or clinician. She functions interdependently with a high level of independent practice. Her practice includes diagnostic level decision making with the individual, family, and community. She may work in a neighborhood health center, long term facility, or other setting with a large agency population. She may serve as an educator, practitioner, and/or preceptor.

Through continuing education, associate degree, diploma, and baccalaureate nurses may become geriatric nurse practitioners. They will function in an interdependent manner as members of a health team. Settings in which the geriatric nurse practitioner works include nursing homes, long term care facilities, and official and voluntary agencies.

NURSES AS ADVOCATES

Nurses working with elderly clients should possess the professional expertise to intervene on their behalf. This means not only negotiating within the health delivery system but also working to change policies within health agencies to bring about more humane treatment of older people. Building the case for advocacy can be accomplished through the use of the nursing process as a systematic method for problem solving and the utilization of the Standards of Practice for Gerontological Nursing as a basic guide for evaluating health agency amenity for change.

Nurses possess the power and potential to plan and deliver more effectively appropriate health and nursing intervention in the surveillance and management of health care needs of older people. We are changing from an industrialized society to a human service oriented society. Nursing can and should have a front-line position. The future belongs to those who help shape it.

REFERENCES

1. Fowles, Donald G.: "Some Prospects for the Future Elderly Population," in *Statistical Reports on Older Americans*. U.S. Department of Health, Education and Welfare, Office of Human Development, Administration on Aging, National Clearinghouse on Aging, January 1978.
2. Havighurst, Robert: *Developmental Tasks and Education*. David McKay Co., Inc., New York, 1973.
3. Brocklehurst, John: "Aging and Health," in Hobman, David (ed.): *The Social Challenge of Aging*. St. Martin's Press, New York, 1978.
4. U.S. Department of Health, Education and Welfare, Public Health Service: *The Practitioner and the Elderly, Working with Older People: A Guide to Practice*. Washington, D.C., April 1970, pp. 11–21.
5. Christakis, George (ed.): "Levels of Nutritional Assessment for the Elderly," in *Nutritional Assessment in Health Programs*. The American Public Health Association, Washington, D.C., 1973.
6. Lawton, M. Powell: "The Functional Assessment of Elderly People," in Brown, M. (ed.): *Readings in Gerontology*, 2nd ed. The C. V. Mosby Co., St. Louis, 1978.
7. Williams, T. Franklin: "Assessment of the Geriatric Patient in Relation to Needs for Services and Facilities," in Reichel, W. (ed.): *Clinical Aspects of Aging*. Williams and Wilkins Co., Baltimore, 1978.

BIBLIOGRAPHY

Brown, Mollie (ed.): *Readings in Gerontology*, ed, 2. C. V. Mosby Co., St. Louis, 1978.
Christakis, George (ed.): *Nutritional Assessment in Health Programs*. The American Public Health Association, Washington, D.C., 1973.
Hobman, David (ed.): *The Social Challenge of Aging*. St. Martin's Press, New York, 1978.
Reichel, William (ed.): *Clinical Aspects of Aging*. Williams and Wilkins Co., Baltimore, 1978.

CHAPTER 19

NURSING ROLE IN COMMUNITY MENTAL HEALTH

JANICE STEVENSON BERNS, M.S.N., R.N., AND MARGARET SMITH HAMILTON, M.S., R.N.

Mental health problems have grown to critical proportions within the United States. Over 10 percent of the population has some form of mental or emotional illness that would benefit from professional help. Twenty-one million families, one in four, are affected by the mental illness of someone in their immediate family.[1]

In 1963, President Kennedy stated:

"Mental illness and mental retardation are among our most critical health problems. They occur more frequently, affect more people, require more prolonged treatment, cause more suffering by the families of the afflicted, waste more of our human resources, and constitute more financial drain upon both the Public Treasury and the personal finances of the individual families than any other single condition."[2]

It was his personal inspiration and political negotiations that so greatly influenced mental health services in this country. With the passage of the Community Mental Health Centers Acts in 1963, the community mental health movement began to set the pace for comprehensive health care for all.

Community mental health is an interdisciplinary approach to meet the mental health needs of a group of people within a geographically defined area. It is concerned with the promotion of mental health, the prevention of mental illness, and the care of the mentally ill. Leininger states:

"The primary intent of the community health movement is to provide comprehensive psychiatric services for individuals, families, school children, workers in industrial centers,

319

and other groups in a variety of community and cultural settings. An underlying assumption of this movement is that individuals and families having emotional problems will seek help with less reluctance and at an earlier time when comprehensive psychiatric services are easily accessible to them."[3]

Nurses, psychologists, psychiatrists, social workers, and ministers are team members.

The community mental health nurse, with educational and clinical preparation, provides comprehensive nursing services to meet community mental health needs at preventative, acute, and rehabilitative levels. Community mental health nursing is a specialty within the American Nurses' Association, Division of Psychiatric and Mental Health Nursing Practice, which defines psychiatric and mental health nursing as:

" . . . a specialized area of nursing practice employing theories of human behavior as its science and purposeful use of self as its art. It is directed toward both preventive and corrective impacts upon mental disorders and their sequelae and is concerned with the promotion of optimal mental health for society, the community, and those individuals who live within it. Psychiatric and mental health nursing is practiced in a variety to settings, on a continuum from institutions characterized by high levels of team-work and technology, to community-based, noninstitutional settings where the nurse practices on a highly independent, self-directed basis."[4]

HISTORICAL DEVELOPMENT
OF COMMUNITY MENTAL HEALTH

Mental health and nursing have their roots deeply embedded in man's societal development. In order to have an understanding of the evolution of the community mental health movement and the role of the community mental health nurse, an understanding of their historical development is necessary (Table 19-1).

Primitive man believed that illness was caused by possessions or evil spirits. Medical folklore abounds with stories of invisible spirits which caused disease. People focused upon demon possession and witchcraft as explanations for all types of sickness. Any disease and ultimately death were viewed as punishments for an offense against the gods. Protection

TABLE 19-1. Major milestones in the development of community mental health[5,6,8]

Date (approximately)	Concept
400 BC	Mental illness defined and classified by Greek medicine
1200 AD	Religious institutes used for treatment
1600s	Causes of mental illness sought
1700s	Mental illness viewed as a treatable illness
1750s	First hospital for the mentally ill
1800s	Psychiatry developed as a medical specialty
1880s	Emphasis on prevention of mental illness
1900s	Organized preventive medicine in the community
1930s	Recognition of early treatment in childhood
1940s	Group therapy, stress tests, treatment of neurosis and psychosomatic illness
1960s	Government and community support, acceptance, and education

against any illness was thought to have been provided by the gods who had control of the evil processes and could ward off evil spirits.[5]

When faced with sickness or death, man developed remedies that were rooted in religion and magic. When these remedies did not work, the sick were rejected. The mentally ill were often outcast and left to survive by themselves. Many of these historical developments have fostered beliefs that still linger today. Superstitions, miracle cures, and beliefs that man's life is predetermined by the gods are often encountered in today's society. Even physical rejection of the mentally ill remains in modern times through the use of state institutions and employment discrimination.

The Egyptians believed that astrology influenced health and disease and that the gods determined man's destiny. When Egyptian gods were displeased, they punished mankind with illness and plagues. The art of healing was practiced by the Egyptian priesthood. The physician would cast spells and incantations to placate the gods. The temple was the place where the evil spirits were exorcised from the ill. The mentally ill were treated as the physically ill for the removal of the demonical possession.[6]

Early Greek medicine followed Egyptian ideology by considering mental illness as demonical possession. Again, the temple was the place of healing. But the Greeks differed from other early cultures in that they tried to label the differences between physical and mental illness.[7] Hippocrates tried to separate medicine from religion. He also tried to define mental illnesses. As Greece developed into a nation, the theory and practice of medicine for the mentally ill also developed. Mental disorders were classified and specific treatments were formulated. Perhaps the greatest contribution of this period was the identification of the brain as the center of activity and the concept of mental illness as a natural phenomenon.[8]

The belief that disease was punishment for sin was also held by the early Sumerian and Oriental nations. Illness and disease were studied in relation to the moon and stars. Incantations were used to eliminate evil spirits found in the water, air, and earth. Harmony of the body prevented mental illness. These beliefs of man remained unchanged through the Eastern Roman period, and the Mohammedan and Jewish cultures followed Greek ideas into the Medieval period of medicine.[5]

In the medieval period, the mentally ill were seen as heretics or witches and punished or burned at the stake. However, during this time, the roots for humane treatment of the mentally ill began to appear. Although mental illness was still thought to be caused by evil spirits, steps to help the mentally ill were initiated through the organized efforts of the Catholic Church. Priests and theologians classified and defined mental illness. Religious institutions were used as the first hospitals and provided for the confinement of the mentally ill.[6] Although this was a beginning, treatment was sometimes cruel and punitive. People would be put in chains for several weeks and given diets of water and bread. Late in the period, institutions for the insane began to develop throughout Europe. Some understanding of the mentally ill was evident, but treatment of their illness remained poor and conditions within the asylums were deplorable, with overcrowding and hygiene being major problems.

During the 17th and 18th centuries, man became concerned with the real causes of mental illness and its treatment. In the late 17th century, physicians and philosophers spoke against witchcraft and spirit possession and the inhumane treatment of the mentally ill. Modern psychiatry was developing into a medical specialty. Writings and interest in the mentally ill increased and correlations between the emotional life and the environment were developed. People considered the mentally ill person as sick and therefore deserving of and needing treatment. So, in this age of theory and reason, human thought reigned supreme.

This represented a major change in thought. Attempts for social reform to help the mentally ill were begun by dedicated people who brought the subject of poor treatment of the mentally ill to the attention of the community. People such as Pinel in France, Tuke in England, and Todd in the United States stimulated this reform.[9]

During the 18th and 19th centuries, community mental health advanced significantly in the United States. During the mid-18th century, Benjamin Franklin opened a hospital in Philadelphia which provided for the mentally ill. A decade later in Williamsburg, Virginia, a hospital exclusively for the mentally ill was opened. Dr. Benjamin Rush brought to a scientific level the study of mental illness in the United States.[6] The roots of modern medicine were firmly implanted. Psychiatry developed as a separate specialty in medicine. Various types of mental disorders were identified, described, and classified. Social concerns and issues were gaining momentum. State supported mental hospitals were established across the United States. Although their intent was good, these hospitals provided minimal care and were generally overcrowded. Dorothea Dix called attention to the poor conditions in these institutions and organized a crusade for better treatment. She stimulated public concern and lobbied before state legislatures for congressional passage of bills supporting the humane treatment of the mentally ill.[10] In 1844 the Association of Medical Superintendents of American Institutions for the Insane was developed. Later this organization became the American Psychiatric Association.[11] Towards the end of the century, psychiatry concentrated on the prevention of mental illness, improved treatment of the ill and of the less severely disturbed.

The early 20th century produced the movement toward organized preventive medicine. Although the public was reluctant to accept the mentally ill within the community and often placed them in institutions that provided substandard care, substantial developments were in progress. Psychiatry was developing within the community. A new humanistic interdisciplinary community approach with goals of prevention, treatment, and followup care was developing. Public education emphasized the need to change community attitudes towards mental illness and to promote a better understanding of community mental health. The idea that it was possible to prevent mental illness was being recognized. A strong interest in social change, social problems, and community involvement developed. With the development of a body of knowledge about mental illness, the public demanded changes in conditions through the legislative process to provide for the obvious social and physical needs of the mentally ill. Prevention was the dominant theme of the legislation.

During the 1920s and 1930s, further improvements were made. In the First World War, attention was given to soldiers with emotional disorders such as shell shock and depression. At the same time the problems of young children were analyzed with the belief that early treatment would prevent problems in adulthood. Child Guidance Clinics were developed for this specific purpose. The economic depression of the 1930s brought about even more social interest as the era of the New Deal began. In 1935, the United States government passed the Social Security Act, the first nationwide governmental entry into the health field. In general, more services within the community were made available to the mentally ill.[12] In fact, communities began defining their own needs. Health care was being thought of as a right of all rather than the privilege of a few.

After World War II, there was a readiness for the community mental health movement. Several developments strengthened this movement. Psychiatry developed new trends during the war years. For the first time, inductees were screened for the stresses of military service and combat. Treatment of neuroses and psychosomatic illnesses was advanced. Group therapy was utilized to treat large numbers of military men at one time. Psychiatry was accepted by the medical community. During this time period, legislation provided monies for training in various mental health related fields.[13] In 1946 Congress passed the National Mental Health Act which focused on mental health problems and deficiencies and provided for construction of mental health facilities and grants to states for research and training of personnel. In 1949 Congress created the National Institute of Mental Health which had enormous influence on the expansion of the community mental health field. In 1955 Congress passed the Mental Health Study Act which developed the Joint Commission on Mental Illness and Health. The Commission's final report was the 1961 Action for Mental Health which discussed the problems in the public mental hospitals and called for certain changes. These changes included more community outpatient clinics, more inpatient psychiatric treatment within the general hospital, and changes in the public mental hospitals.[10] President Kennedy also presented a report on mental illness and mental retardation which called for a new approach to the problems of the mentally ill and a shift to a broader definition of mental illness and health. Federal funds increased the number of community level mental health services available which in turn decreased the number of patients in the state institutions. Numerous mental health bills followed, including the Community Mental Health Construction Act of 1963, the Hospital Improvements Programs, the Inservice Training Programs, the Mental Health Benefits of the Social Security Amendment of 1965, the Mental Health Amendment of 1967, the Community Mental Health Center Amendment of 1970, and the Social Security Amendment of 1973.[6] Table 19-2 indicates the rapid growth in mental health legislation during recent times.

HISTORICAL DEVELOPMENT OF COMMUNITY MENTAL HEALTH NURSING

A great many forces and developments shaped community mental health nursing as we know it today. Organized nursing activities began during the Middle Ages when the Catholic Church cared for the wounded during the Crusades. Nursing consisted of charitable services

TABLE 19-2. Twentieth century mental health legislation[6]

Date	United States legislation
1908	The National Committee for Mental Hygiene
1922	The International Congress for Mental Hygiene
1935	Social Security Act
1946	National Mental Health Act
1949	Mental Health Study Act
1960	Joint Commission on Mental Illness and Health
1961	Action for Mental Health Report
1962	Mental Illness and Mental Retardation Report
1963	Community Mental Health Centers Construction Act
1963	Hospital Improvement Program
1963	Inservice Training Programs
1965	Mental Health Benefits of the Social Security Amendment
1967	Mental Health Amendment
1970	Community Mental Health Centers Amendment
1973	Social Security Amendment
1975	Community Mental Health Centers Construction Act Amendment
1977	President's Commission on Mental Health

to the poor until the late 19th century when trained psychiatric nurses were first available.[6] The first training school for psychiatric nurses was opened in 1882 at McLean Hospital in Belmont, Massachusetts.[13] Several additional psychiatric training programs opened during the next decade. However, psychiatric nurses were not properly utilized even at the beginning of the 20th century. The nurses who were employed in hospitals were generally responsible for routine tasks such as housekeeping and patient hygiene.

The 1930s and 1940s saw a major change in the role of psychiatric nursing. Institutional care was expanding rapidly and increased numbers of patients were being placed in psychiatric institutions. In order to handle the patient load, psychiatrists needed experienced psychiatric nurses to assume more direct care of patients in the mental institutions.[14] Nurses worked primarily with chronic psychotic clients who may have been institutionalized for several years with little or no treatment. Their role was to provide for the basic needs of the patients.

During this time, increased focus was being placed on specialized psychiatric training. The majority of nursing schools had already offered psychiatric nursing in their curricula. However, the National Mental Health Act of 1946 provided substantial federal funds to initiate, improve, and expand training programs in psychiatric nursing. In 1952 psychiatric nursing training was made a requirement for state registration.[13] The National League for Nursing, in 1953, published a statement entitled "A Study of Desirable Functions and Qualifications for Psychiatric Nurses." This provided a major impetus to community mental health nursing by concluding that special training was necessary for psychiatric nursing.[6]

In the mid-1950s, psychotropic drugs were made available, thus more clients became amenable to treatment and more nurses were therefore required to provide therapy.

With the passage of the community mental health legislation of the 1960s, the psychiatric nurse's role expanded rapidly in the community. The traditional role as a team member in a psychiatric hospital was expanded to outpatient departments, neighborhood health centers, and ambulatory settings.

The 1960s saw the emergence of the community mental health nurse as a unique community worker. Treatment of the mentally disturbed was being shifted back to the community. Community care programs were begun and they utilized professional nurses who were already accustomed to working with the mentally ill in the home setting. Many nurses working in this field wrote about their work, describing their role and helping other nurses understand community mental health nursing. One study in 1965 described the role of several community nurses in home care programs for chronic schizophrenics. This was an early demonstration of the role of nurses in community mental health programs. Their role consisted of providing medication, counseling and supportive guidance, continual reassurance to the patient and his famiy, and advice on the management of the patient's difficult behavior for the family.[15]

During this time period, nurses moved into the ambulatory and outpatient clinics in psychiatry. They had to define for themselves and the other mental health professionals exactly what they could offer as mental health clinicians and what contribution could be made to the community.[16]

Thus, nurses took on the role of liaison person, linking the hospital and the community. One program with public health nurses was successful in providing more continuity of care for patients because the hospital and the community had a better understanding of each other's approach and philosophy of patient care.[17]

In 1970 the American Nurses' Association held a conference on community mental health nursing sponsored by a grant from the National Institute of Mental Health. Nurses described and defined their roles in community involvement, staff development, treatment modalities, and organizational and administrative issues in community mental health. The distinct roles of the nurse as therapist, team member, and liaison person with communities were discussed.[18]

The community mental health nursing role is ever expanding, due in some part to the shortage of psychiatrists. In 1973 only 2300 psychiatrists were practicing in the United States, and one-half of these were located in five states. Amazingly, two-thirds of all counties in the United States did not have even one practicing psychiatrist.[1]

The development of psychiatric nursing was very similar to the development of public health nursing. Since manpower was scarce, both the public health nurse and the psychiatric nurse developed their roles to function independently within the community for the care of the client. These nurses moved into collaboration with other disciplines, again expanding the nurse's role. Both public health nursing and psychiatric nursing evaluated the needs of the community by studying the problems of the community and its ability to cope with these problems.

THE ROLE OF THE COMMUNITY MENTAL HEALTH NURSE

Community mental health nursing is a comprehensive approach to mental health services for individuals, families, children and adolescents, the elderly, and groups in various community settings. The focus of nursing care is on traditional methods and innovative designs in the preventive care and treatment of mental health problems as they touch all aspects of human living. The community mental health nurse is a nurse theoretically and clinically prepared to deliver mental health care to people in the community. Operating with the philosophy that the availability of mental health services is the right of the community, she or he views clients as individuals, members of families, and community members, deserving of competent and comprehensive nursing care. The nurse is someone who is educated and experienced in the planning, delivery, and evaluation of mental health services. Work performance is often a reflection of the level of education and the types of clinical preparation and experience she or he has had.

When community mental health nursing was in its early stages, starting in the 1960s, there was little differentiation between the various levels of nursing. There were nurses practicing in community mental health nursing with an assortment of educational backgrounds and levels of experience. Some nurses came with psychiatric inpatient experience and others from a public health background. Educational backgrounds ranged from a nursing diploma to a master's degree. As the role of the community mental health nurse evolved, the nurse assumed more clinical responsibility and the role became more complex and often unclear. The need for defining and clarifying the role of the nurse and professional nursing standards in community mental health nursing became necessary. Today the American Nurses' Association, Division on Psychiatric and Mental Health Nursing Practice has set forth standards of nursing practice in a statement on psychiatric and mental health nursing.[33] Both of these have helped define the role of the community mental health nurse within the context of professional psychiatric and mental health nursing. However, there are still some discrepancies in the conceptualization of the role of the community mental health nurse. Significant factors that influence the definition of the nurse's role are personal identity and clinical skills; type of practitioner, based on education and clinical work experience; the nurse's role as a team member working with her/his professional colleagues; the model of mental health services (primary, secondary, or tertiary preventive mental health approaches);

and the philosophy, policies, and politics of the mental health setting where the nurse is employed.

PERSONAL IDENTITY AND CLINICAL SKILLS

An important component of the role of the community mental health nurse is personal identity. This is how she or he identifies and understands herself or himself in the process of work. Understanding can be an arduous task. It is a very important and necessary characteristic of a competent community mental health nurse. Dealing with people and their personal difficulties, struggles for personal change, and growth can tax any individual. Because of this, the nurse needs to understand her/his own limitations and capacity to work with troubled individuals and their families.

When the decision is made to work in this kind of setting there are certain qualities and attributes the nurse should have. They include:

1. Consistency. Giving the same message all the time.
2. Creativity. Using one's imagination for new and different approaches and designs at work.
3. Value clarification. To understand the people of the community and the services they need without imposing one's beliefs on them. To avoid harsh judgments because of one's own prejudices.
4. Respect. The ability to treat all individuals with dignity and worthiness regardless of their beliefs and life styles.
5. Independence. A good sense of one's nursing identity so one is able to make decisions, judgments, and clinical diagnoses.
6. Patience. Ability to wait for results, changes, and noticeable progress.
7. Genuineness. The ability to be sincere and one's real self.
8. Empathy. The ability to understand the other person's situation on an intellectual and feeling level.
9. Warmth. The ability to communicate the feeling of concern, intensity, and caring.
10. Self-criticism and self-evaluation. To examine one's professional work objectively and with an open mind.

Crucial to community mental health nursing is the aquisition of professional and clinical skills. The foundation for such clinical skills is often laid during the educational process. These are refined and improved through advanced clinical and work experience. Often a role or job description for a community mental health nurse will require professional skills ranging from very specialized mental health treatment techniques to highly developed talents in community relations. Such professional competencies include the following:

1. Basic communication skills. Facilitating effective verbal exchange of thoughts and feelings.
2. Community knowledge. This is knowing the community and the culture. Surveying or assessing can help provide a good view of the community.
3. Treatment modalities. Direct services to clients include crisis intervention, individual psychotherapy (supportive and insight oriented), play therapy, couple and family therapy, and group therapy.
4. Medication dispensing. This may involve supervising patients on medications and observing for side effects.
5. Mental health consultation. This is the collaborative effort of the community mental

health nurse and the agency whom she or he is advising. Usually the nurse assists the agency with identifying and understanding mental health concepts as they relate to the work of the agency. The nurse also helps resolve questions and problems the agency has in her or his areas of specialty.

6. Teaching and education on mental health concepts. The nurse is often called upon to share her/his knowledge of a holistic approach to mental health care and to educate community groups such as the Parent-Teacher Association, scouting organizations, youth groups, and church groups through lectures, seminars, and discussions on relevant mental health topics.

7. Liaison work. This is the working together, planning, and organizing approaches to patient care with other community agencies.

8. Community organization, planning, and research. This can often be the most creative area of community mental health nursing. The planning, organizing, and research that each nurse becomes involved in is dependent on the needs of the community and the individual's particular skills and interests.

LEVELS OF PRACTITIONERS IN COMMUNITY MENTAL HEALTH NURSING

There are a variety of nurses working in community mental health. They come from an assortment of educational backgrounds and clinical nursing experiences. Basically they can be divided into three major catagories: community mental health nurse I; community mental health nurse II; and the clinical nurse specialist in community mental health (Table 19-3).

COMMUNITY MENTAL HEALTH NURSE I

A community mental health nurse I is a licensed registered nurse who has attended a two or three year academic program, either a hospital school of nursing or an associate degree college course in nursing. Both types of programs provide the fundamentals of community mental health nursing. At some point during her/his nursing education the nurse receives the basic didactic presentation and conceptual approaches to community mental health nursing. Some clinical experience in this area may have been part of a psychiatric nursing course. This nurse, after a minimum of one year experience in psychiatric nursing, may work as a beginning community mental health nurse I under the direct supervision of a clinical nurse specialist or other skilled mental health professional.

The category of community mental health nurse I also includes the college graduate nurse with a bachelor's degree in nursing. This is the nurse who received academic and clinical preparation for working in community mental health. This includes in-depth concepts in psychiatric nursing theory, good interpersonal techniques and communication skills, crisis intervention approaches, and community liaison work. The nurse may have received additional clinical experience during educational preparation, particularly if the nursing program offered the opportunity for senior clinical specialization in the area of the student's choice. She or he is the beginning practitioner.

Kathryn Gardner, a clinical nurse specialist, describes a similar model for nursing roles in community mental health.[19] She states that the skills a beginning practitioner should have are:[19]

1. Interviewing techniques and skill in interpersonal relationships based on the principles of psychiatric nursing.

TABLE 19-3. Levels of community mental health nursing

Practitioner	Community Mental Health Nurse I	Community Mental Health Nurse II	Clinical Nurse Specialist in Community Mental Health
Education and experience	Nursing diploma or associate degree with minimum one year of psychiatric nursing experience Baccalaureate degree graduate	Baccalaureate degree plus two years of clinical experience	Master's degree in psychiatric/mental health nursing
Professional responsibilities	Interviewing techniques, interpersonal relationship skills, basic knowledge of prevention, assess client's level of functioning, observations/data collection, facilitate and use community resources	Mental health educaton, supportive therapy, behavioral management of psychiatric disorders, therapeutic one-to-one relationship, crisis intervention technique, assessment of patient's functioning, knowledge of family theory, group dymanics, personality development, sociopsychological principles, theories, methods of mental health treatment	Insight oriented psychotherapy, family therapy, group therapy, psychoanalytic theory, psychopathology, diagnostic evaluation, community organization, mental health consultation, supervision, eclectic approach to mental health and treatment
Licensure and certification	Professional licensure by state	Professional licensure by state, American Nurses' Association Certification as Psychiatric and Mental Health Nurse	Professinal licensure by state, after two years of clincial experience: eligible for American Nurses' Association Certification in Psychiatric and Mental Health Nursing; adult or clinical specialist in psychiatric and mental health nursing—children and adolescent
Employment settings	Community mental health centers, community nurse for psychiatric in-patient setting, preventive programs.	Community mental health centers, crisis intervention teams, high risk populations—child abuse, rape, drug abuse, preventive programs	Community mental health centers, crisis intervention/multi-service center, mental health consultant and/or supervisor, private mental health facilities, individual private practice, administration, teaching, research.

2. Understanding of the concept of preventive mental health care and ability to assist in community preventive programs.
3. Ability to communicate with other professionals and community agencies regarding client care.
4. Ability to assess the client's level of functioning.
5. Nursing observation and data collection that may be helpful for better client care.
6. Ability to facilitate client use of community resources.

The community mental health nurse I is most often found as a team member at large community mental health centers. She or he is sometimes the community nurse for an inpatient setting, helping to find community placements for hospitalized patients who need a nursing home or an alternative housing or a halfway house. The nurse may be in charge of community followup on medication for previously hospitalized psychiatric patients and may give weekly injections of medication to psychiatric patients in the community or at the mental health center. She or he may also work in preventive programs such as a maternal-infant clinic as a nursing observer and health educator.

COMMUNITY MENTAL HEALTH NURSE II

The community mental health nurse II is the second type of practitioner. She or he is a licensed professional baccalaureate degree nurse with at least two years of clinical experience. Usually the experience is inpatient psychiatric nursing but can be in supervised community mental health work. Gardner[19] again outlines clinical skills appropriate for this nursing role. They include:

1. Knowledge of therapeutic intervention skills and communication.
2. Behavioral management of psychiatric disorders.
3. Establishment and use of a therapeutic nurse/patient relationship and primary responsibility for a few patients.
4. Principles of clinical psychiatric nursing and clinical psychopathology.
5. Assessment of patient's level of functioning.
6. Crisis intervention techniques.
7. Short term and long term supportive psychotherapy. Supportive psychotherapy is described by Weiner[20] as a professional relationship that helps the patient deal more effectively with real world problems without uncovering or exploring his unconscious conflicts and concerns. Its goal is to assist the patient in understanding and controlling those thoughts and feelings he is already dimly aware of.

The Division on Psychiatric and Mental Health Nursing of the American Nurses' Association describes a community mental health nurse II as a psychiatric-mental health nurse when she or he is capable of demonstrating professional standards of knowledge, experience, and quality of patient care through a formal review process.[4] The means for this kind of formal review of professional and clinical competency for the community mental health nurse II is through the American Nurses' Association certification program for the psychiatric and mental health nurse.

The American Nurses' Association states that this nurse should demonstrate the following:

1. Knowledge of theories on personality development.
2. Knowledge of sociopsychological principles.
3. Knowledge of family theory and group dynamics.

4. Mental health teaching and education for individuals, families, and communities.
5. Knowledge about what other professionals contribute to mental health care.
6. Theories and methods of treatment for mental health care within the framework of the nursing process (assessment of patient, plan nursing action, implementation, and evaluation).

This nurse, the community mental health nurse II, is found in most community mental health centers. Functioning as a member of an interdisciplinary team, she or he does work with chronic psychiatric and rehabilitative patients in the community, providing medication services when necessary. She or he may have a caseload of clients, doing supportive and educational therapy. More recently this nurse is found working with people and families in crisis and may be a member of an emergency or crisis team of a mental health center or employed by a crisis intervention center. Rape, child abuse, drug abuse are all areas covered. Like the community mental health nurse I, she or he also is involved in community preventive programs. This includes such areas as mental health education to the community, maternal-infant projects, and geriatric programs working toward more socializing for the elderly.

CLINICAL NURSE SPECIALIST

The clinical nurse specialist is the third type of nurse practitioner in community mental health nursing. This is the type of practitioner most often seen in community mental health. She or he is a clinical specialist in psychiatric and mental health nursing and has received academic and clinical preparation during a graduate level nursing program. This includes a clinical placement during the master's program with supervision in the treatment of clients and their families. In addition to graduate education, this nurse is also distinguished by a depth of knowledge, competence, and practice in an eclectic approach to individual psychotherapy, group therapy, and family therapy techniques, mental health consultation, and community organization. The American Nurses' Association now certifies this type of community mental health nurse under the certification program as a clinical specialist in psychiatric and mental health nursing.

The academic preparation for this clinical specialist derives its theoretic component from the social, behavioral, and biologic sciences as well as the nursing, medical, and psychological theories of psychotherapy.[4] Examples of some theoretic sources commonly included in a clinical specialist's program are: general systems theory, communication, learning and interpersonal relationship theory, personality theory, psychoanalytical theory, crisis intervention techniques, group process and therapy techniques, theory and practice of family therapy, research techniques, consultation, and organization strategies. Leininger,[3] in an article on community mental health nursing, suggests that in addition to the standard and traditional theoretic components, some concepts and theories that should also be integrated into graduate education are: concepts on the nature and definition of a community and community and social organizational theories; cultural, cross-cultural, and ethnologic aspects of mental health; an emphasis on prevention aspects and criteria for assessing causes of mental illness; and resources that support optimal mental health in various communities.

The focus of the clinical preparation of the nurse specialist in community mental health is twofold. The first is to assume primary psychotherapeutic responsibility and provide direct care service to all clients. Second, she or he provides indirect nursing care through clinical supervision and consultation and community education and research.

Direct nursing care in community mental health means that the nurse is highly competent in the various treatment modalities. The type of treatment utilized most frequently is psychotherapy. This denotes a formal, contractual, and structured relationship between the nurse-therapist and the client for the explicit purpose of effecting a change in the client.[4] The nurse specialist is supervised in the clinical practice of psychotherapy during graduate education and for several years after graduation.

Some of the techniques of psychotherapy are as follows:

PSYCHOANALYTIC PSYCHOTHERAPY

This is insight oriented treatment based on "psychoanalytic understanding of human behavior . . . (an) attempt to modify behavior by such psychological methods as confrontation, clarification, and interpretation . . . introspection by the patient and empathic understanding by the therapist."[21]

SHORT TERM PSYCHOTHERAPY

This is a short term therapy technique aimed at resolving an individual's difficulty within a given timetable. The therapeutic relationship can be defined as supportive or time limited. Supportive therapy focuses on the individual who usually is having an emotional crisis and needs professional help to decrease anxiety, increase coping ability, and prevent further depression and psychopathology. Time limited therapy, a technique defined by James Mann,[22] is based on an agreement between client and therapist to focus on one central problem for a limited period of time. Although this treatment incorporates all the important psychoanalytic concepts, it is based on the recurring life crisis of separation-individuation.

GROUP PSYCHOTHERAPY

Group therapy is a therapeutic experience occurring in formally structured groups. Members are approximately chosen, placed in a group, and guided by a trained therapist for the purpose of helping each other. The goals of this therapy are to relieve psychic pain, to bring about personality changes, and to provide a "corrective emotional experience"[23] for group members. The group leader uses a variety of techniques and interpretations of group members' interactions to bring about this change.

FAMILY THERAPY

This is a variety of techniques using different therapeutic approaches aimed at bringing about change in the structure and process of a family. The basic premise of family therapy is that the difficulty does not lie with one individual but is the problem of the family's system of interaction.

PLAY THERAPY

A clinical specialist may specialize in child treatment in community mental health. The mode of therapeutic expression used with individual children is play. Virginia Axline states that:

"non-directive play therapy . . . may be described as an opportunity that is offered to the child to experience growth under the most favorable conditions since play is his natural medium for self-expression. The child is given the opportunity to play out his accumulated feelings of tension, frustration, insecurity, aggression, fear, bewilderment, confusion. By playing out these feelings he brings them to the surface, gets them out in the open, faces them, learns to control them or abandon them."[24]

Other forms of direct clinical nursing services that the nurse should be skilled in according to the American Nurses' Association statement[4] are mental health counseling and education, intake and diagnostic evaluation, medication surveillance, home visits when indicated or in a crisis situation. As a primary clinician she can be found in most any community mental health center, multiservice agencies, outpatient departments, private mental health facilities, community health centers, and sometimes in court clinics, drug abuse centers, alcoholism prevention centers, crisis intervention centers, and independent private practice.

Where the clinical specialist works also is determined by the specific age group chosen as a specialization. The majority of nurses work with the adult population. However, there are nurses who specialize in the treatment of children, adolescents, or geriatric clients. There are also nurses who specialize according to their area of interest, such as child abuse, drug abuse, problem pregnancy counseling, crisis intervention work, alcoholism, chronic patients in the community, or preventive approaches with infants and mothers.

A clinical nurse specialist in community mental health also provides nursing services to the community indirectly as an administrator, consultant, and educator. This nurse is seen operating in an administrative capacity in mental health centers, some mental health facilities, and influential governmental positions within state mental health departments. As a consultant she or he is employed by community health nursing organizations, public health nurse departments, school systems, residential schools, maternal-infant care programs, and other similar federal grant projects on mental health. The clinical specialists whose focus is primarily education are seen as members of university and schools of nursing faculty where they specialize in community mental health nursing.

A significant component of the role of the community mental health nurse is professional identity, that is, her or his relationship with other mental health professionals and what she or he uniquely contributes to the field of community mental health. Often those working in mental health or those involved in mental health systems ask why nurses work in this area and what they contribute to the field. To understand why a nurse is a crucial member of any mental health team it is important to understand the professional nurse. She or he is a unique individual who functions both as a generalist with a broad health background and health knowledge and also as a specialist with clinical skills and knowledge in her area of expertise. As a member of a mental health team she or he is often the only professional, other than a psychiatrist, who is a health resource person and who has knowledge of psychotropic medications and their reactions and side effects.

The nurse is a provider of knowledge of general health matters and the physical as well as psychological aspects of illness. In an article on the role of the community mental health nurse, Harris and Solomon state that in addition to being a medical resource person the nurse is a clinician trained to be supportive, tolerant, and the bearer of TLC (tender loving care) for those difficult and overly dependent patients.[25]

Suzanne Lego talks about how nurse-therapists are different and identifies their holistic approach to patient care and their crisis orientation to clients. Having dealt with life and death situations throughout their formative educational years in nursing, they are capable and comfortable with their total patient care approach. In another study done in Colorado on the role of the community mental health nurse, other professionals were asked how they viewed the nurse. They stated that she/he possessed something different, called the "X factor," that distinguished her/him from other mental health professionals. DeYoung and Tower state:

> ". . . there seemed to be an X factor in the nurse's relationship to the patient. After that statement the nurses began trying to define the uniqueness of a nurse as they saw it. The *medical background* of the nurse was an important part of the equation. An additional factor was the *eclectic nature* of the nurse's educational background. The nurse specializes to some extent but is still *generalist* enough to see the whole patient. It was agreed that nursing education puts more emphasis on the *total patient* than does current medical education. One of the more elusive qualities of nurses' background is the fact that they have dealt intimately with the *basics of life and death*. Perhaps as a result of this, the nurse has learned to assess the *realistic and practical aspects* of situations. Another important factor identified by the panelists was that the nurse's basic orientation to the patient is guided also by the *ethics* learned as part of the profession—the 'something holy.' The ethics involve, ideally, a profound *respect* for the individual, *integrity and honesty* (particularly when mistakes are made), and a willingness to sacrifice one's own comfort, especially sleep, in order to provide service to the patient. These ethics are taught (or more often absorbed) during nurses' training."[27]

The ANA[4] states that the nurse in this area distinguishes herself or himself by her or his commitment to holistic and continuous patient care, the integration of both medical and social system models in clinical work, and the use of the nursing process as an accountable, systematic approach to comprehensive patient care.

By understanding her contributions and her role, the nurse can foster professional working relationships with psychiatrists, psychologists, and social workers in community mental health. The nurse needs to be aware of the various philosophies, roles, and expectations of the other professionals. This will facilitate a collaborative working relationship and a higher level of both independence and interdependence with her professional colleagues. Leininger[3] identified the three types of working situations of mental health professionals that are seen by community mental health nurses. She describes the setting where roles are undifferentiated. The roles of the various disciplines in this situation are open, flexible, and based on the individual clinician's interest and experience. The nurse truly works side by side with other professionals and it is difficult to distinguish between the professionals. A setting like this may be a multiservice agency or a liberal community mental health center.

The second is the differentiated role model. Here each profession is considered for its different contributions and is viewed as complementing the others. The role of the clinician is based on the individual's profession. This would occur in a traditional mental health setting such as a hospital-based program.

The last setting is the ambivalent viewpoint of professional roles. There is uncertainty and confusion among the professionals about their roles. They often vacillate between the undifferentiated role and the traditional role model. Some settings where this occurs are drug abuse programs and neighborhood health centers.

LEGAL CONSIDERATIONS

Nursing is legally defined by Nurse Practice Acts. These acts have been passed by all state legislatures. These are the statutory bases for the profession of nursing in the United States. A state's Nurse Practice Act states the duties a nurse carries out, defines requirements for licensing a professional nurse, and creates a Nursing Registration Board.[28] This is the administrative state agency that oversees the licensure process. All nurses, regardless of their education or specialty area, must first pass the standard nursing examination boards and be registered and licensed in order to practice any nursing. There is only one basic licensure process. All registered nurses in community mental health nursing are licensed. There is no additional license given for nurses educated or experienced in a specialty area.

Licensure

Presently all licensing occurs through the various state Nursing Boards of Registration. However, there has been much discussion and some attempts in the past to abolish special registration boards in nursing and allocate the licensing process to the various institutions that employ nurses. Licensing of this nature, called *institutional licensure,* would require that the nurse be accountable for her professional practice to the institution rather than to a professional licensing authority (nursing board). The individual nurse would certainly lose some autonomy and have less input should institutional licensure occur. Some of its proponents say it would reduce the financial cost of health care, offer better utilization and distribution of health care providers, and reduce fragmentation of the delivery of health care services.[29] Although these sound like valid consumer oriented reasons, they can easily be challenged and have failed to be motivating factors for the impetus toward institutional licensure. Any attempts to implement institutional licensure, such as the proposal to abolish the Board of Registration in Nursing in Massachusetts in 1973, have been met with strong protests from the nursing profession, including several resolutions passed by the National League of Nursing during their 1973 national convention[29] and avid demonstrators at public hearings.

Although institutional licensure is not a current threat to the practice of community mental health nursing, it is helpful to understand how it could affect the practice of nursing. A clinical specialist in community mental health is able to treat patients and families because of clinical skills in psychotherapy. This nurse also is able to work with these clients because of the Nursing Practice Act and licensure under this act. Should an institution regulate this practice, it may restrict the practice of nursing therapy according to its needs rather than the role or expertise of the clinical specialist.

Certification

The American Nurses' Association has instituted a comprehensive certification process. Since 1973 the association has been instituting, developing, and improving its professional certification process. The ANA Interdivisional Council on Certification, including representatives of all the ANA divisions on practice and the boards of certification, has defined the process as follows: "Certification is the documented validation of specific qualifications demonstrated by the individual registered nurse in the provision of professional nursing care in a defined area of practice."[30]

Certification differs from licensure. Stachyra[31] elaborates on the difference by stating that licensing a professional defines that practice of the licensed person and prohibits by law others from performing functions restricted to the license. That is, all nurses can practice what is legally defined by their state's Nurse Practice Act. Certification, however, is a national professional process and does not prohibit uncertified nurses from performing the same acts a certified nurse does since the professional organization that certifies does not have the legal regulatory power. However, such certification is the beginning of more professional accountability and self-regulation. So a clinical specialist in community mental health nursing who is not certified can still perform direct care services in therapy, supervision, and consultation, but should the nurse continue practicing without starting the process of certification once eligible, eventually her or his professionalism will be challenged and competency questioned.

Certification by the ANA has several purposes. They include: 1) The chief purpose is to validate quality performance. Its main focus is one of quality assurance. Certification allows a nurse to "demonstrate that she has achieved a level of performance which allows her to validate qualification for rendering specialized nursing care of high quality."[32] It gives recognition of public, professional and consumer concern for professional accountability and quality assurance of services above and beyond the basic licensure process. 2) Economic and third party payments. A system of certification can allow for new methods of payments in nursing. If nurses are to be reimbursed for services delivered according to clinical competence and expertise, the profession must have a means for identifying those nurses and regulating the quality of advanced nursing practice on this level. 3) Recognition of an individual's professional accomplishments and quality of practice through achieving national credentials.

According to the ANA by-laws adopted during the 1976 convention, each ANA division on nursing practice is required to "provide for the recognition of professional achievement and excellence in its area of concern."[30] Each division of nursing practice decides in what areas nurses should be certified. The Division of Psychiatric and Mental Health Nursing offers two different certifications. They are: 1) certification as a psychiatric and mental health nurse and 2) certification as a clinical specialist in psychiatric and mental health nursing. This level of certification offers specializations in adult practice and in child and adolescent practice.

A nurse practicing in community mental health falls into one of these two areas. Each certification process is comprehensive and takes several months. The Division of Psychiatric and Mental Health Nursing makes the final decision to certify, based on the individual candidate's credentials and performance. Certification for the two sections includes the items listed in Table 19-4.

ACCOUNTABILITY

Accountability means that a nurse is responsible and liable for her own nursing actions. Nurses have primary responsibility for the competency and quality of nursing care that they provide. All nurses in community mental health nursing are accountable to the guidelines of Professional Nursing Standards established by the Division of Nursing Practice. The nurse integrates the standards formulated by the Division of Psychiatric and Mental Health Nursing into her practice of community mental health nursing.[33]

The following is a case example of how these standards are applied to nursing practice.

Marie, a 15-year-old female adolescent, walks into a youth crisis center in her hometown. She is anxious, upset, and fears that she is pregnant. She speaks with the nurse, a clinical specialist and member of the crisis team working at the center that evening. Marie tells the nurse that she has been concerned about her possible pregnancy for a few weeks now but that she has been afraid to discuss the situation with anyone. She states that she has been especially reluctant to mention her concerns to her parents.

Nursing intervention according to the established nursing standards is shown in Table 19-5.

TABLE 19-4. Requirements for certification as a psychiatric and mental health nurse

	Psychiatric and Mental Health Nurse	Clinical Specialist in Psychiatric and Mental Health Nursing
Proof of eligibility	Licensed R.N.	Licensed R.N. plus master's degree
Examination	Passed written comprehensive examination in pyschiatric and mental health nursing	Passed written comprehensive examination in specialty area of adult or children/adolescents clinical specialist
Clinical practice	Direct nursing care for at least two years, with a minimum of four hours a week. Nurse is directly responsible and accountable for care.	Direct nursing care for at least two years post-master's for eight hours a week. Nurse is the therapist in two kinds of treatment.
References and case presentation	Endorsement by colleagues, professional references, evidence of supervision, evidence of clinical work by case presentation	Endorsement by colleagues, professional references, evidence of supervision, evidence of clinical work by case presentation

FINANCIAL ASPECTS

Presently, the financial structure of community mental health nursing is dependent on and defined by the various mental health centers and institutions that employ nursing personnel. How an employing agency is funded, whether it is a private or public facility, the availability of federal funds and federal grants, and contracts for payments from third party payers, including insurance companies, are all factors that influence funding and monies available to mental health facilities and community mental health nurses.

Community mental health facilities are financially defined as private, public, or partnership agencies. A private mental health facility receives no public, federal, or state funding on a regular basis. The facility is supported by fees for services by clients, reimbursements from third party insurance payments (Blue Cross-Blue Shield, Aetna, etc.), and possibly by private endowments. An example of this kind of facility would be a mental health outpatient department of a private general hospital. Although such an outpatient department would be serving the mental health needs of the community and functioning somewhat independently of the large hospital structure, it is still financially accountable to the hospital comptroller and administrator. Chances are that if such a mental health outpatient department did not stay within its financial budget or prove to be financially solvent, the staff would be cut back or some services would be discontinued.

Another example would be a mental health facility in the community that offered private services in the various therapies to the public. Facilities of this nature have a set fee for client services and depend on client payment. If a client cannot pay the established fee, they are referred to another agency with a more negotiable fee, such as a sliding scale, where people pay according to their income.

A mental health facility that is supported through public funding is usually funded by the state in which it operates. All states have some mental health facilities as part of their public service programs. Historically these facilities have been the larger, archaic state mental

TABLE 19-5. Nursing standards and nursing intervention

Standards	Nursing Intervention
I. Data are collected through pertinent clinical observations based on knowledge of the arts and sciences with particular emphasis upon psychosocial and biophysical sciences.	The nurse observes for possible teenage pregnancy. She proceeds with pregnancy testing while continuing to observe Marie's reactions and responses to discussion of her situation.
II. Clients are involved in the assessment, planning, implementation, and evaluation of their nursing care program to the fullest extent of their capabilities.	The nurse questions and explores with Marie on what she wants for herself and what she thinks her options are, if she is pregnant.
III. The problem solving approach is utilized in developing nursing care plans.	The nurse reviews with Marie her history, getting a sense of her personal characteristics and capabilities. She learns Marie has a history of a recent therapeutic abortion and doesn't want to go through another. Together they discuss alternatives.
IV. Individuals, families, and community groups are assisted to achieve satisfying and productive patterns of living through health teaching.	Marie returns to the crisis center the next day. The pregnancy test is positive. She is adamant about carrying the baby to term and keeping the baby. The nurse does some basic prenatal teaching and instructing.
V. The activities of daily living are utilized in a goal directed way in work with clients.	Marie is still in school and wants to continue. The nurse holds family meetings to discuss with Marie and her family her future as well as her day-to-day functioning now and how she will continue with a normal life-style and stay in school.
VI. Knowledge of somatic therapies and related clinical skills are utilized in working with clients.	Even though Marie seems depressed, no medication is prescribed for this. She is referred to the prenatal clinic where all medical and somatic therapies for pregnancy are screened and evaluated.
VII. The evnironment is structured to establish and maintain a therapeutic milieu.	The nurse evaluates the inpatient unit of the community mental health center for management of a pregnant teenager, so if Marie needs psychiatric hospitalization, she will know where she can receive therapeutic care within a therapeutic milieu (environment).
VIII. Nursing participates with interdisciplinary teams in assessing, planning, implementing, and evaluating programs and other mental health activities.	The nurse organizes and plans a multidisciplinary conference with all the professionals involved with Marie (prenatal, school, etc.) to plan a comprehensive approach to assisting Marie and her family.
IX. Psychotherapeutic interventions are used to assist clients to achieve their maximum development.	Family therapy is recommended for Marie and her family. Another community mental health nurse specialist at the center is the professional who will provide the treatment.
X. The practice of individual, group, or family psychotherapy requires appropriate preparation and recognition or accountability for the practice.	The nurse, prepared in family therapy, contracts with the family for short term treatment with the goal of improving their family pattern of interaction in an effort to help Marie with her difficulties.

TABLE 19-5. Continued.

Standards	Nursing Intervention
XI. Nursing participates with other members of the community in planning and implementing mental health services that include the broad continuum of promotion of mental health, prevention of mental illness, treatment, and rehabilitation.	The nurse discovers that Marie is not the only pregnant teenager the center is dealing with. At the same time there is an increase of problem pregnancies at the high school. She initiates and facilitates community meetings to investigate methods of addressing this issue.
XII. Learning experiences are provided for other nursing care personnel through leadership, supervision, and teaching	The nurse supervises other members of the crisis center team who are dealing with similar client situations.
XIII. Responsibility is assumed for continuing educational and professional development and contributions are made to the professional growth of others	The nurse attends conferences with other professionals, discussing new trends in teenagers and the facilities available for them for treatment of a teenage pregnancy, birth, and early infant care.
XIV. Contributions to nursing and the mental health field are made through innovations in theory and practice and participation in research.	The nurse decides to investigate on a formalized basis this increase in teenage mothering. She starts a research project.

hospitals. Since the 1960s many hospitals have closed larger sections and many patient wards. A broader community approach to mental health services has been adopted. With this approach came community clinics and satellite settings based in the community but still designed and dependent on the financial structure of the larger state hospital system. These community mental health settings are still financially limited by the amount of state tax dollars allocated to the programs in the annual fiscal budget.

A partnership agency is a mental health facility that is a federal-state-local partnership. This agency receives funding from all three sources or from governmental sources and the private, local mental health association. Unitl 1963 all funding supports for mental health centers depended on state and local sources. With the Community Mental Health Center Act in 1963, monies were legislated for federal financial support for the construction of mental health centers. Funding was determined by the population size and the socioeconomic condition of each state. In 1965, legislation adopted by Congress authorized federal support for community mental health personnel staffing. In 1970 a series of amendments was added to the 1963 legislation allocating up to 90 percent of the funding for construction in poverty areas.[34] With this kind of federal assistance, many mental health centers were able to build and staff new programs and expand old services. The National Institute of Mental Health (NIMH) is the federal agency responsible for the management of grants and the development of policies. Regional offices are established throughout the country, and these regional centers are actively involved in grant review and approval and fiscal management of programs. The local mental health association is usually a private, nonprofit corporation that is concerned with the mental health of a particular geographic community. Its funding comes from several sources, mostly private contributions. As can be seen, the federal level and the local level work together to provide strong financial bases for community mental health facilities.

There are two concerns about funding that are commonly raised by fiscal administrators.

One is where the responsibility for funding assistance should lie—with the federal government or the local government. Local financial assistance often provides the sense of community interest and participation that federal assistance does not, yet federal assistance is not subject to the whims and personal interests of local politicians.

The second issue is the justification of funding a mental health program that is not financially solvent. An example is long term care and intensive therapy programs with very sick schizophrenics in the community. As mental health moves more towards financial independence and dollar for dollar accountability, preventive and long term programs are being asked to prove their economic justification regardless of their therapeutic value. What was once assumed emotionally helpful for people will be viewed as economically unhelpful for the mental health facility and will be discouraged or eliminated. Schumacher, an economist, noted how these kinds of situations are viewed in the world.

> "If an activity has been branded as uneconomic, its right to existence is not merely questioned but energetically denied. Anything that is found to be an impediment to economic growth is a shamful thing, and if people cling to it, they are thought of as either saboteurs or fools."[35]

The financial funding for the community mental health nurse is defined by one of the above facilities. That is to say that she or he is salaried by the fee for service received from direct care services in a private mental health facility; has a state allocated position with a set salary in a public mental health facility; or is either on a state salaried position or salaried by federal grant money in a partnership setting in mental health. More recently, nurses have been supporting themselves in community mental health through private practice. As nurses become highly competent and skillful in their treatment techniques, several have been working with small private client caseloads. The future direction of this movement will depend on the development of a national health insurance plan and when nurses will be reimbursed by third party payments for independent nursing services.

SCOPE OF SERVICES

The scope of community mental health nursing practice has expanded and matured as nurses have grown with new and challenging responsibilities in prevention, intervention, and rehabilitation. According to the American Nurses' Association, these three areas comprise the chief goals of the mental health delivery system and form the parameters of the scope of contemporary community mental health nursing practice.[4] These same concepts form the preventive approach to mental health care that is the foundation of the community mental health movement. The thrust of the community mental health movement, since its inception, has been on prevention. The preventive approach as a level of health intervention was originally derived from the public health field. Leavell and Clark wrote on preventive medicine in 1953, identifying the approaches to preventive medicine as primary prevention, secondary prevention, and tertiary prevention.[36] These are the same concepts Gerald Caplan, a psychiatrist, adapted and applied to an approach to understanding community mental health. He states:

> " 'Preventative psychiatry' refers to the body of professional knowledge, both theoretical and practical, which may be utilized to plan and carry out programs for reducing (1) in-

cidence of mental disorders of all types in a community ("primary prevention"), (2) the duration of a significant number of those disorders which do occur ("secondary prevention"), and (3) the impairment which may result from those disorders ("tertiary prevention")."[37]

It has been this concept of prevention that nurses have used as a conceptual way of viewing and understanding their role in community mental health. This is a structured and serviceable way of viewing health and the necessary prevention, intervention, and rehabilitation when there is mental distress. The community mental health nurse is constantly applying these concepts to his or her own clinical work. In describing the work and the specialty areas involved in, his or her services will be organized and conceptualized according to primary, secondary, and tertiary approaches to community mental health.

Primary Prevention

In community mental health nursing, this is the level of health intervention that focuses on the prevention of mental illness and the education of the public on mental health concepts. The prevention of mental health problems is accomplished by working with people before they are in crisis situations. This is accomplished by planning, organizing, and operating preventive programs concentrating on populations that may be considered high risk, that is, those persons who by virtue of their circumstances may be placed in stressful situations or are more susceptible to mental illness. By understanding individual, family, and community needs, conflicts, stresses, and strains, the nurse can identify potentially harmful situations and develop methods to assist clients in increasing their capacity to deal with the problems and hassles of everyday life.

PREVENTIVE PROGRAMS

These programs are usually initiated by the nurse or the clinic she or he works with. They often are started by someone who has a particular interest in one cluster of people. For example, the nurse in community mental health nursing who also has an interest in maternal and child health may choose to work with pregnant women concerning the issues of being pregnant and preparing for the baby's arrival. She/he may also work with a group of women who have young infants about the adjustment a family needs to make with a newborn. By encouraging and assisting the parents in identifying what changes they will need to make, the nurse is providing anticipatory guidance to a young family. Kilker and Wilkerson[38] address this in their article on the anticipatory guidance of the expectant family. They discuss how a pregnant woman and her family may feel and experience the pregnancy and the period immediately after the birth. They identify how a nurse can assume that most people in this position will experience some stress and that by preparing clients and talking to them about what they may experience, some stress can be alleviated. Pregnancy and the postpartum period is historically an area of primary prevention work for professionals, and the nurse is no exception. Pregnancy and childbirth, although a very joyous time, can also be a time of a developmental crisis. Many individual and family adjustments need to be made. The community mental health nurse is prepared to identify problems in this process and provide treatment if it is indicated. Education for expectant and new parents is an important component of the nurse's role. Educational and supportive groups are one way of accomplishing this. This same concept can also be applied to parents of older children and to nonparenting young adults. Betty Glenn Harris describes a course she designed for young people to help them assess the demands of being a parent, as compared to other life committments, and their capacity to meet those demands.[39]

MENTAL HEALTH EDUCATION

The community mental health nurse provides educational programs for clients, other professionals, and people interested in mental health. What she/he teaches and how depends largely on her or his area of expertise, level of comfort with groups and speaking, and the requests of those seeking educational services. Religious groups, civic organizations, and school or community groups are examples of some people who may request lectures, seminars, or discussions on mental health. These are also examples of the types of organizations the nurse can approach if interested in providing this kind of educational service to the community.

Sometimes the nurse will organize and lead time-limited educational groups for parents of children of a particular age, i.e., parents of toddlers or parents of adolescents. Parents can be educated to improve family and parent/child interaction through presentation of ideas and theories by professionals and through the experience of the group discussion of similar concerns with other parents.

Another population that could greatly benefit from the nurse's services in preventive care is the elderly. The elderly have special community mental health needs. Because they are at times less demanding about the kind of services they should receive, they are overlooked. The aging process is something we all face and for some people it can be a lonely experience, crippled with many loses. Berezin[40] describes the psychodynamics of the aging process in terms of external and intrapsychic realities. The external realities are the environmental and societal aspects. An elderly person is treated as an aged individual by the rest of society. There is no control over this, only control over this kind of philosophic thinking. The internal or intrapsychic realities refer to the individual personality. The self-image of the elderly person, his perception of how others see him, and his adaptation to the aging process are all important components of the elderly person's personality. Understanding this makes it possible for the nurse to intervene on a psychological level. There is little she or he can do on an economical, social and physical level. The way to reach some elderly people is by showing a special and concerned interest in them as separate unique individuals with something worthwhile to offer in a relationship.

An area of preventive work with the elderly is preretirement education and counseling. This is becoming more popular with several community and retirement groups and some mental health centers. It is the preparation of working adults for a major upheaval in their daily routine and the loss of self esteem through job accomplishment. A study done on preretirement counseling and education stated:

"... there are superb opportunities for utilizing preventive services and intervention techniques in the clearly predictable crisis in health status, retirement, the loss of loved objects, role relationships, and financial distress. Despite the predictability of age-related crisis, however, research, planning, and program implementation of these events are still not frequent in mental health settings."[41]

Secondary Prevention

In community mental health nursing this is the level of health intervention that focuses on treatment of mental illness and the prevention of associated complications. The steps involved in the treatment of someone with a mental health problem include identification of the problem, intervention when there is a crisis situation, diagnosis and evaluation of the mental health status, providing the recommended therapeutic care plan, liaison work with other agencies and professionals to facilitate a holistic approach to the care of the individual when necessary, and evaluation of the nursing services provided whenever possible.

INDENTIFICATION AND CASE FINDING

The astute community mental health nurse is skilled at identifying when an individual has a mental health problem. She also is available to help others in this process of identifying and referring someone for mental health services. When early identification and intervention are practiced, they can often prevent the long term and chronic debilitating effects of mental illness. Some factors that a nurse takes into consideration in early identification are request for therapy, decreasing ability to cope with life on a day-to-day basis, any increasingly stressful stiuation, and any signs of psychosis (disorganized thinking, inappropriate affect, delusions, hallucinations).

CRISIS INTERVENTION

This is the therapeutic management of a person in the state of acute disequalibrium. It is work toward a healthy psychological resolution of a person's distressful situation. It is believed that intervention at the time of a crisis with a healthy resolution can restore a person to his usual level of functioning, if not a higher level. An unhealthy resolution can leave a person functioning on a level lower than his precrisis state.

The feeling of being in crisis is familiar to all of us. Few of us escape situational crisis during our lifetime, and all of us experienced developmental crisis as part of our growing up and aging.

A *situational crisis* is a distressing event or a stressful experience that threatens our sense of well-being. It disrupts our physical, emotional, and social balance and equilibrium. Losing a job, a family divorce, and accidental death or even severe property damage are all examples of a situational crisis. Burgess identifies the *victim crisis*.[42] This is a crisis or stressful experience that threatens the individual physically or psychologically because they are traumatized, injured, or destroyed in some way. Rape is an example of this. National disasters, such as a flood, are also examples. The Disaster Relief Act of 1974 (Public Law 93-288) gave recognition to the need for mental health services for people in crisis during any national disaster.[43]

A *developmental crisis* is equally as threatening to our overall sense of well-being. But because it is so much a part of our everyday living, we are not as likely to think of it in terms of a crisis. Such major life changes and adjustments as adolescence, marriage, the birth of a first child, and retirement are all considered developmental crises.

Once the crisis is identified, the nurse can begin the management of the client's situation. Donna Aquilera and her collegues describe specific steps to be taken in crisis intervention.[44]

They include:

1. Assessment of the individual in crisis and what his problem is. Identifying the cause of the crisis early is the key to resolving the crisis.
2. Planning therapeutic nursing interventions. The more appropriate the intervention, the more effective it will be on the individual's overall adjustment.
3. Intervention. The nurse helps the individual gain an understanding of his situation, aids him in expressing himself and his feelings about his situation, and explores with him ways he can cope with his situation.
4. Resolution. This is the settling of the disruption caused by the crisis and the planning and anticipatory guidance for the future.

DIAGNOSTIC EVALUATION

This is the intake evaluation done on clients seeking help through a mental health center. In a few interviews with the client, the nurse collects information, family history, and current concerns from the client. Based on the results of this psychological evaluation, a diagnosis, disposition, and recommendations for treatment are made.

TREATMENT

When mental health services are recommended, a therapeutic treatment is developed by the nurse. A community mental health clinical specialist is skilled in various types of treatment. They include individual psychotherapy, play therapy when working with children, group therapy, family and couples therapy. Therapy is the facilitation of personal growth through identification of problems and difficulties and changing one's behavior in order to relieve one's psychological pain. The type of therapy, therapeutic goals set by the client, and length of treatment all depend on the kind of treatment that is initially recommended. Because the nurse is responsible for her or his clients from admission through discharge and accountable for competencies in treatment, she or he is doing *primary nursing*. [45] Just how the nurse works and the kind of therapy done depends on how comfortable she or he is with the various treatment modalities. Some nurses are psychoanalytical, others use behavior modification, transactional analysis, and the Rogerian approach. One approach that some nurses in community mental health have used is what they describe as the "social network approach." [46] This technique allows the nurse to take a more complete view of the client and his problems. She interviews all those important people in the client's life. She has a meeting with those significant persons and together they decide and plan with the client for his future.

LIAISON AND REFERRAL

In keeping with the nursing tradition, the nurse in community mental health often finds herself the coordinator of services rendered to specific individuals and families in the community. The planning of a comprehensive care plan for some necessitates open communication among all professionals and agencies involved with the family. The nurse can facilitate such communication and collaborative working together by organizing and participating in conferences and planning with other agencies. It is equally important for community agencies to know how, when, and why they should refer clients to a mental health center.

One agency the nurse works closely with is the social welfare department because they are frequently the agency that sees so many of our high-risk community individuals and families. She or he assists the social welfare staff in identifying a client in emotional crisis and those troubled individuals needing mental health services. The social welfare system has been described by Milton Wittman as follows:

"The social welfare system is a network of interlinked public and voluntary services to people. It supplies basic economic needs for the dependent segment of the population, for people with no income or limited income. It provides rehabilitation for those with physical, mental, and social limitations. Within the scope of its concern would fall every conceivable variation of social pathology which appears on the American scene. Illustrative of the most pressing problems which challenge and burden the social welfare system are those of poverty, family breakdown, divorce, desertion, illegitimacy, interpersonal conflict, delinquency, crime, mental disorders, racial strife, and urban decay."[47]

MENTAL HEALTH CONSULTATION

Mental health consultation is a collaborative interaction between two or more people. They include the consultant (specialist in community mental health nursing) and the consultee (any working professional who asks for the specialist's help with a problem). The consultee seeks input and suggestions from the nurse because of her or his work and knowledge in mental health. The consultee applies the data obtained from the consultant to his day-to-day activities as a caregiver in the promotion of mental health and in the prevention and treatment of psychological disorders.

The purposes of mental health consultations are promoting primary prevention, fostering independent problem solving with the consultees, improving their work as professionals when dealing with mental health issues, and effecting overall planning and changes in the agency or system when indicated.

As a consultant, the mental health nurse must have her/his services requested by the consultee. The nurse establishes a relationship with the consultees, guarantees confidentiality on the topics they discuss, and is supportive yet objective during the discussion and consultation process. Consultation can be based on the model of the nursing process: assessing who is the client and what the problem is; planning goals and objectives in the problem solving; implementing and trying out the proposed solution; and evaluating with the client if the consultation has been helpful.

Professionals with whom the community mental health nurse consults include school personnel, nursery and day care personnel, staff members of nursing homes and chronic care facilities and also with other nurses, especially public health nurses, Visiting Nurse Associations, and general hospital nurses. As both a consultant and a nurse, she or he understands that the stress of illness and hospitalization can increase a patient's anxiety and may even trigger emotional problems. As a consultant she or he assists nurses in understanding this process, particularly with the difficult, demanding, or withdrawn patient.

The nurse sees patients on the wards, the medical and surgical units, pediatrics and maternity, special units such as CCU and ICU, respiratory units, and shock trauma units. These are patients that have been identified as problematic or high risk by the nursing staff. Lisa Robinson describes one example in which the psychiatric nurse consultant met with the staff nurses to assist them in identifying the patients' difficulties.[48] Together they planned nursing care and nursing interventions that would be most effective with those difficult patients.

Consulting with community health nurses, she or he often focuses on the management of the chronic psychiatric patient in the community and the identification and appropriate use of mental health concepts in their casework. Dorothea Hover, in her work as a consultant with public health nurses, stated that the nurse promotes "skilled intervention at early stages of family disequilibrium to prevent further emotional breakdown and to enchance the positive resources within the family.[49]

The process of mental health consultation is one of the most difficult and complex processes of community mental health nursing. The essence of successful consultation lies in the adequate preparation, training, and experience of the nurse. Nurses without such preparation should not attempt the consultation process with other community caregivers and professionals.

In addition to the treatment of individuals and families and consultation to the community, the nurse in community mental health must be aware of and knowledgeable about nursing interventions for some target populations of the community. They include the following.

CHILD ABUSE

This is the physical, sexual, and/or psychological abuse or neglect of a child. Parents who abuse or neglect their children usually have a history of being abused themselves as children.[50] This is why a total family approach is taken and why the abused child and the abusing parent are both viewed as victims. The nurse's role in situations where there is child abuse consists of the following:

1. Knowing the signs and symptoms of abuse, identifying cases, educating other mental health professionals.
2. Reporting, by law, any cases she knows of to the proper authorities.
3. Encouraging referrals in potential child abuse cases to do preventive work with the family.
4. Treating the parents and families of the abused child.

SUDDEN INFANT DEATH SYNDROME

SIDS is the sudden, unexpected, unexplained death of an apparently normal healthy infant. Such dealths have occurred since early civilization. Yet only in the last few years have we begun to identify it, fund research for its cause, and provide help to the families of these young victims. The community nurse has been the key professional working with the followup and counseling of these SIDS families. Some reasons given at the joint conference of the National Foundation for SIDS and the National Institute of Mental Health are the following:[51]

1. The nurse works in the community, makes home visits, and has easy accessibility to the family.
2. The nurse, by virtue of her or his education, is familiar and comfortable in dealing with the matter of death and dying.
3. The nurse is experienced with the medical terminology, and can explain SIDS and any pathologist's report to the family in a way they can understand.

The community mental health nurse is also involved in counseling SIDS families. More importantly, she is available to the community nurse for consultation, assisting a grieving family and helping them with grief work, and recognizing when the family could benefit from therapy. Commonly, she/he is one of the few mental health professionals who is knowledgeable about sudden infant death syndrome.

ADOLESCENCE

Halfway between childhood and adulthood, adolescence is indeed a tumultuous time. Some adolescents seek therapy on their own when they are having a difficult time. However, most seek help indirectly. For example, an emotionally upset 16-year-old will surely throw the entire family into a chaotic state. At this point, some parents will seek help for their adolescent, themselves, or the entire family. Another critical entry point is through sexuality counseling (venereal disease counseling, illegitimate pregnancy counseling, pre- and postabortion counseling) and substance counseling (drugs and alcohol). Neighborhood health centers, multiservice agencies, and ambulatory settings often have a medical clinic that treats these concerns. It is through the collaborative work with these other professionals that the nurse's help can be therapeutic with these troubled young aspiring adults.

An example of how a nurse can utilize counseling and medical skills would be with a group of adolescent unwed mothers. Here the nurse could help the young women deal with individual and interpersonal problems on a therapeutic level and have some sessions centered around the direct demonstrations of proper infant care.

MIDDLESCENCE

No age is without its difficulties. As one approaches middle age, there are increased responsibilities, self-evaluation, and the giving up of those unattainable goals. One nurse-author describes her own experience with this stage of middlescence.[52] She talks freely about her difficulties with the death of a parent and the placement of a parent in a nursing home. The community mental health nurse will often see clients during this period seeking help for themselves in the form individual therapy.

Suicide is a problem for all ages, but the highest range of statistics is during the adult years. The key to the reduction of the suicide rate lies in the recognition and diagnosis of predictable signs. Some mental health centers work closely with the area's suicide prevention center. Together they discover clues to the potential suicide risk person. Once a person has attempted suicide, the nurse has a clear role in intervening. She does followup care and treatment when possible. It has been suggested[53] that there be consistent suicide followup available.

> "It might be well to pattern the followup procedure for suicide attempts roughly after that of health educators working with VD or TB follow-up, and look forward to the time when suicide attempts follow-up can be built into routine health services. The follow-up could be seen as "post crisis follow-up" and would be a legitimate aspect of a comprehensive approach to suicide prevention. It is known that the most dangerous period with relation to suicide is within three months after a suicidal crisis."[53]

Another aspect of suicide work for the nurse is in the situation in which a suicide has occurred. The nurse can be available to the victim's family, who face grief and prolonged guilt reactions. No other kind of death in our society creates this type of deep emotional shame and scarring for the surviving family.

THE ELDERLY

Secondary prevention and intervention in the care of the elderly can be addressed through the nurse's involvement with crisis intervention programs, nursing homes, and outpatient group psychotherapy.

Crisis Intervention and Emergency Programs

Through these programs a nurse can reach out to the elderly with a mental health problem. Providing these services and permitting intervention in the home or wherever necessary can be an alternative to hospitalization.

Nursing Homes

The nurse establishes relationships with the nursing homes in her area. She consults with the staff of the nursing home about difficult patients and teaches them techniques for dealing with them. She maintains primary responsibility for following patients placed in the nursing home after a psychiatric hospitalization.

Outpatient Group Psychotherapy

Groups for the elderly have been successful in a variety of settings. One nurse organized a therapy group for the community's elderly when they found the elderly misused the emergency room with vague psychosomatic complaints.[54] Many elderly were using the emergency room for attention for themselves and to relieve their loneliness and isolation.

Another setting was the mental health center. Ambulatory patients from nursing homes met at the center on a monthly or bimonthly basis. This gave them the opportunity to express their feelings and be supportive of one another, but it also proved to be a great source of socialization.

Tertiary Prevention

In community mental health nursing this is the level of health intervention that focuses on the rehabilitative process. The goals of working with people who have experienced mental health problems or psychiatric illness are prevention of long lasting and debilitating effects, restoration to their optimal level of health, and returning to community living or community after-care programs for those who were hospitalized.

COMMUNITY AFTER-CARE PROGRAMS

This is a program sponsored by the psychiatric team designed to meet the hospitalized patient's individual needs for community living. The community mental health nurse provides assistance in the activities of daily living during this transitional period and acts as the liaison for the patient and his community resources. Available for supportive therapy, she or he is also capable of providing instruction and counseling in health and hygiene, vocational and economic referrals, accessibility to social and religious groups, and methods of decision making. She provides medication, supervises self-administration when possible, or may even run medication groups for a number of patients. Throughout this assistance, instruction, and counseling, the nurse encourages and prepares the patient for independent living and self-reliance.

During this time the nurse also assists the patient's family with the complexities they face. These families are under tremendous stress, can become isolated from social network and support systems, and experience a decreased decision making capacity. They are in need of assistance and support in problem solving and planning for the future and direct and realistic anticipatory guidance as their family member reenters the community.

ALTERNATIVE HOUSING

There has been a marked increase in the number of mental health and psychiatric patients who have been discharged into the community. The long-term hospitalization of patients is an outdated form of treatment. It is believed that the sooner a person can return to the community the better his chances are at making a healthy adjustment. Several factors have contributed to this process. They include: 1) The growing belief that realistic rehabilitation cannot take place in the isolated hospital setting. 2) The belief that the community is designed to meet many social, personal, and economic needs of patients. 3) The realization that illness can be treated effectively in the community, especially through the use of medication.

As patients return to the community they need a place to live. Some of the more common living arrangements in the community, or community residences as they are called, are halfway houses.

Halfway houses are facilities that house a number of people with mental health problems. Some are financially subsidized by the state, and some are solely supported by the people who live in the house. A typical house would have 10 to 15 people with 1 or 2 house parents. These are usually mental health workers who receive supervision from a professional at the mental health center. At times these will be community mental health nurses.

Not only emotionally troubled persons live in a halfway house but also drug and alcohol abusers, delinquent youth, the mentally retarded, and the elderly. The nurse's role is often one of supervisor or consultant to the paraprofessional who lives at the house. She or he may work with several individuals around supportive therapy or medications.

Some community residences have been successful endeavors. They provide the emotional and social support that is necessary to sustain an individual in community living. Although community residences have proved to be a viable alternative to hospitalization and have a history of working well, many communities are opposed to them. The nurse and other professionals are frequently faced with the problem of community acceptance.[55] Many people are frightened by the establishing of such a residence in their own community. Ignorance and lack of knowledge about such alternative living arrangements are the major reasons for opposition. Special zoning is necessary and good community education and relations with the people are a must.

Community Mental Health Center

In understanding the nurse in community mental health, it is important to have a clear view of the scope of nursing services. It is also important to understand the system that allows for that variety in scope of nursing services. Although the nurse is found in a variety of community settings, she or he is most frequently located in a community mental health center or an affiliated agency.

The community mental health center provides mental health services and psychiatric services for a population in a specific community called a *catchment area*. This concept, fundamental to public health, means a selected area and population of 75,000 to 200,000 within a geographic boundary. The state is divided into catchment areas in order to facilitate and organize the delivery of mental health services.

The Community Mental Health Centers Construction Act of 1963 first awarded federal funds totaling 150 million dollars to community mental health centers. This funding was provided in the form of construction grants which encouraged the building of comprehensive community mental health centers nationwide. Subsequently, additional funds have been available in the form of construction and building grants and staffing grants for centers. In order to qualify for such grants, a center must meet the standards set by the federal government and the CMHC Act.

In 1963 these standards required CMH centers to provide the following five essential services:[56]

1. *Inpatient care.* This is total patient care of a client who needs psychiatric-mental health hospitalization. Such a mental health unit must be accesible to any community person seeking hospitalization on a 24 hour basis.
2. *Outpatient.* This is a program of psychiatric mental health services available to all ages on an outpatient basis. Such psychiatric treatment would include individual, group, and family therapy.
3. *Partial hospitalization program.* This is a service of day or night treatment programs available for those persons who need some hospitalization but not necessarily 24 hour coverage. It includes day hospital programs which offer a psychiatric service during the day and allow the patient to return home at night and night care programs which allow a hospitalized patient to maintain a job and return to the hospital at night.
4. *Emergency services.* This is the 24 hour coverage that a CMH center offers. This makes it possible for a community person to seek help at any time. Each center establishes its own system for emergency services, either by Hot Line, a walk-in center, or crisis intervention teams who are on call.
5. *Consultation and education.* The CMH centers consult and provide education to other professionals and other community agencies on a variety of mental health issues. This involves working with the school systems, neighborhood health centers, and local hospitals.

In 1975 the Community Mental Health Center Amendment PL94-63[57] was passed. This revised the requirements of the comprehensive community mental health center by adding seven more essential components. They include:

6. *Followup care services.* This is an established and ongoing program that continues to be concerned about the mental health care of patients after their discharge from the mental health center.
7. *Program of transitional halfway house services.* This is a setting for mentally ill patients not requiring hospitalization but also not able to live in the community on their own.
8. *Specialized services for the mental health of children.* This is a full range of diagnostic, treatment, liaison and followup services for children and adolescents.

9. *Specialized services for the mental health of the elderly.* This is a full range of diagnostic, treatment, liaison, and followup services for the elderly.
10. *Assistance to courts and other agencies.* This is a prescreening process for patients considered for referral from the judicial and other systems to mental health units.
11. *A program for the prevention and treatment of alcoholism and alcohol abuse and for rehabilitation of alcoholics and alcohol abusers.*
12. *A program for the prevention and treatment of drug addiction and abuse for the rehabilitation of addicts, abusers, and drug dependent persons.*

LEGISLATION

Public interest in mental health services has led the way to various legislative changes. Legislation introduced by Senator Daniel Inouye of Hawaii proposes to amend the present CHAMPIS Program. (The present program provides health care for dependent and other beneficiaries of our military personnel). This bill would provide for expanded, independent roles for qualified psychiatric nurses in the Medicare and Medicaid programs and for the reimbusement of such services.[58]

Ned Kellog writes: "Legislation now before Congress would go a long way toward establishing registered nurses as independent professinals . . . making it possible for them to receive fee for service payments covered by Medicare and Medicaid . . . (and) would help assure equal consideration of nurses in any future national health insurance program."[59]

Martha Mitchell, Chairperson of the Division on Psychiatric and Mental Health Nursing Practice has recommended that "qualified psychiatric nurses determine the necessary services (for patient care) as part of their standard nursing practice and (that) these be permissible reimbursements as recognized by CHAMPIS."[60]

The President's Commission on Mental Health

President Carter established the President's Commission on Mental Health in 1977. The purpose of this commission was to assess the needs of the mentally ill and provide recommendations for types of research the government should support. This is the most extensive review of the nation's mental health needs since 1961. The Commission issued its final report in April 1978. The report's recommendations focused on eight major areas:[61]

1. Improving community support systems (families, neighbors, community organizations).
2. Community based services as the keystone of the mental health system.
3. National health insurance to include appropriate coverage for mental health care.
4. Increase the number of mental health professionals.
5. Establishment of a center for prevention in the National Institute of Mental Health with primary prevention as the priority.
6. Protection of basic human rights.
7. Increase mental health research.
8. Education of the public.

"Nurses are specifically mentioned in sections addressing reimbursement, manpower shortages at state mental hospitals, and mental health education for primary care practitioners. . . . The report affords nursing a recognition long needed in such high level documents. . . . Nurses are specifically named as one of the four types of mental health care providers in organized settings whose services should be reimbursable (the others being physicians, psychologists, and social workers). . . . This is the first time an official document of this level unequivocally includes nurses in its discussion of insurance reimbursement. The recognition acknowledges the role of nurses in mental health care and gives visibility to their professional competence."[61]

PERSPECTIVES ON COMMUNITY MENTAL HEALTH NURSING

The community mental health nurse of the future will continue developing from the traditional roles of both the psychiatric nurse and the public health nurse. The nurse will be committed to the overall mental health of the individual within the community and will provide direct care or supervise that care through the use of community members. The community mental health nurse will assume the role of advisor or consultant to the community. Other responsibilities will include the planning of the educational and social programs related to mental health in conjunction with community leaders.

As nurses develop their community mental health roles, a more independent practice will develop. In order to develop these roles, nurses need to perform more research to increase the body of nursing theory. Any community mental health nursing advances in the future will rely heavily upon the level of nursing research presently performed.

The community mental health nurse will encounter a vast number of community concerns for research. The major areas will include drug abuse, family disorganization, mental retardation, children and minority concerns, integration of public and private mental health care, national health insurance, manpower, reforms of federal health legislation, systems integration, and service delivery.

The current public interest in community mental health nursing emphasizes prevention. This includes earlier and more effective detection of the psychiatric conditions which cause social maladjustments and the explorations of the sources of those conditions. The community is changing its concepts and attitudes. Partly because of public education, the public now believes that a patient deserves good care, even if he cannot recover from his particular malady. The concept of health has expanded to include emotional factors associated with most types of illness. The ultimate goal of community mental health nursing is the attainment of an emotionally mature, well-adjusted individual.

REFERENCES

1. *Facts about Mental Illness.* National Association for Mental Health, 1972.
2. Kennedy, John F.: "Mental Illness and Mental Retardation." Presented at the 88th Congress, 1st Session. House of Representatives Document 58. Washington, D.C., 1963.
3. Leininger, Madeleine: "Community Psychiatric Nursing: Trends, Issues, and Problems." *Perspectives in Psychiatric Care,* 7(1):11, 1969.
4. "Statement on Psychiatric and Mental Health Nursing Practice." American Nurses Association, Division on Psychiatric and Mental Health Nursing Practice. ANA 1976, PMH-3 10M-12/76.
5. Garrison, F. H.: *An Introduction to the History of Medicine,* 4th ed. W. B. Saunders Company, Philadelphia, 1967.
6. Burton, Lloyd, and Smith, Hugh: *Public Health and Community Medicine.* The Williams & Wilkins Company, Baltimore, 1975.
7. Saunders, J. B.: *Transitions from Ancient Egyptian to Greek Medicine.* University of Kansas Press, Lawrence, Kansas, 1963.
8. Schneck, J. M.: *A History of Psychiatry.* Charles C Thomas, Springfield, Ill., 1960.
9. Bellak, L.: *Handbook of Community Psychiatry and Community Mental Health.* Grune & Stratton, New York, 1964.

10. Deloughery, Grace, et al.: *Consultation and Community Organization in Community Mental Health Nursing.* The Williams & Wilkins Company, Baltimore, 1971.
11. Graham, T. F.: *Parallel Profiles.* Francisan Herald Press, Chicago, 1966.
12. Gardner, M. S.: *Public Health Nursing.* The Macmillan Company, New York, 1931.
13. Burgess, Ann, and Lazare, Aaron: *Psychiatric Nursing in the Hospital and the Community.* Prentice-Hall, Inc., Englewood Cliffs, N.J., 1973.
14. Noyes, A. P.: "Nursing Needs in the State Mental Hospitals." *American Journal of Nursing,* 33:787,1933.
15. Scarpitti, Frank R., et al.: "Public Health Nurses in a Community Care Program for the Mentally Ill." *American Journal of Nursing,* 65:89, June 1965.
16. Fischelis, Mary C., and Errera, Paul: "Psychiatric Nurse in an Outpatient Clinic." *Nursing Outlook* 16:68, April 1968.
17. Grafeh, Mehadin, et al.: "Linking Hospital and Community Care for Psychiatric Patients." *American Journal of Nursing* 68:1050, May 1968.
18. "Community Mental Health Nursing." *American Journal of Nursing,* 70:1019, May 1970.
19. Gardner, Kathryn: "Levels of Psychiatric Nursing Practice in an Ambulatory Setting." *Journal of Psychiatric Nursing and Mental Health Services,* 15(9):26, Sept. 1977.
20. Weiner, Irving: *Principles of Psychotherapy.* John Wiley and Sons, New York, 1975.
21. Stewart, Robert: "Psychoanalysis and Psychoanalytic Psychotherapy," in Freedman, A. M., Kaplan, H. I., and Sadock, B. J. (eds.): *Comprehensive Textbook of Psychiatry/II.* The Williams & Wilkins Company, Baltimore, 1975.
22. Mann, James: *Time-Limited Psychotherapy.* Harvard University Press, Cambridge, 1973.
23. Yalom, Irvin D.: *The Theory and Practice of Group Psychotherapy.* Basic Books, Inc., New York, 1970, p. 21.
24. Axline, Virginia: *Play Therapy.* Ballantine Books, New York, 1969.
25. Harris, Michael, and Solomon, Kenneth: "Roles of the Community Mental Health Nurse." *Journal of Psychiatric Nursing and Mental Health Services,* 15:35, Feb. 1977.
26. Lego, Suzanne: "Nurse-Psychotherapist . . . How Are We Different?" *Perspectives in Psychiatric Care,* 11(4):144, 1973.
27. DeYoung, Carol D., and Tower, Margene: *The Nurse's Role in Community Mental Health Centers.* The C.V. Mosby Company, St. Louis, 1971.
28. Smith, Carol Gibson: "Legal Dimensions of Nursing," in Burgess, A. W. (ed.): *Levels of Health Intervention.* Prentice-Hall Inc., Englewood Cliffs, N.J., 1978.
29. Kelly, Lucie Young: "Institutional Licensure." *Nursing Outlook,* 21(9):566, Sept. 1973.
30. "ANA Funds Certification Program for Two Years: New Areas Added." *American Journal of Nursing,* 78(4):534, April 1978.
31. Stachyra, Marcia: "Self-Regulation through Certification." *Perspectives in Psychiatric Care,* 20(4):148, 1973.
32. Editorials: "Certification—Assurance of Quality." *The American Nurse,* March 15, 1978, p. 4.
33. *Standards of Psychiatric and Mental Health Nursing Practice.* American Nurse Association. Developed by Executive Committee and the Standards Committee of ANA Division on Psychiatric and Mental Health Nursing Practice. Kansas City, MO., 1973.
34. Weston, Donald W.: "Development of Community Psychiatry Concept," in Freedman, A. M., Kaplan, H. I., and Sadock, B. J. (eds.): *Comprehensive Textbook of Psychiatry/II.* The Williams and Wilkins Company, Baltimore, 1975.
35. Schumacher, E. F.: *Small is Beautiful.* Harper and Row, New York, 1973.
36. Leavell, Hugh R., and Clark, E. Gurney: *Preventative Medicine for the Doctor in his Community: An Epidemiologic Approach,* 3rd. ed. McGraw-Hill Book Company, New York, 1966.
37. Caplan, Gerald: *Principles of Preventative Psychiatry.* Basic Books, Inc., New York, 1964.
38. Kilker, Rosemary, and Wilkerson, Betty L: "Anticipatory Guidance of the Expectant Family," in Hymovich, D. P., and Bannard, M. U. (eds.): *Family Health Care.* McGraw-Hill Book Company, New York, 1973.
39. Harris, Betty Glenn: "Learning About Parenting," *Nursing Outlook,* 25(7):457, July 1977.
40. Berezin, Martin A., and Stotsky, Bernard: "The Geriatric Patient," in Golann, Stuart E., and Eisdorfer, Carl (eds.): *Handbook of Community Mental Health.* Appleton-Century-Crofts, New York, 1972.
41. Green, M. R., et al.: "Pre-retirement Counseling, Retirement Adjustment, and the Older Employee (An experimental study measuring the interrelationship of factors affecting retirement

adjustment, resistance to retirement, and the effectiveness of the older employee)," in Golann, S. E., and Eisdorfer, C. (eds.): *Handbook of Community Mental Health*. Appleton-Century-Crofts, New York, 1972.

42. Burgess, Ann Wolbert, and Holmstrom, Lynda L.: *Rape: Victims of Crisis*. Brady Company, Baltimore, 1974.

43. Brownstone, Jane, et al.: "Disaster-Relief Training and Mental Health." *Hospital and Community Psychiatry*, 28:30, Jan. 1977.

44. Aquilera, Donna, Messick, Janice M., Farrell, Marlene S.: *Crisis Intervention*. The C.V. Mosby Company, St. Louis, 1970.

45. Eisenman, Elaine Pivnick: "Primary Care in a Mental Health Facility." *Nursing Outlook*, 24(10):640, Oct. 1976.

46. Garrison, John, Kulp, Carolyn, and Rosen, Sherryl: "Community Mental Health Nursing: A Social Network Approach," *Journal of Psychiatric Nursing and Mental Health Services*, 15:32, Jan. 1977.

47. Wittman, Milton: "The Social Welfare System: Its Relation to Community Mental Health," in Golann, Stuart E., and Eisdorfer, Carl (eds.): *Handbook of Community Mental Health*. Appleton-Century-Crofts, New York, 1972.

48. Robinson, Lisa: "A Psychiatric Nursing Liaison Program." *Nursing Outlook*, 20(7):454, July 1972.

49. Hover, Dorothea: "Mental Health Consultation with Public Health Nurses, Using Transactional Analysis as a Tool." *Journal of Psychiatric Nursing and Mental Health Services*, 14(6):15, June 1976.

50. Kempe, C. H., and Helfer, R. E.: *The Battered Child*. University of Chicago Press, Chicago, 1968.

51. Miles, Margaret S. (ed.): "The Mental Health Aspects of Sudden Infant Death Syndrome (SIDS). Conference Report from the National Foundation for Sudden Infant Death, Inc. New York and the National Institute of Mental Health Dept. HEW, July 30, 1975.

52. Weaver, Barbara R.: "Halfway to Ninety," in Hall, Joanne E., and Weaver, Barbara R. (eds.): *Nursing of Families in Crisis*. J. B. Lippincott Co., Philadelphia, 1974.

53. Shneidman, Edwin S.: "Prevention of Suicide: A Challenge for Community Science," in Golann, Stuart E., and Eisendorfer, Carl (eds.): *Handbook of Community Mental Health*. Appleton-Century-Crofts, New York, 1972.

54. Duetsch, Christine B., and Kramer, Nancy: "Outpatient Group Psychotherapy for the Elderly: an Alternative to Institutionalization." *Hospital and Community Psychiatry*, 28(6):440, June 1977.

55. Cupaiuolo, Anthony A.: "Community Residences and Zoning Ordinances." *Hospital and Community Psychiatry* 28(3):206, March 1977.

56. Community Mental Health Center Acts of 1963.

57. Community Mental Health Center Amendments of 1975. Public Law 94-63, Title III 2-5, 2-6.

58. Congressional Record. Senator Inouye. Senate Bill #617, 618. February 3, 1977.

59. Kellog, Ned: "Will Congress Declare Independence for Nurses?" RN, 38(7):30, 1975.

60. ANA testimony presented by Martha Mitchell, Chairperson, Division on Psychiatric and Mental Health Nursing Practice on CHAMPIS Regulations DOD 6010 8-R, before Department of Defense. September 7, 1977.

61. Hadley, Richard: "President's Commission Sets National Mental Health Goals." *The American Nurse*, 10(6):1, June 15, 1978.

CHAPTER **20**
NURSING ROLE
IN CONTINUING CARE

PHYLLIS J. GOODHUE, M.S., R.N.

Continuing care services provide a multidisciplinary approach to early screening, assessment, planning, and followup which meets peoples' needs through coordinated community efforts that enable maximum health levels to be reached. It is the responsibility of a continuing care service to provide continuity of optimal medical and nursing care for the patient needing discharge planning. Continuity of care considers the patient's short term and long term needs and relates his medical and nursing requirements to the psychosocial needs that affect his recovery. To be effective it must consider the assessment of the patient's level of care need, the spectrum of services available, and implementation of an appropriate plan to meet the patient's total care needs.

HISTORICAL DEVELOPMENT

Prior to the 1940s and World War II, the acute care needs of patients were met by the general practitioner at home or in the hospital and the patient was returned to his community. Not much thought was given to where the patient was going and how he would provide for his continuing care needs. It is not easy to trace the evolution of discharge planning. There were societal changes during the 1940s and early 1950s, i.e., more women going to work, increase in births, and the building of smaller houses. Fewer older people were living with their grown children and were living instead in small apartments in older houses in the cities while their children moved to the suburbs. The extended family became the nuclear family. During World War II, medicine began to focus on discharge concepts. Medical care studies were concerned with costs, including readmissions and the increasing recognition of a patient's lack of choices on discharge.[1]

In the 1950s, discharge planning was beginning to be thought of as a necessity for quality of care. The 1961 White House Conference on Aging presented statistics showing that advances in health care had extended the life expectancy of our population and had placed new challenges on the health care delivery system.[2] With the increase in the life span, an increase in chronic illness and disability also occurred as increasing medical research resulted in the ability to treat certain disease processes which prior to this had been fatal. There was greater demand for acute care beds which led to early discharge. Many patients being discharged no longer needed acute care but were not being cared for adequately when returned to their prehospital setting.[3]

By the 1960s, a crisis, defined as patients in trouble because of an imbalance between problems faced and resources available, had occurred. Social work services and community health nursing which had been available since the early nineteenth century were over-extended. It was obvious that new resources must be made available with a unification of effort between the hospitals and the community to prevent duplication and increase in cost.[1] Instant discharge planning and crisis management were prevalent as hospitals began to recognize that their responsibility for health care extended outside of their health care facilities. The possibility of discharge planning units was assured when the federal government created a major impact on the delivery of health care by the introduction of Public Law 89-97 (the Social Security Amendments of 1965).[4] It was complicated and consisted of two major titles. One was Title XVIII, Health Insurance for the Aged (Medicare), which became effective July 1, 1966; the second was Title XIX, Grants to States for Medical Assistance Programs (Medicaid), which became effective January 1, 1966. Four other titles, Titles I-IV, were modifications of existing provisions. The availability of health insurance for older people would allow them choices for provision of health care which they did not have prior to the enactment of this legislation. They were now assured of short term inpatient protection with semiprivate coverage. For many, it meant no longer having to go to the county or city hospital unless it was their CHOICE. They were no longer "charity" patients. It was anticipated that in the long run there would be a decrease in use of the acute hospitals when alternative programs were put into effect.[5]

Medicare did increase the demand on the physician's time, and many physicians felt that the hospital was the logical place to center their practice. Fewer physicians were based in the community. Patients came to the physicians at their offices in the hospitals or to clinics. Clinic visits were paid for, as was diagnostic testing. Although Medicare was originally a health insurance program for people 65 and older, it is now available for people under 65 who have been disabled for two years. It is a federal government program run by the Health Care Financing Administration.[5] It has two parts, hospital insurance and medical insurance. Medicare hospital insurance (Part A) helps pay for medically necessary inpatient hospital care and, after a hospital stay, for care at home or as an inpatient in a skilled nursing facility. Medicare medical insurance (Part B) can help pay for doctor services, outpatient clinic, physical and speech therapy, and other medical services and supplies that are not covered by the hospital insurance part of Medicare. Payments also are handled by private insurance organizations, i.e., Blue Cross-Blue Shield, under contract with the government. Organizations handling claims from hospitals, skilled nursing facilities, and home health agencies are called *intermediaries*. Organizations handling claims from doctors and other suppliers of services covered under the medical insurance part of Medicare are called *carriers*. For people with very low incomes, the Medicaid program in their state may pay the amount Medicare does not pay and may pay some health care expenses not covered by Medicare.

The Continuing Care Coordinator needs to be aware of the rules and regulations and how they affect patients. A great deal of interpretation is necessary for patients and their families as to what their insurance pays for posthospitalization care. Care for the treatment of an illness or injury must be reasonable and necessary.[5] For example, care would not be covered if a physician placed a patient in a skilled nursing facility when an intermediate care facility would serve as well. Some health care services are not generally accepted by the health community as being reasonable or necessary for diagnosis and treatment, i.e., acupuncture. Services must be generally recognized as safe and effective by the health community.

Medicare does not cover custodial care. When the purpose of a patient's treatment plan is primarily to meet personal care needs and could be provided by persons without professional skills or training, it is considered custodial. A patient may not be able to dress, feed, bathe himself, or take oral medications, but a licensed (skilled) person is not required to do these things for him. People believe that if the home health agency or health care facility participates in the Medicare program, everything should be covered; however, only skilled care is covered.[5] When Medicare was first introduced, it was seen by many health professionals as a panacea for the elderly. It was not immediately realized that only acute care and immediate postacute care needs were addressed. The nursing profession was not active in defining skilled nursing. All nursing is skilled. The definition used by Medicare is care that can only be performed by or under the supervision of licensed nursing personnel. There are six conditions which must be met if Medicare hospital insurance is to help pay for home health visits.[5] These conditions are: 1) a stay in a qualifying hospital for at least three days in a row, 2) home health care is for further treatment of a condition which was treated in a hospital or skilled nursing facility, 3) the care needed includes part-time skilled nursing care, physical therapy, or speech therapy, 4) the patient is essentially homebound, 5) a doctor determines the need for home health care and sets up a home health plan within 14 days after the discharge from a hospital or participating skilled nursing facility, and 6) the home health agency providing services is participating in the Medicare program.

There are five conditions which must be met if Medicare hospital insurance is to help pay for care in a skilled nursing facility.[5] These conditions are: 1) a hospital stay of at least three days in a row before a transfer to a participating skilled nursing facility, 2) a transfer to the skilled nursing facility because care is required for a condition which was treated in the hospital, 3) an admission to the facility within a short time (generally within 14 days) after hospital discharge, 4) a doctor certifies that there is a need for skilled nursing or skilled rehabilitation services on a daily basis, and 5) the facility's Utilization Review Committee or a Professional Standards Review Organization does not disapprove the stay. Medicare medical insurance can help pay for home visits if four conditions are met: 1) There is a need for part-time skilled nursing care or physical therapy or speech therapy, 2) a doctor determines the need for the services and sets up a plan for home health care, 3) the patient is essentially homebound, and 4) the home health agency providing services is participating in the Medicare program.[5] It is extremely distressing for patients and their families to be told that their insurance is not going to pay for care which they feel is their right. It is less traumatic if they are confident of the continuing care coordinator's knowledge of health care rules and regulations, payment mechanisms, and the coordinator's ability to find alternatives.

NURSING ROLE

Appropriate discharge planning for continuing care does not just happen, it requires planning and organization. Some states have mandated specific rules and regulations such as Massachusetts in August, 1971:[6]

1.0 PLANNING FOR CONTINUING CARE

There shall be an organized multi-disciplinary service to aid the attending physician and his patient in planning for continuing care upon discharge from the hospital. The continuing care service shall be designed so as to facilitate the transfer of the patient from the hospital setting to an appropriate independent living arrangement or to another institution or level of care therein.

1.1 The hospital administrator in conjunction with the Director of Nursing and Social Service shall designate a specific individual to be known as the "Coordinator of Continuing Care" or designate a specific unit for this purpose.

     1.1.1 Wherever an individual is designated as the "Coordinator of Continuing Care," the individual shall be a social worker or public health nurse and shall have particular competence in carrying out this responsibility based on education, experience, and knowledge of community resources.

     1.1.2 Wherever a specific unit is designated, there shall be at least a nurse and social worker assigned to the unit to assess patient needs and to plan together for continuity of patient care.

1.2 The coordinator shall be responsible for the coordination of the plan for continuing care under the direction of the physician and in cooperation with the patient, the family, and other members of the professional staff.

1.3 A mechanism shall be established, operative, and described in writing, for early screening of patients to determine whether continuing care planning will be necessary.

1.4 The individual or unit responsible for coordination of planning for continuing care shall maintain in writing a current description of out-of-hospital resources which shall be available to the attending physician and other members of the professional staff.

1.5 The Coordinator of Continuing Care shall be responsible for the timely transfer of appropriate information from the hospital to the posthospital institution or agency in order to insure continuity of patient care.

     1.5.1 When a patient is transferred to another institution, a patient care referral form approved by the Department shall be completed and accompany the patient.

     1.5.2 When a patient is discharged and referred to a community agency for continuing care, a patient care referral form approved by the Department shall be completed and sent to the agency prior to, or at the time of, patient discharge.

     1.5.3 The medical discharge summary shall be sent by the hospital no later than 72 hours following discharge of the patient to an institution or community agency.

1.6 The hospital shall give notice of anticipated or impending transfer of the patient to the community agency or institution at least 24 hours prior to discharge and shall assist in making arrangements for safe transportation.

1.7 The coordinator shall assist the utilization review committee in its consideration of the appropriateness of continuity of patient care.

1.8 Written records shall be maintained which contain sufficient information to enable the coordinator or unit to prepare periodic reports which shall include the number of patients for whom coordination of continuing care was provided and the types of placement made.

EDUCATIONAL PREPARATION

The reference to a "public health nurse" means one with a baccalaureate degree in nursing which guarantees community health nursing preparation. Many continuing care nursing coordinators have a master's degree in community health nursing. It is expected that a minimum of two years' nursing experience be required—one year in the hospital setting and one year in the community. When a continuing care nurse acts as a consultant it is recommended that he or she have a master's degree in community health nursing and five years of nursing experience, some of which was in a leadership position. A study done with the Los Angeles County Health Department in which the community health nursing consultant reviewed charts retrospectively for necessity of followup planning showed that only 4 of the 88 she assessed as needing followup had been referred to outside agencies.[3] A study done by Baltimore City Hospital in 1970 showed that only 60 percent of medical patients discharged had adequate medical followup.[7] We have medical care plans, social care plans, and nursing care plans. By 1970, the trend in medicine was toward specialization which resulted in fragmented care plans. Orientation of physicians has not been toward continuing care; staff nurses have found it time consuming, adding to their overextended workload. The rules and regulations for continuing care are written mainly in nursing terms, and the professional nurse is seen as the coordinator of the care plan. The continuing care nurse is the one nurse directly concerned with the continuity of care for a patient moving from one service to another within the facility, for one being discharged, and for any patient needing followup after discharge.[8]

SCOPE OF SERVICE

The organized continuing care office or discharge planning office or transfer office is staffed according to the size of the health care facility and the need for the service. The models which I have observed or been told about are:

1. A continuing care nurse or nurses who do the patient assessments and communicate them to the social worker who does the discharge plan.
2. Continuing care nurse as a freestanding coordinator or discharge planner.
3. A continuing care nurse and a social worker as discharge planners.
4. A continuing care nurse as a consultant and coordinator of the discharge plan.

In many hospitals, the office includes several nurses who, with the physician, the unit nurses, the social workers, and other professionals, assist the patient and his family in planning for the discharge. The trend in some places is toward "Patient Services." This would include a discharge planning nurse (continuing care), social worker, professional standards review coordinator (for utilization), and a patient relations representative. In large skilled nursing facilities (SNFs) there is frequently a continuing care nurse and a social worker. The smaller homes may rely on their consultant social worker.

Discharge planning has not been well addressed by the Joint Commission on the Accreditation of Hospitals or by the American Nurses' Association for nursing standards.

Objectives of a continuing care office include the following:

1. Provide for continuity of care from a health care facility to community through planning for the patient's next level of care.

2. Facilitate the transfer of patients from a health care facility to home environment or to another facility.

3. Help physicians and allied hospital staff recognize and provide for the total post-hospital needs of the patient.

4. Make optimum use of hospital beds.

5. In addition to discharge arrangements, make followup visits to patients placed in other health care facilities or evaluate their continuing needs if they have their medical followup in the hospital clinic.[9]

Discharge planning for continuing care requires thorough evaluations of the medical, emotional, and psychosocial needs of the patient, the family, the home, and an extended care facility, if one is necessary. It is important to avoid premature discharge. It is particularly important to avoid uprooting a person from familiar surroundings without careful preparation for such a move. Sudden shifts may undermine a person's defenses and create so much anxiety that personality deterioration may result. The concept of planning with a person rather than for that person often is difficult for families and especially for the professionals to accept. Requests for outside help develop only because patients can no longer solve their problems through their own efforts. The staff in a discharge planning office must proceed with the conviction that most human beings wish to operate to the maximum of their capabilities throughout their lives and that this wish does not diminish or disappear as one's physical and emotional resources dwindle. One of the basic functions of the discharge planning office is to present all of the possible alternatives for continuing care to the patients and their families and allow them to accept responsibility for making the decisions. When the patient is mentally incompetent and there is no family, the approach would be for the various members of the staff to make a decision for the patient.

The people usually considered when describing the need for continiung care are the elderly and the chronically ill. Others may include any person who requires recuperative care or rehabilitative care. Care within the acute general hospital is expensive and is unsuited to meet the total medical, emotional, and psychosocial needs of patients after their acute illness has passed. In teaching hospitals, interns and residents focus on acute care and often see long term care as unexciting. Long term care has begun to attract the attention it requires from the health professions. A patient is entitled to a reasonable assurance that the admitting hospital will have a working relationship with other health care facilities and agencies and to expect that patient care plans planned and initiated in the hospital will be continued. Certainly hospitals must implement a workable plan for not only diagnostic workup, evaluation, and treatment but also rehabilitation and an ongoing plan of total care.

In order to achieve an ongoing plan of care, the continuing care coordinator must be skilled in:

1. *Case finding.* This is particularly important if the position is a new one. Personal observation and rounds with other nursing personnel are the most obvious ways to case find. If there are enough nurses in the continuing care unit, a formal system of Kardex rounds once a week or joining with social service for patient care rounds could be managed. The active participation of the physician in these formal discussions depends on the type of facility. In some teaching hospitals, the interns come to the rounds and present their patients to the other disciplines; others have the charge nurse present rounds. The majority

of referrals would be obtained in this manner, and often patients can be screened out at this time because of sharing information. The social worker may have known a patient from previous admissions and is continuing the same plans. These rounds provide a multidisciplinary approach to discharge planning by reviewing each patient's current status and projecting discharge planning needs. This approach sensitizes all disciplines to the problems being faced by the patient and provides an avenue for communication and coordination of care. If the continuing care coordinator is on her own, a perusal of the Kardex may be necessary to avoid overlooking patients with needs and avoid last minute plans.

2. *Assessment of continuing care needs* of patients and their families. The nurse giving direct care will have initiated an assessment before the continuing care nurse gets the referral. This is built upon and discussed, becoming another method of screening. The continuing care nurse is responsible for evaluating patients early in their stay to assess their nursing needs, activities of daily living, and their understanding of their medical conditions. The assessment is written in the patient's record. This leads to

3. *Coordinating information from a multidisciplinary team.* The continuing care nurse shares her assessment with the physician and other members of the team, which include, when possible, patients and their families. This can be done by arranging team conferences to include family. Each individual is assisted in making a plan to meet care needs in the setting which is most conducive to maximizing that individual's potential for living. Initial short term and long term goals are set, and the type of care that appears to be most suitable to meet the individual medical, nursing, and psychosocial needs of the patient is determined. In order to do this, the continuing care nurse must

4. Have an *on-going knowledge of community resources* by assessing the services offered and keeping a resource file which is readily available to anyone in the facility. The assessment is best done with followup of patients and face-to-face contact with other community agency personnel to build professional relationships. Extended care facilities should be visited so that patients can have the facility described and the programs explained to them. It becomes particularly important when the family is unable to do this for them. Once it has been established which resources are available, the continuing care nurse is responsible for

5. *Implementing the discharge plan* by matching the total patient needs with the available resources. Every effort is made to return patients to their homes when possible. Human integrity is more easily achieved in the individual's home setting, and continuity of care means maintaining the life-style of a patient as much as possible. If they are unable to return home, alternative housing should be explored, i.e., elderly housing, foster homes. Many patients can have a home plan after a transfer to an extended care facility for rehabilitation or recuperation. When a nursing home is the inevitable discharge plan, patients must be given time to adjust. It is here that the continuing care nurse and the social worker collaborate most closely. The continuing care nurse has a psychosocial orientation to patient care and is ever alert to the need for social service referral. Determination of what level of care patients need requires professional judgment which includes knowledge of their psychosocial needs, their potentials, and the measures necessary to attain or maintain optimal health status. This data, along with the more obvious physical needs, must be matched against the capability of a facility to meet the individual's needs. In this process, the continuing care coordinator is continually aware of

6. *Developing and maintaining cooperative working relationships* with other disciplines. The integration of services with a written plan is the responsibility of the continuing care coordinator, although the actual writing is done by the disciplines involved. This act of

coordinating the written plan is an excellent way to develop relationships with other disciplines. It is important to make staff members aware of referral channels and the appropriate time to initiate the referral. The continuing care coordinator should not need a referral from a private physician to initiate discharge plans. Unfortunately, some physicians do not understand the concept of continuity. In teaching hospitals this can be resolved by in-service orientation as the new house officers arrive. If offered only five minutes, take it; the time will expand with questions. With private physicians, a letter explaining what you can do for patients or asking for an appointment to explain what you have to offer patients will help. Nursing administration should insist that the coordinator needs no formal referral. Comprehensive discharge planning can only be achieved through an organized team approach which includes administration. As the coordinator case finds and screens, one of the team members she or he will contact will be the physician.

One area of the acute care hospital which has many continuing care problems is the emergency room and its holding unit area (patients are admitted for under 72 hours for observation). The following case study illustrates the concept of continuing care starting in a busy city emergency room.

Case Study

Mr. G., 80 years old, is a typical patient for whom a continuing care nurse would provide intervention. He presented in the emergency ward on a Friday morning with a history of having fallen two days previously in his apartment. His family had been unable to reach him by telephone and subsequently notified the police, who brought him to the hospital.

Review of his hospital record showed a visit to the primary care clinic two weeks prior to this visit. Chief complaint had been fatigue of approximately six months duration. A medical workup on an ambulatory basis revealed no specific causes. The problem list included chronic obstructive pulmonary disease, benign prostatic hypertrophy, left inguinal hernia, congenital strabismus, and bilateral cataracts.

Initial examination revealed multiple abrasions and fracture of the eighth rib. He was neurologically intact although he was unable to maintain himself in a sitting position; his gait was not tested. The doctor talked with the patient's niece by telephone and found that he lived alone. The niece and the patient's sister lived 30 miles away and, although they were interested in his welfare, they were unable to take him into their home at this time. The doctor felt that medically the patient could be discharged, but because his ability to care for himself at home alone was questionable, the continuing care nurse was called to assist with discharge planning.

Initial interview with Mr. G. revealed a disheveled appearing man with multiple abrasions, lying on a stretcher. He was oriented and able to carry on a conversation, but he appeared drowsy and his speech was somewhat slurred. He said that he lived alone in a third floor apartment, ate his meals out, and had been able to care for himself independently. When he was told that he might have to go home alone, he seemed to have no clear idea of his current limitations. He remembered falling in his apartment and being unable to get himself up. When asked how he thought he would be able to manage, he replied that he had neighbors who would be able to look in on him and his relatives also would be available.

The nurse in the emergency ward had ordered a lunch for Mr. G. and we were now able to observe his functional ability. When the stretcher was rolled to an upright position the patient fell to the left and had to be braced in order to sit up. He was able to feed himself using his right hand, but it was quite awkward for him. While attempting to ambulate him, we found that he required the assistance of two people to transfer from the bed to the chair and, although able to sit alone, was unstable.

It now was clear that it was impossible for Mr. G. to return home alone. When his niece was contacted she stated that her mother, Mr. G.'s sister, had recently been hospitalized and that she was kept quite busy with visiting her mother and managing her own household. However, she was concerned about her uncle and said that she would be able to take him into her home at least until nursing home placement could be arranged. She would come to get him in the late afternoon when her husband returned from work.

This seemed to be the only solution to the problem of how to care for Mr. G. if he was to be discharged. There was concern, however, because it was felt that the niece was not really aware of how much physical care Mr. G. required. There was a long weekend coming up, and the visiting nurse in the niece's community was not available for three days.

The physician was informed of the discharge plan and the reservation that it was not satisfactory. The emergency ward nurse also shared these reservations. We inquired about the possibility of a neurology consult which the doctor had at first felt was not necessary. However, with our assessment of Mr. G.'s functional ability and the history we had obtained from the family which seemed to indicate a marked change, he agreed that a neurology consult would be appropriate.

A more complete workup was then instituted including electroencephalography (EEG) and electrocardiography (ECG). Based on findings from the EEG and neurologic examination, the neurologist's impression was of a nondominant right hemispheric lesion. It was decided to admit Mr. G. for further evaluation and treatment.

He was admitted at 6 P.M. and at 8 P.M. was noted to be having difficulty breathing and increasing abdominal distention. Nasal gastric aspiration revealed coffee ground, guaiac positive material. After surgical consult he was taken to the operating room where he underwent closure of a perforation in the pylorus and extensive abdominal irrigation. Several hours postoperatively he developed density over the left lung field and underwent bronchoscopy and lavage and was on a respirator for 24 hours. When his condition stabilized he returned to his unit where he had an unstable postoperative course complicated by fever, pneumonia, and vomiting.

After about a month, his condition stabilized and he was reassessed for a discharge plan.

Mr. G. had some rehabilitation potential but had not been able to demonstrate it due to his unstable condition. The nursing assessment showed a left hemiparesis upper and lower extremity and left hemiopsia. He was not aphasic but required much stimulation to be responsive. Physical therapy and occupational therapy had begun treatment.

During the next few days through informal discussions with staff, it was shown that Mr. G. had many nursing problems. The input from the nursing staff is always invaluable in assessing a patient. Often it is the key information from the direct care givers on the patient units that is so important to determine 1) what the patient can do, 2) what nursing problems may be present for discharge, and 3) what needs to be communicated to any agency or facility as nursing priorities.

One of Mr. G.'s nursing problems was that he had an inadequate fluid intake; his foley was on a clamping schedule, but his output had dropped in response to his intake. He was still not participating in his care or transfers and was still lethargic. The nursing staff was trying hard to push fluids to maintain his intake and output. They were also trying to provide stimulation by bringing him to the nursing station for several hours a day.

Mr. G.'s case was presented at patient care rounds with the neurology residents, continuing care, social service, and physical therapy where he was seen as a diposition problem by the neurology staff. Concern was expressed at the seeming lack of potential Mr. G. showed in terms of planning for discharge.

Every patient has some "rehab potential," but not every patient is appropriate for a rehabilitation center, although most patients have the ability to attain a somewhat higher level of functional ability. For one patient, this may mean learning to feed himself after a long investment by a staff member—an investment taking months. When considering a patient for a rehabilitation center, the goals are more intensified. Is the patient able to cooperate, to follow commands? Will he benefit from intensive physical, occupational, and/or speech therapy? Is he too fragile or weak for therapy two times a day? Can his functional ability be maximized within a relatively short period of time?

Mr. G.'s physical therapist described him as being lethargic, with poor sitting balance and not able to follow commands. The occupational therapist agreed and noted that passive range of motion had begun on his left upper extremity. We were urged by the neurology residents to have Mr. G. transferred as soon as possible, but we felt that it was too early to initiate direct action. Mr. G. needed time to respond to nursing care, physical and occupational therapy. He was not a good candidate for the rehabilitation facility nearest his relatives because of his nursing care problems and his lethargy. It was appropriate for him to spend more time in the acute care facility. We explained this to the neurology residents; they agreed and we documented the plan in the record for the Professional Standards Review Organization. Continuing care's priority now was observing how the patient responded and increasing communications with his family.

A nephew of Mr. G.'s telephoned and expressed a sincere family interest and willingness to help with discharge plans. Within two days, two nephews and Mr. G.'s sister came to the continuing care office to make plans. Although social service had reviewed financial coverage with the family, they asked to have Medicare benefits for posthospital care and particularly for rehabilitation explained. They were told that Medicare would pay for an active on-going rehabilitation program in full for the first 20 days following discharge from an acute care facility and a major portion from the 21st to the 100th day, and that part of an active, on-going rehabilitation program was the patient's ability to respond and make progress in such a program. We asked the family to try and stimulate Mr. G., encourage him to eat and drink, to try to feed himself, and to pull himself up in bed with his active extremity. They, in turn, gave us additional information regarding Mr. G.'s life. He had been a policeman, married to a devoted wife, and had no children. They had lived in the same community all their lives. Fifteen years ago, just after he retired, Mr. G.'s wife died. He withdrew into their apartment, letting no one but the delivery boy in and not venturing out himself. The family was allowed to maintain contact by telephone and mail.

This information was shared with the rest of the staff immediately. This man was essentially a loner and we had him in the middle of a large unit. We were disappointed because he was not responsive and he probably was withdrawing from the noise and confusion of the large unit. We were not able to change his location but would change our approach to a more private one.

Within a day or two, Mr. G.'s sister called to tell us that many in her family had low thyroid and were treated with thyroid replacement. Perhaps this was part of her brother's problem and lack of responsiveness. She asked if the doctors could check on this and was assured it would be communicated to them. It was, and the neurology resident drew T4 and RT4s which were normal. She was reassured when told this.

During this period, the patient had not progressed too well. He continued to have varying levels of alertness, difficulty in maintaining his oral intake, and at one point required some I.V. fluids for hydration. He also had developed a decubitus ulcer which did not help his physical therapy treatments for sitting balance. The only thing in Mr. G.'s favor was that he seemed to have some return of function in his left leg.

Again Mr. G.'s case was presented at patient care rounds with the neurology staff. The residents were concerned with his lack of progress and were going to reexamine data available to see if there was a medical problem which they had overlooked that might be causing his lethargy and lack of progress.

The neurology staff was also very concerned about progress regarding his disposition because if Mr. G. checked out medically, then he did not need an acute care facility and must be discharged. We assured the residents that we would continue to follow Mr. G. and institute action when it was appropriate. We again explained that the patient needed a little more time, especially in view of further medical workup. It was fairly certain that if Mr. G.'s case was presented now to the particular facility most appropriate for his needs, he would not be accepted. It is part of the role of a continuing care nurse to affect the best discharge plan for the patient even in view of physician pressure to move the patient. The plan was documented in the patient's progress notes.

Within the next day or two, Mr. G.'s hematocrit dropped and it was questioned whether there was gastrointestinal bleeding. He was given blood transfusions, and x-rays of his gastrointestinal tract were scheduled.

During this time, we met with his nephew and sister and explained what had happened to Mr. G., why he was getting blood, and why he was scheduled for x-ray studies. They, of course, were very concerned, and Mr. G.'s sister continued to visit almost every day. We explained to them that this might account for Mr. G.'s lethargy and that when he stabilized we would need to again think about a discharge plan.

The upper gastrointestinal and barium enema tests were negative for any repeat gastrointestinal bleeding. Mr. G. seemed more responsive; he was taking fluids better, his decubitus ulcer was healing, and his foley catheter was out although he required a condom catheter. We felt it was time to initiate contact with the rehabilitation center. Arrangements were made for the screening nurse to come and see the patient within the week. This was communicated to various members of the team including Mr. G.'s family.

Mr. G. was seen by the screening nurse from the rehabilitation center and accepted for their program. The patient seemed to be gladdened by this news. His family was happy and said they had tried hard during those last several days especially to give him encouragement and a few "pep" talks.

Mr. G. waited a short period of time for a bed and was discharged to the center where he did very well. When the continuing care nurse at the center arranged for home care services, he decided to return to his old neighborhood. Mr. G. was no longer a recluse and soon came to know his neighbors. For his return appointment to clinic he was referred by the neurology resident to a nurse practitioner who soon had him involved with an elders action group.

CONCLUSION

Pressure to keep beds free for acutely ill patients has become one focus in explaining the development of discharge planning offices. The other focus is to meet the needs of patients who are physically or emotionally disabled, who have no home or have no one at home to help them. As one works with the problems of continuing care, there develops an awareness and sensitivity that there are two distinct yet interdependent aspects. The first deals with the staff who are responsible for the continuing care of patients and the system set up for the planning and delivery. The second deals with a more complex subject, namely, the health service of our country and its cost and availability of resources to meet the needs of the people today.

Additional legislation which affected the continuing care nurses' role was Public Law 92-603, popularly called the Social Security-Medicare-Medicaid Bill of 1972.[10] The President of the United States called it "landmark legislation" when he signed it. It was forecast that the measure would prove to be one of the most historic and far-reaching pieces of social legislation since the original Social Security Program was passed. There were 95 changes in the Medicare-Medicaid laws with implication for the entire health care community. One mandate was the federal monitoring of patient care evaluation—specifically, the establishment of the Professional Standards Review Organization (PSRO).

The PSRO provision created a nationwide network of locally based physician groups for reviewing the necessity, quality, and appropriateness of institutional care provided under provisions of the Social Security Act. Its purpose is to promote effective and economical health care services by requiring professional review of these services, making sure they are medically necessary and are performed in the kind of facility deemed most appropriate.[10] There were, and still are, existing quality review systems, i.e., medical audit, nursing audit, quality assurance programs. The continuing care service should have representation on these committees. If that is not possible, then at least they should have some say in the decision making processes. It is an absolute must to have representation on the PSRO or utilization committee. This legislation forces accountability by virtue of demanding written documentation of continuing care involvement and discharge planning. The continuing care coordinator and PSRO coordinator (who is often a nurse) need to have close communication so that a patient's stay is not denied when the stay is appropriate. They must consider underutilization as well as overutilization and inefficient use of resources.

The role of the continuing care nurse coordinator, particularly in the form of discharge planning, is a vital component in comprehensive health care. The technique is evolving. There is a great need for research, study, and commitment. Future trends are emphasizing home care with services at home a choice for patients rather than an alternative. Home care can save money if it prevents or shortens hospital or extended care facility stay, but home care is a complex service which must be carefully assessed and monitored.

REFERENCES

1. National Commission on Community Health Services, Report of the Commission: *Health Is a Community Affair.* Harvard University Press, Cambridge, 1967.
2. *The Nation and Its Older People.* White House Conference on Aging, U.S. Government Printing Office, Washington, D.C., 1961.
3. Hansen, Johanne, et al.: *Continuity of Nursing Care from Hospital to Home.* National League for Nursing, New York, 1966.
4. "The Coming Impact of Medicare: A Symposium." *Hospitals,* March 16, 1966, p. 51.
5. U.S. Department of Health, Education, and Welfare, Social Security Administration: *Your Medicare Handbook.* Government Printing Office, Washington, D.C., 1978.
6. The Commonwealth of Massachusetts, Department of Public Health, Massachusetts General Laws, Chapter III, Section 53, (13 Aug. 1971).

7. LaRocco, A.: *Planning for Hospital Discharge: A Bibliography with Abstracts and Research Reviews.* National Center for Health Services Research and Development, Rockville, Md., 1970.
8. David, Janis H.: "Liaison Nurse." *American Journal of Nursing,* 69(10):2142, Oct. 1969.
9. Gonnerman, Alice: "After Hospitalization, What? Discharge Planning Offers Answers." *Journal of American Hospital Association,* 69(4):81, April 1969.
10. "Public Law 92-603—Professional Standards Review Organization," American Medical Record Association, 1973.

BIBLIOGRAPHY

American Hospital Association: *Discharge Planning for Hospitals.* The Association, Chicago, 1974.
Bristow, Opal, Stickney, Carol, and Thompson, Shirley: *Discharge Planning for Continuity of Care.* National League for Nursing, New York, 1976.
David, Janis, Hansen, Johanne, Madden, Barbara, et al.: *Guidelines for Discharge Planning.* Staff Associative Ranchos Los Amigos Hospital, Cal., 1968. Charles B. Slack, Inc., Thorofare, N.J., 1973.
David, Janis H.: "Liaison Nurse." *American Journal of Nursing,* 69(10):2142, Oct. 1969.
Deakers, Lynne Power: "Continuity of Family Centered Nursing Care Between the Hospital and the Home." *Nursing Clinics of North America,* 7(1):83, March 1972.
Delberg, Andre, Gustafson, David, and Van de Ven, Andrew: *Group Techniques for Program Planning.* Scott, Foresman and Co., Glenview, Ill, 1975.
Department of Community Health Services, School of Public Health, University of Michigan. *Coordinated Home Care Manual,* 1966.
Fry, Ronald E., Plovnick, Mark S., and Rubin, Irwin M.: *Improving the Coordination of Care: A Program for Health Team Development.* Ballenger Publishing Co., Cambridge, Mass., 1978.
Gonnerman, Alice M.: "After Hospitalization, What? Discharge Planning Offers Answers." *Journal of of the American Hospital Association,* 69(4):81, April 1969.
Hamilton, Constance, Pratt, Mary, and Groen, Marion: "The Nurse's Active Role in Assessment." *Nursing Clinics of North America.* 4(2):249, June 1969.
Hansen, Johanne: *Continuity of Nursing Care From Hospital to Home.* National League for Nursing, New York, 1966.
Juntti, Jeanette M.: "Problem Solving in Arranging for Comprehensive Home Care." *Nursing Forum,* 8(1):103, Jan. 1969.
LaMontagne, Margaret, and McKeehan, Kathleen: "Profile of a Continuing Care Program, Emphasizing Discharge Planning." *Journal of Nursing Administration,* 5(8):23, Oct. 1975.
LaRocco, A.: *Planning for Hospital Discharge: A Bibliography with Abstracts and Research Reviews.* National Center for Health Services Research and Development, Rockville, Maryland, 1970.
Mitch, Anna D., and Kaezola, Sophie: "The Public Health Nurse Coordinator in a General Hospital." *Nursing Outlook,* 16(2):34, Feb. 1968, pp. 34-36.
Moreland, Helen J., and Schmitt, Virginia C.: "Making Referrals Is Everybody's Business." *American Journal of Nursing,* 74(1):96, Jan. 1974.
National Commission on Community Health Services. Report of the Commission: *Health Is a Community Affair.* Harvard University Press, Cambridge, 1967.
National League for Nursing, Council of Hospital and Related Institutional Nursing Services: *Patient Discharge and Referral Planning—Whose Responsibility?* National League for Nursing, New York, 1973.
Oregon State Health Division, Community Health Nursing Section: *Home Health Agency Advisory Committee Reference Guide.* Oregon, 1972.
Peabody, Sylvia R.: "Assessment and Planning for Continuity of Care." *Nursing Clinics of North America,* 8(2):307, June 1969.
Phillips, Harry T., and Larkin, Mary C.: "Staff Education for Continuity of Care." *Hospitals,* 46(4):54, Feb. 1972.
"Public Law 92-603 Professional Standard Review Organizations." American Medical Records Association, 1973.
Schwartz, Doris: "Communication Between Hospital Staff and Community Agencies: A Study of Referrals to the Public Health Nurse." *American Journal of Public Health,* 50(8):1122, Aug. 1960.

"The Coming Impact of Medicare: A Symposium." *Hospitals,* 40(6):51, March 1966.

The Commonwealth of Massachusetts, Department of Public Health, Massachusetts General Laws, Chapter III, Section 53, 13 Aug. 1971.

U.S. Department of Commerce, National Technical Information Service: *Planning for Hospital Discharge: A Bibliography with Abstracts and Research Reviews.* Springfield, Va., 1970.

U.S. Department of Health, Education, and Welfare, Health Resources Administration, Bureau of Health Services, Research and Evaluation: *Patient Classification for Long Term Care.* December 1973.

Virginia, Sister: "Extended Care Closes Gaps in Continuity of Care." *Hospital Progress,* Sept. 1968, p. 78.

Walter, Judith Bloom, Pardee, Geraldine, and Malbo, Doris: *Dynamics of Problem Oriented Approaches: Patient Care and Documentation.* J.B. Lippincott Company, Philadelphia, 1976.

White House Conference on Aging, 1961: *The Nation and Its Older People.* Government Printing Office, Washington, D.C., 1961.

Willard, Harved, and Kase, Stanislav: *Continuing Care in a Community Hospital.* Harvard University Press, Cambridge, 1972.

UNIT **III**
MAJOR DISEASES AFFECTING COMMUNITY HEALTH

The focus of community health nursing is the promotion and maintenance of health and healthful living. Disease prevention, whether at the primary, secondary, or tertiary level, is necessary to meet this goal. These chapters are included to orient the nurse to major causes of illness in the United States and the role community health nurses can play in their control and/or elimination.

These diseases are of particular importance because they cross many social, economic, cultural, age, and educational barriers. Individuals, families, or communities experiencing any of these conditions or at risk to develop them can be encountered by the community health nurse regardless of the role and site at which she works. Knowledge of disease impact on health status and intervention at any one of the prevention levels is imperative in the delivery of effective nursing care.

CHAPTER 21

CARDIAC AND CIRCULATORY DISEASES

ROSALYN JONES WATTS, M.S.N., R.N.

For centuries, clinicians have relentlessly searched for the multifaceted causes of heart and circulatory disturbances. Although large sums of money are allocated for cardiovascular research, ultrasophistocated diagnostic techniques, and avant-garde therapeutic modalities, heart disease remains the number one killer in the United States.

To the layman, however, the heart may be perceived as the "fountain of life," a powerful, pulsating, rhythmic force which keeps a person alive. Indeed, the lament, dispair, and anguish of a broken heart has been expressed by artists and writers. As a symbolic core of interpersonal interaction and intimacy, the heart is uniquely distinguished as the affective center for feelings and emotions.

This chapter synthesizes concepts of cardiovascular disease and psychosocial adaptation of the sick individual within the contextual framework of a systems model. More specifically, it addresses 1) dimensions of cardiovascular disease, 2) adaptation of the individual, spouse, and family to devastating illness, and 3) role of the community health nurse in preventing heart and circulatory disorders.

DIMENSIONS OF CARDIOVASCULAR DISEASE

The cardiovasular system is a highly complex, sophisticated, and closed circuited unit which consists of the heart and circulatory system, containing about 60,000 miles of blood vessels. Innumerable genetic, prenatal, physiologic, psychosocial, and environmental factors contribute to the progressive destruction and deterioration of the cardiovascular system. Each structural component of the heart, for example, may be subjected to dysfunction. This includes coronary arteries, pericardium, myocardium, endocardium, cardiac valves, and the conduction system. In addition, diseases of the blood vessels often cause damage to the major target organs, i.e., heart, brain, eyes, and kidneys. This paper focuses on the major cardiovascular disorders of coronary artery disease, hypertension, stroke, and rheumatic heart disease.

Epidemiologic Data

GENERAL STATISTICS

In 1975, the National Center for Health Statistics reported 994,514 deaths from cardiovascular disease. This excessive mortality rate is extremely high when comparing death rates from other diseases such as cancer (365,693), accidents (103,030), pneumonia (55,664), and diabetes (35,230).[1,2] In other words, more than half the deaths in the United States, some 53 percent, are attributed to disorders of the heart and blood vessels. The following data are reported regarding the percent of all deaths due to cardiovascular disease according to age group: 35-44 (27 percent), 45-54 (39 percent), 55-64 (47 percent), and 65-74 (55 percent). In other words, as the individual gets older, his chances of dying from cardiac and related disorders greatly increase. In terms of prevalence, it is estimated that 29,000,000 Americans are afflicted with cardiovascular disorders.[1,3] In summary, the estimated economic costs of cardiovascular dysfunction are projected at $28.5 billion in 1978. Such costs are attributed to loss of manpower in labor, industry, and overall health care expenditure.

SPECIFIC STATISTICS: THE MAJOR CARDIOVASCULAR DISEASES

Death due to cardiovascular disease may also be categorized according to the major type of disorder. These include: heart attack—642,719 (64.6 percent); stroke—193,038 (19.5 percent); hypertensive disease—17,327 (1.7 percent); and rheumatic heart disease—12,930 (1.3 percent).[1,2] It is essential to note that prevalence of hypertensive disease exceeds that of coronary artery disease by six to one.

HYPERTENSION

Of the estimated 24 million Americans with high blood pressure, about 20 million are white and 4 million are black. When reviewing this prevalence data in terms of the total population in the United States, hypertension is found in 15 percent of whites and 27 percent of blacks.[4] More specifically, the increased incidence of hypertensive heart disease and higher mortality rates is greater in blacks than in whites for the same age and sex groups. Furthermore, mortality and prevalence rates increase with age.

CORONARY ARTERY DISEASE

Although second to hypertension in terms of prevalence, the heart attack remains the number one killer in this country, claiming 642,719 deaths in 1975.[3] In addition, 50 to

60 percent or 350,000 of the overall cardiac deaths occur instantaneously or within 24 hours of onset of acute symptoms. This phenomenon known as *sudden death* afflicts many Americans (200,000) under 65 years of age.[5] In other words, a large percentage of the patients die at home, en route, or before entry into the health care system.

Mortality rates from ischemic heart disease are far greater for middle-aged men, both black and white, in contrast to white females. A decade later, during the menopausal years, the risk and incidence of heart disease increase for the white female. The higher mortality rates for black females are due to the greater incidence of high blood pressure in this group.[2]

Coronary artery disease must be viewed within the context of associated risk factors which are not necessarily the cause of the disease but may contribute to the proliferation of the pathophysiologic process. The major risk factors identified include hypertension, hyperlipoproteinemia, cigarette smoking, diabetes or impaired glucose tolerance, stress, and a sedentary life style. Most of these epidemiologic data were obtained during an extended health survey of the inhabitants of Framingham, Massachusetts.[2] When risk factors are combined, e.g., cigarette smoking and hypercholesterolemia, or perhaps cigarette smoking, elevated cholesterol, and hypertension, the tendency for a heart attack or stroke greatly increases.

STROKE

Mortality rates from cerebral vascular disease numbered 194,038 in 1975.[1] It is also believed that some 1,840,000 Americans are disabled by a stroke, having survived the initial insult. This disorder frequently results from sustained hypertension. In addition, cerebral vascular disease continues to be the most frequent neurologic admission to the hospital.

RHEUMATIC HEART DISEASE

Although only 12,930 deaths from rheumatic carditis were reported in 1975, this disease continues to afflict 100,000 children and 1,700,000 adults.[1] The cardiac manifestations of rheumatic fever are well documented in the literature. Rheumatic fever develops in children between the ages of 5 and 15. The clinical syndrome results in only 3 percent of the cases which develop sore throats. Deaths from rheumatic heart disease have decreased considerably with the utilization of antibiotics since the mid-1940s.[3,7]

Etiologic Factors

CORONARY ARTERY DISEASE

Recent clinical evidence suggests that sudden death results not from myocardial infarction but from a disturbance of cardiac rhythm. Such data were reflected in those persons who were successfully resuscitated and did not show electrocardiographic evidence of myocardial damage.[5] A colloquium on sudden coronary death also identified the characteristics of "recovered" heart patients who die suddenly. Such persons would display 1) ventricular bigeminy or early coupled ventricular premature beats, 2) previous heart attacks, and 3) coronary prone age.[5,8]

The development of atherosclerosis, however, is a progressive, long-termed multifactorial pathogenic process which begins with injury to the arterial intima. Other factors which contribute to the proliferation of coronary atherosclerosis are flow and pressure changes within the arteries, autonomic influences, decreased cardiac output, and alteration of the coagulation factors within the blood.[9] Eventually, the arterial lumen becomes roughened and narrowed by fatty deposits. It is now recognized that coronary thrombosis is an acute event which results within a pathologic milieu of preexisting coronary lesions. Finally, the blood supply to the myocardium is disrupted resulting in myocardial infarction. It should also be emphasized that healing of the damaged heart is facilitated through the development of collateral circulation. In approximately 6 to 12 weeks, healing and scar maturation take place within the damaged myocardium.

Let us now identify the major risk factors which continue to the generation of the atherosclerotic process and ischemic heart disease.

Lipid Abnormalities

Cholesterol, triglycerides, and phospholipids circulate in the blood as chemical aggregates known as lipoproteins. According to the lipid infiltration theory, increased proliferation and infiltration of lipids into the intimal and medial arterial walls lead to the formation of atheromas.[3]

Cigarette Smoking

Inhalation of large quantities of nicotine triggers an increased sympathetic response resulting in tachycardia, elevated blood pressure, enhanced cardiac output, and peripheral vasoconstriction. In addition, high concentrations of carbon monoxide displace oxygen from hemoglobin, thus interfering with oxygen transport at the tissue level.[10]

Diabetes

Underlying mechanisms of increased sensitivity of diabetics to heart attacks have not been pinpointed. "Silent infarcts" and cardiac arrest may be attributed to severe diabetic neuropathy.[11]

Stress

Prolonged stress potentiates cardiovascular and metabolic response resulting in 1) release of catecholamines from the adrenal medulla and subsequent mobilization of glucose and fatty acids and 2) release of aldosterone from the adrenal cortex and antidiuretic hormone from the posterior pituitary resulting in a conservation of salt and water.[12] Eventually the entire cardiovascular system, i.e., heart and vasculature, is stressed due to increased cardiac load. In addition, an increased and then decreased fibrinolytic response has been documented in patients with myocardial infarction.[12]

HYPERTENSION

In terms of etiology, hypertension is classified into two categories. These are called primary or essential hypertension and secondary hypertension. This latter classification refers to hypertension of known etiology, e.g., glomerulonephritis, renal vascular disease, coarctation of the aorta, and Cushing's disease. The etiology of primary hypertension, about

90 percent of the hypertensive population, is therefore unknown. Other clinical investigators have attempted to subclassify this group into high, normal, and low renin hypertensives. More specifically, they contend that individuals displaying high renin activity levels exhibit a greater increase in peripheral vascular resistance and cardiac output. [13] It should be emphasized that no single, isolated etiologic factor has been identified in causing hypertension. Multidimensional factors such as heredity, age, race, obesity, and sodium ingestion contribute to the development of sustained high blood pressure. In the long run, systemic hypertension causes pathophysiologic deterioration of the vasculature within the heart, eyes, kidneys, and brain, i.e., major target organs.

CEREBROVASCULAR ACCIDENT

The consumer term "stroke" refers to a disruption of the blood supply to the brain. This inadequate cerebral perfusion may be manifested by several mechanisms. These include 1) cerebral embolism—floating blood clot lodges in an atherosclerotic cerebral artery, resulting in cerebrovascular occlusion; 2) cerebral hemorrhage—bursting of a cerebral blood vessel or aneurysm resulting in bleeding into brain tissue and clot formation; and 3) compression —external pressure in a cerebral vessel by a space occupying lesion, resulting in disruption of blood flow and cerebral impairment. In an effort to repair this process, neighboring arteries enlarge in order to deliver a sufficient blood supply in the damaged area. [1,14]

RHEUMATIC HEART DISEASE

The relationship between rheumatic fever and Group A streptococcal pharyngitis has been firmly established. It should be emphasized that all sore throats are not due to streptococcal insult. Moreover, only 3 percent of streptococcal sore throats result in rheumatic fever and subsequent rheumatic heart disease. In addition, subclinical exposure of patients to the organism without clinical manifestation of pharyngitis is also possible. Furthermore, the Group A betahemolytic streptococci consist of more than 50 types, based on a serologic grouping systems, thus increasing the probability of repeated episodic attacks in susceptible persons. [15,16]

The cardiac manifestations of rheumatic fever vary with different clinical investigations. Several mechanisms are attributed to the destruction of cardiac tissue. These include: 1) direct invasion of the tissue by the streptococcal organism, e.g., Aschoff bodies found in many autopsy resorts; 2) elaboration of toxic antigens by the organism, e.g., streptolysin S; 3) progressive development of an autoimmune reaction. In some persons, rheumatic carditis develops resulting in a variety of cardiac murmurs, congestive heart failure, cardiomegaly, and pericarditis. In addition, persons with evidence of rheumatic valvular heart disease are further subjected to attacks of bacterial endocarditis. [2,7]

Clinical Characteristics of the Major Cardiovascular Disturbances

Let us examine the typical clinical profile of a client with the major cardiovascular disturbances of coronary artery disease, hypertension, stroke, and rheumatic heart disease. In terms of case finding, identification of potential problems, and clinical assessment, Table 21-1 will help the community health nurse identify the various clinical syndromes or characteristics of each disorder. More specifically, this chart presents information such as the targeted age group, common symptomatology, and standard treatment routines

TABLE 21-1. Client profile of major cardiovascular disorders*

	Coronary Artery Disease	Hypertension	Cerebrovascular Accident	Rheumatic Heart Disease
Age group	Middle age and older (40–59)	Young adult, middle age and older	Middle age and older	Children (5–15 yrs.) Adults
Synonym	Ischemic heart disease Coronary thrombosis Myocardial infarction	Silent killer High blood pressure	Stroke C.V.A.	– – –
Symptoms	*Warning signs* Uncomfortable pressure, fullness, squeezing, or pain in center of chest lasting 2 minutes or more. Pain not relieved by nitroglycerine. Pain may spread to shoulders, neck, or arms. Severe pain, dizziness, fainting, sweating, nausea, or shortness of breath. Symptoms may subside and and then return.	*Warning signs* No warning signals in majority of patients. Early detection and screening essential. A few patients may describe: dull occipital headache in a.m., weakness, fatigue, palpitation, hematuria.	*Warning signs* Sudden temporary weakness or numbness in face, arm, leg, or one side of body. Temporary loss of speech. Difficulty in understanding speech. Temporary dimness or loss of vision in one eye. Unexplained dizziness. Sudden falls. Recent change in personality or mental ability.	*Major manifestations* Polyarthritis Chorea Erythema marginatum Subcutaneous nodules Carditis Cardiomegaly Congestive heart failure Pericarditis Cardiac Murmurs: Mitral stenosis, Mitral insufficiency, Aortic stenosis, Aortic insufficiency *Minor manifestations* Previous rheumatic fever Fever
Medical management during postacute period	*Cardiac rehabilitation* Return to optimum levels of functioning Medications: vasodilators, diuretics, digoxin Dietary restrictions	*Drug management* Thiazide diuretics Sympatholytics Hydralazine Beta blockers Dietary control	*Stroke rehabilitation* Relearning ADL (Activities of Daily Living) Facilitating independence	*Continuous antibiotic prophylaxis* Benzathine penicillin G.I.M. Penicillin G. Oral or Sulfadiazine Oral
Nursing intervention	Clinical assessment Client and family education	Monitoring blood pressure Client education Facilitating patient compliance with medical routine	Clinical assessment Individual patient and family education re: illness and potential for optimal recovery	Clinical assessment Health screening, promotion, and consumer education

*Synthesized from American Heart Association literature.[1,6,9]

which facilitates the nurse's understanding of the spectrum of clinical disorders and anticipated methods of nursing intervention.

In summary, it should be emphasized that the typical "coronary prone" male is middle-aged or older and afflicted with single or multiple risk factors. Some of these risk factors cannot be changed, e.g., family history, race, and age. Other risk factors, however, can be changed with sufficient medical and nursing intervention. For example, abnormal elevations of the following clinical findings could be altered: [1,9]

1. Hypertension: greater than 140/90.
2. Lipid abnormalities: serum cholesterol of more than 260 mg. percent; fasting triglyceride of more than 250 mg. percent.
3. Uric acid levels: greater than 7.5 mg. percent.
4. Abnormal glucose tolerance and diabetes: elevated blood sugar or glucose tolerance test.

Finally, risk factors such as cigarette smoking, diet, stress, and exercise can be changed by the person at risk who is well informed about the clinical disorder and highly motivated to assume responsibility for his own health.

Unfortunately, the hypertensive patient does not realize that he can be symptom free and walking around with sustained, elevated blood pressure. Health screening programs conducted within the community or indeed multiphasic screening programs by the American Heart Association may help with case finding. It has also been established that half of the hypertensive population are aware of their disorder and less than half of this number are adequately treated. [13] The potential for the hypertensive consumer to develop a stroke has also been well documented. Some of these persons may develop Transient Ischemic Attacks (T.I.A.), i.e., display transient neurologic symptoms which last from a few seconds to several hours. Others may present with a progressive stroke over a period of days, thus exhibiting increased neurologic deterioration. Still others may be incapacitated with rapidly destructive cerebral impairment.

Finally, patients with rheumatic valvular heart disease are susceptible to virulent bacterial endocarditis. These individuals need additional prophylactic antibiotic therapy whenever they undergo surgical or dental procedures. In addition, as persons with rheumatic heart disease approach the third and fourth decade of life, progressive valvular deterioration and hemodynamic changes in the myocardium are evident. These persons are potential candidates for cardiac surgery and replacement of the diseased valves with prosthetic devices.

CURRENT TREATMENT MODALITIES

The utilization of the coronary care unit since the early 1960s has helped to reduce in-hospital mortality rates. Patients die from complications of myocardial infarction such as dysrhythmias, congestive heart failure, and profound cardiogenic shock. Many patients will be successfully treated in coronary or critical care units and thus survive initial or repeated coronary insults. Such treatment includes standard drug therapy with electrocardiagraphic and hemodynamic monitoring. Patients will spend three or four days in an ultrasophisticated, highly technologic environment and later are transferred to a stepdown or progressive care unit. Most patients with uncomplicated myocardial infarctions will complete a hospital stay of ten days to two weeks.

Coronary artery bypass surgery is considered to be a reasonable therapeutic option for patients with coronary artery disease. The primary objectives of this surgery are to 1) provide symptomatic relief of angina, 2) improve left ventricular function, 3) prevent myocardial infarction, and 4) prolong life. For many individuals, symptomatic relief from anginal pain has helped to improve the quality of life. Promotion of longevity continues to be investigated by clinicians by utilizing prospective randomized studies or retrospective matched studies. It should be emphasized that all heart attack victims need not be treated with surgery. Appropriate candidates for coronary artery bypass surgery should include individuals with unstable angina pectoris unresponsive to medical management, Prenzmetal's angina (chest pain at rest), main left coronary artery disease, and immediate post-infarction patients with unstable angina. [17]

Individuals with rheumatic heart disease may eventually undergo open heart surgery during the adult years. Such persons may have inserted prosthetic devices or heterographs to replace diseased mitral or aortic valves.

In summary, community health nurses must recognize that consumers with cardio-vascular diseases may become ill from a heterogeneous group of disorders. Some of these patients have been subjected to medical and/or surgical therapeutic modalities, whereas others have failed to enter any health care system.

ADAPTATION TO ILLNESS: A SYSTEMS PERSPECTIVE

Let us now explore the adaptation of the sick individual within the contextual framework of a systems theoretical perspective. More specifically, let us use the typical coronary prone middle-aged, married family man in presenting our case.

The Systems Model

Systems theory is currently utilized as a conceptual framework by many scientists from a variety of disciplines. [18] This orientation perceives the world as a holistic unit, a constellation of suprasystems and subsystems, which recognizes the interplay of innumerable components within and outside each system. Most social scientists believe that man, the family, and the community are open systems with the capacity for growth and maturation. [19] The human being may be viewed as a system possessing both physiologic subsystems and psychosocial value systems. A person does not function as an isolated entity within an amorphous environmental vacuum but actively interacts with others within the context of dyadic, familial, and community suprasystems. Normal life cycle changes or superimposed crises may disrupt the equilibrium or homeostasis of the personal, marital, and family systems. Application of the general systems model to the social context of relationships may help clarify the pervasive impact of illness on the individual and significant others in his life.

Normative Developmental Life Cycles of the Individual – Marital and Family Systems

Research on the psychosocial development of the adult has identified predictable, characteristic, age-specific events through which the individual, the marital relationship, and family life progresses. These critical periods are intricately interrelated and intertwined and thus should not be viewed as separate entities. From a systems perspective, the intrapersonal turmoil of the coronary prone male affects his attitudes, emotions, and behaviors, thus eventually disrupting equilibrium within marital and family systems.

Normative Life Cycle During Adulthood

The stages of psychosocial development throughout the lifespan of man have been postulated by Erickson.[20] In other words, the eight ages of man extend from the period of basic trust vs. mistrust until the final period of ego integrity vs. despair. Other investigators such as Lidz,[21] Gould,[22] and Levinson[23] have pinpointed psychosocial developmental tasks of adulthood which must be dealt with by every person. More specifically, Levinson divided adulthood into seven distinctive stages from pulling up roots (18 to 21 years) until older age (60 years and over). No person progresses through life unperturbed or unruffled but must confront such issues as autonomy, intimacy, commitment, and ordering of priorities. The coronary prone person may be struggling with the conflicts of midlife explosion during his 40s or aspiring for greater intimacy during the mellowing years of the 50s.

MARITAL LIFE CYCLE

Berman and Lief[24] identified the critical stages of marital life which range from shifting from the family of origin to new commitment until the final stage of mutual support for productivity and fulfillment in the aging couple. Dyadic relationships deal with interpersonal struggles such as power, intimacy, and inclusion or exclusion of persons within the marital system. Ironically enough, although divorce rates are soaring in this country, many persons continue to marry and remarry.

FAMILY LIFE CYCLE

Duvale[25] has proposed a longitudinal view of family development which extends from a beginning family (married couple without children) to the aging family (retirement or death of both spouses).[26] The primary tasks of the family are to provide basic physical needs, establish a marital unit, and enhance the personality development and enculturation of offspring. Most family therapists view the marital unit, a subsystem of the family system, as the executive unit, facilitator and orchestrator of family life. Structural family therapist Minuchin[27] asserts that the parental coalition must be maintained in addition to generational boundaries between parents and children. The development of gender identity and appropriate sex-linked roles is facilitated within the context of family interactional patterns. One can readily see that neurotic, disorganized, and chaotic family life frequently results if the marital unit is dysfunctional. Such disorder eventually affects each person in the family system.

In summary, having reviewed the normal sequential development of crises within the individual, dyadic, and family systems, we must assume that each system is interrelated to the other. Table 21-2 is an encapsulated summary of the developmental stages, tasks, and description of each system, as the individual progresses through adulthood.

Attitudes and Behavior of Cardiovascular Patients

CORONARY PRONE PERSONALITY

The concept of a coronary prone personality is not a 20th century invention. Sir John Hunter in the 18th century and Sir William Osler, leading cardiologist in the 19th century,

TABLE 21-2. Developmental stages of adult life: a perspective from each system

System	Individual stages	Marital stages	Family stages
Source	Levinson,[23] Gould,[22] Lidz,[21] and Erickson[20]	Berman and Lief[24]	Duvale[25] Glick and Kessler[26]
Stage: 1 (18–21 years)	Pulling up roots Developing autonomy	Shift from family of origin to new commitment	Beginning family: married couple without children
Stage: 2 (22–28 years)	Provisional adulthood Developing intimacy Occupational identification	Provisional marital commitment Uncertainty about marital partner Stress over parenthood	Child bearing family: oldest child up to 30 months
Stage: 3 (29–31 years)	Transition at 30 Deciding on commitment to work and marriage	Commitment crises Rates of individual growth may diverge Restlessness	Families of preschool children: oldest child 30 months to 6 years
Stage: 4 (32–39 years)	Settling down Deepening commitments Pursue long range goals	Productivity: children, work, friends, and marriage Each spouse has different way of achieving productivity	Families with school children: oldest child, 6–13 years
Stage: 5 (40–42 years)	Mid-life transition Search for place between aspirations and environment	Summing up: evaluation of successes, failures, goals Tenuous intimacy Power conflicts	Families with teenagers: oldest child, 13–20 years
Stage: 6 (43–59 years)	Middle adulthood Reordering priorities Search for intimacy	Resolving conflicts and stabilizing the marriage Different rates of emotional growth Intimacy threatened by boredom	Families as launching centers during the middle years First child gone and last child leaving home Empty nest to retirement
Stage: 7	Dealing with aging process Retaining zest for life	Supporting/enhancing the other Fear of loneliness, sex, failure	Aging families Retirement to death of both spouses

attributed arterial degeneration to occupational stresses and life style. [28] Recent investigators, such as Friedman and Rosenman, [29] integrated psychological and behavioral factors which contributed to the proliferation of coronary artery disease. For example, Friedman describes the classic type A coronary prone personality as:

"... a characteristic action emotion complex which is exhibited by those individuals who are engaged in a chronic struggle to obtain an unlimited number of poorly defined things from their environment in the shortest period of time ..."[29]

At the opposite end of the continuum is the type B individual who is described as relaxed, unhurried, and mellow. [28] Jenkins further delineated clinical cues for identifying type A and type B persons. It should be emphasized that few, if any, persons are pure type A or type B, but many show a clustering or preponderance of behavioral patterns of each designated type. Table 21-3 summarizes the distinguishing features of the polarized behavioral styles.

PREADMISSION BEHAVIOR

As stated in a previous section, the majority of cardiac patients, at least 60 percent, die of sudden death before reaching the hospital. Therefore, delay in seeking medical help or, indeed, the prolonged decision time accounts for the high percentage of preadmission deaths. In fact, the hospital arrival time for most patients ranges between 2.5 and 4 hours. [30] Other investigators report that factors such as educational background, occupation, and socioeconomic class are not significant in determining whether or not persons

TABLE 21-3. Comparison of Type A and Type B behavioral patterns*

	Type A	Type B
Values	Inner directed	Less competitive, enjoy sports
	Competitive; crave recognition and power	Deny desire for power
	Conscientious, responsible	
Style of thought	Do many things simultaneously	Relaxed, nonhurried
	Achievement oriented	Values socialization
	Vigilant in expression and posture	Notices environment, astute observer
Interpersonal relationships	Self-centered	Interested in others
	Anger easily aroused	Less frustrated at work
	More frustrated in work situation	
	Aggressive sexually—"loves the chase"	
Overt behavioral characteristics	Talks loudly, rapidly, and with emphasis	Uses gratifying phrases, may circumvent a point
	Interrupts	Listens intently
	Tense, energetic movements	Looser style
	Clench hands	Takes time to generate full smile
	Flash momentary tense smile	Slow rhythmic breathing
	Hearing sighing	

*Synthesized from Jenkins, [28] Rosenman, [48] and Friedman. [29]

attempt to get to the hospital. Older patients, however, will attempt to seek medical help more so than younger individuals.[30] Furthermore, Moss and associates have identified a progression of three separate cognitive functions involved in the decision making process. In other words, the patient must 1) perceive presenting symptoms, 2) recognize the severity of the symptoms, and 3) realize or acknowledge that medical care is indicated.[30,31] Other investigators have also indicated that denial is the primary defense mechanism operating during the preadmission phase. Finally, it is now recognized that self-medication and also delay on the part of the physician in advising patients to seek hospitalization contributes to the overall delay.[31]

Impact of Illness on the Individual and Family

INDIVIDUAL ADAPTATION

Most critical care nurses are familiar with the severely ill coronary patient who is incapacitated by intense pain, fear of death, and an overall display of anxiety in the highly technical, sophisticated milieu of the coronary or intensive care unit. He then progresses to a period of denial in which it is difficult for him to believe that he had a heart attack. Finally, around day 3 or 4, the patient may become profoundly depressed and thus devastated, perplexed, and angered by the realization of a heart attack. Cassem and Hackett,[32,33] further assert that premorbid abrasive personality traits become evident by day 5 or 6. In addition, his diminished self-esteem, sense of masculinity, or, as described by Cassem, "ego infarction" are manifested when he reflects on the innumerable psychosocial and socioeconomic losses which result because of the cardiac insult.[33] It is important to note that, although efforts are made to encourage self-involvement and independence as patients improve and become less dependent on nursing care while hospitalized, the individual must adapt to this anxiety provoking situation. Moos and Tsu[34] have categorized the major adaptive tasks upon the hospitalized patient. These illness related tasks include dealing with pain and incapacitation, hospital environment and treatment intervention, and developing relationships with professional staff. They describe more general adaptive tasks as preserving emotional balance, self-image, and relationships with family and friends. More importantly, however, preparing for an uncertain, unpredictable, and questionable future tends to be a major source of anxiety.

ADAPTATION OF THE SPOUSE AND FAMILY

In viewing the middle-aged, coronary prone male within the context of his developmental, marital, and family life cycles, one can readily perceive that the devastating aftermath of a myocardial infarction may be viewed as a grieving process which involves the individual and his entire family. Most studies indicate that anxiety, irritability, and most of all depression were common in patients during the convalescent stages.[35] In terms of the marital relationship, many wives are confused and conflicted in relating to a husband, a former breadwinner, protector, dominant force, and decision maker, who must modify his role within the marital and family systems. Many husbands feel trapped and angered over the oversolicitousness and overprotectiveness of the spouse. The wife, on the other hand, may feel guilty in causing her husband to have a heart attack. In other words, the profound depression, fatigue, and significant shift in marital and family roles result in disequilibrium and subsequent marital and family stress. Fear of resuming sexual intercourse may also help to foster a feeling of inadequacy and decreased masculinity. If a relationship was characterized by power struggles, mistrust, and a lacking of intimacy, then resumption of sexual activity may be more difficult during the postcoronary period. [36] Many investigators report that regardless of the quality of the relationship, marital conflict developed during the convalescent period primarily due to misunderstanding about ischemic heart disease, misinterpretation of instructions, lack of information, and poor patterns of communication. [35,36] Kasl [37] further describes the paradoxic dilemma confronting the recovering cardiac patient who is neither severely ill or extremely healthy. Situated in a twilight state of ambiguity and perplexity, the "at risk" role of the heart patient is characterized by an indefinite life span, reduced social obligations, and lack of continuous reinforcement from health professionals.

Community Implications

Return of the patient to optimal levels of physiologic and psychosocial function is the primary aim of cardiac rehabilitation. The most essential variable in measuring and projecting appropriate vocational and physical adjustment is the patient's perception of his own health. Factors which influence patient perception of the pervasive effects of a heart attack include his past personal biases and experiences, understanding of his illness, and communication with his physician. Self-esteem, self-worth, and an overall feeling of well-being are enhanced when a cardiac patient is successfully rehabilitated and thus returns to work. A comprehensive medical evaluation system for returning to work should include a review of clinical course of the patient, updated physical examination, appropriate blood studies, chest x-ray, and resting electrocardiogram. Stress testing is also emphasized by some cardiologists. The exercise electrocardiogram helps to identify readiness or nonreadiness for employment and psychologically reduces ambiguities regarding work capacity. These tests may begin 7 to 11 weeks after myocardial infarction. (See section on cardiac rehabilitation).

The committee on Stress, Strain, and Heart Disease of the American Heart Association [9] recommended that the community become more informed about the nature and scope of heart disease and the overall employment potential of the cardiac victim. Such key community persons include physicians in clinical and industrial practice, lawyers, insurers, employers, union representatives, and workmen's compensation lawyers. They also suggested that the American Heart Association assume a more active role in facilitating [9] 1) modification of practices which may inhibit the reemployment of heart patients, all of which could be accomplished by enhancing communication between concerned groups, 2) wider application of second injury compensation laws to heart victims, 3) greater enforcement of the Vocational Rehabilitation Act of 1973 which is applicable to cardiac patients and encourages increased employment opportunities through "affirmative action" programs.

Other Significant Research on Consumer Health

We have already established that normal developmental changes occur within the individual, marital, and family life cycles. In addition, having examined the impact of illness on the individual and his family, let us now review how significant life changes may negatively affect the health of the consumer. It is now recognized that a clustering of events within the life of an individual may evoke a psychophysiologic reaction and thus precipitate illness in a susceptible person. Clinical investigators Holmes and Rahe [38] have ranked 43 life events in a social readjustment rating scale and assigned a mean value to each one of these happenings. Examples of such events include:

#1 rank: Death of a spouse   Mean value = 100
#11 rank: Change in health of family member   Mean value = 44
#25 rank: Outstanding personal achievement   Mean value = 28

In addition, a person is administered a questionnaire entitled "Schedule of Recent Experience" which lists specific critical events which have occurred within the last six months. From the data, the researcher can tabulate and quantify a sum commonly called life change units (LCU). Clinical investigations now indicate that a person with more than 300 LCUs has an 80 percent probability of getting sick in the near future. Prospective and retrospective European studies have corroborated these findings in cardiac patients by noting the life change units were significantly higher in fatalities from myocardial infarction than in survivors.[39] In addition, the exacerbation of other illnesses has also been associated with increased life change units. These include diabetes, duodenal ulcers, fractures, athletic injuries, and traffic injuries.[38]

Such information is vital for community health nurses in counseling patients to modify or postpone a cluster of stressful life events. In addition, this data reflects the necessity for assessing the client within the context of his marital and family situation.

DIVERSIFIED ROLE OF THE COMMUNITY HEALTH NURSE IN PREVENTION OF DISEASE

The role of the community nurse in providing optimal health care is extremely diversified and multidimensional. She or he may be perceived as a change agent who directly administers nursing care to clients in the community or as a health facilitator, utilized primarily as a consultant, coordinator, educator, and researcher of community problems.

Let us examine the various intervention strategies which may be used by the nurse in promoting health and preventing disease. Health professionals have categorized the prevention of disease according to three levels of primary, secondary, and tertiary prevention.[40] *Primary prevention* focuses on the prepathogenic period and deals with concepts of health promotion and specific measures to forestall disease or injury. *Secondary prevention* is directed toward forestalling or disrupting the already established decrease process by means of early diagnosis, prompt treatment, and limiting the disability through the formulation of realistic goals. *Tertiary prevention* concentrates on the rehabilitative aspect of illness with nursing activities directed toward restoring the patient to optimal levels of physiologic, psychosocial, and vocational functioning. The community health nurse, therefore, plays a vital role in preventing the major cardiovascular diseases of coronary artery disease, hypertension, stroke, and rheumatic heart disease.

Primary Prevention

HEALTH APPRAISAL OF THE COMMUNITY

Before undertaking any program of health promotion, education, or screening, community health nurses should become more informed about the total health concerns of the community. In other words, health appraisal of the specific community should precede any screening program for cardiovascular disturbances. The community, therefore, is treated as "the patient" with specific needs, interests, and problems.

The community health nurse may be involved in assessing the health status of the target population or group.[2] Several group health indicators may provide these data. These include:

1. Symptoms and complaints—home, school, work
2. Risk factors—blood pressure, cholesterol
3. Disease categories—heart disease and others
4. Mortality
5. Level of social functioning—work and school attendance, ability to do housework, disability
6. Measures of population growth—birth, fertility, death rates, life expectancy, drug and alcohol abuse
7. Measures of health care utilization

Such data may be obtained by questionnaire, interview, clinical observations, records of health care facilities, records of reportable diseases, and community vital statistics. Once this information is obtained directly or indirectly by the community health nurse, she or he may be involved in designing and implementing a cardiovascular screening program which would be meaningful to the target group. A hypertension screening program, for example, in a black community may take place in a hospital lobby, community health center, mobile unit, church educational building, shopping center, and so forth. Subsequent strategies for further health planning, intervention, and evaluation would follow the screening program.

MODIFYING THE RISK FOR CARDIOVASCULAR DISEASE

It has already been stated that risk factors such as heredity, sex, race, and age cannot be changed. Since the majority of Americans living in a highly mobile, technologic, stressful society are almost destined to die of cardiac and related disorders, efforts should be made for modifying potential risk factors which could be changed. These include: cigarette smoking, diet, stress, and sedentary living. In addition, consumers need to be more informed about the potential hazards of a streptococcal sore throat.

The public health nurse may be used as a health educator in the school or community. Programs of family life education could be offered within a community center, local YMCA, consciousness raising groups, or church groups, or as continuing education courses in local high schools and colleges. The primary philosophy of this health education approach is to emphasize the concept of self-care and self-help. In other words, each person is responsible for himself and must become informed about his health status and potential changes in his body. The content of these courses should include information about anatomy and physiology, nutrition, dangers of cigarette smoking, concepts of mental health, and referral options. Audiovisual materials, patient education, handouts, and consumer oriented American Heart Association films frequently reinforce the concepts presented in didactic lectures. In addition, small group discussions may help participants deal with feelings and anxieties of young adults in the process of parenting. Health education, therefore, begins at home prior to schooling. Such community based health education programs are nonexistent in most areas of the country. It is now recognized that most health curricula in public schools should discuss the hazards of smoking, inadequate dietary habits, the importance of exercise, and other health issues.

FAMILY HEALTH RECORD

Community health nurses are frequently involved in case finding. For example, prevention of initial attacks of rheumatic fever requires that clients recognize and secure proper treatment of upper respiratory tract infections. It is difficult for parents or patients to recall not only symptomatology associated with rheumatic fever but also other important health data related to the medical history of the individual and the family constellation. For these reasons Sehnert[41] has recommended the compilation of a family health record. The major components of this record include:

I. *Emergency numbers:* family doctor, dentist, pharmacist, ambulance, emergency hospital, poison control center.
II. *Birth information in nuclear family:*
   1. Listing of father, mother, and each child
   2. Pertinent data on each person—birthday, birth weight and height, mother's health during pregnancy, delivery (normal/abnormal), condition at birth, blood type.
III. *Family History* (family of origin and nuclear family):
   1. Grandparents, uncles, aunts, parents, and children
   2. Data regarding specific disease—cancer, diabetes, heart, hypertension, stroke, allergies, alcohol or drug abuse, age of death and cause of death
IV. *Drug record for each person:* name of drug, reason for usage, allergic reactions.
V. *Record of laboratory tests and procedures:* x-rays, electrocardiograms, blood work, pap tests.
VI. *Accidents, surgery, hospitalization record:* name of person, date, age, what happened, severity and complications

SECONDARY PREVENTION

EARLY DIAGNOSIS AND PROMPT TREATMENT

Once the individual has become afflicted with a cardiovascular disease, this person and significant others within the family system should become knowledgeable about the early warning signals of heart attacks and impending strokes. In addition, community health nurses should instruct these persons about medications, treatment options, and alternatives in adapting to the specific illness. (See Table 21-1 for the overall client profile of major cardiovascular diseases.) Some authorities have recommended that family members learn the basic lifesaving technique of cardiopulmonary resuscitation. Although some communities have mobile life support units or ambulance services, immediate intervention by a family member may prevent sudden death. Such consumer oriented cardiopulmonary resuscitation (CPR) programs have been sponsored by the American Heart Association.

HEALTH PROMOTION MEASURES FOR LIMITING DISABILITY

Community health nurses may be instrumental in designing, implementing, or facilitating intervention strategies in an effort to promote health. Many persons, for example, participate in behavior modification programs, relaxation techniques, and physical exercise programs. The advantages and benefits of such regimens are as follows:

1. *Behavior modification* refers to a systematic application of the principles of learning to the analysis and treatment of problematic, disturbing, and destructive behaviors. These techniques are used in a variety of clinical settings in the treatment of such disorders as alcoholism, phobias, and sexual problems. These techniques may also be useful in modifying such maladaptive behavioral risk factors as cigarette smoking and overweight. [42] Clients may be referred to outpatient clinics which utilize a behavioral approach.

2. *Relaxation techniques* have been practiced by the Eastern and Western religious mystics for centuries. The secular world, however, has also been exposed to the techniques of self-hypnosis, transcendental meditation, and progressive relaxation as proposed by Jacobson. [42] The relaxation response may be defined as a hypometabolic condition in which the individual achieves a tranquil state of generalized diminished psychophysiologic activity. Attainment of such a state may be helpful in counteracting highly stressful, anxiety provoking states within the cardiovascular patient. The relaxation response, according to experimental evidence, elicits decreased muscle tone, blood pressure, heart rate, and respiration. Relaxation techniques have been used as a therapeutic modality in treatment of alcohol and drug abuse. Other clinical investigators have successfully used such techniques in lowering the blood pressure of hypertensive patients. [43] Community health nurses could also consider such methods for clients as adjuncts to therapy.

3. *Exercise and physical fitness programs* have been emphasized within the last several years. Middle-aged, coronary prone individuals and persons who have recovered from a myocardial infarction may benefit from participation in supervised community physical fitness programs. It should be noted that phase IV of cardiac rehabilitation represents the period of recovery in which the individual is able to carry out the activities of daily living and returns to work. Before any exercise program is initated, the cardiac status of the individual should be evaluated by stress treadmill testing. After such a procedure, an individualized exercise prescription is written which defines the target heart rate, duration, frequency, and recommended activities. The psychologic benefits of exercise training after recovery from a heart attack are an improvement in well-being, self-confidence, and diminished anxiety and depression. Physiologic benefits reported include a lowering of heart rate, systolic pressure, and cardiac output. For many persons the severity of arrhythmias and anginal episodes is also decreased. Once again, community health nurses could refer their clients to well-supervised, medically controlled programs in such settings as the YMCA, Jewish community centers, community athletic clubs, and so forth. Exercise programs are contraindicated in patients with progressive angina pectoris, uncontrolled congestive heart failure, uncontrolled hypertension, arrhythmias, and uncontrolled diabetes. [44,45]

Tertiary Prevention

HEALTH APPRAISAL OF CLIENTS WITH CARDIOVASCULAR DISEASES

Health assessment of the chronically ill patient is essential for the community health nurse to determine if the client is maintaining the status quo or developing further complications. Most schools of nursing have incorporated health assessment skills into their curricula. Such skills are useful to the nurse who may be seeing the client in a community health center or in the home. The following outline identifies the major systems which should be assessed in monitoring the status of patients with heart and circulatory diseases. It is also assumed that the reader is already familiar with the basic concepts and approaches to the history and physical examination.

I. Data base: name, address, phone number, and referring physician or referring clinical agency
II. Referral summary
III. Listing of medical and nursing problems
IV. History:
   1. Family history
   2. Past medical history:

Congenital heart disease	Diabetes	Obesity
Rheumatic heart disease	Hypertension	Smoking
Angina pectoris	Cerebral vascular accident	Other stress factors
Myocardial infarction	Hyperlipoproteinemia	

   3. Significant life changes or events in the last six months
   4. Inquiry about significant symptoms:

Chest pain	Palpitation	Cyanosis	Fatigue
DOE	Cough	SOB	Weight gain
Orthopnea	Nocturia	Hemoptysis	Syncope
Edema	Phlebitis	PND	Pallor

   5. Inquire about stroke related symptoms—difficulty with balance, weakness, paralyses, memory lapses, difficulty in speaking
   6. Review of other systems if necessary
V. Physical examination:
   1. Vital signs
   2. Neck:
      Venous jugular system and arterial system: engorgement of veins, presence of normal/abnormal pulsation, scars, bruit, graduation of carotid pulsation
      Thyroid: enlarged, nodular, bruit
      Trachea: position, midline/deviated
      Lymph nodes: anterior and posterior cervical, pre- and postauricular, supraclavicular
      Salivary glands: enlargement of parotoid, submaxillary
   3. Chest and lungs:
      General inspection: contour, symmetry, expansion, rate and rhythm, use of accessory muscles
      Percussion: resonance, flatness, comparison of symmetrical areas, diaphragmatic level, and movement
      Auscultation: character and intensity of breath sounds, duration of inspiration and expiration, rales, friction rub, and adventitious sounds
   4. Heart:
      Inspection: abnormal impulses, point of maximal impulse (P.M.I.)
      Palpation: check forceful, sustained, displaced left ventricular impulse; check for thrills
      Auscultation: cardiac rate and rhythm, intensity of S_1 and S_2, physiologic splitting, extracardiac sounds (S_3 and S_4), murmurs and their location, timing, intensity, quality, configuration, and duration

5. Nervous system:
    Gait posture
    Motor system: examination for weakness
    Sensory system: pain, touch, dermatome distribution
    Deep tendon reflexes, superficial reflexes, and pathologic reflexes
    Assessment of cranial nerves
    Mental status: orientation, memory, aphasia
VI. Formulation of a nursing diagnosis

Once the nurse completes the health appraisal she or he could determine if the clinical status of the client is stable or if further consultation is warranted. In addition, the nurse should compare the findings with the verbal or written report from the referring agency.

CARDIAC REHABILITATION

This section will concentrate on rehabilitation of heart patients. The reader should consult medical-surgical texts for a full discussion of rehabilitation of the stroke victim. Restoration of the client to optimal levels of physiologic and psychosocial functioning is the primary goal of rehabilitation. Cardiac rehabilitation, currently categorized into four distinct stages, begins the day after hospitalization. These phases, according to Wenger,[45] consist of: phase I—coronary care unit; phase II—remainder of hospitalization; phase III—convalescence; and phase IV—period of recovery or maintenance. The community health nurse, however, will usually have contact with clients during convalescence and recovery when the individual has returned home. Although a large number of hospitals have designed patient education programs or discharge planning for cardiac patients, many persons return to the community without receiving adequate instruction or teaching about their illness. The following teaching outline may be utilized by nurses with individuals or groups of clients with heart disorders. In other words, areas of course content should include: 1) concepts of cardiac rehabilitation; 2) atherosclerotic disease process—nature of a heart attack; 3) risk factor modification; 4) nutritional information; 5) understanding medications; 6) exercise and heart disease; 7) psychosocial adaptation to illness; and 8) guidelines for patients during the convalescent and recovery period.[46] Inclusion of family members in any teaching program is beneficial to the client and the entire family.

Community Resources

More community resources are available to clients and families with cardiovascular disturbances. Group discussion for families of stroke victims and sessions for cardiac patients and their spouses are also proliferating. Harding and Morefield[47] describe group meetings with the wives of patients with myocardial infarction. Such issues as depression, grieving, communication, work, and sexual fears were discussed in an open, accepting, and therapeutic setting. Many projects are also sponsored by the local chapters of the American Heart Association. In addition, many lay organizations help clients and their families deal with innumerable psychosocial and economic problems which devastate family functioning. For example, chapters of groups such as "Sharing and Caring" and "Smokenders" are located in many communities throughout the United States.

SUMMARY

Heart and circulatory disease remains the number one killer of Americans who live in a highly complex, sophisticated, and anxiety provoking society. This chapter explored the dimensions of cardiovascular disease. In order to clarify the scope and magnitude of the problem, epidemiologic data, etiologic factors, clinical presentation, and current treatment modalities were reviewed.

Also examined were the impact of illness on the sick individual, his spouse, and family. The use of a systems theoretical framework helped to explain how dysfunctioning in one person will eventually disrupt the equilibrium within the total family system. Finally, the diversified role of the community health nurse at the primary, secondary, and tertiary levels of health prevention was also described.

REFERENCES

1. American Heart Association: *Heart Facts 1978.* The Association, New York, 1977.
2. Hogue, C.: "Epidemiology per Distributive Nursing Practice," in Hall, J., and Weaver, B. (eds.): *Distributive Nursing Practice—A Systems Approach to Community Health.* J.B. Lippincott Co., Philadelphia, 1977.
3. Wintrobe, M., et al.: *Harrison's Principle of Internal Medicine,* 6th ed. McGraw-Hill Book Co., New York, 1970.
4. Smith, W. McFate: "Epidemiology of Hypertension." *Medical Clinics of North America,* 61:467, May 1977.
5. *Cooper Colloquium on Sudden Coronary Death.* KPR Information/Media Corporation, Cooper Laboratories, 919 Third Avenue, New York, New York, 10022, May 1973.
6. American Heart Association: *Diagnosis and Management of Stroke.* The Association, New York, 1968.
7. Committee on Rheumatic Fever and Bacterial Endocarditis of the Council on Cardiovascular Disease in the Young: *Prevention—Rheumatic Fever Prevention.* American Heart Association, New York, 1967.
8. Roberts, W.: "Pathology of Sudden Cardiac Death as Acute Myocardial Infarction," in Gordon, M. (ed.): *Self Assessment in Clinical Cardiology.* Yearbook Medical Publishers, Chicago, 1974.
9. American Heart Association: "Report of the Committee on Stress, Strain, and Heart Disease." *Circulation* 55:825A, May 1977.
10. Fuhs, M.: "Smoking and the Heart Patient." *Nursing Clinics of North America* 11:361, June 1976.
11. Naughton, J.: "Neuropathy Cited as Playing Role in Heart Disease." *Diabetes Outlook,* 12:1, November-December 1977.
12. Gilmore, J.: "Physiology of Stress," in Eliot, R. (ed.): *Stress and the Heart.* Futura Publishing Co., New York, 1974.
13. Gunnells, G.: "Hypertensive Vascular Disease—General Comments," in Gordon, M. (ed.): *Self Assessment in Clinical Cardiology.* Yearbook Medical Publishers, Chicago, 1974.
14. McHenry, L.: *Essentials of Stroke Diagnosis and Management.* Smith Kline Corporation, Philadelphia, 1973.
15. Jawetz, E., Melnik, J., and Adelberg, E.: *Review of Medical Microbiology.* Lang Medical Publications, Los Altos, California, 1968.
16. Wannamaker, L.: "Perplexity and Precision in the Diagnosis of Streptococcal Pharyngitis." *American Journal of Diseases of Children,* 124:352, 1972.
17. Perloff, J.: "Treatment of Coronary Heart Disease." Presented at Cardiology Conference, Hospital of the University of Pennsylvania, Fall, 1977.
18. Von Bertalanffy, L.: "General System Theory and Psychiatry," in Arieti, S. (ed.): *American Handbook of Psychiatry,* Vol. III. Basic Books, New York, 1966.
19. Anderson, R., and Carter, I.: *Human Behavior in the Social Environment: A Social Systems Approach.* Aldine Publishing Co., Chicago, 1974.

20. Erickson, E.: *Childhood and Society*. W.W. Norton and Company, New York, 1963.
21. Lidz, Theodore: *The Person*. Basic Books, New York, 1968.
22. Gould, R.: "Phases of Adult Life." *American Journal of Psychiatry*, 129:5, November 1972.
23. Levinson, D.: *The Seasons of a Man's Life*. Alfred A. Knopf, New York, 1978.
24. Berman, E., and Lief, H.: Marital Therapy from a Psychiatric Perspective: An overview. *The American Journal of Psychiatry*, 132(6):583, June 1975.
25. Duvall, E.: *Family Development*. J.B. Lippincott Company, Philadelphia, 1967.
26. Glick, I., and Kessler, I.: *Marital and Family Therapy*. Grune and Stratton, New York, 1974.
27. Minuchin, S.: *Families and Family Therapy: A Structural Approach*. Harvard University Press, Boston, 1974.
28. Jenkins, D.: "The Coronary-Prone Personality," in Gentry, W., and Williams, R. (eds.): *Psychological Aspects of Myocardial Infarction and Coronary Care*. The C.V. Mosby Co., St. Louis, 1975.
29. Friedman, M., and Rosenman, R.H.: *Type A Behavior and Your Heart*. Alfred A. Knopf, New York, 1974.
30. Moss, A.J., and Goldstein, S.: "The Pre-Hospital Phase of Acute Myocardial Infarction." *Circulation*, 41:737, 1970.
31. Tjoe, S.L., and Lauria, M.H.: "Delays in Reaching the Cardiac Care Unit: An Analysis. *Chest*, 61:617, 1972.
32. Cassem. N.H., and Hackett, T.P.: "Psychological Aspects of Myocardial Infarction." *Medical Clinics of North America*, 61:77, July 1977.
33. Cassem, N.H., and Hackett, T.P.: "Psychological Rehabilitation of Myocardial Infarction Patients in the Acute Phase." *Heart and Lung*, 2:382, May-June 1973.
34. Moos, R., and Tsu, V.: "The Crises of Physical Illness: An Overview," in Moos, R. (ed.): *Coping with Physical Illness*. Plenum Medical Book Company, New York, 1971.
35. Wishnie, H., Hackett, T.P., and Cassem, N.H.: "Psychological Hazards of Convalescence Following Myocardial Infarction." *J.A.M.A.* 215:1292, February 1971.
36. Watts, R.: "Sexuality and the Middle-Aged Cardiac Patient." *Nursing Clinics of North America*, 11:349, June 1976.
37. Kasl, S.: "Issues in Patient Adherence to Health Care Regimens." *Journal of Human Stress* 1:5, 1975.
38. Holmes, T.H., and Rahe, R.H.: "The Social Readjustment Rating Scale." *Journal of Psychosomatic Research*, 11:213, 1967.
39. Theorell, T., and Rahe, R.H.: "Life Change Events, Ballistocardiography, and Coronary Death." *Journal of Human Stress*, 1:18, 1975.
40. Beland, I., and Passos, J.: *Clinical Nursing*. Macmillan Publishing Co., New York, 1975.
41. Sehnert, K.: *How to Be Your Own Doctor*. Grosset and Dunlap, New York, 1975.
42. Benson, H., Greenwood, M., and Klemchuk, H.: "The Relaxation Response: Psychophysiologic Aspects and Clinical Applications." *International Journal of Psychiatry in Medicine*, 6:87, 1975.
43. Stone, R., and DeLeo, J.: "Psychotherapeutic Control of Hypertension." *The New England Journal of Medicine*, 294:80, 1976.
44. Naughton, J.: "The Contribution of Regular Physical Activity to the Ambulatory Care of Cardiac Patients." *Postgraduate Medicine*, 57:51, April 1975.
45. Wenger, N.: *Coronary Care—Rehabilitation After Myocardial Infarction*. American Heart Association, New York, 1973.
46. Niccoli, A., and Brammel, H.L.: "A Program of Rehabilitation in Coronary Heart Disease." *Nursing Clinics of North America*, 11:237, June 1976.
47. Harding, L., and Morefield, M.: "Group Intervention for Wives of Myocardial Infarction Patients." *Nursing Clinics of North America*, 11:339, June 1976.
48. Rosenman, R.H., and Friedman, M.: "The Relationship of Behavior Pattern A to the State of the Coronary Vasculature." *American Journal of Medicine*, 44:525, 1968.

BIBLIOGRAPHY

Bruce, R., and Lerman, J.: "Exercise Testing and Training in Relation to Myocardial Infarction." *Postgraduate Medicine*, 57:59, April 1975.
Crawshaw, J.E.: "Community Rehabilitation after Acute Myocardial Infarction. *Heart and Lung*, 3:258, 1974.

Freeman, Ruth: *Community Health Nursing Practice.* W.B. Saunders, Philadelphia, 1970.

Goldstein, S., and Heideman, E.: "Sudden Death and Coronary Heart Disease." *Cardiovascular Nursing,* 12:11, July-August 1976.

Gulledge, A.D.: "The Psychological Aftermath of a Myocardial Infarction," in Gentry, W.D., and Williams, R. (eds.): *Psychological Aspects of Myocardial Infarction.* The C.V. Mosby Co., St. Louis, 1975.

Kark, Sidney: *Epidemiology and Community Medicine.* Appleton-Century-Crofts, New York, 1974.

Petrich, J., and Holmes, T.H.: "Life Changes and Onset of Illness." *Medical Clinics of North America,* 61:825, July 1977.

Sutherland, John: *A General Systems Philosophy for the Social and Behavioral Sciences.* Braziller, New York, 1973.

Sutterly, Doris, and Donnelly, Gloria: *Perspectives in Human Development: Nursing Throughout the Life Cycle.* J.B. Lippincott, Philadelphia, 1973.

U.S. Department of Health, Education, and Welfare: *The Development and Implementation of a Curriculum Model for Community Nurse Practitioner.* DHEW Publication No. HRA 77-24, August, 1977.

Wynn, A: "Unwarranted Emotional Distress in Men with Ischaemic Heart Disease." *Medical Journal of Australia,* 2:847, 1967.

CHAPTER 22
CANCER

CAROL ANN BINGHAM, M.S.N., R.N.

The word cancer elicits more emotional response than perhaps any other disease which afflicts mankind. The diagnosis of cancer is perceived as a great tragedy. Patients can expect an outpouring of sympathy, compassion and pity because of the anticipated disfiguring, debilitating and painful effects of the disease. Family members are perceived as victims of the financial and emotional drain caused by the effects of chronic illness and death. Health care professionals who provide services to cancer patients and families can anticipate that others will view their work as being extremely depressing and unpleasant. These rather typical responses indicate that the community's collective attitude and behavior toward cancer is an expression of fear.

DEFINITION

Cancer is the lay terminology for a variety of different malignant growth processes. Malignant cells can arise from any tissue; however, these cells no longer perform the specified functions of the parent cell and therefore do not serve any useful, physiologic function. The most significant characteristic of malignant cells is a rapid, uncontrolled, and disorderly growth. Metastasis is the process by which cancer cells spread to surrounding tissues or are transported to new locations causing a secondary tumor growth.

ETIOLOGY

It is known that cancer is caused by a cellular dysfunction although the exact etiology still remains a mystery. Evidence, to date, suggests that there is no one single answer. Instead the presence of malignant cell growth probably involves several factors which, either alone or in combination, are responsible for the development of tumors. The factors most frequently implicated with tumor development include genetic factors, hormonal factors, carcinogens, immunologic factors, and psychological factors.

Genetic Factors

Certain types of cancer have been transmitted from parent to child. Retinoblastoma, a malignant glioma of the retina which only occurs during childhood, has been identified as a hereditary disease. The Philadelphia type chromosome 21 has been isolated in many patients with chronic myelocytic leukemia. Inherited cancers are characterized by early onset and a multiplicity of primary tumors.[1] Although certain cancers can be traced to genetic transmission, all cancers have the potential to occur by heritable and nonheritable forms.

What is frequently referred to as inheritance is the tendency toward the development of cancer in certain families. There seems to be some genetic susceptibility associated with familial tendencies; however, the precise mechanism has not been determined.[2]

Hormonal Factors

The evidence that links hormonal use and cancer is inconclusive. There is no increased evidence of breast cancer among oral contraceptive users.[3] A prolonged level of hormone use may be potentially carcinogenic; recent studies have established a possible association between estrogen intake in postmenopausal women and an increased risk of endometrial cancer.[4] Diethylstibestrol taken by women 15 to 20 years ago is now causing vaginal cancer in the female offspring.[5] More research is needed to conclusively establish the link between hormone use and tumor development.

Carcinogens

A carcinogen is any physical, chemical, or biologic substance or factor which increases the probablilty of tumor development. Each day new evidence is presented implicating yet another substance as a potential cancer producer, thus making it more and more difficult for individuals to avoid contact with offending substances. Unfortunately, many of the research findings are inconclusive because the studies were done on laboratory animals which received doses in extreme excess of anticipated normal use. The best gauge for the wary consumer is that the effects of most carcinogens are dose related. In those instances where the substance in question seems to pose a potential, significant health hazard, the government has imposed regulations concerning accessibility, acceptable levels, warning labels, and so forth. Carcinogens can be classified as either chemical, radiation, or virus. Table 22-1 summarizes some of the known carcinogens in man.[6]

TABLE 22-1. Carcinogens in man*

auramine	melphalan
asbestos	mycotoxins
busulfan	nickel carbonyl
betel nut	pitch
benzene	radiation:
coal tar products	ionizing
creosote	ultraviolet rays
cutting oils	nuclear fission products
chlornaphazine	uranium
chewing tobacco	radon
chromates	radium
dimethyl sulfate	soots
hormonal imbalance?	shale
mineral petroleum	smoke:
magenta	cigarette
mustard gas	cigar
	pipe

*Compiled from Weisburger, pp. 45-90,[6] and Baldonado and Stahl, p. 17.[8]

Immunologic Factors

Many scientists now believe that the body is continually manufacturing neoplastic cells which are subsequently destroyed because of a natural immunity. The immune system acts as a surveillance mechanism searching out foreign cells (i.e., cells that are different from the normal body cells). Through a complex series of reactions, the immune system kills or modifies any foreign substance of extrinsic or intrinsic origin. If the immune system functions improperly or is overwhelmed by a massive invasion, the tumor cells will continue to grow unchecked.[7] The immune system becomes ineffective at removing tumor cells if:

1. The tumor has grown beyond 100 million cells.
2. The body has an insufficient number of stem cells.
3. The thymus gland has been removed or dysfunctions.
4. The tumor cells contain a membrane impermeable to the circulating antibodies.
5. Insufficient nutrients are available to manufacture the necessary antibodies.
6. The immunologic system is depressed due to age, disease, infection, drugs, alcohol or stress.[8]

Psychologic Factors

There seems to be a causal relationship between negative life experiences and cancer. Malignant disease may therefore be the end result of ineffective coping mechanisms. Frequently cancer victims are found to be tense, rigid, inner directed, authoritarian, ambitious, and overstriving beyond their personal resources.[9] Because they are more inhibited in their outward responses, they appear to be apologetic, acquiescent, and polite. Bahnson and Bahnson[10] found that individuals with neoplastic disease have repressive ego defenses. In another study of patients with lung cancer, the subjects were described as having a "poor emotional outlet."[11] The evidence seems to indicate that there is a correlation between personality types and the development of malignant neoplasms. In addition, prolonged frustrations and prior life events influence susceptibility to disease.[12] Of significant importance is the loss of a relationship or history of bereavement.[13] The risk increases significantly when the loss is manifested with feelings of despair, hopelessness, and helplessness.[14] Other predisposing factors include unresolved tension or conflict with parents or childhood experiences and an inability to express emotional feelings, particularly anger.

STATISTICS

Cancer plays no favorites. It affects people at any age, of either sex, of all races, and from any ethnic, social or economic background. Although cancer may strike anyone at any time, there are some variables which have a bearing on who may or may not get cancer.

Age

Cancer kills more children between the ages of 3 and 14 than any other illness. According to figures presented by the American Cancer Society, over 200 children under the age of 15 died during 1975.[15] The figures indicate that the incidence of cancer increases in frequency with age. Between the ages of 15 and 34 the mortality rate rises to about 4,000. This increases to 36,000 deaths between the ages of 35 and 54 and to 123,000 for those in the 55 to 74 age bracket. The rate for those who are older than 75 years is approximately 66,000. This last figure does not indicate a drop but a smaller percentage of the population within this age range.

Sex

More men than women die of cancer each year, although cancer is the leading cause of death for women between the ages of 30 and 54. The most frequent site of cancer in men is the lung, while cancer of the breast is the most common type of cancer in women.[15]

Ethnic

The cancer incidence rate for blacks is higher than for whites; blacks also have a higher cancer mortality rate than do whites. Blacks had significantly higher incidence and mortality rates associated with cancer of the lung, colon-rectum, prostate, and esophagus. Early diagnosis, when the disease is localized and therefore curable, occurs more frequently in whites than in blacks. It is felt that social, economic, and cultural variables and not biologic differences account for the variation between black and white cancer rates.[15]

Behavioral patterns and geographic location are perhaps the two most significant social variables associated with cancer. Socially acceptable behavior may encourage 1) estrogen ingestion to combat menopausal symptoms and the aging process, 2) cigarette smoking, 3) alcohol consumption, 4) the use of hair dyes, 5) convenience foods containing large amounts of chemicals as additives and preservatives, and 6) excessive sun exposure to attain a "healthy glow."

Economic

Cancer is an extremely costly illness in terms of both direct and indirect costs. Direct costs include hospital bills, outpatient charges, home care nursing, and nursing home costs. Statistics published by the Health Insurance Institute show that in 1975 the daily costs in a community hospital averaged $151 which totaled $4,228 for a 28 day hospital stay.[15] Total costs will vary according to the type of cancer, the course of the disease, and individual needs but will probably range between $5,000 and $50,000.[16]

The annual economic expenditure for cancer including direct and indirect costs is estimated between $15 and $25 billion yearly.[15]

Cultural

Cultural habits and the environmental factors may also affect the development of particular types of cancer. Table 22-2 summarizes the cultural and/or geographic locations that are associated with specific types of cancer.[17]

Political

Congressmen also dread cancer and therefore consistently allocate large amounts of money for cancer research. Few legislators would publicly oppose efforts aimed at curing cancer. However, the current focus within political circles is on relieving the economic plight of cancer victims by a national health insurance. Senator Edward Kennedy has proposed a plan under which "employers would pay the major share of health insurance for employees and dependents, the federal government would pay for the poor and unemployed, and medicare would provide benefits for the elderly."[18]

SCOPE OF THE PROBLEM

Cancer is the second leading cause of death in this country. Approximately 700,000 people were diagnosed as having cancer during 1978. According to the present rates, one-in-four Americans can expect to eventually develop cancer. Over 3 million Americans have a history of cancer. One out of every six deaths is from cancer. This averages out at 1,070 cancer deaths per day and an estimated 390,000 for 1978. More recently the figures seem to be leveling off. Four out of every six cancer patients die; however, this figure could be decreased to three if every individual had the benefit of earlier detection and prompt treatment.[15] Cancer continues to be a substantial health care problem. Although most cancer patients can expect periods of hospitalization, the trend is toward management in the home and community. Home health care, with the support and guidance of the community health nurse, allows the cancer patient to remain an integral part of the family and community through the preventive, diagnostic, therapeutic, and terminal phases of illness.

IMPACT OF THE DISEASE

It is difficult to make any generalized statements about cancer. Each type of cancer has specific disease manifestations, suggested treatments, and an expected course. Cancer may, however, be described as a disease which can potentially affect every body system and all aspects of life and living. How any one person responds to cancer is governed by

TABLE 22-2. Cultural and geographic factors in cancer*

Type of Cancer	High Incidence Location	Comments
Mouth	Bombay, India	Associated with chewing betel quid. Alcohol & tobacco implicated in other locations.
Nasopharynx	South China	Genetic predisposition, will occur even after migration.
Esophagus	Rhodesia	Associated with alcohol, seems to have a synergistic role with tobacco.
Stomach	Latin America and Japan	Incidence decreases as immigrants adjust to a new country.
Colon-rectal	United States	Unknown etiology.
Liver	Mozambique (Bantu)	90% occur in chirrotic livers caused by exposure to synthetic chemical agents.
Gallbladder	Japan	Associated with cholelithiasis.
Pancreas	New Zealand	Unknown etiology.
Bronchus	Liverpool, England	Associated with urban living, cigarette smoking, occupations involving contact with radiation, chromates, nickel, hematite, asbestos; air pollution.
Breast	North American (Hawaiian, Caucasian)	Associated with upper income, family history, obesity, nonchild bearing.
Cervix	Colombia	Ethnic groups who generally have circumcised male sexual partners have a lower incidence (i.e., Jewish, Muslim). Associated with age at first intercourse and the number of sexual partners (e.g., higher in prostitutes, lower in nuns).
Prostate	United States (blacks)	Associated with married men and contact with cadmium.
Testis	Denmark	Questionable genetic influence.
Penis	Africa	Associated with phimosis due to infection due to smegma in noncircumcision.
Kidney	Sweden	Seems to be some carcinogenic factors in the urine of cigarette smokers.
Bladder	United States	Associated with tobacco and occupational carcinogens.
Malignant melanoma	New Zealand and Europe	Incidence increased in those who have greater exposure to the sunlight.
Skin	El Paso, Texas (non-Hispanic)	Associated with occupations involving contact with tar or mineral oil, contact with ultraviolet radiation especially in the South, chronic ulceration.
Brain and nervous system	Israel	Associated with environmental factors.
Thyroid	Colombia	Associated with ionizing radiation in childhood.
Bone	Rumania	Unknown etiology.
Lymphosarcoma and reticulosarcoma	Israel (non-Jews)	Associated with malarial stimulation of the reticuloendothial system.
Leukemia	Eastern Europe and United States (Jews)	Questionably due to genetic influences, radiation, chemicals.

*Compiled from Higginson and Muir, pp. 241-306. [17]

the multiple variables and combination of variables that make the person a unique individual. Cancer is perhaps the most anxiety producing disease known to man. Although the impact of cancer on the patient, family, and community will vary considerably from situation to situation, in most instances the disease will not permit noninvolvement. The pervasive nature of the disease requires active participation to prevent or mitigate the otherwise catastrophic effects that cancer can produce for the patient, family, and community if allowed to grow unimpeded. The community health nurse must try to understand the meaning of cancer to that patient, family, and community in order to anticipate and interpret the impact of the disease.

Individual

From the appearance of the first symptoms through diagnosis, treatment, metastasis, and death the cancer patient can probably expect major alterations and stress in every significant aspect of life. The patient will encounter many conflicts both within himself and with others as he attempts to cope with the disease restrictions, changing goals, and altered expectations. The adjustments which the patient must make in his daily living routines and relationships may result from the disease, the treatment, or a combination of the two. Following is a discussion of those areas which are generally most stressful for the patient.

ADAPTATION TO CHRONIC ILLNESS

Cancer patients are faced with an ever-increasing list of disturbing physical symptoms which frequently become more intense in severity and duration as the disease progresses. The patient's whole orientation changes from one of wellness with periodic interruptions of illness to illness with ever-diminishing periods of time when he feels physically well.

The treatment procedures, such as radiotherapy, chemotherapy, and surgery, add to the physical exhaustion of the patient and therefore reinforce to the patient that he is indeed a sick person. The surgery, depending upon the location and extent, will necessitate temporary or permanent activity restrictions and may produce an alteration in the patient's daily routines. If the surgery is disfiguring or disabling, the patient is then not only sick but is also disabled or freakish and therefore not normal. The patient may find that the community accepts the sick person much more readily than the "abnormal" person.

If chemotherapy and radiotherapy are given on an outpatient basis, the patient must alter his routine to accommodate the treatment schedule. Generally this requires regularly scheduled visits to the hospital clinic or x-ray department during the course of radiation therapy or chemotherapy. Each visit to the hospital reinforces to the patient that he is sick. The illness may in fact become very acute during the treatment period. The nausea, vomiting, mouth ulcers, and general malaise that the patient experiences may in some cases be worse than the disease symptoms.

As the disease progresses the weakness and debilitation may become profound. One of the most distressing symptoms for the patient is the lack of energy leading to such extreme exhaustion that he becomes unable to perform even the most basic personal hygiene tasks without experiencing fatigue. As the patient loses ability to function, he also loses control of his environment and is placed in a dependent position.

CHANGE IN SELF-CONCEPT AND BODY IMAGE

Loss of function for cancer patients may be related to the disease process or may result from surgery or treatments. Donovan and Pierce[19] define body image as "the sum total of the feelings and perceptions an individual has about his body." The loss of function or body part and the meaning which that has to the patient is related to the visibility of the loss, the extent of functional impairment, and the meaning or emotional attachment to the affected part. The patient's perception of the magnitude of the loss will have a direct bearing on his ability to adapt and to incorporate the loss into an altered body image. Loss of a limb, mutilating tumor growth or surgery, loss of a bodily function (colostomy), loss of ability to communicate (laryngectomy), and loss of sexual identity (mastectomy) will necessitate a permanent alteration in body image. Less obvious and temporary body changes can occur as a result of cancer treatments and can also be very upsetting to the patient who is forced to deal with so many changes all at one time. These may include alopecia as a result of chemotherapy, severe acne from steroids, and hirsutism associated with hormone therapy. The altered body image may cause feelings of self-hatred, self-pity, rejection, anger, depression, and isolation until the individual is able to incorporate the altered body image into his concept of self.

Self-concept is best described as the sum total of the individual's perceptions about himself—who he is, what he is, what he believes in, his goals, dreams, and fears. In addition to body image, the self-concept includes roles and relationships, sexuality, and production capabilities.

Frequently the disease process will dictate what roles the patient is able to maintain; however, other roles which the patient would prefer to keep and is capable of keeping may be taken from him. In an attempt to relieve the cancer victim of needless worries and stress, the patient may find himself in a useless, nonproductive position because of the presumed good intentions of family and friends. Other people begin to take over responsibility for the roles which the patient had been assuming up until the time of illness. The patient then is no longer able to think of himself within that context and begins to perceive himself as being nonproductive and useless. If the people who share the patient's environment are uncomfortable with the full significance of what is happening, they will unknowingly begin to isolate themselves from the patient to avoid confrontation of the issues. Standing by and watching someone deteriorate creates many helpless feelings. As the roles change so do the relationships which were constructed over a period of time as a result of the responsibilities of the assigned role. As the relationships deteriorate, the patient begins to be excluded more and more thus leading to the feeling that he has been abandoned and therefore must be useless.

Feelings of uselessness and nonproductivity become critical when the patient is no longer able to perform his life's work and therefore fulfill his financial and/or service obligations. Husbands and fathers who cannot financially support the family and mothers who cannot care for their children tend to feel worthless and guilty because of their inability to meet their obligations. The patient must feel that he is making a useful contribution in order to have a positive self-concept.

One of the roles which cancer may interfere with is that of being a successful and/or desirable sexual partner. Sexuality involves physical, emotional, and functional components. Alterations in any one of the areas will affect the relationship with a sexual partner. An ostomy patient may avoid further sexual encounters because of fear of odor. A woman may think of herself as an undesirable partner after a mastectomy. The development of a meaningful sexual relationship involves more than penile insertion into the vagina; however, many couples will need help and encouragement to explore other sexual techniques and to rediscover that they are indeed sexually desirable and attractive.

FEAR OF PAIN

Cancer, in the minds of many people, is associated with pain—excruciating pain—that is uncontrollable. The anticipation of pain increases the anxiety as the patient musters all of his energies to brace himself against the onslaught of pain. This will lead to anxiety and tension in all the other areas of the patient's life and will decrease his overall ability to cope with the disease. Although pain is a very real problem for some cancer patients, there are many other patients who experience little or no physical pain.

FEAR OF DEATH

The diagnosis of cancer for many people is synonomous with death—an agonizing, prolonged death that will completely destroy the individual. Although the patient may not in any way indicate outwardly that death is a possibility, chances are that he has thought about it. Fear of death might be more appropriately stated as fear of the dying process and fear of being abandoned by those he loves.

COPING MECHANISMS

The manner in which a person copes with any stressful situation, and specifically with cancer, is based upon the sum total of that person's experiences and his previous patterns of coping. Lipowski[20] defines coping as the "cognitive and motor activities which a sick person employs to preserve his bodily and psychic integrity, to recover reversibly impaired function and compensate to the limit for any irreversible impairment." Some patients will adjust quite well to the stresses and adaptations which cancer may impose, while others are completely devastated by the experience and seem to be in a continual state of crisis.

Family

Cancer changes not only the patient but the patient's family. Any serious illness will cause some amount of family tension and adaptation. How the family copes with cancer will depend upon the coping styles of each member and how they deal with crisis as a family unit. The areas which create the most stress for the patient are also the areas which are most difficult for the family to cope with. Adaptation to chronic illness, role changes, financial burdens, and grief are the most frequently encountered family stresses.

ADAPTATION TO CHRONIC ILLNESS

It is very difficult for the family members to watch their loved one slowly succumb to the ravaging effects of cancer. Family members experience a feeling of helplessness and loss of control when they are useless to help prevent the spread of the disease or to arrest any of the patient's disturbing symptoms. The pain which the patient suffers is transmitted to the family, and until the patient's pain is under control they cannot be comfortable either.

Family members may need to make alterations in their schedules to accommodate the patient. This may mean time away from other commitments to transport the patient for treatment, adjusting the living arrangements or sleeping patterns to provide space and someone to care for the patient, and it may mean that the family cannot enjoy doing things as a family unit if someone must stay home with the sick family member.

If the family members are living away from home, the stresses and feelings of help-lessness may be exaggerated. Adult relatives with families of their own are torn between obligations and responsibilities to their spouses and children while wanting to be close and able to help their sick relative during times of need. As families become scattered across the country, the distance can create another stress. Trips to visit the cancer patient or to assist other family members may be costly, time consuming, and difficult to arrange because of other commitments and obligations. Family members who are located at distances from the cancer patient are always in the uncomfortable position of being unaware of what is happening and of knowing that it may be impossible for them to arrive in time should something happen.

The disease process is frequently a long one encompassing several years during which time the condition will cycle through periods of crises, improvements, and plateaus. Family members who are encouraged by the patient's improvement soon learn that these periods are short lived, and they must always be emotionally braced for the next crisis which generally indicates disease progression. Certainly there are exceptions to this rule; there are patients whose disease appears to be cured, but these cases do not fall under the category of chronic disease. It is the chronicity which is most difficult to deal with, to the point that some family members might wish that the disease would run its course and get it over with. That appears to be easier to deal with than the long drawn-out process that never seems to end and which is so difficult to deal with, because each encouraging event will eventually be replaced by an equally discouraging one. Family members may also have to face the reality of more cancer. The appearance of cancer in one family member may increase the anxiety for others that they, too, may eventually be cancer victims.

ROLES AND RELATIONSHIPS

Serious childhood disease imposes a great emotional burden on the parents and will affect their response to the sick child's siblings. If the serious illness is cancer, the parents must face the fact that the child will die prematurely or may require painful, long term treatment, and perhaps disfiguring surgery. It becomes difficult not to set that child apart and give him special attention to compensate for the pain and suffering the child must endure as a result of the disease process. The child may not be able to attend school or enjoy other childhood activities and is thereby deprived of the fun times that his siblings have. The siblings can feel neglected or unloved if the parents focus too much attention on the sick child.

The cancer patient, because of limitations imposed by the disease, may not be able to fulfill many of his family responsibilities and the family will have to improvise or look elsewhere for assistance. If the cancer patient was the financial provider, another family member may need to provide the financial support or the family may be forced to draw upon their savings or receive government assistance. If the cancer patient was caring for small children, it may be necessary for another family member to assume that respon-sibility or to bring in help from the outside. All of the family based activities and relation-ships are affected. Who will drive the children to ball practice and music lessons? Who will paint the house? Who will walk the dog? All these become important issues if the task in question was the responsibility of the cancer patient.

The alterations and adaptations occur not only for roles of responsibility but also in the relationships that exist within the family. The disease may necessitate changes in the sexual practices between husband and wife, father and son may have to find a new way of discussing problems if father can no longer take the fishing trips where these discussions occurred, and the whole family may begin to resent the disruptions to their life and routines which occur as all the attention is focused on the sick family member.

FINANCIAL BURDENS

The cost of any chronic illness can be quite expensive, but the cost of all cancer related items—drugs, supplies, and physician services—tends to be higher. In addition to the direct cost, there are many indirect costs which greatly increase the financial burden of cancer. Wigs, special clothing, labor saving devices, comfort items, structural modifications, and loss of income or decreased productivity by the cancer patient and/or a family member can impose overwhelming financial burdens.

Frequently insurance coverage is exhausted long before the financial obligations are met. Other patients are ineligible for health insurance because of a history of cancer. Some insurance policies carry a rider excluding coverage for cancer treatment. As the costs continue to mount, a family's entire savings can be completely wiped out. If this money was being set aside for college, a family excursion, or a new car, all family members must share in the loss and disappointment that cancer has brought upon them.

GRIEF

Families are also aware that the diagnosis of cancer may mean premature death. In general, the families are much slower at coming to a realization that the disease has run its course and that death is a possibility. The process by which a family copes with grief closely parallels the stages of dying as defined by Kübler-Ross.[21] First there is denial both of the disease and later of the terminal nature of the disease. This is followed by anger that this is happening. The anger seems to be related to the total sense of helplessness to do anything to affect the eventual outcome. Eventually the family begins to make bargains in hopes that by changing various things (attitudes, behavior, etc.) they can affect the outcome. The motivation is frequently guilt that they have not been good or have not done everything within their power to change the course of the disease. When they finally realize that nothing they do will change the inevitable, there is a sense of extreme depression. The depression is replaced by acceptance when they can face the reality of the situation.

COMMUNITY

The community helps to form the attitudes which are then reflected in the community's behavior in response to that particular issue. The community's attitude toward cancer is best described as that of fear. The response to fear is either flight or fight.

Many people flee from cancer because they still believe it is a contagious disease. People also flee from cancer because of the uncomfortable feelings which are generated by being placed in a helpless position. Cancer patients and their families are pitied because they have become victims of a disease which is uncontrollable and spreads like a fire through the forest. People also avoid cancer because they believe that they may be subjected to unpleasant sights and odors. As the community isolates cancer and its victims, the cancer patient is pronounced socially dead far in advance of biologic death. Industry is particularly guilty of creating social deaths. Many cancer patients are denied employment based only upon the fact that they have a diagnosis of cancer, without any consideration of the type of cancer, the treatment, interval since diagnosis, prognosis, or present physical condition. Records show that many rehabilitated cancer patients have more productive years and are more physically capable than are persons with other chronic illnesses.

The health community shares many of the same fears about cancer. Health care providers are frequently guilty of withholding information from a patient because they believe that the information is too upsetting, and the patient therefore needs to be protected. Those individuals who choose to work with cancer patients are questioned by their colleagues, "How can you work with those people? Isn't it depressing?"

The fight against cancer is best symbolized by the Sword of Hope—"a double-edged blade with twin serpent caduceus to emphasize the medical and scientific aspects"[15] of the American Cancer Society, "a voluntary organization of about 2.3 million Americans united to conquer cancer."[15] The organization provides programs in research, education, patient service, and rehabilitation from a budget in excess of $125 million which is obtained by fund raising and from bequests and legacies. The work that is being done through this organization has touched the lives of many cancer patients and their families.

In some instances, the fear and flight becomes a fight. For example, nonsmokers who fear that inhaling smoke may cause cancer and other respiratory diseases have waged a fight for public space that is smoke-free and have, as a result of their campaigns, created smoking and nonsmoking sections in restaurants, on public transportation, and have, in some instances, prohibited smoking entirely in public buildings.

PREVENTION

Prevention of cancer primarily involves avoiding contact with known carcinogens and following good basic health practices including regular physical examinations. The responsibility for cancer prevention includes the individual, the family, and the community and especially the government, industry, and health care providers.

Manufacturers who use or produce carcinogens must provide adequate safeguards so that employees are not exposed to carcinogens in quantities that will produce cancer. Although most industries willingly accept their share of responsibility for the health of their employees, there are always a few for whom the monetary rewards preempt consideration for others. In other instances the research data are inconclusive and do not clearly prove that a substance will produce human cancer. If the evidence is doubtful, industry is hesitant to make costly operational changes or remove the product from the market. This has led to many debates and law suits and an ever increasing number of government imposed regulations to assure a safe environment for employees and safe products for consumers. There are, however, many gray areas where the individual must weigh the consequences of accepting employment in an area which may increase his risks of getting cancer. The individual must also make the decision to use or not use products which carry warning labels indicating that use of the products may cause cancer. Avoidance of carcinogens will not guarantee that the individual will not get cancer; it will, however, eliminate a known risk factor.

Routine physical examinations will not prevent cancer but will provide the advantage of early detection so that treatment can begin while the disease is localized. Survival rates are greatly influenced by early diagnosis and prompt treatment. As part of the public education program of the American Cancer Society, this organization has compiled a set of seven warning signals. Appearance of any one of the warning signals should prompt a visit to the doctor because the individual *may* have cancer. For many people knowledge of the warning signals has meant early diagnosis; however, a certain number of people avoid consulting a physician out of fear that their suspicions will be confirmed.

Research into the causes and treatment of cancer have lead to the development of various screening techniques which have been successful in detecting cancer during its earliest stages. A nationwide breast screening program funded by the American Cancer Society and the National Cancer Institute was initiated in 1971. The program has been the subject of much criticism surrounding the use of routine x-ray screening in asymptomatic women between the ages of 35 and 50. Table 22-3 summarizes the cancer screening techniques.

Scientists have recently discovered that cancer victims have a substance in their blood that is absent in healthy people. The chemical, galactosyltransferase isoenzyme II (GTII), can be detected in the blood months before the patient shows any signs of cancer.[22] It is too early to tell, but this may be the answer to cancer mass screening programs.

Until a mass screening program is available, selective screening should specifically focus on those individuals or groups of individuals at risk. These would include those individuals who are routinely exposed to carcinogens (smokers, industry workers, radiology personnel), people living in areas with a high cancer incidence, individuals with a family history, individuals with "cancer personalities," or those who have recently been exposed to large amounts of stress.

Regular physical examinations and self-examinations are the most important preventive measures that any individual can do to assure early detection and consequently early treatment with greater chances for affecting a cure.

DIAGNOSIS

The techniques most frequently used to detect or confirm cancer include radiology studies, immunoassays, biochemical tests, and cytology tests.

Cytologic studies involve the microscopic examination of specimens to detect any abnormal cell growth. Specimens can be obtained by aspirating fluid or by a needle or

TABLE 22-3. Cancer Screening

Breast	Self-examination
	Mammography*
	Thermography
Cervical	Pap smear
Colon-rectal	Guaiac test slide
	Proctosigmoidoscopy
Lung	Sputum cytology
	Fiberoptic bronchoscopy
	Chest x-ray

*May induce breast cancer in women under age 50.

surgical biopsy. The test can detect the presence of malignant cells and can even detect cancer *in situ*. During this extremely early stage of cellular change, the patient does not clinically have cancer. However, before the organ is completely overtaken by malignant cells, the epithelial cells of that particular organ will show nuclear abnormalities. Detecting cancer *in situ* is associated with very high cure rates. This makes the cytologic examination a valuable tool for detection of early cancer and for determining the amount of cellular involvement with later stages of cancer growth.

There are several biochemical tests which may be elevated in the presence of malignant disease. These include some enzymes, zinc, copper, and plasma proteins.[23] The serum acid phosphate level may be elevated in cancer of the prostate, while the serum alkaline phosphatase level is elevated in cancer of the liver or bone. It is also possible that tumor cells may produce alkaline phosphatase. Metastasis to the liver and biliary system is associated with hyperbilirubinemia, an elevated SGOT, and an elevated alkaline phosphatase. Metastasis to the skeletal structures causes high calcium levels and an elevated alkaline phosphatase.

TREATMENT

Surgery

Surgery is the oldest form of treatment and is the treatment of choice for breast, lung, gastrointestinal, endometrial, cervical, ovarian, head and neck, thyroid, sarcoma, melanoma, and renal cancers. Baldonado and Stahl[8] report that 80 to 85 percent of the curable cancers are treated with surgery. More recently, however, surgery has become part of an interdisciplinary treatment approach. Cancer surgery is frequently radical surgery, but when used in combination with other treatments it is hoped that a more conservative surgical approach can be taken. Cancer surgery is indicated to remove a tumor mass; depending upon the type and location of the tumor this may have disfiguring results. In some instances, reconstructive surgery can minimize the effects of earlier mutilating surgery. Oophorectomy and adrenalectomy are surgical procedures which may be used to manipulate hormonal balances. Palliative surgery is done to relieve distressing symptoms, to give the patient a more comfortable existence, or to prevent deterioration. Surgical intervention (e.g., cordotomy) is also sometimes indicated for pain control.

Radiation Therapy

Radiotherapy is indicated for treatment of localized tumors. Rapidly dividing cells, which are characteristic of cancer cells, are most sensitive to the effects of radiation. By altering the atoms in the chemical system of the cell, radiotherapy can cause cell destruction. The amount of destruction will vary according to the dose and intensity of the radiation (i.e., alpha, beta, or gamma rays) and the site to be irradiated. Areas with a higher percentage of tissue oxygenation will be more responsive to radiation. The longer an area is exposed to radiation, the greater the effects will be. However, radiation destroys normal cells along with the cancer cells. Giving the radiation in fractionated doses will allow normal cells to recover between doses. Table 22-4 lists the cells which are most sensitive to radiation.

In addition to the destruction of tumor cells, radiation can produce effects in the body

TABLE 22-4. Cells sensitive to radiation*

Epithelial cells	Testes	Lymphocytes
	Intestinal crypts	Erythroblasts
	Ovaries	Myeloblasts
	Skin	Endothelial
	Secretory glands	Connective tissue
	Lungs	Tubular cells of kidney
	Bile ducts	Bone
		Nerve
		Brain
		Muscle

*Compiled from Baldonado and Stahl, pp. 67-68.[8]

that limit its usefulness in treating cancer. It can cause skin dermatitis with scaling, weeping, erythemia, and dry skin; in extreme cases it is responsible for radiation burns and ulcerations. Radiation can also result in permanent skin changes such as increased pigmentation, atrophy, and thickening. The effects on the mucous membranes include ulceration, diarrhea, bleeding, dry mouth, changes in taste, sore throat, and dysphagia. The hematopoietic system responds with a decrease in the number of circulating red blood cells, white blood cells, and platelets. Radiation may also produce sterility and be responsible for bone necrosis and fractures. After radiotherapy, patients complain of nausea, vomiting, fever, loss of appetite, and a general malaise.

Radiotherapy may be used as a palliative treatment to relieve bone pain and to minimize the symptoms of brain metastasis.

Chemotherapy

The use of naturally occurring or synthetic drugs either alone or in combination is what is referred to as chemotherapy. Chemotherapeutic agents act on the cell cycle and are classified according to their mode of action.

Antimetabolites interfere with the metabolic pathways of dividing cells and substitute abnormal components for the essential metabolites. Because the drug closely resembles normal cell metabolites, it enters the cell where it interferes with DNA synthesis. The cell is unable to reproduce and therefore dies. Antimetabolites include antifolics, antipurines, and antipyrimidines.

Alkylating agents alter DNA by binding the chains together or breaking the chains. Alteration of the DNA molecule will inhibit cell growth and division.

Natural products can affect cancer cells in a number of different ways. Included in this group are antibiotics, alkaloids, and enzymes.

It is not yet known how hormones affect tumor growth, but it is known that some cells are dependent on hormonal support for metabolic activity. It has recently been found that some cells have a receptor in the cytoplasm which combines with the hormone. The receptor protein is specific for each hormone. Individuals who have hormone receptors are more likely to respond to hormone therapy than are individuals without the hormone receptor.[24] There are also a number of miscellaneous agents that act by inhibiting either DNA, RNA, or protein synthesis.

Table 22-5 lists the most commonly used chemotherapeutic agents and the types of

TABLE 22-5. Commonly used chemotherapeutic agents*

Drug	Indications for use
Antimetabolites	
cytosine arabinoside (antipyramidine)	Leukemias, acute and chronic
fluorouracil (antipyramidine)	Bladder, breast, gastrointestinal, liver, lung, oropharynx, ovary, prostate, uterus
mercaptopurine (antipurine)	Leukemias, acute and chronic
methotrexate (antifolic)	Leukemia, acute; choriocarcinoma, lymphosarcoma, mycosis fungoides, osteogenic sarcoma, solid tumors
thioguanine (antipurine)	Leukemias, acute and chronic
Alkylating agents	
busulfan	Leukemias, chronic; polycythemia vera
carmustine (BCNU) (nitrosurea)	Brain, gastric, Hodgkin's lymphoma, melanoma, renal
chlorambucil	Breast, Hodgkins disease, leukemias, chronic; lymphoma, ovary, testicular
cyclophosphamide	Hodgkin's lymphoma, leukemias, acute and chronic; lymphoma, rhabdomyosarcoma, solid tumors, Wilm's tumor
lomustine (CCNU) (nitrosurea)	Brain, gastric, Hodgkin's lymphoma, melanoma, renal
melphalan	Breast, myeloma, ovary, testicular
mitomycin C	Breast, bronchogenic, cervical, colon, gastric, head and neck, malignant melanoma, pancreas
nitrogen mustard	Breast, bronchogenic, Hodgkin's lymphoma, ovary
Natural Products	
actinomycin D (antibiotic)	Choriocarcinoma, lung, rhabdomyosarcoma, sarcoma, testicular, Wilm's tumor
adriamycin (antibiotic)	Breast, genitourinary, Hodgkin's disease, leukemia, acute; lung, neuroblastoma, sarcoma, thyroid
bleomycin (antibiotic)	Lymphoma, sarcoma, testicular, urinary
daunomycin (antibiotic)	Leukemias, acute and chronic; neuroblastoma
L-asparaginase (enzyme)	Leukemia, acute
vinblastine (alkaloid)	Breast, Hodgkin's disease, lymphoma, reticuloendothelial
vincristine (alkaloid)	Choriocarcinoma, leukemia, acute; lymphoma, neuroblastoma, rhabdomyosarcoma, solid tumors, testicular, Wilm's tumor
Hormones	
androgens	Breast
estrogens	Breast (postmenopausal), prostate
prednisone	Breast, hematologic, Hodgkin's disease, leukemias, acute and chronic; lymphoma, myeloma, ovary, prostate
progesterones	Breast, endometrial, renal
Miscellaneous	
hydroxyurea	Leukemia, chronic; malignant melanoma
procarbazine	Hodgkin's disease, lymphoma, lung, myeloma, ovary

*Compiled from Baldonada and Stahl, pp. 45-47.[8]

cancers they are used to treat. Chemotherapeutic agents can be quite toxic to normal cells. By using the drugs in combination and by timing the administration, it is possible to minimize the toxic effects of many of the agents.

The toxic effects that occur most frequently and are of most concern to the patient include stomatitis, nausea, vomiting, alopecia, parasthesia, liver damage, right sided heart failure, pneumonitis, and myelosuppression affecting the white blood cells, red blood cells, and platelets.

Immunotherapy

The goals of immunotherapy are to challenge the immune system in order to achieve a more efficient immune response, to augment the immune response, and to alter the tumor cell surface to make it more immunogenic.[8] Immunotherapy or alteration of a depressed immune system is accomplished by one of the following methods.

Active Specific Immunization

Tumor cells or antigens are reinjected into the patient in an effort to stimulate the patient to produce antibodies.

Active Nonspecific Immunization

Antigens such as BCG are given to stimulate the immune system to become more active.

Passive Immunization

The patient is given lymphocytes from another patient who has been cured. This includes bone marrow transplantation between histologically identical persons.

Adaptive Immunization

The patient is injected with blood leukocytes from a donor who has been grafted with the recipient's tumor.

Immunotherapy may be used as an adjunctive therapy with surgery, chemotherapy, and radiotherapy. The initial therapy reduces the tumor size, then immunotherapy is used to remove the remainder of the tumor cells.

Treatment of Systemic Effects

In addition to treatment of the disease, the patient may need treatment of a variety of systemic effects of either the disease or the disease treatment. Table 22-6 summarizes some of these other treatments.

Quackery

Cancer patients may resort to the use of unproven methods of therapy for a variety of reasons. The devices, diets, and drugs generally appeal to the ignorant, those who are fearful of the effects of the proven treatment measures, those who are impatient with the

TABLE 22-6. Treatment for systemic effects

Anemia	Blood transfusions, folic acid, multivitamins, supplemental iron, decreasing oxygen consumption, and activity
Fever and infection	Hypothermia, antipyretics, antibiotics, antifungal therapy
Hypercoaguability	Ambulation, heparin, oral anticoagulants
Hypercalcemia	Restrict calcium intake, hydration, steroids, mithromycin, thyrocalcitonin, phosphates, diuretics
Anorexia, nausea and vomiting	Sweeten foods, avoid unpleasant odors, antiemetics, deep breathing, swallowing, liquids
Cachexia	Hyperalimentation

slow progress of traditional methods, or those who cannot accept that the proven methods will not cure the disease and are looking for a miracle.

PROGNOSIS

Although cancer is a very serious disease and one that is associated with premature death, not all people will necessarily die from their cancer. The American Cancer Society[15] reports that about one-third of all the people who get cancer will be alive for at least five years. In 1930 only one in five patients could expect to survive beyond five years,[8] so progress is being made. In fact, cancer patients may outlive cardiac, diabetic, and stroke patients.

As the disease progresses, 60 to 80 percent of all cancer patients will develop metastasis.[8] The lung is the most common site for metastasis. Other metastatic sites include the bone, which causes pain and pathologic fractures; the spinal cord, causing compression; the liver, causing metabolic and enzymatic alterations and ascites; effusions (the accumulation of fluid) frequently found in the lung, pericardial space, and peritoneal cavity; the gastrointestinal tract, causing obstruction; and the brain, causing personality and behavioral changes.

The combined effects of the disease and the treatments can lead to a wide variety of systemic alterations which, if left unattended, will greatly increase morbidity and mortality. Generalized body reactions include the following: Anemia may be due to hemolysis from the treatment. An autoimmune hemolysis also occurs with leukemia and the lymphomas. The anemia can also result from blood loss or a reduction in red blood cell production due to bone marrow depression. Nutritional deficiencies, especially an insufficient intake of iron and folic acid, may also produce anemia. Cachexia is a problem for most cancer patients. The generalized wasting which frequently occurs is created by the ever increasing metabolic demands of the tumor.

Some tumor cells release a thromboplastic substance into the blood stream which causes hypercoaguability and can lead to disseminated intravascular clotting. Other patients have a bigger problem with bleeding tendencies caused by thrombocytopenia as a result of drug induced bone marrow depression. Bone metastasis and an ectopic production of parathormone cause hypercalcemia in about 10 percent of all cancer patients.

Pain, anorexia, nausea, and vomiting are less life-threatening effects but can be extremely annoying and uncomfortable for the patient. The pain is frequently caused by pressure of the growing tumor on the visceral organs but may also result from a reflex stimulation.

Chemotherapy and radiotherapy account for much of the anorexia, nausea, and vomiting. They may also create abnormalities in the taste sensation so that the patient has a higher threshold for sweets and a lower threshold for bitter tastes.

Fever is a common symptom with the hematologic malignancies. Infection results from a defect in the immune system (e.g., leukopenia associated with malignancies of the hematopoietic and reticuloendothelial systems) or is created by the treatments that depress the defense mechanisms (i.e., chemotherapy, radiotherapy). Surgery incurs a risk of developing infection, and long-term steroid therapy suppresses and masks the symptoms of infection and increases the patient's vulnerability to fungal and yeast infections. Antibiotic therapy increases the infection risk for opportunistic or drug resistant infections in patients with a defective immune system. Opportunistic infections are caused by resident organisms normally found in the mouth, colon, skin, vagina, urinary tract, or upper respiratory tract. Cancer patients, because of a defective immune system, are very susceptible to varicella (herpes zoster) and vaccina (chicken pox) and should avoid contact with anyone who has recently been vaccinated or who has any type of disease. The most common sites for infection are the skin, blood stream, perineum, bladder, kidney, respiratory tree, lungs, and mouth. Infection is a very serious problem for cancer patients and is directly responsible for many cancer deaths.

COMMUNITY HEALTH NURSING CONCERNS

It is frequently difficult to single out problems that apply specifically to the individual and to the family. Rogers[25] has developed a theoretic framework for nursing that considers the wholeness of man that cannot be understood when it is reduced to particulars. The community health nurse, in planning care for the cancer patient, should think in terms of a patient-family unit because neither functions in isolation of the other. It therefore becomes difficult to separate approaches to the patient versus approaches to the family. Following is a summary of some of the major concerns that a community health nurse would assess when planning care for the cancer patient.

Individual

Whenever possible the cancer patient should remain at home following the same routines and maintaining the same roles and relationships that existed prior to illness. This will allow the individual to remain part of what is meaningful to him. The patient should remain at home except for brief periods of hospitalization through all phases of the disease up to and including the terminal phase. The emphasis should be on maintaining wellness, not perpetuating illness.

As the disease progresses, the patient may find that more and more energy is consumed in merely accomplishing the normal activities of daily living. When the patient is faced with diminishing energy levels, he must begin to recognize his physical limitations and to set realistic goals to live within those limits or to find acceptable alternatives. The community health nurse, in planning care, must consider the patient's value system, usual patterns, the interruptions in life style which were necessitated by the disease, and how the patient perceives the alterations. Under all circumstances, the patient must remain in control of his life and must be consulted in any decision regarding him.

NUTRITION

One of the most important things that the cancer patient can do for himself is to maintain an adequate nutritional intake. The well-nourished patient will have the energy necessary to withstand the treatment (surgery, chemotherapy, radiotherapy) and will be able to tolerate the occasional bouts of nausea, vomiting, and decreased intake without becoming wasted. In addition, the patient will have better results from the chemotherapy[26] and will provide sufficient protein for the immune system to function optimally.

Souchon and coworkers[27] found that cancer patients who received an adequate amount of calories and protein survived longer. The loss of appetite and apathy associated with cancer may be due to lipid metabolites, which are the by products of lipid catabolism.[28] Vitamins and particularly vitamin C will assure adequate functioning of the immune system.

Vomiting, diarrhea, and a draining fistula can result in electrolyte losses (i.e., sodium, potassium, and chloride) in addition to the water loss. Elevated calcium levels are a problem caused by destruction of bone and release of calcium into the blood.

Giving the patient responsibility for providing his body with sufficient quantities of the proper nutrients is one way of allowing the patient to remain in control. High protein, high calorie foods are recommended with vitamin supplements if the patient is not able to tolerate the vegetables and fruits to meet the recommended daily requirements. Commercially prepared preparations are available which contain all of the essential nutrients in a readily absorbable form. For those patients for whom normal digestion is a problem, these preparations may be beneficial, but intake of familiar foods which are particularly enjoyable for the patient should be encouraged and used if possible. Small frequent feedings are better tolerated and may be less tiring if the patient has difficulty conserving energy. Brushing the teeth and rinsing the mouth may help make the food more appetizing. Petroleum jelly will help to heal cracked lips.

The real challenge comes when the community health nurse must help the patient maintain an adequate nutrition when eating or absorption is a problem. The most frequent nutritional problem is nausea and vomiting. This is most often associated with chemotherapy. Some individuals rarely experience nausea and vomiting while others will have severe bouts of nausea each time they receive chemotherapy. If nausea and vomiting is a problem, the community health nurse may assist the patient in arranging the hours of medication administration (i.e., late afternoon or after the evening meal) so that fewer meals will be lost, and so that, hopefully, the patient will be recovered by the morning and able to eat breakfast. Antiemetics may be necessary to relieve the nausea. Compazine and Torecan generally seem to be more effective than Tigan. Elevating the upper torso can also help relieve the nausea. Sour ball candy or breath fresheners can restore a pleasant taste in the mouth after vomiting. Certain drugs seem to cause an alteration in taste sensations. This seems to be particularly pronounced in relation to proteins (e.g., meat, fowl, and fish). Serving these foods cold or choosing other foods with a less distinctive aroma and taste seems to be somewhat helpful.

Radiotherapy will also affect the patient's ability to eat. Swelling, irritation, and mucosal changes account for most of the radiotherapy problems. Moniliasis and ulcerations of the mouth cause such pain on mastication that food is avoided. As therapy continues these symptoms extend down the alimentary tract. Symptoms may become so severe that the patient will not eat at all. Until the symptoms subside, the patient should limit intake to soft foods and liquids. Acidic juices such as orange juice or spicy foods can be irritating to mucosal linings and should be avoided. Sucking on ice or using a local anesthetic may help to numb sensitive areas.

There are some very specific nutritional problems associated with cancer located along the alimentary track. Cancer of the head and neck causes difficulty with mastication and swallowing. Esophagectomy may create a malabsorption of fat and gastrectomy can cause a dumping syndrome with related vitamin B_{12} and iron deficiencies.

Severe nutritional problems associated with the cancer, surgery, radiotherapy, or chemotherapy may require intravenous therapy, a tube feeding, supplemental dietary liquids, or hyperalimentation to correct or control the problem. Although these are useful and necessary management approaches, finding methods that closely assimilate the patient's previous eating patterns and behaviors is most desirable. Gastric feedings of blenderized foods are preferable to the expensive, commercially prepared variety and allow the patient to control what he eats, while also allowing the individual to gradually adjust the strength. Preparing foods with MCT oil (a medium-chain triglyceride) will control steatorrhea for patients with absorption problems,[28] but will not necessarily require major dietetic alterations. The goal is to provide all of the basic nutritional requirements in a form that is appropriate to that individual's altered needs while still adhering to that individual's previous dietary patterns.

ELIMINATION

The major problems with elimination seem to focus around diarrhea, constipation, urinary incontinence, and surgical diversion.

Diarrhea is believed to be caused by a hormonal secretion.[19] When diarrhea is a problem, the patient should avoid eating those foods which caused loose stools in the past (e.g., raw fruits and vegetables, whole grain foods, coffee, tea, nicotine, alcohol). Tranquilizers and antispasmodics to decrease peristalsis may be needed. If diarrhea exists for any length of time, the anal region can become quite tender and excoriated and may require sitz baths, creams, or local anesthetics to relieve the discomfort.

Constipation can be a very big problem for patients receiving opiates or vincristine. This is one instance where the patient can no longer rely on his previous patterns and methods for maintaining regularity. Stool softeners, mineral oil, or a laxative must be taken daily and the patient must be acutely aware of the interval between bowel movements. An enema or suppository should be taken every three to four days if the patient has not passed stool within that period of time. Patients on strong narcotics can become impacted quickly. It is extremely uncomfortable to be disimpacted and can be avoided by strictly adhering to a daily laxative program.

Although indwelling urinary catheters are discouraged because of the high incidence of infection and loss of bladder tone, it is the treatment of choice if keeping the individual dry restores him to society. If fear of accidents prevents an individual from becoming an active, functioning person again, then that is the goal, not maintaining the integrity of the urinary system.

Urinary and fecal diversion are included among those surgical procedures which can totally destroy the individual's body image. To expel waste materials on the abdomen is a repugnant idea for some. Concern about accidents, odor, or noises, and altered appearance can become the overriding considerations and thus prevent the "ostomy" patient from ever seeing himself as a normal person, living a typical life. The goal is living, not performing a function.

With perhaps minor changes in routine, the ostomy patient should fit into the family's routine schedules without any problem. If an irrigation is required, the time chosen to perform this should be based upon previous bowel habits, the time that the patient leaves for work, the needs of other family members (particularly for the bathroom), the time of day large meals are generally eaten, and the length of time required to irrigate. Gas and odor can generally be controlled by avoiding troublesome foods (e.g., onions, beans, cabbage, fruit juices, concentrated sweets, and uncooked fruits and vegetables cause diarrhea; eggs, fish, coffee, and garlic cause odor). Oranges and orange juice, parsley, cranberry juice, and buttermilk help to control odor. Marshmallows will help to give consistency and formation to the stool. Cranberry juice and pulverized aspirin tablets added to the drainage bag will help to acidify the urine and cut down on odor for ureteroileostomies. Urinary calculi are generally due to a poor fluid intake in an attempt to keep the output scanty.

TERMINAL CARE

The community health nurse may be consulted at various times for various reasons throughout the cancer disease course. However, when the patient reaches the terminal phase of the disease, it is frequently the community health nurse who becomes the primary health care provider. It is to the community health nurse that the patient and the patient's family turn to during this most difficult time.

There are no magic answers of how to give care to dying patients. It is extremely difficult work which can quickly drain the care provider of all physical and emotional strength. There are no substitutes for the care and compassion which are required to provide the dying patient with quality days, not a quantity of days. Keeping the patient comfortable while permitting him the freedom to do what he wants, when he wants may require much ingenuity.

One of the biggest problems for terminally ill cancer patients is pain. Not all cancer patients have pain, but for those who do, every effort must be made to relieve it. McCaffery[29] defines pain as "whatever the person experiencing pain says it is and exists whenever he says it does." This definition relates well to the gate control theory of pain[30] which describes pain as a complex perceptual experience whereby sensory input is altered by a distinctive but interacting neural system before the input evokes pain perception and response. Therefore, the pain producing situation, the individual's unique history of pain, and the person's present state of mind will each influence the individual's reaction to and perception of pain. Large diameter fibers located in the spinal cord can block the pain from reaching the brain. These large diameter fibers on the surface of the skin are stimulated by vibration, scratching, rubbing, and so forth.

The community health nurse can use the gate control theory to manage a patient's pain. Vibration, rubbing, scratching, back rubs, massage, hot or cold applications, and measures to allay anxiety and occupy the mind are all effective methods for reducing the patient's pain. These techniques can be used either alone or in combination with other pain management methods to relieve pain. The nonchemical procedures for relieving pain are neurosurgery, electrostimulation, biofeedback, acupuncture, hypnosis, and radiotherapy.

The goals of analgesic pain management are to: 1) provide pain relief without clouding the sensorium, 2) control pain whenever possible with oral medications, and 3) devise a schedule which usually provides pain relief for at least four hours.[31]

In planning a pain management program for the terminally ill, it must be remembered that terminal cancer patients have chronic pain which does not diminish with time and may, in fact, become worse. If the pain is not controlled, it will become the center of one's life and the meaning of existence for that patient. Uncontrolled pain will quickly drain all of the patient's physical and mental resources. If the patient is being controlled with narcotic analgesics, tolerance will develop. "Tolerance is characterized by a decreased duration and intensity of the effect of the drug on its repeated administration."[32] As tolerance develops, a larger dose is necessary to produce the same effect. This is different from the physical dependence which is manifest by withdrawal symptoms and abstinence behavior.

The most frequent mistakes made in medicating for pain are 1) not giving doses large enough to relieve the pain, 2) giving the medication too infrequently without sufficient knowledge of the duration of effective action, 3) assuming that the oral dose is equivalent to the parenteral dose, and 4) neglecting tolerance as a valid reason for increasing the dosage.

Brompton's cocktail (a potent oral analgesic liquid containing morphine, cocaine, alcohol, simple syrup, and an aromatic elixer)[33] is not a miracle drug that will solve all the pain management problems. Perhaps the drug's most significant feature is that it is given every three to four hours around the clock thereby preventing pain, not merely keeping it in check. Advocates of heroin believe that pain control cannot be achieved until this drug is legalized, however, drugs that are readily available now are capable of relieving pain if used in the correct doses and given before the pain returns. The nurse is not doing the patient in pain any service by suggesting that he "tough it out" awhile longer under the misguided assumption that too much strong medication will cause addiction—a situation to be avoided at all costs!

Giving nursing care to terminally ill patients does not require an arsenal of supplies, equipment, machinery, drugs, and advanced technical knowledge. It does require a nurse who is skilled in providing good basic nursing care, who can listen to what the patient is saying and can respond to the patient's wishes. Making the patient comfortable is the goal. This sounds quite simple, but all too frequently the goal becomes an adequate intake, a daily bath, getting out of bed, taking the prescribed medicine, avoiding skin breakdown, and so forth because "the patient needs it" or "it would be good for him." Instead the patient needs someone to be with him when he wants it and someone who is willing to allow him to say or do what is most meaningful for him. Eating may not be important, and the patient doesn't care if he dies with an open sore on his buttocks, but it is very important that his wife understand his burial wishes or that he take a drive in the country to see the autumn colors one last time. Nurses talk about individualized patient care and responding to the patient's needs, but only when these are in agreement with the nurse's preestablished plan of care. It is very difficult to watch a patient starve himself, but dying is the last thing this patient can do by himself and he should be allowed to do it his way.

It is not necessary that all patients reach the stage of acceptance[21] prior to death. It is important that the community health nurse recognize the specific behaviors which indicate that the patient is progressing through the stages. For example, the nurse who can do absolutely nothing that pleases the patient should not defend these actions or request a reassignment but should recognize that the patient is ventilating his anger about what is happening to him. If the patient seems unusually depressed, the community health nurse should not try to cheer him up or recommend mood elevators. Both the anger and the depression are appropriate, normal behaviors during the dying process and should be recognized as such. The goal of the community health nurse is not to force the patient to progress through the stages (this will only end in failure) but to provide an atmosphere of open communication and understanding so that the patient is given the opportunity to progress at his own pace to the stage which is best for him.

Family

The family of the cancer patient will, at times, assist the community health nurse to provide care to the patient and will, at other times, be the focus of the nurse's intervention. The family's needs and reactions will closely parallel, in type and in number, the needs of the cancer patient. When the disease is quiescent and the patient is an integral member of the family, the disease is forgotten or at least relegated to a position of less importance. This is not the time to constantly remind the patient that he is not well but should be the time when the patient and family prepare physically, emotionally, and financially for the future. Unfortunately, most families do not use this time to honestly and openly make plans. Consequently, as the disease progresses, each significant change has the potential for precipitating another crisis. While the patient's energy reserves dwindle due to the treatments and disease, the family begins to lose energy too by trying to take on too much responsibility and by failing to set realistic limits. They must be encouraged to conserve their energy and to use it wisely over what may be an extended illness period. They must recognize and appropriately utilize the strengths of each individual member and the collective strengths of the family unit. Most importantly, they must not feel or be encouraged that they can or should even try to do it alone. They must realize that help is available and that asking for help does not mean admitting defeat. All family members should, whenever possible, be consulted regarding family decisions, and the individual family member should be consulted regarding decisions which directly affect that member. Family members cannot know what is best for the patient without consulting him. It is not a service to anyone to make decisions regarding that person's life under the assumption that it would be too upsetting to consult the person. This is the most dehumanizing and frustrating thing that could be done to any thinking, feeling being. Families must be cautioned not to make the patient's decisions.

NUTRITION

Overcoming anorexia can be a challenge for the patient and his family. Whenever possible the patient will probably eat better if he is able to follow the behaviors and patterns which are most enjoyable to him. Cocktails and wine before meals may stimulate the appetite. Food that is served attractively (flowers, napkins, china, silverware, etc.) may serve as an invitation to eat. If the patient is accustomed to eating with his family, they may arrange to eat in his room with him when he is unable to join them. The patient may attempt to try a small portion of his favorite foods when nothing else seems appealing. Sometimes altering the recipe may allow the patient to eat foods that would otherwise be contraindicated. The family plays a major role in making meals enjoyable, attractive, and consequently encouraging the patient to eat.

Eating and health are closely entwined. When the patient does not or cannot eat, the family may try to force foods on him so that he will feel better or perhaps even get better. This could create conflict as the family tries harder to induce eating when the patient is unable or has no desire to eat.

ELIMINATION

Elimination is generally perceived as a private function, however, it may become a family concern if the patient is unable to meet his own needs. The bedridden patient with urinary or fecal incontinence may become a burden to the family trying to keep the patient clean and dry. The community health nurse may be able to suggest some labor saving techniques (bedside commodes, rubber sheeting, indwelling catheter, etc.) that will help to conserve the energy of the family and still allow the patient some control. Family members may need to learn techniques to irrigate a colostomy or change the bags.

Assisting someone with personal hygiene specifically in relation to waste materials may be an unpleasant task for some family members. Their behaviors and facial expressions may convey this message to the patient which can reinforce to the patient that he is a burden.

TERMINAL CARE

Most people, given the choice, would prefer to die at home. But caring for terminally ill cancer patients may, at times, be very difficult. Families who make the commitment to honor the patient's request will need help, support, and encouragement from the community health nurse and the community at large.

The biggest mistake made by families wishing to keep the patient at home is in underestimating the amount of care required and the energy capabilities of the person(s) providing the care. No one family member can assume responsibility for providing care on a 24 hour basis. That individual needs both physical and emotional rest away from the patient, otherwise the person is sleeping with one eye and one ear open waiting for the patient to call. The primary caregiver needs the opportunity to get away from the house and do something different—go to the beauty parlor or play cards with the "boys." Outlets away from responsibility for the patient will allow the primary caregiver to rejuvenate and return refreshed and ready to start working again. Without these breaks the primary caregiver can quickly be drained of all energies and therefore be unable to respond to the patient at a time when he may most need help. Reductions in family size and increasing family mobility may mean that there are few family members among whom primary care giving responsibilities can be shared. When this is the situation, the family may need to rely upon other supports (e.g., friends, neighbors, church members, colleagues). This may be difficult for some people who pride themselves on being able to do for themselves without asking for help. The community health nurse will be one of those supports and can relieve the primary caregiver for certain periods of time. However, the community health nurse cannot be the only backup support; it is a responsibility of the nurse to assist the patient and family to identify that support system and establish how, when, and why they will use the system.

After the family has made the decision to keep the patient at home, there may come times when they question the correctness of that decision and suggest that the patient may receive better care in a hospital or nursing home. The community health nurse must reassure the family that the decision was a good one and that the care they are providing is no different than what would be done in an institutional setting. Praise and reassurance of a job well done may be the most important thing that the community health nurse does for the family.

The nurse must assess the needs of family members during this time. While all energies are directed toward the dying patient, family members may be neglecting their own needs. These might include physical, psychological, spiritual, educational, social, or financial needs. Each family member also has other obligations and responsibilities which cannot be ignored. The community health nurse may need to offer polite reminders, thereby giving the person permission to attend to nonpatient activities. This may be especially necessary when the activities might be interpreted as light or frivolous.

The community health nurse must assess the patient and try to anticipate what his needs may be during the periods between visits. If the family has been alerted to anticipate a particular problem and has been given some suggestions of what to do, they will be in a better position to cope with the situation. When it becomes apparent that the patient will die soon, the nurse should discuss with the family how death might occur. The nurse will also want to review with them what to do after death—who needs to be notified and whom within the family has been designated to do what.

The family will undoubtedly have questions and concerns that need immediate attention and cannot wait until the community health nurse's next visit. The family should have the name and phone number of someone who is available to provide help and support 7 days a week, 24 hours a day. Frequently the concern can be handled during a telephone call, while at other times the family may need the physical presence of someone who is willing to respond to them in their hour of need. Hospice home care programs are designed to specifically meet the needs of terminally ill patients and their families.

Although it is ideal for the patient to die at home, some families are not able to cope with and accept responsibility for the care of their dying member. The patient is then usually admitted to an acute or chronic hospital or skilled nursing home. More recently inpatient hospice care is being made available in this country. Here, in a homelike environment, the patient is permitted to remain in control of his life and his destiny while receiving professional care to keep him comfortable and pain free.

The job of the community health nurse does not end with the death of the patient. The period of bereavement is a particularly difficult one and is associated with significantly higher morbidity and mortality rates.[13] The amount of grief is not necessarily proportional to biologic ties, however, grieving is a normal reaction for those who have experienced a loss. The grieving process and the psychological stages of progression are very similar to those associated with dying. Engel[34] identifies the stages as shock and disbelief, developing awareness, restitution, resolving the loss, and idealization. The individual must be permitted to grieve before being able to resolve the loss and begin living without the lost person. The process is lengthy, generally requiring 12 to 18 months for the loss of a significant person. There is no one correct way to grieve (e.g., tears need not be shed). The community health nurse cannot develop any preconceived ideas of how the grieving family members should behave; in most instances it will vary from individual to individual.

Anniversaries, holidays, and special family days are particularly difficult and the grief during these times is extremely intense. The community health nurse can reassure the family that their behavior and feelings are normal and must be expressed before the grief is resolved.

Pathologic grief is grief that is greatly exaggerated in intensity or duration which affects the individual's ability to function. The person may exhibit symptoms of mental illness or self-destructive behavior. The community health nurse must recognize pathologic grief and assist the person in getting appropriate professional help.

The community health nurse must pay particularly close attention to the needs of grieving children because they are frequently forgotten grievers. Families will attempt to shield children from death and dying. The child is confused by what is happening around him, his questions are answered in vague generalities, and he is isolated from the events associated with death. The child is placed in an awkward position of grieving when he has supposedly been sheltered from all the unpleasantness and consequently is left to grieve alone. The mystery and unknown which surrounds death for the child may cause that individual to fear death rather than perceiving death as a part of living.

Community

The community health nurse, perhaps more than any other health care professional, is knowledgeable about available community resources and how to correctly use them. The community health nurse is also in a unique position to know and understand the specific needs of the cancer patient. Therefore the community health nurse should be an active, vocal participant when community services are planned. The cancer patient and his family will probably need assistance with food costs and preparation, living and health care costs, transportation, equipment and supplies, spiritual needs, facilities accessible to the handicapped, readily available and cheap special care items (e.g., mastectomy bras), child care, rehabilitation items, terminal care, and funeral arrangemets.

Perhaps one of the most useful and some of the best community services available for cancer patients and their families are the self-help groups composed of other individuals experiencing the same problems. Laryngectomy, mastectomy, and ostomy patients have self-help groups available to help them adjust to the unique aspects related to their diseases and surgery. Make Today Count, the Candlelighters, and the Widow-to-Widow programs are designed to help the dying and bereaved. These groups provide a perspective and service that will augment the services offered by the community health nurse.

The community health nurse is in a unique position to provide valuable guidance and assistance to developing hospice programs. Hospice care must be viewed as an extension of existing services and facilities and not the creation of new services and facilities which are costly and may duplicate available services.

EDUCATION

Public Education

The American Cancer Society sponsors many programs which are designed to help people protect themselves against cancer. These programs include clinics to help smokers learn effective ways to break the habit, teaching techniques of self-examination, developing awareness of available screening methods, and teaching and reviewing good health practices.

Many hospitals and professional health organizations offer public educational programs to help develop community awareness of cancer prevention, screening, and treatment approaches.

Professional Education

The goal of professional education programs is to share the latest developments in cancer to the health community. Conferences, meetings, and workshops are available on a national and local basis to disseminate information on the detection, treatment, and rehabilitation of cancer. There is a wide variety of films and publications which are specifically geared to those health care professionals involved in cancer care.

The American Cancer Society and the National Cancer Institute spend millions of dollars yearly to train physicians, dentists, nurses, and allied health care professionals in the diagnosis and treatment of cancer. Specially approved teaching centers and hospitals provide the environment and equipment so that those giving cancer care can learn the latest techniques which ultimately result in better patient care and improved cancer morbidity and mortality rates.

RESEARCH

The National Cancer Institute has developed a comprehensive program of clinical research centers which are involved in cancer research. The American Cancer Society also provides a large amount of money which is earmarked for cancer research. Cancer research projects include studies to determine the causes of cancer, human behavior and personality traits associated with cancer, genetic factors, carcinogens, risk factors, prevention and screening techniques, treatment methods, rehabilitation, immunology, hormonal factors, relationship to viruses, cancer cell differentiation, radiology techniques, nutritional factors, pain management, symptom control, terminal care concerns, and alternative methods of care (i.e., hospice).

Much time, money, and professional knowledge has gone into cancer research. Cancer remains in the forefront of public and professional attention, because the knowledge to irradicate the disease is not yet available, however, each year significant advances are made in prevention, treatment, and rehabilitation methods.

The role of the community health nurse is to interpret prevention, treatment, and rehabilitation advances to the cancer patient, the patient's family, and to the community with the goal of allowing the cancer patient to remain, whenever possible, an active member of his family and of his community.

REFERENCES

1. Anderson, D.E.: "Genetic Varieties of Neoplasia," in *Genetic Concepts and Neoplasia.* Symposium on Fundamental Cancer Research, 1969, present at the University of Texas. M.D. Anderson Hospital and Tumor Institute at Houston. The Williams & Wilkins Co., Baltimore, 1970.
2. Fraumeri, J.F., Jr., "Genetic Factors," in Holland, J.F., and Frei, E., III (eds.): *Cancer Medicine.* Lea & Febiger, Philadelphia, 1973.
3. Hertz, R.: "Evaluation of Current Information Concerning the Relationship between Hormonal Usage and Cancer." *Clinical Obstetrics and Gynecology,* 20:165, 1977.
4. Lipsett, MB.: "Estrogen Use and Cancer Risk." *J.A.M.A.* 237:1112, 1977.
5. Herbst, A.L., Ulfeder, H., and Poskanzer, D.C.: "Adenocarcinoma of the Vagina: Association of Maternal Stilbestrol Therapy with Tumor Appearance in Young Women." *New England Journal of Medicine,* 281:878, 1971.
6. Weisburger, J.H.: "Chemical Carcinogenesis," in Holland, J.F., and Frei, E., III (eds.): *Cancer Medicine.* Lea & Febiger, Philadelphia, 1973.
7. Silverstein, M.J., and Morton, D.L.: "Cancer Immunotherapy." *American Journal of Nursing,* 73:1178, 1973.
8. Baldonado, A.A., and Stahl, D.C.: *Cancer Nursing: A Holistic Multidisciplinary Approach.* Medical Examination Publication Co., Garden City, N.Y., 1978.
9. Gengerelli, J.A., and Kirkner, F.J.: *The Psychological Variables in Human Cancer.* University of California Press, Los Angeles, 1954.

10. Bahnson, M.B., and Bahnson, C.B.: "Ego Defenses in Cancer Patients." *Annals of the New York Academy of Sciences,* 164:623, 1969.
11. Kissen, D.M., Brown, R.I.F., and Kissen, M.: "A Further Report on Personality and Psychosocial Factors in Lung Cancer." *Annals of the New York Academy of Sciences,* 164:535, 1969.
12. Holmes, T.H., and Rahe, R.G.: "The Social Readjustment Eating Scale." *Journal Of Psychosomatic Research,* 11:213, 1967.
13. Parkes, C.M.: *Bereavement.* International Universities Press, New York, 1972.
14. Seligman, M.E.P.: "Giving up on Life." *Psychology Today,* 80, May 1974.
15. *Cancer Facts and Figures, 1978.* American Cancer Society, 1977.
16. *The Impact, Costs, and Consequences of Catastrophic Illness on Patients and Families.* Cancer Care, Inc., New York, 1973.
17. Higginson, J., and Muir, C.S.: "Epidemiology," in Holland, J.F., and Frei, E., III (eds.): *Cancer Medicine.* Lea & Febiger, Philadelphia, 1973.
18. Staihar, J.: "Health Care in Canada vs. Medical Bills Here." *The Washington Post,* Tuesday, October 10, 1978, A-9.
19. Donovan, M.I., and Pierce, S.C.: *Cancer Care Nursing.* Appleton-Century-Crofts, New York, 1976.
20. Lipowski, Z.J.: "Physical Illness, the Individual and the Coping Processes." *Psychiatry in Medicine,* 1:91, 1970.
21. Küber-Ross, E.: *On Death and Dying.* Macmillan, New York, 1969.
22. Podolsky, D.K., Weiser, M.M., Isselbacher, K.J., et al.: "A Cancer-Associated Galactosyltransferase Isoenzyme." *New England Journal of Medicine,* 299:703, 1978.
23. Reynoso, G.: "Biochemical Tests in Cancer Diagnosis," in Holland, J.F., and Frei, E., III (eds.): *Cancer Medicine.* Lea & Febiger, Philadelphia, 1973.
24. Rosen, P.P., Menendez-Botet, C.J., Nisselbaum, J.S., et al.: "Pathological Review of Breast Lesions Analyzed for Estrogen Receptor Protein." *Cancer Research,* 35:3187, 1975.
25. Rogers, M.E.: *An Introduction to the Theoretical Basis of Nursing.* F.A. Davis Co., Philadelphia, 1970.
26. Bingham, C.A.: "The Cell Cycle and Cancer Chemotherapy." *American Journal of Nursing,* 1978:1201, 1978.
27. Souchon, E.A., Copeland, E.M., Watson, P., et al.: "Intravenous Hyperalimentation as an Adjunct to Cancer Chemotherapy with 5-Fluorouracil." *Journal of Surgical Research,* 18:451, 1975.
28. Burkhalter, P.K.: "Theories of Causation," in Burkhalter, P.K., and Donley, D.L. (eds.): *Dynamics of Oncology Nursing.* McGraw-Hill Book Company, New York, 1978.
29. McCaffery, M.: *Nursing Management of the Patient With Pain,* J. B. Lippincott, Philadelphia, 1972.
30. Melzack, R., and Wall, P.D.: "Pain Mechanisms: A New Theory." *Science,* 150:971, 1965.
31. Beaver, William. Pharmacology Consultant, The Washington Home Hospice: Personal Communication, 1978.
32. Houde, R.W.: "The Use and Misuse of Narcotics in the Treatment of Pain," in Bonica, J.J.: *Advances in Neurology,* Vol. 4. Raven Press, New York, 1974.
33. Davis, A.J.: "Brompton's Cocktail: Making Good-Byes Possible." *American Journal of Nursing,* 78:611, 1978.
34. Engel, G.L.: "Grief and Grieving." *American Journal of Nursing,* 64:93, 1964.

CHAPTER 23
DIABETES MELLITUS

DIANA W. GUTHRIE, M.S.P.H., R.N., F.A.A.N., AND RICHARD A. GUTHRIE, M.D., F.A.A.D.

Diabetes mellitus is a chronic disease that has been recognized for centuries. It has been classified as both an endocrine disease and as a disease of metabolism. The cause of this disease is still unknown although it has been associated with a deficiency in the production and/or release of the hormone insulin, which is secreted by the beta cells of the pancreas. These beta cells are a part of the clusters of cells found throughout the pancreas called the *islets of Langerhans*.

Diabetes mellitus is characterized by abnormal, elevated blood glucose levels frequently accompanied by glucose passing into the urine. Diabetes is usually hereditary in origin although other causes such as viral infections, stress drugs such as steroids, other hormonal based diseases such as acromegaly, tumors of the pancreas, or blood based disease, such as hemochromatosis, are sometimes associated with diabetes.

The cardinal symptoms of diabetes are the three "polys": polydipsia or frequent thirst, polyphagia or frequent food intake, and polyruia or frequent urination. These symptoms are found in the insulin dependent type of disease called juvenile diabetes mellitus. Tiredness, obesity, changes in vision, or sores that do not heal in an appropriate length of time are found in the noninsulin dependent type of disease called *maturity onset diabetes*. The new terminology for these two forms of diabetes mellitus is type I diabetes (juvenile type) and type II diabetes (maturity onset type) and these two designations will be used in this chapter. Diabetes can be quite dangerous and life threatening. It may cause alterations in body chemistry that may lead to electrolyte imbalance and, if intervention does not occur, to acidosis and death. In the more chronic state, neuropathy, retinopathy, nephropathy, and/or angiopathy may develop. The chronic problems can result in loss of feeling or pain, blindness, kidney failure, hypertension, impotency, atony of the bladder, and other problems.

The derivation of the words "diabetes mellitus" are from the Greek and Latin. Diabetes is a Greek work meaning to siphon or to pass through while mellitus, the Latin word, means sweet tasting or honeylike. In diabetes mellitus, the ancient Greeks noted the weight loss and frequent urination. They reported the "melting down into the loins." The Egyptians wrote about this disease on a papyrus dating from the second millennium B.C. They noted that the urine attracted insects. The Romans perhaps tasted the urine and added the mellitus to the descriptive term, diabetes. Dated material from India and China also noted the phenomena of frequent urination, thirst, and sweet tasting urine, leading to death. The other diabetes is called *diabetes insipidus*. Diabetes insipidus is a disease of the posterior pituitary gland resulting in a deficiency of antidiuretic hormone and the inability of the body to retain fluid—the passing of large volumes of flat or insipid tasting diluted urine.

It was not until the late 19th century that diabetes was demonstrated in animals. Before this time during the 18th century with the timely discovery of the microscope, Langerhans was able to see and describe the islets named after him a few years later. Minkowsky was the first to hypothesize that the pancreas and diabetes were somehow related. Although he was the first one to surgically cause diabetes in dogs, he was unable to isolate the hormone, insulin. It was not until the summer of 1921 that Frederick Banting, a surgeon, and the soon to be doctor, Charles Best (Best was then a medical student), devised a method to preserve the beta cell function outside the body so that insulin could be obtained for those cells.[1] Up to this time, diet was the only treatment for diabetes. Everything from programmed fasting periods to choices of foods, such as rancid meat and vegetables cooked three times in their own water, are examples of some of those initial treatment choices. When life saving insulin was discovered, all believed that a cure for the disease had been found. What actually had been found was a treatment that truly was life saving but also had the potential of opening the door to other life threatening problems.

Insulin is a life saving drug, of that there is no doubt. It has been refined, modified, and concentrated but no other breakthrough as dramatic as the discovery of insulin has occurred since its discovery. The 1950s did bring us the oral hypoglycemic agents which are pills, such as the sulfonylureas, which cause the pancreas to secrete as much insulin as possible or the biguanides, another class of drugs with a different mechanism of action, which were removed from the market in the fall of 1977. In the 1960s, Berson and Yallow developed a method of determining insulin levels in the blood by the discovery of radioimmunoassay. The electron microscope also expanded our world of understanding of diabetes. In the 1970s, glucagon, a hormone discovered in 1922 which is synthesized from the alpha cells of the pancreas, was studied and began to come into its own as a contributing factor in some of the problems of type I diabetes. Glucagon causes the liver and muscle cells to release stored glucose into the blood stream. Somatostatin, a hormone from the delta cells of the pancreas, shows potential as a regulatory hormone for the release of both insulin and glucagon.

Insulin deficiency is the key factor in the causation of diabetes mellitus. Insulin's action on glucose, a primary fuel for the body, is to permit the entrance of glucose into muscle, fat, and liver cells. By this action, insulin thus facilitates the use of glucose for body energy, prevents the mobilization of fats, and allows amino acids to enter the cells for protein systhesis. Insulin is not needed for glucose to enter into the nerve cells or the living cells of the intestinal wall. Normal blood glucose levels are between about 50 mg/dl and 150 mg/dl. Variations above and below this range most often cause noticeable effects on the body.

The action of insulin on cells is influenced by enzymes. Hexokinase and glucokinase are the two most active enzymes. Glucokinase aids in glucose storage in the liver. Hexokinase is involved in breaking down glucose in most of the other cells. This action is specific to muscle cells for the formation of energy and to fat cells for the formation of fats. Enzyme action is also involved in the conversion of glucose to fat. All this is controlled by the so-called *second messenger*, cyclic adenosine monophosphate or CAMP[2] (the *first messenger* is RNA or ribonucleic acid which is responsible for signaling protein synthesis including synthesis of insulin in the beta cells). The main stimulus for insulin to be released from the beta cells is the blood glucose level although other stimuli may be involved. These stimuli could be other hormones, sulfonylureas (such as found in oral hypoglycemic agents), ketones, and vagal stimulation. Stress will allow more glucose to be available to the body. The release of epinephrine during stress will cause the diminishing of the secretion of insulin. Insulin secretion may also be diminished by the action of thiazide diuretics, starvation, and decreased oxygen availability to the brain. Injected insulin may also cause a decrease in endogenous insulin.

When insulin is deficient or defective and the body is unable to transport glucose into the cells, body mechanisms are set into motion to try to compensate for the deficiency. Free fatty acids, an important source of energy for the cells, now increase in availability to the liver which, in turn, converts them into the ketone bodies—betahydroxybutyric acid, acetoacetic acid, and acetone. Amino acids, no longer able to enter the cell, also develop increasingly elevated levels in the blood system. All this action results in hyperglucosemia and glycosuria especially if the blood glucose is above the renal threshold (160 to 180 mg/dl in most children and 180 mg/dl or above in adults). Ketonemia and ketonuria (which may be seen in the urine no matter what prevents glucose from entering the cell—gastroenteritis, dieting, or not enough insulin) and elevated amino acids concentrations may also be seen. Hyperglucosemia leads to an osmotic gradient in the kidney resulting in polyuria and dehydration with an intracellular to extracellular redistribution of the body fluid. Hunger is an outcome of the body's inability to fulfill the cellular needs. Even in the presence of hunger and excess food intake, weight loss will occur. As dehydration increases and the electrolytes become unbalanced (pH lowered, CO_2 lowered, sodium lowered, serum potassium elevated, total body potassium lowered, and serum bicarbonate lowered), diabetic ketoacidosis results.

Even though we know the chemical composition and the molecular structure of insulin, much mystery still remains. Insulin deficiency may be partial or absolute. Insulin deficiency may be caused by the inability of the body to synthesize insulin or the failure of the pancreas to release insulin from the beta cells once it is synthesized. There is also the possibility that diabetes may be caused by the inability of insulin to act on the cell membrane's receptor sites or by a deficiency of receptor sites (type II diabetes). The etiology of diabetes is certain when part or all of the pancreas has been destroyed by tumor, surgical removal, or inflammation. In obese individuals, there are greater than normal amounts of insulin output. The excess insulin sercretion is thought to be due to overeating. The excess insulin, in turn, appears to induce a decrease in insulin receptors on the cell membrane by a mechanism as yet not elicited. A decrease in insulin receptors induces a state of insulin resistance which causes hyperglycemia which in turn induces greater insulin secretion, a further decrease in receptors, and a vicious cycle.

ETIOLOGY

The two major theories of the development of diabetes are the hereditary theory and the viral theory. Diabetes is thought to be inherited as a recessive gene. If both parents have diabetes of the adult type (type II), there is about a 100 percent chance of the child developing diabetes. If both parents have insulin dependent diabetes (type I), the child's chance of developing insulin dependent diabetes is between 45 to 65 percent, not 100 percent as we believed in the past. Fraternal twins have the same chance of developing the disease as if they were born independently.[3] Identical twins have an increased chance of developing the disease but not, as previously thought, a 100 percent chance of developing it especially if they have type I diabetes. The failure to demonstrate 100 percent concordance in identical twins with type I diabetes suggests that the cause of this form of diabetes is multifactorial and that the hereditary predisposition is acted upon by environmental factors.[4] One of these environmental factors may be viral infection. The present theory is that what the diabetic inherits is the inability to exclude specific viruses which may attack the beta cells. Antigens develop against these invaded beta cells resulting in an autoimmune phenomenon. When enough beta cells are destroyed, the body's metabolic balance is altered and the disease process becomes revealed by means of glucose tolerance testing or by symptomatology.

CLASSIFICATION

Diabetes can be classified in a number of ways. One classification is as follows: prediabetes, chemical diabetes (called prediabetes by some), and overt diabetes (Table 23-1).[5] Prediabetes is a state of genetic susceptibility and is more of a historical term until an adequate genetic marker for diabetes is found. Women who have babies weighing over nine pounds at birth or numerous unexplained still births and/or miscarriages are suspected of being prediabetic. Certain individuals with a strong family history might also be placed in this category. Chemical diabetes is a state of abnormal carbohydrate chemistry and is best characterized by the glucose tolerance test. The fasting blood glucose is normal with the rest of the glucose tolerance test abnormal. An early chemical diabetic may have a response of a rapidly elevated blood glucose followed by a sharp decline. This would be paralleled by a delayed but rapid rise and often over-response of insulin secretion almost concurrent with a rapid drop in glucose levels. The resulting symptoms of hypoglycemia (sweatiness,

TABLE 23-1. Classification of diabetes mellitus*

Prediabetes	Chemical Diabetes	Overt Diabetes
Strong family history	Normal tasting blood glucose	Abnormal fasting blood glucose
Nine pound babies or over	Oral glucose tolerance test	Oral glucose tolerance test
Frequent unexplained still births and/or miscarriages	(abnormal insulins and/or glucose)	(abnormal insulins and glucose), but not needed
Obesity	No signs or symptoms	Developing signs and symptoms
No signs or symptoms		
No positive laboratory tests		

*With permission from Jackson, R.L.: "The Child with Diabetes." *Nutrition Today* 6:7, March/April 1971.

pallor, nausea, shakiness, etc.) occur an hour or two after the ingesting of the concentrated glucose solution. Chemical diabetes may then progress from a mild state in which the fasting blood glucose in normal and the OGTT only mildly abnormal to a severely abnormal test. Overt diabetes may be manifest when symptomatology occurs but is actually apparent as soon as fasting blood glucose becomes abnormal (110 mg/dl or higher).

Another method of classification is that of primary and secondary diabetes mellitus (Table 23-2). Primary diabetes is broken down into two categories: ketosis prone (juvenile or type I diabetes mellitus) and ketosis resistant (adult, maturity onset or type II diabetes). Ketosis prone diabetes most commonly occurs during childhood or adolescence. This results in an insulin dependent type of diabetes that is unstable. These individuals are most often completely dependent on outside insulin. The beta cells are replaced by hyalinized tissue. Ketosis usually follows uncontrolled hyperglycemia, leading to ketoacidosis and, if unchecked, to coma and death.

Nonketosis prone or ketosis resistant diabetes is mainly found in individuals who are over 40 years of age. This type of diabetes is often manifest by excess release of insulin as determined by the glucose tolerance test with insulin measurements. The resultant diabetes is usually stable with little change in the beta cells. Microvascular diseases are more often seen as a complication of ketosis prone individuals whose diabetes is not well controlled. Macrovascular disease is more frequently seen in the individual who has the ketosis resistant type of diabetes.

Secondary diabetes mellitus is caused by a loss of or damage to pancreatic tissue resulting in a lack of insulin. There is also a stress diabetes resulting from an increased insulin need that cannot be met. The diabetes caused by burns or hyperalimentation falls into this category and is reversed once the stress is removed. Excess secretion or administration of counterregulatory hormones such as growth hormone, glucagon, or adrenocorticosteroids may also produce a reversible diabetic state.

STATISTICS

Age appears to have some importance in the diabetic syndrome. Maturity onset (type II) diabetes is usually seen in individuals who are over 40, and insulin dependent (type I) diabetes is seen mainly in individuals under 40 years of age. Still, type II diabetes has been

TABLE 23-2. Classification of diabetes mellitus

Primary Diabetes	
Ketosis prone	*Ketosis resistant*
Juvenile diabetes mellitus	Maturity onset diabetes
Usually under 40 yrs. of age	Usually over 40 yrs. of age
Unstable	Stable
Beta cells changed	Beta cells unchanged
Insulin dependent	Noninsulin dependent

Secondary Diabetes
Due to loss or damage of beta cells
Surgery
Infection
Drugs
Alteration in hormone release

documented in children and type I diabetes is found frequently in the elderly. Insulin dependent diabetics do grow up and as their disease is better controlled, they will become older. On the other hand, those with ketosis resistant type II diabetes may eventually lose their ability to make the low quality of insulin they produce and eventually need to be given insulin. Because of the overlapping of the age groups, we prefer the newer classification of type I and type II diabetes as previously defined.

Approximately 2 percent of the American population has diabetes. About 5 to 10 percent of the diabetic population are insulin dependent adults, while 80 percent or so are maturity onset or type II diabetics with approximately seven-eighths of this population overweight.[6] Roughly, one out of every 600 school age children has the disease.[7,8] The prevalence appears to increase with age with over two-thirds of the diabetes population over 55 years of age. The majority of known diabetics are at least 45 years of age and the chance for diabetes doubles with every ten years of life.

There is a predominance of women with diabetes. Over 55 percent of those with diabetes are female, and women are 50 percent more likely to have the disease than men.[6] Nonwhites are more likely than whites to have diabetes. There is an increased incidence noted in black women and this has apparently increased dramatically over the last ten years. Native Americans have a significantly higher incidence of the disease than the general populations. The majority of these people have type II diabetes. It has been estimated that 20 percent more nonwhites than whites develop diabetes. The prevalence of the disease in nonwhite populations appears more related to economic than to social class or to race, per se. The level of stress related to social adjustment may play a part as an environmental factor in this disease, but to date no firm studies have determined the specific figures to confirm this relation to the disease process. The best correlation in these individuals is with obesity.

Social stresses, such as employment problems brought on by fear in employers who perhaps have had bad experiences with previous employees with diabetes, may contribute to a worsening of the diabetic syndrome. Employer fears are unfounded. There are data to show that those patients with well-controlled diabetes are often more disciplined individuals and therefore better employees in the long run.

Economic aspects of this disease are great. Supplies alone for an insulin dependent person, who is well managed, are several hundred dollars per year. People with low income are three times more likely to develop the disease. Fourteen percent of the population are bedridden for an average of 1.5 months per year. Many insurance companies drop an individual once that individual is diagnosed as having the disease. Without considering the costs of chronic complications of the disease, the National Commission reported that more than $5 billion per year is lost from the direct and indirect costs of this disease to our nation.[6]

Diabetes is officially the fifth leading cause of death by disease. In some methods of classifying statistics, it may actually be the third leading cause of death by disease. The American Diabetes Association, the major voluntary organization for diabetes, and the Juvenile Diabetes Foundation are actively supporting legislation to gain support for much needed research monies and monies for education and for the funding of diabetes centers for the education of professionals. These groups are also pressing for improvement in the management of patients with this problem in order to reduce the devastating toll of this national and international problem. At an increase in incidence of diabetes of 6 percent per year, by 1980 13 million people will have diabetes. There are over 600,000 diabetics diagnosed each year. It is perhaps easier to comprehend this fact when we recognize that one out of four families has a history of diabetes and that one out of every

20 people will develop diabetes in their lifetime. Perhaps what is most shocking is that perhaps as many as one-half of all heart attacks, three-fourths of all strokes, four-fifths of all gangrene are caused by vascular disease resulting from diabetes. Diabetes is also the leading cause of new cases of blindness. Three hundred thousand or more deaths are attributed to diabetes each year. Once a person develops insulin dependent diabetes, the individual, especially without good control of the disease, is said to have only about 30 years to live. Diabetics are believed to have only one-third the life span of a nondiabetic. A 50 percent increase in the prevalence of diabetes has occurred between the years of 1965 and 1973 alone. The statistics show that those with diabetes are 25 times more prone to blindness, 17 times more prone to kidney disease, 5 times more prone to gangrene, and twice as prone to heart disease than the nondiabetic. The chance of being diabetic doubles with every 20 percent increase in body weight. There is the chance that one-half of the children with the disease will die from renal disease within 25 years to 30 years after the diagnosis of the disease. Prior to the age of 40, many of these children will face the prospect of blindness and/or death by renal failure. In the population studied by the National Diabetes Commission, those children followed 15 years or longer had eye disease 63 percent of the time, high blood pressure 20 percent of the time, and nearly 100 percent of the time became afflicted with scarring of the glomeruli of the kidney.[6]

SCOPE OF THE PROBLEM

Since the discovery of insulin in 1921, few dramatic changes in therapy have occurred. Even with the in-depth research that has occurred and is presently going on, neither a cure nor the prevention of the disease is immediately in sight. The 33,000 deaths indirectly attributed to diabetes in 1975 made diabetes the fifth leading cause of death by disease. Diabetes and its complications (especially vascular disease) are responsible for over 300,000 deaths annually and result in a not proud ranking as the third leading cause of death behind heart disease and cancer. We are now not only looking for a prevention or a cure but also to develop better methods of treating the disease and preventing complications. The scope of this disease becomes even wider as it is recognized that this syndrome may affect every part of the body in some way or another. Diabetes may affect every organ, every organ system, and eventually every cell of the body. Other problems which are not life threatening can also have serious consequences.

The psychological impact of having a chronic, potentially crippling disease can be disastrous. Peridontal disease may be as much as three times higher in diabetics than in nondiabetics, even though the chance of dental caries is no higher. Nerve cells may also be involved, resulting in either a peripheral or autonomic neuropathy or both. Damage to the nerve cells can lead to decreased innervation of muscle tissue including the nerves to the bladder or the hand. Pregnancy is now possible for the diabetic woman, but the increased stress of pregnancy in an already diseased individual suffering from complications of the disease increases the possibility of further damage. The eyes can be involved with the development of cataracts and/or retinal disease and blindness. The kidney may also develop damage through the thickening and therefore weakening of the basement membranes surrounding the glomerular capillaries.[9] Since over $5 billion is spent each year on diabetes and one-half of that is directed to health care costs, it is surprising to find that only $46 million was spent on research in the United States in 1975.

Diabetes involves many facets of care. Great emphasis is needed in each facet including patient care, patient education, and patient research as well as biochemical research for that elusive cure and prevention of a most devastating disease. From infancy on to death, this disease may plague the individual and/or the whole family. The responsibility and challenge of having a child or adult in the family with the disease, especially if the person is insulin dependent, can be quite an adjustment. Many families are unable to cope with the impact of the disease. The challenge to the community health nurse can almost become beyond comprehension as the nurse attempts to direct and deliver quality health care.

IMPACT

The Individual

The impact of the diagnosis of a chronic disease can be a very profound event in the life of an individual. The denial, anger, bargaining, and final resolution may take days to years to complete. A person may never adjust to the fact that the disease will last a life-time. Fear of loss of body functions may become the uppermost thought in the mind of a diabetic. Experiences may heighten this fear—an aunt who lost a leg, an uncle who went blind, seeing someone who has had a severe insulin reaction, and so on. The statistics as found in the National Diabetes Commission's report will not be comforting. A child might have a life span of 30 years after diagnosis or one-third that of the nondiabetic. The possibility of developing terminal renal disease in 25 years and blindness in 10 to 15 years is psychologically overwhelming. The impact of controversy is also felt. From one side they learn that control does make a difference, but then they may hear a speaker who still believes that complications are concomitant with the disease. Who are they to believe? How does this affect their decision making? The American Diabetes Association's pronouncement of March 1976[10] stating that control is important in the prevention of vascular disease is certainly one of the most supportive statements an individual can read. Education certainly will assist in the decision making process, but there is still the doubt. If the person becomes blind or otherwise incapacitated, does that person really want to keep on living? For the teenager, this is almost too much in the attempt to adjust from adolescence to adulthood. If the individual is the only one known to have diabetes in the school or at work, that individual has a tendency to feel different. Especially during the teenage years, feeling different may be more than can be tolerated. Fearful employers may not hire an individual with known diabetes. Employers might fire an employee or perhaps make a decision that would alter the work responsibilities, often resulting in a pay decrease, when diabetes is discovered. In total, the individual will have feelings of fear of loss, of being alone, or of being confined to the management he or she is directed to follow. Care must be taken that the response to these feelings is not self-destructive behavior or increased tensions leading to further difficulties in family interaction.

The Family

It is difficult enough to find out that a spouse has diabetes but to learn that your own child has the disease can lead to intense feelings of guilt, fear for self and for the individual, and resentment for the confining atmosphere that the disease management may impose upon the household. There may also be a feeling of rejection as their "perfect" child is now imperfect. Blame may be placed on the child or the other parent as the "cause" of the problem. Self-doubt may arise: "Am I the right kind of parent, or did I do something wrong to deserve this?" Families may respond to various feelings in a variety of ways. This response may be by overprotection, by neglect, or by harrassment. In the over-protection syndrome, the parents may not let the child out of their sight or they may be quite fearful when the loved one is out of sight. In the neglect syndrome, the parents may even deny the disease or ignore the disease in the children as it is "their disease." Anger (or love or annoyance) may be expressed by constant harrassment of the individual to. "Do this," "Take that," or "I'm going to tell the doctor," or, worse, "If you don't do that, you will die." If the parent is single, then one parent may blame the child for the family pressure that led to the divorce or, if the individual alone is involved, he or she may be fear-ful about being along and/or blame the disease for all problems. Family feelings may become unrealistic as they experience crisis episodes with the diabetic person. As has been inferred, this disease may result in family disunity and further disorganization.

The Community

The community impact of diabetes is presently an indirect problem. The impact of the disease could and does affect work placement, knowledge about the disease, training facilities for those that may become handicapped, and financing to establish education and care programs as well as research into this disease. The first and foremost problem is lack of public information about detection, patient education, patient management, and job discrimination. The increase of the impact of this disease may be felt in greater intensity if more people that have diabetes marry and have children. If the incidence has increased more than 50 percent since 1965, then the potential for the next 10 years would result in an even greater effect on industry. Those whose diabetes is poorly controlled will miss work days. This disease causes more days in bed among the noninstitutionalized population than any other disease.[6] If the individual becomes blind or needs renal dialysis, the cost to the community is greatly increased as the involved individual would in no way be able to afford the total cost of care and treatment that are part of the rehabilitation process or just part of the life support process alone. The National Commission reports that the economic impact of diabetes today is more than double what it was reported to be eight years ago. The community may then be faced with the burden of taxes to allow funds to be distributed in order that treatment and care may be given when needed.

There is the need for early diagnosis . Perhaps with early diagnosis, problems may be prevented. The rehabilitation of the individual and/or family in the community might then be less expensive. If adequate care is given, the chance then for these well-controlled individuals to live longer lives means an increased need for adequate nursing care in various levels of nursing homes. If skilled nursing is needed for those with complications, the cost will become far greater. The problems related to the community then compound the needs for time, information, and money.

PREVENTION – TREATMENT APPROACHES

The Individual

This disease syndrome requires the approach by the nursing process.[11] Assesssment is a must before any planning may be started. The plans must be individualized to fit into the life style of the person or family with the disease. As the plans are implemented, the evaluation process must also be individualized. Although the assessment has an emphasis on environmental facilities, the physical assessment of the individual will take priority. This would include the capabilities and limitations of the individual both mentally and physically. Everything from pedal pulses to the history of sexual function needs to be included in the physical assessment.[12] The overall nutritional status of the individual as well as other impressions made by the physical and mental assessments will direct the community health nurse to coordinate with the physician to refer the client to appropriate resources if they are not already included in the care plan. Treatment and approaches to such should be based on the preventive aspects of care.

To date, we do not know how to prevent the disease. We also do not know exactly how to mimic mother nature when the disease is overtly recognized. The detection of an individual in the chemical diabetes state may allow some possibility for the prevention of the progression of the disease. This may perhaps be accomplished with weight control adequate for height, the prevention of obesity, and with the restriction of concentrated sweets as a part of daily food habits.

Tissue typing has given us some insight as to the potential for developing the disease. Researchers are pursuing retrospective studies utilizing new tools such as tissue typing, and we hope there will be increased opportunity for the use of this knowledge. Chromosomes have been noted to have specific configurations for some specific diseases. On the number six chromosome are antigenic sites known as the HLA (Human Lymphocyte Antigens) system. Maturity onset diabetes has been found to have no definable pattern of HLA. There is a characteristic HLA typing pattern in juvenile diabetes. If individuals who subsequently may develop diabetes can be identified by HLA typing and the cost of the typing becomes more realistic (at present, tissue typing costs about $700), then perhaps in the identified individual ideal nutrition can be stressed, etiologic environmental factors can be diminished, and the onset of the disease perhaps delayed until a cure or prevention, such as a vaccine, may be developed.

If an individual develops diabetic ketoacidosis, treatment may be by a combination of intravenous and subcutaneous or intramuscular administration of insulin along with supportive fluid and electrolyte therapy. Another method of approach is the perfused insulin technique in which small amounts of insulin are administered intravenously and continuously over a period of several hours. As blood glucose is lowered and stabilization is reached, the patient is transferred to subcutaneous insulin. During the acute period of care, the patient should be monitored carefully. The state of hydration, the body chemistry, the vital signs, cardiac monitoring for indications of potassium alterations, checking of urinary glucose, and monitoring the administration of insulin, in whatever form, are parameters that should be monitored during this most acute time.

Further management of the disease is based on life-style, insulin actions, and knowledge of self-care. Insulinization needs to be adequate to cover the needs of the body throughout the 24-hour period. Therefore, knowledge of insulin action is a must (Table 23-3). Insulin may be detected in the blood stream but may not be available in quality or quantity sufficient to be able to fill the receptor sites during the entire 24-hour period. Insulin may act differently in different individuals and in different age groups.

Medication and/or diet should be prescribed around the individual and the individual's life-style, not the individual around the regimen. In most individuals, adequate insulinization on a 24-hour basis requires two or more doses of combinations or singly of intermediate and rapid acting insulins. Long acting insulins are used in some programs. Treatment is adequate only if flexibility and 24-hour insulinization are possible under the chosen

TABLE 23-3. Action of medications. The most recently published figures on insulin and oral agent action in adults and children.

Rapid Acting Medication			
Drug	*Onset*	*Peak*	*Duration of Activity*
Adults			
Oral agent [13]			
Tolbutamide (Orinase)	(half life 4-5 hrs)	5-8 hrs	6-12 hrs
Insulin [14]			
Regular	1/2-1 hrs	2-3 hrs	5-7 hrs
Semilente	1/2-1 hrs	4-7 hrs	12-16 hrs
Children and adults—effective duration of action [5]			
Insulin			
Regular	1/2 hr	2-4 hrs	6-8 hrs
Semilente	1/2 hr	2-4 hrs	8-10 hrs

Intermediate Acting Medications			
Drug	*Onset*	*Peak*	*Duration of Activity*
Adults			
Oral agents [13]			
Acetohexamide (Dymelor)	(half life 6-8 hrs)		12-24 hrs
Tolazamide (Tolinase)	(half life 6-8 hrs)	4-8 hrs	10-15 hrs
Insulin [14]			
NPH (Neutral Protamine Hagedorn)	1-2 hrs	8-12 hrs	18-24 hrs
Lente	1-4 hrs	8-12 hrs	18-24 hrs
Children and adults—effective duration of action [5]			
Insulin			
NPH	1-2 hrs	6-8 hrs	12-14 hrs
Lente	1-2 hrs	6-8 hrs	14-16 hrs
Globin	1-2 hrs	6-8 hrs	12-14 hrs

Long Acting Medications			
Drug	*Onset*	*Peak*	*Duration of Activity*
Adults			
Oral agents [13]			
Chlorpropamide (Diabinese)	(half life 35 hrs)		40-60 hrs
Insulin [14]			
PZI (Protamine Zinc Insulin)	4-8 hrs	14-20 hrs	36+ hrs
Ultralente	4-8 hrs	16-18 hrs	36+ hrs
Children and adults—effective duration of action [5]			
Insulin			
PZI	4-6 hrs	18+ hrs	36-72 hrs
Ultralente	4-6 hrs	8-12 hrs	24-36 hrs

regimen. Diet or meal planning should include spacing of meals and snacks to meet the timing of the insulin, oral medication, and/or activity. For many who work, coffee breaks are written into the contract and one often eats a bite before going to bed—a three meal, three snack pattern. This plan is appropriate for children, also. Most children have shorter glycogen storage time and, therefore, need frequent feedings, such as three meals and three or more snacks. As a person becomes more elderly, less food is needed just as when a child is growing into adulthood, more food is needed. Food intake must be based on a known plan that should be constantly watched and changed to meet changing needs. If the child is growing as he or she should, the baseline of medicine should gradually be increased as food intake is increased. The goal is to keep the urine as sugar free as can be tolerated without any undue episodes of low blood sugar (hypoglycemia). Variations should be planned for increases and decreases of food intake when activity is increased and decreased over and above the usual activity level. If food intake is to capacity or if the individual is overweight, then a decrease in insulin may be the choice of approach rather than an increase in food.

The Family

Once an individual in a family is diagnosed as having diabetes, the other family members should be tested in order to belay apprehension. It is recommended that the glucose tolerance test with the addition of insulin values for testing be used. Any abnormal glucose tolerance tests should be watched closely by repeated testing in six months to a year. If any abnormality is noted, the family should be directed to plan food intake so that weight will become commensurate with height and to remove all concentrated sweets from the meal plan.

The family should become involved in the education process as part of the total treatment. Meal preparation, injections, urine testing, and record keeping are aspects of care that all family members may assist with at one time or another. Input from other family members may be needed just during illness in some patients while in other patients, especially when the child is very young, family support may be needed at all times. The family should help the individual to become independent as age and maturity warrants. An example of this is the answer to the most asked question about the insulin dependent child. When should the child be able to give his/her own insulin? The reply is always the same, "When the child shows readiness by interest in doing such."

Some families may be under such emotional strain that having a person with diabetes in the family may just be too much to handle. When this occurs, the family interaction becomes abnormal, resulting in not only mentally sick individuals but also mentally ill families. Counseling may be needed to assist the family in determining its coping ability. Education is needed to understand the mechanisms of the disease, its treatment, and ramifications so that the family may know on which problems to pinpoint their fears and plan their counseling needs. Families should also be aware of how diabetes is used by some people or children to gain attention. Families should therefore learn best how to support the individual in positive ways rather than negative ways induced by the disease.

One should also attempt to determine the food needs, including likes and dislikes of the total family. The family schedule should also be taken into consideration. Alternate choices to changing likes, dislikes, and family schedules could be determined by role playing and/or interview techniques. Resources should be identified for alternative choices during times of crisis for intervention, continuing education, financial support, and counseling. The family, not just the individual, should be encouraged to join the Diabetes Association as one source of support and continuing education. The family should be encouraged to work together in both crisis and noncrisis situations.

The Community

Public education is the most valuable use of both time and money. The community as a whole should learn to determine the danger signs so that the medical intervention may be early rather than late (in a crisis type of intervention). Detection programs may be the best method to gain attention concerning the information each person should know about the disease. One or two hour postglucose load blood glucose levels would be a better screening device for diabetes, but almost as helpful would be one or two hour postprandial (postmeal) tests, provided the calorie intake and carbohydrate load are standardized. The results should be adjusted for age (Table 23-4).

Professionals in the community should be frequently exposed to findings about the disease. Education should be on a continuing basis so that the health workers will feel comfortable and able to try new developments and procedures found by nursing or medical research and to be more adequate in bringing about optimal patient care.

PROGNOSIS

Prevention

Methods of prevention of diabetes are minimal or nil at present. Improvements of glucose tolerance may be seen with weight loss but not significantly by use of any medications. Basic good nutrition with adequate food intake, not too much or too little for the amount of activity, may perhaps be the only overall deterrent of the disease. Certainly, the absence of or limit of inappropriate stress would be one of the other factors associated with the possible prevention of the problem. Education would certainly be a must for the individual and/or family to determine body needs such as the limitation of concentrated sweets, adequate rest, exercise, and appropriate nutrition for total body needs. Before prevention becomes practical, a method of identification of those susceptible will be needed, i.e., a genetic marker. No such marker is presently available.

TABLE 23-4. Effects of age on glucose tolerance*

Plasma Glucose†	Fasting	1 hour	2 hour	3 hour
Standard values	130	195	140	130
Ages 50 to 60	130	205	150	140
Ages 61 to 70	130	215	160	150
Ages 71 to 80	130	225	170	160

*Shuman, C.R.: "Outpatient Management of Diabetes Mellitus." *Consultant* 18:29, Feb. 1978, with permission.
†All glucose values are expressed in mg/dl. Plasma values are 15 percent higher than whole blood values.

Treatment

The prognosis for this disease, especially if the disease has not been well controlled, is poor. For the most part, treatment and prognosis will vary depending on the complications. The complications are divided into three basic groups: acute complications, intermediate complications, and chronic complications.

The acute complications of diabetes mellitus are *diabetic ketoacidosis* and *hypoglycemia.* Diabetic ketoacidosis is as dangerous to man as is severe hypoglycemia. These are the opposites in the scale, from too high blood glucose to too low blood glucose. Diabetic ketoacidosis may begin with hyperglycemia (elevated blood glucose levels), followed by glycosuria (glucose found in the urine), and progress to diabetic ketosis (glucose as well as ketones are found in blood and urine accompanied by mild dehydration). Diabetic ketoacidosis is all of the above phenomena plus electrolyte or chemical imbalance. In diabetic ketoacidosis, insulin must be given as soon as possible. If the individual is in the emergency room, insulin and fluids should be started even before the individual is moved to intensive care especially if the ketoacidosis is severe. Profound diabetic ketoacidosis would be exemplified by the presence of coma and Kussmaul type (heavy, labored) respiration. A plasma expander, by intravenous feeding, should concurrently be administered along with the insulin. Blood would be drawn to determine the level of the glucose, bicarbonate, sodium, and potassium as well as the acetone level in the blood. D-5-W or D-10-W with appropriate electrolytes would be administered once the dehydrated state is reversed. Insulin is continued every four to six hours until normal blood glucose levels are reached. [15]

Hypoglycemia may occur in either a mild, moderate, or severe form. Mild hypoglycemia may be treated by food, in amounts from 40 to 80 calories or 10 to 20 grams of carbohydrate. Rest is encouraged and treatment may be repeated in 10 to 15 minutes. Moderate insulin reactions are accompanied by definite symptomatology such as dilation of pupils, perspiration, shakiness, strong, rapid pulse, and/or headache. Treatment requires 10 to 20 calories (2.5 to 5 grams of CHO) in children and 20 to 40 calories (5 to 10 grams of CHO) in adults as a concentrated sugar. Treatment may be repeated in 10 to 15 minutes or followed with small amounts of food before activity is resumed. Severe hypoglycemia (insulin reaction or insulin shock) may result in the individual becoming comatose, extremely drowsy, or convulsive. Fifty percent glucose (20 percent glucose in infants) in graduated amounts depending on the body surface area of the person is the treatment of choice to be administered intravenously. Home treatment would be the administration of 1 mg glucagon IM or subcutaneously for those over three years of age and 0.5 mg glucagon for those children three years of age and under. Seizure precautions should be taken. Simple sugar may be administered by enema or in the buccal pouch if other methods of treatment are not available. Once the individual becomes alert, simple sugar solutions should be administered until any nausea subsides. Then food may follow before activity may be safely resumed. [16,17]

Hyperglycemia may be caused by too much food or too little insulin. Diabetic ketoacidosis may be caused by too little insulin or infection or other stresses which increase the need for insulin. The major causes of hypoglycemia are too much insulin, too little food, or too much activity without enough extra food or a decrease in insulin. Damage may occur to various body organs by extremely elevated blood glucose. Death may result from cerebral edema associated with diabetic ketoacidosis and/or aspiration associated with seizures resulting from low blood glucose levels (Table 23-5).

TABLE 23-5. Symptomatology

Specific to Diabetic Ketoacidosis

1. Thirst
2. Dry skin
3. Fruity smell to the breath
4. Kussmaul respiration (heavy and labored breathing)
5. Glucose in urine
6. Acetone in urine

Specific to Hypoglycemia

1. Shakiness
2. Excessive sweating
3. Large pupils
4. Nervousness
5. Weakness
6. Faintness
7. Loss of speech
8. Paralysis
9. Convulsions
10. Urine glucose free by second specimen
11. No ketones in urine

Found in Both Diabetic Ketoacidosis and Hypoglycemia

1. Personality change
2. Inability to concentrate
3. Irritability
4. Hunger
5. Blurred or double vision
6. Restlessness
7. Headache
8. Nausea
9. Numbness and tingling
10. Staggering gait
11. Confusion
12. Drowsiness
13. Coma

Intermediate complications are varied and include psychological maladjustment, surgery, illness, and pregnancy. Psychological maladjustment in a noncoping individual may lead to suicide by either socially acceptable or nonacceptable forms. Socially acceptable suicide in the diabetic is by such means as overeating with hyperglycemia and obesity, failure to watch control by urine testing, failure to follow a meal plan, or compensating for changes in activity. Socially unacceptable suicide is by drugs, alcohol, or other self-inflicted overt injury. The stage of denial or anger may become too prolonged, leading to deviations of behavior that may result in physical stress on self or family. The prognosis is good if family support is evident and counseling is begun in time. [18]

Surgery should only be undertaken if the individual's blood glucose is within acceptable levels, except in emergencies. There is an increased hazard if the blood glucose is out of control, for surgery acts as a stress which will elevate the blood glucose further. Even more important, the healing process will be impeded when the blood glucose level is elevated. The retarded healing process will lead to a greater chance of postoperative infection. Regular insulin in proportionate amounts should be administered before surgery along with the planned intravenous fluids. Insulin should not be placed directly in the 250 ml or larger volume flask unless albumin or other similar agent is first placed in the intravenous solution, to prevent insulin binding to the container. Regular insulin should continue to be administered in sufficient amounts on a continuous basis or in appropriately spaced subcutaneous or intramuscular injections until the individual is stable in the postoperative period. [19]

During illness, adequate amounts of supplemental insulin should be administered so that the infection may run its course without interference of the diabetes. Medication should be administered to meet the needs of the infection and increased insulin given to control the blood glucose elevation that may be caused by the stress of the disease and/or the medication used. Gastroenteritis should be recognized for the problems it may cause. This disease may result in a lack of absorption of food from the intestines. Insulin may need to be decreased if there is poor absorption or if inadequate calories are obtained from the clear liquids ingested.

Pregnancy progresses most satisfactorily if the control of the diabetes is closely managed. If damage has already occurred to the body, the stress of pregnancy can become quite damaging. For example, if retinal damage is already apparent, the increased stress of pregnancy might cause rupture of the blood vessels in the retina, especially if the woman is allowed to deliver vaginally. Delivery is most often by cesarean section at 36 to 37 weeks gestation, although normal delivery practices would be possible for the mother with well controlled disease. [20,21] Control of the blood glucose in pregnancy would also decrease the possibility of an overweight baby. Increased blood glucose in the mother may result in hyperglycemia in the infant with increased beta cell development and insulin secretions. There will then be subsequent storage of the excess glucose received through the placenta resulting in infant obesity. On delivery, the sudden cessation of elevated glucose levels may result in hyperinsulinemia and hypoglycemia episodes in the infant. The hypoglycemic episodes may be controlled by immediate treatment with 10 to 20 percent glucose by vein by continuous intravenous perfusion. [22] Occasional, periodic administrations of Susphrine is needed only in the most severe cases of refractory hypoglycemia.

Chronic complications are divided into the categories of kidney disease or nephropathy, eye disease or retinopathy, nerve disease or neuropathy, and blood vessel disease or angiopathy. [9] Kidney disease is the most severe of the chronic complications since it may cause uremia and death. Kimmelstiel-Wilson disease is the final stage of diabetic nephropathy and consists of a nodular sclerosis of the glomeruli in the kidney. Treatment, when end stage kidney disease is reached, is by kidney transplant or by renal dialysis. Retinopathy may involve retinal detachment, retinal hemorrhage, deposits of exudate on the retina, clouding of the vitreous humor, and, although not involved directly with the retina, cataracts. Laser treatments are used to coagulate the bleeding vessels seen on the wall of the retina. Lens removal will alter the translucency caused by the glycosylation of protein [23] in the lens (seen in diabetic cataracts). Retinal detachment may be surgically corrected and the use of vitreophage will remove and replace the cloudy vitreous in front of the retina.

Neuropathy may be quite serious also. Neuropathy may result in atony of the bladder or paralysis of the muscles of the extremities. Sensation may become more acute or increasingly less sensitive. Autonomic neuropathy may result in lack of action of sphincter muscles, such as in the openings of the bladder, the anus, the pylorus, or lack of sensation of the genital organs such as the penis or the clitoris. Control of the blood glucose level may result in marked improvement in sensation. Pain often is present during the healing phase of diabetic neuropathy and patients need to be so warned. The pain may last anywhere from six months to a year or longer. Gastrostomies, ureterostomies, or other such surgery may become necessary for the treatment of sphincter problems caused by autonomic neuropathy. Silastic implants in males with neuropathic impotence may permit sexual functions to continue.

Angiopathy is manifest in a number of ways affecting either the large or small blood vessels. It may lead to coronary disease, atherosclerosis, retinal and kidney disease, as well as gangrene or stroke. Bypass surgery in the heart or extremities may permit better circulation to prevent further damage, angina, or in the extremities better healing of ulcers and the prevention of gangrene.

Improvement in blood glucose has been shown to improve blood vessel pathology as manifest by capillary or basement membrane thickening, the pathologic lesion of diabetes small vessel disease. Studies by Maurer[24] have shown, in both the animal and human models, that normalized blood glucose will alter and normalize vascular tissue in the kidney. If a damaged kidney is placed in the nondiabetic rat, the damaged kidney will improve. In humans, if rigid standards of diabetic control are met, the individuals have a decreased chance of succumbing to heart disease, stroke and other problems resulting from blood vessel disease, and kidney failure.

COMMUNITY HEALTH NURSING CONCERNS

The Individual

Since the success of diabetic control is closely related to the 24-hour balance of diet, exercise, and medication, and the individual's ability to cope as well as the ability and willingness to participate in a regimen, the community health nurse can be most helpful in assisting in the overall understanding and adjustment to the disease. The patient contact sessions should include basic assessment of needs before developing the individual's particular education program. Group sessions may then need to be arranged so that a sharing of problems and ideas concerning all aspects of care is available. Since diet plays a large part in the management, these sessions might also involve food buying and food preparation as well as problems or typical situations that would challenge anyone on a daily basis.

Assessment in the home is critical. How much is the individual (and family) able to spend for food? How is the food prepared? How are portion sizes of the food intake determined? Where is the insulin (oral agents) kept? How are the syringes handled? Where is the urine testing equipment kept? Where are the results of the urine tests, medications, changes in food, and physical responses kept? How accurate is the record? How does the individual relate to other members of the family (nuclear and/or extended family members)?

The community health nurse should also be involved in assisting the person with diabetes to be aware of resources for both acute and chronic needs. The nurse should help the person with diabetes to learn about all aspects of health care, not just the diabetes. Included could be information on general safety and health as well as dental, eye, and skin care. Assistance in helping an individual to become independent will not allow the nurse to actually make the community contacts needed for assistance but should allow the individual the freedom and the courage to choose to contact these resources himself. For example, the nurse might direct the patient to have the number of the doctor or nurse by the phone so that valuable time is not wasted in an emergency. Direction might be given for contacting the nearest Diabetes Association. Have the individual (or parents) chosen a dentist and an ophthalmologist? Who is the family physician? How is the individual integrating exercise into the daily plan? Not only must the community health nurse assist the individual in recognizing the community health resources, but she or he also should feel responsible for assisting the individual in coordinating the community services to meet the greatest number of physical and mental needs.

The Family

The family in essence holds the key to total diabetic control, whether this is a family of one or many. If the individual that has diabetes does not have self- or family support, the chances of following a regimen adequately for good control are very much in doubt. As the community health nurse assesses the individual needs, the community health nurse must also assess the total family needs. Are the family members able to communicate well? Are the parents able to supply the support and guidance of the child both physically and mentally? Are the family members overprotective or underprotective? Are the parents and/or siblings fearful about the disease and its manifestations? Is counseling needed to improve the family's interaction and communication? Are the family members able to identify and use community resources accurately and appropriately? Are the family members coping with the impact that one of their loved ones has a chronic disease? All the preceding is a necessary part of the total family assessment.

The family must be encouraged to take part in the total care of the patient in actual or nonactual (supportive) means. Part of this challenge is to involve the family in the self-care of the client which will certainly allow some interaction even if only verbally. Hopefully, this is done in a supportive, nonharassing manner. The family must be aware of the possibility of other family members developing the disease themselves. Therefore, community nurses should be involved in seeing that the family is familiar with the signs and symptoms of the disease. They should encourage good nutrition practices. These practices should lead to general health care practices such as good nutrition, adequate skin and hair care, plenty of exercise in relation to physical abilities, and appropriate amounts of rest. The family should be guided in recognizing the stresses placed on the individual with the disease and how it may alter the behavior patterns. The family should be educated to deal with crises, should they occur. The family should know at what point the health professional should be called and which crises may actually be prevented.

The approach of the community health nurse should be in a calm, continuing, knowledgeable format that provides the avenue for the family to be guided to make better health care decisions and therefore add to the potential life span of the individual with diabetes.

The Community

The integral part the community health nurse plays in the community cannot be overemphasized. In assessing the needs of the community, this person would determine the scope of the problem in the catchment area. Once the scope of the problem has been determined, then the resources should be listed. Is there an association specific to meet the needs of the diabetic and the family? Is the community mindful of the impact of the disease on life, on the economy, on the biopsychosocial adjustment? Are adequate resources available so that the community might become familiar with the signs and symptoms of the disease? Are methods of detection available either through history or blood testing? Are alternate resources available if the community is small enough not to have such readily available resources? Is professional and patient education present in hospitals and/or offices of the community? Are there ways to develop continuing education within the community?

Perhaps the most frustrating problem in the community is the problem related to inadequate management. The nurse may be convinced of the need for regulated control of the diabetes, but the physician(s) in the community may not see this as a priority. They may also not see the need for education both of professionals or the lay public. Education alone will not improve the control of the disease.[25] The main purpose of education is to provide the basis of safe, close management of the blood glucose and the understanding that leads to compliance and/or the motivation to follow a regimen that would result in a healthier, more stable physiologic response. Methods of improving physician support may be through the distribution of medical journals, appropriately placed articles (such as on bulletin boards, in hospital lounges), and by continuing education. More often than not, when education is made available to the professionals, the professionals who need it most often are the ones who do not attend. Another method of approach is the statement, "I read (or heard) that intermediate acting insulin is only effective in duration (or some other provocative statement) for 14 hours or so. Have you read anything about this lately?" or "Are you familiar with this information?" Perhaps negative replies will be the result, but perhaps the stimulus to read, learn, and compare may be instigated in the professional and perhaps change will then follow.

RESEARCH

With the discovery of insulin in 1921, the disease was thought to be cured. Little did we know that Pandora's box had been opened. With insulin people live longer and therefore have time to develop the complications that have caused so much sorrow. Our humane attempt to decrease the number of injections of insulin needed per day by using longer acting insulins contributed to the problems. We saw fewer complications when multiple injections of regular insulin were used.

During the last decade, there have been more changes in diabetes knowledge than in the previous 40 years. The impetus for the new changes has been found through biomedical research. Radioimmunoassay, for which Berson and Yalow[26] received the Nobel Prize in 1978, allowed the finite measurement of various hormones, such as circulating insulin, which could not be accurately measured before. The use of radioimmunoassay and other techniques has led to new information concerning the synthesis, secretion, transport, action, and degradation of insulin. All this must be understood before a prevention or a cure can be found.

Through the use of the electron microscope and radioactive labeling techniques, along with radioimmunoassay, Lacy and others[27] have increased our knowledge as to the steps in insulin production. Steiner and associates[28] have performed research which led to the discovery of proinsulin, the precursor of insulin, and preproinsulin, a chain of eight amino acids that allows the embryonic insulin molecule to enter into the Golgi apparatus. In the Golgi apparatus, cleavage of the molecule occurs. Initially the eight amino acid prechain is released. Then through enzymatic action, the connecting peptide (C-peptide) is separated from the 28 amino acid chain (A chain) and the 31 amino acid chain (B chain) of the definitive insulin molecule. Knowledge of the C-peptide fraction gives the researcher a tool to use to measure the insulin secreting ability of the beta cells. Previous to this discovery, interfering antibodies made it difficult to distinguish endogenous from injected insulin. Endogenous insulin is found quite frequently in the early recovery or "honeymoon" period of diabetes. The fact that a diabetic can recover endogenous insulin, even temporarily, after initial diagnosis should act as a challenge to the physician to institute a therapeutic regimen that protects beta cell function for as long as possible.

Spiro's work on basement membrane biochemistry has led to the increased understanding of the need for adequate insulinization of the body cells.[29] With insufficient insulin there is an increase in enzymes called glucosyltransferase and galactosyltransferase. These enzymes add glucose and galactose to the amino acids forming the concentric circles of proteins that make up the composition of the basement membrane. This glycosylation process causes the separation of the protein layers of the capillary basement membrane and leads to the thickening. This thickening leads to increased pore size and results in leakage of protein into the tissue or the urine. Thickening also permits the weakening of the walls of the blood vessels so that less stress is needed to rupture the wall.

Siperstein and associates[30] through their choice of study subjects came to the conclusion that thickening of capillary basement membranes was a concomitant with the disease, was genetically predetermined, and was unalterable by control of the blood glucose. Williamson and Kilo[31] demonstrated the normal progression of the thickening of capillary basement membranes and concluded that basement membrane thickening is based on duration of the disease and control of the blood glucose. Jackson and others[32] have been able to demonstrate in humans that improved control of the blood glucose not only stabilizes the basement membrane but also causes some thinning of the membrane, i.e., a reversal of the vascular disease.

The thickening of basement membrane has been a key point in the argument for or against normalization of the blood glucose. One theory states that there is no value in controlling the blood glucose because the vascular disease as manifest by capillary basement membrane thickening is a genetic concomitant of the diabetes. The other theory states that vascular disease may be prevented or at least delayed by appropriate treatment methods. Until the data are conclusive, the only hope for the diabetic is the best control possible to prevent the greatest possible damage.

Perhaps another interesting research race is on. This race is between the development of an artificial pancreas and the perfecting of the techniques of pancreas transplants. Transplantation has been tried in various settings, mainly in the animal model. Whole pancreases, islets of Langerhans, or just beta cells have been transplanted. Beta cells have been placed beneath the skin, in the peritoneal cavity, injected into the liver through the portal vein, or into the spleen. The need for immunosuppressant drugs is the major problem, for blood glucose levels have been normalized by this approach. Tissue rejection, however, soon occurs. Fistula formation secondary to exocrine secretions may occur when the whole pancreas is transplanted. On the other hand, the artificial pancreas, once thought to be the easiest answer to the problem of complete diabetic control, has developed problems of its own. The glucose sensor becomes covered with fibroblast cells soon after implantation so that in three to four months the sensor is no longer able to function. Short term use of the machinery (sensor, computer, pump, and insulin filled reservoir) has been found useful during surgical procedures and delivery. Information derived from the Space Sciences Division at the Whittake Corporation used by Soeldner and Bessman has made smaller more portable models possible.

There are many other aspects of diabetes that are under study. One of these new studies involves the use of an oil-water-oil immulsion of insulin to allow an oral route for administration of insulin. Much study is being done in the area of nutrition as well as treatment of diabetes complications. Studies of the usefulness of somatostatin for the stabilization of blood glucose are underway. Somatostatin is a hormone originally found in the pituitary gland that is responsible for the cessation of the release of growth hormone. It now appears to also be a regulator of the release of glucagon and insulin. If, in the insulin dependent diabetic, this hormone were added to the insulin to be injected, it might suppress glucagon secretion and improve diabetes control. The hormone has limitations, however, since it has a very short half life and would also suppress growth by concurrently suppressing growth hormone. Work is underway to solve both these problems.

Further research is needed to find new ways of controlling the effects of the disease on the individual. Research should include methods of education as well as planning and overall management. Better methods for permitting a smoother psychosocial adjustment are also needed. Those with diabetes must then be kept informed of the progress being made in diabetes research so that they do not lose the hope that a cure is possible. Whether it is 1 year, 10 years, or longer, we are closer to the answer than we were at the time of the discovery of insulin, and patients should be taught to maintain as good diabetes control as possible until the answer to their disease is found.

EDUCATION

The biggest charge for the community health nurse, besides assistance in psychosocial adjustment to diabetes, is the education component of diabetes care. The psychosocial adjustment can easily be a part of the education process, which is in turn intertwined with management. Even though the management may not be adequate, the education process may assist the individual and/or family to recognize the specific needs that would improve the overall control of the disease in the afflicted person. Education should then consist of many parts and an attempt made to plan for avenues of continuing education.

Before starting any education program that is formal, the patient/client and family must be ready. Informal education by discussion should be readily available to answer immediate questions and to assist in the psychological adjustment until the time when formalized education may be started. The education should also be based on the appropriate educational level for the best learning possible. The material should then be repeated in a variety of forms to assist in the learning process.

There is a myriad of information that should be learned. The immediate information should help the family or person survive until more in-depth information can be presented to assist in home management and family living (Tables 23-6 and 23-7). The total or basic program should include various aspects of self-care, understanding of the need for certain procedures, and what to do in event of an emergency (also what constitutes an emergency). The information should then note what the disease is and what we know about the causes. Methods of communication with members of the support group or team should be listed. Who should they call if questions arise outside the counseling sessions or the classroom? They should be given guidance on what to tell the professional, significant others, and why. They should be given a list of the supplies they will need for care and suggestions on where the supplies may be obtained and how much they will cost.

Insulin is a life saving hormone whether it is made available to the body internally or externally. The mysteries of what insulin is and how much is known about it will act as a basis for further study or reading. The introduction to medications should then include their action and expected dosage parameters. The side effects should then be disclosed in order that the patient and/or family will be aware that the medications are not a cure, but all phases of management must be respected.

The mechanics of self-care may sometimes be controversial. Should the angle of the syringe be 45° or 90°? Should the urine test be on a single or a double voided urine specimen? As these individuals read, they can become quite confused.

The goal for teaching the mechanics of injection, urine testing, record keeping, and meal planning should be to perform the procedures as safely and accurately as possible. The angle of the needle should be related to the thickness of the skin. The method used to tighten the skin should also be in relation to its thickness. The length of the needle

TABLE 23-6. Teaching outline

Session I
  A. An introduction to the manual.
  B. What is diabetes?
    1. What has happened and why?
    2. What is known about the disease?
  C. How to contact team members.
  D. What to tell the teacher, employer, friend, and spouse.
  E. Purchase and care of supplies.
Session II
  A. What is insulin?
  B. What insulin products are available?
  C. The effective time action of various insulin preparations.
  D. What are the oral agents available?
  E. The time action of various oral agents.
Session III
  A. How to withdraw insulin.
  B. How to rotate an injection.
  C. How to give an injection.
  D. How to care for reusable and disposable syringes. (Alternate topic—Implications of diabetes on daily living.)
Session IV
  A. Mixing of insulin in a syringe.
  B. Mixing of insulin in a vial (as appropriate).
    1. U-100 insulin
    2. U-50 insulin
    3. U-25 insulin
    4. U-10 insulin
  C. Untoward reactions of insulin.
    1. Atrophy
    2. Hypertrophy
    3. Rash—localized
    4. Rash—generalized
    5. Insulin resistance
  D. Hygiene and exercise. (Alternate topic- If insulin mixture information is not needed, this session may be all on hygiene and exercise.)
Session V
  A. Urine tests for glucose
    1. Clinitest
    2. Diastix
    3. Testape
    4. Clinistix
  B. Urine tests for ketones.
    1. Ketostix
    2. Acetest
  C. Other methods of testing urine (as needed).
    1. For the partially sighted.
    2. For the blind.
  D. The parameters of control.
    1. The double void.
    2. The single void.
    3. The fractional.
    4. The 24 hour urine.
    5. A_1C Hgb.

Session VI. Acute Complications
  A. Hyperglycemia, diabetes ketosis, and diabetes ketoacidosis.
  B. Cause of hypoglycemia (mild, moderate, severe).
  C. Prevention of hypoglycemia.
  D. Treatment of hypoglycemia.
  E. Use of glucagon.
  F. When and what to report to the physician.
  G. The importance of identification.
Session VII. Intermediate Complications
  A. Diabetes and illness.
  B. Symptoms and treatment of illness.
    1. Meal plan.
    2. Variation in 2 dose insulin or other medication.
    3. Supplementing with regular insulin.
  C. When to call for medical assistance.
  D. The Somogyi effect.
  E. Surgery.
  F. Pregnancy.
Session VIII. Intermediate Complications (cont.)
  A. Emotional adjustment.
  B. The effect of stress.
  C. How to handle stress.
Session IX. Chronic Complications
  A. Nephropathy
    1. Treatment
    2. Research
  B. Neuropathy
    1. Treatment
    2. Research
  C. Angiopathy
    1. Treatment
    2. Research
  D. Retinopathy
    1. Treatment
    2. Research
Session X
  A. Record keeping.
    1. Filling out the record.
    2. Interpreting a record (self-management).
  B. Scheduling of activities.
  C. Self-management.
    1. What the record means.
    2. When to call the physician.
Review
  A. Urine testing
  B. Insulin procedures and/or oral agents
  C. Treatment of hypoglycemia
  D. Meal planning
  E. Record keeping
  F. Social adjustment
  G. Self-management

TABLE 23-7. Dietary teaching outline

Session I
  A. Dietary history of diabetes.
  B. Introduction to meal planning—importance of carbohydrates, protein, and fat.
Session II
  A. Normal nutrition. (What is a balanced diet?)
    1. Composition of carbohydrate, protein and fat.
    2. Minerals and vitamins.
  B. Normal diet (the diabetic meal plan).
Session III
  A. Insulin in relation to food.
  B. Exchange groups.
Session IV
  A. Discuss meal plan book.
  B. Other approaches to meal planning.
Session V
  A. Sample meal plan.
  B. Weighing food.
Session VI
  A. Develop two days' menu.
  B. Relation of exercise to food intake.
Session VII
  A. Use of the record in relation to diet.
  B. How to interpret records in relation to changing exercise levels.
Session VIII
  A. Diet for illness (total available glucose vs. calories for calories).
  B. Variations of diet for illness in relation to specific illness.
    1. Clear liquids in vomiting and diarrhea.
    2. Intake as tolerated.
    3. 20 percent less calories.
Session IX
  A. Birthday and school parties
  B. Dining out
  C. Late meals
Session X
  A. "Going home" meal plan
  B. Dietary resources

should be one-half the thickness of the skin fold, again related to the thickness of the skin. The speed of the injection should be in relation to the feelings of the individual. Methods of cleanliness should be observed.

The untoward reactions of having to take insulin should be known. Hypoglycemia as a specific topic may be introduced here and then discussed in more depth later. Methods and rules to use in mixing or not mixing various insulins should be presented and illustrated. In the injection procedure itself, a slower nonpressure approach appears to be more appropriate with children while a "shock" type of approach appears to work best with adults. One finds that the longer the adult thinks about the injection, the more difficult it seems to be to self-administer the insulin. Most children and perhaps adults will go through a cycle of rejection of self-administration of insulin one to two weeks after the start of self-administration of insulin. This will be started by the administration of an uncomfortable injection. If supportive practice and noncommital encouragement of the continuing of self-administration of insulin is not encouraged, then a negative block against the "needle" is apt to occur.

The use of hygiene and exercise should become a part of the mechanics of daily life. Everything from foot care to hair care and dental hygiene to planning exercise should be included in the instruction. The individual should be made aware of the fact that as he or she is first a *person* and second that he or she has a disease called diabetes. It should then be recognized that the individual should be treated as a whole person. Therefore, the whole body should receive attention, not just the disease.

The importance of urine testing, as a guide and/or warning of what is happening and/or what is to come, will give the individuals and families the assurance that they are in control of the medication and the disease and indeed their total selves. The various urine tests that are used in assessing diabetic control all have problems of one sort or another. The committee on therapeutics of the American Diabetes Association released recommendations on the use of urine testing products in 1978.[33] Included in this section of the educational program should be the types and timing of various urine testing methodologies.

One, two, and five drop methods of urine testing may be confusing, but the use of such tests, especially the two drop method, is highly recommended in the insulin dependent person. The stick or tape tests for urine sugar are felt to be adequate for the noninsulin dependent person. The teaching should include information as to the interpretation of the single voided test, the double voided test, the use of fractional urines, and how fractionals closely approximate the single voided test. (Comparisons between the single and double first and second voided urine tests have been made. Sixty-three percent of the time, the second voided specimen may falsely indicate a better degree of control than is actually there. The valuable information of the first voided test supported by the timely information of the second voided test, where indicated, should be strongly considered.[35]) Education should also included how to collect and interpret the 24-hour urine, the use of the hemoglobin A_1C as a measurement of control,[34] and, when needed, methodologies of testing useful to the handicapped.

Education should include knowledge of the acute complications, hyperglycemia, and hypoglycemia. Various methods of treatment for various physiologic responses should be part of survival techniques. Knowledge of the use of alternate methods of treatment are a must. Recognition of signs and symptoms of diabetic ketoacidosis and hypoglycemia will help the family or patient to differentiate between the two.

Identification as a diabetic should be worn at all times but often is not worn or is worn with embarrassment. This simple insurance policy, the wearing of identification, should be dealt with in a positive vain. It should be taught that positive identification of a diabetic in an emergency will allow others to recognize that necessary measures should be instituted to control the emergency. This is especially true for hypoglycemia where recognition will allow the use of glucagon in time (in cases of severe insulin reactions) to prevent further problems.

Intermediate complications are the problems of psychosocial adjustment, illness, the Somogyi phenomenon, pregnancy, and surgery. Points should be included in the educational program on how to recognize the problems of illness and what measures must be taken or what should be reported. The Somogyi effect or overinsulinization should be taught so that early recognition may be made and proper alterations made in management. The history of the spilling of sugar in the urine after increased exercise without noticeable alterations in food or insulin is an easy sign of the Somogyi phenomenon to interpret in the learning process. What to do at the time of surgery or when specific types of illness occur will give information helpful for greater control over the disease. Variations, caused by more acute alterations in activity levels, may be confused by the addition of other stresses both physical and mental and may lead to a compounding of the psychological response. Instruction in how to handle stress by means of relaxation or other coping mechanisms will assist in both the overall adjustment to diabetes as well as in the immediate adjustment to the classroom.

Chronic complications can be most difficult to put into perspective. Certainly one does not want to build up feelings of fear, rather those of understanding by guiding the individual in making choices as he or she progresses through life. Including methods of treatment of complications in the educational program may assist in alleviating feelings of anxiety. Although some professionals may fear the mental image information about complications might instill, ethically the patient has a right to know that such information does exist. The saddest tale of all is the individual, blind from diabetes, who states that if she had been told such problems might occur, she would at least have had the choice to work for or not to work for better control of the disease.

Record keeping of the results of diabetes management is really a key adjunct to good self-care. If a particular management program does not allow the person to actually make the changes in management that are needed, good record keeping still allows excellent guidelines as to when to call the physician for possible changes in the regimen. Patients can be taught that if the spill of glucose in the urine gradually or quickly increases, that more insulin or less food is needed. They can be taught that if a spill occurs at a certain time of day, that something preceding those times of spillage of glucose in the urine should be changed. The change could be less food, more exercise, or more insulin. Patients should be taught that if hypoglycemia becomes frequent, less insulin or more food is needed. They should be taught the use of supplemental insulin and the choices of amounts and types of foods to ingest for various types of illnesses (i.e., clear liquids containing regular sugar to be used when gastroenteritis is apparent).

Patients should be goal oriented. When well, they should wish to see that the urines are as sugar free as possible without symptoms of serious insulin reactions. When ill, to maintain about 0.5 to 1 percent sugar in the urine with the urine acetone free is the goal.

Meal planning should accompany each educational session in some form. Whether it is discussing the diet for illness or for everyday activities, the meal plan can become a useful teaching tool. Eating during special occasions should be considered and the patient should be taught how to eat during times of stress such as illness, depression, or extra activity. Before the patient goes home, practice sessions in developing meal plans and choices of foods should be held for the patient and the family. Whatever the method used to determine the food intake, it should fit individual needs. Meal planning using exchange lists provides various food choices from specific food groups. The meat group (7 grams of protein, 2.5, 5, or 7.5 grams of fat—55, 75, or 95 calories respectively) gives a variety of lean to fatty meats as well as beans, cheeses, eggs, and peanut butter. The vegetable group has a listing of eight foods to be used as desired (the lettuces, radishes, and watercress) while the rest of the foods on the list must be counted in half-cup serving sizes (5 grams carbohydrate, 2 grams protein—25 calories). Fruits are available in 32 kinds (10 grams carbohydrate—40 calories). The bread list is composed of a variety of breads, pastas, and high carbohydrate vegetables (15 grams carbohydrate, 2 grams protein—70 calories). Fats include nuts as well as oleo, butter, olives, and avocadoes (5 grams fat—45 calories). Skim milk (80 calories with no fat) is the reference substitute for the milk group although 2 percent (120 calories) or whole milk (10 grams carbohydrate, 8 grams protein, 10 grams fat—160 calories) may also be used.

Another food system, called the point system, is sometimes taught. The point system is based on 75 calories per point. Meal patterns are spelled out by simple numbers rather than exchanges. For example, if the individual were receiving 1800 calories, this would be divided by 75 to equal a total of 24 points. These points would be distributed, as would the exchanges, throughout the day. A listing of foods would be available by calorie points. Carbohydrate points can be calculated too, if desired (15 gm CHO divided into the total amount of CHO to equal the points for that day, i.e., 15 into 180 gm CHO equals 12 points which would be distributed with the calorie points). A combination of the two systems can be accomplished by calorie points if one considers 1 calorie point for a medium fat meat, a bread, or a skim milk serving and 0.5 calorie point for the fruit, the vegetable, or the fat serving. Whatever the method chosen, the stress is on individualization, no restriction on calories unless overweight, and restriction of concentrated sweets except in cases of emergency.

CONCLUSION

Teamwork is needed to adequately meet the needs of the person with diabetes. The community health nurses are the team coordinators who have the ability to assist the individual with diabetes toward better health both mentally and physically. Coordination of the team's efforts must be evident in order to prevent or to handle various problems as they arise. Without cooperation of all the team members, with the patient and the family being key people on the team, this cannot be accomplished.

The goal for ideal control is normal glycemia, normal lipid levels, weight adequate for height, no disturbing hypoglycemia episodes, urines free of glucose, acetone, and protein, and no developing complications. In children, there should be normal growth. There are three links in the chain of good control. With the loss of any one of these links, control cannot be achieved. These three links are 24 hour insulinization of the cells, education of the patient and family, and patient cooperative participation in the treatment regimen. This does take effort, but the results of the outcome are well worth the time taken to achieve the results. Burton has stated that "Diabetes is . . . the most important of the metabolic disorders."[36] Priorities concerning case load and time should then be properly proportioned so that those clients with diabetes may receive optimal care and guidance.

REFERENCES

1. Leibel, B.S., and Wrenshall, G.A.: *Insulin.* University of Toronto Press, Toronto, 1971.
2. Smith, M.: "Intermediary Metabolism," in Guthrie, D.W., and Guthrie, R.A. (eds.): *Nursing Management of Diabetes Mellitus.* C.V. Mosby Co., St. Louis, 1977.
3. Wilner, D.M., Walkley, R.P., and Goerke, L.S.: *Introduction to Public Health.* Macmillan Publishing Co., New York, 1973.
4. Tattersall, R.B., and Fajans, S.S.: "A Difference Between the Inheritance of Classical Juvenile Onset and Maturity Onset Type of Diabetes of Young People." *Diabetes* 24:44, 1975.
5. Jackson, R.L., and Guthrie, R.A.: *The Child with Diabetes Mellitus in Current Concepts.* The Upjohn Co., Kalamazoo, Mich., 1976.
6. *Report of the National Commission on Diabetes,* vol. 3, part 2. U.S. Government Printing Office, Washington, D.C., Dec. 1975.
7. Goswitz, K., Howen, G., and Thompson, T.: "The Prevalence of Diabetes in Michigan School Age Children." *Diabetes,* 25:128, Feb. 1976.
8. Kyllo, C.J., and Nuttall, F.Q.: "Prevalence of Diabetes Mellitus in School Age Children in Minnesota." *Diabetes,* 27:57, 1978.

9. Jordon, J.: "Chronic Complications of Diabetes," in Guthrie, D.W., and Guthrie, R.A. (eds.): *Nursing Management of Diabetes Mellitus.* C.V. Mosby Co., St. Louis, 1977.

10. Cahil, G.F., Etzwiler, D.D., and Frenkel, N.: "Blood Glucose and Control in Diabetes Mellitus." *Diabetes* 25:237, March 1976.

11. Orem, D.E.: *Nursing Concepts of Practice.* McGraw-Hill Book Co., New York, 1971.

12. Schumann, D.: "Mastering the Art of Assessment," in Chaney, P.S. (ed.): *Managing Diabetes Properly.* Nursing 77 Book Intermed Communications, Horsham, Pa., 1977.

13. Boyden, T.W.: "The Proper Place of Oral Hypoglycemics in Diabetes Management." *Drug Therapy* 8:67, March 1978.

14. Bressler, R., and Galloway, J.A.: "The Insulin Pharmacology and Uses." *Drug Therapy* 8:44, March 1978.

15. Guthrie, D.W., and Guthrie, R.A.: "Breaking a Vicious Cycle," in Chaney, P.S. (ed.): *Managing Diabetes Properly.* Nursing 77 Book Intermed Communication, Horsham, Pa., 1977.

16. Jordon, J.: "The Acute Care of Diabetes," in Guthrie, D.W., and Guthrie, R.A. (eds.): *Nursing Management of Diabetes Mellitus.* C.V. Mosby Co., St. Louis, 1977.

17. Schumann, D.: "Insulin Reactions: Fighting Fear and Fact," in Chaney, P.S. (ed.): *Managing Diabetes Properly.* Nursing 77 Book Intermed Communications, Horsham, Pa., 1977.

18. Desimone, B.S.: "Psychosocial Implications of Diabetes," in Guthrie, D.W., and Guthrie, R.A. (eds.): *Nursing Management of Diabetes Mellitus.* C.V. Mosby Co., St. Louis, 1977.

19. Dye, L.: "Surgery and Diabetes," in Guthrie, D.W., and Guthrie, R.A. (eds.): *Nursing Management of Diabetes Mellitus.* C.V. Mosby Co., St. Louis, 1977.

20. Sheets, C.: "Pregnancy and Diabetes," in Guthrie, D.W., and Guthrie, R.A. (eds.): *Nursing Management of Diabetes Mellitus.* C.V. Mosby Co., St. Louis, 1977.

21. Garofano, C.: "Pregnant Diabetics: Dispelling Myths," in Chaney, P.S. (ed.): *Managing Diabetes Properly.* Nursing 77 Book Intermed Communications, Horsham, Pa., 1977.

22. Guthrie, D.W., and Guthrie, R.A.: "Infant of the Diabetic Mother," in Guthrie, D.W., and Guthrie, R.A. (eds.): *Nursing Management of Diabetes Mellitus.* C.V. Mosby Co., St. Louis, 1977.

23. Koeny, R.J., and Peterson, C., et al.: "Correlation of Glucose Registration and Hemoglobin A_1C in Diabetes Mellitus." *New England Journal of Medicine,* 295:417, 1976.

24. Mauer, S.M., et al.: "Studies of Rate of Regression of the Glomerular Lesions in Diabetic Rats Treated with Pancreatic Islet Transplantation." *Diabetes,* 24:280, 1975.

25. Etzwiler, D.D., and Robb, J.R.: "Evaluation of Programmed Education Among Juvenile Diabetics and Their Families." *Diabetes* 21:967, Sept. 1972.

26. Berson, S.A., and Yalow, R.S., et al.: "Insulin Metabolism in Human Subjects: Demonstration of Insulin Binding Globulins in Circulation of Insulin Treated Subjects." *Journal of Clinical Investigation,* 35:170, 1956.

27. Lacey, P.E.: "Beta Cell Secretion—From the Standpoint of a Pathologist." Banting Memorial Lecture, 1970, *Diabetes* 19:895, Dec. 1970.

28. Steiner, D.F., Hollan, O., Rubenstein, A., et al.: "Isolation and Properties of Proinsulin Intermediate Forms and Other Minor Components From Crystalline Bovine Insulin." *Diabetes,* 17:725, 1968.

29. Spiro, R.D., and Spiro, M.J.: "Effect of Diabetes on the Biosynthesis of the Renal Glomerular Basement Membrane. Studies on the Glycosyl Transferase." *Diabetes,* 20:641, 1971.

30. Siperstein, M.D., Unger, R.H., and Madison, L.L.: "Studies of Muscle Capillary Basement Membranes in Normal Subjects, Diabetic and Pre-Diabetic Patients." *Journal of Clinical Investigation,* 47:1973, 1968.

31. Kilo, C., Vogler, N., and Williamson, J.R.: "Muscle Capillary Basement Membrane Changes Related to Aging and Diabetes Mellitus." *Diabetes* 21:881, 1972.

32. Jackson, R.L., Guthrie, R.A., Esterly, J., et al.: "Muscle Capillary Basement Changes in Normal and Diabetic Children." *Diabetes,* 24 (Suppl. 2):400, 1975.

33. Kohler, E. for ADA Committee on Materials and Therapeutic Agents: "Materials for Testing Glucose in the Urine." *Diabetes Care,* 1:64, Jan.-Feb. 1978.

34. Koenig, R.J., Peterson, C.M., Kilo, C., et al.: "Hemoglobin A_1C as an Indicator of the Degree of Glucose Intolerance in Diabetics." *Diabetes,* 25:230, 1976.

35. Guthrie, D.W., Guthrie, R.A., and Hinnen, D.: "Single vs. Double Voided Techniques for Urine Testing." *Diabetes Care* 2:269-271, May-June 1979.

36. Burton, L.E., and Smith, H.H.: *Public Health and Community Medicine,* William and Wilkins Co., Baltimore, 1975.

CHAPTER **24**
INFECTIOUS DISEASES

NICKI MORINA RICHARDS, M.S., R.N.

A communicable disease is caused by an infectious agent found in the biologic environment. Any communicable disease requires an interaction between the host and agent, direct or indirect transmission from the agent reservoir in the environment to the host, and an appropriate host which can provide adequate living conditions for the infectious agent. The following definitions are critical to an understanding of the communicable disease process:

1. *Host:* Man or animal which provides adequate living conditions for the infectious agent.
2. *Agent:* A biologic organism found in either the internal or external environment of the host capable of causing an infectious disease.
3. *Reservoir:* The environment where living conditions are conducive to the maintenance, growth, and reproduction of the infectious agent.
4. *External environment:* The current surroundings of the host.
5. *Internal environment:* The physical and psychological characteristics of and condition of the host.

In order for any communicable disease to develop, there must be an interaction between a host and an agent within a supportive environment.

THE HOST

The host is the susceptible person or animal which provides adequate living conditions for the invasion of an infectious agent and the development of communicable disease. Three factors which determine the response of the host to such an invasion are 1) general health status, 2) inherent characteristics, and 3) acquired characteristics.

The host's general health status affects the severity of the development of a communicable disease once invasion of tissue has occurred. Age, nutrition, psychological factors, presence of other diseases, and fatigue are aspects of the host's general health which determines the response to the invading agent. Chronic disease, malnourishment, and age can significantly alter the ability of the body to resist invasion and fight off infection. It is assumed that malnourishment or an inadequate nutritional status decreases resistance to infections. However, there is no consistent evidence to support this.[1] Protein deficiencies and amino acid imbalances do appear to influence the severity and duration of illness which develops. The issue of nutritional effect is controversial, complex, and not completely understood. There is evidence, as in tuberculosis, that nutritional deficiencies may reactivate a latent infection.[2] "Among the many odd facts concerning the influence of nutrition on infection is that resistance can be decreased by certain foodstuffs which have high nutritional value . . . paradoxically, nutritional deficiencies can increase resistance under certain circumstances."[2]

Inherent characteristics of defense against invasion or combating infection are *nonspecific* and *specific*. The nonspecific characteristics are the skin, mucous membranes, cilia and body pH, or body secretions which generally protect against invasion of any pathogen. If an organism is successful in breaking through these barriers, the body mobilizes with internal, specific mechanisms such as leukocyte phagocytosis, reticuloendothelial response, and changes in metabolic activity creating an intracellular environment unfavorable to survival or multiplication of the pathogen.[2]

Immunity is the successful resistance of the body to foreign agent invasion. Immunity is either active or passive. Two types of active immunity are humoral immunity and cellular immunity. Humoral immunity occurs when antibodies or immunoglobulins are produced and circulate in the blood. The body produces antibodies in response to specific foreign organisms, thus attacking the invading agent. Cellular immunity is the ability of the lymphocytes to become sensitized to foreign agents.[3] Sensitization occurs because there is an imprint on the cell memory which enables the body to quickly respond to a subsequent invasion by the same organism. The specific antibodies are released when needed to fight off the agent invasion. Passive immunity is the direct transfer of antibodies from another source providing temporary protection. The body is not stimulated to produce its own antibodies. The host is protected for a short and temporary duration and subsequently not able to produce antibodies on another challenge by the foreign organism. An example of this is the placental transfer of maternal antibodies protecting the newborn for about six months to one year of age.

THE AGENT

The infectious agent is a biologic organism from the internal (endogenous) or external (exogenous) environment which is capable of causing disease in man. A specific infectious agent (e.g., *Mycobacterium tuberculosis*) is *essential* to cause a specific disease (tuberculosis). Characteristics of organisms are its pathogenicity, virulence, morphology, reservoir, mode of transmission, portals of entry and exit, and the type and severity of the host response.

The pathogenicity of an organism refers to the ability of the organism to invade tissue and to the ability of the organism to cause illness in a host. Of the many organisms in nature, about 50 are pathogenic or able to cause disease in man. The others are generally nonpathogenic.[1]

Virulence influences the degree of the illness.[4] Virulence can be determined by the number of pathogenic organisms present, the ability of the organism to overcome the body's defenses, and the status of the host's defenses. A strongly virulent organism, however, may be capable of serious illness despite the wellness of the host. For example, unless treatment is received, even a healthy host will contract rabies if bitten by an infected animal.

The structure of an organism is known as its morphology. The structure will determine such characteristics as resistance to destruction, portal of entry, and growth environment needed. Infectious agents range from simple viral particles to higher complex organisms such as bacteria, chlamydias, mycoplasmas, rickettsiae, spirochetes, fungi, protozoa, and viruses.

The reservoir is a place in the environment where living conditions are conducive to the maintenance, growth, and reproduction of the organism. Man, animals, and inanimate objects (soil, water) can be reservoirs.

The mode of transmission is the manner in which the agent leaves its reservoir and is in contact with the portal of entry of a host. This can be by direct or indirect means. Direct transmission is actual or proximal contact such as physical touch, sexual intercourse, direct exposure of tissue, or immediate contact with large droplets carrying an organism (sneeze, cough). Indirect transmission is vectorborne (ticks, mosquitoes), airborne (tiny droplets, aerolyzed particles), or vehicleborne (instruments, dressings). In addition, some organisms are capable of transmission via a variety of modes and not limited to one.

The type and severity of clinical illness which results in the host is often characteristic of certain organisms. As stated earlier, host factors influence the resulting state. Measles virus, for instance, usually causes a mild to moderate degree of clinical symptoms such as fever, conjunctivitis, coryza, and a typical blotchy rash. The host response may vary according to the mechanism of action by the infectious agent, such as its ability to produce toxins, cause hypersensitivity reactions, produce endotoxins, live intracellularly, and stimulate immune response.[4]

THE ENVIRONMENT

Biologic organisms are found in man's internal (endogenous) and external (exogenous) environment. Generally, endogenous organisms peacefully coexist with the host. Exogenous organisms are most often the cause of communicable disease in man. Factors in the external environment which influence the host and agent are physical characteristics, socioeconomic factors, and behavior patterns.

Physical characteristics of the environment include natural boundaries such as rivers, mountains and forests, topography, climate, weather and atmospheric conditions. The more immediate surroundings of the host include the place of residence, work, and recreation. Certain areas and conditions of the environment are conducive to providing reservoirs for infectious agents and maintaining living modes of transmission. An example of a disease dependent on the interrelationships in the environment is characterized by Rocky

Mountain spotted fever (a disease occurring throughout the U.S.). In the temperate climate area during spring and summer near certain wooded areas, there exists a rickettsiae which causes the disease. It is transmitted from infected animals or rodents to man via the bite of the infected tick which carries the organism or contamination of skin with crushed tissues or feces of the tick.[5]

Socioeconomic factors of social class, housing, occupation, employment status, finances, and education influence the environmental setting, making it conducive or nonconducive to the growth and reproduction of organisms. Poverty is a complex state related to socioeconomic factors and behavior patterns. The spread of infectious agents is facilitated by many conditions found in poverty areas[2] such as substandard living conditions, poor sanitation, inadequate finances, crowded conditions, infestations of rodents and arthropods, decrease in available health resources and/or utilization of them, lower educational status, emphasis on short term priorities, sense of powerlessness, crisis situations, and unemployment. The above conditions along with a decreased level of general health provide prime circumstances for increased susceptibility to infection and communicable diseases.

The behavior patterns of the individual are a result of cultural influence. Some examples of behavior are personality, hygienic practices, nutritional patterns, health seeking practices, work and play activities, and social interactions. Behavior may increase exposure, make the host more susceptible, or interfere with proper treatment. A person with diabetes increases exposure to local and later systematic infections such as staphylococcus if he does not follow aseptic technique when preparing and administering the injection of insulin. Further, if he interferes with his own therapy by not adhering to a special diet or not monitoring his urine for sugar, he is likely to increase his susceptibility to infection in addition to risking direct complications of the diabetes.

Inadequate immunization histories for children, poor nutritional practices, and improper wound care can increase chances of contracting infections or communicable diseases. In attempting to change any health practices, the nurse must be aware of cultural mores and attitudes of the population with which she or he works.

THE INTERACTION

There exists an ongoing and dynamic interaction between man and his environment. Since the infectious agent also exists in man's environment, there is the potential for contact between the two. Once this contact is made, there are a variety of host responses which include 1) colonization, 2) inapparent or latent infection, 3) mild, moderate, or severe illness possibly resulting in death, and 4) carrier state.[4] The communicability of a communicable disease is variable during the disease process.

The status of both the host and agent at the time of contact determines the degree of illness. The virulence of an organism alters in an ebb and flow manner. This virulence seems to decrease over time.[2,6] Man individually and holistically increases resistance by continually adapting to environmental exposures with infectious agents. Some of this resistance is apparently passed on genetically to others. If a group or race has never had contact with an infectious agent in the past, it is likely severe disease will result on exposure to a new pathogen. Nonpathogenic organisms or weakly virulent infectious agents may exist in a latent state within the host. Illness may result only if the host susceptibility increases.[2]

Colonization is the growth and reproduction of an organism without invasion of tissue or host reaction. For example, colonization may occur as in the case of *Escherichia coli* (a normal body organism) colonizing the mucous membrane of the gastrointestinal tract. It becomes important if there is a sudden change in the general health status of the individual. Illness could then result.

Inapparent or latent infection is characterized by no detectable symptoms (subclinical) at any stage of the disease. However, the disease may be transmitted and cause serious disease or damage in another host who is not resistant. Those with inapparent or latent infection are unlikely to seek medical care and are not easily identified because of inadequacies of diagnostic tests. Gonorrhea has been diagnosed in both males and females who do not have any symptoms of the disease such as a purulent discharge and urethritis but still are able to transmit the infectious agent.[7,8]

Illness caused by an infectious agent may have mild, moderate, or severe symptoms such as fever, rashes, anorexia, lethargy, immobility, and organ impairment. Although mild cases may not be diagnosed or treated, persons with moderate and severe clinical symptoms are often seen by a doctor or other health professional. Severe illness may require hospitalization and even result in death.

Carrier states occur when a person is infected by an organism, does not have clinical symptoms, but is a potential source of infection for others.[4] Carrier states are periods of communicability whether or not a person ever becomes symptomatic. Chronic carrier states may persist for indefinite periods of time. Some persons without symptoms are carriers of beta hemolytic streptococcus which causes throat infections and possibly rheumatic fever in others. Food handlers should be tested for typhoid carrier states before being hired to prepare or serve food.

The degree of illness or the type of symptoms whether mild or severe is not necessarily an indication of the communicability of the disease. The communicable period is the length of time the disease can be transmitted directly or indirectly from an infected man or animal to another host.[5] There may be a characteristic communicable period for diseases such as during the beginning incubation period, the prodromal period, the acute illness, or the later convalescence.

SCOPE OF THE PROBLEM

The problem of communicable disease still persists today. Although the threat of death from communicable disease has decreased over the years, morbidity (illness rate) has not. The status of the host, alterations in the infectious agents' characteristics, and inadequacies in interventions contribute to this phenomenon. Proposed DNA research for the future has stirred much debate because of the fear of new untreatable diseases.

The threat of mortality due to communicable diseases has significantly decreased due to the usual course of waning virulence of infectious agents (pathogens), man's adaptive responses, and advances in public health, science, and medicine. Indeed, chronic diseases such as heart disease and cancer are more prevalent and the leading causes of death in the U.S. today.[9]

The morbidity (illness rate) caused by communicable diseases, however, has not significantly decreased. In fact, for some diseases, such as those caused by viruses, morbidity has increased. "The paradox is that the percentage of hospital beds occupied by patients suffering from infection is now as high as it was 50 years ago. Today as in the past, moreover, disorders of the respiratory and digestive tracts with a microbial etiology constitute the most frequent causes of absenteeism from school, office, factory, or from training in the armed forces."[2]

Host susceptibility and resistance are variable. Host status affects the degree of infection by an organism (microbe) and determines the extent and severity of the disease symptoms. Although not always predictable, groups of persons can be identified as risks to contracting disease. Persons inadequately immunized, elderly persons in poor health, those with chronic disease especially if there is altered immune response (cancer, chemotherapy, irradiation), and those of low socioeconomic groups (poverty) are examples of higher risk populations. Current life-styles increase exposure to different settings and persons, thereby increasing the likelihood of exposure to a wider variety of infectious agents. The percentage of persons adequately immunized to the childhood diseases is currently under close scrutiny. This of course varies in each community. There is a nationwide effort to assess and immunize the school children in the U.S. There are 46 states which require specific immunization for school entry but these laws have not been consistently enforced. In Cincinnati, Ohio in the fall of 1974, only 60 percent of the 63,000 primary school children were adequately immunized. The Boards of Health and Education worked conjointly to enforce the Public Health Law and excluded from schools those children not adequately immunized. At the same time, immunization clinics were set up in a variety of preexisting clinics in the city. In two years, 91 percent of children from kindergarten to tenth grade were immunized.[10]

Alterations of infectious agents' characteristics producing mutant strains may result in organisms which are virulent, pathogenic, and resistant to known therapies for prevention and treatment. It was reported, for instance, at the World Health Organization scientific meeting in 1976, that there existed a penicillin resistant strain of *Neisseria gonorrhea* (penicillin being the drug of choice). In addition, in a penicillin resistant case it was found that the organism was also resistant to the alternate drug, spectinomycin.[11] The occurrence of new and virulent organisms is a potential threat. This is demonstrated by the sudden occurrence of a respiratory illness (Legionnaire's disease) at a convention of the American Legion in Philadelphia in August 1976, which was responsible for 26 deaths and over 100 ill persons. Because of the sudden onset and fatal outcome, there was a great deal of publicity nationwide. During a 16 month period from August 1976 to December 1977, a total of 150 sporadic cases around the country were confirmed. Of these, 32 persons died. As of April 1977, systematic investigation had identified a bacterium as the infectious agent in this pneumonialike illness. Pertinent data such as mode of transmission, natural reservoir, and predisposing host factors are still unknown. In November 1978, an international conference was planned so that persons involved in studying varying aspects of this disease could meet, share their findings, and update existing knowledge.[34] Could this be the result of environmental change, increased susceptibility of the host, a new or mutant infectious agent, or a combination of all of these?

Inadequate interventions because of insufficient knowledge, limited funds, or decreased involvement may contribute to an increase of any communicable disease. Incomplete immunizations plus the inaccurate timing or scheduling of them is demonstrated in the following example. The incorrect administration of the measles vaccine contributed to the nationwide epidemic in 1977. The beginning 18 weeks of 1977 showed that in persons younger than 18 years of age, there was an increase of almost 52 percent over the same period of 1976. This was a 93 percent increase over the median of the previous five years. It also was determined from the data that the efficacy of the vaccine was lower for those receiving it before 1966 when it was given at nine months of age. Because of the potential

interference of remaining maternal antibodies and the decreased attack rate for children*
who received it after one year of age, it is now recommended that measles vaccine be given
at 15 months of age.[35]

A current controversial issue is the genetic research of recombinant deoxyribonucleic
acid (DNA). This is the manipulation of genes to produce different organisms. DNA is
found in the nucleus of the cell. It is responsible for overall cell function and makeup of
the genes which carry hereditary characteristics.[3] Since cell growth and reproduction
intimately involve DNA, a grave concern about laboratory experimentation is the evolution of highly infectious, virulent strains with previously unknown properties which may
escape from the lab and cause disease. Those in favor of this DNA research believe it
offers a great deal to understanding hereditary characteristics and immunity. They feel this
risk is of small concern since lab strains easily become attenuated and lose their pathogenicity. In addition, measures of strict controls and containment are planned.[12]

IMPACT ON THE INDIVIDUAL

Communicable diseases potentially affect the physical, psychological, and socioeconomic
status of the individual. The degree of illness and the person's response vary. In order to
understand the impact of communicable disease on the individual, objective and subjective data about the person's illness and circumstance must be considered.

The physical status of an individual is affected by the type, stage, communicability, and
severity of the disease. Factors which influence an individual's experience with the
communicable disease are age, developmental stage, and general health status. The type
of symptoms depends on the extent of infection and the body systems involved. They are
either localized, isolated to a larger area, or generalized. The variety of symptoms associated with respiratory illness, for example, are coryza, cough, congestion of mucus, and
difficulty in breathing. A generalized response includes symptoms from a variety of systems such as fever, pruitic rash, coryza, malaise, and anorexia. The stage of illness and
degree of communicability also influence the individual's experience. Prodromal or the
initial period of time during which an illness is developing may be experienced as a feeling
of "coming down with something." The illness may range from mild clinical symptoms to
severe acute ones with variable duration. The convalescent period or the recovery time
may also vary with character and duration. When recovering from the flu, it may take
weeks to feel like oneself again. In contrast, tuberculosis may take several months or
chickenpox may be a matter of a few days. The degree of communicability may require
certain precautions to avoid the spread of the infectious agent to others. A person may
feel perfectly fine but be a reservoir of a highly infectious organism. When gonorrhea is
asymptomatic, the individual is still able to spread the pathogen on contact but does not
have any symptoms and may be totally unaware of the infection.

The age of the person is a significant factor in terms of body response to invasion and
illness. Frequency of viral illness is higher in younger children versus adults whereas the
severity of the same disease is often greater in adults. Infectious mononucleosis in childhood is often unrecognized or nonspecific because of mild symptoms. The only evidence
of past disease is an antibody titre to Epstein-Barr virus which is the virus known to cause

---

*Attack rate is the number of children receiving the immunization after one year of age divided by the
total number of children immunized.

this disease. Those exposed to this same virus as older teens have more severe symptoms and illness and are usually diagnosed and treated by a physician.[13,14] The developmental stage of the individual can be a factor. The occurrence of rubella (German measles) is often a mild febrile illness with minimal symptoms in a three year old. However, the occurrence of rubella in a pregnant woman especially in the first trimester can be extremely risky and traumatic. It is associated with perinatal loss and malformations of the developing fetus such as congenital cataracts, cardiac defects, anomalies of the middle ear, microcephalus, and mental retardation.[15]

Psychological status of the individual depends on the host's knowledge of the disease, level of education, perception of circumstances, previous experiences, and need to alter his life-style. An individual's knowledge of the disease causation may influence his psychological response. For instance, he may be anxious, fearful, embarrassed, or guilty. One may feel guilty about exposing others to a communicable disease such as hepatitis. This is particularly true when an individual may be the primary source (index case) which causes an epidemic of the disease. When a person is ill, his life-style alters as he assumes a sick role. "In this role he exchanges freedom, autonomy and self-direction for control, but at the same time he gains protection, freedom from responsibility and care."[16] This may be desirable or undesirable depending on the individual's perception of the role and past experience. A person who is usually in a position of power and control may have difficulty in this dependent role.

The socioeconomic status of the individual is affected to the extent that role changes are required. Aspects of socioeconomic roles are interpersonal relations, economic status, and environment. An individual assumes a variety of roles in society such as parent, spouse, worker, friend, student, or member of an organization. Some persons assume more roles than others. Each of these roles has responsibilities which are carried through by the individual. The extent that communicable disease or the threat of communicable disease interferes with an individual's ability to carry out these roles is varied. Interactions with others may need to be altered. If there is a chance to transmit an infectious agent, precautions need to be taken even if the individual feels fine. An individual with confirmed venereal disease (gonorrhea, syphilis) has a social responsibility to abstain from sexual contact until he or she no longer is a source of infection. The economic status is affected when time, energy, and money are drained because of inability to work at one's occupation or fulfill the necessary and meaningful tasks of caring for a home and family. This is significant if a person is the only one fulfilling this role under usual circumstances. The environment of the house or work may very well be the source of contact for the individual. The individual may still be at risk of exposure. This problem may be overwhelming as with rodent infestations of an apartment building. The cooperation of the landlord and even neighborhood persons is necessary to rectify the situation. To mobilize such a group or the person responsible may be beyond the individual's ability or motivation.

In understanding the impact of communicable disease on the individual one must be sure to consider both objective and subjective data. Objective observation and examination of the clinical symptoms are necessary. Further, the individual's personal interpretation of the illness as it affects his psychological and socioeconomic circumstance is essential.

IMPACT ON THE FAMILY

Those persons the individual interprets as family include both the primary group and significant others who must be identified. From birth the socialization process influences an individual's behavior patterns. A communicable disease, as any other disease, may cause hardship to the family resulting in disequilibrium to their usual functioning state. Their own risk of developing the same disease due to similar causative factors, their perception of the illness, and the need to alter family roles all impact on the family.

The family is defined as a primary, intimate group which is an open system that grows, develops, and evolves.[17] The primary family is the one into which one is born. In addition to the primary family, significant others are those persons immediately outside the primary group who occupy a rank of high status to the individual.[18,19] Therefore, they are able to participate in the meaningful interaction of the family group. They can be relatives, close friends, or health care providers (visiting nurse, doctor, or others). For the purpose of this section, family refers to the broader intimate group including significant others.

Socialization is a process which occurs within the primary family. Socialization is the means by which the human organism acquires the behaviors, values, norms, and attitudes of the social units of which he is a part.[19] One is then socialized to a particular culture with behavior patterns which have been reinforced by the members of the primary family.

The disequilibrium within the family group which results from a communicable disease may begin with the reality of exposure to others. People at risk include family members and persons with whom one is living, working, or playing. If the individual remains at home and needs to be cared for, it is likely that family members will participate in that care. Their knowledge of causal factors, modes of transmission, ways to carry out care, treatment, and rationale for control measures are very important.

The family's understanding and interpretation of the disease is based on its culture. Its perceptions may elicit a variety of psychological reactions such as anxiety, embarrassment, or guilt. If a family's interpretation of the disease is that it is a punishment for some wrongdoing, it may believe that the individual must atone for this and make retribution for the wrongdoing.

It is important to understand the extent that a communicable disease affects the family as a group. In addition to determining the structure of the family group, it is necessary to identify the roles of each member and their manner of interaction. Alterations in family roles may be necessary. Their life-style patterns may change either temporarily or permanently. They may need to be flexible to assume new roles and responsibilities in addition to those normally carried out. Finances may be drained because of medication, therapy, and hospitalization. Because the breadwinner may be the person who is ill, this role may have to be assumed by others in the family group or community resources sought out. In any event, the impact a communicable disease has on a family will be influenced by such factors as culture, etiology of disease, member of family affected, need for role changes, and financial losses. All factors need to be analyzed to reduce the severity of the impact experienced as a result of the disease.

IMPACT ON THE COMMUNITY

For the purpose of this chapter, the community refers to a place which is designated in political units by census tracts. Aspects of disease surveillance are identified by the community in order to understand the impact that communicable diseases have on it. Subdivisions of the community are the people, geographic environment, and political influence.

A community has many characteristics and can be defined in several ways. It is a social entity where the organization of social activities afford people daily access to those areas of activity which are necessary in day-to-day living.[20] A community is a place, a social system, and a collection of people. A school, ethnic group, and church membership can be considered communities. The boundaries of census tracts "are usually established jointly by local committees and the Bureau of the Census to achieve some homogeneity of such population characteristics as economic status and living conditions."[1]

Disease surveillance is the systematic collection of pertinent data related to all aspects of the occurrence, spread, and effective control of a disease.[5] This information is usually summarized by giving the rates of disease occurrence in specific areas. The morbidity, mortality, and distribution of the disease are examples of the rates of communicable disease occurrence. The morbidity rates of a community are expressed as incidence and prevalence rates. In order to determine the significance of communicable disease in a community, it is necessary to understand these terms. The following are formulas used to calculate the rates:[22]

$$\text{Incidence rate (per 1000)} = \frac{\begin{array}{c}\text{Number of new disease cases in a}\\ \text{population during a specified time period}\end{array}}{\begin{array}{c}\text{Number of persons exposed to}\\ \text{disease risk during that period of time}\end{array}} \times 1000$$

$$\text{Prevalence rate (per 1000)} = \frac{\begin{array}{c}\text{Number of disease cases in a}\\ \text{population at a specified time}\end{array}}{\begin{array}{c}\text{Number of persons in a popula-}\\ \text{tion at that specified time}\end{array}} \times 1000$$

The difference between incidence and prevalence rates is that incidence refers to the number of *new* cases during an *interval* of time. Prevalence rate is the number of *existing* cases including the new ones at a particular *point* in time. For example, during a two week period there may be an incidence rate of 15/1000 of new cases of hepatitis in a community. But, a total of 36/1000 cases of hepatitis are prevalent in that same community, having been diagnosed previous to those two weeks. Mortality rates due to communicable diseases are measured in various ways. The most common one includes three elements: the population group who were exposed to the risk of disease; a time factor; and the number of deaths occurring in the exposed population during a certain period.[22] The distribution of disease occurrence is the identification of the location by geographic boundaries and demographic characteristics. This may uncover a population at risk for developing a communicable disease, missed or unreported cases of a communicable disease, or carriers of the infectious agent. For example, an increased incidence of hepatitis may be traced to a certain restaurant in a community where an infected worker continues handling food. He then becomes a primary source (index case) for patrons of that restaurant who are thus at risk of developing the disease. An epidemic is likely to result. Certain diseases may be present at a consistent rate in a community. This rate is used as a frame of reference for that community to determine the significance of changes. Also, this rate is also compared to the state, region, and nation. For rare diseases such as cholera, one case in a community is quite significant and may represent an "epidemic."

The demographic characteristics of the people as a group are age, sex, religion, occupation, educational level, and location in the community. Information such as life-style patterns, recreational activities, and cultural behaviors help to increase understanding of the persons in the community and help to identify causative or contributing factors. Segments of the population which seem to maintain and foster the growth of infectious agents may be identified by analyzing the characteristics and distribution of groups in the community. Religious beliefs may prevent a family from receiving immunizations which are required.

The environment of the community is its surroundings. This includes the natural boundaries, topography, climate, weather, atmospheric conditions, and residential and work settings. Reservoirs within the natural environment which provide ideal conditions as breeding grounds of pathogens and vectors and other vehicles of transmission must be identified. Areas of substandard housing with unsanitary conditions may be infested with disease carrying rodents or arthropods. Stagnant water which is used for recreation can foster the growth and transmission of organisms. The irresponsible dumping of waste products into waterways or near the drinking supply potentially exposes many persons to infectious agents.

The political influence in the community depends on the inhabitants, the officials, and the decision making process. Health regulations are established to protect the public. The community has responsibilities as a result of them. The political atmosphere influences priorities established and the ability of the community to keep its population healthy. The responsibility for health regulation enforcement is shared by consumers of health care as well as health care providers (who are also consumers!). Health regulations are established by each state. Currently, the state public health departments have the right and responsibility on the local level to enforce the laws. The state departments do so also upon request of the community or an adjacent community if it is indicated. It is necessary to maintain enforcement and vigilance of health regulations. Some examples of community services are periodic restaurant inspections, water quality control of public and private facilities, housing inspection, sewage and garbage collection, and sanitation. At some times there may be a tendency to ignore, relax, or close one's eyes to violations of the health code. This is to the detriment of the population. For example, if a community depends economically on the tourist trade, they may be unwilling to publicize the occurrence of a communicable disease for fear of jeopardizing that income.

A community's wealth, resources, and ability to alter factors in the environment vary. It is critical, however, to remain vigilant and persistent in the identification of disease and disease factors. Protection of the public health is every citizen's responsibility.

PREVENTION AND TREATMENT

The goals or expected outcomes of interventions are focused on altering the factors of the host, agent, or environment. There are three levels of prevention: primary, secondary, and tertiary. Since interventions also entail undesirable effects, the benefit-risk ratio is a critical consideration in choosing the best alternative. It is possible to initiate effective measures before knowing all the causal factors of a particular disease.

The goals of interventions are the decrease of host susceptibility or the increase of host resistance, the alteration of environmental threats, and the establishment of barriers to host-agent contact. The interventions must be based on sound rationale and follow a systematic collection and analysis of data. This analysis enables the identification of the problems and needs of the client whether it be an individual, family, or community. It is very important that the client participate in all the planning stages of intervention, including the establishment of goals, course of action, and evaluations.

Prevention refers to those measures which inhibit, interrupt, or slow the progression of disease.[4] Interventions are geared toward prevention, treatment of the disease, and restoration of the individual. Primary prevention measures are employed before the disease occurs to alter host susceptibility such as immunizations or to reduce exposure to the infectious agent as with asepsis. Secondary prevention involves the early diagnosis and treatment of a communicable disease, such as screening for syphilis, in order to alter the course, cure the disease, and prevent further complications. After the occurrence of a disease resulting in disability, tertiary measures such as physical therapy are geared toward the limitation of the disability, rehabilitation, and management of convalescent states.[4] Those measures considered in this section are unique to communicable disease but in no way minimize other measures of care which also can be applied to diseases of a noninfectious nature.

Short or long term effects from interventions are not always desirable, for some side effects can be worse than the disease itself. In identifying the alternative measures of intervention, the benefit-risk ratio should be determined.[23] The risk of treatment must be weighed against the benefit of that treatment. This deliberation includes the likelihood of exposure to a specific communicable disease, the consequence of that disease, and the effectiveness of the treatment. The alteration of indications for smallpox vaccination is a result of this process. Smallpox vaccination was once required as a part of immunization practice in the U.S. The last outbreak here was in 1949. In 1967 a worldwide program to eradicate smallpox was initiated. As a result of this program, smallpox is the first communicable disease to be eradicated worldwide. Prior to this, the vaccine was given to persons in the United States only if they were traveling to countries where the disease still existed, since complications from the vaccine, although rare, presented more of a threat than the disease itself. Since smallpox is transferred only by contact with an infected person, its reappearance is not anticipated.

It is not always possible to anticipate effects from interventions. Since interventions can interfere with the balance of nature, a resultant disturbance may occur. The indiscriminate use of antibiotics for minor problems may result in decreased effectiveness or agent resistance in the face of more serious disease. An example of such intervention is Gullain-Barré syndrome, which is a self-limiting paralysis. It occurs in 10 out of 1 million persons who have been vaccinated against influenza, within eight weeks of the injection. Before the swine flu vaccination program in 1976, this syndrome was not recognized as a reaction to this particular measure. Of the persons who experienced the Guillain-Barré syndrome, 5 to 10 percent were left with residual weakness and 5 percent died.[24]

PREVENTION AND TREATMENT FOR THE INDIVIDUAL

Prevention and treatment of communicable diseases in the individual are implemented through the three levels of prevention. Measures of primary prevention in the individual are health promotion, immunization and chemotherapy. Early diagnosis and treatment, the prevention of spread of communicable disease to others, and restoration measures are aspects of secondary prevention. Tertiary measures of prevention are not necessarily indicated unless there is resultant disability. Measures attempt to reduce the disability, to provide rehabilitation efforts, and to seek out resources to aid in altered life-style patterns.

Primary prevention is an effort to prevent communicable diseases before they occur. Health promotion is accomplished through health education and anticipatory guidance. First, an individual must perceive himself vulnerable to an invasion by an infectious agent.

In addition, he must perceive that the result of that contact is of serious consequence to him. If he believes that he is capable of altering the occurrence of a communicable disease and the cost of his action is not greater than the benefit, he is likely to be motivated to act in behalf of prevention of the disease. Increased awareness, a trigger to action, and adequate knowledge are more likely to result in action by the individual.[25] This action may require a behavior change on the part of the individual. Critical aspects of this are that the individual is motivated, ready to learn, and able to do so.

Primary prevention includes both active and passive immunization. This increases host resistance by enhancing normal body defenses. Active immunity, which is developed as a result of immunization with a specific vaccine, is a method of protection. Vaccination is available for approximately 25 communicable diseases. The following are recommended for the routine immunization against childhood diseases: diphtheria, tetanus, and pertussis (DTP); polio; measles, mumps, and rubella (MMR) (Tables 24-1 and 24-2).[26] Other immunizations are given when one may be at risk of the disease because of the type and setting of work or travel to areas of the world where exposure to an infectious agent is a possibility. When traveling to certain areas, immunizations against typhoid, yellow fever, and cholera are necessary. The Public Health Service Advisory Committee on Immunization Practices (ACIP), the American Public Health Association, and the Committee on Infectious Diseases of the American Academy of Pediatrics make statements and recommendations about vaccines and immunization practices.

Passive immunity occurs when antibodies are directly injected or infused into the individual from another source. Man or animals (commonly the horse or rabbit) are other sources which have produced antibodies to a specific infectious agent. The individual's body does not produce its own antibodies and therefore it is only a temporary protection. It is used when a person has been exposed or is at risk of exposure to an infectious agent. It has been successful in preventing infection or minimizing illness. The various immune globulins from man and the antisera and antitoxins from animals are measures of passive immunity. Immune globulins are derived from pools of human blood plasma. It is important that immune serum globulin is given as soon as possible (at least within two weeks)

TABLE 24-1. Recommended schedule for active immunization of normal infants and children*

2 mo	DTP	TOPV
4 mo	DTP	TOPV
6 mo	DTP	TOPV (optional)
1 yr		Tuberculin test
15 mo	Measles, rubella	Mumps
1½ yr	DTP	TOPV
4-6 yr	DTP	TOPV
14-16 yr	Td (repeat every 10 yrs)	

*From Report of the Committee on Infectious Diseases, 18th ed., p. 3, American Academy of Pediatrics 1977, with permission.
  DTP = Diphtheria and tetanus toxoids combined with pertussis vaccine.
TOPV = Trivalent oral poliovirus vaccine.
  Td = Combined tetanus and diphtheria toxoids (adult type).

TABLE 24-2. Primary immunization for children not immunized in early infancy*

Under 6 yrs of Age	
First visit	DTP, TOPV, tuberculin test
Interval after first visit	
1 mo	Measles, mumps, rubella
2 mo	DTP, TOPV
4 mo	DTP, TOPV
10-16 mo or preschool	DTP, TOPV
Age 14-16 yr	Td (repeat every 10 yr)

6 Years of Age and Over	
First visit	Td, TOPV, tuberculin test
Interval after first visit	
1 mo	Measles, mumps, rubella
2 mo	Td, TOPV
8-14 mo	Td, TOPV
Age 14-16 yr	Td (repeat every 10 yrs)

*From Report of the Committee on Infectious Diseases, 18th ed., p. 11, American Academy of Pediatrics 1977, with permission.
DTP = Diphtheria and tetanus toxoids combined with pertussis vaccine.
TOPV = Trivalent oral poliovirus vaccine.
Td = Combined tetanus and diphtheria toxoids (adult type).

after exposure to the infectious agent. If it is used as prophylaxis (preventive measure) in a person working closely with blood products or traveling to high risk areas, the immune serum globulin should be repeated every four to six months since it is only a temporary protection.[27] Zoster or varicella immune globulin (ZIG or VIG) is prepared from the plasma of healthy donors who are convalescing from herpes zoster infection (shingles) or varicella (chickenpox). It is used in children with leukemia who, because of treatment, have suppressed immune systems. Upon exposure to chickenpox (for which there is no vaccine available) they receive passive immunity with ZIG or VIG. It has been successful in preventing or modifying the disease and thus protecting these immune deficient children from disseminated and possible fatal infection. It is critical that it is administered within 72 hours of contact. The supply is intermittent and therefore insufficient.[28] Antisera and antitoxins are derived from the serum of animals who have been challenged with an infectious agent or specific toxin of a disease. Antibodies are present against that specific disease and most inactive substances are removed. Because it is derived from an animal source, there is always the potential for a severe reaction like serum sickness or anaphylaxis. This is not likely to occur on the first innoculation but on subsequent ones after the body has been senitized with the foreign protein and has produced allergic antibodies against that protein. Antisera are used when there is no other source available because of the likelihood of severe allergic reaction. It is available for diphtheria, botulism, and gas gangrene. These are used as prophylaxis or in the early stages after exposure to an infectious agent. It must be remembered that the critical time period varies with each communicable disease.

Therefore, the critical time period dictates when the immune serum is administered. The temporary protection usually lasts from one to six weeks.[26]

Antimicrobial therapy or chemotherapy has been used as prophylaxis and direct therapy. If a person is predisposed to communicable disease or if a communicable disease is likely to result in severe illness, medication including antibiotics, antivirals, or antimalarials may be given in lower doses to provide adequate blood levels to prevent or inhibit infection.

Early diagnosis of communicable disease enables prompt treatment for the individual and prevention of spread to others. These are aspects of secondary prevention. Part of early diagnosis is the determination of the status of the communicability of the disease. The ability to grow pathogens in culture media from material taken from the host is one way of doing this. Another is ascertaining from the recent literature the known period of communicability and mode of transmission. In order for the individual to be diagnosed early, he must seek care and be identified through screening or on interview of a known contact person. The blood test required for marriage licenses identifies individuals with syphilis. Contacts are often identified through careful interview and then notification of those with a communicable disease is made by health personnel. During the process of providing direct care and restoring the individual to his previous health status, measures to protect others are implemented. Direct measures may be provided by the individual, family, friends, or health care providers such as the nurse or her assistant. Some examples of these measures are bedrest if indicated, adequate fluids and diet, specific medication, and assistance with activites of daily living. If the individual is either severely ill or circumstances are not conducive to his recovery or the prevention of spread to others, hospitalization may be required.

Other measures of secondary prevention are disinfection, isolation, and quarantine. Disinfection, the killing or inhibiting growth of infectious agents by physical or chemical means, is concurrent or terminal. Concurrent measures are employed on an ongoing basis during the infectious or contagious stage of the illness. Terminal disinfections are the thorough measures employed after the person is removed or ceases to be a source of infection. Isolation separates a contagious host (man or animal) from others during the period of communicability to prevent direct or indirect spread of the agent. Quarantine is distinct from isolation as it limits movement for the incubation period of well hosts who have been exposed to a communicable disease.[5] (Incubation period is the time between exposure to an infectious agent and the first signs of prodromal symptoms.)

Tertiary measures are not always indicated. If an individual with a communicable disease recovers but is left with some form of disability such as paralysis, an alteration in his lifestyle is necessary. Physical therapy and counseling are measures which may help to reduce the disability. Rehabilitation includes all aspects of physical, psychological, occupational, social, and spiritual implications. Altered approaches to a previous life-style or direct changes in life-style may require the assistance of other specialized professionals in the community in addition to the nurse. An adult male may benefit from counseling when a mumps infection with an orchitis results in sterility. A person convalescing from tuberculosis may need to change occupations and lead a less active life.

PREVENTION AND TREATMENT FOR THE FAMILY

The family of the individual with a communicable disease may or may not be affected by the disease. Primary preventive measures involve the identification of family members at risk, the implementation of protective measures, and the promotion of health. If the ill individual is unable to care for himself, family members may be involved with secondary and tertiary interventions.

Once a communicable disease has been diagnosed in an individual, it is important to identify those persons, including family members, who are at risk of exposure and development of the same disease. Those persons who have not been adequately immunized to the childhood diseases need to be immunized. If family members have already been exposed to the communicable disease, measures of passive immunity can be employed if they are available and indicated. For example, persons exposed to hepatitis A can receive an injection of gamma globulin (a specific immune globulin) which will provide antibodies to protect against the disease. If the source of the infectious agent is common to family members, it should be identified and removed from the environment. Should this be impossible, family members should take precautions to protect themselves. Some diseases such as chickenpox or influenza are difficult to prevent once exposure has occurred. A family may then need to watch, wait, and avoid exposing others to the same disease.

Health promotion of family members is accomplished through health education and anticipatory guidance. As is true for the individual, the family must be motivated and ready and able to learn, especially if the goal causes alterations in long established behavior patterns. The family's culture must be considered. This is best done by involving the family (including key members) in the identification of problems and needs, the planning of goals, and the choice of interventions at all levels of prevention. If an intervention is not acceptable because of beliefs, values, attitudes, and so forth, it will be very difficult if not impossible to implement. The Papago Indians of southern Arizona have a high incidence of tuberculosis. They initially seek treatment from the tribal medicine man. When they are finally diagnosed and treated by a medical doctor, they have a high rate of noncompliance to medical treatment. Often they discharge themselves from the hospital before completing treatment because it is very stressful for them to be separated from their family and friends.[29] If the individual, family, and even the medicine man could be included in the planning of care, perhaps their compliance with therapy and the effectiveness of that therapy will improve.

Family members may be involved with both secondary and tertiary levels of prevention. The effectiveness of interventions depends on the understanding, ability, and motivation of the caretaker and the amount of direct or indirect support provided by other family members and significant others. Critical to nursing care by family members is their readiness, understanding, and knowledge of the disease, modes of transmission, methods to protect themselves, and methods to prevent spread to others. They may need to be taught measures for comfort, restoration, and rehabilitation. The interventions need to be individualized to the circumstance and meet the particular needs of the family as well. Examples of measures are physical therapy, family and individual counseling, financial aid, and diversional activity. Family members may also suggest some innovative and sound ideas for health care based on their cultural values. This should be encouraged by the nurse and other health care providers in an atmosphere of mutual exchange of ideas and realities.

PREVENTION AND TREATMENT IN THE COMMUNITY

Input from various disciplines is involved with planning and implementing interventions on all levels of prevention. Community intervention occurs with aggregates or groups of persons. Information from vital statistics and disease surveillance provides valuable on-going data with implications for future interventions in a particular community. Program evaluation is necessary to insure effectiveness, competency, and relevancy of programs and avoid duplication of services.

The health problems of a community are often complex because several social systems within the community are affected. Input from various disciplines includes health, social, and political systems. In order to ensure that community needs and interests are addressed, citizens who are not health personnel should be included in identifying health problems and planning programs. The health professional provides his skill, expertise, and judgment in making recommendations. The action, however, must be meaningful to the community members in order for them to participate and support any health programs.

Community health involves aggregates and groups of persons. These groups often have similar characteristics or interests which serve to designate them as a group. In addition to persons living in the community, those who travel daily to and from school, work, play, and commerce should be kept in mind. In terms of communicable diseases, they may be a source of an infectious agent or also be exposed to one which is a threat to the community.

Public health laws are established with the intent of protecting the public. Local community officials are designated as having the right and responsibilities to enforce these laws. Community activities which serve the public and protect it against communicable disease are sewage and garbage disposal, chlorination of swimming pools, purification of the water supply, eradication of animals, rodent and arthropod control, inspection of food and food handling and the inspection of housing, immunizations, health education and screening programs, and casefinding through interviews and followup. These methods help to identify susceptible persons, contacts, or carriers of specific communicable disease or the health hazards in a community.

The community collects data on itself through vital and health statistics. This is a method of systematically recording such vital events as births, deaths, and illness in the population.[22] Disease surveillance is a systematic collection and analysis of information regarding the occurrence of communicable disease. It depends on the cooperation of all persons in the community. Early detection, reporting, and treatment may prevent spread of an infectious agent and complications from the disease process. It is not easily accomplished since reporting is often a problem. Communicable diseases which are mild and not associated with serious consequences are not always reported. Usually those more serious and rare ones such as cholera or rabies are consistently reported. [30,31] The U.S. Public Health Service has established a list of notifiable diseases (Table 24-3).

The collection, analysis, and dissemination of data concerning communicable disease are done through the Public Health Department on the local, state, and national level. The Center for Disease Control in Atlanta, Georgia is the national central office and is under the Department of Health and Human Services, Public Health Service. A weekly report is published and distributed with current information on communicable disease known as the *Morbidity and Mortality Weekly Report.*

Through the World Health Organization, worldwide surveillance and dissemination of information to and from all countries are achieved. The data collected may trigger epidemiologic investigation in attempting to uncover probable causes and factors of communicable disease. The worldwide surveillance of disease enables decisions on international regulations and recommendations. The Bureau of Epidemiology at the Center for Disease

TABLE 24-3. Specified notifiable diseases in the United States

Amebiasis	Plague
Anthrax	Poliomyelitis, total and paralytic
Aseptic meningitis	Psittacosis-ornithosis
Botulism	Rabies in man and animals
Brucellosis	Rubella
Chickenpox	Salmonellosis
Cholera	Shigellosis
Diphtheria	Smallpox
Encephalitis, 1′ infectious	Tetanus
Encephalitis, postinfectious	Trichinosis
Foodpoisoning (outbreaks)	Tuberculosis
Hepatitis A	Tuleremia
Hepatitis B	Typhoid fever
Hepatitis, unspecified	Typhus, fleaborne (murine)
Leprosy	Typhus, tickborne (Rocky Mt. spotted fever)
Leptospirosis	Venereal disease:
Malaria	Syphilis
Measles	primary
Meningococcal infections	secondary
Mumps	Gonorrhea
Pertussis	Yellow fever

Cholera, plague, smallpox and yellow fever are covered by international regulations by International Quarantine Agreement. Some states may have additional diseases which are reportable in their specific areas.

Control publishes a yearly booklet on *Health Information for International Travel*. This is supplemented with a weekly "Blue Sheet" giving information on the quarantinable diseases and occasionally issues an "Advisory Memorandum" with information on newly identified health problems. Anyone traveling internationally can consult this booklet or contact their local health department at least two weeks before departing. The intent of these regulations is to protect the individual and to prohibit the spread of infectious agents to and from countries. This intelligence system has aided in the compilation, analysis, and dissemination of information as it affects the entire world. The process of disease surveillance has contributed greatly to the knowledge and understanding of multicausal mechanisms of disease occurrence and points for intervention. It enables the continued study and research to build on the knowledge so far acquired and points in a direction for further investigation.

There are a variety of existing health programs and agencies in most communities. Program evaluation is important to determine the effectiveness, competency, and relevancy of them. The focus of evaluation is the structure, the process, and the outcomes of the program.[21] Outcome evaluation of existing or proposed programs depends on explicitly stated goals. Evaluation may uncover indications for a new focus, programs, and methods. It may also demonstrate a duplication of services which is unnecessary and costly to a community.

PROGNOSIS

Although it is difficult to generalize about the prognosis of communicable diseases, there has been a trend. The prognosis of the disease depends on its natural history, the availability of effective treatment, and the prevention of complications and the compliance of the host.

As long as man is part of the ecology, there will always be the risk of disease caused by infectious agents in the environment. So far, man has been successful in decreasing the incidence and mortality of most communicable diseases and the trend seems to be maintained. Two diseases which are exceptions to this downward trend are gonorrhea and Rocky Mountain spotted fever.[30] A once fatal disease such as smallpox has been eliminated.

The natural history of the communicable disease depends on aspects of the infectious agents, host response, and environmental influence. The pathogenicity and virulence of an organism may change as a natural event. Man adapts to environmental changes with increased exposure to organisms resulting in alterations in resistance which seems to be passed on genetically. Since the environment is ever changing, new organisms, diseases, and adaptive responses will evolve.

The existence, availability, and early effective treatment are critical for some diseases to alter the course of disease and enhance host defenses. During the course of illness, prevention of further complications insures a quicker and more complete recovery. Methods of prevention and control have enabled man to interfere at several points of causation, thus interrupting disease occurrence and spread. Primary prevention of disease is easier in most cases and less expensive than treatment of a disease. Immunization for the childhood diseases has been successful in decreasing the incidence of these diseases. Mumps virus vaccine was introduced in December 1967 and since that time has become a part of routine immunization practices. In 1968, almost 88 cases/100,000 were reported. This is a conservative number since mild cases may not be diagnosed and reporting may not have been optimal since it only became a reportable disease in 1968. Compare that figure to the 1976 data of almost 18 cases/100,000.[30] That is quite a significant difference and indicates to some extent the effectiveness of the vaccine in the prevention of mumps.

Control measures have been effective in interrupting host-agent contact. Personal hygiene such as handwashing before handling food and after excretion and defecation, proper refrigeration and storage of food, and spraying with effective insecticides are all measures to obstruct interactions of host and agent. Chemotherapy such as antibiotics, antivirals, and antimalarials have contributed to the prophylaxis and cure of many communicable diseases. As mentioned, many forms of interventions such as drugs have undesirable effects. The benefit-risk ratio needs to be considered since more severe reactions than the illness may result from the intervention. Drug resistant strains of pathogens have developed.

Lastly, host compliance with measures of prevention and treatment is critical to the prognosis and outcome of many diseases. For some diseases, there may be little or nothing one can do and it is necessary for the disease to run its own course. Motivation for prevention is highly variable. The host must perceive himself as susceptible and able to increase his resistance. If new information is integrated into behavior patterns, there is good potential for decreased severity, incidence, and fatality due to communicable diseases. Man has come far in the fight against communicable diseases, but there remains his responsibility to continue to pursue new avenues of prevention and treatment and to remain vigilant.

RESEARCH

Research builds on current knowledge and produces new knowledge. Areas of research which have implications for communicable diseases are scientific, psychosocial, and behavioral.

Current scientific study includes organism characteristics, adaptive responses of the host and agent, host defense factors, the development of effective drugs, new vaccines, and review of the efficacy and safety of existing vaccines. To facilitate the last, the record keeping for immunizations has expanded to include, in addition to personal information, the following: the vaccines given by name, manufacturer, and lot or other identifying number as well as dose, site, and route of administration. Any undesirable reactions are also noted and recorded.[26] Continual disease surveillance and investigations of epidemics often uncover essential information such as causative factors, persons at risk, and needs for prevention and control. The National League for Nurses (NLN) has outlined guidelines for the investigation of an epidemic (Table 24-4).[32]

Psychosocial and behavioral research has been quite productive in this century. Family and cultural research can help uncover some of the variables which greatly influence the individual, family, and community. It can expand knowledge and understanding of various

TABLE 24-4. Guidelines for investigation of disease outbreaks or epidemics*

1. Confirm the existence of an epidemic.
   a. Must have knowledge of the usual incidence of the "event" within the institution.
   b. Does the number of new cases of the "event" clearly represent an increased incidence? What is the attack rate?
2. Identify the scope of the investigation.
   a. To control the epidemic is the primary task.
   b. To gain additional knowledge of disease causation is a secondary objective.
3. Identify the disease or "event."
   a. What is the clinical picture?
   b. What do laboratory tests show?
4. Define who is involved ("case-finding").
   a. Identify as many cases of the "event" as possible.
   b. Determine populations and areas that are at risk of having the "event" occur.
5. Orient cases of the "event" as to place, time, and person.
   a. Define what kind of people became ill, when they became ill, and where.
   b. Look at circumstances of exposure, life-style, habits, age, and prior susceptibility.
   c. Look for patterns in occurrence of the "event."
   d. Look for factors which differentiate groups where the "event" occurred from groups where the "event" did not occur.
   e. Calculate the incidence rate for subgroups of population in order to identify those at highest risk of having this "event" occur.
6. Design appropriate control measures.
7. Report results to appropriate health authorities.
   a. Infection control committee.
   b. Community health department.

*From NLN Pub. No. 20-1582, *Infection* Control, 1975, pp. 51-52, with permission.

ethnic and cultural groups and discourage stereotyping and ineffective methods of interventions. It may also promote a reevaluation and reorganization of the health services to meet the needs of these cultural groups. Increased study of health behaviors may help identify critical factors in changing attitudes and behaviors enabling the improvement of methods of health promotion and teaching. Self-care and family care activity have been recently revived and studied as alternatives to current health practice. Patient education studies continue to provide valuable information which enhances the effectiveness of that particular method of intervention. Program evaluation is a more recent endeavor where the structure, process, and outcome of programs are analyzed to determine efficiency, effectiveness, and relevancy. Methods to accomplish this process of evaluation are currently underway.

EDUCATION

The purpose of health education is to share knowledge, increase awareness, and change attitudes and behavior. All health care personnel have the opportunity to participate in teaching but do not always do so. Many attempt it but do not have the understanding or tools to be effective. The federal government defines health education as "not only knowledge transmission but also the range of practices designed to motivate, stimulate, and provide skills to help people live longer, free from disease and disability."[33]

Health care providers (nurses and doctors) begin to acquire a scientific and psychosocial background in their basic education programs. They develop a process of learning which is continuous. Many participate in informal self-learning activities and continuing education programs, but that knowledge base does not necessarily include critical aspects of providing education, that is, the methods and strategies to promote effective learning. The health professional as a teacher needs not only to transmit applied knowledge in terms that the consumer understands, but also facilitates a behavior change. The task of the health educator is to "make it easier to follow healthful practices and less desirable to choose unhealthful behavior."[33]

Areas which need to be further developed or included in educational programs of health care providers are teaching-learning principles, impact of cultural influences, methods of promoting behavior change, and understanding the factors in health behavior practices. With communicable diseases, the aspect of a specific etiology often overshadows the reality of interactive factors involved with disease causation. A more "ecologic" perspective needs to be pursued in the identification of multicausal factors in the occurrence of communicable diseases. In addition, the health professional needs to understand and know how to evaluate the effectiveness of his interventions, including teaching. This is critical. One should have expected outcomes or goals in providing education so that the effect of knowledge acquisition on attitudes and behavior can be evaluated, also the methods and strategies used to reach those goals are evaluated. Health care providers must include information to consumers, keeping in mind their perceptions and values. In addition, since the effect of health education is to effect specific change in behavior, the consumer should have the opportunity to acquire the techniques and skills needed to bring about and maintain that change.[33]

Health consumers should be a part of the education program from the beginning of the planning stages. In this way their needs, interests, and specific characteristics can be included and addressed. This is essential if one desires their support and participation. Settings can be informal or formal, planned or spontaneous, individual or groups. Health education can be incorporated into the curriculum in the school system or offered as special classes. Mass media such as TV, radio, newspaper, community organization networks, and hot lines are all possibilities of reaching the public. Finances may be an issue for some programs. Often local, state, and federal support is available but this varies. If the topic is of current interest and a priority, there is more opportunity for funding. An example is the venereal disease campaign in the last few years. If finances are not available, fundraising activity may be necessary before an education program gets underway.

Communicable diseases impact on all strata of our society. Even with many advances in immunizations and treatments, they continue to be a threat. Through a thorough study of people, cultures, attitudes, values, beliefs, scientific inquiry, and education, the morbidity of the communicable diseases may be reduced as with the mortality rates.

REFERENCES

1. Holprich, Paul D. (ed.): *Infectious Diseases,* 2nd ed. Harper and Row, New York, 1977.
2. Dubos, Rene: *Man Adapting,* 11th ed. Yale University Press, New Haven, 1975.
3. Guyton, Arthur C.: *Textbook of Medical Physiology.* W.B. Saunders Co., Philadelphia, 1976.
4. Mausner, J.S., and Bahn, A.K.: *Epidemiology: An Introductory Text.* W.B. Saunders Co., Philadelphia, 1974.
5. Benenson, Abram S. (ed.): *Control of Communicable Diseases in Man,* 12th ed. American Public Health Association, Washington, 1975.
6. Thomson, Daniel: "The Ebb and Flow of Infection." *JAMA,* 235(3):269, Jan. 19, 1976.
7. Judson, F.N., Miller, K.G., and Schaffnit, T.R.: "Screening for Gonorrhea and Syphilis in the Gay Baths, Denver, Colorado." *American Journal of Public Health,* 67(8):740, Aug. 1977.
8. Braff, E.H., and Wibbelsman, C.J.: "Asymptomatic Gonococcal Urethritis in Selected Males." *American Journal of Public Health,* 68(8):779, Aug. 1978.
9. USDHEW/PHS/Health Resources Administration/National Center for Health Statistics: *Comparability of Mortality Statistics for the 7th and 8th Revisions of the International Classification of Diseases,* U.S. Rockville, Md., Oct. 1975.
10. Anthony, N., Reed, M., Leff, A.M., et al.: "Immunization: Public Health Programming through Law Enforcement." *American Journal of Public Health,* 67(8):763, Aug. 1977.
11. USDHEW/PHS/CDC: *Morbidity and Mortality Weekly Report (MWWR).* 26(5):29, Feb. 4, 1977.
12. "Recombinant DNA Hearing at Harvard, Nine Scientists Disagree." *Boston University Journal,* 24(3):5, 1976.
13. Evans, A.S.: "Infectious Mononucleosis in University of Wisconsin Students." *American Journal of Hygiene,* 71:342, 1960.
14. Sutton, R.N.P., et al: "Aspects of Epstein-Barr Virus Infection in Childhood." *Archives of Disease in Childhood,* 49:102, 1974.
15. Pritchard, J.A., and MacDonald, P.C.: *William's Obstetrics,* 15th ed. Macmillan Publishing Co., New York, 1975.
16. Bell, R.R.: "The Impact of Illness on Family Roles," in Spradley, B.W. (ed.): *Contemporary Community Nursing.* Little, Brown and Co., Boston, 1975.
17. Rapoport, A.: "Modern Systems Theory: An Outlook for Coping with Change." *General Systems,* 15:22, 1970.
18. Mead, George: *Mind, Self, Society.* University of Chicago Press, Chicago, 1934.
19. Stryker, Sheldon: "Symbolic Interaction as an Approach to Family Research." *Marriage and Family Living,* Vol. 21, May 1959, p. 115.
20. Warren, Roland L.: *The Community in America,* 2nd ed. Rand McNally College Publishing, Chicago, 1972.
21. Tinkham, C.W., and Voorhies, E.F.: *Community Health Nursing Evolution and Process,* 2nd ed. Appleton-Century-Crofts, New York, 1977.
22. Lilienfeld, A.M.: *Foundations of Epidemiology.* Oxford University Press, New York, 1976.

23. Top, Franklin H., and Nehrle, Paul F.: *Communicable and Infectious Diseases.* C.V. Mosby Co., St. Louis, 1972.
24. *MMWR.* 26(24):199, June 17, 1977.
25. Becker, Marshall H. (ed.): *The Health Belief Model and Personal Health Behavior.* Charles B. Slack, Inc., Thorofare, N.J., 1974.
26. *Report of the Committee on Infectious Diseases,* 18th ed. American Academy of Pediatrics, Evanston, Ill., 1977.
27. *MMWR.* 26(52):427, Dec. 30, 1977.
28. *MMWR.* 26(43):359, Oct. 28, 1977.
29. Winn, Mary C.: "A Proposed Tuberculosis Treatment Program for Papago Indians," in Brink, P.J. (ed.): *Transcultural Nursing: A Book of Readings.* Prentice-Hall, Englewood Cliffs, N.J., 1976.
30. USDHEW/PHS/CDC: *MMWR Annual Summary 1976.* Atlanta, Georgia, 1976.
31. Marier, Robert: "The Reporting of Communicable Diseases." *American Journal of Epidemiology,* 105(6):587, Jan. 1977.
32. *Infection Control.* National League for Nursing, New York, 1975.
33. Cooper, Theodore: "Present HEW Policies in Primary Prevention." *Preventive Medicine.* 6:200, 1977.
34. *MMWR.* 26 (2):9, Jan. 14; (6):44, Feb. 11; (14):111, April 8; (27):224, July 8; (52):443, Dec. 30, 1977; and 27 (21):176, May 26, 1978.
35. *MMWR.* 26 (14):109, April 8; (21):175, May 27; (29):233, July 22, 1977.

BIBLIOGRAPHY

Donovan, M.I., and Pierce, S.G.: *Cancer Care Nursing.* Appleton-Century-Crofts, New York, 1976.
Graham, Saxon: "The Sociological Approach to Epidemiology." *American Journal of Public Health,* 64:1046, Nov. 1974.
Katz, S.H., and Wallace, A.F.C.: "An Anthropological Perspective on Behavior and Disease." *American Journal of Public Health,* 64:1050, Nov. 1974.
McInnes, Mary Elizabeth: *Essentials of Communicable Disease,* 2nd ed. C.V. Mosby, St. Louis, 1975.
Milio, Nancy: *The Care of Health in Communities Access for Outcasts.* Macmillan Publishing Co., New York, 1975.
Wardwill, Walter I.: "Population Density and Mobility." *American Journal of Public Health,* 64(11): 1052, 1974.
U.S. Bureau of Census: *Statistical Abstract of the U.S., 1972.* Government Printing Office, Washington, D.C., 1972.
USDHEW/PHS/CDC: *Morbidity and Mortality Weekly Report.* Atlanta, Georgia, Jan. 1976–April 1978.
USDHEW/PHS/CDC: *Health Information for International Travel 1977.* Atlanta, Georgia, 1977.
USDHEW/PHS/CDC/Bureau of State Services: *U.S. Immunization Survey, 1974.* Atlanta, Georgia, April 1975.

25
CHRONIC OBSTRUCTIVE LUNG DISEASE

SUE DRISCOLL, M.S., R.N.

   Chronic obstructive pulmonary disease has become a major health care problem interrupting personal and family goals. The care of individuals with chronic obstructive lung disease necessitates a multidisciplinary approach. Coordination of acute hospital care with home health care planning is critical to effective patient management. The focus of this discussion is directed toward exploring the elements of maintaining effective home health care.

Chronic obstructive lung disease is defined by the American Thoracic Society as diseases of uncertain etiology characterized by a persistent slowing of airflow during forced expiration.[1] Most commonly, disorders included in this definition are chronic obstructive bronchitis and chronic obstructive pulmonary emphysema. When the specific disease entity cannot be isolated as chronic bronchitis or emphysema or if the disorder is a combination of both, then the term chronic obstructive lung disease or COLD is utilized. Chronic obstructive pulmonary disease or COPD is a synonymous term for COLD. The term COLD will be used throughout the remainder of this discussion.

Asthma is also included in pulmonary disease states characterized by obstruction to the flow of air. Asthma is simply defined as an increased airway response with concomitant narrowing of the internal diameter of the airways.[1] This reaction by the airways is in response to various specific external or internal stimuli. The clinical picture is often manifested by wheezing with the respiratory effort, edema of the airways, inflammation of the airways, increased mucus production, and cough. Asthma can be well controlled by the judicious use of desensitization of environment, allergy shots, and thorough patient education. The airway obstruction noted in the patient with asthma is often reversible with continuous use of bronchodilating drugs and careful use of steroids. Thus the individual can have complete or almost complete remission of symptoms between attacks with appropriate medical management.

Other disorders commonly discussed in the category of chronic obstructive lung diseases include bronchiectasis and cystic fibrosis. Cystic fibrosis or mucoviscidosis is not a primary obstructive lung disorder. Rather it is an inherited disease of the exocrine glands. Cystic fibrosis affects primarily the sweat glands, respiratory system, and digestive system. One system may be more acutely involved in one person than in another person.

One of the earliest changes in the lung is a dilatation and hypertrophy of the bronchial glands with an increase in mucus production. Subsequent to this change, mucus plugging of peripheral airways with obstruction of the airways, chronic respiratory infections, and tissue damage to the lung structure results. This process continues with increasing loss of lung function and culminates in death. The diagnosis is usually made in early childhood. Until recent years the average age of death was 12 years old.[2] Presently, individuals can live well into young adulthood and beyond with careful medical management.

Development of bronchiectasis can be a complication of cystic fibrosis. Bronchiectasis is simply defined as an abnormal dilatation of the airways secondary to inflammation and ulceration.[3] These dilated portions of the airways collect large amounts of mucus that must be expectorated. The development of bronchiectasis is often associated with recurrent and severe respiratory infections such as pneumonia. The clinical picture is one of coughing large amounts of thick purulent sputum especially in the early morning. The treatment is directed toward control of superimposed respiratory infections and a continuous program of measures to promote clearance of secretions from the airways.

The scope of this discussion is limited to exploration of the health care management of COLD including chronic bronchitis and emphysema. Specifically included will be coverage of populations at risk, contributing pathophysiology as it relates to modalities of care, survey of disease management including education and research, and the role of the community health nurse in prevention and treatment. The emphasis is directed toward promotion of the development and maintenance of home health care programs. The reader is advised to review anatomy and physiology of the lungs for a clearer understanding of concepts of basic pathophysiology of COLD.

PREVALENCE AND PREDISPOSITION

Specific epidemiologic data regarding both chronic and acute respiratory illness are continually being collected. Correlation of the information is at best two to five years behind in some areas due to the complexity and scope of data being collected. The Social Security Administration's current economic figures show the cost of COLD is continuing to rise sharply. Figure 25-1 shows the rise in paid benefits. Disability benefits paid to individuals and their dependents for the calendar year 1977 reached a record $750 million. Benefits paid to the individual were a staggering $625 million in 1977.[4] This compares to $100 million paid in Social Security Disability Benefits for respiratory disease in 1966 and an estimated $400 million paid in 1970.[5] These figures are related to chronic disorders excluding neoplasms (carcinoma) of the lung.

There are an estimated 185,000 to 200,000 individuals with chronic obstructive respira-

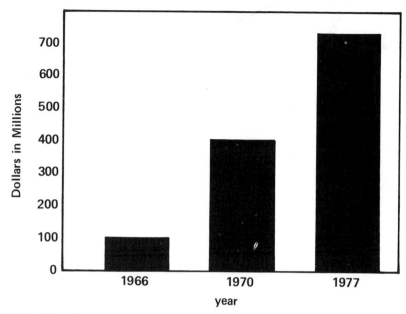

FIGURE 25-1. Social Security disability benefits paid. The increased cost related to COLD benefits presents a formidable economic burden to all. The role of inflation cannot be discounted when looking at these figures.

tory diseases on the Social Security Disability roles.[4] Chronic respiratory illness ranks sixth nationally as a disabling disease.[4] A National Health Survey conducted in 1970 by the Public Health Service estimated that almost 8 million persons were diagnosed with emphysema or chronic bronchitis and that an additional 6 million persons were diagnosed with asthma. Thus almost 14 million known Americans were affected by one of these three chronic respiratory conditions at that time. In other words, 3 percent of the U.S. population was diagnosed with a form of chronic lung disease. No doubt the figure has risen over the past 10 years and there is speculation that the increase will continue.

The economic and human loss figures are equally impressive. The National Center for Health Statistics of the Public Health Service estimated that in 1976 there were 4,490 deaths attributed to chronic bronchitis which figured to 2.1 per 100,000 population. Emphysema was attributed to 17,550 deaths or 8.2 deaths per 100,000 population. The term chronic obstructive lung disease has become more widely used since 1976 and has documented 21,472 deaths or 10 persons per 100,000 population. Thus over 43,000 persons died in 1976 as a result of chronic bronchitis, emphysema, or a combination of these disorders—COLD.[5]

Further investigation of these figures noted that approximately three-fourths of these individuals were white males. The age groups were divided into those persons under 45 years of age and those persons 45 and over. The 1976 figures showed that over 5500 males between the ages of 35 and 64 died, representing an estimated economic loss in earnings of almost $376 million. This compared to over 300 women who died with an estimated $24 1/2 million economic loss. Nonwhite males and females were also extrapolated from the total. Included in the figures were 2361 nonwhite males and 116 nonwhite females. This represented an estimated economic loss of over $38 million and

$3 million respectively. The loss of human resources due to a chronic debilitating disease has a negative impact on the gross national product. The decrease in output is coupled with an added increase in the total economic burden through usage of national, state, and local financial support networks.

Investigations have been conducted in an attempt to identify those persons with a predisposition to development of chronic respiratory disease. Two examples follow which were reported in the American Review of Respiratory Disease. In the first study by Higgins, Keller, and Metzner,[6] smoking, sex, social and economic status, as well as educational levels were investigated as contributing factors in the incidence of chronic respiratory disease. In a town in Michigan, 4699 men and women between 25 and 64 years of age were surveyed. Previous studies quoted had indicated that there was a higher prevalence of lung disease among laborers and semiskilled workers as compared to workers at other occupational levels. Other conclusions made are subsequently noted. Such information is useful as an indicator of higher risk populations. In addition, such findings may be beneficial in patient history taking and evaluation of the patient and family environment. The incidence of COLD was noted to be higher among lower socioeconomic groups. The overall prevalence of chronic bronchitis was found to be decreased among white collar workers as opposed to blue collar or agricultural workers whether they smoked or did not smoke. Cigarette smoking was related to a higher incidence of chronic bronchitis. This finding was more prevalent in those who smoked one or more packages of cigarettes per day. The principal conclusion when looking at all levels of smoking habits combined was that the incidence of chronic bronchitis was lower among college educated men. Among women, those with the least education had the highest prevalence of chronic bronchitis and the greatest change in lung function regardless of smoking habits.[6]

The prevalence of chronic bronchitis was essentially unrelated to the level of income when smoking habits were not incorporated. In general, the mean lung function was found to be best in those men in high income brackets and least in men rated in the lower income brackets regardless of smoking habits. No associations could be quantitatively stated between income and prevalence of chronic bronchitis.

There does seem, however, to be a relationship between employment associated with high density dusts, metals, and synthetic fiber occupations and the incidence of lung disease. Two possible correlations are of interest. 1) Cigarette smoking is more prevalent in poor socioeconomic circumstances. 2) Blue collar workers are most often employed in working conditions associated with chronic respiratory irritation. The combination of personal pollution (smoking) and occupational exposure may be a factor in the development of respiratory dysfunction. The reader must keep in mind that while these conclusions are of interest they should be used to generate further study. Replication of research adds reliability and validity to the findings.

In the second study by Lieberman, Gaidulis, and Roberts,[7] race as it related to genetic predisposition to COLD was explored. The study surveyed 1841 seventh grade students. A genetic factor (alpha$_1$-antitrypsin) found in the blood and known to predispose to an early onset of emphysema was tested. Blood samples were drawn from each student participant. A deficiency of the enzyme alpha$_1$-antitrypsin was found in 3 percent of the white subjects as opposed to 0 percent of the nonwhite subjects.

Further studies conducted to identify specific populations at risk would be helpful to health care personnel in counseling as well as for prevention or retardation of the progression of COLD. For example, in a health maintenance clinic white males with an identified genetic predisposition to emphysema would be advised not to smoke nor seek employment in job settings considered to be a high pulmonary risk.

In summary, the prevalence of COLD is found more frequently among white males. Smoking and job environment are related predisposing factors. Women continue to be less likely to develop lung disease. However, this trend is changing with more women smoking and more women entering the labor force at all levels. There is no question that chronic lung dysfunction presents an economic burden to the individual, the family, the community, and the country as a whole. Further study is certainly necessary to provide valuable data to health care personnel toward prevention and treatment of the spectrum of chronic respiratory disease.

ETIOLOGIC FACTORS

Knowledge of various factors having a precipitating influence on the development of chronic lung dysfunction is beneficial in working toward health care prevention and maintenance. Longitudinal survey studies and well controlled physiologic research studies have isolated certain predisposing factors contributing to the development and/or progression of the COLD. The first of these, cigarette smoking, unquestionably contributes to both the incidence and progression of chronic respiratory dysfunction. The Advisory Committee of the Surgeon General's office compiled a massive volume of data and in a 1964 report indicated that cigarette smoking was indeed linked to the development of acute and chronic lung dysfunction.[8] Following that report all cigarette manufacturers were required to place the following statement on each package of cigarettes: "Warning: The Surgeon General Has Determined That Cigarette Smoking Is Dangerous to Your Health." Several years following this report there was a noted decline in the number of cigarettes consumed. A ban on cigarette advertising on national television (although cigars and tobacco advertising are still allowed) was enacted. In recent years, however, a rise in cigarette consumption has been noted among women and teenagers. Specific reasons are speculative and involve discussion of complex and changing social mores.

The effects of second-hand smoke (nonsmokers exposed to a smoking environment) have also been documented. One known component of cigarette smoke is carbon monoxide. With smoke inhalation the carbon monoxide combines more quickly than oxygen with hemoglobin in the blood forming carboxyhemoglobin. This combination reduces the amount of available oxygen to the tissues. Sufficient amounts of carboxyhemoglobin act in effect to suffocate the cells. Clinically, the carboxyhemoglobin blood levels of non-smokers exposed to a nonventilated smoking environment rise significantly. Nonsmokers can thus have similar health "benefits" heretofore attributed only to the person who smokes.

A recent educational pamphlet by the American Cancer Society notes that women who smoke while pregnant have a higher incidence of spontaneous abortion. Their babies also tend to have lower birth weights than babies born to mothers who do not smoke. Cigarette smoke in the mother's bloodstream alters the heart rate and blood pressure and affects the oxygen supply as well as the acid-base balance of the unborn infant.

Reasons people continue to smoke are varied. "My mother had emphysema and she never smoked." "I had an uncle who smoked, and he lived to be 90." "You've got to die of something." "I'll gain weight." "It calms my nerves." "Everyone else in my group smokes." "My parents smoke." "My doctor smokes." "It's too late. I already have emphysema."

Health care personnel at every level need to assume an active role in health education as well as support and promote prudent health care legislation. Smoking habits of health care professionals must also be investigated and evaluated. These individuals are often utilized by the public as role models for follow through in health care maintenance.

Proper public health education must be directed toward exposing rationalizations for what they are—excuses. The reasons some people develop lung disease and others do not is presently not well understood. It is known that smoking tends to potentiate the development and increase the severity of symptoms which in turn accelerates resultant functional disability of the lungs.

While it is certainly true that everyone must die of something, the prospect of living many years with a severe debilitating disease is a sobering thought. The effects on the individual and his family are a heavy burden to carry. One could also say that in Russian roulette there is only one chance in six of getting the bullet. The thought processes seem to be on similar levels.

Weight gain is not an automatic consequence of smoking cessation. There is no specific physiologic connection presently identified. Personal eating habits and need for oral gratification may be more plausible reasons. Dietary counseling may be necessary as a supportive measure to the exsmoker. A variety of activities which give the mind and the body alternative activities is beneficial. Exercise helps depress appetite and should be encouraged. Verbal reward and encouragement are also helpful in assisting the individual through those first few days after smoking cessation. Family support and understanding including no smoking in the house as well as temporary avoidance of high smoke density places is beneficial. It is not unusual for the individual to be more jittery, pace, and consume many packages of gum.

Physiologically, smoking does not calm nerves. Psychologically the individual may believe this to be a fact. A biofeedback educational program sponsored by one state lung association demonstrates this fact to teenagers throughout schools within the state. One test has the student place the lead of a pencil into a small hole. If the sides of the hole are touched a buzzer rings. The student then smokes a cigarette and attempts the same maneuver. The results demonstrate that after one cigarette the steadiness of the hand in deliberate sensitive maneuvers is less (the buzzer sounds), and the point is graphically made.

The social pressure of initiating smoking habits is a prime factor in influencing the beginning smoker. Friends are a big influence as well as parents. Among teenagers who smoke, a high percentage of their parents also smoke. Girls tend to follow their mothers' smoking habits more than that of the father. The sharpest increase in smoking seems to be among teenagers in general and girls specifically.[9] The need to feel accepted socially, peer pressure, and the association of smoking with adulthood are identified reasons for smoking. Support through preventive educational programs initiated by the students themselves is being encouraged and supported by state lung associations and the American Cancer Society around the country. Younsters are also beginning to have an effect on decreasing parental smoking habits.

Benefits are noted if a person does quit smoking regardless of whether chronic lung disease is present. The most immediate benefit is often a cessation of chronic intermittent cough and a reduction in sputum production. The risk of developing lung neoplasms (cancer) is decreased. There is an improvement in the lung's defense mechanisms toward prevention of infection and removal of foreign debris from the bronchial airways. This factor helps reduce potential for upper respiratory infection which often causes loss of work days. Many people actually are able to admit that they generally feel better and have more physical energy after smoking cessation.

The long term chronic effects of cigarette smoking may take 20 or more years to develop into a specific clinical consequence such as chronic bronchitis and/or emphysema. The following physiologic reactions are noted after smoking one cigarette: increase in heart rate, increase in systolic blood pressure, interference with the oxygen-carbon dioxide exchange in the lung, increase in airway irritation, paralysis of the ciliary clearance mechanism which assists in removal of bacteria and debris from the airways, and constriction of peripheral capillary blood flow reducing skin temperature of extremities.

Legislative action to reduce smoking in public places as well as efforts by national organizations and community sponsored groups are making strides toward changing social attitudes regarding smoking habits. A myriad of written literature is available for public distribution as well as various audiovisual materials and community hospital sponsored quit smoking clinics. These efforts have not gone unnoticed as 30 million people have quit smoking.

Besides being affected by the personal pollution of smoking, the lung is also affected by air pollution from other sources. Identified sources such as emissions from automobile exhausts and industrial pollution from smokestacks emitting sulphur dioxide in combination with other compounds into the air produce what is commonly referred to as air pollution. Government, state, and local agencies are looking at measures to decrease air pollution. California, for example, is one state with very stiff automobile emission laws. Heavily industrialized cities and states are enacting legislation dictating the amount of toxic emissions allowed from industrial smokestacks. It is not uncommon for certain large industrialized cities to broadcast warnings to citizens with respiratory diseases to stay indoors on identified high ozone days to prevent further respiratory compromise. Ozone is a combination of various air pollutants which occurs often in highly industrialized and populated cities.

There are numerable chemically identified air pollutants. The two most widely known are carbon monoxide and a group known as sulphur oxides. Two sources from which carbon monoxide is emitted are auto exhausts and cigarettes. Carbon monoxide has approximately 200 times the affinity for the hemoglobin molecule as does oxygen. The rate of diffusion of oxygen from the gas exchange units into the blood is thus decreased. Consequently the oxygen tension in the blood and the availability of oxygen for tissue use is lessened. A high density automobile city which also experiences a stagnation of air on a given hot day often produces minor respiratory irritations in healthy individuals. This same situation could send a person with COLD to the hospital with severe compromise of respiratory function.

Air pollution from various sources can increase mortality specifically with respect to the elderly and those with a chronic form of cardiopulmonary dysfunction. The role of air pollution in aggravating the symptoms of those with chronic respiratory disease is established, but its effect as a cause of emphysema and/or chronic bronchitis is not as clear. On the basis of epidemiologic work completed outside the United States such an effect is highly suspect.

Occupational air pollution from various industrial sources exposes a certain portion of an estimated 80 million workers to constant and potentially harmful dusts, particles, and/or fumes. A detailed occupational history is a part of pulmonary evaluation. For example, in recent years asbestos has received much publicity as a carcinogenic agent while coal worker's disease has long been a known occupational lung disorder. Some persons who develop lung disorders secondary to coal dust deposition in the airways of the lung also develop emphysema. This seems to be a more common occurrence in those workers who also smoke.

Chronic obstructive airway disorders other than COLD most commonly associated with occupational exposure are allergic forms of chronic bronchitis and occupational asthma. The diagnosis is most often suspect after a detailed occupational history. For example, chest tightness and/or coughing attacks may have a temporal relationship to work exposure. The absence of such attacks during days off and vacation periods is usually found. Various dusts and/or chemical fumes can also mediate lung dysfunction of an acute and/or chronic nature. Once the diagnosis is established, avoidance of the causative irritant is necessary.

Studies have not conclusively demonstrated that chronic obstructive lung disease is caused by any specific occupational exposure. In descriptive research studies variables such as smoking habits and general environmental exposure are difficult to control. Therefore, the resulting lung dysfunction is believed to be mediated by a number of interrelated factors. The most often associated disorders with occupational exposure are acute episodes of pneumonia, changes in chest x-rays indicative of various scars from past lung insults, and transient mild respiratory symptoms (running of eyes and nose, cough, and transient fever).[10]

Certain allergic responses which may be closely associated with asthmatic symptoms may be able to be controlled well by medication. Vocational rehabilitation may be necessary as part of the treatment regimen. The object is to decrease exposure to respiratory irritants and arrest deteriorating lung function. Federal, state, and local governmental agencies are very concerned about health and safety in job settings. The government agency known as OSHA (Occupational Safety and Health Administration) is responsible for finding hazards, setting standards, and enforcing regulations.

Normal alterations in the environment such as temperature and humidity can also contribute to increased symptomatology. It is not uncommon for those individuals with COLD to be more short of breath or have increased symptomatology on hot humid days or cold windy days. Avoidance of weather extremes can be helped with "weather" counseling. For example, the use of air conditioning in the summer is advised. A mask over the nose and mouth when outside on cold days is beneficial. Dryness of winter air can cause an increase in cough and a drying of mucous membranes. Increased dryness can cause difficulty in expectoration of mucus. Use of added humidity is helpful to keep secretions more liquified and less tenacious.

The final etiologic factor to be discussed is genetic predisposition to lung disease. In recent years it has been discovered that an inherited deficiency of an enzyme inhibitor alpha$_1$-antitrypsin increased the likelihood of rapidly progressive emphysematous changes in young adults.[11] Further research is being conducted in the area of enzyme deficiency as well as excess concentrations of certain enzyme groups and their resultant effects on lung structure and function. The answers to the role of various naturally occurring enzymes and the development of lung disease may hold keys for the improving diagnostic and treatment measures in the future.

A detailed familial history is necessary to help in the diagnostic process relative to those individuals who have greater potential for the development of chronic lung disorders. A detailed personal history assists in guidance and counseling in areas such as vocational interests and appropriate job placement. Genetic counseling can also be of assistance in the care of two individuals who each carry the chromosomal predisposition for chronic lung disease. For example, genetic counseling is usual for parents who have a child with cystic fibrosis.

In summary, contributing factors in the development of chronic respiratory disorders are multifocal. The most commonly recognized factor is long term use of cigarettes. Certainly external environmental as well as occupational exposure to irritating compounds have a fluctuating contributory role. Inherited traits are yet to be fully explored, but familial tendency does seem pertinent in development and progression of certain chronic respiratory diseases.

Increasing consumer awareness through health education by national as well as local community sponsored programs has a distinct function in both prevention and treatment of respiratory disorders. Generating political activism by an informed and concerned society is needed to help develop reasonable and prudent health care legislation.

PATHOPHYSIOLOGY

A basic foundation incorporated into the treatment program of all individuals with chronic lung disease is an understanding of how the lung functions as well as an explanation of what is wrong with the lungs. An in-depth analysis of the alterations in structure and function of diseased lungs is beyond the limits of this discussion. A comparison and contrast of dysfunction in chronic bronchitis and emphysema is presented.

Certain commonalities exist between chronic bronchitis and emphysema. This is especially true in the late stages of both diseases. Both have an insidious onset. The alterations in pulmonary structure and function are present long before clinical symptoms are apparent. The major functional abnormality of both chronic bronchitis and emphysema exists in the peripheral small airways which ordinarily contribute little resistance' to the flow of air into the normal lung. Considerable disease must be present in these small airways before airway resistance becomes subjectively perceived by the victim. Many individuals who develop either chronic bronchitis or emphysema are or have been one or more pack per day cigarette smokers for more than 20 years. Excessive mucus in the airways is not an uncommon finding in both diseases. The individual with a primary diagnosis of emphysema may not be as aware of this mucus and therefore not perceive mucus production as an integral aspect of his problems. Lung structure is illustrated in Figure 25-2.

With advanced disease the coexistence of chronic bronchitis and emphysema (COLD) is a more common occurrence. Research into both of these disorders encompasses both the search for accurate testing measures of lung function and dysfunction as well as investigation into specific factors mediating the onset of small airways disease. In the transition between health and chronic bronchitis and emphysema, it is believed there is a stage where substantial obstruction in the peripheral airways exists with little or no influence on lung function.[12] Investigators are looking at populations of cigarette smokers and conducting various tests related to lung function. The hope is to be able to diagnose beginning phases of dysfunction through specified pulmonary function studies.

Current thinking is that cessation of smoking may reverse the beginning stages of small airway obstruction. If this proves true then it may be valuable to routinely incorporate testing of pulmonary function in the physician's office. Subsequent health care interventions interrupting the sequence of events toward end-stage chronic bronchitis and

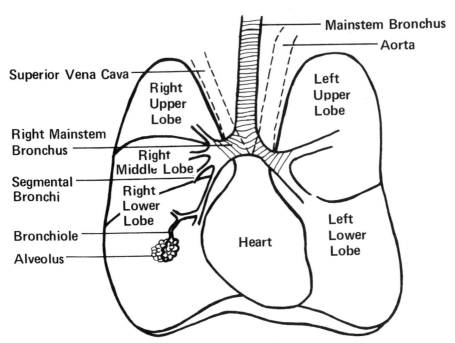

FIGURE 25-2. The lungs consist of right and left sides. The right lung is divided into the upper, middle, and lower lobes. The left lung is divided into the upper and lower lobe. The conducting airways leading to the gas exchange units (alveoli) become progressively smaller in diameter (less than 2 mm in internal diameter). The mainstem bronchus divides into the right and left mainstem bronchus. These bronchi further divide into the upper, middle, and lower segmental bronchi. This subdivision continues to the point at which the blood capillary interfaces with the surface of the alveolus where the actual gas exchange is completed.

emphysema (COLD) may then be possible. Presently, conclusive evidence is not available regarding early detection measures and long term followup studies are still necessary.

At present then, diagnosis and treatment begins when the patient enters the health care network. The individual most commonly presents to his physician with unexplained shortness of breath and/or a persistent cough with or without mucus production. Treatment begins with accurate data collection by medical history and by accurate assessment of presenting symptomatology. Tests of pulmonary function, arterial blood gas analysis (oxygen, pH, and carbon dioxide), chest x-rays, electrocardiogram, and physical exam are also routinely utilized.

In contrast to pulmonary emphysema, chronic bronchitis is an airway disease involving the peripheral bronchioles to a greater extent than the alveolus itself. The extent of lung involvement dictates to some degree the presenting symptomatology. There is usually an associated chronic cough as well as chronic sputum production. Structurally there is an increase in size of the tracheobronchial mucous glands which line airways at the level of the terminal bronchiole. These glands which line the bronchial wall secrete most of the mucus. Individuals with chronic bronchitis tend to have excess mucus in their peripheral airways. The overall internal diameter of the airway is also narrowed as a result of inflammation. Since peripheral airways less than 2 mm in internal diameter contribute little to overall resistance to airflow, the most significant area of increased airway resistance most likely occurs at the level of what are known as segmental bronchi. At the segmental bronchial level, the total cross-sectional area of the airways is at its smallest, and mucous glands contribute a high proportion of the lining of the bronchial wall. Increased mucous gland size (hypertrophy) and increases in the number of mucous gland cells (hyperplasia) contribute to the increased resistance to airflow.

The presence of airway edema, inflammation, and mucous gland cellular (goblet cell) alteration (metaplasia) can be anticipated in chronic bronchitis. However, the generalization of these findings to all individuals with chronic bronchitis is not possible. Each individual must be treated according to his or her symptoms and the physician's clinical findings. Generally, treatment is directed toward optimal bronchodilatation, control of secretions, prevention and control of superseding infections, maintenance of physical exercise, proper diet, and prevention of heart failure which is a late complication of long standing chronic bronchitis. The role of the nurse is integral in this program as will be discussed in the next section.

Pulmonary emphysema is a result of alteration of the structural units of the lung. Specifically, the structure involved is the acinus. This is the unit structure of the lung when gas exchanges (oxygen for carbon dioxide) take place. The structure of the acinus is presented in Figure 25-3. Emphysema is a permanent, abnormal enlargement of any portion of the acinus, with accompanying destruction of the integrity of this structure.[13] While there are several types of emphysema which have been identified, the important concept to keep in mind for this discussion is the general mechanism by which emphysema affects lung mechanics.

Loss of elastic recoil is the primary functional abnormality in emphysema.[13] Simply stated elastic recoil is the normal tendency of the lungs to try to collapse to their resting state (expiratory phase) after an inspiratory effort. The chest wall (thorax) has a natural tendency to want to spring outward. These two forces are held in apposition in the intrapleural space as shown in Figure 25-4. Inspiration is an active process using muscular effort supplied by the diaphragm and to a lesser extent intercostal muscles of the thorax. Expiration is normally a passive process involving the elastic recoil of the lung. With the loss of elastic recoil, the inward retractive force of the lung is diminished and a state of chronic lung hyperinflation exists. This is often referred to clinically as barrel chest. Barrel chest, however, also includes skeletal abnormalities of the thorax. The more correct term is hyperinflation of the chest.

Airway size is also affected by loss of recoil. Dimension of airways is determined to a great extent by the recoil pressure applied to them. Consequently, at a given volume of inspired atmospheric gas, the airways in an emphysematous lung are already narrower than in a normal lung, thus the total resistance to the flow of air is greater. Clinically, then, the ability of a person to expel the air he or she inspires is decreased and air tends to be "trapped" in the bronchi. The term "flabby airways" is sometimes used to describe this loss of airway function. Alterations in the flow of air affect the distribution of gas to the various lung compartments or lobes. The destruction of portions of the acinus results in a loss of portions of the surrounding vascular bed. This capillary bed is the systemic contact for oxygen pick-up from the alveoli and carbon dioxide transfer from the red blood cells into the alveoli. Emphysema can also be diagnosed in part by testing the effectiveness of diffusion of gases from alveoli into the blood. Diffusion is the process by which oxygen moves from the alveoli into the capillary and carbon dioxide moves from the capillary into the alveoli. Decreased diffusion capacities are more common in emphysema than in mild cases of chronic bronchitis.

The patient with a higher proportion of emphysematous changes often presents to the

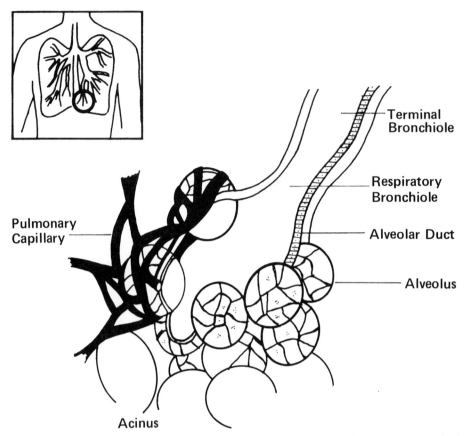

FIGURE 25-3. The acinus is the portion of the airway peripheral to the terminal bronchiole. It resembles a grapelike structure. The acinus is the actual gas exchange portion of the lung. Within this structure are three succeeding orders of respiratory bronchioles which become more impregnated with alveoli. The alveoli are the saclike air cells clustered within the alveolar duct. The pulmonary capillaries cover the alveolar surface. Gas exchange occurs by diffusion of gas from the alveoli into the capillary blood and vice versa.

physician with a complaint of dyspnea associated with mild to moderate activity. Treatment is directed toward improvement of gas exchange by use of breathing retraining, breathing and physical exercises, and in late stages low flow chronic home oxygen therapy (prescribed when the arterial oxygen saturation and partial pressure are insufficient to meet systemic demands).[14,15] Adequate oxygenation is essential to reduce myocardial work and to meet basal metabolic tissue needs. Prevention of infection and physical therapy measures are utilized to improve the efficiency of the process of respiration. Bronchodilators are also given a trial use to see if there is a bronchodilating response and thus a reversible component of obstruction.

While it is helpful in increasing understanding to be able to identify distinguishing characteristics as well as to understand functional disparities, the clinical distinction between these two disease processes is not always clear. Many patients have features of both disorders and are thus diagnosed with COLD.

To summarize then, two common forms of chronic obstructive airway disease are

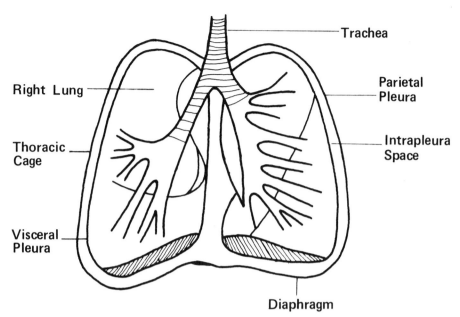

FIGURE 25-4. The natural tendency for the lungs to collapse and the chest cage to spring outward is opposed by a thin fluid lining between the surface of the lung (visceral pleura) and the inner lining of the chest wall (parietal pleura). The fluid lining in this potential intrapleural space functions to maintain the integrity between the two surfaces and to provide lubrication for the expansion and contraction of the lungs.

chronic bronchitis and pulmonary emphysema. The first is defined in functional terms with chronic sputum production. The second is defined anatomically as a varying degree of destruction of select portions of lung structure. Due to the fact that the major functional abnormality in both disorders occurs in the smaller airways, considerable dysfunction must exist before actual airway resistance is subjectively perceived. The clinical picture may vary somewhat from individual to individual, but treatment is directed toward early detection measures, maximal dilatation of the airways, improvement in the gas exchange process, effective secretion clearance, prevention of infections, removal of known airway irritants, psychological support measures, improved patient knowledge of disease process, prevention and/or retardation of the progression of lung dysfunction. The role of various health care professionals is integral in this endeavor.

NURSING INTERVENTION

The intensive need for consistent outpatient followup is difficult for the physician alone to provide. The management of chronic lung disease is time consuming and can be fraught with frustration. A shared responsibility by the physician with other members of the health care team (nurses, physical and respiratory therapists, and social service) ensures earlier recognition of patient deterioration. The development of home health care rehabilitation programs and utilization of all health care personnel in providing maintenance therapy is essential.

Chronic obstructive lung disease is a family treated disorder. The presence of a chronic disorder interrupts one's goals and life ambitions. This factor alone presents a formidable challenge with which to cope. Added to this is the financial burden placed on the individual and the family. If the victim is in the peak wage earning years, his job may be in jeopardy. The need for the spouse to work in order to augment income may become necessary. The ability to send the youngsters to college, to pay off the mortgage, and to have a "nest egg" for retirement are all affected by a chronic debilitating disease. Consistent interface with the health care system is essential to help the patient and family meet changing needs.

For some individuals insurance coverage benefits may be dropped or decreased after a specified number of hospitalizations in one calendar year. Participation in ongoing rehabilitation programs has been demonstrated to reduce the number of hospitalizations in both the Petty and Burrows studies.[16] Medicare usually covers 80 percent or more of approved outpatient costs. A list of these approved costs is available through state offices of health and social services. In certain instances patients with insufficient funds may also have to explore their eligibility for medical assistance. Many states are now trying to lobby for both federal and private insurance coverage for services of nurse practitioners as well as more complete coverage of community health nursing care services. Strides are being made but must continue to be supported both at a national and local level.

Maintenance of employment and to a lesser extent vocational rehabilitation is part of a total treatment program. Successful job retention is related to the energy expenditure necessary in performance of the job, the individual's level of exercise tolerance, and the ease with which the individual can change jobs within the company. Working with employers to increase their understanding of the employee's capabilities can be assistive in promoting job retention. Avoidance of stigmas attached to chronic disease is a part of the counseling process. Employers are sometimes reluctant to hire a person with a known chronic disease. The concerns range from excess use of sick leave to social reactions to coughing, sputum expectoration, and watching someone with obvious breathing difficulties. Employers in the local community can be a positive resource in assisting the individual toward a more productive life-style. Appropriateness of job placement, individual skills, and internal motivation toward productivity are essential.

The loss of personal motivation and a feeling of hopelessness expressed by those with COLD is an ever present barrier to both the patient and family in any rehabilitation program. Most individuals equate chronic lung disease with a progressive downhill course. Indeed they can see and feel the change in their activity tolerance and sense of well being.

The psychological effects of COLD are varied and complex. There may be some feeling of being punished for smoking all those years. Faced with the prospect of a decreasing ability to perform in a variety of social roles, the individual resorts to coping mechanisms such as withdrawal, denial, or anger. Helping the individual to adjust to the possibility of role reversal in the family is difficult. The further prospect of not being able to function in the accepted sexual role of husband or wife is also an area which needs to be addressed. The assistance of other members of the health care team may be indicated. Family therapy can be beneficial. Support and guidance by the nurse is helpful as the individual moves through changes in his self-concept and perceived relationship changes within the family.

Physical Measures of Rehabilitation

Physical rehabilitation is more successful with active participation by the family as well as the patient. Goals cannot and should not be made for the patient and family. The internal motivation coupled with external motivation factors is directly related to perceived control over one's self-care program. The nurse can provide positive reinforcement, make suggestions, assist in problem solving, and help find necessary resources, but the responsibility for care lies primarily with the patient and his family.

Maintenance of physical capability is very important. Suitable leisure time pursuits within the person's capability are to be encouraged. Helping the individual find acceptable alternative choices can contribute to retention of a positive self-image as well as functional capability. Fishing is usually a sport which can be maintained even if supplemental oxygen therapy becomes necessary. Various hobby crafts are often taken up by both men and women. A person who feels he has some measure of control over his condition and believes he has choices to make tends to be more positively oriented.

Home health care evaluation is essential in helping the patient and family make necessary adjustments in their daily living patterns. Increasing difficulty in completion of personal hygiene is not unusual. Showering with the bathroom door closed may give a sense of suffocation or exacerbate coughing as the environment becomes more steamy. Energy expenditure in taking tub baths may promote its postponement. Assistance in bathing by a family member may eventually be necessary. Shaving and brushing the teeth may also become increasingly energy consuming. Pacing of such activities with periods of rest helps.

Dressing to comfort with an emphasis on loose clothing and avoidance of tight belts which restrict diaphragmatic movement and thus chest expansion is advised. Bending over to tie shoes may also induce shortness of breath. Slip on shoes may be more advisable. Counseling on spacing activities with periods of rest helps conserve personal energy.

Meal times can be exasperating for both husband and wife. Typically if the husband has COLD his wife tries to prepare all "his" favorite foods to encourage eating. The very process of eating becomes fatiguing. In such instances it may be more advisable 'to prepare five small meals daily as opposed to three large meals. Facing a plateful of food can be psychologically overwhelming. Foods that are easier to chew and digest also facilitate eating. Resting for an hour or so after meals aids in the digestive process. Persons with COLD may present undernourished in appearance or in an overweight status. Excess weight can be a problem. Extra pounds increase cardiovascular workload, affect breathing patterns, and act to restrict diaphragmatic movement. An overweight condition contributes to decreased activity patterns.

Exercise is an important component of the rehabilitation program. Various physical exercise regimens have been utilized over the years. The emphasis of these exercises has been to strengthen abdominal muscles by various knee-chest maneuvers and modified abdominal resistance exercises (i.e., placing a book on the abdomen while breathing). Patient compliance for these exercises is not necessarily consistent. Many people do not enjoy routine exercising. Creative alternative patterns need to be explored. For example, use of a swimming pool facility. The water helps buoy the person up while practicing arm and leg exercise at various levels of perceived strain.

Promoting mobility with selected activities requiring use of different muscle groups attains the objective of building and/or maintaining strength and flexibility. A patient's exercise tolerance can be measured by use of a sophisticated exercise stress test which measures oxygen consumption against oxygen availability as well as the ability of the cardiopulmonary system to respond to increased oxygen demands and increased physical strain. In the home setting the patient can be taught to monitor his pulse rate with activity. The resting pulse is counted. A specified activity is completed. The pulse rate is taken immediately after the activity and at prescribed intervals until resting pulse is again attained. The patient keeps a record of his perceived cardiopulmonary stress during exercise as well as changes in pulse rate and breathing pattern. Periodic followup evaluation can be completed in the physical therapy outpatient department and recommendations for exercise modifications made. Walking, golf, light housework, fishing, and swimming are examples of varying energy consuming activities. Capabilities vary from individual to individual. Eventually, however, for some ambulation from the bed to the easy chair may be fatiguing. At this point the patient must carefully set priorities in selecting his activities based on available energy and the energy expenditure that the activity requires.

For example, stair climbing becomes increasingly difficult. Solutions are varied depending upon the household space, finances, and patient capabilities. Initially, proper breathing techniques are taught with respect of efficient use of oxygen. Alterations in living patterns may become necessary. For example, a second floor bedroom may be placed on the first floor. If financial status allows, an automatic chair lift can be installed on the stairway. Suggestions made for altering living space and activity must be realistic in terms of personal and financial capabilities.

Sleeping habits are also altered. The patient may go to bed earlier and sleep later or wake up intermittently throughout the night. Determining the cause of this arousal is helpful in distinguishing between an underlying physiologic or psychological cause. Careful questioning related to level of dyspnea, increased cough, feelings of suffocation, and signs of congestive heart failure need to be explored.

Cessation of smoking is critical. Various smoking clinics are available in communities to assist patients and family members to quit. If the patient fails in his or her efforts to quit, chastisement is not suggested. This behavior tends to cause the patient to avoid the health care person. Consistent encouragement for efforts made such as smoking less each day, changing to a low tar brand, quitting during an upper respiratory infection, and use of cigarette filters reinforces and encourages further attempts to decrease cigarette consumption which may eventually lead to smoking cessation.

Liberal alcohol consumption is also to be avoided. Alcohol is considered a respiratory depressant and excess amounts tend to decrease the effectiveness of the lung defense mechanisms against invading organisms.[17] One or two beers a day or a cocktail with dinner is not considered excessive.

The nurse's role in assisting the patient as he moves through various changes in daily activity capabilities cannot be overemphasized. The patient most vividly sees and senses his physical deterioration by his ability to "do" for himself.

Improvement in Breathing Coordination

Shortness of breath is a common symptom of COLD. The patient is often taught coordinated breathing patterns during hospitalization. The emphasis is placed on decreasing the use of accessory muscles of the neck and chest wall. Relaxation techniques applied to various muscle groups can help reduce muscle tension and in certain instances promote a general state of relaxation. This is conducive to a more coordinated breathing pattern. These techniques are not unlike yoga or meditation forms of exercise.

The patient is also instructed in a coordinated breathing pattern using abdominal muscles as much as possible. The usual pattern is to breathe in slowly on a count of two and out slowly on a count of four. Exhalation is done through pursing the lips. Pursing the lips creates an artificial resistance against the exhalation of air and helps keep airways from excessive narrowing and collapse on exhalation. This maneuver allows for a more complete exhalation of air and thus less trapping of air in the lungs.

The use of intermittent positive pressure breathing (IPPB) devices, as a mechanism to insure deep breathing and promote a more even distribution of air, has been less highly regarded in recent years in favor of breathing coordination reeducation and routine health care followup. This pattern of thinking has helped free many persons from electrical outlets. The trend away from routine use of IPPB in the home has also helped decrease respiratory infection. An IPPB machine which is not meticulously kept clean can harbor bacteria which in turn are blown into the patient's airways with the treatment. The result is often a pseudomonas pneumonia. If the patient does not desire to part with his machine, daily attention must be paid to appropriate cleaning measures. The use of one-half strength white vinegar and water on removable parts on a daily basis is necessary.

Secretion Clearance

Retained secretions are a problem as they promote infectious processes and obstruct airways. The initial concern in effective secretion removal is adequate hydration. Therefore encouragement of at least 1500 to 2500 ml of fluid per day is recommended. This helps liquefy secretions which aids in their removal.

The adjunct use of aerosal therapy may be of benefit in instances when prolific, thick, tenacious sputum production is a problem. Aerosol is the suspension of water particles in a gas stream. The aerosal is produced by a nebulizer device. The patient inhales this steam for a specified time prior to initiation of vigorous maneuvers to remove secretions. Aerosal therapy can be performed in an outpatient department of a hospital or in the home. Purchase costs of equipment do vary and insurance coverage for such devices also varies. The equipment may also be rented from a hospital supply company. A doctor's signature that this therapy is essential to maintenance of patient health is usually requested in obtaining third party payer funds.

Postural drainage, percussion, and vibration are techniques utilized to assist the patient in the removal of secretions that are difficult for him to mobilize. The patient's spouse or other family member is taught the technique. The idea is to utilize gravity and vibration technique over various lobes of the lungs to loosen secretions from the walls of the bronchi and thus facilitate mucus removal. This technique is generally most effective when practiced in the morning and evening. Secretions accumulate in the lungs throughout the night, thus tending to be thicker and more prolific by early morning. It is also not uncommon for secretions to appear darker in color in the morning as compared to the middle part of the day. Maximal clearance of the airways prior to bedtime helps reduce nighttime accumulation of secretions. Initially, the technique may be taught in a hospital inpatient or outpatient setting by physical therapists, respiratory therapists, and/or registered nurses. The most important component to retaining the information is home care followup. The patient and family can learn to modify the procedure based on sputum production and exacerbations of respiratory infection.

An ineffective cough pattern reduces the effectiveness of sputum removal. Energy expenditure and shortness of breath are increased. The patient must be taught how to cough effectively while expending the least amount of physical effort. A strong forceful cough is not recommended as the pressure generated causes premature collapse of "flabby" airways and subsequent air trapping. Short bursts of coughing are more effective.

Patients are also instructed on how to evaluate color, amount, and consistency of sputum. If the color changes from clear or white to yellow, green, or brown and becomes increasingly difficult to raise, the physician should be notified. Such changes often indicates presence of an infection. In climates where dryness or decreased humidity is a problem, added humidity is advised to facilitate less viscous sputum. Proper cleaning and maintenance of any humidifying device is stressed.

Medications

The role of medications is specific to the underlying disease as well as patient response. Bronchodilators are employed to facilitate maximal airway diameter and thus reduce airflow resistance. The patient must be cautioned in use and abuse, side effects, and in certain cases how to evaluate the need for specific dose adjustment.

Antibiotics are utilized in treatment of upper respiratory infection. The patient may have standing instructions from his physician when to initiate a course of antibiotic therapy. A record should be kept of the number of respiratory infections as well as the infection's response to a given antibiotic. The patient should take the full 7 to 10 day course even though he or she may feel better after three or four days. If no improvement is noted then the antibiotic may need to be changed. Antibiotics should not be stored for long periods of time as their potency may be decreased. Chemical make-up of a drug may change with long storage time (greater than one year or as specified). A periodic check of the medicine cabinet can avoid use of outdated and potentially dangerous medication.

Corticosteroids are employed on a short term basis to assist in reduction of inflammation and edema of the airways. The patient must be cautioned not to abruptly stop the drug but follow the physician's advice in gradually reducing the dosage as prescribed.

Sedatives and hypnotics (e.g., Valium) are not recommended as these drugs tend to further depress an already compromised respiratory center. The respiratory center is the generator for the initiation, rate, and depth of respiration.

Annual flu shots are recommended for these so-called high risk persons. Community health agencies sometimes conduct free shot clinics. The pneumococcal vaccine is also recommended as a deterrent to development of pneumococcal pneumonias, a common source of infection for the patient with COLD.

The final medication employed is low flow oxygen. When the patient's cardiopulmonary system reaches a point of dysfunction where sufficient oxygen cannot be supplied to maintain tissue demands, then additional inspired oxygen concentrations are necessary. Various systems are available for home use. The standard oxygen tank is still used in many areas. This form of oxygen delivery cuts down on the patient's mobility as he or she can only travel as far as the tubing allows. This is an omen to many that the end is near, and they seem to give up prematurely. More recently a liquid oxygen system has been made available to patients. This type of oxygen system offers portability and added safety features over oxygen cylinders. The most recent advance is called an oxygen liberator. This device utilizes room air, removing the nitrogen from the air, leaving oxygen as the primary end product. The consistency of delivery of preset oxygen concentrations is currently being tested and evaluated. The advantage of such a system is that oxygen could be obtained from room air as opposed to storage in a reservoir. The disadvantage is that the device runs on electricity and requires an electrical source. This decreases the patient's mobility. The cost of continuous oxygen therapy can range from $100 per month up to $300 to $400 per month. Medicare pays up to 80 percent of such costs in most cases.

In the event no insurance coverage is available, the nurse needs to be creative in finding sources of funding when the patient is unable to pay. In some instances local community groups such as the Lions Club or Jaycees may be resources. In other instances the town treasury itself may be a source of funding for one of its community members.

The judicious use of medications cannot be overemphasized. Caution must be taken in purchase of over-the-counter drugs and inhalants. Synergistic relationships may exist with certain drugs taken together. For example, two prescription drugs, lasix and digitalis, when taken together can deplete the body's potassium level. Patients on these drugs should be asked to increase their dietary potassium intake. Orange juice and bananas are good sources of potassium. Periodically serum blood levels are drawn to check for possible toxicity to a given drug. Examples are digitalis and theophylline (aminophylline) blood content. The patient and family need to be alert to side effects of excess medication.

CONCLUSION

COLD has become one of today's major public health problems. There is a significant impact on the economy, morbidity, and psychosocial integrity of the family unit. Advances in knowledge of the physiology of respiration and mechanisms which interfere with the lung function are important components in the care and management of COLD. There is no known cure for COLD and lung transplants are presently unsuccessful in animal models. Advances in knowledge have helped find ways to prevent progression of the underlying disorder and to control to varying degrees the functional disturbances present. Numerous well-organized multidisciplinary rehabilitation programs are necessary. Lertzman and Cherniak[18] stated the concept of rehabilitation most concisely and completely. Rehabilitation is "restoration of the individual to the fullest physical, medical, mental, emotional, economic, social and vocational potential of which he is capable." Home care programs provide continued health care assessment as well as support and encouragement to the patient and family.

Well integrated home health care can result in fewer hospital admissions and maintenance of self-care for a longer period of time. This tends to promote positive feelings about self with resultant improvement in a sense of psychological well being.

REFERENCES

1. Burrows, B.: "Pulmonary Terms and Symbols." *Chest,* 67:585, 1975.
2. Wood, R.E., Boar, R.F., and Doersuk, C.F.: "Cystic Fibrosis." *American Review of Respiratory Disease,* 113:834, 1975.
3. American Lung Association: *Introduction to Lung Disease.* American Lung Association, New York, 1973.
4. Lerner, P., Social Security Administration, Personal Communication, 1978.
5. National Health Survey, PHS, Hyattsville, Md., Series 10, Number 115, March 1977.
6. Higgins, M.W., Keller, J.B., and Metzner, H.L.: "Smoking, Socioeconomic Status, and Chronic Respiratory Disease." *American Review of Respiratory Disease,* 16:403, 1977.
7. Lieberman, J., Gaidulis, L., and Roberts, L.: "Racial Distribution of a_1-Antitrypsin Variants Among Junior High School Students." *American Review of Respiratory Disease,* 114:1194, 1976.
8. U.S. Department of Health, Education, and Welfare: "Smoking and Health. Report of the Advisory Committee on Smoking and Health to the Surgeon General of the Public Health Service." Public Health Service Publication #1103, 1964.
9. Ayres, S.M.: "Cigarette Smoking and Lung Diseases—An Update." *Basics of RD,* 3:2, 1975.

10. Jones, R.N., and Weill, H.: "Occupational Lung Disease." *Basics of RD,* 6:1, 1978.
11. Burrows, B., Knudson, R., and Kittel, L.J.: *Respiratory Insufficiency.* Yearbook Medical Publishers, Chicago, 1975.
12. MacKlem, P.J.: "Disease in Small Airways." *Basics of RD,* 4:4, 1976.
13. Thurlbeck, W.M.: "Chronic Bronchitis and Emphysema—The Pathophysiology of Chronic Lung Disease." *Basics of RD,* 3:3, 1974.
14. Stewart, B.N., Hood, C.I., and Block, A.J.: "Long-Term Results of Continous Oxygen Therapy at Sea Level." *Chest,* 68:486, 1975.
15. Brannin, P.K.: "Oxygen Therapy and Measures of Bronchial Hygiene." *Nursing Clinics of North America,* 9:114, 1974.
16. Petty, T.L. (ed.): "Rehabilitation of the Pulmonary Cripple: A Symposium." *Chest,* 60:25, 1971.
17. Šarić, M., Lučić-Palaić, S., and Horton, R.J.M.: "Chronic Nonspecific Lung Disease and Alcohol Consumption." *Environmental Research,* 14:14, 1977.
18. Lertzmann, M.M., and Cherniak, R.M.: "Rehabilitation of Patients with Chronic Obstructive Pulmonary Disease." *American Review of Respiratory Disease,* 16:1146, 1976.

BIBLIOGRAPHY

American Cancer Society: "When a Woman Smokes." Publication #2051-LE, 1975.

American Lung Association: "Disability Benefits for Chronic Lung Disease Patients—The System is Uneven and Often Unfair." *American Lung Association Bulletin* 64:7, Jan./Feb. 1978.

Baum, G.L.: *Textbook of Pulmonary Diseases,* ed. 2. Little, Brown & Company, Boston, 1974.

Beland, I.L., and Passos, J.Y.: *Clinical Nursing Pathophysiological and Psychosocial Approaches,* ed. 3. MacMillan Publishing Company, New York, 1975.

Black, L.F., and Mitchell, M.M.: "Evaluation of a Patient Education Program for Chronic Obstructive Pulmonary Disease." *Mayo Clinic Proceedings,* Vol. 52, pp. 106-111, Feb. 1977.

Blancher, G.: "Caring for the Patient with Advanced Emphysema." *RN,* 37:41-45, Aug. 1974.

Block, A.J.: "Low Flow Oxygen Therapy Treatment of the Ambulant Outpatient." *American Review of Respiratory Disease* (Supplement Conference on the Scientific Basis of Respiratory Therapy), 110:71, 1974.

Burrows, B. (ed.): "Symposium on Chronic Respiratory Disease." *Medical Clinics of North America,* 57:545, May 1973.

Dirschel, K.M.: Symposium on the Patient with Long-Term Illness, "Respirations in Emphysema Patients." *Nursing Clinics of North America,* 8:617, Dec. 1973.

Dudley, D.L., Wermuth, C., and Hague, W.: "Psychosocial Aspects of Care in the Chronic Obstructive Pulmonary Disease Patient." *Heart and Lung,* 2:389, May-June, 1967.

Foss, G.: "Postural Drainage." *American Journal of Nursing,* 73:666, April 1973.

Fuhs, M.F., and Stein, A.M.: "Better Ways to Cope with COPD." *Nursing 76,* 6:28, Feb. 1976.

Gloor, E.M.: "Chronic Obstructive Pulmonary Disease and the Role of the Public Health Nurse in Instituting a Programme of Home Care Service." *International Journal of Nursing Studies,* 10:111, May 1973.

Gold, W.M.: "Asthma." *Basics of RD,* 4:1, 1976.

Goldsmith, J.R.: "Health Effects of Air Pollution." *Basics of RD,* 4:1, 1975.

Hass, A.H., and Rusk, H.A.: "Rehabilitation of Patients with Obstructive Pulmonary Diseases. The Role of Enriched Oxygen." *Postgraduate Medicine,* 39:612, 1966.

Herron, Sister C.: "Home Care of the Patient with C.O.L.D. *Nursing 76,* 6:81, Feb. 1976.

Lagerson, J.: "Nursing Care of Patients with Chronic Pulmonary Insufficiency." *Nursing Clinics of North America,* 9:165, 1974.

Lanser, J., and Pancoast, A.: "Caring for the Asthmatic at Home, in School, and on the Job." *Nursing 73,* 3:62, Nov. 1973.

Manners, B.T., et al.: "Smoking and Chronic Non-Neoplastic Broncho-Pulmonary Diseases." *Public Health Reviews,* 2:215, May 1973.

Michaelson, E.D.: "Oxygen Therapy and Delivery in Obstructive Pulmonary Disease." *Heart and Lung,* 7:627, July/Aug. 1978.

Mullins, E., et al.: "Patient and Family Education in Respiratory Care." *Respiratory Care,* 19:273, April 1974.

Nield, M.A.: "The Effect of Health Teaching on the Anxiety Level of Patients with Chronic Obstructive Lung Diseases." *Nursing Research,* 20:537, 1971.

O'Dell, A.J.: "The Administration of Airway Humidification." *Nursing '74,* 4:66, April 1974.

Moody, L.E.: "Nursing Care of Patients with Asthma." *Nursing Clinics of North America,* 9:195, March 1974.

Petty, T.: *Intensive and Rehabilitative Respiratory Care.* Lea and Febiger, Philadelphia, 1971.

Petty, T.L., and Finigan, N.M.: "Clinical Evaluation of Prolonged Ambulatory Oxygen Therapy in Chronic Airway Obstruction." *American Journal of Medicine,* 45:242, 1968.

Pierce, A.K., and Saltzman, H.A.: "Conference on the Scientific Basics of Respiratory Disease." *American Review of Respiratory Disease,* 110:1, Part 2, 1974.

Rau, J., and Rau, M.: "To Breather or Be Breathed—Understanding IPPB." *American Journal of Nursing,* 77:613, 1977.

Secor, J.: *Patient Care in Respiratory Problems.* W.B. Saunders Co., Philadelphia, 1969.

Sedlock, S.: "Detection of Chronic Pulmonary Disease." *American Journal of Nursing,* 72:1407, Aug. 1972.

Stanley, L.: "You Really Can Teach COPD Patients to Breathe Better." *RN,* 41:43, April 1978.

Taylor, C.M.: "Caring for the Chronically Ill—One Day at a Time." *Nursing 78,* 8:59, Sept. 1978.

Traver, G.: "Assessment of Thorax and Lungs." *American Journal of Nursing,* 73:467, March 1973.

Traver, G.: "Chest Assessment." *American Journal of Nursing,* 73:467, March, 1973.

Waterson, M.: "Teaching Your Patients Postural Drainage." *Nursing 78,* 8:51, March 1978.

Willims, M.H.: "Symposium on Pulmonary Disease." *The Medical Clinics of North America,* 61:1163, 1977.

CHAPTER 26
ARTHRITIS

MACKEY P. TORBETT, Ph.D., R.N., AND GERI C. BUDESHEIM, M.N., R.N.

RHEUMATOID ARTHRITIS

Definition and Etiology

Rheumatoid arthritis (RA) is a chronic systemic disease characterized primarily by inflammation of the synovial membrane in joints but can involve any connective tissues of the body. Connective tissues which might be involved include: bone, periosteum, cartilage, blood vessels, bursae, dermis, joints, fascia, tendons, tendon sheaths, and ligaments.

The disease begins as an inflammation of the synovium. This inflammation produces edema, vascular congestion, fibrin exudate, and infiltration of leukocytes. Often the amount of synovial fluid increases, becomes turbid, and has a decreased viscosity. The synovium thickens and grows out and over the articular cartilage eventually destroying this cartilage and destroying the bone beneath it. With destruction of cartilage, bony surfaces may touch and progress to a state where these surfaces adhere together, creating a state of bony ankylosis. Tendons, ligaments, and muscles are often weakened resulting in instability and/or partial dislocation (subluxation) of the joints. Deformities are common, giving RA a reputation of being the "crippling type of arthritis." RA often starts in the smaller joints of the hands or feet and progresses in a centripetal pattern to involve the larger joints. In contrast to osteoarthritis, RA involves joints symmetrically. For example, a proximal interphalangeal joint may be involved on each hand, but not necessarily on the same finger on each hand.[1]

In 1859 RA was described as a separate disease entity. Since that time, many theories as to the cause of the disease have been postulated. No specific microorganism or virus has been identified as the cause of the inflammatory response. Rheumatoid synovial cells show a decreased sensitivity to infection by Newcastle disease virus and the rubella virus. This finding lends support to the theory that RA may be caused by a slow or persistent virus infection. However, no specific virus particles have been identified.

The American Rheumatism Association has established criteria for the diagnosis of rheumatoid arthritis.[2] For a definite diagnosis of RA to be made, the following five signs or symptoms must be continuous for six weeks:

1. Morning stiffness.
2. Pain or tenderness in at least one joint (observed by a physician).
3. Swelling (soft tissue thickening or fluid, not bony overgrowth alone) in at least one joint (observed by a physician).
4. Swelling (observed by a physician) of at least one other joint (any interval free of joint symptoms between the two joints involvements may not be more than three months).
5. Symmetrical joint swelling (observed by a physician) with simultaneous involvement of the same joint on both sides of the body. Terminal phalangeal joint involvement will not satisfy this criterion.

Malaise, weakness, loss of weight, and anemia are general symptoms that are often reported by patients with active RA. Small, nontender subcutaneous masses called *rheumatoid nodules* are found in 20 to 25 percent of patients. These nodules are usually found over bony pressure points such as the elbow and exterior surface of the forearm, but may occur in the lung, myocardium, pericardium of the heart, spleen, larynx, and dura mater of the brain. RA nodules are seen more commonly in patients with severe disease and high rheumatoid factor titers.

The most popular theory of etiology is that the disease process is the result of an autoimmune response. A specific antibody called *rheumatoid factor* (RF) has been identified in the serum of 30 percent of adult patients with RA. RF has also been found in high titers in a number of other diseases such as subacute bacterial endocarditis, sarcoidosis, leprosy, and syphilis. Present opinion is that RF plays a role in perpetuating disease activity as it reacts to the patient's own IgG, but that the disease process is triggered by some other agent or mechanism. Whether this is a metabolic reaction or a specific virus continues to be a mystery.

The following clinical factors support the hypothesis that RA is an autoimmune disease:

1. An immunoglobulin called rheumatoid factor (RF) exists in the serum of 30 percent of patients with RA.
2. The synovium is infiltrated by lymphocytes and plasma cells. Antigen and antibody particles are also found in the cells of the synovial exudate.
3. The complement levels of synovial fluid are lowered. (Complement works with antibodies to bring about an immune response). If complement is low, then it is presumed that it has been partly used up in an immune reaction.[2,7]

Statistics

AGE

RA can occur at any age but most commonly affects young adults between 20 to 40 years of age.

SEX

Women are affected with RA three times more frequently than men.[2] A specific genetic marker HLA-B27 has been associated with ankylosin spondylitis and Reiter's syndrome.[5] No specific genetic marker has been identified with rheumatoid arthritis, although it is possible that such a marker or markers do exist.[4] A study of 28 sets of monozygotic twins, one of whom had RA, failed to provide evidence of genetic transmission or predisposition to the disease.[2]

RACIAL

RA has not been found to have an affinity to affect a certain race of people.

SOCIAL AND ECONOMIC

According to 1970 statistics of the Arthritis Foundation, there were 3.4 million disabled persons at any one time and 205 million days of restricted activity annually; 12.2 million days were lost from work (regular job) each year.[3] The 1977 statistics show that $4.5 billion are lost in wages and $4 billion spent on medical care. The total annual cost to the national economy due to arthritis in 1977 was $13 billion.[4] There have been some studies which indicate that the onset of rheumatoid arthritis is preceded by some life crisis event (death of spouse, divorce, and so forth) in a significant percentage of patients.[6]

CULTURAL

RA is a rare disease in tropical climates. It occurs more commonly in Britain than in the United States. The incidence is about the same in the United States and Canada.[8]

POLITICAL

Fifteen percent of all Social Security Disability income paid by the government is paid to individuals disabled because of some type of arthritis. Arthritis affects the political arena because it affects the way tax dollars are spent. Congress must decide on funding for arthritis research through the National Institutes of Health.[4]

Scope of the Problem

At least 5 million Americans have rheumatoid arthritis.[9] This represents 3 percent of the total U.S. population.[2]

Individual Impact

RA affects young adults in the prime years of their lives (ages 20 to 55). During these years, young adults are completing their education, choosing a spouse, rearing children, and are involved in community activities. The impact on the individual will depend on the stage of their disease and the level at which they are able to function.[2] Often, some alterations in the patient's life-style must occur for optimum response to therapy.

It is a shock to an individual's body image and self-esteem to tell them they have a chronic disease for which we presently have no cure. A patient responds to this news in varying ways. He may cry, deny it, or minimize the significance of the disease. He may have one or more of the following reactions: fear, anxiety, dependency, and/or anger.[10] The individual may fear invalidism, loss of his job, and becoming a burden on his family. It is important that good communication exists between the patient and the health care providers. The rationale for treatment must be explained to the patient consistently until he begins to grasp how he can contribute to the management of his disease. With the initial news of his diagnosis, the individual probably retains very little of what he is told.

Family Impact

Every individual is also a part of some kind of family unit. The patient's state of health, therefore, has multiple effects on the significant others in his life. If the affected individual is the sole economic supporter for the family and he must reduce his work to a parttime status or become unable to work, this presents an economic crisis for the entire family. A college age child may have to work a year in order to continue his education. The affected housewife may have to negotiate with family members in order to give up certain household responsibilities which she can no longer perform.

Family members need to be aware of the cyclic nature of RA. Otherwise, they may feel the patient is malingering. Family members need to be told that the patient may display anger at them as a defense against their own feelings of dependency and depression. The patient's spouse and/or children need to be able to vent their feelings and receive support from health professionals. Too often there is no contact between the primary physician and the patient's family. Even if the family accompanies the patient to the physician's office or clinic, they are often left in the waiting room.

Prevention and Treatment Approaches

INDIVIDUAL

The goals of treatment are the relief of pain, prevention of deformity and control of the inflammatory process in order that the patient may attain and/or maintain his highest level of independence.

The basic treatment program consists of education of the patient and his family, heat, therapeutic exercises, rest, and salicylates at therapeutic doses.

Education

If the patient does not understand the rationale of the treatment program, he probably will not comply with it. Written materials such as pamphlets available free from the Arthritis Association can give the patient something to read later at home. Health care providers must remember that "telling" is not "teaching." The patient's understanding of his disease and rationale for treatment need to be checked out periodically.

Heat

Heat is helpful in reducing muscle spasm which is often a part of the patient's pain. Patients are advised to sleep under an electric blanket (all year if they have air conditioning in the summer) in order to reduce morning stiffness. Heat can also be applied by taking a hot shower, local application of moist hot packs, or by use of a heating pad. Paraffin baths using a ratio of 3 oz. of mineral oil to 1 lb. of parrafin can be prepared and used to provide pain relief for hands and feet. Each hand is slightly flexed and dipped five or six times into the parrafin then wrapped in a towel for 20 minutes. Afterwards, the paraffin is peeled off and placed back in the container for the next use.

Exercise

Therapeutic exercises are necessary to maintain joint mobility and prevent deformities. Rest and exercise are important in the treatment of arthritis. Patients need specific guidelines in order to be able to gauge their own day-by-day activities.

In our clinic, three levels of therapeutic exercises are prescribed:

Level I. Do one full range-of-motion (ROM) of all major joints. This level is the only exercise the patient should do if his joints are *hot* and *swollen.* Too much exercise to acutely inflamed joints can cause joint damage. However, it is important that *one* full range-of-motion be carried out each day in order to prevent contractures.

Level II. Do five repetitions of range-of-motion to all major joints. In addition to one brief maximal exercise (BME). This is done by lifting a 1 or 2 lb. weight, can, or sandbag with the foot or hand (if prescribed for arm strengthening) and hold 5 sec. or to the count of 5. Level II exercises should be performed when most of the pain and swelling has disappeared.

Level III. Do ten repetitions of ROM and do progressive resistive exercises (PRE). The amount of weight lifted is gradually increased and number of repetitions are increased up to 15 times. Level III should be performed when the patient has no acute joints although morning stiffness may be present.

General principles to remember are:

1. Exercises or activities which repeatedly put stress on a specific joint should be avoided. One example of this is a patient who has difficulty with his knees should not bicycle or perform an exercise such as this because it can put stress on the knee joint.
2. Swimming is generally a good exercise since the joints are exercised supported by the weight of the water.
3. Any exercise or activity which keeps the joints in the same position for an extended period of time is not ideal. For example, crocheting and knitting keep fingers in a flexed position. Patients who do these activities should be encouraged to take 10 or 15 min. rest each hour and *extend* their fingers.
4. Application of *cold* compresses *after* exercise may reduce inflammation or irritation of the joint due to the exercise. Some patients find cold rather than hot is more beneficial in relieving pain also.

5. Any exercise or activity which produces joint pain afterwards for longer than 30 min. should be avoided. Pain is a warning signal that too much stress has been placed on that joint.

Rest

Ten hours of sleep at night is recommended. If the patient can not sleep this long, he should still go to bed as this will rest his joints even if he cannot sleep. In addition, two rest periods during the day should be taken. Obviously, patients who have full time jobs can not always do either of these recommendations. Patients who work should be encouraged to lie down if possible or at least elevate their feet and legs during their scheduled breaks at work. Since naps during the day may not be possible, it is suggested that when they arrive at home, they lie down for at least 30 min.

Pacing of activity and rest is a concept which needs to be taught to the patient. If the patient plans to go out for the evening, he must learn to rest prior to going out. Without proper rest, the patient may find himself overtired and in pain before the evening is over. The pattern of rest and activity must be very individualized depending on the patient's activities and responsibilities.

Salicylates

Therapeutic doses of aspirin for an anti-inflammatory effect ranges from 12 to 24 aspirins a day. Patients are usually started on two aspirin four times daily and asked to add one aspirin a day until 14 or 16 are being taken. A blood salicylate level can then be taken (should be around 1.5 hours after last dose of aspirin). Twenty to thirty mg./dl. is the therapeutic range for the blood salicylate level. Patients should be instructed to take their aspirin in the middle of their meals to reduce gastric irritation. An antacid can also be taken with the aspirin if the patient complains of gastric distress. Patients should be told that if tinnitus occurs, to continue the aspirin but reduce the dosage by one aspirin a day until tinnitus is no longer present.

It is important for patients to understand that aspirin is one of the best drugs available for the treatment of arthritis. Aspirin is such a common drug that patients often feel nothing is being done for them unless they are on a "prescription" drug. The merits of aspirin need to be explained to patients a number of times. They must understand why it is important to take it at the proper intervals.[11] Aspirin tends to inhibit normal platelet aggregation. This factor needs to be remembered especially if a patient is also taking an anticoagulant.

For patients who cannot tolerate aspirin, there are many nonsteroidal anti-inflammatory drugs (NSAID) on the market. Some of these are fenoprofen, ibuprofen, tolmetin, and naproxen. Patients should know what drugs they are taking and what adverse effects should be reported to their nurse or physician. All of the NSAID drugs as well as aspirin can cause gastric irritation. Patients need to know when to take the drugs in relation to eating. Any gastric distress or melena should be reported to the physician or nurse. Fenoprofen, unlike most drugs used in the treatment of arthritis, must be taken 30 min. before or 2 hrs. after meals for proper absorption to take place.

Success of the treatment program is usually measured by looking at several outcomes. Parameters most often used to help determine disease activity are: sedimentation rate, morning stiffness, joint count, and grip strength.

Initially, the sedimentation rate may be high. Normal is less than 20 mm/hour in adults and less than 10 mm/hour in children. When a patient has many inflamed joints, his sedimentation rate is often high. If the anti-inflammatory drugs are effective, the sedimentation rate should decline.

Joint count, or the number of painful joints present when compressed during the musculoskeletal exam, should decrease. For example, when a patient's RA is very active, the joint count may be 20, but as the disease is brought under control the joint count may be 0 to 5.

Morning stiffness is the time it takes the patient to "limber up" after getting out of bed in the morning. It is *not* the time when all discomfort is gone but the period from time of arising until it is easier for him to move around. With very active diseases, a patient's morning stiffness lasts two to three hours or longer. With response to therapy, this time should decrease. If a patient's time of morning stiffness has decreased to less than 30 min., it is one indication that he is improved and treatment is effective.

Grip strength is a good outcome to measure because RA often involves the small joints of the hand. This is measured by rolling up a blood pressure cuff, pumping up the mercury to 20 mmHg, and asking the patient to squeeze the cuff using their most powerful grip one hand at a time. A control or "normal" reading can be obtained by the examiner independently squeezing the cuff. As the patient responds to treatment, grip strength should increase.

A subjective measure can be used by asking the patient to rate himself. For example, ask the patient to rate himself on a scale of one to ten if one is the best and ten is the worst he can feel. Although this is a subjective measure, it can give the nurse or physician the patient's perception of whether he is improved.

If the patient is on a program to gain or lose weight, measurement of weight on each visit can be obtained to determine the patient's progress. It the patient is anemic, periodic measurement of hemoglobin can determine the patient's status. It is important to check the blood pressure of all patients on each contact because a certain percentage will have problems with hypertension. Patients on corticosteroids are particularly prone to develop hypertension.

If the basic program of education, heat, therapeutic exercises, rest, and salicylates is not effective in controlling the patient's RA, other modes of treatment are implemented. (See stepping stones of treatment, Fig. 26-1.)

The occupational therapist (O.T.) is a valuable member of the arthritis team. The O.T. can assess the patient to determine what activities of daily living the patient is having difficulty performing. The goals are to teach the patient joint protection in order to prevent unnecessary stress on small joints and help prevent contractures. The therapist can assist the patient in planning his daily activities to simplify and organize tasks and help him modify usual ways of performing tasks to minimize stress on joints. Four Ps are stressed: pacing, planning, priority setting, and positioning. The therapist can acquaint the patient with assistive devices which will allow the patient to remain independent rather than depending on others. The *Self-Help Manual for Arthritis Patients* which was prepared by the Allied Health Professions section of the Arthritis Foundation in 1973 has excellent pictures of assistive devices available and the names of companies from whom these devices can be ordered.

Assistive devices should not be used in lieu of assisting the patient to attain the ability to do the task without an assistive device. In other words, if the patient can regain through

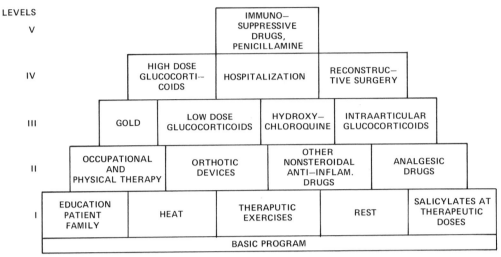

LEVELS

V — IMMUNO–SUPPRESSIVE DRUGS, PENICILLAMINE

IV — HIGH DOSE GLUCOCORTI–COIDS | HOSPITALIZATION | RECONSTRUC–TIVE SURGERY

III — GOLD | LOW DOSE GLUCOCORTICOIDS | HYDROXY–CHLOROQUINE | INTRAARTICULAR GLUCOCORTICOIDS

II — OCCUPATIONAL AND PHYSICAL THERAPY | ORTHOTIC DEVICES | OTHER NONSTEROIDAL ANTI–INFLAM. DRUGS | ANALGESIC DRUGS

I — EDUCATION PATIENT FAMILY | HEAT | THERAPUTIC EXERCISES | REST | SALICYLATES AT THERAPEUTIC DOSES

BASIC PROGRAM

FIGURE 26-1. Management of rheumatoid arthritis. (Modified from Smyth, Charles J.: Postgraduate Medicine 51(6):31-39, May 1972 and prepared by rheumatology staff physicians, University of Kansas Medical Center.)

exercise the ability to do a task, he should not become dependent on a device rather than working on the exercises.

The occupational therapist is often the team member who makes orthotic devices such as splints, although in some hospitals this service is provided by the physical therapist. Splints are often ordered to rest a specific joint such as the wrist. These are referred to as "resting splints" and may be ordered to be worn only at night. A "working" or "functional splint" may be worn on a part such as the hand to provide support even though the fingers can still be used. The patient needs to understand the purpose and directions for use of any orthotic devices ordered.

If the patient needs additional pain relief not provided by aspirin or a NSAID, a non-narcotic analgesic is ordered. Narcotics should be avoided since addiction could easily occur in a patient who has chronic pain. If a patient continues to have progressive disease despite the basic treatment program, the next treatment modality is gold (chrysotherapy) therapy.

When corticosteroids first made their advent into the treatment of arthritis, it was thought a "cure" had been found. Patients demonstrated dramatic response to cortico-steroid therapy. However, it was soon apparent that only the symptoms were relieved and that withdrawal of therapy meant exacerbation of symptoms. In addition, time has demonstrated that prolonged corticosteroid therapy can cause a multitude of problems for the patient. The lowest dosage of corticosteroid needed to control the acute inflammatory process is recommended when corticosteroids are used. This is usually no more than 20 mg every other day and preferably lower. Some common problems experienced from long term corticosteroid therapy and the reasons the problems occur are listed in Table 26-1.[12]

Adrenal suppression and atrophy can be reduced by placing the patient on every other day therapy rather than daily therapy and by having the patient take his corticosteroid between 6 and 8 A.M. rather than later in the day.[10,12] It is always a goal of therapy, when possible, to get the patient off the corticosteroid and on another drug which will not cause such systemic side effects.

TABLE 26-1. Problems associated with long term corticosteroid therapy

Side effects	Reason
Susceptibility to infection	Decrease in small leukocytes Fever suppressed
Osteoporosis	Increased glomerular filtration Increased excretion of calcium
Psychological disturbances such as euphoria, insomnia, depression, manic-depressive psychosis	Cause? Possibly cerebral edema
GI irritation and ulceration	Increased secretion of hydrochloric acid and pepsinogen by the stomach.
Diabetes mellitus	Gluconeogenesis increases 6-10 fold. Slightly decreased glucose utilization by cells.
Myopathy	Due to catabolic effect, negative nitrogen balance resulting in muscle atrophy, weakness of proximal muscles of the arms, legs, shoulders, and pelvis.
Hypokalemia	Increased production of aldosterone causes retention of sodium and excretion of potassium.
Hypertension	Exact mechanism unknown. May be caused by increased sodium and water retention.

Occasionally, an injection of a glucocorticoid directly into the joint space will provide dramatic relief of the inflammation and thus relieve the patient's pain. Rheumatologists differ as to the frequency at which such injections should be repeated. Some feel that repeated or too frequent injections to the joint can contribute to joint damage.

The treatment may progress to a trial of hydroxychloroquine (Plaquenil) if the patient has been unresponsive to other drugs. This drug requires eye exams every three to four months by an ophthalmologist since retinal damage with loss of vision can occur. The first sign of retinopathy is decreased visual fields and thus the periodic exam by the ophthalmologist should prevent serious retinal damage.

More aggressive treatment is used in patients with systemic manifestations such as vasculitis when, for example, high dose glucocorticoids might be indicated. Hospitalization with daily intensive physical therapy, teaching, and medication regulation is used by some physicians for all newly diagnosed patients with active RA.

Reconstructive surgery of many types is now available. Silicone joint implants can be inserted into the hands of patients with ulnar or radial deviation of the fingers. Total joint replacement is indicated in patients with severe bony joint damage which is often accompanied by impaired joint mobility, pain and subluxation, or ankylosis. The hip was the first joint to be replaced surgically and has been the most successful. In about 15 to 20 percent of the patients having knee joint replacements, loosening of the prothesis has occurred. This problem is being studied to determine if it can be prevented and how it can be best treated once it has occurred. Total shoulder and elbow replacements are presently the newest types of replacements being performed and very little data are available regarding their success. Many factors must be considered to determine if the patient is a good candidate for surgical treatment. Some of the factors are: Have all conservative methods of treatment been tried? Is the patient's general health such as to enable him to be a good surgical risk? Is the patient well motivated to assist in all the exercise required in the postsurgery rehabilitation program?

At the top of the treatment program is the use of immunosuppressive drugs. Drugs such as penicillamine, cyclophosphamide (Cytoxan), and azathioprine are presently being studied for the results of their use in the treatment of patients with RA. Levamisole is said to be an immunostimulant drug and, according to a British study, is as effective as penicillamine.[11] Patients on these drugs need close monitoring as serious side effects can occur. Due to this factor and to the fact that their value and safe dosage levels in the treatment of RA patients is still being studied, the use of immunosuppressive drugs for RA should be conducted by university treatment centers.

FAMILY AND COMMUNITY

As previously stated, the family needs to be involved in the education and the planning of care for the patient. The diagnosis of a chronic disease can put an added strain on family relationships. If the relationships within the family are strong and stable, the illness of a family member is usually accepted and the patient receives much support from family members. The patient and his family need to have realistic expectations of each other. No one is *always* supportive or always understands.

If family relationships are unstable or some members are easily threatened, the illness of a family member can create a crisis situation. Unrealistic fears of being burdened with an "invalid" may cause disruption of relationships. Health professionals need to be sensitive to the emotional climate and offer support and/or professional counseling when desired.

Communities can offer support in many ways. Employers can make special working hours and provide appropriate rest periods for employees with arthritis. Persons within communities can offer support through the giving of money to the Arthritis Foundation. They can give time as a volunteer to provide transportation for medical care or shopping. This latter service is often needed by older persons with arthritis. Individuals are often unaware of services needed. Communities must be educated as to the needs of persons with arthritis, for example, providing elevated commodes and doors to accommodate wheelchairs in public buildings.

Prognosis

The course of RA is difficult to predict. Patients with similar initial symptoms and lab values respond to modes of treatment differently. In addition, because the disease is characterized by remissions and exacerbations, it is impossible to say with absolute certainty whether response is due to treatment or to the natural course of the disease.

A couple of variables studied have indicated a poorer prognosis. First, patients with initial high rheumatoid factor titres in their serum seem to have a more rapid progression of their disease. Second, bony erosive changes developing early and progressing rapidly in the first 18 months of the course of the disease are usually considered a bad prognostic pointer.[13]

Community Health Nursing Concerns and Approaches

ASSESSMENT

The nurse who visits the patient in his home environment can assess many factors which can contribute to or deter the patient's successful response to treatment. The following interview outline in Figure 26-2 is one method of obtaining essential data for planning patient care.

Good baseline data with problem identification and outcome criteria can make followup visits more productive and efficient. The history will also be helpful to the nurse as she communicates with other health team members. During the interview, the nurse can assess the patient's understanding of his illness and treatment regimen including his medications, exercises, and rest as well as special treatment modalities such as splints. The nurse can also observe the patient's environment for special problems. For example, does the patient have her kitchen arranged in such a manner as to conserve time and energy and minimize stress on small joints? Does the patient have difficulty with activities of daily living such as bathing or dressing? If so, is the help of an occupational therapist needed in helping the patient solve these problems?

In assessing the patient's joint mobility, the nurse can use her own normal joints as a gauge for determining if the patient has lost any range-of-motion. Muscle strength can be assessed by observing the patient getting up and down from a chair and walking. If quadricep muscles are weakened, the patient will have difficulty getting out of a chair without the use of his hands.

Family interaction may also be observed to determine if the patient is receiving supportive or nonunderstanding treatment from family members, or are family members being overprotective?

NURSING DIAGNOSIS (PROBLEM IDENTIFICATION)

If a specific problem list is kept current, the nurse will be aware of which problems have been resolved and which continue to be problems.

OUTCOME CRITERIA

These are specific objectives written in terms of the behavior changes the nurse and the patient expect to see if the problem has been improved or alleviated.

NURSING INTERVENTION

Plans for nursing care should be specific. For example, if you plan to teach the patient why exercise is important, state the steps of your teaching. Check off or state those completed so that at the next visit you can evaluate the effect of your teaching.

I. DEMOGRAPHIC DATA

Name _____ Age _____ Sex _____ Ht. _____ Wt. _____
Address (Street & City) _____ Race _____
Occupation _____ Marital Status _____
Medical Insurance _____
Source of Referral _____ Children _____

II. SOCIAL, FAMILY DATA

A. Role in family
B. Usual lifestyle
C. Hobbies
D. Type of housing
E. Usual hours of sleep or rest periods
F. Family support (including spouse or significant others' understanding of patient's illness)

III. PAST MEDICAL HISTORY

A. Childhood diseases
B. Other illnesses
C. Surgeries
D. Family history of connective tissue diseases
E. Drug allergies

IV. HISTORY OF ARTHRITIS SYMPTOMS

A. Preceding illnesses
B. Data of onset of first symptoms
C. Description of first symptoms and progression of symptoms since onset:

   1. First joints affected.
   2. Presence of swelling, pain, redness, extent of limitation of motion, symmetry of joints involved.
   3. General pattern of joint involvement since onset.
   4. History of alopecia, malar rash, photosensitivity, Raynaud's phenomenon.

D. Factors which aggravate symptoms.
E. Amount, location, and duration of morning stiffness (onset; when stiffness lessens), history of fever, anorexia, or weight loss.

V. PAST TREATMENT

Name of drugs and/or treatments, how long used, why discontinued, evidence of sensitivity or reaction.

VI. PRESENT MEDICATIONS AND TREATMENT
(including exercises and supportive devices)

VII. SIGNIFICANT LAB AND X-RAY DATA
(Rheumatoid factor, ANA, Sed Rate, CBC, x-rays)

VIII. MEDICAL DIAGNOSIS
Nursing Diagnosis (list patient problems)

CARE PLAN

PROBLEM	OUTCOME CRITERIA	NURSING INTERVENTION	EVALUATION

FIGURE 26-2. Interview outline for planning patient care. (Compiled by Geri Budesheim.)

Research

During the past five years research has focused on the etiology of RA and other connective tissue diseases. The current research is focused in the area of the immune response and autoimmunity. Many studies have centered around the role of T-lymphocytes and B-lymphocytes in the immune response. If RA is an autoimmune response and researchers can determine what triggers or turns off such responses, a cure may be found for RA.

Education

Many people believe arthritis is one of those disorders you live with but that nothing can really be done about it. Only through education within the health professions and among the general public can this erroneous thinking be eliminated. Proper treatment and exercise can reduce joint destruction and the accompanying deformities characteristic of RA. The Arthritis Foundation suggests that the general public be educated regarding the warning signals of arthritis which can be any one of the following:

1. Persistent pain and stiffness upon arising in the morning.
2. Pain or tenderness in one or more joints.
3. Swelling in one or more joints.
4. Recurrence of these symptoms, especially when they involve more than one joint.
5. Pain and stiffness in the neck, lower back, knees, or other joints.
6. Tingling sensations in the finger tips, hands, and feet.
7. Unexplained weight loss, fever, weakness, or fatigue.

JUVENILE RHEUMATOID ARTHRITIS

Juvenile rheumatoid arthritis (JRA) is the term applied to RA which develops before the age of 16.[2] The peak incidence of onset was between ages 2 and 3 and the mean age was 5.5 on a study of 88 children with JRA.[14] It affects girls two times more often than boys. In the United States 250,000 children have JRA.

Three distinct subclasses of JRA have been identified as the following:

1. *Systemic JRA* is characterized by intermittent fever, skin rash, and multiple joint involvement as well as anemia and leukocytosis. This is the most serious of the subclasses.
2. *Pauciarticular JRA* describes those patients who have less than five joints involved. Fever, anemia, and leukocytosis are uncommon and crippling arthritis rarely occurs. This type affects 40 percent of children with JRA. Usually joint involvement is asymmetrical and affects the large joints such as the hip or knee. Fifty percent of children will be serum positive for antinuclear antibodies and will have chronic iridocyclitis which is more likely to occur in this group. Iridocyclitis can only be diagnosed by slit-lamp examination by an ophthalmologist. Ten to twenty percent of children affected with pauciarticular JRA will have ocular damage from iridocyclitis. The iridocyclitis may cause redness or burning or can progress insidiously and cause cataracts. For this reason some doctors recommend slit-lamp examination

of the eye every six months in patients with juvenile rheumatoid arthritis and every three months if the disease involves one or more joints.[16]

3. *Polyarticular JRA* describes the intermediate type between systemic and pauciarticular. More than five joints are involved but systemic manifestations occur less frequently. This subclass can be further segregated into those children who are rheumatoid factor positive and those who are negative for rheumatoid factor.

A characteristic rash occurs in 20 percent of children affected by JRA. The rash occurs most often toward evening on the extremities and is aggravated by heat such as produced by fever or hot bath. The rash is maculopapular with the lesion being about 10 mm in diameter, pale red with an area of central clearing. Occasionally the rash will be pruritic.[15,17]

Prognosis and Course of Disease

Good prognostic signs are early age onset, absence of nodules, no bony erosions, and serum negative for rheumatoid factor. Though bony erosions are less common than in the adult, bony ankylosis is more common in JRA.[15] Joints affected are the same as in the adult with RA except the cervical spine, temporomandibular, and distal interphalangeal joints are more commonly affected in JRA.

The diagnosis of JRA must be differentiated from rheumatic fever, joint infection, and neoplastic diseases such as leukemia.

Etiology

JRA was initially thought to be an infectious process but no organism has been isolated despite the fact that infections precede or concur with the onset in one-third to one-half of the cases. Immunologic factors as well as physical trauma have been suggested as potential causal agents.[14] A couple of studies have found a significant psychodynamic problem within a year before the onset of JRA. Divorce or marital separation of parents was reported most frequently.[14]

The treatment of JRA is essentially the same as for adults. Aspirin remains the safest and best drug. It should be prescribed in dosages to maintain a salicylate blood level of 20 to 30 mg percent. Aspirin 100 mg/kg of body weight in four divided doses with food is generally adequate to maintain such blood levels. If aspirin does not control synovitis, gold is usually the second drug tried. Gold dosage is 1 mg/kg of body weight/week up to a body weight of 25 kg. Maintenance dosage is given for 20 weeks and then spaced out to every 2 to 4 weeks. Signs of gold toxicity are rash, proteinuria, and leukopenia, the same being true for the adult on gold therapy. Corticosteroids should be prescribed with caution since they do not prevent joint destruction and can cause stunting of growth in the child. Corticosteroids are indicated to prevent loss of vision due to iridocyclitis or in cases of vasculitis. They should always be prescribed in the lowest dosage necessary to suppress the inflammatory process.

Physical therapy as well as occupational therapy is often necessary to maintain joint mobility and prevent muscular weakness and contractures. With children exercise should be structured using play activities. Although contact sports may be contraindicated, swimming provides good exercise. Children should not be needlessly restricted from activities and should live as full and normal lives as possible. Parents of children with chronic arthritis tend to overprotect their children. This can inhibit the child's normal progress toward independence and have a negative effect on his personality. The community health nurse can observe the child-parent interaction in the home and can guide parents toward a more realistic and constructive approach to their child's illness. Children need to continue their education with other children in public school whenever possible in order to develop intellectually and emotionally. Special counseling may be necessary to determine long range goals and approaches with children with severe disability due to arthritis. As soon as the child is able, he should assume responsibility for taking his medication, doing exercises, and so forth. The nurse can be creative in helping children devise ways of remembering to do exercises and take medications.

DERMATOMYOSITIS AND POLYMYOSITIS

These disorders are characterized by inflammation of striated muscles primarily affecting proximal muscles of the legs, arms, neck, and pharynx. Arthritis occurs in 40 percent of patients and most commonly affects the MCP and PIP joints of the hands and the wrist bones. Joints are affected bilaterally and symmetrically. Symptoms experienced by the patient are joint pains with morning stiffness, malaise, and weight loss (commonly occurs), weakness of proximal muscles, and muscle pain or tenderness in 60 percent of patients. Skin lesions occur in 60 percent of patients and are characterized by a lilac-colored facial rash in butterfly distribution and on the upper neck and limbs, often photosensitive and sometimes tender. The rash may be accompanied by edema. On the upper eyelids a peculiar dusky lilac suffusion may occur, called heliotrope rash, and is pathognomonic of dermatomyositis. A small percentage of patients develop intestinal disturbances and pulmonary fibrosis. Seventeen percent of adults with a visceral malignancy will have an associated polymyositis or dermatomyositis.[2] However, dermatomyositis occurring in children is not associated with malignancy.[18] Calcinosis, which is subcutaneous deposits of calcium, occurs in 20 to 40 percent of children in later stages of the disease. These lesions may ulcerate and drain and/or become infected.

These disorders can occur at any age but more frequently occur in persons 50 and 60 years of age, affecting females twice as often as males. There is no hereditary factor known in causing these disorders. No race is particularly prone or immune nor is geographic area significant. Incidence has been approximated as one case per 280,000 population per year.[2]

Etiology of these disorders is unknown. A hypersensitivity mechanism or an underlying humoral immunodeficiency coupled with over activity of cell mediated immunity have been postulated as etiologic factors.

Diagnosis is made by clinical manifestations and by ruling out other connective tissue disorders through lab and x-ray tests. The sedimentation rate is abnormal in 50 percent of patients, and serum aldolase is raised in 75 percent of patients in the active phase and is useful in monitoring response to treatment. Myography is usually abnormal but nonspecific.

Treatment consists of physical therapy to maintain or increase muscle strength. Corticosteroids are administered orally to suppress the inflammatory process. Serum enzyme levels should decrease and the patient's muscle strength should improve with response to therapy. Adult dosages of corticosteroids during the acute stage range from 40 to 60 mg daily. For children 1.5 to 2 mg/kg of body weight/day is ordered in the acute stage. Seventy-five percent of patients improve with treatment. If no improvement occurs, the patient should be thoroughly studied for a malignancy. Some adult patients will respond poorly to corticosteroids but usually improve with the addition of methotrexate injections weekly in dosages of 25 to 50 mg.[2]

Prognosis has improved greatly with the use of high dose corticosteroid therapy. The disease is characterized by remissions and exacerbations, therefore, extended followup care is essential.

Early symptoms of fatigue and proximal muscle weakness are often vague and can accompany many viral illnesses. Low grade fever, general misery, and muscle weakness are complaints of children with the disorder. A public health nurse may help in encouraging adults and children with proximal muscle weakness to seek medical attention. She can also monitor patients' response to therapy by grossly testing muscle strength. In addition the nurse can help in teaching the patient and his family about the disease and its treatment.

ANKYLOSING SPONDYLITIS

Ankylosing spondylitis is a chronic connective tissue disease affecting primarily the spine and sacroiliac joints. The inflammatory process progresses to calcification of spinal ligaments which restricts spinal mobility. There is a family history of the disorder in 6 percent of patients affected. There is a greater incidence of HLA B-27 (human leukocyte antigen) in patients affected. The disorder occurs in males 90 percent of the time and affects 0.4 percent of all males. It occurs between the ages of 15 to 30 but seldom earlier or later.[2]

Symptoms experienced by the patient are low backache and/or pain in both buttocks and morning stiffness. In about 10 percent of patients pain may radiate in the sciatic distribution. One-fourth of patients may complain of fatigue, weight loss, or iridocyclitis or iritis. Some patients will have peripheral joint arthritis of shoulder and hips (40 percent), knees (15 percent), ankles (10 percent), feet (5 percent), wrists (5 percent), and rarely in fingers. Eighty percent of patients affected will have an elevated sedimentation rate. As the disease progresses, the following characteristic changes may be seen on x-ray: 1) blurring, sclerosis, or fusion of sacroiliac margins and 2) formation of syndesmophytes (bony growth) along the anterior and lateral margins of the vertebrae leading to a "bamboo spine" appearance on x-ray.[10]

The course of the disease is quite variable and frequent remissions and exacerbations are common. In some patients the disease may remain limited to the sacroiliac joints. In other patients the disease progresses over 10 to 20 years to the "poker" or stiff back which is diagnostic of this disorder. Kyphosis with forward carriage of the head may occur. In addition, over time there is limitation of chest wall expansion due to involvement of the costovertebral joints.

Treatment consists of: 1) reducing stress to the spinal column by rest periods or vocational change to a sedentary type work: 2) drug therapy with phenylbutazone and indomethacin, steroids should be avoided; 3) exercises to maintain as full mobility as possible; 4) proper positioning to prevent flexion contractures. Firm mattress with no pillow under the head is best to prevent forward flexion of the cervical spine.[2,10]

The community health nurse can encourage patients with characteristic symptoms to seek early diagnosis and treatment. In diagnosed patients, the nurse can monitor and encourage patients to adhere to their treatment program as well as teaching the patient about the disorder and its treatment in order to minimize flexion contractures.

GOUT

Gout is a disease which affects the joints and may in some cases damage the kidney. It most likely is due to a genetic defect in purine metabolism. It is now well known that the purine bases adenine and guanine are necessary elements for deoxyribonucleic acid (DNA) production in the cell. They also play an important part in protein production as well as other cellular biochemical processes. Consequently, they are vital to the organism for proper cell functions. On the other hand, the end product of purine metabolism is uric acid. In patients with gout, hyperuricemia is usually present. This can be due to defects in more than one enzyme system. The uric acid normally is excreted by the kidney and to a lesser degree degraded in the gastrointestinal tract. Hyperuricemia may be caused by incomplete destruction of uric acid, an increase in urate production, or decreased urinary excretion of uric acid. If, for example, the uric acid is not adequately excreted by the kidney, it may be deposited in joint tophi.

Talbott and Yü give a good description in defining the typical primary gout episode:

"The development of acute and severe arthritis in one or more joints of the extremities in a male without a history of previous joint distress is the usual presenting feature of gout. The onset is sudden, the cardinal signs of inflammation, heat, redness, swelling, and tenderness are present, maximum distress is reached within a few hours, and with subsidence of each of the signs, either spontaneously or drug induced, the affected member becomes normal and the only residual evidence of morbidity may be an elevated serum uric acid concentration. Gout usually appears in males after puberty and females after menopause."[21]

Also, Kelley states:

"The typical attack involves one joint in the lower extremities, the more distal the joint, the more typical. Initial attacks often have a nocturnal onset. Patients may be awakened at night by the pain or they may notice joint pain upon arising in the morning. In the early stages, attacks last only a day or so. In the course of the untreated disease, attacks increase in frequency, duration, and severity. Typically, patients describe the pain of gouty arthritis as the worst they have ever experienced. For some, the slight pressure of a bedsheet or of a breeze on the affected joint may be intolerable; one patient told me in all seriousness that his joint was so severely affected that it hurt when somebody pointed at it."[22]

Gout is a disease that has been alluded to in the literature for centuries. There is some controversy about whether or not King Asa of Judah (915-875 B.C.) did indeed have gout or some other malady. Some historians are of the opinion that he did in fact suffer from gout.[23] The patient with gout is typically depicted in the cartoons as being overweight, on crutches, with a huge bandage around the foot to protect the swollen great toe. He is usually very unhappy about the situation and in obvious pain.

Gout is more common in men than women. The ratio of men to women is at present an unsettled question, however, there is evidence to support a greater occurrence in men. The onset occurs most commonly during the middle decades of life with a mean age of 44 years.[21] Gout affects all races and seems to be widely distributed throughout the world. Historically gout has been associated with royalty and in the past decade with intellectual performance and achievement; however, it is not restricted to such individuals;

the vigorous but impoverished may develop gout as well as the effete or affluent.[22] In 1973 it was estimated that 0.2 to 0.3 percent of the population was affected, or approximately 500,000 persons in this country had the disease.[24]

The impact of gout on the individual need not be devastating. Even though an acute episode can be extremely painful it need not be allowed to persist. The joint distruction which can accompany chronic tophaceous gout should no longer occur. It is one of the few rheumatologic diseases in which a well defined diagnostic test exists. The treatment, though not curative, will prevent symptoms in a compliant patient.[25] Because gout can be controlled with adequate drug therapy it need not be classified as a disease that can cause an economic loss to the family or put a burden on the community.

Even though gouty arthritis has been a known disease for ages there is still difficulty in some cases of differentiating it from other forms of arthritis. Consequently, a subcommittee of the Diagnostic and Therapeutic Criteria Committee of the American Rheumatism Association was given the task of collecting data to be used to develop criteria for classifying arthritis due to gout. Their conclusions were that the best way to classify a patient as having acute gout is to demonstrate characteristic sodium urate monohydrate crystals in the joint fluid.[26] In the absence of either joint fluid or tophaceous sodium urate crystals, six or more of the following items serve as reasonable criteria for gout.[26]

1. More than one attack of acute arthritis.
2. Maximum inflammation developed within one day.
3. Monoarthritis attack.
4. Redness observed over joints.
5. First metatarsophalangeal joint painful or swollen.
6. Unilateral first metatarsophalangeal joint attack.
7. Unilateral tarsal joint attack.
8. Tophus (proved or suspected).
9. Hyperuricemia
10. Asymmetric swelling within a joint on x-ray or examination.
11. Subcortical cysts without erosions on x-ray.
12. Joint fluid culture negative for organisms during attack.

After the diagnosis of gout is made, there is more than one drug available for treatment. Colchicine can be given by mouth or intravenously but is usually used only for acute episodes and with the patient hospitalized. Gastrointestinal side effects of nausea, vomiting, diarrhea, and intestinal cramps indicate toxicity of the drug and it should be stopped. It is of the utmost importance to instruct patients as to the occurrence of these symptoms so they will know it is usual and can be reversed by withdrawal of the drug. Other drugs which do not give GI upset are phenylbutazone and indomethacin. All three drugs can be ulcerogenic so the patient with an active ulcer may experience more severe GI problems. Phenylbutazone can cause fluid retention and should not be given to patients with hypertension and congestive heart failure. Indomethacin may cause severe headache and other CNS disturbances.[22]

After the acute attack, hyperuricemia may be treated with allopurinol which is an inhibitor of purine biosynthesis.[22] Uricosuric drugs, such as probenecid may be given to increase renal clearance of uric acid. These can contribute to renal calculi. The nurse's responsibility lies in the area of proper instruction to the patient. The teaching plan should include:

1. The cause of the disease.
2. Why the joint is so painful (the inflammatory process).
3. The availability of treatment.
4. The action of the drug.
   a. Importance of adhering to dosage.
   b. Importance of taking the medicine at times prescribed.
5. Side effects of drug and what action to take.

Historically, gout has been associated with strong drink (alcohol) and rich foods. It is true that some foods are high in purine and that gout is the result of an error in purine metabolism. However, its association with the intake of alcohol and purine rich foods in moderation does not seem to contribute to an acute attack. The fasting which usually accompanies overconsumption of spirits may have a potentiating effect on uric acid metabolism and in this manner is frequently associated with seizures of gout.[27]

Although purines can be produced in the body by denovo synthesis, any additional intake in food could add to the production of uric acid from their metabolism. The foods patients should be advised to avoid are those rich in purines such as meats, spinach, and the Leguminosae family (e.g., soybeans, peas, peanuts).[28]

Perhaps one of the most important nursing tasks is to dispel the legendary tales about gout and see that the patient adequately understands the disease in order to cope with it. Acute attacks will continue to occur at times, but with proper medical management crippling should not result and the patient should not be incapacitated from pain or deformity.

In the community the nurse will see many patients with arthritic complaints. By using the criteria listed she can make a good nursing assessment and give attention to the specific needs according to her nursing diagnosis. After the diagnosis of gout has been made and medical management is involved, the nurse must continue to work with the patient for maintenance and supportive purposes to see that acute attacks are diminished and deformity is eliminated.

OSTEOARTHRITIS

An estimated 40.5 million Americans or 37 out of every 100 adults have osteoarthritis by x-ray examination. About 12 million of them have it seriously enough to cause painful problems. Ninety-seven percent of all people over 60 show signs of the disease.[29]

The disease affects women more often than men. It is a disease of the joints and is sometimes referred to as degenerative joint disease. There are also other names like osteoarthrosis and hypertrophic arthritis that are sometimes used interchangeably.

The cause is unknown and there is no cure at present, but it can be controlled. It has been called a wear and tear disease that affects joints that get the most use during a lifetime. It is more commonly found in the age group over 60, but can occur before that age. Because of pain and immobility it can cause loss of work time and cause a considerable economic burden.

There is difficulty sometimes in differentiating osteoarthritis from the other rheumatic diseases such as gout and RA. The onset is usually insidious, it usually affects the distal interphalangeal joints, hips, and knee joints and need not be symmetrical.

Pain is increased with use, there are bony enlargements, the ESR is normal, and there are no serum abnormalities in 95 percent of the patients. There are no special features found in the synovial fluid. [30] Visual prominences on the distal interphalangeal joints known as Heberden's nodes have a much higher frequency in females. [31]

In order for the nurse to give proper assistance to the patient with osteoarthritis, she must first do a thorough assessment of the patient, the support group, i.e., those living with the patient, and the environment. A number of factors will determine what is to be done. Some of these are age, weight, education, and degree of motivation. An assessment of the amount and location of pain is of the utmost importance. The patient's pain must be dealt with before he or she can be encouraged to increase activity. Limits in activity should be evaluated so new ways of doing necessary activities can be introduced to the patient. The primary objectives in the treatment are relief of pain and return of activity through a proper rehabilitation program. After a medical regimen has been established there may need to be surgical restoration of some joints that show almost total destruction. Surgery for replacement of the hip and knee joint has been increasingly successful in the past few years.

Since this is a disease of the joints with no other systemic involvement such as in RA, the nurse must focus her attention on the relief of pain and to allow the patient as much mobility as possible. The nursing care of joint involvement for osteoarthritis would be the same as that for joint involvement in rheumatoid arthritis.

REFERENCES

1. Pearson, Donald A., and Sharp, John T.: "The Etiology of Rheumatoid Arthritis." *Bulletin of Rheumatic Diseases,* 27(3):891, 1976-77.
2. Rodman, Gerald P. (ed.): *Primer on the Rheumatic Diseases,* 7th ed. American Medical Association, 1973.
3. "Arthritis—The Basic Facts." National Arthritis Foundation, New York, 1970.
4. *Annual Report, 1977.* Arthritis Foundation, Atlanta, 1977.
5. Bluestone, Rodney: "Immunogenetics and Ankylosing Spondylitis." *Clinics in Rheumatic Diseases,* 3(2):255, Aug. 1977.
6. Hoffman, Agnes L.: "Psychological Factors Associated with Rheumatoid Arthritis." *Nursing Research,* 23:218, May-June 1974.
7. Fudenberg, H.H., Stites, D.P., Caldwell, J.L., et al.: *Basic and Clinical Immunology.* Lange Medical Publications, Los Altos, Calif., 1976.
8. Hollander, Joseph Lee, and McCarty, Daniel J.: *Arthritis and Allied Conditions.* Lea and Febiger, Philadelphia, 1974.
9. *Annual Report, 1978.* Arthritis Foundation, Atlanta, 1978.
10. Ehrlich, George E.: *Total Management of the Arthritic Patient.* J.B. Lippincott, Philadelphia, 1973.
11. Decker, John L.: "The Management of Rheumatoid Arthritis." *Medical Times,* 106:28, Nov. 1977.
12. Blunt, Mary, and Kinney, Anna Belle: "Chronic Steroid Therapy." *American Journal of Nursing,* 74:1626, Sept. 1974.
13. Hart, Dudley F.: "Presentation of Rheumatoid Arthritis and Its Relation to Prognosis." *British Medical Journal,* 2:621, Sept. 1977.
14. Henoch, Garica Jean, Batson, Jean W., and Baum, John: "Psychosocial Factors in Juvenile Rheumatoid Arthritis." *Arthritis and Rheumatism,* 21(2):229, March 1978.
15. Huskisson, E.C., and Hart, Dudley F.: *Joint Disease: All the Arthropathies.* Williams and Wilkins, Baltimore, 1973.
16. Healey, Louis A.: "Juvenile Rheumatoid Arthritis—Earlier Diagnosis." *Consultant,* 13:185, March 1973.
17. Schaller, Jane G.: "Diagnosis and Treatment of Arthritis in Children." *Medical Times,* 106:65, Nov. 1977.
18. Lell, Mary Elizabeth: "Dermatomyositis of Childhood." *Pediatric Annals,* 6:115, March 1977.

19. Sigler, John W., et al.: "Gold Salts in the Treatment of Rheumatoid Arthritis." *Annals of Internal Medicine,* 80:24, Jan. 1974.
20. Pennys, Neal S., Ackerman, Bernard, and Gottlieb, Norman L.: "Gold Dermatitis." *Archives of Dermatology,* 109:374, March 1974.
21. Talbott, John H., and Yü, Ts'al-Fan: *Gout and Uric Acid Metabolism.* Stratton Intercontinental Medical Book Corp., New York, 1976.
22. Kelley, William N.: "Current Therapy of Gout and Hyperuricemia." *Hospital Practice,* 11:5, 1976.
23. Rosner, Fred: "Gout in the Bible and The Talmud." *Annals of Internal Medicine,* 86:6, 1977.
24. Barth, Werner F.: "Gout." *American Family Physician,* 8:5, 1973.
25. Gall, Eric P.: "Modern Management of Gout." *Arizona Medicine,* 35:7, 1978.
26. Wallace, Stanley L., et al.: "Preliminary Criteria for the Classification of the Acute Arthritis of Primary Gout." *Arthritis and Rheumatism,* 20:3, 1977.
27. MacLachlin, Margaret J., and Rodman, Gerald P.: "Effects of Food, Fast, and Alcohol on Serum Uric Acid and Acute Attacks of Gout." *American Journal of Medicine,* 42:38, 1967.
28. Sodik, Farid, et al.: "Understanding Gout." *Journal of the American Pharmacy Association,* 17:2, 1977.
29. *Osteoarthritis, A Handbook for Patients.* The Arthritis Foundation, Atlanta.
30. O'Duffy, J. Desmond: "Differential Diagnosis of Rheumatic Disease in the Elderly." *Journal of the American Geriatrics Society,* 25:2, 1977.
31. Wright, Erna: "Osteoartrosis." *Clinics in Rheumatic Diseases,* 2:3, 1976.

IV

MAJOR MENTAL HEALTH ISSUES AFFECTING COMMUNITY HEALTH

As the society in which we live becomes more complex, individual and group coping mechanisms can become impaired with pain, injury, and even death the eventual outcome. Stress from many sources has become the norm for living rather than the exception. In providing nursing care to clients in the community, the nurse is often an initial professional observer of emotional fragility or breakdown. Her ability to identify normal from abnormal coping patterns, to identify stress factors, and to be familiar with community resources which can aid in supporting individuals and families through emotional turmoil is essential in providing comprehensive care. These chapters are included to sensitize the reader to some of the issues she or he may encounter, their etiology and treatment approaches, and the role the nurse may play in assessing and intervening appropriately in such situations.

CHAPTER **27**
FAMILY CRISES AND EMOTIONAL DISORDERS

FREDDA HERZ, PH.D., R.N.

In the past several decades, the behavioral science disciplines have made quantitative leaps in their ideas regarding human behavior and emotional disorders. The field has shifted from considering a psychiatric symptom as an expression of an individual independent of his or her context to viewing psychiatric symptoms as a function of relationships between people, particularly those intimately connected to one another. The idea that psychiatric symptoms are an expression or a symptom of family distress began with the early research on schizophrenic family systems and now enjoys fairly wide acceptance. Both behavioral scientists and clinicians have begun to accept the notion that the family system is a primary force in determining human behavior. The family provides the context for understanding emotional disorders and the arena for the prevention and treatment of these disorders.

One may ask "What makes the family so important in determining human behavior?" Although there is no simplistic answer to this question, one aspect of the family's importance is related to the fact that we all grow up in families of one form or another and that most of us continue to live in families during our adult lives. Another aspect of the family's importance is related to the nature of the family's relationships over time. In contrast to other social systems, the family's organization and process appear to derive from the emotional ties of multiple and continuous generations. Haley[1] believes that the continuity of generations distinguishes not only different human systems but also the total human species from other animal species.

During most of the previous decade, there has been great interest in defining and understanding the family processes which influence and/or maintain psychiatric symptomatology. Although there is by no means agreement or a full understanding of these processes producing human difficulties, there appears to be a shift toward understanding the normative processes of family life.[1-3] One aspect of this shift in focus is an increased interest in the family life cycle and a new emphasis on the relationship between the family's life cycle and the development of psychiatric symptomatology. This shift in focus has been elaborated in a family life cycle framework.

According to this framework, psychiatric symptomatology can be viewed as instances of disruption in the course of the family life cycle. The family life cycle consists of a series of developmental phases. The developmental crises differentiating these phases are a series of family emotional issues. Difficulty in resolving these issues, due to dysfunctional family process or situational crises, results in the disruption of that life cycle phase. This disruption or interference in life cycle resolution is expressed by the development of psychiatric symptoms in one (or more) family members.

Statistics regarding specific psychiatric symptomatology are not useful to this framework for two reasons. First, these statistics group symptoms according to traditional diagnostic classifications which are influenced by the context of the diagnosis. Secondly, these statistics often do not discriminate the diagnoses by age, sex, or type of symptoms making the results difficult to interpret.

The purpose of this chapter is to present the community health nursing student with a framework for understanding emotional disorders or psychiatric symptoms as disruptions in the family life cycle. Toward this end, six family life cycle phases will be discussed with reference to the emotional task(s) of each. The second part of the chapter will focus on specific family processes which tend to impede life cycle resolution. The last part of the chapter will explore the utilization of this framework for the assessment of family needs and the planning of appropriate direct and indirect nursing interventions. The' type or nature of the symptom seems to depend on the family's history and the intensity of the family process.

THE FAMILY LIFE CYCLE

The family life cycle can be divided into six phases, each with its own emotional task: 1) the unmarried young adult; 2) the couple without children; 3) the family with young children; 4) the family with adolescents; 5) the family with grown children; and 6) the family with elderly (Table 27-1). Since families are self-perpetuating, a discussion of the life cycle phases can begin at any developmental phase. For the sake of selecting a starting point, we will begin our discussion with the young unmarried adult.

The Young Unmarried Adult

In general, people are older when they marry than their counterparts of several decades ago.[4] In terms of the family life cycle, later marriages mean a lengthening of the life cycle phase between leaving the family of origin and establishing one's own nuclear family, and although some young adults are choosing not to marry, marriage is still the norm of our culture. Therefore it will be considered the end point of this life cycle phase. In contrast to previous generations, the young adults of today do not leave the parental home

TABLE 27-1. Family Life Cycle Phases, Tasks, Symptoms

Family life cycle phase	Family life cycle emotional task (major ones)	Family member or system level where symptom appears	Types of symptoms
1. Young un-married adult	To establish self singularly in adult world while maintaining relationship to family.	Young adult Couple	Schizophrenia Peripheral adult conflict
2. The couple without children	To form and work out details of an intimate relationship be-tween two.	Couple Spouse	Separation and/or divorce Depression, depen-dency, any number of variations
3. The family with young children	To establish a new subsystem as parents. Or renegotiate marital and extended family relationships.	One of the spouses	Depression, work, post-partum psychosis, alcoholism
4. The family with adolescents	To begin treating children as adults (adjust hierarchy) while maintaining parental relation-ship. To renegotiate marital relationships and change re-petitive ways of behaving toward each other.	Couple Adolescent	Separation/divorce, antisocial symptoms Alcohol, drug abuse, sexual promiscuity
5. The family with grown children	To readjust to being a family of of two. To relate to grown children while maintaining separate boundaries.	Couple Young Adult	Usually a period of relative harmony. May find the young adult with difficulty establishing self extra-familially in career, etc.
6. The family with the elderly	To remain connected to suc-ceeding generations. To die with dignity.	Spouses	Physical symptoms of aging get worse.

only to marry, but rather they leave to begin establishing themselves singularly in the adult world.

In order to accomplish this task, those in their twenties must define their status in relation to peers, work, and the opposite sex. The end of this life cycle phase is traditionally marked by the decision to marry and the committment to a mate through marriage. For those who choose not to marry, this choice may mark the end of this phase. The process is one of taking hold in the world, working out the externals of life, and beginning to set a life pattern. There is always the conflict between the need for a safe structure, like the family, and the need to explore and experiment with changing structures.

The family forms the backdrop for this process both internally and externally. In establishing their view of the world and themselves in the world, young adults often utilize an internal model of their parents' life pattern as a base for comparison and growth. The goal is to be different from the parent(s), to break away from their parents' life pattern. At the same time, the family is the safe external structure to which the young adult can and will rebound in time of anxiety or need. The family must not only permit the child entrance and exit, but must at times expel the recalcitrant child. The parental dilemma is one of balancing their wanting to hold the child in time of need but also wanting the child to move on and become independent. The successful resolution of this life cycle phase entails achieving an intricate balance so that adulthood is achieved without a cutoff from family.

An inadequate resolution of this life cycle phase occurs when the young adult and his or her family do not perceive the task as balancing involvements but rather as an either/or choice. That is, when the young adult cannot adequately maintain relationships with both family and the adult world, the life cycle task is unresolved. Although psychiatric symptoms can occur in any one of the central participants, they usually express themselves in the individual most affected by the lack of resolution, the young adult. The range and form of the symtomatology are varied and influenced by factors such as the intensity of the family process, the psychiatric history of the family, and the length of time the issue remains unresolved. Part of the form of the symptomatology depends on the tipping of the emotional scale. That is, certain forms of symptomatology are related to being unable to leave one's family and others and to being unable to remain connected to them. In general, when the young adults are too intensely involved with their families, they often become peripheral adults. At its greatest intensity, there are those young adults who have a schizophrenic episode during this phase. At a somewhat lesser intensity are those young adults who are unable to be responsible by obtaining jobs and supporting themselves. These young people often develop an irresponsible life-style and expect the family to be financially and emotionally responsible for them. The following is a clinical example of the latter type of situation.

The client, a 29-year-old male, was the first born in a family of two children. He had a younger sister. After numerous attempts to establish himself outside the family, this young man was living at home with his parents. After a somewhat stormy adolescence in which he had done poorly in school, he had gone away to college. He had finally finished his college education after several extended rebounds into the family for emotional and financial support. He had lived at home briefly after college while seeking a teaching job. He was fired from the teaching job because of his irresponsibility and became a shoe salesman. Between these two jobs, he had lived at home and was again supported by his parents. He got married to a high school sweetheart shortly after the second job began. The marriage ended with his wife leaving him after three years because of his poor working and spending habits. He lost the second job and again went home to live with his parents. His parents again supported him and began to pay for a graduate education. He found a third job and moved out again. When he was bored with this job he quit and came home again. At this point, his parents, who had always believed their son needed support because of his insecurity, began to become concerned about his inability to make it on his own and also to resent his demands on their personal lives. The family then sought assistance for their difficulties.

Families of physically ill or handicapped young adults experience difficulties similar to the family described above. In general, the more severe the disability or illness, the greater the young person's difficulty in establishing himself in an adult world. Frequently, it is not the child's actual disability which impedes the life cycle task resolution, but rather the family's fear and anxiety about the actual or imagined effects of extrafamilial contacts.

When inadequate resolution of this life cycle phase derives from the young adults' inability to remain connected to their families, the emotional consequences can also be harsh. Generally, the young adults' inability to remain connected to their families while establishing themselves in the adult world derives from the same type of emotional intensity which leads other young adults to remain overinvolved with their families. The difference appears to be in the method of resolution. The tendency for young adults to achieve independence by cutoffs or disassociating from their families is supported culturally. The difficulty with this type of task resolution, as with the other, is that is does not solve the emotional task of simultaneously establishing independence while remaining connected to the family.

The Couple Without Children

The young adult phase is ended by the selection of a mate and the decision to marry. Although the terms selection and decision imply a rational process, several authors suggest that the process is mostly emotional or irrational.[1,5-6] Many people, especially the young, might argue that the decision to marry is more likely to be rational with more young couples now living together before marriage. However, the national marriage and divorce statistics[4] illustrate that the rate of divorce is still higher than ever during early marriage. Haley[1] believes that no matter how long couples live with one another, the very commitment to marriage changes the nature and intensity of the relationship. The author's own clinical research and experience support this idea.

Whether the decision to marry is based on rational or irrational processes, marriage is a state of prolonged unreserved intimacy. The young couple must not only work out their boundaries as individuals but also the external details of living together as a married couple. They must decide how to make decisions, how to handle disagreements, and how to handle each other's sensitivities. In addition, they must make decisions regarding finances and living arrangements. In essence, they must learn how to handle the unreserved intimacy of living with a mate. While they are working out their boundaries as individuals within a marriage, they are establishing boundaries in terms of systems. They must decide which peers they will see and when they can be seen. Since marriage involves the joining of two families, the couple must also begin to define their boundaries and relationships with their extended families.

In terms of the extended families, marriage does not mean that the young adult is no longer the parent's child, but someone else's husband or wife. While previously most of each spouse's emotional connection was to their families, it now is to one another. The effort to establish their relationships while at the same time maintaining their emotional connections to the extended family (and other significant people) is the major struggle the young couple faces individually and together. Reciprocally, their families struggle to redefine their relationships with their children.

When one considers the increased complexity of this life cycle phase in comparison to the previous one, it is not only a wonder that anyone gets married but that they stay married. In fact, many do not. Many couples divorce by the end of the second year of marriage.[4,7] Divorce tends to occur when the couple is unable to work out some aspect of their relationship as a couple. Psychiatric symptoms, if they occur, are likely to be in the spouse who is most emotionally pulled between the extended family and marriage.

If at the end of two years the couple has remained married, they are often confronted with the decision of whether to have children. Childbearing and rearing, once considered the natural consequences of marriage, is now becoming a matter of choice. The increased cost of childrearing, the increased focus on the use of environmental resources, and the desire of many women to pursue careers are a few of the societal changes contributing to the notion that child bearing and rearing is a matter of choice. Since the majority of couples are still choosing to have children,[4] there has been little opportunity at this time to study the life cycle of those couples who opt to remain childless.

The Family With Young Children

The arrival of a child denotes the arrival of a new generation and marks the beginning of other role and relationship changes in the previous generation. Just when the couple thought they had their game of two worked out, they embark on a game of increasing complexity. Spouses become parents and their parents, grandparents. Whether the birth was welcomed or viewed with difficulty, there will be repercussions throughout the system. In terms of marital relationships, these repercussions are related to the fact that the arrival of a child means a new level of commitment and responsibilities to one another. Whatever uncertainties remain about the marriage, they are intensified or at least brought to attention with the birth of a child.

The responsibilities and demands of parenthood force the couple to shift their relationships in various ways, some subtle, some drastic. The emotional intensity once shared by two must now be expanded to permit the entrance of a third member. That is, the couple must shift their marital relationship to permit the establishment of a new set of parental relationships.

In terms of the extended family relationships, the arrival of a child brings them closer to the extended family while at the same time setting them apart. As parents, each of the couple are now more individuated as adults and are viewed less as children by their parents. However, the birth of a child also brings them more into the network of relatives. New boundaries must be devised in terms of grandparent visitation, babysitting, and/or caretaking arrangements. Oftentimes working out these new boundaries leads to disagreements between young couples or between the spouses and the extended families. Problems or psychiatric symptoms at this phase are usually related to the rapid changes in the roles and relationships at all system levels. It is not uncommon for a symptom to be expressed in the young mother who may become tired, depressed, demanding, or even psychotic.[1] However, she may be responding to the demands of a new baby, a husband who feels trapped, and/or an overinvolved extended family. The following is an example of a woman pulled in all directions.

> A couple, married for three years, had just had their first child three months before. The wife, 32 years old, was joyous in the hospital but upon arrival at home had become steadily depressed. The husband, 33 years old and an only child, had asked his mother to come and assist the baby nurse in caring for his wife and their child. She arrived immediately upon the mother and child's discharge from the hospital. The husband spent an increasing amount of time in his law practice. His mother, anxious to be a good grandmother, did not let the wife care for the baby. For the next several months the wife's depression continued to increase until hospitalization was considered.

Just viewing the wife's depressive symptoms separate from the context would simply lead to a diagnosis of postpartum depression. But such a diagnosis does not explain her symptoms nor does it suggest a solution. Her symptoms are an understandable response to an untenable situation. This woman's depression could only be treated by dealing with her isolation from her husband and her baby. Dealing with this isolation would involve removing the well-intentioned grandmother.

Traditionally, the raising of young children posed a special problem for women. While women were taught to believe that childbirth and childrearing were self-fulfilling, they often experienced themselves as being isolated from the adult world. Since raising young children can often be frustrating by itself, being cutoff from the adult world, in which husbands were very involved, only increased the intensity of the experience. Women would often place increasing demands on their husbands to provide them with adult contact and/or relief from the children. Although this traditional role presented particular difficulties for women (and some for men), the new breed of career-minded mother is not without its own set of problems. While the traditional roles of mother and father were well defined, the new breed of parents must redefine marital and parental roles and juggle space and time to permit the simultaneous involvement of both in career and family.

For example, a couple I was recently seeing in treatment clearly illustrates the problems for a dual career family. The wife, who had reinitiated her career after a brief period of childrearing, was finding herself overworked with home, family, and job responsibilities. During my initial meeting with her and her husband, it became obvious that a relationship renegotiation was necessary to permit both the time and opportunity to engage in their active careers. On a simple level, informing each other of their weekly calendar helped to organize their time together. On a relationship level, they had to redefine who was to do what at home and with their children.

Whether or not the couple functions in the traditional childrearing roles, problems during the latter part of this life cycle phase tend to center around balancing marital and parental roles. When there is an imbalance in these roles, such as when one of the couple is more a parent than a spouse, problems tend to arise with one or more of the children. Problems with the children will arise during normally stressful periods such as when the child (or children) start school. Environmental or situational stresses may also influence symptom development in the child.

The Family With Adolescents

During this family life cycle phase, there are generally no additions to the nuclear family. That is, the family cast is not changing. However, this is often a period of great turmoil due to the changing hierarchial or structural arrangements in the family. In terms of the parent-child relationships, the parents' major task is to begin the shift to treating the children as peers while at the same time being responsible to them as parents. The typical adolescent upheaval or rebellion can be viewed as a struggle to change the family organization to permit more "adult" or mature behavior.[1] In general, the more parents attempt to rigidly adhere to the previous organization, i.e., treat the adolescents as children, the greater the struggle. At the same time, parents who go to the other extreme and treat their children as adults may experience similar difficulties as those who utilize a rigid structure. In either case, adolescents may escalate their negative behaviors. If the hierarchy is rigid, they will challenge it; if the hierarchy is too fluid, they may escalate their behavior to have the parents define limits to the behavior. Either parental behavior may result in psychiatric or emotional symptoms in the adolescent, the most common of which relate to drug and alcohol abuse.[8] In essence, what often begins as an experiment becomes a symptom when it remains uncontrolled.

At the same time parents are dealing with the changing family hierarchy, they are also dealing with numerous marital issues. Symptoms of marital difficulties during this life cycle phase appear to be related to the family focus shifting from parenting to spousing. For the first time in a number of years, the couple is not busy with young children. The husband's success struggle is often complete, or there is a realization that his goals are unreachable, i.e., if he is going to be successful, it is usually by this time. The wife, if she hasn't been working, begins to have the time to do so. At the same time, the marital relationship patterns have often become fixed. That is, the couple has worked out some rigid or repetitive ways of dealing with their conflicts.

One of the major repetitive patterns may have been to deal with marital conflicts through the children. As the children reach the teenage years, these mechanisms may not work any longer and the couple may be forced to reexamine their relationships. The fact that the family cast is not changing serves to decrease the fluidity of the system and further increase the strain on the marriage by decreasing the options for tension reduction. Sometimes couples resolve their marital issues by adding to the cast of the family, that is, they "decide" to have one last child. If this tension is dealt with through a child, the child becomes symptomatic. If it is not for whatever reason, marital strain, conflict, or extramarital affairs will often be the developing symptom. The tension and the resulting reexamination of the marital relationship may also result in renegotiation of commitment to the relationship or a decision to terminate the marriage.

Part of the difficulty for the parents as individuals relates to the shifts in the extended family relationships. Often during this life cycle phase, the parents' parents are entering retirement and aging. Each of the spouses is forced to deal with his or her parents' eventual death. Increasingly throughout this phase, they may be required to parent their own parents as they become more elderly and ill. The actual caring for their own parents and the experience of their parents as an elderly couple may further increase the tendency toward reexamination of the marital relationship.

The Family With Grown Children

By describing this life cycle phase as "Weaning Parents From Children," Haley[1] describes the parental part of this family life cycle phase. Sheehy's[9] description of this life cycle task as "Pulling Up Roots" describes the part the emerging adults play in this family drama. The process of leaving the parental home is a mutual and often painful task for the late adolescent and the parents.

Although the task of the family with adolescents is preparation for this phase, it seems that all families enter a period of crisis when the children begin to leave home. The outcomes of the crisis vary not only from family to family but also within families. In some families, the anxiety gets progressively worse until the youngest child leaves home. In other families, the upset progressively decreases as each child leaves. The intensity of the crisis (and the severity of the outcome) are dependent upon a number of factors, the most significant of which appears to be the family's degree of child focus. That is, if the couple have viewed themselves mainly as parents, they will tend to have difficulty adjusting their marital relationship and the family tension will be high. The couple must return to being a family of two. It is not uncommon for issues put aside when the children were born to enter the forefront again. Oftentimes couples experience some degree of conflict.

It is not by chance that schizophrenia most frequently occurs in young adults during this life cycle phase. The young adult is expected to pull up his roots and the family is thrown into turmoil. In those families with severe turmoil, oftentimes the only way the child can deal with the situation is through severe symptomatology. The harder it is for the family (including the child) to separate, the greater the likelihood of psychiatric symptomatology developing in the child. Most commonly, the children leave home angrily in the midst of this turmoil and attempt to achieve their separation or individuation by cut-offs from their family.

The Family With Elderly

There is increasing national interest in this life cycle phase which begins with the children leaving home and ends with the death of the spouse. In actuality, this life cycle phase consists of two subphases, one extending from the children leaving home to the retirement of one of the spouses and the second extending from retirement to death.

In terms of the first subphase, if a couple has succeeded in weaning their children while maintaining their marriage, they enter a period of relative harmony. This harmony is relative in the sense that there are fewer family members to deal with and because the couple has decided to remain together. However, the couple must adjust to being two again, including the practicalities of how much food to prepare, whether to remain in their home, and how to deal with the emotional issues of how and what to say to one another. The more child-focused the family has been and the longer the period of childrearing, the more likely the spouses will experience difficulties being alone with one another.

Upon the retirement of one spouse, the couple must adjust to being together all of the time. Oftentimes they are bored, feel useless, and are increasingly isolated. In a culture that is very youth oriented, growing old often means hopelessness and death. In some instances, where one spouse is feeling particularly useless and hopeless, the other spouse's physical illness or emotional upsets give a purpose to life. Often, each spouse cares for the other and shares in the household responsibilities. Certainly the economics of being old also has profound effects on their lives. In most instances, a poor economic situation can mean a miserable retirement rather than the "glorious" one the couples had planned for themselves.

When the elderly become too ill to care for themselves or when one spouse dies, the children often take on the role of parenting. The family must decide what to do with the ill or remaining parents. For them, this is often a period filled with sorrow, guilt, anxiety, and turmoil. Symptoms such as depression or behavioral symptoms may develop in the child who becomes the caretaker or perhaps in the grandchild closest to that grandparent. For remaining spouses, the death of a spouse often means their own death is near. In fact, it has been found that spouses often die within a year of one another.[2] The issue for all elderly couples is how to die with some degree of dignity.

In summary, life cycle tasks are the normal crises of family life. All families experience more or less stress in the resolution of their life cycle tasks. The amount of stress families experience is related to the degree of difficulty they are having resolving the task of a particular life cycle phase. The more difficulty the family is having, the more likely it is that emotional symptoms will develop in one or more of the family members. Although numerous factors can influence the family's ability to resolve the life cycle tasks, dysfunctional family processes and stressful situational life events appear to be of importance.

Family Process, Situational Events and the Life Cycle

The term dysfunctional family processes is used here to describe those family dynamics which interfere with a family's functioning. The most common process of this type is the triangle. Although there are numerous variations of a triangle, it is defined broadly as a dysfunctional relationship in which the relation of any two depends on the relationship with a third. Briefly, the dysfunctionality of a triangle is associated with the fact that direct open relationships are not possible between any two parties when the tension increases between them. A frequent variation of a triangle occurs when the spouses' relationship depends on their relationship to a child. Often one child is more involved in the process, but it is possible for all of the children to be involved to some extent. The more the spouses' relationship is dependent upon the child, the greater the difficulty they experience when this child goes to school, goes to college, and/or gets married.

Other variations of the triangle may involve the extended family. A common one is when one of the spouses relates to his or her parents through the other spouse. Or the spouse may refuse to see his or her parents because the other spouse does not like them. Although these triangles are more frequent in early marriage, they often remain in the same form after the arrival of children. Most frequently the form of the triangle shifts to involve the children. Here the grandparents may interfere in parenting or they may relate to their children only as the parents of the grandchildren. Sometimes the parents and the families attempt to work out their relationships through the children. The difficulty with these triangles (as with all triangles) is that no two people relate directly to one another but always do so through a third.

The second major influence on life cycle task resolution is the stress related to situational life events such as divorce and remarriage, and physical illness or death of a family member. Since the effects of these life events could alone be the subject of a chapter, the general effects will be briefly described here. In general, these and other life events increase the family stress and change the family structure. For instance, divorce may make it more difficult for a mother to let her child go off to school. Remarriage when children are present often means working out early marriage issues at the same time as working out other life cycle issues. At the same time depending on the life cycle phase, these life events may be experienced differently and have different effects on the family. For example, the death of a father in a family with young children creates different issues than it does for the family with grown children. For the family with young children, the death of either parent leaves a major gap in the functioning of the family. Adults at this life cycle phase have major responsibilities to self and others. In contrast, the death of either parent with grown children, although disruptive, does not create a major gap in family functioning.

THE APPLICATION OF THE FAMILY LIFE CYCLE FRAMEWORK TO COMMUNITY HEALTH NURSING PRACTICE

The idea that emotional disorders are signals of system distress in resolving life cycle tasks is consistent with the focus of nursing practice in general and community health nursing practice particularly. The focus of nursing practice is the maintenance and promotion of human systems. Nursing practice is accomplished through the application of an abstract body of knowledge concerned with the life processes of human systems[10] as they relate in a complex hierarchy of families, groups, social organizations, communities, and societies.[11] The specific areas of nursing practice derive from the situations in which nursing knowledge is applied to practice. Generally, these areas include clinical, teaching-learning, and research situations. Although traditionally the health setting has denoted the specialty areas of nursing practice, there is an increased focus on the body of knowledge and practice skills common to all areas of clinical practice.

All areas of nursing practice are concerned with meeting the health care needs of human systems throughout their life cycle. This concern is related to the increasing realization that episodes of illness are disruptions of limited duration in the total life experience and that health care must be focused on decreasing these episodes through an emphasis on health promotion and maintenance. This emphasis necessitates a shift from viewing in isolation to viewing them in the context of systems of which they are an integral part. Concurrently, this emphasis demands a shift in the definition of client populations to include not only those who seek help but also those who do not.

The unique position and contribution of community health nurses derives from several areas. First, community health nurse practitioners have a visible/available position as members of a community. Second, from this position these nurses are more able to view the home health care needs of both help-seeking and nonhelp-seeking client populations in the context of the client's daily existence. Third, in terms of community mental health needs, community health nurses are able to utilize their nursing knowledge and their knowledge of family and community life to plan appropriate interventions in the community context. Utilizing their unique positions and knowledge, community health nurses have a significant function in the treatment and prevention of mental health difficulties. By providing an understanding of emotional disorders in context, the family life cycle framework presented in this chapter can be utilized by community health nurses in the assessment and intervention with numerous client populations. Since nurses are concerned with both help-seeking and nonhelp-seeking client populations, assessment and intervention utilizing the family life cycle knowledge will be discussed with reference to both these populations.

Help-Seeking Populations

These clients are those who identify themselves as in need of assistance. If one views a mental health difficulty as a signal of symptom distress, then the symptomatic individual can be defined as the identified patient and the client is the family. One way to begin to incorporate this view of the family as the client into practice is to organize record keeping and note taking by family. Toward this end, all initial contacts with help-seeking clients, identified patient, or other family members should include the construction of a family "map" or *geneogram*. The geneogram can be standardized on a form and completed in initial meetings as illustrated in Figure 27-1. This geneogram should contain data about the family membership and structure over three generations. The ages, names of all family members who live at home, and the dates of significant life events should be recorded. (See Table 27-2 for key symbols utilized for the geneogram and Table 27-3 for significant life events to be recorded.) If routinely completed on all help-seeking clients, this form can become a general information sheet about the family for the client charts. Additionally, such

THE GENEOGRAM

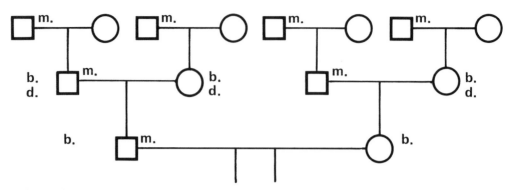

FIGURE 27-1. The geneogram gives a map of the family membership and structure over time. Beginning on the bottom with the nuclear family and proceeding upwards, list the names, ages, sexes, significant life events, and ethnic backgrounds of the three generations.

TABLE 27-2. Key symbols for a family geneogram

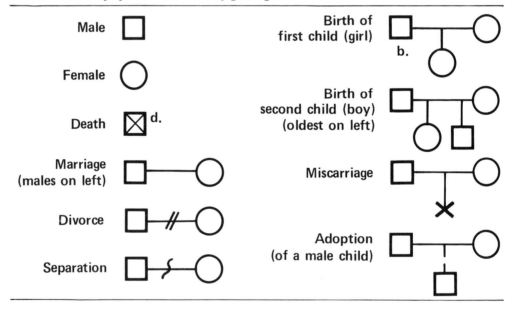

TABLE 27-3. Life events to be recorded on family geneogram

A. Marriages, separations, divorces
B. Births, miscarriages, adoptions
C. Deaths and causes of death
D. Geographic location of extended family
E. Geographic moves of family
F. Major illnesses, disabilities, or handicaps
G. Ages, sibling positions of offspring

information provides a ready source of data for any agency research or health planning with regard to characteristics and/or family structure of the client population.

All initial contacts with help-seeking families should also include an assessment of the family mental health needs in terms of information community health nurses may be interested in obtaining at some time during her initial visits with a family. In general, this information is organized around the following three question areas nurses may ask themselves with reference to a particular family: (1) What life phase is this family in? (2) What are the major emotional tasks of this phase? and (3) Are there any indications the family may be having difficulty, i.e., are any symptoms present within the family or in their interface with other symptoms? (See Table 27-1.) This information may assist community health nurses not only in planning direct mental health interventions but also in intervening with other health care needs.

Assessment of family mental health needs can be more broadly utilized in determining populations at risk and neighborhood or group mental health problems. The family data collected by community health nurses in their contacts with help-seeking clients can serve as a source for determining a commonality in the neighborhood needs or as hypothesis testing for exploration of such needs on a larger scale. For instance, if the community health nurses have had contacts with numerous single parent families at one life cycle phase experiencing similar difficulties, this may serve as the basis for planning a larger scale intervention program. At times, community health nurses can perform mental health assessments at the request of a different help-seeking population. These populations can be community agencies, schools, or industries which define a mental health need of a particular client population. Community health nurses may be approached by these social agencies to do assessments of the mental health needs and to plan appropriate interventions.

The major roles community health nurses utilize in their intervention with help-seeking populations are as consultants and educators. Nursing interventions with mental health problems are organized to promote family responsibility for dealing with the problems and to utilize community supports to maintain the identified patients or symptomatic family members in the community. General intervention guidelines are as follows:

1. *Know the limitations of one's capabilities.* Community health nurses (as well as all other nurses) must utilize their clinical judgment to determine if they have the knowledge or capabilities to deal with a problem. A number of factors will affect the nurse's decision about whether to intervene, the most important of which are: a) the size of the caseload, b) the family's response/resistance to initial assessment, c) the availability of other community resources to handle the problem, and d) the nurse's reactions to dealing with a particular problem. Generally speaking, the more long term and intense the family difficulty, the more likely outside referral sources are necessary. If referral is made elsewhere, the community health nurse can and should function as the case manager or coordinator.

2. *In direct interventions, remain calm and provide structure and community support.* When families seek help with their difficulties it is usually after they have made numerous attempts to deal with the issue(s) themselves. Therefore, they are often experiencing a great deal of stress when a nurse gets involved. If nurses remain calm and structure their contacts with the family, they assist in decreasing the family stress. At the same time, providing community supports through friends, neighbors, and extended family also helps to relieve the family's stress.

3. *Maintain the symptomatic family member in the community.* Research on the effects of institutionalization suggests that this process only freezes family difficulties and increases the sick "patient" label of the symptomatic family member. It is important to remember that the client is the family and all members participate in the difficulties. Families may need to be assisted in this redefinition of a situation. Often, utilizing support groups (as mentioned above) can assist the family in maintaining the symptomatic member by providing material and personal support. If the client needs medication to be maintained, the nurse can assist the family in seeking the resources to get such medication. The underlying question always is what has to happen for this person to not be further labeled "patient."

Nonhelp-Seeking Population

These are client populations which are unknown entities to community health nurses, i.e., those clients who may not be experiencing difficulties or who may not, by virtue of their culture and/or social class, view help seeking as acceptable to their family. Considering the size of the U.S. population and the number of patient mental health contacts per year,[8] there is a large client population who may be experiencing difficulties or who are at risk for difficulties who will not seek assistance or label themselves as patients. A great deal of professional time and energy has begun to be devoted to providing services to these populations. Because of their knowledge regarding the subpopulations in the community, community health nurses have a major role as mental health needs assessors and family life educators with these populations.

In terms of mental health assessment, community health nurses can assess the neighborhood mental health needs by determining the life cycle characteristics and potential problems and risks of that population and the community resources available to deal with them. Often, the types of problems noticed by social agencies such as schools, the police, churches, and service organizations are good indicators of a broader mental health need of the total neighborhood. Community health nurses must not only utilize the resources of these agencies for assessment but must provide family life information to these agencies to assist them in dealing with mental health problems.

Nursing interventions with nonhelp-seeking client populations often are preventive and educational in nature. The general purpose of these interventions are two-fold: 1) to provide knowledge about dealing with family issues and 2) to encourage families to seek help when they need it. Once specific needs are determined by the community mental health assessment, guidelines of nursing interventions are as follows:

1. *Utilize an educational approach rather than treatment approach to the population.* These clients do not define themselves as patients and therefore will tend to not participate in anything that defines them as such. Just as clinics have been more successful by defining themselves as "health" clinics, educational programs which focus on family life and health will increase the likelihood of reaching a target population.
2. *Utilize cosponsorship with another nonhelp defined agency for the educational program.* In addition to not wanting to be defined as a patient population, most of the nonhelp-seeking population will attend programs, workshops, and so forth only when they are not sponsored by a known mental health agency. Likelihood of participation is increased when programs are offered through churches, social groups, or schools.

Sometimes when there is a well defined target population, educational or support groups existing in the community may be able to offer such a program in conjunction with the community health nurse.

3. *Utilize a topic of general interest to all families.* Although the selection of a topic is based on community need, there are some general areas that always spark community interest, for instance, parenting, drugs, women, career, divorce. In choosing a title for the program, selecting one that implies an educational focus that will be fun and will promote discussion is helpful.

4. *Establish the details of the experience several weeks in advance so advertisement is possible.* In establishing the details of the program, characteristics of the population must be considered. If children are to participate, an after school time is necessary. If only parents are to participate, not only must evening hours be chosen, but babysitting provided. After these details are decided upon, free advertisements in community sections of newspapers and stores can be initiated. Often local radio stations will also advertise such public-minded programs free of charge.

5. *Utilize audience participation in the program.* Generally audiences learn more from programs in which they are active participants. Any number of techniques involving small group process or plenary sessions can be utilized.

6. *Evaluate the program and determine audience interest in furthering such programs.* This is an essential part of the nurse's educational function. Once you have the population, you need to have their assistance in evaluating the effectiveness of the program in terms of the goals and in planning future programs in terms of their needs. Often this can be accomplished by utilizing a brief evaluation form.

CONCLUSION

Community health nursing is of major importance in assessing and intervening with community mental health needs. Part of the community health nurse's unique position in this regard evolves from her visibility/availability in the community and ability to view human problems in the context of daily life. A family life cycle framework which defines emotional disorders as difficulties in the family developmental life cycle provides a contextual view of stress and emotional disorders. This view, when applied to community health nursing practice, defines the family as the smallest unit of client assessment and intervention and nurses as family life educators and consultants to all community populations.

REFERENCES

1. Haley, J.: *Uncommon Therapy: The Psychiatric Techniques of Milton Erickson.* Ballantine Books, New York, 1973.
2. Holmes, T.H., and Masuda, M.: "Life Change and Illness Susceptibility," in *Separation and Depression.* AAAS, 1973.
3. Carter, E., and Orfanidis, M.: *The Family Life Cycle.* Gardner Press, New York, 1980.
4. Glick, D.: "Updating the Life Cycle of the Family." *Journal of Marriage and the Family,* February 1977, pp. 5-13.
5. Lederer, W.J., and Jackson, D.D.: *Mirages of Marriage.* W.W. Norton and Co., Inc., New York, 1968.
6. Duvall, E.M.: *Marriage and Family Development.* J.B. Lippincott, Philadelphia, 1977.
7. HEW: "Statistical Notes 100, Marital Stress, Living Arrangements and Family Characteristics of Admissions to the State and County Mental Health Hospital and Outpatient Psych. Clinics."

Department of Health, Education and Welfare, Public Health Service, National Institute of Mental Health, 1973, 1974.

8. NIMH: "Statistical Note 100," February 1974; "Statistical Note 92," 1971; "Statistical Note 148," May 1978. Department of Health, Education and Welfare, Public Health Service.

9. Sheehy, G.: *Passages: Predictable Crises of Adult Life.* Bantam Books, New York, 1976.

10. Rodgers, M.E.: *An Introduction to the Theoretical Basis of Nursing.* F.A. Davis Co., Philadelphia, 1970.

11. Hall, J.E., and Weaver, B.R.: *A Systems Approach to Community Health.* J.B. Lippincott Co., Philadelphia, 1977.

12. American Psychological Association: *Publication Manual,* 2nd Ed. American Psychological Assoc., Washington, 1977.

28

SUBSTANCE ABUSE: DRUGS AND ALCOHOL

VIRGINIA TROTTER BETTS, M.S.N., J.D., R.N. AND
ANNE WETZEL SALETTA, M.S.N., R.N.

The idea of substance abuse as a health problem is certainly not unique. In the past decade there has been increasing awareness among health professionals and the lay public alike that drug and alcohol abuse is a serious problem within our society. Awareness grew as the incidence of abuse increased until the mid 1970s at which time incidence of abuse continued to be high but public and professional focus on this problem tended to decrease because other social/health problems such as physically abusive behavior, rape, and veneral disease received more attention. Despite these other health problems, substance abuse including both alcohol and drugs continues to be a major health problem in the United States as evidenced by high rates of incidence, significant psychological and physiologic disabilities of the abusers, and major family disruptions consequential to substance abuse. As a major health problem, substance abuse and its consequences will be frequently seen by the community health nurse (CHN). This chapter will attempt to provide information needed by the CHN to facilitate the assessment of the abuse problem, the planning and implementing of care for the abuser and his family, and the evaluation of current levels of care for this problem within the context of the nurse's community.

DEFINITIONS

To facilitate understanding of the problems of substance abuse, the CHN needs a working knowledge of the following definitions. These definitions are important for the ability of the CHN to communicate professionally about the severity of the problem involved and to decrease the social stigma aroused by the words "drugs," "addiction," and "alcoholism."

Drug use is the use of drugs following orders of a physician or experimental use without a prescription that has no long range negative consequences for the individual.

Drug abuse is the use of drugs with or without a prescription over a period of time that leads to behaviors that cause the individual familial, social, occupational, financial, medical, or legal problems.

Drug addiction is the use of drugs for a sufficient duration of time and in sufficient dosage that the individual's body develops tolerance and dependence upon the chemical.

Tolerance is the physiologic need for a drug in ever increasing amounts to achieve the same psychological effect while *dependence* is the body's physiologic need for a drug in order to function. Removal/discontinuation of such a drug causes withdrawal symptoms.

Alcoholism is the use of alcohol over a period of time that leads to behaviors that cause the individual familial, social, occupational, financial, medical, or legal problems.

Substance abuse is a term seen with increasing frequency in the literature to describe the use of any chemical, drug or alcohol, that is causing the individual familial, social, occupational, financial, medical, or legal problems. This term is useful in describing a similar set of problematic behaviors of the abusers but, because of the disparity in the legalities of alcohol and drug use, separating drug use from alcohol use or abuse is frequently necessary to adequately discuss the topic.

COMMONLY ABUSED DRUGS

Alcohol

Alcohol is a drug. Its availability as a consumer product, unconnected to either the medical prescription system or to the illicit drug traffic system, gives it a unique image in the eyes of society. This image—one of an acceptable concomitant of social interaction—obscures the true pharmacologic properties of alcohol.

Alcohol is the most abused drug in the United States. Its usual route of ingestion is oral. It is a CNS depressant that leads to intoxication and psychomotor disturbances. Drinking alcohol gives the individual an almost immediate feeling of calmness but it does not produce euphoria. Alcohol is physically addictive and withdrawal without medical treatment can lead to death. Prolonged ingestion of alcohol can produce severe pathophysiologic conditions including cirrhosis of the liver, CNS damage, and peripheral nerve damage.

Marijuana and Hashish

Marijuana and hashish are illicit drugs whose use is widespread especially in the population under age 25. The usual route of administration is by inhalation and sometimes by oral ingestion in foods or tea. Marijuana and hashish are depressant drugs that decrease anxiety and are intoxicating. They produce mild euphoria in some users under some circumstances. They are nonaddictive.

Hallucinogens

This class of illicit drugs includes LSD and mescaline among others. These drugs are used for thrills or sprees and are rarely used on a daily basis. The drugs are orally ingested and act to alter perception, jumble senses, and produce hallucinatory-like experiences. Hallucinogens have produced irrational behavior and psychosis in some individuals but there is no physiologic dependence upon them.

Barbituates, Sedatives, and Tranquilizers

These legal drugs are widely available through prescription or black market channels. Frequently abused drugs in these classifications include Seconal, Nembutal, Quaalude, Valium, and Equanil. These drugs are CNS depressants and are used prescriptively to decrease anxiety, control behavior, and produce sleep. The usual route of administration is oral ingestion, but some abusers inject these drugs intravenously. These drugs are physically addictive and uncontrolled withdrawal can result in death. Overdose leading to death is a real threat with many drugs in this category especially if taken in conjunction with alcohol which increases these drugs' depressant action.

Amphetamines

These are legal drugs which include Dexedrine, Benzedrine, and Methedrine among others. The usual route of administration is oral but some "speed freaks" inject the drug intravenously. The drug produces feelings of euphoria, power, and omnipotence and stimulates physiologic functioning. Prolonged use of amphetamines results in weight loss, insomnia, and physical dehabilitation. Amphetamines are not physically addicting but are highly reinforcing and easily produce psychologic dependence. While there are no physical withdrawal symptoms, a severe depression follows discontinuance of amphetamine use.

Narcotics

The drugs in this category are the most widely recognized drugs of abuse. Some of the drugs in this category include Morphine and Dilaudid which are legal drugs and heroin which is illicit. The usual route of administration is by "snorting" or "shooting" including both intravenous and intramuscular injections. Narcotics are CNS depressants which produce immediate euphoria and intoxication. Narcotics are addictive but the narcotic withdrawal syndrome is not life threatening and can be safely accomplished without medical supervision.

SCOPE OF THE PROBLEM

Incidence

There is a high incidence of substance use and abuse in America today; however, it is often difficult to obtain accurate statistics on the illicit use/abuse because of the legal consequences of such use, especially drug use. In 1977 almost 3 out of 4 adults used alcohol and it is estimated that 10 million Americans abuse alcohol.[1,2] Alcohol is the most widely used drug in America today. In most states it is legal for those 18 years and older to drink and society condones such drinking. In some respects, drinking is almost a rite of passage to adulthood in this culture.

Use of other illicit substances has increased markedly. Of these, marijuana/hashish use has had the most significant increase. Incidence of usage of all substances varies with age, sex, race, sociocultural patterns, geographic patterns, educational patterns, socio-economic patterns, occupation, family life, and peer influence.

Age

Age is a major factor in substance use and abuse. Substance usage begins in the 12 to 17 year old age group, peaks in the 18 to 34 year old group, and decreases in the 35+ year old group. The 18 to 25 year old group consistently has a higher incidence of substance use than any other age group.[1,2] Tables 28-1, 28-2, and 28-3 show how usage of alcohol and marijuana/hashish has increased since 1972. Note that usage of alcohol continues to be high until age 35 while usage of marijuana/hashish peaks at ages 18 to 25, then has a marked decrease in use after age 25.

Sex

Although men continue to be the majority of substance users and abusers, women are narrowing the gap. Incidence of substance use is on the rise in females and there has been a marked increase in both the use of alcohol and marijuana/hashish since 1972.

Race

Race is not a significant factor in substance use at this time, as Tables 28-1 and 28-2 indicate.

Sociocultural Patterns

Studies have indicated that culture influences substance abuse. Unfortunately, little data are available about cultural effects on illicit drug use and abuse and more research is needed in this area. However, research data are available for effects of culture on alcohol abuse.

Ethnic and religious backgrounds both affect alcohol abuse. Rates of alcohol abuse tend to be lower among cultures that have religious or social sanctions about alcohol abuse. For example, the Italian and Jewish cultures have low rates of alcohol abuse, even though alcohol consumption is an integral part of the culture. However, as second and third generations grow away from the original cultural roots, alcohol abuse increases.[3,4] Another example is the Irish culture. The Irish are noted for large, frequent consumption of alcohol and a higher incidence of alcohol abuse than either Italian-Americans or Jewish-Americans.[4]

Those individuals who attend church on a regular basis and/or are involved in many church related activities also have a lower incidence of alcohol abuse.[3]

TABLE 28-1. Comparison of current drinkers in 1972 and 1977 *

Current Drinkers	1972 %	1977 %
Age		
12–17	24	31
18–21	65	71
22–25	66	70
26–34	62	70
35 +	46	50
Sex		
Male		
12–17	27	37
18–35 +	65	67
Female		
12–17	21	25
18–35 +	42	50
Race		
12–17		
White	24	33
Nonwhite	19	23
18 +		
White	52	59
Nonwhite	58	51

*Extracted from National Survey of Drug Abuse: 1977, p. 104.[2]

TABLE 28-2. Lifetime prevalence and use of marijuana/hashish in 1972 and in 1977 *

Category	1972 %	1977 %
Youth (12–17)	14	28.2
Male	14	33
Female	13	23
Race		
White	16	29
Nonwhite	5	26
Adults		
18–25	48	60
26–34	20	44
35 +	3	7
Sex		
Male	22	30
Female	10	19
Race		
White	15	24
Nonwhite	21	27

*Extracted from National Survey of Drug Abuse: 1977, pp. 48–49.[2]

TABLE 28-3. Comparison of marijuana/ hashish in past month in 1972 and in 1977*

Category	1972 %	1977 %
Youth (12-17)	7	16.1
Male	9	19
Female	6	13
Race		
White	8	17
Nonwhite	9	12
Adults		
18-25	28	28
26-34	9	12
35+	less than 0.5	1
Sex		
Male	11	11
Female	5	6
Race		
White	8	8
Nonwhite	9	8

*Extracted from National Survey of Drug Abuse: 1977, pp. 52-53.[2]

Geographic Patterns

Substance use and abuse occur more frequently in metropolitan and suburban areas and are more prevalent in the Far West and the Northeast sections of America than in the Middle West or South.[1-3] Rural areas and small towns seem to have a decreased proportion of substance abusers and an increased proportion of abstainers.[1,3]

Educational Patterns

There appears to be a direct relationship between educational level and substance use. The higher the educational level the greater the chance that one has used either alcohol or an illicit drug.[1,3]

Socioeconomic Patterns

Socioeconomic patterns are also related to substance use and abuse. Those from the middle and upper class are more likely to use/abuse both illicit and legal drugs.[1,3]

Occupations

There is a lack of data in this area. However, research that has been done has shown that professionals and businessmen have a higher percentage of alcohol use than do farmers.[4]

Family Life

One of the most influential factors on substance use and abuse is family life. Children tend to adopt the attitudes, beliefs, and practices that they observe their parents using. Recent research[1] indicates that teenagers are more likely to use both illegal and legal substances if their mothers smoke cigarettes, are moderate drinkers, or have ever used psychotherapeutic drugs. Minimal levels of teenage substance use occur in families where the mothers do not meet any of these three criteria. Interestingly enough, there is little, if any, evidence to show any correlation between fathers' substance use and sons' and daughters' substance use.[1] Thus the mother's behavior is a persistent influence on the child's behavior into the teenage years.[1]

Older siblings also influence substance use among younger siblings. Teenage substance use is significantly higher in families where an older sibling has used drugs, and youths with older siblings are more prone to illicit substance use than those who are the eldest or only child.[1]

Marriage also affects substance use and abuse. Attitudes and beliefs about such use may change to coincide with that of the spouse. In our society, the wife's attitudes tend to change to reflect the husband's beliefs and practices.[5] At all age levels, married adults and/or those with children in the home are less likely to use illicit drugs than those who are not so immediately involved in such relationships.[1]

Peers

Peers also influence substance use and abuse. They may help determine attitudes about drugs and usage of drugs. Friends, coworkers, and companions influence where and when, how often, and amount of substance used. People generally respond to peer pressure in regard to substance use and abuse and tend to associate with those who share similar attitudes and practices.[2,5]

HISTORICAL PERSPECTIVES ON SUBSTANCE USE/ABUSE

1776-1900

Substance abuse is not a new problem. It has existed since the colonizing of America. Alcohol has been used since the days of the Pilgrims and was the major drug used until the middle 1800s. Drinking beverages such as beer, wine, and sometimes rum was an accepted part of Colonial life. Occasional drunkenness was condoned but not encouraged, but frequent drunkenness, a fairly common occurrence, was severely punished.[1,3]

Later, waves of immigrants brought their drinking patterns and habits with them to America. During the late 18th and early 19th centuries, drinking moved out of the home and into the taverns. Alcohol use became more associated with male behavior and gradually became morally unacceptable behavior for "respectable" women, an attitude that still exists today.[5]

Drinking behavior changed as the West was settled. The West was a vast, wild, untamed land with few vestiges of "civilization." Heavy drinking occurred there, especially in the mining towns, logging camps, and cattle towns. The legends and myths surrounding the frontiersman, cowboy, and seaman painted a picture of a rough and ready, hard-drinking man and further contributed to the concept of alcohol use as a "manly" thing to do.[5,6]

Although alcohol use continued, drug abuse began to be a major problem after the Civil War. There were three factors that were instrumental in creating the situation of drug abuse at this time.

The first was the invention of the hypodermic syringe developed in 1856. It provided a relatively simple, safe way to inject morphine under the skin, thus providing effective, fast pain relief. Morphine became the drug most used to treat dysentery and pain among Civil War soldiers. Because of its indiscriminate use by well intentioned physicians, thousands of soldiers became physically addicted to morphine.[7]

The second major factor was the importation of the Chinese to help build the railroad across the West. Like earlier immigrants, they brought their culture and pleasure habits with them; however, instead of drinking alcohol, the Chinese smoked opium. Use of opium (by smoking) became a widespread fashion by the 1890s.[7]

The third factor was the widespread use of patent medicines during this time, most of which contained addicting substances such as opium and alcohol. This was probably the most important factor of the three. By the turn of the century, it is estimated that 1 out of 500 Americans was a substance abuser.[7]

During this time religion exerted pressure to control substance use and abuse. In particular, organized religion preached temperance and abstinence from alcohol. The churches' influence and war on "demon rum" gathered speed and culminated in the Temperance Movement. This war began as a condemnation of excessive drinking and drunken behavior. It moved gradually toward condemning all drinking.[5] Unfortunately, since patent medicines were accepted even by churchgoers, this major source of substance abuse as well as opium use was largely ignored by the Temperance Movement during this time.

1900-1960

In the early part of the twentieth century, the major substance abused was opium and its derivatives. In 1906 the passage of the Food and Drug Act required that contents of patent medicines be listed on the label. This was the beginning of the end of patent medicines and the start of federal intervention in substance use and abuse.[7]

By 1914, the Temperance Movement had managed to have alcohol banned in many states. However, in 1914 an estimated 1 out of 400 Americans were substance abusers of opium and its derivatives.[7] Until this time the selling of opium was not illegal. The Harrison Act of 1914 made the selling of narcotics to users illegal, thus forcing users to buy the drug illegally and in fact creating a "black market" for drugs.[7]

In 1919 the prohibition amendment was passed, prohibiting the sale of alcoholic beverages on a national level. This amendment did for alcohol what the Harrison Act of 1914 did for narcotics—it created a thriving black market. Prohibition lasted until 1933 when it was repealed. It was most unsuccessful in controlling alcohol use and has left a legacy of emotional turmoil that in part accounts for the present confused, ambivalent attitudes Americans today have about substance abuse.[5]

Until the 1930s, use of opium and its derivatives was the primary interest of federal legislation. Legislation was aimed at controlling the importation and manufacture of opium and its derivatives. However, in the 1930s marijuana use began to be perceived as a major problem. Marijuana had been in use in the country for several years prior to the 1930s, but its use had spread during the prohibition era. Marijuana began to be linked with criminal activity and was then included as a narcotic in federal drug legislation in 1937.[7]

Until the 1940s laws were aimed at controlling importation of drugs, not at domestic control. Thus poppies and marijuana could be and were legal crops in America. In 1942, the Opium Poppy Control Act was passed and the growing of opium poppies within the U.S. controlled.[7]

Throughout the first half of the twentieth century, substance abuse continued to be a growing problem with the major drugs of abuse being alcohol, heroin, morphine, and cocaine. However, in the 1960s the type of substances used shifted and began to include substances which alter mood and consciousness.[7]

TRENDS IN SUBSTANCE USE

1960 - Present

Before 1962, those citizens with a lifetime experience of substance use were limited to 2 percent of the population.[1] Between 1962 and 1967 an increasing number of youths and young adults began using marijuana, primarily in regions of the country other than the South. Stronger substance use remained low.[1,7]

From 1967 to 1972 dramatic changes occurred in the use of marijuana and stronger substances. Those individuals admitting to having taken a substance during their lifetime doubled and in some instances more than doubled. Use of marijuana/hashish increased at a greater rate in whites than nonwhites, eradicating the racial differences observed in earlier years. While lifetime use of marijuana/hashish has increased substantially for all populations, lifetime experience with hard drugs (Morphine, heroin, Demerol) has decreased.[1]

Substance use has continued to climb since 1972. By 1977 more than half the young adults reported using marijuana at least once, as did more than a quarter of all youth (see Table 28-2). The most recent increases were in the metropolitan areas. There has been an increase in marijuana/hashish use among the 15 to 17 year olds and women. Research[1] indicates that those who did not experiment in the past are now increasingly likely to do so. Thus since 1972 there is a broader spectrum of the population who has used marijuana/hashish at least once.[1]

Upward trends in lifetime experience with substance use which began in the late sixties continues as marijuana/hashish use spreads through a larger, more varied segment of the population. This pattern may affect the social climate for substance use and abuse in our society.[1,7]

As mentioned earlier, substance use is directly related to age and the type of substance used. Current use rates may increase gradually as present youths and young adults mature.[1]

It is interesting to note that individuals born in different decades have a great diversity in their substance use history. For example, few of those born in the 1920s or 1930s have ever used marijuana/hashish either as a youth or young adult. Very few of those born in the 1940s ever used marijuana/hashish as a youth; those who have used it were in their 20s when they began use. A third of those born in the 1950s have first used marijuana as youths. This example illustrates the rapid pace with which this social change has taken place.[1]

Substance use is practiced by more people today than ever before. As substance use becomes a more common event, social attitudes toward use will change and become more liberal. As social climate becomes less negative and more resigned towards substance use, barriers to such use will begin to erode. Beginnings of this trend can be seen in the current move to legalize or decriminalize the use of marijuana.[1]

If this chain of events does occur, it could cause not only an increase in substance use but also a change in the pattern of such use. Today substance use is seen primarily among those under 25 years of age. Many young people "quit" using when they reach adulthood. However, if the barriers to use are reduced, such people may be less inclined to discontinue usage and substance use will be less identified with a developmental stage. Also many persons now are occasional users. With the reduction of use barriers, such people may increase the amount and/or the frequency of their use. Therefore, in the future, changes in substance use patterns could be much greater than they were in the 60s.[1]

To summarize, trends in illegal and legal substance use have occurred during an era of major social change. During the past 20 years, women's role and the standing of minorities have undergone major modifications; sexual mores and attitudes have become more liberal; individual rights have been emphasized; America has been involved in an unpopular war; and the nation has undergone a leadership crisis. Because of these factors the society has been in disequilibrium with social roles and expectations in a state of flux. Research shows that when such societal disequilibrium occurs, substance use and abuse increase.[1,5-7] As substance use/abuse increases, it could cause a major change in substance use/abuse as we know it today. A change that is even more significant than the one American society witnessed in the 60s.[1]

ETIOLOGY

The causes of substance abuse have been explored by researchers for years. The results of the research have been varied and far from definitive. The most familiar abuse etiology theories are those of genetic predisposition, biochemical abnormalities, sociologic determinates, and deviant behavior as response to stress.

As needed research in the area of substance abuse etiology continues, the CHN needs a model to help conceptualize the reasons for clients' abusing behaviors. One simplistic but helpful model is shown in Figure 28-1.

The P^{2}RSR model seems a realistic one for viewing 1978 society. Certainly all individuals experience the increased availability of drugs and alcohol. Legal drugs to relieve

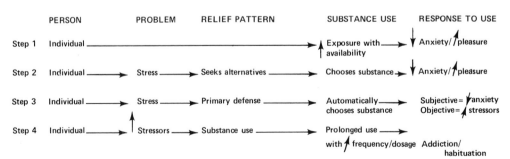

FIGURE 28-1. Person Problem Relief Substance Response Model (P^{2}RSR). A substance abuse etiology model. (Designed by Virginia T. Betts.)

anxiety, produce sleep, increase energy, and eliminate pain are frequently prescribed and prescriptions are easily refilled. Most cities and towns of moderate size and sophistication have some drugs available on an illicit market especially marijuana/hashish, cocaine, PCP, and some heroin and other narcotics. Alcohol use is widespread with the legal drinking age lowered to 18 in most states. Thus, Step 1 of the model in Figure 28-1 happens with ever increasing frequency—an individual is exposed to a psychoactive substance and receives a pleasurable response in the form of relief of anxiety or the thrill of excitement.

Step 2 of the model demonstrates the consequences of increased substance use. In Step 2, an individual is faced with stress. If that individual has been exposed to substance use, there is a tendency for the individual to choose substance use as an alternative solution to his stressful situation.

The use of alcohol or drugs is accompanied by feelings of relief, pleasure, and freedom from hurt. In Step 3, the individual begins to choose substance use as a primary solution for stress. Subjectively substance use is a positive solution, for the individual's anxiety level decreases in the face of stress. Objectively it is no solution for his behavior engenders consequences that add to, not eliminate, his stress. Step 3 therefore demonstrates that for many vulnerable individuals in the population, as the incidence of use increases the likelihood of abuse also increases.

Step 4 of the model demonstrates that the individual's abuse pattern can lead to addiction. The individual's whole life revolves around alcohol or drugs, and he has increasing problems with family, friends, employees, teachers, neighbors, and/or the police. These problems increase the stress faced by the individual leading to increased prolonged substance intake. The individual is now either psychologically and/or physically dependent upon his substance of choice.

IMPACT

Individual

The impact of substance abuse upon the individual can be ascertained somewhat from the definition of the term. The abuser experiences a multifaceted set of problems—many very painful and many of his own making.

Psychologically the two major concepts operating within the substance abuser are low self-concept and dependence. Despite the outward aura of sociability and adept interpersonal skills, the substance abuser is burdened with a low sense of self-worth which forces him to obtain need gratification through skillful use of covert dependence behaviors.

Internally the individual who is abusing drugs or alcohol is an individual who is filled with self-hate, depression, and despair when he is "straight" and who is numb, oblivious to reality, and egocentric when he is "high." Neither state connotes well being for the abuser, and he is restless and unhappy, yet most fearful of change. Returning to a "straight" or sober life-style is a goal that is frequently verbalized but difficult to achieve especially with the abuser's fear of change and his lack of skills in satisfactorily handling his own life.

Behaviorally the abuser appears intent on self-destruction. He is irresponsible and impulsive which, when coupled with substance intake that is out of control, results in enormous social and physical injury to himself. Whereas alcohol abuse causes more severe physical disability for the abusers, drug abuse causes more social disability. The reason for this variation is that alcohol in any amount is legal *per se* while the use of drugs, other than on a strict prescription basis, is illegal. The legality of alcohol abuse, except when the abuser becomes violent or a safety risk to others such as in drunk driving, allows for a prolonged period of drinking for the abuser, thus frequently increasing physical injury and disability before other social problems erupt.

The illegality of drug abuse creates social problems of great impact for the abuser, for drug provision is risky and expensive. The expense involved leads to a radically changed life-style that many times involves criminal activity such as drug dealing, robbery, male and female prostitution, and partial or total involvement with a drug oriented subculture. The drug abuser more quickly disrupts his preabuse patterns of living than the alcohol abuser. Family, occupational, and legal problems become frequent and familiar to the drug abuser.

It is difficult to determine which substance of abuse has a harsher impact. It seems sufficient to say that the substance abuser is an individual with many problems and few answers—an individual in crisis with depleting support.

FAMILY

The impact of substance abuse upon the family can best be conceptualized in terms of systems theory. As one member of the family experiences change (substance use becomes substance abuse), the whole family experiences change. Within the family, roles are reordered and communication patterns are altered. Within the community, interpersonal relationships deteriorate and family status decreases. The family experiences these resultant changes as painful disequilibrium. In this state of disequilibrium the family members attempt to adjust to achieve homeostasis. They use denial of the problem, aggression toward the abuser, self-isolation of the family from the community, and, many times, a temporary or permanent separation of the core family as means of achieving family equilibrium. Whatever mechanisms the family uses to cope with a substance abusing member, the family feels guilty, shameful, and inadequate.[8] Family members are frequently embarrassed by neighborhood knowledge of incidents of alcohol intoxication leading to accidents and violence or incidents of drug-related arrests leading to publicity and imprisonment. The economic welfare and general health of the family usually declines, and members who previously functioned well in the community begin to experience problems of their own. Children of substance abusing parents are particularly adversely affected by family disequilibrium. A drop in grades at school, an increased difficulty in peer relationships, and an increase in delinquent behaviors including alcohol or drug use are not unusual. Like the individual abuser, the substance abuser's family experiences the abuse problem as crisis.

Community Impact

The substance abuser has an increased rate of accidents and suicide and dies earlier than a person who is not an abuser. Also perhaps fifty percent of all homicides and fatal accidents involve the use of alcohol or other drugs.[9] The absentee rate for substance abusers is also greater. They earn less than the nonabuser, thereby providing less money for them and their families to spend.[9-10] (Spouses of substance abusers also have an increased rate of illness, accidents, and absenteeism due to the stressful situation in which they live.[9]) This situation results in loss of wages for the abuser and his family, loss in production of goods for his employer, and a decrease in the amount of goods for the consumer to buy.[8]

The substance abuser and his family members impact on the other community systems in which they normally function. As mentioned earlier, if the spouse works, his/her job performance may decrease; the children often have trouble with school work or run awry of the law; and the abuser may also run afoul of the law, his employer, or may infringe upon the rights of his neighbors by his behavior. It is difficult to quantify the impact of these situations on the community and more research needs to be done in this area.[9,10] For every instance of abuse, it is known that three people are adversely affected by the abusing behavior.[11]

However, the economic impact of substance abuse is possible to estimate. In 1975, the approximate cost in dollars from alcohol abusers alone was $45.75 billion, an increase of $25.84 billion since 1971.[9] Business production losses are estimated at $15.47 billion, 35 percent of the total.[9] Because of the illegality of drug abuse, no adequate studies of economic impact are available.

Not included in the above amount is the cost to the company or firm of poor or wrong decisions made by executives, managers, or foremen who were hungover, intoxicated, or "high" when they made decisions. This also does not include the cost of poor workmanship by the abusers. This can ultimately cost businesses and the public billions of dollars.[10]

Substance abusers also have an impact on other community services. Since they are prone to accidents and illness, they benefit more from programs such as workman's compensation insurance and health insurance. Since their absenteeism is greater, they and their families are more likely to be on public welfare than their nonabuser counterparts. So not only is their loss of productivity costly to the consumer but it also is costly in terms of taxes the consumers pay to provide support services for these abusers.[9,10]

TREATMENT APPROACHES

The substance abuser has many choices of treatment modalities when, by choice or coersion, he is ready to begin treatment. However, choices are limited by resources: 1) community availability of programs, 2) financial resources for payment for treatment, and 3) policies of the referring authority, especially if treatment is a nonvoluntary placement.

Alcohol

For the alcohol abuser, inpatient detoxification is usually a first step if the abuser is addicted. During this inpatient stay not only is withdrawal from dependence upon alcohol properly medically managed, but other health problems such as nutritional deficiencies and liver, heart, and peripheral nerve disease are diagnosed and treated. Detoxification can be followed by an inpatient rehabilitation stay lasting from three weeks to six months, involving individual, group, and family counseling plus alcohol education and vocational counseling.

If long term inpatient rehabilitation is not affordable or desirable due to continuing involvement of the alcoholic with his job and/or his family, detoxification can be followed by alcohol counseling and education through local community mental health centers. As a concomitant to the counseling, the alcoholic can be involved in Antabuse therapy. This is a chemotherapy approach where the alcoholic daily takes disulfiram, a drug which produces nausea if alcohol is later consumed. Antabuse therapy provides the alcoholic with an added impetus to decrease impulsive drinking. Another community treatment resource for the alcoholic is Alcoholics Anonymous (AA), a self-help group of exalcoholics who provide support, information, and motivation to former abusers. AA chapters are available in most cities and moderate-sized towns and AA members may make initial contacts with the abuser while he is still being detoxified in the inpatient unit.

Drugs

For the drug abuser, the drug of abuse determines the treatment modality. If the individual is addicted to Demerol, barbituates, sedatives, and/or tranquilizers, detoxification should be done on an inpatient unit due to the need for careful medical supervision. Likewise, withdrawal from amphetamines produces such a severe depression that inpatient detoxification is the modality of choice. Narcotics withdrawal, while uncomfortable, is not life threatening, but can still best be accomplished on an inpatient basis when the immediate goal is a drug free state. No detoxification is needed for the abuser of hallucinogens, marijuana/hashish, or cocaine.

When addicts are detoxified and abusers begin to be drug free, there are several modalities available. Therapeutic communities emphasize learning to live with stress without drugs for extended periods of time within groups of other exabusers. Inpatient residential programs with an emphasis upon counseling are also available. Community programs through community mental health centers and drug and alcohol clinics offer intensive counseling, drug education, urine screening, and vocational rehabilitation programs for abusers who have sufficient support systems to facilitate community living. Halfway house living arrangements are available in some localities.

A community program not previously mentioned that is available to narcotics abusers is methadone maintenance. These programs switch an addict from his narcotic drug of abuse to an equivalent dosage of methadone without the detoxification process. Methadone is given to the addict daily at the clinic under a formal set of rules with many federal controls. Usually counseling and vocational services are provided through the clinic.

Family

Families of substance abusers receive treatment from many sources. Family and individual counseling is usually available in most settings where the abuser is receiving help as well as being available in private clinics and community mental health centers. The most effective treatment for substance abusers with an intact family is family therapy. Such therapy benefits the abuser and each of the family members. Anger, guilt, and denial are decreased in family therapy, and positive approaches to substance abuse behaviors are elicited. Likewise communications, relationships, and here and now difficulties are addressed and worked through, thus giving each member a healthy model for problem solving when therapy is terminated.

The families of alcoholics have the added support of the Al-Anon and Ala-Teen programs. These are self-help groups formed from families of alcoholics and recovered alcoholics to aid the family in its recovery from a member's alcoholism. Nationally there are no comparable family support groups for the families of drug abusers although such groups sometimes exist on a local level.

Industry

Industry ignored the problem of substance abuse among employees for many years.[10,12] It was not until the 1940s that programs began to appear to help employees with substance abuse problems. There were reasons for this. Management was not aware of the problem, its scope, or its impact on industrial operations. Substance abuse was often a hidden problem because of the social stigma attached to it and companies feared having that stigma attached to them. Also rapport between management and labor was missing and neither was aware of the benefits working together could bring to both.[10]

Today industry has begun to realize that the substance abuser is often a skilled worker who has been with the firm for many years. The firm has invested much time and money in training him. He is a valuable person in terms of this investment and in terms of his on-the-job experience.[10]

Although there is still room for improvement, many companies today participate in rehabilitative programs for the substance abuser. Such programs have increased in number and scope since the 1940s (50 programs in 1944, almost 500 by 1973[13]).[10]

This increase is due in part to recognition of the problem and in part to an increased interest in the problem by the federal government. Funding from public and private foundations has also increased for substance abuse programs in industry. Also these programs have been shown to be cost effective to the company. For example, the cost of one program was estimated at $12,315. It provided a net savings of approximately $218,759 to the company.[14]

Many models of treatment are available now but most programs share these common features: identification of the offending behavior and its effect on the person's job performance; referral to a program coordinator who talks with the person (may confront the person) and offers help; and referral for treatment if necessary. Programs presently functioning assure the abuser of confidentiality. His employer usually maintains the abuser on the job while he is undergoing treatment. However, if the employee refuses treatment and his job performance does not change, he is often fired.[3,10] Follman[10] tells of a company that instituted an alcoholic rehabilitation program. One hundred and eighty employees were referred to the program, but 80 percent of them refused to go. After being suspended for a short period of time and warned that the next step would be termination, all those who had initially refused to attend agreed to go. This program had a 78 percent recovery rate.

Many experts believe that programs of this type are successful because they result in early identification of substance abusers and can intervene early in the cycle before the abuser has lost everything. The early substance abuser still has an investment in his life. His job may be of primary importance to him. He is still fairly socially stable, i.e., has a family, a home, and a job. He has a stake in the recovery process that is lacking later on in the cycle.[10]

It is interesting to note that at one time experts felt that the abuser must be internally motivated and volunteer for treatment. Research[3,8,10] indicates that there is no significant difference in outcomes between those clients who volunteer for treatment and those who are drafted.

PREVENTIVE APPROACHES

The prevention of social/mental health problems is a difficult task. Gerald Caplan's work delineating the focus of primary, secondary, and tertiary prevention models is of great help in conceptualizing where, when, and toward whom certain prevention activities should be focused.[15] In the P[2]RSR model for Substance Abuse Etiology (see Fig. 28-1), it seems clear that a focus of prevention for the CHN upon Step 1 would be futile. Prevention of substance use is not really the issue. The real focus for prevention would be upon Step 3—to prevent the progression of individuals from substance use to substance abuse. This prevention could be approached by two methodologies—specific and nonspecific prevention strategies.[3]

Specific Strategies

Specific strategies are those activities aimed solely at preventing substance abuse. The activities include drug and alcohol education in schools and in the community, early screening programs specific to drug and alcohol use for identified "at risk" populations, proposing responsible state and local legislation that would decrease some of the detrimental effects of drug use (i.e., treatment as an alternative to imprisoning substance abusers), and seeking limitations on the advertising and promotion of alcohol and drug use.

Nonspecific Strategies

Nonspecific strategies are those activities aimed at preventing some of the stresses impacting on individuals resulting in their moving from substance use to substance abuse. As Step 3 in Figure 28-1 indicates, individuals with poor coping skills facing stress are more likely to move to substance abuse. Thus, some nonspecific prevention activities include improving parenting skills in families in the community, increasing self-concept and personal growth of individuals in the school setting, improving access to counseling during major life crises such as adolescence, retirement, and at death of loved ones, and reducing social problems such as poverty and unemployment. In other words, the specific strategies would focus on responsible use of alcohol and drugs in the society and the nonspecific strategies would focus on promotion of positive mental health.

COMMUNITY HEALTH NURSING APPROACHES

The CHN has several roles. Three of the predominate roles include the public health nurse, the school nurse, and the occupational health nurse. In practicing within these three roles, the CHN will have opportunities to use skills in dealing with substance abuse.

When the individual abuser is the CHN's focus, a primary role is *assessment*. Substance abuse is usually at least verbally covert. The CHN must be able to observe and interview accurately if substance abuse cases are to be found in time to prevent severe disability. When the CHN finds an individual who is losing days from work or school, whose behavior is becoming increasingly erratic, who has somatic/sleeping complaints, and/or who has visible signs of intoxication, euphoria, or mental dullness, an appropriate *nursing diagnosis* could be substance abuse. If further inquiry supports this assessment, then the CHN should make a *referral* to a local drug/alcohol treatment center. The CHN must be aware of drug/alcohol *treatment resources*, their scope, and their approaches so that appropriate referral can be made. Following up on the client's response to the referral is essential as denial of the abuse problem is a major defense mechanism of the abuser. Decreasing the denial and getting the client into treatment is a major intervention step.

Following treatment, the CHN can play a vital role in the abuser's *followup care*. Substance abuse is a chronic illness and as such is characterized by remission and exacerbation. Followup, contact, *supportive interaction,* and *motivating* the client through the difficulties of the "cure" process are nursing activities of the highest value.

The CHN can provide needed care for the family of the substance abuser. She can provide *drug or alcohol education* to the family and, through this process and *supportive therapy,* help the family to understand that the problem they face is a family one. The CHN can provide crisis intervention therapy to the disorganized family and aid them in their goal to *restore equilibrium* to the family system. The CHN should encourage the family to participate actively in *family therapy* to insure the progress of the abuser and to increase the mental health status of each of the other family members.

Community Needs

There are first of all not enough preventive programs presently functioning. Secondly, treatment facilities for substance abusers are inadequate to meet the needs. Curricula in primary and secondary schools often do not include information about substance use and abuse. Teachers are not comfortable with the subject matter and tend to gloss over it, if it is even mentioned. Parents also are uncomfortable with the topic and use denial to deal with their feelings. Parents and teachers need educational programs to learn about and update their knowledge about current substance use and abuse and how to handle their children's questions.

Agencies that work with substance abusers are often overburdened and cannot meet the needs of those who turn to them for help. Programs that work with the family and the abuser exist but there are not enough of them. Unfortunately, funding for such programs competes with funding for other programs such as battered wives and child abuse. At present, programs for dealing with substance abuse are low on the priority list for federal support.

Nurse's Role in Community

As stated, community agencies to help the substance abuser do exist; however, they are often filled to capacity and have a waiting list. How can the CHN help with this dilemma? In addition to her role as a resource person, the CHN can be a valuable leader in the community. Because of her education and background she can speak out authoritatively about community needs and local problems. She can take a public stand supporting prevention programs and responsible approaches to establishing community treatment centers that can deal with the substance abuser. Finally, she can mobilize public interest groups within the community to work towards establishing prevention and treatment programs.[13]

RESEARCH

The research available currently in the literature to state prognoses for either treatment or prevention does not appear to be highly reliable. Methodology is scantily discussed and treatment success rates running as high as 90 percent seem skewed and self-serving.

   Much more research in the substance abuse field needs to be done especially at the local level. Each community needs a study to assess the levels of substance use and abuse it faces in order to facilitate appropriate community intervention. Research of the area of substance abuse is difficult in terms of getting valid data due to the social stigmas attached to abuse and due to the legal ramifications involved in the area of drug abuse. Despite the difficulties, such studies are essential to valid planning and allocation of resources for prevention/treatment.

REFERENCES

 1. National Institute on Drug Abuse: *Highlights from the National Survey on Drug Abuse: 1977.* U.S. Department of Health, Education and Welfare, Washington, D.C., 1977.
 2. National Institute on Drug Abuse: *National Survey on Drug Abuse: 1977, Volume 1.* U.S. Department of Health, Education and Welfare, Washington, D.C., 1977.
 3. Banonis, B.: "The Community Health Nurse as an Agent in Primary Prevention," in *The Community Health Nurse and Alcohol Related Problems.* National Institute of Drug and Alcohol Abuse, U.S. Government Printing Office, Washington, D.C., 1978.
 4. Estes, N., and Heinemann, M.: *Alcoholism: Development, Consequences, and Interventions.* The C.V. Mosby Company, St. Louis, 1977.
 5. Kendal, E.: "Effects of Attitudes on Delivery of Health Care," in *The Community Health Nurse and Alcohol-Related Problems.* National Institute of Drug and Alcohol Abuse, U.S. Government Printing Office, Washington, D.C., 1978.
 6. Cahalan, D., and Cisin, I.: "Drinking Behavior and Drinking Problems in the United States," in Kissin, B., and Begleiter, H. (eds): *Biology of Alcoholism,* Vol. 4. Plenum Press, New York, 1976.
 7. Ray, D.: *Drugs, Society, and Human Behavior.* The C.V. Mosby Company, St. Louis, 1974.
 8. Goodman, L.: "Support for the Family with Alcohol-Related Problems," in *The Community Health Nurse and Alcohol-Related Problems.* National Institute of Drug and Alcohol Abuse, U.S. Government Printing Office, Washington, D.C., 1978.
 9. Abernathy, M.: "Alcohol-Related Problems: A Perspective," in *The Community Health Nurse and Alcohol-Related Problems.* National Institute of Drug and Alcohol Abuse, U.S. Government Printing Office, Washington, D.C., 1978.
10. Follman, J.F., Jr.: *Alcoholics and Business: Problems, Costs, Solutions.* American Management Associations, New York, 1976.
11. Research Training Institute. Project Number 23U1611. Reseach Training Institute, Research Triangle Park, N.C., October 27, 1978.
12. Urban, M.: "Drugs in Industry," in *Drug Use in America: Problem in Perspective,* Vol. 1. U.S. Government Printing Office, Washington, D.C., 1973.
13. Archer, J.: "Occupational Alcoholism," in Schramm, C.J. (ed.): *Alcohol and Its Treatment in Industry.* Johns Hopkins University Press, Baltimore, 1977.
14. Anonymous: "Can Companies Afford to Help Alcoholic Employees?" *Rep. Alcoholism* 34(2):26, 1976.
15. Caplan, G.: *Principles of Preventive Psychiatry.* Basic Books, New York, 1964.

CHAPTER 29
VICTIMOLOGY

PATRICIA M. DISABATINO, M.S., R.N.

One has only to pick up a newspaper or turn on a television to be reminded of the violence that exists in society today. This is not something new, but what has emerged in recent years is a concern and interest in the victim of this violence. Hence, the term victimology has come into usage, as ways of understanding and helping the victim of violence have been sought. The instances where the potential victim is particularly vulnerable are of special concern for health care professionals and will be focused upon in this chapter. Of particular interest are the victims of rape, child abuse, wife abuse, suicide, and homocide. In each of these cases both physiologic and psychological trauma is involved. Also in each of these instances a single act of violence may create several victims. In addition to the direct recipient of the violent act, family members, friends, observers, or the person who is responsible for committing the violent act all may be appropriately called victims. It helps to consider the act itself as the thing which creates the victims, and not who or whatever causes that act to happen. By looking at violence from this point of view, it is possible, for instance, to define both the child who is abused and the parent who does the abusing as victims.

An essential part of the study of victims is the feeling of powerlessness on the part of the person who is being harmed. In the case of rape, wife abuse or child abuse where the victim is apt to be a woman or child, there is a real physical sense of powerlessness due to the victim usually having less physical strength than the attacker. Part of this helpless feeling is that there is no sure prevention for becoming the victim of an act of violence. Also, powerlessness may be the result of the victim's feeling that there is no alternative or recourse for avoiding being victimized.

Often, such violence may involve pathologic family relationships. Not only may such problematic family functioning be the direct cause of such victim producing acts as suicide, homocide, wife abuse, or child abuse, but the stress generated by a family member becoming the victim of another member of the family may be such that additional trauma occurs. This is because of the breakdown of support systems which are needed for successful resolution of the issues resulting from acts of violence. This can happen with the victim or other members of the family who are caught up with the pathologic response of the family to the violent act. For instance, the child who is present when his mother is beaten by his father is also a victim. The child is horrified by what he sees and will probably not have the opportunity to discuss his feelings with either parent satisfactorily due to their own preoccupation with trying to cope with their own feelings regarding the event. Thus the child also becomes a victim, although he was not the direct object of the physical abuse. When there is more than one victim in a crisis situation, this presents more complex problems for the nurse and other health care workers. An example of this would be an abused wife and abused children in the same family, or more problematic still, an abused wife abusing her children.

Even when the family unit displays no outward coping difficulties under normal conditions, the stress of a family member becoming victimized, by a rape or mugging for instance, can lead to such a stressful situation that usual coping mechanisms and lines of support do not function. This leads to interruption of the resolution of the trauma resulting from the act of violence. The family members of a rape victim may have such tremendous feelings about the event that they are unable to help the victim when she most needs it. In a larger sense they too need assistance with coming to grips with their feelings in order to resume a normal life.

Obviously, there are many issues involved with the study of victims and their problems which speak to the necessity for understanding and intervention by health care professionals. It is specifically necessary to examine the role of the nurse. Working with the victims and their families is an important aspect for nursing. This may be accomplished in several ways. The nurse is a practitioner who works with the client to deal with the physical and emotional trauma that is the result of a client being the victim of an act of violence. The nurse is a client advocate who will help the client negotiate the maze of legal, social service, and societal networks that victims must often be confronted with. The nurse is a change agent who recognizes the need for public education to dispel the many prevalent misconceptions that exist about victims of violence and the implications of being victimized. The nurse as change agent realizes that these misconceptions may hinder a victim's seeking help and, indeed, discourage preventive measures against further acts of violence. The nurse has a role as a researcher to investigate the causes and effects of violence on people, to establish the best ways to help the victims of that violence, and to institute preventive measures against the recurrence of such acts. The nurse has a role as a manager in the coordination of providing care to the victims of violence and their families. Finally, the nurse has a role as teacher in educating clients and the public at large about the implications and consequences of becoming a victim of violence.

In a discussion of what victimology is, it is necessary to examine the acts which create a victim and who is at risk to become one. In addition to the acts of violence mentioned previously, an individual or a group of individuals could be victimized by a variety of circumstances, like accident or illness, for example. In this chapter, however, the discussion will be limited to those violent events which, generally, result from and generate stress on the family unit, namely, rape, suicide, homocide, wife abuse, and child abuse.

When a violent act is committed, there is a target for that violence. That target becomes a victim. There are factors which make some individuals more vulnerable as potential victims. An individual may be at risk for becoming a victim by virtue of physical size or strength (e.g., women, children, the elderly), location (e.g., on a dark stairway, alone in a parking garage, in a high crime area), or circumstance (e.g., lack of protection, appearance, economic situation, domestic situation). Not all acts of violence have as their victims individuals who are identifiably at risk. In the case of random acts of violence, it is impossible to predict a potential victim.

RAPE

Rape is a violent crime in which sexual assault is only the primary mechanism by which the violence is perpetrated. It has been documented that the rapist's motivation is not, generally, sexual.[1] Frequently serious physical injury accompanies forced intercourse. Anal or oral sex may be part of the experience for the victim. Generally, rape has two components: that the sexual act took place and that it was without the consent of the victim. Rape victims range in age from infants to the very aged. The only thing they seem to have in common is that they were in the wrong place at the wrong time and were not able to avoid being raped. Because rapes are frequently not reported to the police, it is difficult to estimate the extent to which they occur. However, it has been estimated that only one rape in five is reported.[2] In 1973 the Federal Bureau of Investigation reported 51,000 cases of rape or attempted rape.[3] If this is the case, there were conceivably a quarter of a million cases of rape that year.

A woman may be reluctant to report a rape for fear of reprisal on the part of her attacker or for feelings of humiliation and shame. Many of these feelings are due to widespread misconceptions about rape and its victims. Women do not provoke rape. It is not always, or even usually, possible for a woman to avoid rape by struggling with her assailant. Since women are usually at a physical disadvantage with a potential rapist, the attacker will often threaten bodily harm if the woman resists him. There is often a weapon to back up that threat. Thus, resisting may increase the possibility of the victim incurring physical injuries. It may even lead to the rapist killing his victim. All women are potential targets for the would-be rapist. Although there are some common sense preventive measures that can be utilized to decrease the possibility of being raped, no woman is exempt from being the target of the rapist, regardless of age, appearance, status, or location. A sizable portion of reported rapes occur in the victim's own home. If a woman is going to be raped, it is hardly likely that she will "relax and enjoy it." Rape is a brutal assault and not a pleasurable experience by any stretch of the imagination.

Bringing charges against a rapist is a trying, difficult procedure for a woman to endure and she may choose to avoid additional stress by dropping or not pressing them. Due to the low arrest and conviction rate for rape, the victim may consider the whole process futile, in any event.

Recently much has been written of the consequences of rape. Burgess and Holmstrom[1] coined the phrase "rape trauma syndrome" to describe the impact of rape upon the individual. Victims experience considerable physical and emotional trauma from a rape. There are two phases of reaction. In the first or acute phase, which lasts several days following the rape, the victim may exhibit any of the following somatic complaints: specific or generalized soreness, disturbed eating or sleeping patterns, exaggerated emotional responses, increased irritability, and feelings of anger, anxiety, guilt, or shame.

During the second or resolution phase, the victim may change residences several times, have nightmares, develop phobias which are frequently related to the circumstances of the rape (being alone, being in the dark), or experience sexual dysfunction. As with all victims of violence, the woman who has been raped describes tremendous feelings of helplessness while being attacked.

The impact of rape on the family and friends of a victim varies. If the victim is a child or young adolescent, there are tremendous feelings of rage and guilt on the part of the parents. Fathers, particularly, describe wanting to kill or maim the rapist. There is almost always the feeling that there was something they could have done to prevent the rape on the part of the parents. Grief at loss of innocence is also a frequently voiced emotion by parents.

When the victim is an adult, anger and guilt are also present in the family's reaction, but the woman may also have to cope with other types of feelings. Was there something which the victim did to provoke the attack or some way in which she could have avoided it? The husband may have altered feelings about his wife's sexuality or morality which cause problems for both partners.

There are some measures which will decrease the probability of the woman becoming the victim of rape. Since it is always preferable to prevent such an occurrence rather than deal with its aftermath, these measures should be part of a nurse's health teaching wherever possible.

First, be aware that the environmental circumstances can be an invitation to the rapist. For instance, remove all evidence that suggests a residence is occupied by a woman alone, like telephone listings and names on a mailbox. List first initial and last name only. Keep a dog for protection, if possible. Install safety locks on doors and windows. Open door only when the caller is known. Insist on identification from repairmen, meter readers, and the like before admitting them to the home. Have a neighbor that could be signaled in the case of possible attack. Have hallways in apartment buildings and all doorways adequately lighted. Do not fumble for keys at the doorway, have keys ready before the door is reached.

Avoid dark, unlighted places, like parking garages. Always check the back seat of a car before entering it. If walking alone on a street, walk in the middle of the street, if possible. Avoid lonely streets. If there are people in the vicinity, a rapist is less likely to attempt an attack. Do not enter an elevator with someone who appears suspicious. When in an elevator, stay near the control panel so the emergency button can be reached if necessary. Avoid going anywhere alone. Do not wear chains around the neck, they can be used to choke or strangle. Weapons should be used with extreme caution. Do not use anything the attacker could grab and use. Avoid any clothing that could restrict movement.

If a confrontation with an attacker is suspected, it is most important to remain calm. If it is possible, avoid the situation by seeking a place with other people or that is well lighted, a store, for instance. Acting in an unexpected manner can sometimes prevent an attack, but use fighting and screaming cautiously. This type of behavior could further excite a rapist. Self-defense maneuvers should be used only by those who are familiar with them. If a blow fails to incapacitate an assailant, it may provoke further violence or injury. A good rule of thumb is to evade rather than fight off a rapist. Measures of self-protection should be planned whenever possible.

Finally, if attempts to avoid rape prove futile, try to remember everything possible that would enable the police to apprehend the rapist. Physical appearance plus distinguishing characteristics like birthmarks, scars, tattoos, jewelry, clothing, and the manner of speaking would be most beneficial to help identify the rapist. This also gives the victim some feeling of being able to control the situation. If she is able to gather some information which will help catch the rapist, she is not as apt to feel quite so helpless.

The nurse's role in disseminating this type of information is crucial and can involve all public health nurses, especially those in schools and industry.

Nurses may have several roles in treating a rape victim. There are two important aspects of care, physical and psychological. There is the added dimension of the legal ramifications, which the nurse should be cognizant of when caring for a rape victim. The first contact the nurse may have with a woman who has been raped is in the emergency room of a hospital. The victim may come in alone or with friends or be brought to the hospital by ambulance or by the police. She may be quite emotional and verbal or she may be withdrawn and display little affect. Sometimes a victim will call the hospital before arriving.

If this should be the case, it is important that the victim be made aware of the need for evidence should she decide to press charges against her assailant. One of the first things many women want to do after being raped is to change clothes and bathe. This destroys some of the physical evidence of the rape (presence of seminal fluid in the vaginal canal, for instance) and is therefore undesirable until after she has been examined by a physician, who may testify to his findings at a court proceeding. A woman may not be able to make a decision about this just after she has been raped, but advise the woman to come to the hospital immediately and bring the clothes she was wearing with her. Since the police may want them for evidence, it is desirable that the victim bring another change of clothing with her, if possible. Aside from the legal implications, the victim may be so immobilized from the trauma she has sustained that she may be unable to get to medical attention for any injuries she might have incurred. Advise her to contact a friend or family member to accompany her to the hospital or offer to contact someone for her if she seems unable to do this herself. If there is no one readily available to bring her to medical attention, suggest that she call the police or offer to do it for her.

The first concern when a rape victim seeks medical attention is treatment of any physical injury such as lacerations, broken bones, and internal injuries. Note carefully the client's appearance including contusions, swellings, abrasions, dirty or ripped clothing, and any stains present. This information is also very important for consideration of any legal action. Some hospitals have special forms to record this information for rape victims.

It is crucial to have a staff member with the victim at all times. In a busy emergency room, it is easy to understand that priorities might easily exclude staying with a quiet, withdrawn rape victim, when there is an automobile accident victim in shock next door and a heart attack victim down the hall. However, the rape victim's needs are just as great, if not as immediately life threatening. Emergency room personnel are becoming more aware of this. A staff that seemingly ignores the plight of the woman who has been raped may compound her trauma and heighten her sense of being alone and abandoned. Therapeutic intervention should be initiated as soon as possible. Assessing the client's needs for communication is the first step. The nurse should encourage the client to verbalize her feelings about her experience while being very supportive.

The emergency room treatment can be very stressful to an already exhausted, anxious client. This is due to the number of physicians, police, and other personnel who examine or interview the victim while she is in the emergency room. At many institutions there is a set procedure or protocol that is the standard for treating rape victims. Such protocols may vary somewhat from hospital to hospital but usually include several basic components. Assuming that there are no physical injuries which require immediate attention, a general physical examination is performed to ascertain whether there is any trauma which is not obvious. A gynecologic examination is done to look for any injury or physical evidence of rape, such as presence of seminal fluid in the vagina or tissue trauma. If the rape involved oral or anal intercourse, a detailed oral or rectal examination would be included. A prophylactic course of antibiotics, to prevent the development of venereal disease, is usually part of the medical protocol. While controversial, in view of the long and short term side effects, an antipregnancy medication, diethylstilbesterol (DES), may be offered. This is a difficult decision for a woman to make, but she should be aware of all the implications of this medication before she chooses whether or not to take it. DES is definitely contraindicated in a client with an established pregnancy due to the high incidence of cervical cancer in the daughters of women who were given DES during pregnancy. There is also frequent occurrence of severe nausea and vomiting as a side effect of the medication while it is being taken.

The nurse who is aware of the implications of rape trauma syndrome realizes that counseling and emotional support are a large part of the intervention necessary for the rape victim. If the nurse is with the victim immediately after the rape, it is beneficial to encourage the client to verbalize her feelings about the experience. Often the client will try to suppress the whole event saying, "I just want to forget the whole thing," or "I can't stand to even think about it." This delays working through the client's feelings surrounding the rape and will hinder the resolution of those feelings. It may result in an increase of the severity of somatic complaints. While encouraging expressing feelings about the experience, it is crucial that the nurse be very supportive of the client. Reinforce the expression of emotions. The victim may have difficulty making simple decisions and mobilizing herself. The nurse-counselor may help by making sure that the woman has someone to stay with and someway to get there. She may offer to get in touch with family or friends so that the client will have someone to be with.

Often friends or relatives have such strong reactions to rape that they feel uncomfortable in discussing the experience with the victim. This could result in the victim's having no outlet for expressing reactions and receiving support. This is another instance which requires intervention on the part of the nurse. Time should be set aside to talk with the friends or relatives who will accompany the client home and to explain to them the client's needs for someone to talk to about her experience and for support. A list of possible somatic complaints should also be included in teaching the family members about the aftermath of the rape experience. In addition, the family should be included in plans for followup treatment so that the impact of the rape upon family members can be assessed and dealt with. Followup care is an important aspect of treatment of the rape victim. At many hospitals there are now specific counseling programs for rape victims. They allow the victim to have immediate counseling while she is still in the emergency room and will followup on the client by means of telephone contact and scheduling appointments to see a counselor.

It may be difficult for the woman to envision feelings she will continue to experience as an aftermath of the rape experience. As a result of this she may not feel the necessity for counseling immediately after the rape. In such cases telephone contact a few days after the assault may be more effective in getting the client into counseling. If there is no specific rape counseling program available in any given institution, referral to an outpatient mental health clinic or a private therapist may be appropriate. In any case there are large volunteer networks, such as WAR (Women Against Rape), which have branches in most areas to which a victim may be referred.

Before the woman is discharged from the emergency room, she should have some understanding of what to expect from the phases of the rape trauma syndrome, and that such reactions are part of the normal resolution of the trauma she has incurred. She should be encouraged to seek professional help with trying to cope with her experience. If the assailant is apprehended and the victim chooses to prosecute charges, additional counseling may be needed to help her through this stressful time. Since there is a backlog of cases in many courts, the trial may take place months or years after the rape has taken place. Even if the trauma of the attack has been successfully resolved, the court proceeding often serves to make the victim relive the experience and the trauma.

CHILD ABUSE

There are several factors related with the incidence of child abuse. All of these are a function of some pathology in the parent's coping styles and relationships. Chief among them are stress, the parents' own childhood experiences, the parents' self-esteem, and the preparation they have had to become parents. Child abuse can include such injuries as lacerations, contusions, fractured bones, burns, or internal injuries. This trauma can be the result of direct action or the outcome of neglect. Frequently, these abusive acts come out of the frustration and anger on the part of the parent at his or her own inability to cope with a given situation. Child abuse, like rape, is frequently not associated with the victim's behavior and may be very difficult to predict. Child abuse occurs in every socio-economic group. Race and ethnicity do not appear to be factors. Child abuse occurs in families where parents are not prepared for their roles and have histories of pathologic relationships in their own upbringings. Abusing parents have "usually perceived their own parents as unloving, cruel, and brutal."[4] Many of them have been abused children themselves.

Child abuse is symptomatic of a malfunctioning family situation. Abusive parents, if they realize there is a problem, are reluctant to seek help because of the stigma attached to being labeled a child abuser. Many abusive parents have had childhood experiences which make establishing trust difficult. Frequently, parents will try to conceal the real reasons for a child's injury for fear of the reaction they would elicit. Therefore, diagnosis of child abuse is often incidental. Abusive parents lack sufficient self-esteem to seek help. Abuse or neglect may derive from ignorance of how to parent. An abused child may be one whose parents do not have adequate knowledge to provide proper diet, clothing, or safety precautions for children. Since abusing parents have frequently been abused as children, often they have not had adequate role models to develop the skills of parenting successfully.

A child cannot defend himself so the impact of child abuse is also associated with a tremendous feeling of helplessness on the part of the child. In addition, if he is abused by his parents, he will not be able to develop a sense of trust and his psychosocial development will be impaired.[5] Abused children demonstrate a higher incidence of mental retardation and speech difficulties.[5] They typically have a poor self-concept. The child may be used as a scapegoat for parental anger and frustration. Abused children tend to react physically, rather than verbally, and often the response is out of proportion with what triggered it. Hyperaggressive behavior frequently follows abuse. Since the role model of the parent is apt to be poor, the child has poor self-control. An abused child may harm a younger sibling or destroy an inanimate object. Behavior in school may also be problematic.

Abusing parents tend to have unrealistic expectations of a child's behavior. An example would be that of an abusing parent perceiving a two month old infant's crying as a deliberate action on the part of the child to annoy the parent. These unrealistic expectations may take other forms. If there are several children in a family, the eldest may be expected to assume traditional parenting functions at a very early age. In one study,[5] there is documentation of three and four year olds taking responsibility for younger siblings. Indeed, there is evidence of role reversal with the child acting as parent to the mother or father. This can lead to a mutigenerational pattern of child abuse where roles are not clearly defined, and a vicious cycle of abused child growing into abusing parent evolving.

The reactions of outsiders to the abusive family is generally one that encourages secrecy and discourages attempts by the family to seek help by failing to provide any support systems. Abused children may be encountered by the nurse in the hospital, if the child has sustained an injury severe enough to warrant the parents seeking medical attention for the child. School nurses may encounter battered children in the community through referral, as can public health nurses. The parent will frequently lie about the cause of the injury in an attempt to conceal the fact that abuse is taking place.

If a case of child abuse is suspected, the nurse has a professional and legal obligation to report this to the authorities. This may vary somewhat from state to state due to differing laws. Who may report a case of suspected child abuse varies from physician to hospitals, nurses, school teachers, social workers, and others.[6] The nurse should be cognizant of the local regulations affecting the handling of such reports. If the nurse does have the responsibility for reporting a case of suspected child abuse, a detailed description of any injuries, including the size and location of cuts, bruises, or burns is required. The report may also need to include descriptions of the child's environment, behavior, and activity, as well as that of the parent.

Since making this kind of report can easily alienate a parent who has difficulty establishing trust to begin with, developing a therapeutic relationship with the family can be hindered. It is important to remember that in a family where child abuse exists all the members of that family can be considered victims of this situation and in need of intervention by health care professionals. The nurse has a unique opportunity in this situation. "Public health nurses bring a variety of skills to aid these families, and in some situations constitute the main therapeutic contact."[7] Although a family where child abuse is present is an extremely complex and difficult situation that can be life threatening for the child, removing the child from the home, temporarily or permanently, can exacerbate the problems that are present. It may lead to total disintegration of the family unit. Since child abuse is indicative of problems in functioning with the entire family, a multidisciplinary approach to treatment with a team of health care workers is usually indicated.

Treatment goals would include immediate behavior modification to limit impulsive and violent actions on the part of the parents. They need to explore with a therapist the reasons for their actions so that they can understand why they behave the way they do under stress. Alternate, acceptable modes of behavior should be reinforced. A mechanism as simple as counting to ten before taking any action when angry has proved to be a useful tool for the abusive parent to utilize. Since the behavior of both the parent and the child in an abusive family tends to be physical rather than verbal, having the parent verbally set limits on behavior that the parent will tolerate will let the child know how the parent will react in a certain situation. This begins to work toward the development of trust.

Long term treatment goals would consist of therapy aimed at improving the self-image of both the parent and the child, programs to teach the skills of parenting, and increasing parent's knowledge of a child's needs and development. Parents and children will require constant reinforcement if the pattern of abusive behavior in a family is to be changed. Helfer and Kempe[7] estimate that, even under the best conditions, only 80 percent of abusive families can be treated with satisfactory results. The implications of this premise is that even if all abusive families were to seek treatment, there would be a sizable number that could not function successfully as a unit, even with help. If these families were then broken up there would be additional trauma to the children and parents and need for further intervention.

One of the most difficult problems for the potential abusive parents is that they feel they have no support systems that will help them when they feel they are likely to lose control and become abusive. Recently, because of the public exposure of the problem of child abuse, groups of volunteers and professionals have formed to provide emergency counseling to abusive or potentially abusive parents. Groups like CAPE (Child Abuse Prevention Effort) and Childline provide free and confidential telephone counseling on a 24-hour-a-day basis. This type of public awareness has to continue to provide somewhere for parents and children to seek help and prevent the occurrence of child abuse.

WIFE ABUSE

There are many similarities between wife and child abuse. They may occur simultaneously and may have many of the same causes. In the case of abuse of the spouse, it is one partner who abuses the other and the victim is usually the woman. The type of physical injuries that can occur with wife abuse are the same as with child abuse, that is, bruises, lacerations, fractured bones, and internal injuries. In addition the abused wife may experience social isolation, ridicule, or economic deprivation. As with child abuse, wife abuse occurs in every strata of society and in all societal groups.

Wife abuse is frequently treated as a "domestic disturbance" by authorities who attempt to intercede as a referee instead of removing the husband from the home. After the police leave, the husband may resume his violent behavior in retribution for his wife's seeking outside aid. Women may be made to feel at fault for precipitating a beating by some action of their own. For these reasons, a woman may be reluctant to seek help. Due to limited resources of support systems, skills, or money, a woman may feel she has no option but to stay in an abusive marriage. This compounds her feelings of helplessness as a victim. As in the case of rape, there are many popular misconceptions which interfere with reporting and treating wife abuse. Generally, women do not derive masochistic pleasure from being beaten. A battered wife may choose to remain with her husband for a variety of reasons. She may fear more severe beatings if she attempts to leave. Her husband may have threatened the children with harm to keep his wife at home. She may have religious reasons to attempt to salvage her marriage. If a woman has no financial resources of her own, she may elect to remain in an abusive situation. Another myth regarding wife abuse is that the woman deserves or provokes the violent behavior of the husband. It is impossible to predict or prevent abuse and the woman is the victim of the violence and not the cause. An event as trivial as failure to pick up a suit at the cleaners may precipitate a beating. In many instances, there is no identifiable event which could be considered even remotely provocative. This is consistent with the fact that the abusive behavior on the part of the husband is his attempt to deal with his own anger and frustration. That anger or frustration may have nothing to do with anything that has occurred in the home, such as the husband who beats his wife as a response to some pressure or problem at his work. As with child abuse, the abusive husband has poor impulse control.

Wife abuse is not a problem that is limited to lower income or poorly educated populations. A battered woman may be young or elderly, married or not, or may or may not have children. The length of marriage or economic status has little correlation to the occurrence of wife abuse. Women are frequently abused while pregnant, and it is often difficult to outwardly identify the family where wife abuse exists.

In a study by Pfouts,[8] coping styles of abused wives were examined. The style that the wife chose depended on her overall evaluation of the benefits and costs of her marital relationship and the alternatives that were available to her. The benefits would include financial security and social approval and the costs might include physical and emotional abuse and negative effects on the children. Four different types of coping styles were found.

The first coping style is when the costs of the marriage outweigh the benefits, and the alternatives outside the marriage are not acceptable. The wife feels trapped in a situation which she feels she can do little to alter. She blames herself for her inability to escape and may come to believe that she deserves the abuse she is receiving. This results in a very poor self-concept in the victim.

When the marriage has benefits that outweigh the costs and she does not have any viable alternatives outside the marriage, the woman is apt to respond with aggressive behavior. This can manifest itself in violence towards her husband; she will fight back. More frequently, however, the children or another outside relationship are what the woman utilizes to release her anger.

If a woman has alternatives that are preferable to an abusive marriage and the benefits of that marriage are low, she is apt to move out of the situation quickly or insist that the abuse cease. If the benefits of the marriage are high and there is also the existence of alternatives outside the marriage, the woman may stay in the relationship for a longer period of time before opting for an alternative. When she does leave, she does so reluctantly.

The first or self-punishing response is easily the most pathologic for the woman. The victim feels the most helpless and has the poorest self-concept. Serious physical injury can occur in any of these situations, but repeated abuse is more likely when the woman has no or poor resources outside the marriage.

The problems of secrecy are just as prevalent with wife abuse as they are with child abuse. The woman may attempt to protect her husband by not seeking help, or she may feel too afraid or helpless to do anything which will alleviate the abusive situation.

The role of the nurse is to provide support and help the woman sort out her feelings and alternatives. She may encounter the battered wife in the hospital or in the community. Since a family where wife abuse exists is indicative of problems with all family members, an assessment of each member is necessary to determine treatment. Traditionally, there has been no place for a woman with limited resources to go if she feels that she must leave her home. Recently, a few temporary shelters have been opened that will house a woman and her children and will provide counseling that will help her resolve what she wishes to do with her life. However, these are few in number and located chiefly in urban areas so that they are frequently filled and not available to rural women.

Grief and guilt are the two main issues that the nurse can help the battered wife work through. An abused wife will experience loss.[9] That is, she will go through the grieving process much the same as that of a death. In a sense her hope, belief, and trust in her marriage and her husband have died. She may deny what has happened to her through repression because she cannot face the reality of the situation. She may exhibit bizzare or inappropriate behavior or disbelief of what has happened. She may think that she has caused her husband's abusive behavior.

As with child abuse, treatment goals should be aimed at improving the woman's self-image and should provide her with resources that will enable her to leave the abusive situation, should she choose to do so. If possible to save the family unit, the husband can be engaged in therapy to examine his own motivations for his actions and explore alternate methods of expressing his feelings. Behavior modification to improve impulse control is the first priority. Children are also victims in a family where wife abuse exists. Whether or not they have been direct objects of physical abuse, they will undoubtedly have been aware of the problem and have been subjected to psychologic trauma.

A woman may not be ready to admit the need for counseling, but, if this is the case, there are some steps the nurse can encourage for the woman's protection in the future. Preventive measures such as planning a possible place to go in the event of a crisis situation would be an important step toward mobilizing the victim and helping her feel somewhat in control. Alleviating some of the helplessness the wife feels in an abusive marriage may give her more bargaining power for altering the marital situation to a more acceptable one for the woman, or allowing her to feel that she can leave it, should that be her choice.

SUICIDE AND HOMOCIDE

Suicide and homocide are both violent crimes that create several types of victims. Within the context discussed in this chapter, not only the people who are killed by suicide or homocide are considered to be victims of those crimes, but families and friends also are defined as victims. The especially violent nature of death in homocides and suicides further complicates the family's coping with the loss of a mother, father, child, or sibling by imposing the additional stress of the violent crime itself.

Many of the previous situations discussed in this chapter can lead to either suicide or homocide. The wife who cannot deal with an abusive marriage and sees no other alternative to that marriage may have such a low self-concept that she may seek to kill herself. Many children have died as a result of beatings inflicted by their parents. Rape victims have been murdered as well as sexually molested. An abusive parent may feel self-destructive.

In these terribly complex and tragic occurrences, there are so many issues that require the intervention of health care professionals. Identifying those persons who need help and the issues that require the attention of the nurse are the first priorities for treatment. The natural feelings of antipathy and revulsion that accompany the parent who has just beaten a child to death must be put in perspective to be able to recognize the tremendous feelings of self-loathing and guilt that that person must be experiencing. The father who cannot bear to be in the same room with his 14-year-old daughter who has been raped is just as much in a crisis state and in need of immediate help as is his daughter. The children of an elderly woman who has been mugged and killed at a bus stop will need assistance in working through the anger that they feel about the injustice of the event.

In each of these circumstances and many conceivable others, the element of shock at the violence and suddenness of the trauma they have experienced may lead to a variety of bizzare and inappropriate behavior. The nurse has the responsibility to provide support for the victim to verbalize the feelings he has about the trauma sustained and explore and define the underlying issues of grief, guilt, anger, or frustration that contribute to the victim's perception of helplessness.

CONCLUSIONS

A victim's feeling of being unable to avoid or escape the situation that is doing him harm is the main concern of the nurse in dealing with the victims of violence. The treatment modalities that the nurse utilizes will depend upon the extent and nature of the trauma the victim has suffered and the coping abilities of the victim on each specific situation.

Another role that the nurse plays in alleviating the problems that victims experience is that of public education of the real needs and concerns of victims of violence. Taking these occurrences out of the closet and providing easy access to treatment without stigma will go a long way to stop and prevent them. Community awareness of the plight of the victim will also provide the support systems that they so desperately need. If a victim knows that there is help available then, perhaps, they will not feel quite so helpless.

REFERENCES

1. Burgess, A.W., and Holmstrom, L.L.: *Rape: Victims of Crisis.* Robert J. Brady Company, Bowie, Md., 1974.
2. Brownmiller, S.: *Against Our Will: Men, Women, and Rape.* Simon and Schuster, New York, 1975.
3. Pepitone-Rockwell, F.: "Patterns of Rape and Approaches to Care." *The Journal of Family Practice,* 3(3):521, 1978.
4. Flanzreich, M., and Dunsavage, I.: "Role Reversal in Abused/Neglected Families: Implications Child Welfare Workers." *Children Today,* Nov.-Dec. 1977.
5. Green, Arthur H.: "Psychopathology of Abused Children." *Journal of Child Psychiatry,* 17:92.
6. Helfer, Ray E., and Kempe, C. Henry (eds.): *The Battered Child,* 2nd ed. The University of Chicago Press, Chicago, 1974.
7. Helfer, R., and Kempe, C. Henry: *Helping the Battered Child and His Family.* J. B. Lippincott Company, Philadelphia, 1972.
8. Pfouts, J.: "Violent Families: Coping Responses of Abused Wives." *Journal of the Child Welfare League of America,* 17:101, 1978.
9. Lieberknecht, Kay: "Helping the Battered Wife." *American Journal of Nursing,* 78:654, 1978.

UNIT V

MAJOR SOCIAL ISSUES AFFECTING COMMUNITY HEALTH

The chapters in this unit have impact on all segments of society. Nutritional issues and grief, dying, and death are directly encountered by all of us. Disabilities, depending to a large extent on the kind and degree of impairment, may or may not be directly experienced. Sensitivity to the influence of these issues will contribute to the degree of nursing intervention chosen. It will be necessary to look beyond the individual or group directly involved and closely examine attitudes, laws, and the environment which may support or impair health enhancing choices. Only by assessing the social and environmental mores, attitudes, assets, and limitations will effective changes be made. Nurses in the community will play an active role identifying and then intervening to provide or enhance health oriented options for the individual, family, and community.

CHAPTER 30
COMMUNITY NUTRITION

THALIA METALIDES, M.S., R.D.

"The nutrition educator must be aware of those culturally accepted norms which affect food ways. Only by working within this established framework can the (health professional) make the appropriate recommendations that will bring about behavioral change. Change is a gradual process and too many recommendations or too drastic a suggestion may overwhelm the individual. The nutrition educator must concentrate on the positive aspects of an individual's diet and encourage the strengthening of these positive habits."[1]

This chapter will acquaint the student with the role of good nutrition in the total health care of individuals and families. It will provide the tools needed to appraise the clients' food practices and to determine their nutritional needs.

INTRODUCTION TO THE SCIENCE OF NUTRITION

Over the centuries man's approach to acquiring food has changed. Originally herbivorous, he became carnivorous as he developed weapons and eventually moved into an agrarian mode of providing food. Food became available all year long as he devised storage methods and learned to process foods to avoid spoilage. Today science and technology seek new agricultural methods to grow, process, and transport food to market, i.e., fertilizers to enrich soil, farm machinery, proper feed for animals, and so forth.

With increasing sophistication and scientific knowledge, humans began to see the relationship of food to the body. They learned that food supplied fuel (known today as kilocalories) and that foods were made up of three main components—carbohydrates, protein, and fat. It was not until the early twentieth century that vitamins and minerals were discovered by their association with deficiency diseases and a new area of science began.

Nutrition can be described as the science and art of feeding the body. The *science* of nutrition is the interrelationship of foods, their nutrients, and bodily functions, which is necessary to maintain health and prevent disease. The *art* of nutrition is the application of the science of nutrition. In order for the health practitioner to apply the science of nutrition, he or she must know the dynamics of culture, environment, religion, economy, and educational levels on the individual. We will explore the impact of these factors on the nutritional status of the individual through the life cycle. Table 30-1 identifies several nutrition resources to be used in meeting client needs at various life cycle stages and will be referred to throughout this chapter.

BASIC PRINCIPLES OF NUTRITION

The most important role that food plays is that of nourishing the body. Foods wisely chosen provide all the nutrients that are necessary for the proper functioning of the body. Foods improperly selected will result in a deficiency of one or more essential nutrients (essential nutrients are those which the body needs and is unable to synthesize).

Nutrients needed daily are carbohydrates, protein, fats, vitamins, minerals, and water. These nutrients supply energy, promote growth, repair tissue, and regulate the body processes (Tables 30-2 and 30-3). Each day selecting foods according to the nutrients they provide helps insure a balanced diet (Table 30-3).

The basic nutrients needed from foods are the same throughout the life cycle, but the amount of nutrients needed changes with growth, pregnancy, lactation, stress of illness, and surgery.

INFANT FEEDING

The feeding practices during infancy are based on a period of rapid growth and reflect developmental milestones, i.e., the infant as a passive suckling gradually developing his active self-feed skills by the end of the first year. In determining the nutritional needs of the young child, it is also important to consider the prevention of future nutrition-related health problems (obesity, atherosclerosis, dental caries, anemia).[2] This is also the time for nutrition education of the mother who helps formulate her infant's food habits. These baseline food practices set the pace for a lifetime of continued optimal nutrition.

Breast Feeding vs. Bottle Feeding

Infants will grow satisfactorily and do well with breast feeding, bottle feeding, or a combination of the two.[3,4] The reasons mothers choose one form of feeding over another reflect culture, social class, economics, and educational level.

TABLE 30-1. Nutrition resources within the community

Program	Eligibility	Program content
Maternal and Child Health	Pregnant women and children of low income families	Free Improved health care services for mothers and children at a clinic affiliated with a specific hospital. Free vitamins, prescription drugs. Includes maternal and infant care, children and youth services, family planning, dental care, intensive infant care, nursing services, nutrition services, and social services
Special Supplemental Food Program for Women, Infants, and Children (WIC)	Individuals at nutritional risk: Pregnant women up to 6 months postpartum. Nursing mothers up to 1 year. Infants and children up to age 5 identified as being at nutritional risk. Must live in geographically determined low income area and be eligible for reduced price or free medical care. Must be certified by WIC staff member. Periodic assessment of risk status.	Provision of supplement foods: <6 months: iron fortified formula and infant cereals, fruit juice high in vitamin C. >6 months: whole fluid milk may be substituted for formula, iron fortified infant cereal, fruit juice high in vitamin C. Women and children: whole fluid milk and/or cheese, eggs, iron fortified hot or cold cereal, fruit or vegetable high in vitamin C. Food distribution: directly from participating agency, via voucher system, or home delivered. Nutrition education is an integral part of program.
Crippled Children's Services	Children with handicapping conditions (such as PKU, cystic fibrosis).	Under Title V. Comprehensive medical, surgical, corrective health serivces (including hospitalization and after care services) aimed at restoration of maximal health. Funds available for purchase of equipment or supplies (Lofenalac for PKU; MCT oil for cystic fibrosis).
Project Head Start	Preschool children age 3 and older.	Year round program. Complete health services, nutrition activities, social services, psychological services, parent involvement in all areas.
School Breakfast Program	All public and nonprofit private schools. Public and licensed nonprofit residential child care institutions.	As set by US Dept of Agriculture: Nonprofit breakfasts meeting nutritional standards. Served free or at a reduced price to children from low income families.

TABLE 30-1. Continued.

Program	Eligibility	Program content
School Breakfast Program (continued)	For needy children or those who travel great distances to school.	Cost to schools reimbursed by federal funds.
National School Lunch Program	All public and nonprofit private school pupils of high school grade or under, some residential institutions and temporary shelters.	As set by US Dept of Agriculture: Nonprofit nutritious lunches offered free or at a reduced price to those who cannot pay. "Type A" lunch follows specified guidelines and meets $1/3$ or more of daily dietary allowance. Schools reimbursed by federal and state funds.
Title VII: Nutrition Program for the Elderly	Those 60 years of age or older and spouses.	1 hot meal/day (offering approximately $1/3$ of day's requirements) 5 days/week. Served in a centrally located group setting in the community.
Meals on Wheels	Elderly over 60 who are unable to leave home.	Centrally prepared meal delivered to home offering approximately $1/3$ of day's requirements.
Food Stamps	Eligibility based on total income, expenses, number being fed in household. Each applicant is considered on an individual basis.	Client should apply at local Food Stamp Office within the community presenting wage slips, sources of income, rent receipts, utility bills. Food Stamps are given free of charge depending on eligibility needs. Used like cash to purchase food at authorized food stores (nonfood items and alcoholic beverages not allowed).

Prior to the twentieth century, breast feeding was the major source of early infant nutrition. Later, however, formula preparations were introduced for infants whose mothers had an inadequate milk supply, who were unable to nurse, or needed to terminate nursing.[5-7] With its initial acceptance and technologic advances (pasteurization, refrigeration, formulation more closely resembling human milk)[5,6] came other reasons for bottle feeding: it became popular in urban settings where mothers had to work and health professionals saw the ready-to-feed formulas on maternity wards as a quick and easy way to feed infants which mothers perceived as an endorsement of bottle feeding.[5-7]

The current trend is toward a "natural" form of feeding. The feeding of choice is breast milk whenever possible and has, in fact, been endorsed by the American Academy of Pediatrics.[6,8] The nutritional advantages of breast milk include: an appropriate nutrient content and distribution of calories necessary for growth and development; an easily absorbed form of fat; a better quality protein; a source of iron which, although insufficient after infant stores are depleted, is better absorbed than the small amount found in cow's milk.[6,8]

There are more than nutritional benefits to breast milk: immunoglobulins secreted into breast milk help protect the infant from infections; to a certain extent breast feeding acts as a natural, though unreliable, contraceptive (ovulation and menstruation being delayed up to six months in some women);[4,6,7] the incidence of breast cancer is lower;[4] there may be an increase in mother-infant "bonding;"[6] and the infant determines the total amounts he will consume with little or no influence from the mother,[5,8] an important aspect in the prevention of future obesity.

Although meeting most of the nutritional needs of the infant up to age six months, human milk is still not "perfect" and needs to be supplemented with iron, vitamin D, and possibly fluoride.[4,8,9]

For the infant whose mother is unable or unwilling to breast feed, a wide variety of proprietary milk formulas is available. The most basic type (evaporated milk with the addition of carbohydrate) still remains in many countries today. It is not as nutritionally adequate as commercial formulas and if used should also be supplemented. All commercial formulas are based on a modification of the carbohydrates, protein, and fat of cow's milk with the addition of vitamins and minerals to more closely resemble human milk. Iron fortified formulas are generally recommended for all infants. To avoid excess feeds, a rough rule of thumb for the amount of feeding is: age in months $+3$ = number of ounces per feeding. Table 30-4 identifies the advantages and disadvantages of bottle feeding.

Vitamin Supplementation

The infant's sole source of nutrients for the first four to six months should be breast milk (supplemented with iron and vitamin D) or formula supplemented with iron. Fluoride supplementation is recommended "shortly after birth in breast fed infants and according to the fluoride content of the drinking water in formula fed infants."[10] However, it is also noted that instituting fluoride supplementation as late as six months of age has been shown to result in a decreased incidence of dental caries while maintaining fluorosis of the enamel at a minimum.[10]

Introduction of Solids

Although tolerated at an early age, the introduction of solid food should be discouraged until four to six months when the infant is developmentally ready.[8,9] There is a decided disadvantage to the early use of solids (earlier than four months) due to a possible increase in calories which can set the stage for infant obesity and childhood obesity as well as permanent adult obesity.[8,9] The mechanism is unclear and may in fact be the result of environment and cultural effects.[10]

When solids are begun, they should be offered one at a time in an appropriate sequence

TABLE 30-2. Major function of nutrients

Sources of energy	Growth and maintenance	Regulation of body processes
Carbohydrate	Protein	Protein
Protein	Mineral elements	Mineral elements
Fats	Vitamins	Vitamins
	Water	Water

to minimize possible allergic sensitivity.[8] Food texture is increased gradually until the infant is able to accept table foods (Tables 30-5 and 30-6).

Nutritional Problems of Infancy

OBESITY

As prevention of obesity is preferable to treatment especially during infancy, parents should be encouraged to offer breast milk or formula as a primary source of nutrients and to avoid "force" (or over) feeding, to consider solid foods as a supplementary source of nutrients at four to six months of age, and to encourage an increase in appropriate physical activity for age. The use of skim milk formulas should be discouraged during the first year as the high energy needs for growth must be met. Only after age one should caloric restriction be considered.[8,9] Vigorous education of the parents, especially the mother as the "gatekeeper," is important including the kind and amount of foods needed by the infant.[11]

IRON-DEFICIENCY ANEMIA

Iron-deficiency anemia is most common among infants and children especially between 6 and 24 months of age.[2,12] It is attributed primarily to the low iron content in human and cow's milk and the poor utilization of the iron in cow's milk. Therefore Fomon[2] recommends 1) that all breast fed infants and infants on evaporated milk formulas receive iron supplementation (7 mg daily as ferrous sulfate or other preparation of similar bioavailability), and 2) that infants fed commercial formulas should be given iron fortified formulas. As the young child takes less milk and more solids, iron fortified cereals and/or foods naturally high in iron should be encouraged (Table 30-7).

DENTAL CARIES

Many children will have some dental caries by the age of two with an increase in incidence with age. The young child who is allowed to go to bed with a bottle is a prime candidate for the *nursing bottle syndrome.* It is the contact of sugar sweetened liquids or juice or just plain milk on the surface of the child's teeth which encourages the destruc-

TABLE 30-3. Food-nutrient profile

Food	Nutrients Supplied	Suggested Daily Amounts*

MILK
milk, cheese, ice cream, yogurt
	protein
	calcium, phosphorous
	riboflavin
	vitamin A
	vitamin D, if fortified
	varying amounts of other
	    vitamins & minerals
		2-4 servings
		1 serving =
		    toddlers: $\frac{1}{2}$-$\frac{3}{4}$ cup × 3
		    children: $\frac{3}{4}$-1 cup × 3
		adolescents: 1 cup × 4
		adults: 1 cup × 2
		pregnant women: 1 cup × 4
		nursing mothers: 1 cup × 4
		elderly: $\frac{3}{4}$-1 cup × 2

MEAT
lean meats, fish, seafood, poultry; dry beans, peas, nuts, peanut butter, eggs,† cheese
	protein
	iron
	B-complex vitamins
	minerals (phosphorous,
	    zinc, magnesium)
	varying amounts of other
	    vitamins & minerals
		2 or more servings
		1 serving =
		    toddlers: 1-2 oz.
		    children: 2-3 oz.
		    adolescents: 3-4 oz.
		    adults: 2-3 oz.
		    pregnant women: 2-3 oz.
		    nursing mothers: 2-3 oz.
		    elderly: 2-3 oz.
		$\frac{1}{2}$ cup legumes = 1 serving

FRUITS and VEGETABLES
include daily 1 serving rich in vitamin C as citrus fruit (orange, grapefruit) strawberries, broccoli
3-4 × /week include a dark green or deep yellow vegetable or fruit (for vitamin A) as carrots, winter squash, spinach, green peppers; other fruits and vegetables as potato, corn, apples, bananas, tomatoes
	vitamin C
	vitamin A
	folic acid
	varying amounts of other
	    vitamins & minerals
		4 or more servings
		1 serving =
		    toddlers: $\frac{1}{4}$ cup or $\frac{1}{2}$
		        medium portion
		    children: $\frac{1}{2}$ cup or
		    adolescents: 1 medium
		    adults: portion as
		pregnant women: apple,
		nursing mothers: tomato,
		    elderly: potato

BREADS and CEREALS
whole grain or enriched breads, cereals, macaroni, noodles, spaghetti, rice, crackers
	B-complex vitamins
	iron
	varying amounts of other
	    vitamins & minerals
		4 or more servings
		1 serving =
		    toddlers: $\frac{1}{2}$ slice bread; $\frac{1}{4}$-$\frac{1}{2}$
		    cup cereal products
		    children: 1 slice bread; $\frac{1}{2}$-1
		    cup cereal products
		    adolescents: 1 slice bread; 1 cup
		    cereal products
		    adults: 1 slice bread; $\frac{1}{2}$-$\frac{3}{4}$ cup
		    cereal products
		    pregnant women: 1 slice bread;
		    $\frac{1}{2}$-$\frac{3}{4}$ cup cereal products
		    nursing mothers: 1 slice bread;
		    $\frac{1}{2}$-$\frac{3}{4}$ cup cereal products
		    elderly: 1 slice bread; $\frac{1}{2}$-$\frac{3}{4}$
		    cup cereal products

*Include larger servings and/or butter, margarine, mayonnaise, oil, sugars for caloric requirements.
†Current information suggests limiting eggs to 3-4 per week.

TABLE 30-4. Advantages and disadvantages of bottle feeding

Advantages	Disadvantages
Convenient	Can be made more concentrated or too dilute
Constancy of nutrients if made properly	Infant encouraged to take more (to finish)
For working mother	Often fed solids earlier because of hunger thus
For mother who is uncomfortable or anxious about breast feeding	increasing total calories
	Hazardous in areas where sanitary conditions
For mother who is a drug or alcohol abuser	are poor
For mother who has chronic illness and/or infection	Early conditioning to sugar
	Expensive (especially ready-to-feed variety)

TABLE 30-5. Feeding guidelines for infants during the first 6 months†

	0-2 weeks	2 weeks-2 mo	2 mo	3 mo	4-5 mo	5-6 mo
Formula						
Per feeding	2-3 oz	3-5 oz	5 oz	6-6$^{1}/_2$ oz	7-8 oz	7-8 oz
Average total	22 oz	28 oz	30 oz	32-34 oz	32 oz	28 oz
Number of feedings	6-8	5-6	5-6	5	4-5	4-5
Food texture	Liquids	Liquids	Liquids	Liquids	Baby soft	Baby soft
Food additions						
Apple juice‡						3-4 oz
Baby cereal, enriched					2-2$^{1}/_2$ tbsp, B & S	3 tbsp, B & S
Strained fruits					1$^{1}/_2$-3 tbsp, B, L, & S	2-3 tbsp, B, L, & S
Strained vegetables					1-2 tbsp, L	2-3 tbsp, L
Strained meats						1-2 tbsp, L
Egg yolk or baby egg yolk						$^{1}/_2$ med or 1 tbsp
Teething biscuit						$^{1}/_2$-1
Total calories	440	560	600	660-680	729-788	791-870
Recommended calories (117 cal/kg)	410	410-608	608	667	725-784	784-878
Oral and neuromuscular development related to food intake	Rooting, sucking, swallowing	Rooting, sucking, swallowing	Rooting, sucking, swallowing	Extrusion reflex diminishes; sucking becomes voluntary	Learning to put hands to mouth; develops grasp	Chewing begins; can approximate lips to rim of cup

*From Scipien, G. M. et al.: *Comprehensive Pediatric Nursing.* McGraw-Hill Book Co., New York, 1979, with permission.

†Calculations based on male growing at the 50th percentile for height and weight.

‡Offer from the cup.

B = breakfast, L = lunch, S = supper

TABLE 30-6. Feeding guidelines for infants 6 to 12 months old*†

	6-7 mo	7-8 mo	8-9 mo	9-10 mo	10-11 mo	11-12 mo
Whole milk						
Per feeding	8 oz‡	8 oz	8 oz	8 oz	8 oz	8 oz
Average total	28 oz	28 oz	24 oz	24 oz	24 oz	24 oz
Number of feedings	3-4	3-4	3	3	3	3
Food texture	Gradual increase	⟶ Mashed table ⟶			⟶	Cut fine
Food items						
Orange juice	4 oz	4 oz	4 oz	4 oz	4 oz	4 oz
Fortified cereal	1/3 cup, B	1/3 cup, B	1/2 cup, B	1/2 cup, B	1/2 cup, B	1/2 cup, B
Fruit, canned or fresh	4 tsp, B, L, & S	4 tsp, B, L, & S	2 tbsp, L & S	2/3 tbsp, L & S	3 tbsp, L & S	3 tbsp, L & S
Vegetables	1 1/2 tbsp, L & S	2 tbsp, L & S	2 tbsp, L & S	2 tbsp, L & S	3 tbsp, L & S	2 1/2 tbsp, L & S
Meat, fish, poultry	1 tbsp, L & S	2 tbsp, L & S	2 tbsp, L & S	2 tbsp, L & S	2 1/2 tbsp, L & S	2 1/2 tbsp, L & S
Egg yolk or baby egg yolk	1 med yolk, or 2 tbsp	1 med yolk, or 2 tbsp	1 med yolk, or 2 tbsp	1 whole egg	1 whole egg	1 whole egg
Teething biscuit or bread	1 biscuit	1 biscuit	1/2 slice bread	1/2 slice bread	1/2 slice bread	1/2 slice bread
Starch—potato, rice, macaroni				2 tbsp, S	2 tbsp, S	2 tbsp, S
Dessert—custard, pudding						2 tbsp, S
Butter		1 tsp	1 tsp	1 tsp	1 tsp	1 tsp
Total calories	859	876	937	974	1037	1069
Recommended calories (108 kcal/kg)	810-864	864-918	918-972	972-1015	1015-1048	1048-1083
Oral and neuromuscular development related to food intake	Begins using cup Sits erect with support ⟶ Feeds self biscuit ⟶			Without support ⟶ Holds bottle	Picks up small food items and releases	Will hold and lick spoon after dipped into food; self-feeding

*From Scipien, G. M., et al.: *Comprehensive Pediatric Nursing.* McGraw-Hill Book Co., New York, 1979 with permission.

†Calculations based on male growing at the 50th percentile for height and weight.

‡Offer small amounts (2-4 oz) when milk is presented from the cup.

B = breakfast, L = lunch, S = supper

TABLE 30-7. Iron rich foods

Best Sources:	meat, fish, poultry (especially liver, kidney, red meats, liverwurst)
Good Sources:	enriched breads and cereals; iron fortified cereals (check labels); dark green leafy vegetables (oxalate content may interfere with absorption); cooked dried beans and peas; dried fruits; molasses
Poor Sources:	milk and milk products

tion of tooth substance especially the upper deciduous teeth.[13] The most obvious solution to this problem is the elimination of the bedtime bottle. Should this prove catastrophic to the child, plain water in the bottle is recommended. The teeth should also be wiped clean with a gauze pad prior to any feeding to eliminate interaction of fermentable carbohydrate with existing placque.[13]

A diet rich in protective foods eaten during periods of tooth formation, maturation, and mineralization can help make a tooth significantly resistant to decay.[14] The most important nutrient is fluoride. Proper fluoridation of public water supplies in areas where the fluoride content is naturally low has been demonstrated to control the incidence of dental caries and is recommended by the Committee on Nutrition, American Academy of Pediatrics.[15]

The control of dental caries includes: 1) fluoridation of public water supplies or the provision of an alternate source of fluoride; 2) a well balanced diet composed of a variety of foods appropriate for age; 3) the elimination of between meal snacks composed largely of sugars; 4) regular daily oral hygiene (including brushing twice daily and using dental floss).

Nutrition Intervention (See Table 30-1)

Nutrition intervention involves the integration of all nutrition resources and programs, including government and community agencies with the inherent needs of the clients to be served:
1. Maternal and Child Health Program.
2. Special Supplemental Food Program for Women, Infants, and Children (WIC).

Nursing Intervention

If certain issues are not addressed, the infant can be at nutritional risk. In delivering health care, the nurse needs to know what to look for. She should consider:
1. The use of vitamin supplementation (whether infant is breast fed or bottle fed).
2. The method of formula preparation used.
3. The appropriate introduction of solids (amount, kind, and texture). (See Tables 30-5 and 30-6).
4. The prevention of dental caries. (Check time of weaning. Is there coke or presweetened powder in the bottle at nap or bedtime?)

THE TODDLER AND PRESCHOOLER

Nutrient Needs

During the second year, the toddler's body needs are still high but energy requirements decrease—his rate of growth has slowed.

Psychosocial Issues

His characteristic small finicky appetite reflects this period of slow progressive growth and often appears as mealtime negativism and "food jags."[16] The toddler has a built-in appetite mechanism which will influence him to eat what he needs, especially if good foods are available. Forcing him to eat is not necessary for him to grow. He eats what he needs even though every meal may not be a balanced meal and he may sometimes go without a meal. An occasional eating jag when he may eat little but chicken rice soup or spaghetti for several days will do him no harm. Forcing often results in more negativism and/or becomes an attention getting device. However, if a major food group is consistently lacking over a period of time, nutrient deficiencies may occur. Since the toddler is unable to handle large portions, nutritious between meal snacks are important (Table 30-8).

By allowing the toddler to explore new textures, new foods, and new feeding techniques (fork as well as spoon), he becomes interested in his food (it is no longer a toy) and is proud of his efforts at self-feeding, although the road to this success may be quite messy.

Nursing Intervention

The nurse needs to help the mother understand that:
1. From a nutritional point of view, the toddler can regulate his intake if the appropriate foods are offered (see Table 30-9 for problem areas).
2. The psychological issues involving the toddler's need for independence and exploration should be respected.

SCHOOL AGE CHILD

Nutrient Needs

Between the ages of 6 to 12, the child's growth rate is still slow yet continuous with occasional spurts and plateaus, climaxing into a final spurt at the end of this period. During this time, continued good food practices assist in the nutritional preparation necessary for adolescent needs.

Psychosocial Issues

The child still imitates his parents and other adults but now wants to mimic his peers as well. Good food practices at home together with positive learning experiences in the classroom and the "new" foods introduced to him in the school lunch program all build on the foundation of sound nutrition principles established during infancy and toddlerhood.

The competition between meal time and play time makes it essential that meals not be skipped and that nutritious between-meal snacks be readily available (Table 30-8).

TABLE 30-8. Nutritious snacks for the young child

Cut up raw vegetables
Fresh and canned fruits
Unsweetened fruit juices
Dried fruits, nuts, seeds:
    raisins,* apricots,* prunes* peanuts, soybeans, sunflower seeds
Peanut butter and/or cream or cottage cheese on crackers
Sliced cheese
Milk; milk puddings
Yogurt

---

*Stick to teeth and may cause caries.

Nutrition Intervention (See Table 30-1)

School Breakfast Program.
School Lunch Program.

Nursing Intervention

The nurse needs to:
1. Help the working mother plan and have available appropriate after school snacks as well as meals to be served by a baby sitter.
2. Help the inactive child find activity interests (to prevent obesity).
3. Suggest alternates to school food programs if any meal is consistently omitted.

ADOLESCENCE

Nutrient Needs

The nutritional requirements of the adolescent are based on sex, age at which growth spurt begins, and the physical stresses placed on the body.

To meet these demands, both boys and girls require an increase in overall calories with a gradual reduction towards the latter period of growth. There is a concomitant need for more good quality protein as well as vitamins and minerals (especially calcium, iron, and iodine).

Psychosocial Issues

It is because of these increased needs that good food practices (hopefully, a carry over from childhood days) should be stressed. However, it is during this time that even the adolescents who have had good dietary patterns tend to adopt poor eating habits. These changes may be due to the growing feeling of independence, the desire to assert their authority, and/or the influence of their peers. Their personal identity is being established resulting in some rebellion over adult control.

TABLE 30-9. Toddler feeding problems

Potential problem Areas	Suggested solutions
Toddler refuses milk	Serve at room temperature (cold milk may be painful to a teething child). Let child pour from a small pitcher; sip through a colored straw. Cook cereals with milk; offer cream soups; milk desserts. Offer cheese, yogurt.
Drinks too much milk	Offer milk after meals only. Offer water if thirsty.
Refuses meat	Minced or ground or bite sized pieces of moist meat or meat that is easy to chew (chicken, turkey). Mild flavored fish (including tuna). Eggs; peanut butter (together with milk); legumes, nuts if able to chew.
Fruits and vegetables	If the child prefers fruits over vegetables, it is better for time being to allow all servings from fruits vs turn him totally against vegetables by forcing. Raw, bite-sized pieces or vegetables cooked crisp vs cooked too long. Add plenty of milk to mashed potato. Mild flavored vs tart fruits. Uncooked dried fruits vs sweets/desserts. Add raisins or fresh fruits to cereals.
Breads and cereals	Serve cooked cereal warm not hot. Add raisins or fresh fruit to cereal. May prefer toast to bread (cut in small pieces).
Too many sweets	Eliminate from home completely. Use "natural" sweets such as fruits. Avoid using sweets as reward or bribe.

Other Hints:
1. Use child size portions.
2. Introduce new foods gradually (without pressure) especially when hungry, followed by familiar foods.
3. Let toddler sit at table that is right height for him with chair that lets him keep his feet flat on the floor or on a foot rest.
4. Offer small portions and let child ask for seconds; use finger foods.
5. Eating with the rest of the family triggers imitation of grown ups (their likes and dislikes, their manners).
6. If toddler seems to be hungry often, offer more protein foods (if weight is up, is he bored?).
7. Offer snacks at regular time each day, not too close to meals; avoid habit of continuous snacking.
8. Parents need to set limits and be consistent but still allow some freedom of control (i.e., respect for his likes and dislikes); parents should take a casual relaxed approach.

Factors Interfering with Nutrient Intake

Many adolescents miss at least one meal a day. When breakfast is omitted one-fourth to one-third of the nutrients needed for the day are lacking and are generally not made up during the day. Reasons include: "I don't have time," "I overslept," "I'm not hungry," "I want to lose weight." Suggestions of nontraditional breakfast foods such as cheese sandwiches and fruit may meet with higher compliance by the adolescent. Nutrients can be obtained from a variety of sources, and nutritional content should be the goal rather than a predetermined "breakfast" food.

Reasons for omitting lunch include: "Don't like what's served at school," "Not enough time," "Lunch period is too early." Although these may be factors beyond the control of the adolescent, the health professional can help him work around the issues, i.e., carry lunch from home eating as much as he can in the time allotted and saving a portion for after school.

The increased nutritional demands of this age cannot be adequately met with the traditional three meals a day. Snacks are also a part of the social life of the adolescent and are often dependent on peer pressures. As hunger is more easily met with high carbohydrate foods, a large proportion of "junk-type" foods (soft drinks, chips, cupcakes) is usually selected, hence the so-called "typical teenage diet."

Nutrient Needs of Adolescent Girls

The girl who is concerned with body image and is more vulnerable to fads stressing slimness may avoid foods which she considers fattening such as milk, bread, and cereals. Her way of reducing may be to skip breakfast and/or skip most of, or part of, another meal (e.g., lunch) with the resultant loss of essential nutrients. Since a girl's caloric requirement is less than a boy's, she cannot eat as often or as much food as he does without gaining weight. Because of their tendency to be more overweight than boys, girls need to be encouraged to take part in physical activity and to eat or drink nutritious foods which supply fewer calories (e.g., fruit, fruit juices, low fat milk).

Other considerations include: 1) increased nutritional needs with oral contraceptives (particularly for pyridoxine, folate, and ascorbic acid),[17] and 2) adolescent pregnancies where increased needs are "superimposed on an immature and far from ideally nourished maternal organism."[17]

Nutrient Needs of Adolescent Boys

Boys are also concerned with body image as regards body building. They too fall prey to the numerous nutrition claims, including high protein supplements as muscle builders. The weight lifter or athlete who feels he must increase his intake of protein foods and take vitamin/mineral supplements to increase muscle mass should be advised that his main needs for athletic performance are proper conditioning, a well balanced (increased calorie) diet, and proper hydration without any supplements.[18] Any consistent changes in overall eating for athletics should be monitored: 1) weight gained can be either fat or muscle; 2) excessive intakes may be the baseline for future obesity; 3) weight reduction diets prior to athletic activities can adversely affect performance resulting in use of calories from protein stores.

Nutrition Intervention (See Table 30-1)

School Breakfast Program.
School Lunch Program.
Maternal and Child Health Program for the pregnant adolescent.

Nursing Intervention

The nurse needs to:
1. Help the adolescent be aware of himself as an individual.
2. Assist adolescents in evaluating food choices.
3. Help adolescents explore alternate food choices considering the need for socialization as well as the need for more nutritious foods (e.g., hamburgers, pizza, milkshakes rather than cola and chips).
4. Encourage regular exercise programs for both males and females.
5. Provide growth and development information and consumer information to the adolescents, teachers, and parents.

PREGNANCY

It can be said with reasonable certainty that the successful outcome of pregnancy is dependent on the good nutritional status of the mother at the time of conception as well as the continued good dietary practices during pregnancy regardless of age. It is also dependent on the total health experiences of both parents and involves their education, economic backgrounds, and sociocultural experiences. Attitudes toward prenatal care are often passed from generation to generation. Current health teaching is toward early ongoing prenatal care with provision for health and nutrition teaching during pregnancy and through the postnatal period.

Weight Gain

Emphasis is placed on the mother's pregravid weight and her weight gain during pregnancy as these are the two parameters which most influence obstetric complications and the infant's birth weight.[19] More importantly considered is the *pattern* of weight gain. The most widely accepted weight gain during pregnancy is 22-26 pounds above prepregnant weight[19-21] with least weight gain during the first trimester (~4 lb) and about 0.4 Kg (0.9 lb) per week until term (Fig. 30-1). Restricting weight gain (as with already overweight mothers) or increasing weight greatly may result in nutritional deficits for both mother and fetus increases the risk of a low birth weight baby, and are thus not advisable.

Nutrient Needs

The complex physiologic changes which take place involve altered dietary needs based on sound nutritional practices. The fetus is dependent on the mother's circulation for its nutrients.

There is a need for additional energy taking into account age, height, prepregnant weight, and activity (which is especially decreased towards the end of pregnancy). The Recommended Dietary Allowances of the National Academy of Sciences[22] recommends an additional 300 calories/day (over nonpregnant needs) during the entire pregnancy. This amount will also insure adequate utilization of good quality protein currently recommended at an additional 30 grams/day.[19-21] Examples of 30 grams of protein and 300 calories: 4 ounces lean meat, fish, or poultry or 4 cups low fat milk or 2 ounces lean meat and 2 cups low fat milk.

PRENATAL WEIGHT GAIN GRID

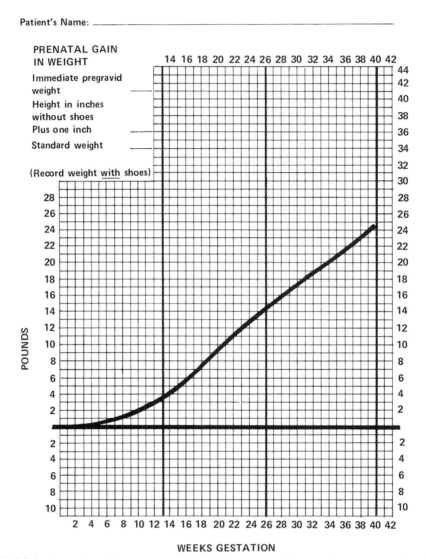

FIGURE 30-1. Normal weight gain pattern during pregnancy. (With permission from Lull, C.B., and Kimbrough, R.A. (eds.): *Clinical Obstetrics*. J.B. Lippincott Co., Philadelphia, 1953.)

Vitamin Supplementation

Although there is some controversy over the recommendation of other nutrient supplements, most authorities agree on routine supplementation of iron and folic acid only.[21] The increased requirements of other nutrients can easily be met through appropriate dietary choices, i.e., one quart of vitamin D fortified milk meets the increased calcium allowance.

Other vitamin and mineral supplements do not appear to be necessary although their routine use has not been found to be harmful.[21] Care should be taken to prevent an intake of excess fat-soluble vitamins. Whether using supplements or not, the mother must be encouraged to continue sound nutrition practices; supplements should not take the place of good eating habits.

Sodium

In the past, most physicians restricted the sodium content in the mother's diet hoping to prevent complications of pregnancy, namely pre-eclampsia. More recently it has been suggested that sodium is an essential nutrient during pregnancy[19] and does not need to be routinely restricted.[20]

Risk Factors in Pregnancy

ADOLESCENCE

The pregnant adolescent under age 17 presents a potential risk on the outcome of pregnancy. Her increased nutritional needs for her own optimum growth potential are compromised by the further requirements of pregnancy.[21] The tendency for poor eating habits including a desire to keep weight down, economic problems, and her emotional immaturity further jeopardize the desirable outcome of pregnancy. There is a higher incidence of low birth weight babies born to these mothers, especially those who are less than 15 years of age.[21]

She should be encouraged to seek early medical care with a good nutritional assessment during her first clinic visit. On the basis of information obtained, a sound nutrition program should be outlined. The adolescent will then need continued understanding and support for good eating habits.

ALCOHOL

Alcoholic intake in any amount during pregnancy presents hazards which should well be avoided. [23] Fetal Alcohol Syndrome (FAS) has long been known to cause low birth weight, physical and/or mental retardation, and brain damage in the infant without the possibility of reversal postnatally (no catch up growth).[24] More recently it has been observed[23] that smaller amounts of alcohol have potentially the same deleterious effect as that found in FAS or, more mildly, may result in behavioral problems. If a mother is suspected of using alcohol to any degree, blood samples may be drawn as proof and mother must be informed of the consequences of continued use during pregnancy.[24]

SMOKING

Women who smoke during pregnancy are at risk for spontaneous abortions.[25] Those who deliver have lower birth weight infants than women who do not smoke with dose related response (the more cigarettes smoked the lower the birth weight).[21]

DRUGS

Along with tobacco and alcohol, maternal narcotic addiction also results in low birth weight infants.[26] Other clinical manifestations include neurologic abnormalities and gastro-intestinal and respiratory symptoms. There appears to be the possibility of a psychological impairment as well.[27]

Nutrition Intervention (See Table 30-1)

Maternal and Child Health Program.
Special Supplemental Food Program for Women, Infants, and Children (WIC).

Nursing Intervention

The issues which the nurse needs to address during pregnancy include:
1. Importance of regular prenatal visits.
2. Age of mother.
3. Mother's pregravid weight and subsequent rate of gain.
4. Adequacy and distribution of calories, protein intake, and vitamin supplements: is mother trying to "diet"?
5. Alcoholic intake, cigarettes smoked, drugs used.
6. Nutrition education aimed not only at the outcome of pregnancy and lactation but at the interval between pregnancies with emphasis on improving her dietary habits as well as those of her children and the rest of her family.

LACTATION

Nutrient Needs

As in pregnancy, the mother's nutrient needs during lactation are again altered. Her appropriate choices will result in a breast milk which is optimum for the growth and development of her infant while taking care of her own needs as well.

There is an additional need of 500 calories/day above prepregnant needs to insure an adequate amount of milk. More than 500 calories is indicated if breast feeding is to continue for longer than three months or if there is more than one infant being fed.[19] Also recommended is an additional 20 grams of protein (~ 3 oz from meat, fish, poultry). The continued intake of 1 quart of milk by the mother insures adequate calcium for lactation. Iron supplementation begun during pregnancy should continue to replace iron lost during pregnancy. Two to three quarts of liquids should be drunk each day to supply the volume of breast milk needed.[28]

Lactating mothers should be made aware of the effect on the infant of certain drugs (including oral contraceptives) and alcohol.[29]

Nutritional Intervention (See Table 30-1)

Maternal and Child Health Program.
Special Supplemental Food Program for Women, Infants, and Children (WIC).

Nursing Intervention

The nurse should:
1. Provide an ongoing evaluation of nutritional intake.
2. Stress the importance of postnatal visits and monitor infant's and mother's progress.
3. Review breast feeding techniques with opportunities for questions from the mother.
4. Discuss guidelines for using bottle feedings during lactation (either mother's milk or commercial formula).

THE MIDDLE YEARS

Nutrient Needs

The nutritional status during this period reflects past and present food practices. A good nutrient intake needs to continue. However, with food consumption remaining the same or increased, with energy needs diminished, and with physical activity generally reduced (due to a more sedentary life style), obesity becomes more prevalent. Diabetes mellitus, atherosclerosis, and coronary heart disease (public health problems of great magnitude) have been associated with obesity and are prevalent in early adulthood.

Because of this phenomenon, the U.S. Dietary Goals[30] were established in 1977 setting forth new guidelines for desirable food patterns to reverse poor habits and prevent them in those who have not adopted them. These suggest:
1. Increase carbohydrate consumption to account for 55 to 60 percent of the energy (caloric) intake.
2. Reduce overall fat consumption from approximately 40 to 30 percent of energy intake.
3. Reduce saturated fat consumption and balance that with polyunsaturated and monounsaturated fats.
4. Reduce cholesterol consumption to about 300 mg a day.
5. Reduce sugar consumption by about 40 percent to account for about 15 percent of total energy intake.
6. Reduce salt consumption by about 50 to 85 percent to approximately 3 grams a day.
7. Reduce if overweight.

Nutrition Intervention (See Table 30-1)

Food Stamp Program.
Screening by American Diabetes Association and American Heart Association.

Nursing Intervention

The nurse should:
1. Do a nutritional assessment.
2. Do an activity assessment.
3. Assist in adjusting diet, taking into account activity level, food preferences, cultural habits, and any disease conditions requiring food modification.
4. Assist in grocery shopping and food preparation activities as necessary.

THE SENIOR YEARS

Although nutrition does not influence aging *per se,* its preventive effect on the complications of aging begins at conception and continues through childhood, adolescence, and the middle years.[31] The good eating habits set down early in life enhance a healthy maturity with the minimizing of certain nutrition-related disorders, i.e., the prevention of obesity may as a result prevent adult-onset diabetes or hypertension. "Prevention of chronic illness by nutritional planning in youth and late maturity promises the greatest rewards in terms of a healthy active old age."[31]

Nutrient Needs

Except for calories, the nutrient requirements are similar to those of early adulthood. The physiologic process of aging as well as reduced physical activity result in a diminished need for calories. However, the total diet must continue to supply all the essential nutrients. Good quality protein is necessary to balance the catabolic processes.

Factors Affecting Food Intake

Malnutrition is common among the elderly for various reasons. Many cannot afford the cost of food and would prefer to choose inexpensive, nutritionally inferior foods—usually high carbohydrate, low protein foods—which are easy to chew and need little preparation. Poor or missing dentition causes them to avoid hard or fibrous foods as meats and vegetables and so they choose bread, potatoes, sweets, tea, and crackers. Adequacy of kitchen facilities (stove, refrigeration), proximity to grocery stores, (limited) mobility, and ability to care for themselves all influence food choices.

Poor appetite is a problem among many elderly. It may be a result of the normal changes in taste and smell causing food to be less tasty. A reduction in GI functioning is seen with increasing age. There is a decrease in the amount of saliva which alters the flavor of food. There is a decrease in digestive enzyme secretions and an overall change in GI efficiency which can also alter appetite.[32] Loneliness due to the loss of a loved one or merely having to eat alone also influences the desire to eat.

Often there is a concern for health and/or longevity leaving the elderly easy prey to food faddism and quackery. Mega doses of vitamins are promoted and are offered as a means of reducing the common cold (vitamin C) and for slowing down the aging process (vitamin E).[31] To date neither claim has been fully substantiated.

In general, the elderly should be encouraged to select a balanced intake from a variety of foods adjusting their calories in accordance with their physical activity with good quality protein, high calcium, and high iron foods emphasized. Six to eight glasses of liquid should be taken daily, such as water, juices, coffee, and tea, and restricted late in the day if nocturia is a problem. They may enjoy eating the dinner meal at noon and/or may prefer frequent smaller meals in place of three large meals (Table 30-10).

Changing old habits into a new life style may be slow and difficult. They are learning new methods of purchasing, preparation, and possibly adjusting to living alone. Range of motion may be impaired resulting in the need for new eating utensils, plates with rim guards, plastic mugs with wide handles, and so forth.

TABLE 30-10. Problems affecting nutrition in the senior years

Potential problem area	Suggested solutions
Poor or missing dentition	Fix teeth; wear dentures. Ground meat; less tender cuts of meat cooked until tender; fish; eggs; cheese; cooked beans/peas. Cooked or canned vegetables and fruits vs raw; fruit or vegetable juices.
Limited funds	Check community resources. Plan ahead, make shopping list, use coupons, check supermarket specials; unit pricing. Food stamps; avoid health food gimmicks. Arrange for leftovers (soups, stews, hash).
Inadequate kitchen facilities	Shop for smaller amounts. Hot plate. Check community resources as Goodwill, churches, etc., for equipment (as refrigerator).
Reduced GI functioning	6-8 glasses liquid/day (limit late in day if enuresis is a problem). For constipation: increase fiber; brisk walk (or some physical activity); avoid mineral oil as laxative.
Poor appetite	Investigate community resources if living alone. Help client prepare more palatable meals.
Weight problem	Total reduction in calories. Frequent smaller meals, well balanced; low fat/skim milk vs whole milk. Nonfood activities.
Limited motility	Calories: skim vs whole milk; less sweets and fats. Food purchasing: easily opened foods with little preparation (frozen vs canned vegetables).
Special diets	Check appropriateness of degree of restriction. Explain clearly and incorporate into present life style.

Special Diets

Special diets are common in this age group and should be worked into the existing life style where possible, keeping in mind such things as ability to chew, alternates to high cost foods, and mobility. Although some conditions require dietary adjustment, drastic food changes may not be necessary. Some diets are unpalatable resulting in a reduced intake and they may be difficult to obtain away from home. An example of this is a salt restricted diet. The use of spices, herbs, and seasonings should be encouraged for increased palatability. Restaurants are only now beginning to accommodate customers on special diets.

Nutrition Intervention (See Table 30-1)

Meals on Wheels.
Nutrition Program for the Elderly (Title VII).

Nursing Intervention

The nurse can:
1. Assess nutritional activity level.
2. Encourage the elderly to include nutritious foods to balance meals taken from community nutrition programs.
3. Assist in budgeting for food, grocery shopping, and food preparation as necessary.
4. Assist in utensil modification improvising with existing equipment where necessary.

INFLUENCES ON FOOD PRACTICES

Ethnic Food Practices

Inherent in each community may be found a myriad of ethnic backgrounds. The cultural food practices which exist may be a close tie with the mother land or a desire to preserve customs handed down (Table 30-11).

The nurse needs to grasp the total situation of the families she deals with. Even if she knows the cultural/ethnic patterns, she should not assume all aspects are practiced. Adjusting foods to the basic pattern is more acceptable than total change. Each family should be viewed on an individual basis avoiding value judgments and projection. Often looking for an understanding of ethnic practices from within the community (not necessarily from a health professional) can be of utmost value.

Economics — Food Budgeting

With the cost of food forever on the increase, helping families purchase the most nutrition possible is a challenge for the nurse. Her background information and appraisal of the family's food practices, resources, and budgeting will enable her to offer appropriate guidance. The following guidelines will assist her in the overall planning:

Consider:
1. Amount of money available and the cost of food.
2. Preplanned menus with plans for leftovers.
3. Total amount of food needed for the family based on food nutrient profile and on availability of foods (allowing for flexibility to substitute within a group of foods).
4. Supplies on hand at home.
5. Infrequent shopping trips (once or twice a month vs. daily or weekly if storage facilities permit.

Recommend:
6. A shopping list thereby avoiding impulse buying and shopping when hungry.
7. Supermarket specials appearing in the newspapers; use of coupons.
8. Store brands vs. name brands.
9. Seasonal fresh produce which may be cheaper per serving than the same canned or frozen food.
10. Less expensive cuts of meat.
11. Avoidance of prepackaged convenience foods such as TV dinners.
12. Label reading to ensure superior nutrition.
13. Unit pricing (cost per portion).
14. Buying only that amount which can be used in a reasonable length of time.

Food Processing

Changes in food supplies and processing have influenced the kinds of food available. Although food processing techniques are employed for a variety of reasons—preservation of foods, improvement of appearance, quality, and nutrition—there has been a growing concern primarily over the use of certain additives. While these are generally monitored by the Food and Drug Administration, the consumer needs to be aware of what is being used and why and contact the appropriate government agency or food companies with any concerns. He should ultimately be responsible for his own food choices and select a well balanced, varied intake.

Food Labeling

The label on a food package is a source of nutrition education and information to help consumers know what is in the products they are buying. Certain information is mandatory: common name of the product, net weight or volume of product contents, listing of ingredients (in descending order of predominance by weight), name and address of the manufacturer or packager.

If a processor makes a nutritional claim in labeling or advertising or if the food is enriched with essential nutrients, further information, in a standard format, is required under Food and Drug Administration regulations: serving size, servings per container, calories per serving, grams of carbohydrate, protein, and fat per serving, protein and a minimum of 7 vitamins and minerals in specific order shown as a percentage of the U.S. Recommended Daily Allowance (USRDA).

Information on cholesterol, saturated and polyunsaturated fatty acids, sodium, and potassium may be included if desired. Other voluntary information may include brand name, price, recipe suggestions, code letters and numbers, dates indicating product freshness, and so forth (Fig. 30-2). The FDA is presently attempting to simplify and effectively communicate information in a manner which will be least costly to the consumer.[33]

Nutrition labeling can help the consumer compare nutrients and cost per serving, select foods appropriate for special diets, and purchase less costly substitutes for higher priced foods.

Food Faddism

The area of nutrition is still a relatively new science and some issues are ill defined. Because of this lack of definition and people's universal interest in food, some new "findings" are distorted into a new fad by the media or self-proclaimed experts. An example would be vitamin E and fertility. The effect of vitamin E on reproduction in rats has been extrapolated to include the same effect on humans, for which there is no basis. Findings in animals or preliminary scientific reports cannot be used as evidence to change food practices.

There are a variety of motivating factors causing people to turn to food faddism. Some are intertwined with culture and religion. Fads become popular in the nutritionally uninformed public. They can be found among people looking for a resolution of their problems through diet and/or among those overly concerned about their health. The poor, the chronically ill, and least educated are most often exploited with unfounded promises.[34]

"Health foods" obtained at health food stores at high cost with the implication of health

TABLE 30-11. Ethnic food patterns*

Food preferences	Puerto Rican	Black ("Soul")	Chinese
Meat	Poultry, pork; salt codfish; dried beans or peas usually mixed with rice.	All meats, fish and chicken usually fried; pig's feet, neck bones; ham hocks; chitterlings (intestines); spareribs; bacon; sausage.	All kinds often mixed with other foods; soybean curd (tofu); eggs, peanut butter.
Milk	In combination with coffee (cafe con leche) or cocoa; cheese.	Limited milk as such; some cheese in combination foods.	Not as beverage although slowly being introduced into diet; some cheese; ice cream.
Fruits and vegetables	Variety of fruits; starchy vegetables (plantains, cassava, sweet potato); salad.	Variety of fruits; vegetables cooked long period of time with salt pork (collard and mustard greens; okra; corn; lima beans; sweet potato).	Large variety used; fruits eaten raw; vegetables cooked crisp.
Breads and cereals	Rice usually seasoned with lard; some bread.	Grits; cornbread; muffins; biscuits; rice.	Rice is the staple; noodles; millet.
Additional foods	Fat pork and lard used in most cooking; sweets.	Sweets; soft drinks; powdered presweetened drinks; gravy.	Soy sauce; MSG.
Nutritional concerns	Obesity	Obesity; hypertension; vitamin losses in cooking.	Diet low in calcium and vitamin D.
Suggestions for concerns	Reduce fat used in cooking; reduce sugar intake.	Reduce snack foods, sweets, fats, salted foods; reduce amount of water and time for cooking vegetables; increase balance of basic foods.	Soybean products, dark green vegetables for calcium; vitamin D supplement may be necessary; check total protein intake.

*Adapted from Herbold, N.H.: "Community Nutrition," from *Nutrition in Clinical Care,* edited by Howard, R.B., and Herbold, N.H. McGraw-Hill Book Company, New York, 1978.

and freedom from disease are a lure to the unwary. There are offers of cures from varying ailments including arthritis, baldness, cancer, and prevention of aging. As a result, the use of these foods may prevent proper medical attention. Some claims are actually harmful, i.e., cures for diabetes, megavitamin dosages for cancer. Imbalances can lead to malnutrition. Examples of health foods include kelp, wheat germ, Brewer's yeast, black-

Japanese	Italian	Jewish
All fish and seafood (fresh, smoked and raw); some meat mixed with other foods; soybean and curd (tofu); eggs.	All meats, fish, chicken; Italian cold cuts (salami, mortadella); Italian pork sausage.	Only meat of divided hooved animals that chew a cud except pork; only fish with fins and scales; poultry; chopped liver; gefilte fish; lox (smoked salmon); herring; eggs.
Little used.	Milk with coffee; cheese (Parmesan, Romano, ricotta, mozzarella).	All types of milk and cheese NEVER taken with meat.
Variety used; fruits eaten raw; vegetables fried in batter or cooked with soy sauce.	All varieties of fruits and vegetables.	All varieties of fruits and vegetables.
White rice; wheat noodles.	All breads; pasta; some rice.	Bagels; egg bread (challah); milk free breads; matzo.
Soy sauce.	Sugar in coffee; pastries; wine; olive oil.	Sour cream; cream cheese; chicken fat.
Diet low in calcium and vitamin D.	Possible obesity.	Foods used tend to be high in cholesterol and saturated fats.
Soybean products, dark green vegetables for calcium; vitamin D supplement may be necessary; check total protein intake.	Reduce fat used in cooking; reduce portion sizes.	Limit egg consumption; use lower fat foods.

strap molasses. These foods in and of themselves are not bad but claiming they have curative powers is misleading and possibly harmful.

Among "health foods" the term "natural foods" has come to mean unprocessed, unrefined, unpasteurized foods. For example, raw vs. canned fruits; whole wheat vs. white flour; raw vs. pasteurized milk. These foods can be expensive and in some instances offer no more than processed foods.

Mandatory Information

Mandatory Information

Voluntary Information

BRAND NAME

PLAIN
LOWFAT
YOGURT

NET WT. 8 oz. (227g)

NUTRITION INFORMATION
(per serving)

Serving Size = 1 Cup   Servings Per Container = 1

Calories.........150   Carbohydrate.....17 gm
Protein..........12 gm   Fat..............4 gm

PERCENTAGE OF U. S. RECOMMENDED DAILY
ALLOWANCES (U. S. RDA) PER SERVING:

Protein..........30   Niacin...........*
Vitamin A........2   Calcium..........40
Vitamin C........*   Iron.............*
Thiamin..........4   Phosphorous......20
Riboflavin.......30   Magnesium........

*Contains less than 2% of the U. S. RDA
of this nutrient.

Ingredients: Cultured, Pasteurized Grade A Lowfat
Milk, 4% Nonfat Milk Solids

PACKED BY
BRAND NAME   ANYTOWN, U. S. A.   12345

CURRY YOGURT DIP

1 container lowfat yogurt
3 T mayonnaise
2-3 tsp curry powder

Blend all ingredients well.
Serve with cut-up raw vegetables.

KEEP REFRIGERATED

FIGURE 30-2. Sample of nutritional label information.

"Organic foods" imply all foods existing in nature. They are foods grown organically without chemical fertilizers or pesticides or additives. The main difference between foods grown organically and those grown in conventional fashion is primarily in the total yield of the crop. The nutrient content does not differ since growing plants do not distinguish between inorganic and organic fertilizers.[34] However, the question of pesticides and health has been the basis of the debate on the use of organic foods to which the Food and Drug Administration has had to respond. People are paying more for natural, organically grown health foods for "safety" reasons yet these foods are not regulated by any law agency.

Vegetarian Diets

Vegetarianism in some communities is a cultural pattern. However, in others it is a fad and may be carried to extremes.

A vegetarian is one who has eliminated some or all animal foods from the diet relying on plant foods primarily. Vegetarianism has been practiced for years throughout the world. Reasons have included economic necessity, religion, culture, and more recently personal choice. The four main categories of vegetarianism include: 1) lacto-vegetarian which includes all vegetables, grains, fruits and nuts supplemented with milk and cheese (lacto) (Milk products add complete protein to this combination and enhance amino acid composition.); 2) lacto-ovo-vegetarian which includes all vegetables, grains, fruits and nuts supplemented with milk and cheese (lacto) and eggs (ovo) (There is no problem securing adequate protein with this diet.); 3) pure vegetarian or vegan which includes all vegetables, grains, fruits, and nuts without any animal foods, dairy products, or eggs (Inadequate protein intake can result.); 4) fruitarian which includes fresh fruits, juices, and nuts (There is a problem obtaining an adequate diet for the strict fruitarian.).

The main concern of the vegetarian should be in receiving adequate protein for growth and maintenance from foods other than meats. Depending on which type of vegetarianism is chosen, this may or may not be difficult.

When planning vegetarian diets, it is important to understand the terms *amino acids,* *essential amino acids,* and *complete protein.* Amino acids are the building blocks of protein. Essential amino acids are those which cannot be synthesized by the body and must be supplied by an outside source. Proteins that contain all the essential amino acids in sufficient quantity and in the right combination for growth and maintenance are known as complete proteins.

If milk and eggs are eliminated from the diet, it is important to achieve greater protein efficiency from vegetables, grains, and nuts by combining them in such a way that the essential amino acids missing from one food can be complemented by that amino acid from another food at the same meal. For example, when rice and dried beans or peas are eaten together, the amino acid efficiency level is higher than when either of these foods is eaten alone. Other combinations are beans and corn; beans and wheat; soybeans, peanuts, and sesame; rice and soybeans; and sesame, soybeans, and wheat (Table 30-12).

There must be adequate caloric intake in the form of carbohydrate or fat so that the protein is not used for calories. There is also a need to eat a larger volume of food to achieve the total calories required; weight changes should be monitored. Supplementing the intake with milk and/or milk products further assures nutritional adequacy in all age groups. When milk and milk products are eliminated, there is a risk of vitamin B12 deficiency. Adult vegans should be encouraged to take a vitamin B12 supplement as

TABLE 30-12. Complementary proteins*

Food	Combination foods

Grains:
  barley
  corn
  oats
  rice
  rye
  wheat
	Peas, beans, lentils, milk, cheese,
	  yogurt.

Dairy:
  milk
  cheese
  yogurt
	Barley, corn, oats, rice, rye, wheat,
	  pumpkin seeds, sunflower seeds,
	  sesame seeds, nuts.

Legumes:
  beans
  lentils
  peas
	Barley, corn, oats, rice, rye, wheat,
	  pumpkin seeds, sunflower seeds,
	  sesame seeds, nuts.

Seeds, nuts:
  pumpkin seeds
  sunflower seeds
  sesame seeds
  almonds
  cashews
  pecans
  peanuts
	Milk, cheese, yogurt, peas, beans,
	  lentils.

*Adapted from Lappé, F.M.: *Diet for a Small Planet.* Friends of the Earth/Ballantine Books, Inc., New York, 1974.

should infants being nursed by vegan mothers.[34] Children do well on fortified soybean milk.[35]

An extreme form of vegetarianism is the Zen-Macrobiotic diet with progressively restrictive stages of food. The diet emphasizes self-discipline and each progressive stage becomes more restrictive. The diet progresses from one containing a variety of foods to one containing mainly cereals and small amounts of fluids. Nutritional deficiencies are common especially at the highest restrictive levels. There have been several reported deaths causing the American Medical Association Council on Foods and Nutrition to "condemn the Zen-Macrobiotic diet as a threat to human life."[36]

Vegetarian diets can be nutritious only if a variety of plant foods are combined to achieve a correct balance of amino acids, vitamins, and minerals. When counseling a vegetarian, the nurse needs to determine the type of vegetarian diet being adhered to. There has to be an understanding of what foods the client will accept so that the diet can be balanced in nutrients but not offensive to the client's principles. An example would be the vegetarian who will accept yogurt as a protein source since it is not considered an animal product. Always the nurse should emphasize the positive aspect balancing the diet around the acceptable foods.

Fad Reducing Diets

Fad reducing diets have exploited obese individuals with promises of "quick weight loss" (Table 30-13). There has been a diet to fit a variety of food preferences—for example, high

TABLE 30-13. Fad reducing diets

Diet	Description	Method of weight loss	Side effects
Atkins Diet	No carbohydrates first week resulting in ketosis. Up to 50 gm carbohydrate/day thereafter as long as ketosis continues. Protein & fat intake unlimited.	Quick weight loss. Weight lost is mainly in form of water. Fewer total calories are consumed usually due to monotony of intake or to already limited caloric content of diet.	Weakness, apathy, fatigue, dehydration, nausea, mineral losses; increase in cholesterol and saturated fat intake has potential for atherosclerosis; kidney involvement (renal malfunction) with decreased fluid intake; increased uric acid levels; rapid weight gain upon cessation of diet.
Stillman Diet ("Quick Weight Loss Diet")	High protein, high fat, no carbohydrate. Unlimited meat, eggs, low fat cheeses. 8 glasses water/day.		
Mayo Diet	High protein, high fat, low carbohydrate. Unlimited eggs, meats, vegetables in 3 meals (no snacks); 1/2 grapefruit at each meal considered the "fat burner").		
Scarsdale Diet	High protein, high fat, low carbohydrate diet. Strict adherence to 14 day meal plan no substitutes.		
HCG (human chorionic gonadotrophin hormone)	125 I.U. HCG 6X/wk for total of 40 injections in conjunction with 500 calorie diet	Weight loss attributed to semistarvation diet.	With reduced caloric intake nutrient intake is low.
Fasting/ Starvation*	Water, tea only	Water loss. Uses body protein to supply glucose to the brain. Burning of fat and muscle protein.	Ketosis, dizziness, fatigue, dehydration, nausea, mineral losses; death if allowed to continue.
Protein Sparing Modified Fast*	1.5 gm protein/kg of ideal body weight in 3 meals (as lean meat, fish, poultry). Multivitamin with iron Potassium and calcium supplement. 2 quarts fluid/day Total nutrition education program. Behavior modification suggested as an adjunct.	Good results as long as dieter stays on program. Insures consumption of body fat sparing body protein. Mild ketosis suppresses appetite. No decisions to make; no choices of food.	Dehydration, nausea, dizziness, emotional depression; increased protein load may trigger kidney complications; improper vitamin and mineral intake can trigger hidden medical problems.
Liquid Protein Diet*	Premeasured powdered protein added to juice, water or milk. Vitamin/mineral supplementation and 2 quarts fluids/day recommended.		

*CAUTION: Fasting, Protein Sparing Modified Fast, and Liquid Protein Diets should NEVER be undertaken without medical supervision.
Comment: These diets do not assist in re-education and maintenance of life time eating habits. Maintenance diets need to be built in to any weight reducing diet.

alcohol diet or diets that encourage eating all the meat or ice cream desired—all with nutritional adequacy in question and with little or no activity included. Most of these diets are nutritionally unbalanced. In some unsupervised cases, deaths have been reported. Often lost weight is quickly regained upon return to the original eating pattern as no nutrition education has taken place.

The most sound approach to weight reduction continues to be an overall reduction in total calories using a mixed diet, an increase in physical activity, and a change in food behavior.

TABLE 30-14. Clinical signs of nutritional status*

	Good	Poor
General appearance	Alert, responsive	Listless, apathetic, cachexic
Hair	Shiny, lustrous; healthy scalp	Stringy, dull, brittle, dry, depigmented
Neck (glands)	No enlargement	Thyroid enlarged
Skin (face and neck)	Smooth, slightly moist; good color, reddish-pink mucous membranes	Greasy, discolored, scaly
Eyes	Bright, clear; no fatigue circles beneath	Dryness, signs of infection, increased vascularity, glassiness, thickened conjunctiva
Lips	Good color, moist	Dry, scaly, swollen; angular lesions (stomatitis)
Tongue	Good pink color, surface papillae present, no lesions	Papillary atrophy, smooth appearance; swollen, red, beefy (glassitis)
Gums	Good pink color; no swelling or bleeding, firm	Marginal redness or swelling, receding, spongy
Teeth	Straight, no crowding, well-shaped jaw, clean, no discoloration	Unfilled caries, absent teeth, worn surfaces, mottled, malposition
Skin (general)	Smooth, slightly moist, good color	Rough, dry, scaly, pale, pigmented, irritated, petechia, bruises
Abdomen	Flat	Swollen
Legs, feet	No tenderness, weakness, or swelling; good color	Edema, tender calf, tingling, weakness
Skeleton	No malformations	Bowlegs, knock-knees, chest deformity at diaphragm, beaded ribs, prominent scapulae
Weight	Normal for height, age, body build	Overweight or underweight
Posture	Erect, arms and legs straight, abdomen in, chest out	Sagging shoulders, sunken chest, humped back
Muscles	Well developed, firm	Flaccid, poor tone; undeveloped, tender
Nervous control	Good attention span for age; does not cry easily, not irritable or restless	Inattentive, irritable
Gastrointestinal function	Good appetite and digestion; normal, regular elimination	Anorexia, indigestion, constipation or diarrhea
General vitality	Endurance, energetic, sleeps well at night; vigorous	Easily fatigued, no energy, falls asleep in school, looks tired, apathetic

*From Williams, Sue Rodwell: *Nutrition and Diet Therapy*, ed. 3. C.V. Mosby Company, St. Louis, 1977, with permission.

The nurse needs to understand the reasons why a particular fad is followed. By recognizing and accepting the client's beliefs, good nutritional principles can be incorporated into the diet without suggesting that the client must change completely to achieve a well balanced diet. Work from where the client is and change only those factors injurious to health.

NUTRITION COUNSELING: A TEAM APPROACH

The efficient interpersonal relationships of the various members of the health team will result in effective nutritional services to the clients to be served. It is a coordinated effort consisting of a mutual respect for one another's services with the ultimate goal of preserving good health within the community.

Because the nurse is most familiar with the community she serves and has close and continued contact with individuals and families, she is best able to appraise their needs and offer guidance in establishing appropriate dietary practices.

The nutritionist consultant who understands the population to be served and its problems can in turn assist the nurse in developing her ability to interview, assess nutritional status (Table 30-14), and direct a nutrition care plan. Continuous communication will expand the overall understanding of the inherent needs avoiding the duplication of services.

Other qualified nutrition resource persons within a community are listed in Table 30-15. Instances where direct referral to a nutritionist is important are listed in Table 30-16.

TABLE 30-15. Nutrition resources in public and private agencies

U.S. Department of Agriculture (USDA)
    State extension services
    Home demonstration agents working with homemakers
    4-H Club agents working with children
Federal government regional nutritionists
State Department of Public Health
State universities with food or nutrition department.
Large general and teaching hospitals.
Voluntary agencies:
    Visiting Nurse Association (VNA)
    Red Cross
    American Cancer Society
    American Diabetes Association (including Juvenile Diabetes
      Foundation)
    American Heart Association
Private and professional groups:
    American Dietetic Association (including state Dietetic Associations)
    American Home Economics Association
    American Public Health Association (including state Public Health Associations)
    National Dairy Council
    Private colleges and universities with food or nutrition department
    Society for Nutrition Education
    Public utility companies
    Food companies

TABLE 30-16. Reasons for referral to the nutritionist

Poor height/weight gain in infants and children
Low stature in children
Overweight
Allergies
Diseases placing body at nutritional risk (for example, malabsorption, cystic fibrosis, celiac disease)
Inborn errors of metabolism (for example, PKU)
Diabetes mellitus
Physical and mental handicaps which might interfere with feeding (for example, cerebral palsy; anorexia nervosa; Prader-Willi syndrome)
Pregnancy and at high risk
Diet abnormalities (qualitative and quantitative)

ACKNOWLEDGMENTS

I would like to acknowledge the technical assistance given by Rosanne B. Howard and the support of Froso Delianides, Jeannette Epstein, and Edith Getchell.

REFERENCES

1. Howard, R.B., and Herbold, N.H. (eds.): *Nutrition in Clinical Care.* McGraw-Hill Book Company, New York, 1978.
2. Fomon, S.J.: *Nutritional Disorders of Children: Prevention, Screening, and Followup.* DHEW Publ. No. (HSA) 76-5612, 1976.
3. Berkelhamer, J.E.: "Distorted Conceptions of Infant Nutrition Among Urban Mothers." *Clinical Pediatrics* 16:986, 1977.
4. Jackson, R.L.: "Long-Term Consequences of Suboptimal Nutritional Practices in Early Life—Some Important Benefits of Breast Feeding." *Pediatric Clinics of North America* 24:63, Feb. 1977.
5. Hambraeus, L.: "Proprietary Milk versus Human Breast Milk in Infant Feeding." *Pediatric Clinics of North America* 24:17, Feb. 1977.
6. American Academy of Pediatrics: "Breast Feeding." *Pediatrics* 62:591, Oct. 1978.
7. Jelliffe, D.B., and Jelliffe, E.F.: "Breast Feeding IS Best for Infants Everywhere." *Nutrition Today* 13(3):12, May/June 1978.
8. Filer, L.J. "Eary Nutrition: Its Long Term Role." *Hospital Practice* 13(2):87, Feb. 1978.
9. Fomon, S.J.: *Infant Nutrition,* 2nd ed. W.B. Saunders Company, Philadelphia, 1974.
10. American Academy of Pediatrics, Committee on Nutrition: "Fluoride Supplementation: Revised Dosage Schedule." *Pediatrics* 63:150, Jan. 1979.
11. Taitz, L.S.: "Obesity in Pediatric Practice: Infantile Obesity." *Pediatric Clinics of North America* 24:107, Feb. 1977.
12. Woodruff, C.W.: "Iron Deficiency in Infancy and Childhood." *Pediatric Clinics of North America* 24:85, Feb. 1977.
13. Nizel, A.E.: "Preventing Dental Caries: The Nutritional Factors." *Pediatric Clinics of North America* 24:141, Feb. 1977.
14. Nizel, A.E.: *The Science of Nutrition and its Application in Clinical Dentistry,* 2nd ed. W.B. Saunders Company, Philadelphia, 1966.
15. Committee on Nutrition: "Fluoride as a Nutrient." *Pediatrics* 49:456, 1972.
16. Howard, R.B., and Herbold, N.H. (eds.): *Nutrition in Clinical Care.* McGraw-Hill Book Company, New York, 1978.
17. Hodges, R.E., in McKigney, J., and Munro, H. (eds.): *Nutrient Requirements in Adolescence.* MIT Press, Cambridge, Mass., 1976.
18. Smith, N.: *Food For Sport.* Bull Publishing Company, Palo Alto, California, 1976.

19. Pitkin, R.M.: "Nutritional Support in Obstetrics and Gynecology," in Schneider, H.A., Anderson, C.E., and Coursin, D.B. (eds.): *Nutritional Support of Medical Practice.* Harper & Row, New York, 1977.
20. Jacobson, H.N.: "Diet in Pregnancy." *New England Journal of Medicine* 297:1051, Nov. 1977.
21. Committee on Maternal Nutrition, Food and Nutrition Board: *Maternal Nutrition and the Course of Pregnancy.* Summary Report, National Academy of Sciences, National Research Council, Washington, D.C., 1970.
22. Food and Nutrition Board, National Research Council: *Recommended Dietary Allowances,* 8th ed. National Academy of Sciences, Washington, D.C., 1974.
23. Ouellette, E.M., et al.: "Adverse Effects on Offspring of Maternal Alcohol Abuse During Pregnancy." *New England Journal of Medicine* 297:528, Sept. 1977.
24. Erb, L., and Andresen, B.D.: "The Fetal Alcohol Syndrome (FAS): a Review of the Impact of Chronic Maternal Alcoholism on the Developing Fetus." *Clinical Pediatrics* 17:644, Aug. 1978.
25. Kline, J., et al: "Smoking: a Risk Factor for Spontaneous Abortion." *New England Journal of Medicine* 297:793, 1977.
26. Madden, J.D.: "Problems Pertaining to the Care of Newborn Infants of Drug-Addicted Women." *Journal of Reproductive Medicine* 20:303, 1978.
27. Cooper, S.: "Psychotropic Drugs in Pregnancy: Morphological and Psychological Adverse Effects on Offspring." *Journal of Biosocial Science* 10:321, 1978.
28. Maternal and Child Health Unit, California Department of Health: *Nutrition During Pregnancy and Lactation,* 1975.
29. Knowles, J.A.: "Excretion of Drugs in Milk—a Review." *Journal of Pediatrics* 66:1068, 1965.
30. Select Committee on Nutrition and Human Needs, U.S. Senate: *Dietary Goals for the United States,* 2nd ed. U.S. Government Printing Office, Washington, D.C., Dec. 1977.
31. Watkin, D.M.: "Nutrition for the Aging and the Aged," in Goodhart, R.S., and Shils, M.E. (eds.): *Modern Nutrition in Health and Disease,* 5th ed. Lea and Febiger, Philadelphia, 1974.
32. Stare, F. J.: "Three Score and Ten Plus More." *Journal of the American Geriatrics Society* 25:529, 1977.
33. Food Labeling Hearings, Department of Health, Education, and Welfare, Food and Drug Administration (Docket No. 78N-0158), 1978.
34. Alfin-Slater, R., and Aftergood, L.: "Food Fads," in Schneider, H.A., Anderson, C.E., and Coursin, D.B. (eds.): *Nutritional Support of Medical Practice.* Harper & Row, New York, 1977.
35. Vyhmeister, I.B., et al.: "Safe Vegetarian Diets for Children." *Pediatric Clinics of North America* 24:, Feb. 1977.
36. Council on Foods and Nutrition: "Zen-Macrobiotic Diet." *Journal of the American Medical Association* 218(3):397, Oct. 1971.

BIBLIOGRAPHY

Deutsch, R.: *The Family Guide to Better Food and Better Health.* Bantam Books, New York, 1973.
Deutsch, R.: *The New Nuts Among the Berries.* Bull Publishing Company, Palo Alto, 1976.
Eschleman, R., and Winston, M.: *The American Heart Association Cookbook.* David McKay Company, Inc., New York, 1975.
Frankle, R.T., and Owen, A.Y.: *Nutrition in the Community: The Art of Delivering Services.* The C.V. Mosby Company, St. Louis, 1978.
Institute of Rehabilitation Medicine, New York University Medical Center: *Mealtime Manual for the Aged and Handicapped.* Simon & Schuster, New York, 1970.
Jordan, H.A., Levitz, L.S., and Kimbrell, G.M.: *Eating is Okay: a Radical Approach to Successful Weight Loss.* Rawson Associates Publishers, New York, 1976.
McWilliams, M.: *Nutrition for the Growing Years,* 2nd ed. John Wiley and Sons, New York, 1975.
Pipes, P.L.: *Nutrition in Infancy and Childhood.* The C.V. Mosby Company, St. Louis, 1977.
Pyke, M.: *Man and Food.* McGraw-Hill Book Company, New York, 1970.
Robertson, L., Flinders, C., and Godfrey, B.: *Laurel's Kitchen: a Handbook for Vegetarian Cookery and Nutrition.* Bantam Books/Nilgiri Press, Petaluma, Calif., 1978.
Stuart, R.B., and Davis, B.: *Slim Chance in a Fat World: Behavioral Control of Obesity.* Research Press Company, Champaign, Ill., 1972.

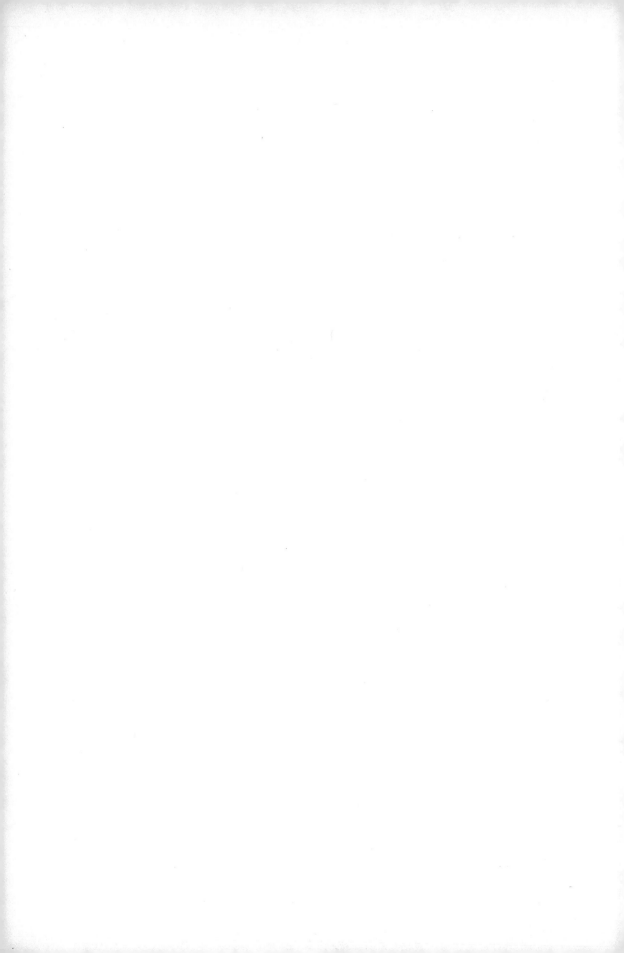

CHAPTER 31
DISABILITIES

LINDA L. JARVIS, M.S.N., R.N.

Disabling conditions can strike any individual or family at any point in the life continuum regardless of social, economic, or racial status. Some disabling conditions are temporary while others are permanent; some are highly visible while others are hidden. Disabling conditions can result from injuries, drugs, genetic defects, aging processes, learning disabilities, emotional trauma, or a myriad of other etiologies. In any event, the individual will experience a condition which will interfere with his or her ability to fulfill personal, social, occupational, intellectual, and/or physical activities and responsibilities.

If disabling conditions can occur to anyone at any time, then exactly what does the term "disabled" mean and who are the people who live and experience this designation? Frank Bowe defines a disability as an impairment which "persists for six months or longer and interferes with a person's ability to do something—walk, see, hear, talk, dress, learn, go to school, work."[1] A person is handicapped when a disability combined with environmental conditions prevents him from performing certain activities. The degree of the disability and the resulting handicap will depend on such factors as extent of impairment, community and family resources, and environmental conditions. An individual confined to a wheelchair with paraplegia from an accident may be able to attend school, obtain a job, raise a family, and enjoy social and recreational activities if attitudes and conditions in the community support this kind of behavior. Unfortunately this is not always the case because our society is perfection oriented with little time or use for the individual who does not meet physical, intellectual, or emotional expectations.

Those with disabilities must continually strive to be heard, acknowledged, and considered in the forward movement of our society. That a disabled person cannot progress at the same rate or in the same manner as a nondisabled person is insufficient reason to be given second class citizenship rights. However, that is often the way it has been.

The need to recognize and aid in the habilitation and rehabilitation of the disabled has increased since the ending of World War I and World War II. Both of these conflicts returned many thousands of young men into a society which was unprepared to meet the needs and demands of this group of men physically and mentally disabled by the wars. Also occurring at this time were advances in pharmacologic treatments for infections so that childhood and adult infections and other conditions were being successfully treated and people were surviving with disabilities as a result of the condition. The disabilities were generally permanent and left many people handicapped. During the decades which have followed, additional advances have been made in antibiotic and other drug therapy and in technology, and longevity has increased so that more people are surviving trauma and illness which earlier had been fatal.

With these advances in drug and technologic therapies, the numbers and scope of disabled persons and disabling conditions has expanded. It is difficult to obtain an exact number of disabled men, women, and children. However, it is estimated that there are approximately 36 million Americans who are disabled and of these members congenital disabilities account for one out of every six disabilities.[1] That means that most people who experience a disability do so between childhood and old age. If 36 million Americans experience some degree of disability, then we need to examine what we are doing to actively deal with the issues, concerns, and problems encountered by this population group.

DISABILITY AS A CRISIS SITUATION

The crisis prompted by a disability is a situational one that has been unexpected. In its simplest terms, a crisis can be defined as a disruption in a person's steady state.[2] The reaction to this crisis by both the patient and family will be of an individual nature. It will be determined by perception of the event, situational supports, and coping mechanisms. Both patient and family will need help in finding ways to deal or cope with the crisis in order to return to the former steady state or to some kind of emotional/psychological compromise. Activities directed toward crisis intervention will include identification of the crisis, stress reduction, nursing interventions, identification and utilization of resources, and evaluation of outcome. The initial crisis situation tends to be short lived, about four to six weeks, and is the prime time for initiating activities to deal with the immediate crisis and lay the foundation for additional interventions as they are necessary.[2]

Nurses need to keep in mind that in caring for clients they may experience crisis situations. This is particularly true when faced with an age peer who has sustained a disability due to illness or accident. It suddenly brings into sharp focus the vulnerability of us all. Janken, in discussing the nurse in crisis, writes about behavior patterns of nurses and interventions needed by them when they are in stress. Behavior patterns include 1) stereotyping of clients, 2) partisanship for or against the client, 3) need for situational supports, 4) coping mechanisms of patient teaching, withdrawal, and projection.[3]

Each of the above behavior patterns can impact on the quality and quantity of care the nurse is able to provide. Stereotyping occurs when the nurse labels the client or family in generalized terms such as "demanding," "lazy," and "uninterested." These labels are not grounded in fact, speak to isolated factors, and hamper the nurse in designing and implementing effective interventions. Although stereotype reactions tend to be negative, they can be positive and still present limitations to effectiveness. Close in hand with the stereotyping of clients and families is the behavior of partisanship. This behavior is characterized by attributing either positive or negative qualities to the behavior and other characteristics of the client or family. It usually involves seeing one as all good and the other as all bad. Effective communication is impossible with this approach.

When self-esteem becomes threatened, it is important that the nurse have available supports which can aid her in returning to the steady state. If this does not occur, her effectiveness will be severely limited and perhaps nonexistent. Defense mechanisms include withdrawal, patient teaching, and projection. Withdrawal involves removal of oneself from a stressful situation. It becomes a negative action when it increases the impact of the problem encountered for both client and nurse. An example would be withdrawal at the birth of a congenitally impaired child. Withdrawal tends to increase both guilt and anxiety. Patient teaching may be used when the client or family is engaging in behavior considered to be detrimental to their health status. If efforts toward reversing or changing the detrimental behavior are not met with success, the nurse will be unable to continue interventions due to frustration with her ineffectiveness. A final coping mechanism is one of projection which occurs when the nurse concludes that the patient/family feels the same way she does and designs nursing interventions based on this assumption. If there is patient/family/nurse agreement concerning perceptions, all will be well; however, if there is a difference in perception, frustration and confusion can severely limit the effectiveness of the nurse.

Because the behavior patterns of the nurse in crisis interfere with her ability to problem-solve with the client/family, efforts at intervention for the nurse are directed toward restoring this ability. Among the steps to be taken are an assessment of the problem situation, evaluation of coping mechanisms, and a plan of action which will allow her to continue functioning, restore self-esteem in her ability to nurse, and aid her in problem-solving successfully with the client/family.

It is very helpful to keep in mind that any disabling condition can represent a crisis for client/family and nurse. The extent to which it is perceived as a crisis will depend on event perception, support systems, and coping mechanisms. Anticipation of the crisis state by the nurse can aid her in dealing with the client/family and establish herself as a helpful resource person. Guiding the client/family through the crisis to a state of equilibrium is the goal.

BARRIERS TO DISABLED PERSONS

Before exploring some nursing interventions to be pursued by the nurse, a few words about barriers are imperative. Bowe identifies six barriers as 1) architectural, 2) attitudinal, 3) educational, 4) occupational, 5) legal, and 6) personal.[1]

The number of *architectural barriers* a disabled person must encounter and deal with is incredible. While rehabilitation on the one hand seeks to achieve the highest level of functioning possible, when the disabled person begins to explore the outside environment, he is met with an almost insurmountable number of odds against him. A tour around your local community can help you identify some of these barriers: crosswalks without wheelchair access, intersections without stop lights or bells, unpaved railroad tracks, poorly maintained streets and sidewalks, buildings with steps but no ramps or ground level entrances, buildings without elevators, rooms with narrow door openings, bathrooms without space for a wheelchair, elevators without raised markings for visually impaired persons, parking places without adequate space, and the list goes on. In short, buildings, transportation facilities, and the layout of the community in general have been with the able-bodied in mind, not with the special accommodations a disabled person might need. When traveling to and from school, work, or play takes so much time and energy, it takes true desire and persistence for the disabled person to endure these obstacles. This is not necessary and could be changed with a commitment by all citizens that access to public and private facilities is the right of all persons, not the privilege of the nondisabled.

Attitudes toward disabled persons are another area of concern. To be sure, there is no one who would want to have a disability. However, people become disabled in a variety of ways and all of us have to deal with this reality. Some of us deal with it by withdrawal as though disabilities were contagious, others are repulsed by the sight of an impaired individual, and others simply ignore or deny the presence of disabled individuals. Some will smile and support disabled people out of fear of offending them, a situation which leads to deceptive practices and may stimulate inaccurate perceptions. There are those who believe that one who is disabled has been possessed by the devil or is paying for the "evil deeds or thoughts" of himself or his family. Still others believe that disabled persons cannot carry out occupational responsibilities or learn or fall in love or have children or, in short, participate in any of the life experiences of human beings. Attitudes and reactions toward disabled persons vary. However, expectations are still stereotyped and far too few steps are being taken to meet the needs of the disabled in education, occupations, housing, relationships, and other endeavors. Whether from insensitivity, fear, or ignorance, we, as a nation, are doing far too little for our 36 million brothers and sisters who are disabled.

Educational rights for disabled persons have been attained as the result of long, hard fights against prejudice and other barriers concerning learning abilities and methodologies. According to Bowe, only about 4 million of the estimated 8 million disabled children and youth are receiving their required educational programming.[1] Special education programs tend to focus on the disabilities rather than the abilities of the children. There is a movement to integrate disabled children into the "normal" classroom. Doing this has the advantage of enriching the learning of the disabled child, exposing nondisabled children to the needs and skills of disabled children and providing an opportunity to deal with prejudices and attitudes about disabled persons at a very basic level. The "disadvantages" include the need to adapt the learning environment to accommodate *all* children, the development of new teaching strategies and methodologies, environmental adaptation, and a reexamination of educational attitudes toward disabled persons by educators and the general population. Educational directions require careful evaluation and scrutiny to determine attitudes toward the educational rights and needs of disabled persons.

Many lay and professional citizens support the pursuit of education in various programs of higher learning. There are many colleges and universities across the country which have made accommodations for disabled students. Southern Illinois University in Carbondale, Illinois, is one university which has constructed its campus and many programs to meet the needs of disabled students. Higher educational pursuits should be encouraged and ways sought to fulfill them.

Occupational barriers, like the others mentioned, present a real problem for disabled persons. Once having learned a skill, one then has to find an employer willing to hire him. The attitude that disabled persons cannot complete jobs, are high risk employees, and utilize a high degree of sick days are without support. Some disabled individuals will need the environment of a sheltered workshop or some kind of vocational rehabilitation program in order to become employed. However, there are many jobs that can be done well by disabled persons and all they ask for is a chance to prove themselves. Because of the difficulty in finding jobs, many disabled individuals who do work find themselves at or near the poverty level in terms of income, hardly an incentive to struggle to attain employment status. However, the drive in most disabled individuals is high and some have stated they have to work twice as hard as their nondisabled peers to prove that they can handle the job. For many, the job represents a real source of satisfaction and personal success.

Legislation to aid disabled persons has been slow in coming and often is implemented with little vigor. There are now laws covering access to public buildings, transportation, civil rights, education, and others.[1] Even with new laws, enforcement is slow or nonexistent with disabled persons having to take action to be heard, often in the form of demonstrations or lawsuits. To be effective in the legal arena, disabled persons will have to become a political force as other minority groups before them have done. Perhaps this kind of approach—increased legal sophistication and political awareness—will aid disabled persons in their quest for human rights. Such action is long past due.

Personal barriers also impact on disabled individuals. Since only one in six is congenitally disabled, the majority have to deal with the impairment after having lived a period of time as a nondisabled person. Depending on the severity and extent of the impairment, activities of daily living, acquisition of an education, maintenance of an income, establishment/maintenance of social relationships, maintenance of the family, and psychological/social adjustments will all be of some concern. With an acquired disability, self-concept, body concept, and self-esteem may all be shattered and require careful nurturing to reestablish themselves in a positive way. The presence and use of a support system will be necessary to assist the disabled person toward optimal rehabilitation. Most importantly the disabled individual needs to come to grips with the impairment as he perceives it and, from that point on, he will be capable of growing if the resources and supports are available.

The preceding is by no means inclusive, however, it does point up some of the very real barriers encountered on several fronts. To be disabled in America is still a difficult state filled with frustrations, hopes, dreams, and reality.

NURSING INTERVENTIONS

The presence of a disabled family member changes dreams, expectations, and roles and impacts on all aspects of family living. The type and severity of impairment, age of onset, high or low visibility of disability, and role in the family will influence the reaction of the client and family. The mother of young children who has a paralyzing stroke will present different problems to be dealt with than if the father in this family had the same condition. Among the problems would be the possible need for role reversals, income insecurity, need for outside assistance to maintain the home, changes in role expectation of the children, and changes in sexual practices. Future plans and goals may have to be forfeited. The impact should either parent become disabled, would be great. The major changes for the mother at home would concern child care, activities of daily living, and household responsibilities. Concerns for the father might be job security, activities of daily living, and an income for the family.

Nurses in community settings come in contact with disabled persons in a variety of settings including schools, occupational sites, ambulatory settings, and visiting nurse agencies. Her effectiveness will depend on her attitudes toward disabled persons, knowledge of community resources, and her willingness to become involved in the support and rehabilitation of the client and family. Her focus should be on the assets of the client and family.

Nursing care for the disabled person and his family will include assessment, case finding coordination, counseling, education, and referral. Before any treatment plans can be designed or recommended, a full assessment, both medical and nursing, will be necessary. Included will be observations of the disabled family member and the family separately and together. This will enable the nurse to determine attitudes and behavioral characteristics about the impairment. Such information will aid in setting priorities and designing nursing interventions. Where possible, school visits should be made to evaluate the setting and observe student/client interactions. Family, social, and financial resources should be identified and explored. Such information will be useful in planning nursing interventions. Transportation facilities and layout of the home environment should be made so that modifications can be suggested and implemented if possible. Occupational evaluation will be needed for rehabilitation planning. This assessment is an ongoing data collection effort and should be updated as new information or observations are available.

Casefinding involves the identification of disabled clients and families. Early casefinding can lead to early diagnosis, treatment, and rehabilitation as necessary. It is important to keep in mind that disabilities can be drug or alcohol related, intellectual, emotional, or behavioral in nature as well as physical. The less obvious disabilities and impairments are the ones often overlooked until difficulties encountered have become dramatic in nature. The perceptive nurse can provide a great service by noting slight deviations which may signal difficulties needing active diagnosis and treatment.

Coordination of care sometimes becomes a real concern as a disabled client and family is seen by a large number of health care providers. The nurse can aid in obtaining some of the care and establish communication channels if a formal system is not in existence so that all involved know what is being done and why. Keeping track of health care activity and information leads to more comprehensive care.

Counseling is carried out by the nurse with both the client and family. This is most often in the form of guidance and support. If the nurse is present during the initial crisis, she may serve to aid the family in reestablishing equilibrium. She can reinforce positive steps taken and make suggestions when a different kind of behavior or approach might be more appropriate. Because she has generally established herself as a trusted health care provider, the nurse may observe behaviors and be told of information which should be shared with others or will impact on the treatment outcome. Her position will enable her to identify this data with the client/family and with them seek appropriate steps to take.

Education will be carried out with the client, family, and community. If the disability was genetic, there may be much need to reassure the parents that they were not "at fault." Reassurance and factual information can help allay some guilt and provide a basis for further exploration and study. Both client and family need realistic information about the disabling condition including etiology and rehabilitation. Self-help and management techniques will need to be taught to both client and family. Particularly with children, it is necessary to provide consistent discipline and parents need input and support in this endeavor. Community education concerning the rights, needs, and facts about various disability conditions can be a start in sensitizing the public to the realities of various conditions and what they mean. Changes in attitudes can begin to be made with educational efforts. Continuous input about disabilities may begin to increase awareness.

The last major nursing intervention will be *referral*. There are a variety of services available in the community, and the community health nurse can help clients and families take advantage of them. Before suggesting utilization of any service, though, the nurse should visit and evaluate it herself. She will then know both assets and limitations and can discuss them openly. The needs of disabled persons cover a wide range including educational, social, recreational, and vocational. Depending on the age of the client, school may be a major concern. A decision will need to be made as to whether public, special education classes, or private schools are most appropriate. It is a difficult question to answer. My bias is that public education classes where the disabled student is part of the regular student body is the goal. This may be difficult in many areas due to facilities, attitudes, and prejudices. However, this barrier will never be broken down without steps taken to break it. Choices of colleges should be made with student access to all parts of the campus and varied learning methodologies as the main criteria. In all cases, referral choices should be carefully made.

Disabled individuals and their families face many barriers. The nurse has a responsibility to involve herself in political/social/educational efforts which will be aimed at breaking them down. Progress for disabled persons can be made when *all* persons are included in the mainstream of life, regardless of their conditions.

People with disabilities have feelings, dreams, concerns, and hopes like all of us. A question which will surely arise, especially as he or she ages, is that of marriage. Whether marriage is a viable choice depends on the disabled individual and mate of choice. It certainly is a possibility and is a decision only the two people involved can rightly make—they know best their assets and limitations.

The community health nurse will be confronted with a variety of disabilities as she performs her job. Her attitudes and those of the general public will determine to a large extent the kind and quality of services provided. Disabling conditions can occur to anyone at anytime regardless of age, race, sex, economic or social status. Disabled persons are with us and deserve the best which can be provided. They desire dignity, respect, and above all a chance to do their best, whatever and however it is fulfilled.

REFERENCES

1. Bowe, Frank: *Handicapping America—Barriers to Disabled People.* Harper & Row, New York, 1978.
2. Barrell, Lorna Mill: "Crisis Intervention—Partnership in Problem Solving." *Nursing Clinics of North America* 9(1):9, March 1974.
3. Janken, Janice K.: "The Nurse in Crisis." *Nursing Clinics of North America* 9(1):18, March 1974.

BIBLIOGRAPHY

Altshuler, Anne, Meyer, Jane, Butz, Marie K.J.: "Even Children Can Learn to do Clean Self-Catheterization." *American Journal of Nursing* 77(1):97, Jan. 1977.
Amundson, Mary Jane: "Nurses as Group Leaders of Behavior Management Classes for Parents." *Nursing Clinics of North America* 10(2):319, June 1975.

Anderson, Beverly, and D'Ambra, Phyllis: "The Adolescent Patient with Scoliosis." *Nursing Clinics of North America* 11(4):699, Dec. 1976.

Barbieri, Winnie Kender: "No Pity." *American Journal of Nursing* 76(9):1482, Sept. 1976.

Barrell, Lorna Mill: "Crises Intervention." *Nursing Clinics of North America* 9(1):5, March 1974.

Bowe, Frank: *Handicapping America—Barriers to Disabled People.* Harper & Row, New York, 1978.

Buck, Barbara, and Lee, Allen D.: "Amputation: Two Voices." *Nursing Clinics of North America* 11(4):641, Dec. 1976.

Bumbalo, Judith A., and Seidel, Mary A.: "Identifying and Serving a Multiply Handicapped Population." *Nursing Clinics of North America* 10(2):341, June 1975.

Burkhalter, Pamela K.: *Nursing Care of the Alcohol and Drug Abuser.* McGraw-Hill Book Company, New York, 1975.

Dubowski, Frances M.: "Children with Osteogenesis Imperfecta." *Nursing Clinics of North America* 11(4):709, Dec. 1975.

Eddy, Mary Elizabeth: "Teaching Patients with Peripheral Vascular Disease." *Nursing Clinics of North America* 12(1):151, March 1977.

Engstrand, Janet L.: "Rehabilitation of the Patient with a Lower Extremity Amputation." *Nursing Clinics of North America* 11(4):659, Dec. 1976.

Farrell, Jane: "Nursing Care of the Patient in a Cast Brace." *Nursing Clinics of North America* 11(4):717, Dec. 1976.

Gordon, Sol: *Living Fully.* A John Day Book, Harper & Row, New York, 1975.

Holmberg, Nola Janine: "Serving the Child with MBD and his Family in a Health Maintenance Organization." *Nursing Clinics of North America* 10(2):381, June 1975.

Janken, Janice K.: "The Nurse in Crisis." *Nursing Clinics of North America* 9(1):17, March 1974.

Kini, Joanne, and Scahill, Mary: "The Institutional Setting: Innovations in Nursing Care." *Nursing Clinics of North America* 10(2):393, June 1975.

Michaux, Louis Arthur: *The Physically Handicapped and the Community.* Charles C Thomas, Springfield, Ill., 1970.

Norris, Geraldine J.: "National Concerns for Children with Handicaps." *Nursing Clinics of North America* 10(2):309, June 1975.

O'Neil, Sally: "Behavior Modification: Toward a Human Experience." *Nursing Clinics of North America* 10(2):373, June 1975.

Pasnau, Robert O., and Pfefferbaum, Betty: "Psychological Aspects of Post-Amputation Pain." *Nursing Clinics of North America* 11(4):679, Dec. 1976.

Pattullo, Ann W.: "The Socio-Sexual Development of the Handicapped Child. A Preventive Care Approach." *Nursing Clinics of North America* 10(2):361, June 1975.

Pfefferbaum, Betty, and Pasnau, Robert O.: "Post-Amputation Grief." *Nursing Clinics of North America* 11(4):687, Dec. 1976.

Pierce, Penny F.: "Gains and Losses of Vascular Surgery Patients." *Nursing Clinics of North America* 12(1):119, March 1977.

Rose, Marion H.: "Coping Behavior of Physically Handicapped Children." *Nursing Clinics of North America* 10(2):329, June 1975.

Segil, Clive: "Current Concepts in the Management of Scoliosis." *Nursing Clinics of North America* 11(4):691, Dec. 1976.

Wright, Joan: "Deaf But Not Mute." American Journal of Nursing 76(5):795, May 1976.

CHAPTER 32
GRIEF, DYING AND DEATH

LINDA L. JARVIS, M.S.N., R.N.

Each of us, in our own way, must deal with the reality of death—it is inescapable. Usually we do not know the time of our anticipated deaths. Those with terminal illnesses or suffering from fatal accidents have a headstart in dealing with the actuality of their own death. For them, their days are more concretely numbered. The community health nurse faces a variety of situations dealing with grief, dying, and death. Her ability to provide supportive nursing interventions will be directly related to her philosophy, experience, and knowledge concerning death and the dying experience. Energy spent early in one's nursing education and nursing career to come to grips with the death experience will provide a foundation for developing increased personal awareness and effective nursing interventions when dealing with grief, dying, and death.

In identifying the type of death one experiences, Pattison[1] lists four distinct categories: 1) *sociologic death*—withdrawal and separation from the patient by others, 2) *psychic death*—the person accepts death and regresses into him or herself, 3) *biologic death*—the organism as a human entity no longer exists, there is no consciousness nor awareness even though the vital organs may continue to function with or without support, 4) *physiologic death*—vital organs such as lungs, heart, and brain no longer function. One may participate in these various categories at different points in time. When one learns that a fatal outcome to a disease or accident is the ultimate result, Pattison describes the reaction as "crisis of knowledge of death."[1] It is at this point that life expectations of the individual and family must be rearranged in terms of time and quality of life. According to Pattison the period

611

from the crisis knowledge of death to the point of death becomes the "living-dying interval" and can be divided into an acute crisis phase, the chronic living-dying phase, and the terminal phase.[1]

Each phase has specific characteristics. The acute crisis phase will be characterized by such experiences as high anxiety, immobilization, conscious state changes, feelings of inadequacy, and various defenses.[1] The chronic living-dying phase will be characterized by fear of the unknown, fear of loneliness, fear of sorrow, fear of losing family and friends, fear of loss of body, fear of loss of self-control, fear of suffering and pain, fear of loss of identity, and fear of regression.[1] The terminal phase is marked by internal signs which the individual responds to. Characteristically there is a withdrawal into one's self perhaps to save energy for the coming event of the actual death experience. It is during the terminal stage that the four types of death mentioned earlier are accomplished. Because the sequence of the types of death can vary, it has lead to many ethical issues such as the use of artificial support when biologic and psychic death have occurred.[1] In any event, the terminal stage can be quite variable in terms of time and quality of life experienced by the individual.

Elisabeth Kübler-Ross in her work with the dying has identified five areas of experience which an individual may undergo during the dying episode. From her early work in 1965 with a group of theology students, she has been a leader in the field of thanatology.[2] The five stages which she suggests a person may go through are 1) denial and isolation, 2) anger, 3) bargaining, 4) depression, 5) acceptance. These stages may be experienced separately or may occur concurrently. It should be kept in mind that these stages are a suggested sequence which the terminally ill person may travel during his illness. However, many people do not follow the pattern suggested or show evidence of shifting between stages at different points of their illnesses.

Both Kübler-Ross and Pattison talk about hope when dealing with the terminally ill patient. The terminally ill seem to hope for some last minute cure or successful drug or treatment protocol, remissions, or arrests which would change their prognoses. Kübler-Ross states "It is this glimpse of hope which maintains them through days, weeks or months of suffering. It is the feeling that all this must have some meaning, will pay off eventually, if they can only endure it for a little while longer."[2] Pattison speaks of an exceptional hope and desirable hope.[1] Exceptional hope deals with expected outcomes such as remissions or arrests in the disease course while desirable hope deals with desired results which have little probability to be realized. Numerous accounts of the experiences of both the terminally ill and their families refer to the persistence of hope, often up to the final moments of life.

The concept of grief has become an important part of the death experience. The terminally ill, the family, and the caretakers all experience grief as a result of the dying and death experience. Weisman defines anticipatory grief as "a phase of coping with inevitable death, to be followed by other forms of mourning and resolution."[3] "Bereavement, of which grief is a part, comprises a series of adjustments in which people realize and reaffirm relationships."[3] Slowly there has developed an awareness that the grief and mourning period is important to the adjustment of the survivors. It is important that people have the opportunity to openly deal with their experience of loss. The funeral ceremony is helpful in allowing people to confront the reality of the death which has occurred. For most people the mourning period is at least a year in length and may cover a longer period of up to three years.[4,5] All parties caring for the terminally ill patient need the opportunity to grieve the loss. If it is not done immediately, it will have to be done at some point in the future. Personal growth cannot take place if the grief process is not allowed to progress to its natural conclusion. Among the behaviors seen at this time are crying, anorexia, insomnia, and movement through activities with little real involvement in them. Personal and community resources need to be available in the form of support—both verbal and personal—if the grief period is to be fully met and resolved. Feifel says "the dead must die before we are able to redefine and reintegrate ourselves into life."[4]

DYING AND DEATH THROUGH THE LIFE CYCLE

The inevitability of death is a fact which all of us will face at some point during our life cycle. The reaction to this fact will depend on factors such as age, past illness/accident experience, culture, past experience with death, religion, and family/peer relationships.

Children and adults react to the dying experience in somewhat different ways. However, there is no conclusive evidence which confirms strict time or developmental parameters to the acknowledgment of death as a finality. Some 3 year olds may see its finality while an 8 year old would not. To a large extent children will react to the dying experience in direct response to their parents' reaction. Regardless of the age at which death is to be encountered, it is a stressful experience for the individual, family, and health providers.

Robert Kastenbaum identifies the following three stages in death perceptions of children: 1) Stage I (until about age 5) finality of death is not grasped, however, there is much curiosity about death and what happens to the body (*separation* between living and dead is the important concept level at this stage); 2) Stage II (from 5 to about age 9) death is now understood as final, there is a tendency to think of death as a person, some think that one can "luck out" and avoid death; 3) Stage III (from ages 9 to 10 onward) death is understood as final as well as *inevitable* and universal; all will die.[6]

For the young child, up to age 5, parents provide the main source of support and security. Children are very perceptive to changes in parental behavior and will respond directly to them. In periods of great stress, there may be role reversal so that the child is the one providing the support and comfort to the parent.[5] Older children realize the impact the illness will have on them and their futures. They are aware of time and fear being different from their peers as a result of their illnesses and required treatments. Time has little realistic meaning for the younger child but is of prime importance to the older child. As the disease progresses and disease remissions become shorter and more difficult to control, there is a tendency to speak less and less of future expectations and to deal more realistically with the present. For the terminally ill of all ages, often there is seen an urgency to utilize time productively and there may be great impatience and anger expressed when requests are perceived as being met slowly.

Young people—adolescent and young adults—are considered low death risk groups. The most common causes of death for this group are from accidents and suicide. This population, in general, has acquired the basic concepts of time, space, and causality and can be expected to have a basic understanding of the concept of death. Cultural expectations such as sex roles, risk taking behaviors, and attitudes toward war and violence will influence the attitudes and behavior patterns of young people in regard to dying and death.

Middle-aged adults tend to perceive death as a life companion.[6] It is often at this age that one experiences the death of parents. As parents die, middle-aged children are left to deal with the reality of death. One tends to think that older persons "should" die but as parents and perhaps older siblings die, the middle-aged person may suddenly see him or herself as the oldest family member. Children's deaths, then, are particularly difficult to accept as young children are not supposed to die. According to Kastenbaum, people establish a "pecking order of death" and establish, at least in their thinking, that the oldest person should by rights die—not younger ones.[6] It is during this period that one begins to acknowledge that, in fact, aging is taking place. People in this age span do tend to die more frequently than was the case perhaps a decade earlier. The onset of various chronic and acute diseases becomes manifest at this age stage. Self-image undergoes changes in the physical and activity realm and there may be either a tendency to cling to youth or to give up. The reaction of the individual will depend on past life experiences, coping mechanisms, and life attitudes.

For the geriatric person, death can, from some viewpoints, be accepted as right and expected. Because of the youth orientation in our society, there has been some difficulty in establishing the age cutoff for being old, with ages like 55, 65, and 70 years being identified. By this stage of life, many people have had direct experiences with death—parents, spouses, and/or children. Occupational retirement is common at this stage. Children are usually grown and have left home. More and more peers are dying which results in further losses, feelings of loneliness, and reinforcement of one's own demise. Plans are often made about distribution of possessions and care in case of disability. Funeral arrangements and burial or cremation decisions are generally made at this time. There needs to be someone or ones with whom the elderly can speak about death concerns. Resolutions of such concerns generally free energy for high quality living within the limits of the individual.

I have mentioned briefly some of the characteristics applicable to various developmental needs. Issues such as communication patterns, religion, family role, economics, type of illness/accident, and time parameters will influence the dying and death experience of the individual and family. If there was marital discord or other family strife present before the mortal event, it will, in general, not be resolved during the crisis. What may happen is that the family will stay together until the death occurs and at that time break apart. For those families who have experienced closeness and support prior to the death experience, they will probably continue or strengthen these bonds.

Once a family member acquires a terminal condition, roles and family expectations often undergo many changes. If the victim is a child, mothers may spend most of their time with the ill youngster. Older siblings may have to assume some parenting activities for younger siblings. There may be feelings of jealousy on the part of well siblings as they see their ill siblings receiving extra attention and perhaps objects such as toys and other gifts. It is important to include siblings in activities of care for the ill child and also allow them to visit the hospital so that they can see what the actual situation is rather than allow their fantasies to fill in the spaces. Efforts should be made by the staff to provide current information to parents, to be available for questions, and anticipate needs for sleep, food, and respites.

Whether to tell a child or adult of the seriousness of the illness has been a much debated question. In general, professionals working in the field of death and dying seem to agree that factual, honest information about the disease, treatment, and prognosis should be done as early as possible and as simply as possible. To try to hide information from the patient or family becomes a burden so great that much of the support and caring needed at this time may be neglected. The explanation and prognosis should be given with the developmental level of the members kept in mind. It will take time for the impact to be fully felt and the same information should be repeated until full understanding is acquired.

As the individual gradually succumbs to the illness or accident, family and staff members may have increasing difficulty in dealing with the death reality. Anger, excessive demands, withdrawal, and evasiveness may characterize the behavior of family and caretakers alike. The communication channels should always be kept open between all parties involved. Breakdown of communication can cause unnecessary feelings of isolation and loneliness—feelings which can be avoided.

Once death has occurred, the family may want to spend some time alone with the deceased. Provision should be made for such time. Where possible, the dying individual should be with family members, if this is not possible, then a staff member should stay with him or her. Touching, caressing, holding, rocking, or other such activities may be fulfilling to both the dying and family member. Common fears as death approaches include experiencing pain or discomfort, being alone when death occurs, and having to take this final journey on one's own. Among decisions which must be made are whether or not to do an autopsy, whether to provide organ transplants, selection of funeral arrangements, selection of casket and dress if appropriate, and the service format.

Funeral services are common in the United States. A funeral can be described as "that experience in which a person can face the reality of what has happened, let memory become a part of the process of grieving and, in the experience, express honest feelings, accept the community support that is freely proffered, and attempt to place the death in a context of meaning acceptable to the individual experience, the trauma of the separation."[7] The funeral experience proceeds through five separate steps: 1) removal, 2) the visitation period, 3) the funeral rite, 4) the procession, and 5) the committal.[7] The removal consists of transferring the deceased to an area for special preparation, such as embalming, usually carried out in a mortuary or funeral home. The visitation period is that period lasting from a few hours to two days in which the body can be viewed by the survivors. It may be held in the funeral home, the family home, church, or public building. During this visitation period with the body present, family and friends begin to deal with the death reality and the active mourning process begins. The funeral rite will vary depending on factors such as culture, ethnicity, religion, and desires of the deceased and family. The funeral rite takes several forms. A religious service consistent with the beliefs of the deceased may be carried out. Others will have secular or humanistic services when the deceased did not embrace a particular religious belief. A memorial service is a funeral alternative which is carried out without the body present and may be religious, secular, or a combination of these approaches. Two other funeral alternatives are direct disposition where the body is cremated or buried without service and body donation.[7] The procession involves the movement of the body from the site of service to the place of interment. Committal involves placement of the body in its final resting place. This process is important because it helps the person face the reality of death and to begin a life without the deceased present.

There is much debate as to the value of funerals as they are practiced in the American society. Among the sources of concern are the use of cosmetics to cover death, the visitation period, a tendency to hurry the gravesite service, use of pillows and fabrics in the coffin which create elaborate resting places, and attempts in some places to modify the expression of mourning. Some funerals are very expensive and there is concern about survivor vulnerability at this time. Many of these issues are important considerations. Any one carried to excess can inappropriately dull the death experience and create guilt, confusion, and anger for the survivor. Support in selection of funeral service and items such as caskets is needed at this time and should be provided when possible.

Before exploring some nursing interventions in the dying and death experience, mention of some of the ethical issues of concern in this area need to be clearly identified. Because of advances in medical technology which can maintain blood circulation and respiration and the increasing use of organ transplants, the exact definition of death has become an ethical, medical, moral, and philosophic issue.

In 1968, an ad hoc committee of the Harvard Medical School presented a report on a definition of irreversible coma which set up criteria which have been used widely in determining whether or not death has occurred. The four criteria which must be met to declare death are: 1) unreceptivity and unresponsivity, 2) no spontaneous muscular movement or spontaneous breathing, 3) no reflexes, and 4) flat EEG (electroencephalogram).[8] This statement came into being because of the increasing number of people who were in comas with heartbeat maintained because they were being ventilated via a mechanical respirator. The question then becomes one of when did death occur? Space does not allow us to explore in great detail the issue of death definition. Although there are many who hold to the Harvard definition of death, there are others who do not and thus the controversy over the medical definition of death continues.[9-11] An agreed upon definition for death will aid treatment decisions, will reduce family grief and guilt, and will open the way for removal of organs for transplant. That such a definition has major implications for the patient, health team members, and the family is precisely the reason that such debate is still relevant and prevalent.

Euthanasia constitutes another large area of moral, medical, and legal concern. Of particular concern is whether or not euthanasia is morally justified and whether or not euthanasia should be legalized so that there is a "right to die with dignity."[2] Arguments for euthanasia usually are for 1) personal/individual liberty, 2) threatened loss of human dignity, 3) efforts to reduce suffering. Arguments against it include 1) sanctity of human life, 2) fear of euthanasia without consent such as infanticide, "wedge argument," 3) fear of probable abuse, obtaining euthanasia consent under inappropriate conditions, and 4) fear of making a wrong diagnosis and the development of new treatment.[12] At its most basic form, euthanasia means the taking of one's life by another—the former being in a state of great suffering from accident or disease. Such action may be active in the case of drug administration or passive as in the withholding of actions which might have prolonged life as in resuscitation. In addition, it may be voluntary when the patient consents to it and involuntary when it occurs while the patient is comatose. In deciding about euthanasia, concern about definitions of death, suicide, and manslaughter become issues of wide concern. It is a difficult decision area and also faces much debate before final decisions are made, if ever. Other issues involve the right of people to know about diagnosis and treatment, informed consent for treatment options, living walls, organ transplants, and suicide. Volumes have been written on each of these subjects and space and time do not permit further exploration. However, as a community health nurse, you will encounter individuals, families, and communities dealing with these issues. Having a position on the issues and being aware of the many perceptions, debates, and philosophic, moral, and ethical points of view will allow you to be supportive and a resource person as people try to sort through the many concerns about the concept of dying and death.

NURSING INTERVENTIONS

Nurses in community health settings may deal with the individual and family coping with the dying and death experience on a variety of levels. She may be present when the diagnosis is made and given to the family as in an ambulatory setting. She may provide ongoing nursing care and support as a visiting nurse as the individual and family deal with the nuances of the disease and treatment in the home. She may serve as a coordinator for the family and patient as various plans are made for placement at home, hospital, or other facility as a continuing care coordinator. It will be necessary for all health care providers, regardless of role and site of service, to maintain open communication among themselves and between themselves and the patient and family.

The nursing process will be the most important tool the nurses use as they deliver care to the patient and family. Through use of this tool, histories will be taken and assessments will be made, goals will be established, nursing interventions implemented and evaluated, and revisions made as necessary. The record will allow nurses to know what interventions have been tried, how successful they were, and what the present nursing care direction is to be.

In coping with the stress of terminal illness or accident, the unpredictability of progress is a constant stress. Will drugs work? If a remission is gained, will it be for an extended period of time? Should heroic measures be taken during the terminal phase? These worries are real and need to be addressed. Community health nurses, because of their work site and the time variable of the terminal condition, are often in key positions to provide meaningful nursing interventions.

A major role is that of resource person. This includes efforts directed at clarifying and restating the medical diagnosis and prognosis if given. Although patients and families are given this information initially, there may be confusion regarding the meaning and such information may have to be repeated several times until it is fully understood and the impact has been incorporated into the reality of all concerned. Because treatment protocols and modalities may be complex and confusing, the community health nurse can aid in explaining the purpose of drugs and treatments, expected response to the drugs and treatments, and any untoward reactions which may occur. Such explanations should be based on the actual and perceived developmental level of the recipient. Supervision in the administration of medication is critical as many drugs are quite toxic and must be very carefully monitored. With both the patient and family, a checklist for drug/treatment administration can be designed as well as a procedure for informing the physician of any untoward reactions. It is of critical importance that the patient and family be supported in drug/treatment procedures so that they see that they can in fact handle the procedure and are more actively involved in the caring/curing process. A third area of resource support is in the finding and utilization of community resources. Whether it is for acquisition of bandages, identification of a support group, or identification of a hospice, utilization of community facilities can aid the patient and family in coping with the illness stress. Resources often are available and they should be tapped so that the family can continue to cope with the dying experience.

An area of repeated need by both the patient and the family is that of support. Part of the role here is to be available in person or by phone. The fear and reality of isolation is valid. It is not always necessary that one talk to either the patient or the family. Sometimes the mere presence, the ability to just sit quietly, is exactly the kind of caring that is needed. It may be that the nurse is the one who will have to seek out the family and determine what the support system is for their unit. Once established, efforts should be directed toward strengthening these ties. As time and the illness progress, these resources will be needed. In offering support, keep in mind that all family members are involved in this dying process and not just the patient and parents or spouse. Children or siblings should be sought and efforts made to discuss with them their fears, concerns and feelings. Where possible, they should be included in the care of the ill child or adult and arrangements made for hospital visits so they can see first hand what is happening. This opens the way for further discussion and provides a reality reference instead of unsupported fantasies.

Because of the many demands required in providing care for the ill member, needed rest, adequate nutrition, and time off may be overlooked. In view of the prolonged period the terminal illness may last, efforts to provide for adequate sleep, food, and recreation should be made. Even if the respite is a walk around the block or an hour's undisturbed nap, relief providers should be sought. Friends, family, and neighbors are often the pool for such support and relief as many people usually have offered such help. As the nurse, you have to identify the need and then set about to find ways to provide the necessary relief.

Decision making at this time is often very difficult. Because future expectations have been mortally wounded with confirmation of a terminal condition, the patient and family find themselves in a period of ongoing adjustment. Difficulties encountered will depend on such variables as prognosis, treatment availability, developmental stage of children, and family resources.

Insofar as possible, family structure should be maintained as before the illness. Children still need to laugh, play, go to school, and be disciplined; all of this should be continued within the limits of the patient's condition. Treatment decisions will need to be made and require nursing support. Help the family determine guidelines to use for when to give medication such as a pain reliever or when to call the doctor to report findings. Having these guidelines will provide criteria and support useful to the family members.

As the terminal phase becomes apparent, a decision will have to be made about dying at home, in the hospital, or in a hospice, if available. This decision should be the family's. Ida Martinson has done some pioneer work in the United States in support of families in their decision to experience a home death.[13] Assistance in modifying the living/sleeping arrangements may be needed. It may be necessary for the nurse to serve as a liaison between the family and the hospital in order to obtain support for home dying. Hospice care, if available, may be requested and the nurse should visit the facility so that she can share with the family services provided. It should be emphasized that decisions concerning the place of death can be changed as desired by the patient and family. This commonly involves a decision to leave the home and go to the hospital but the reverse may also be true. Whatever decision is made, the family should make it and be supported in it.

Pain relief is a source of major concern for both patient and family. A supply of pain medication should be available in anticipation of pain onset. Once started it should be given before it is needed so that the pain level can be controlled. Under no circumstances should placebos be given as it undermines credibility and is generally ineffective. As the nurse, it will be necessary to explain the use of the drug, expected results, and untoward reactions. Family members may have to be taught to give injections. Careful observations concerning drug use and effects should be conducted. Should stronger medication be needed, the nurse can either support the family in requesting the change or act as an intermediary to accomplish the desired result.

The nurse, in working with a family with a terminally ill member, is also a member of a large health team. The nurse's role will depend, as stated earlier, on the site at which she works. Regardless of the setting, she should strive to maintain open channels of communication with the family and the health team. Much misunderstanding and unnecessary loneliness, isolation, and guilt can be avoided if such channels are kept open.

As the patient enters the terminal phase of his illness, emotions on all parts may be volatile. It will be a time when patience and understanding will be of utmost importance. It may be helpful to identify the emotional variability so that it can be discussed and perhaps some relief experienced.

As a team member, the nurse's role will include that of patient advocate. She may be able to act as an intermediary for the patient and family with other health team members and the various resources of the community. The comfort, welfare, and safety of the patient and family will be her main concern.

To work with individuals and families engaged in the dying experience takes time, energy, and courage. Each visit to the physician represents a temporary reprieve or another step toward the inevitable conclusion. In order to be most effective, the nurse should have come to grips with her own philosophy about death and dying. Her ability to support the family throughout the experience will be directly related to her ability to deal with death and dying issues. The satisfaction of aiding a patient and family to a dignified death experience which meets the needs and desires of the principals can be a most rewarding nursing experience. Such an encounter can provide for real personal and professional growth and sensitivity.

REFERENCES

1. Pattison, E. Mansell: *The Experience of Dying.* Prentice-Hall, Inc., Englewood Cliffs, N.J., 1977.
2. Kübler-Ross, Elisabeth: *On Death and Dying.* Macmillan Publishing Co., New York, 1969.
3. Weisman, Avery D.: "The Psychiatrist and the Inexorable," in Feifel, H. (ed.): *New Meanings of Death.* McGraw-Hill Book Company, New York, 1977.
4. Feifel, Herman: "Death in Contemporary America," in Feifel, H. (ed.): *New Meanings of Death.* McGraw-Hill Book Company, New York, 1977.
5. Gyulay, Jo-Eileen: *The Dying Child.* McGraw-Hill Book Company, New York, 1978.
6. Kastenbaum, Robert: "Death and Development through the Lifespan," in Feifel, H. (ed.): *New Meanings of Death.* McGraw-Hill Book Company, New York, 1977.
7. Raether, Howard C., and Slater, Robert C.: "Immediate Postdeath Activities in the United States," in Feifel, H. (ed.): *New Meanings of Death.* McGraw-Hill Book Company, New York, 1977.
8. Report of the Ad Hoc Committee of the Harvard Medical School to Examine the Definition of Brain Death: "A Definition of Irreversible Coma," *JAMA* 205(6): 337, Aug. 1968.
9. Veatch, Robert M.: "Defining Death Anew: Technical and Ethical Problems," from *Death, Dying, and the Biological Revolution 1976,* in Beauchamp, T.L., and Perlin, S. (eds.): *Ethical Issues in Death and Dying.* Prentice-Hall, Inc., Englewood Cliffs, N.J., 1978.
10. Schwager, Robert L.: "Life, Death and the Irreversibly Comatose," in Beauchamp, T.L., and Perlin, S. (eds.): *Ethical Issues in Death and Dying.* Prentice-Hall, Inc., Englewood Cliffs, N.J., 1978.
11. Jonas, Hans: "Against the Stream: Comments on the Definition and Redefinition of Death," from *Philosophical Essays: from Ancient Creed to Technological Man 1974,* in Beauchamp, T.L., and

Perlin, S. (eds.): *Ethical Issues in Death and Dying.* Prentice-Hall, Inc., Englewood Cliffs, N.J., 1978.
12. Beauchamp, Tom L., and Perlin, Seymour: "Euthanasia and Natural Death," in Beauchamp, T.L., and Perlin, S. (eds.): *Ethical Issues in Death and Dying.* Prentice-Hall, Inc., Englewood Cliffs, N.J., 1978.
13. Martinson, Ida: "The Child with Leukemia—Parents Help Each Other." *American Journal of Nursing* 76(7):1120, July 1976.

BIBLIOGRAPHY

Beauchamp, Tom L., and Perlin, Seymour (eds.): *Ethical Issues in Death and Dying.* Prentice-Hall, Inc., Englewood Cliffs, N.J., 1978.
Brewer, Judith: "Sharing a Tragedy." *American Journal of Nursing* 76(5):758, May 1976.
Bunch, Barbara, and Zahra, Donna: "Dealing with Death—the Unlearned Role." *American Journal of Nursing* 76(9):1486, Sept. 1976.
Craven, Joan, and Wald, Florence S.: "Hospice Care for Dying Patients." *American Journal of Nursing* 75(10:1816, Oct. 1975.
Feifel, Herman (ed.): *New Meanings of Death.* McGraw-Hill Book Company, New York, 1977.
Feifel, Herman (ed.): *The Meaning of Death.* McGraw-Hill Book Company, New York, 1959.
Flynn, Eileen D.: "What It Means to Battle Cancer." *American Journal of Nursing* 77(2):261, Feb. 1977.
Foley, Genevieve, and McCarthy, Ann Marie: "The Child with Leukemia—the Disease and Its Treatment." *American Journal of Nursing* 76(7):1108, July 1976.
Foley, Genevieve, and McCarthy, Ann Marie: "The Child with Leukemia—In a Special Hematology Clinic." *American Journal of Nursing* 76(7):1115, July 1976.
Hendrickson, Sharon: "A Philosophy of Death Made Personal." *American Journal of Nursing* 76(1): 90, Jan. 1976.
Jervik, Diane K., and Martinson, Ida M.: *Women in Stress: A Nursing Perspective.* Appleton-Century-Crofts, New York, 1979.
Kübler-Ross, Elisabeth: *Death—the Final Stage of Growth.* Prentice-Hall, Inc., Englewood Cliffs, N.J., 1975.
Marks, Mary Jo: "The Grieving Patient and Family." *American Journal of Nursing* 76(9):1488, Sept. 1976.
Schulz, Richard: *The Psychology of Death, Dying and Bereavement.* Addison-Wesley Publishing Company, Reading, Mass., 1978.
Sonstegard, Lois, Henson, Neva, Zillman, Linda, et al.: "The Grieving Nurse." *American Journal of Nursing* 76(9):1490, Sept. 1976.
Ufemo, Joy K.: "Dare to Care for the Dying." *American Journal of Nursing* 76(1):88, Jan. 1976.
Ward, Barbara J.: "Hospice Home Care Program." *Nursing Outlook* 26(10):646, Oct. 1978.
Wise, Doreen J.: "Learning About Dying." *Nursing Outlook* 22(1): 42, Jan. 1974.

VI

MAJOR ENVIRONMENTAL ISSUES AFFECTING COMMUNITY HEALTH

The quality of the environment is receiving widespread attention. As we experience Love Canal and Three Mile Island damage, community and governmental scrutiny of laws, safety, accountability, and ethics are becoming more intense. The effect environmental decisions have on the quality of life are receiving more debate. People are slowly becoming aware of the impact of industrial, commercial, transportation, and social actions on the status of the environment. As health problems are directly related to various environmental hazards, people are seeking explanations, health treatment, and legislative change which will provide a higher degree of protection.

These chapters are included to provide some basis of understanding of the problems and issues encountered in the area of environmental quality: clients will seek the nurse out to provide facts, answers, and opinions on a variety of these issues. The community health nurse can only be influential as she is knowledgeable and concerned about the actual and potential problems.

CHAPTER 33
POPULATION ISSUES

LINDA L. JARVIS, M.S.N., R.N.

During the last century there has been increasing concern about the growth of the world population. Population can be defined as "the total number of inhabitants of a particular race, class, or group in a specified area" or "all of the people inhabiting a specified area."[1] The study of human populations is called demography and generally addresses such characteristics as size, density, distribution, and vital statistics.

The fact that our national and world population is growing is clearly evident. The growth of any given population will influence a variety of social, political, and environmental areas including economics, occupations, education, housing, resource utilization, land use, health services, population policies, and others. Concerns about the population are complicated by the interrelationship between social, political, economic, health, and environmental forces. This chapter will look at some of the issues surrounding population growth and its impact on the individual, family, and community as relative to the United States.

STATISTICS AND TERMINOLOGY

Population growth or change is dependent on births, deaths, and migration. Changes in any one of these variables will change the population level and will provide both immediate and long range effects. A comparison of population characteristics will help illustrate this. Consider that in the United States in 1790, we had a land area of less than

1 million square miles and a population of under 4 million, representing a density of 4.5 per square mile, while in 1970 the land area has grown to 3.5 million square miles and the population is now more than 200 million with a density of 57.3 per square mile.[2]

When this country was first settled, the population consisted of two main groups—the native Americans and immigrants who represented a wide cross section of ethnic, racial, and religious persuasions. There was much land and the immigrational conquest was on. People were living in either urban or rural settings; suburbs had not come into being. The work effort was largely agricultural, business, and craftsmanship. Life expectancy was low, perhaps 35 years, and infant and child mortality was high, particularly from communicable/infectious diseases. Marriage was the norm and children were generally the result of such unions. Fertility control was low. Children were seen as assets to the family particularly as they were able to aid in the maintenance and growth of the family welfare. Children had family working responsibilities at an early age. As people sought to expand the boundaries of the United States, cultural and ethnic practices often faded but did not disappear as the "melting pot" effect began to be felt.

As we moved into the 20th century and are nearing the 21st century, the life expectancy has been gradually increasing. In 1974 the life expectancy for white males was 69.1, for white females 76.6, for black and other males 63.7, for black and other females it was 71.8.[3] Fertility control is much more attainable. Life expectancy has increased and thus the mortality rate has been reduced. Immigration is fairly well stabilized at about 400,000 per year.[3] The projected population in the United States by the end of the century will be between 245,098,000 and 287,000,000 depending on the fertility rate.[3] All parts of the country are inhabited. We have changed from a rural-urban society to a rural-urban-suburban society. People move from job to job and various geographic locations with little thought to the distances traveled.

The family of today is undergoing many changes. Marriage is still prevalent but childbearing in such unions is often postponed. Where the majority of births once occurred when women were in their 20s, we are seeing increasing numbers of women postponing pregnancies until their 30s. There are also more unmarried women bearing and rearing children. Contraception and abortion are, in general, available. The family structure has become predominantly nuclear rather than extended.

In looking at statistics which examine population projections, the difference in the eventual level will depend, in part, on the birth rate. The replacement requirement is 2.1 children per woman. If the birth rate should fall to 1.8, we would have a population of 251 million by 2000, assuming zero net immigration.[4] A rate of 2.5 children per woman would provide a population of 286 million by 2000.[4] With the absence of immigration at the replacement level the population would stabilize at just under 300 million by 2000 but would exceed 300 million if immigration is permitted.[4]

Another factor which is blatant is that the older population is increasing. There are presently 33 million people drawing Social Security benefits and this number can be expected to increase in the decades ahead. Because there will eventually be fewer people paying into the system due to a smaller working population which must provide funds for a growing population, serious questions are then raised concerning such issues as age of retirement, encouragement of private retirement funds and savings accounts, and reevaluation of the Social Security concept. The proportion of children to the aged is changing and it necessitates a reevaluation of many policies and time held assumptions.

In reading population literature, one is immediately confronted with a great many terms which may be confusing. The ones listed below are commonly encountered:

1. Crude birth rate: births per 1000 female inhabitants per year
2. General fertility rate (GFR): the number of live births per year per 1000 women of childbearing age
3. Age specific fertility rate: births per 1000 women in a single year or five year age group
4. Cohort fertility rate: average number of lifetime births per 1000 women
5. Gross reproduction rate (GRR): replacement rate for all women of childbearing age to replace themselves
6. Net reproduction rate (NRR): the number of females that replace the initial cohort of 1000 females in the course of a generation
7. Replacement level fertility: the level of fertility at which the population would exactly replace itself in the absence of net immigration
8. Natural increase: the excess of births over deaths
9. Life expectancy: the number of years expected to live at the time of birth
10. Age specific mortality rate: deaths per year per 1000 persons of a specific age
11. Crude death rate: deaths per 1000 inhabitants per year
12. Corrected death rate: rate obtained by dividing the life expectancy into 1000
13. Zero population growth (ZPG):
    1) a society in which the age composition is stable and births equal deaths
    2) A society whose population, labor force, and output per worker are all stationary[2-3,5-6]

POPULATION ISSUES AND IMPACT

To discuss the scope of population influence, one has to address environmental issues as well. The relationship between the two—population and environment—is complex and involves a variety of variables. Two groups which hold opposing views are Paul Ehrlich and John Holdren who contend that population levels are directly related to environmental pollution while Barry Commoner, Michael Carr, and Paul Stamler propose that the environmental pollution is due to "the increasing environmental impact per unit of production due to technological changes" rather than the direct influence of population levels or affluence.[7,8] Ehrlich and Holdren propose a total approach in dealing with environmental issues to include population control, the redirection of technology, and the transition from open to closed resource cycles. Commoner, Carr, and Stamler would propose major emphasis on technologic changes to reduce harmful impact on the environment because such environmental damage will continue regardless of population size if such steps are not taken. The preceding statements are, of course, great simplifications of the positions both camps embrace concerning population and environment.

In discussing population impact, seven areas will be covered. These are fertility, life expectancy, resources, education, politics, health, and economics. An effort will be made to discuss the impact on the individual, family, and community of each area.

Fertility

Fertility is the first area of concern. It has been decreasing for several decades except for the period during the late 1940s following World War II and into the 1950s when we experienced a baby boom. We are presently on a track toward replacement level which might be attained sometime during the early 21st century.

There is no way, however, to predict with any degree of certainty that the present trend will continue, the most recent example being the baby boom which increased numbers but was not consistent with the trend in effect at that time. Many factors have influenced, in some way, the present United States population level. One important one is the availability and reliability of contraceptive measures. There is a wide choice including rhythm, condoms, diaphragm, jellies, intrauterine devices, the "pill," and sterilization. The choices are available and have been increasingly so since the passage of the Family Planning and Population Research Act of 1970, although there is much need for expansion of such services. Use of contraception is becoming widespread among the population, including religious groups such as Catholics, which once had a low participation in birth control efforts.

It is also possible for more women to have access to abortion services for the termination of unwanted pregnancies. Since abortions have become legal, increasing numbers of women have utilized this means of terminating unwanted pregnancies. However, access by teenagers and low income groups to such services is still uneven.

The impact such a decision has on the woman and her family is difficult to determine. For some there is guilt, anger, resignation, or relief. The reaction may be related to the circumstances surrounding the conception/pregnancy. Availability and access to the abortion services may influence the reaction as well as the attitude of the health providers who the woman encounters. Although there are those who use abortion as a means of contraception, this kind of usage is of concern and not encouraged. The issues of morality and ethics concerning abortion are still hotly debated and are unlikely to be resolved at any time in the future.

The presence of an abortion center in a given community may result in an increased number of people traveling into the area, a source of dissention among some neighborhood members, or a source of security and stress reduction for others. The reactions will depend on such factors as size of community, religious/ethnic/cultural persuasion, and political bent of the community.

Another factor in population control is that of sterilization. It is done, generally, by tubal ligation for women and by vasectomy for men. The surgical procedure is permanent and usually not reversible. Such procedures are generally voluntary but there have been questions raised about the involuntary use of such procedures on the mentally deficient, minority individuals, and the mentally ill. The true extent of such allegations is probably unknown but fears concerning the involuntary use of irreversible contraceptive measures are founded in fact and extreme caution must be exercised in the sanctioning of such practices to limit the population. Perhaps most vocal in their outspoken opposition to any limit to population growth is the Black Nationalist group. They are striving for a large black population which will be politically powerful and perceive any kind of birth limitation in direct conflict with their growth goal and inconsistent with the woman's role which is perceived as childbearing.[5] Other black groups are suspicious of population limitation but are not so vehement as the Black Nationalists. Their concerns embrace all forms of contraception which include involuntary sterilization, perhaps one of the most fearsome of approaches and one to be evaluated with great caution. Should such activity become accepted, the possibilities for potential abuse are overwhelming.

In the present part of the 20th century, several influences concerning fertility need to be noted. Women are often postponing childbearing/childrearing until their late 20s or into their 30s to pursue education and careers. More women are waiting to marry at a later age or are choosing to bear children outside of marriage. Increasing numbers of women are working which is postponing childbearing or reducing the number of children.

If there develops a trend to postpone childbearing to a later age and still maintain a replacement average of 2.1 per woman, the result will be a change in age distribution of the population.

Whether or not one chooses to practice any birth control measure will depend on a variety of factors including personal maturity level, attitude toward sexual behavior, religious, cultural, and ethnic values, beliefs, and practices. As these factors may change, so might the population growth direction towards either an increase or decline in total numbers. We have no absolute predictor at this time.

Life Expectancy

As the number of older persons has increased, the needs of the population have also increased and changed. Wilbur Cohen, when discussing population, uses the terms "productive" and "dependent."[9] The population is divided into three groups: those 20 to 64 are in the productive group while those under 20 and over 65 are placed in the dependent group. Dependency ratios in 1973 were 86.1 with a child dependency ratio of 67.5 and an aged one of 18.6. Dependency ratios were about 90 during 1960-70 and will be about 65 in the year 2010 and then go to about 80 in the year 2030.[9] Although the Social Security system is being stretched very tightly, if these estimates hold, it may be possible for the anticipated Social Security drain to be less than predicted.

As we are faced with an increasing aging population, many social, political, and health issues must be dealt with. One issue is that of retirement. How will it be handled? Some thought will need to be given to exploring private plans, the encouragement of increased savings plans, and perhaps changes in the retirement age. Decisions which we make should be influenced by such questions as impact on the individual, impact on the work force, and impact on the Social Security system as it is now structured. The rate and impact of inflation will influence decisions.

As the older population increases, there is increased concern with health issues, particularly as we now face the chronic problems of heart, circulatory, pulmonary, and metabolic diseases which focus on the older group. Health service availability and access must be ensured. Steps taken to meet this need can be initiated now so that the services will be more readily attainable in the future.

Housing needs are of prime concern. Elderly housing developments, particularly in urban areas, have not caught up with the present need. Efforts in this direction require careful consideration and planning. Many elderly move out of homes used during their growing years with family and require or desire smaller more efficient housing. This may directly affect a community's tax base.

There are also increasing numbers of people who move to the sun belt areas of the southern United States. This may directly affect such issues as tax base, electoral college vote distribution, health and housing needs, recreation, and transportation needs. As there, is a tendency for more conservative orientation among the elderly, and as they will make up a large proportion of the total voting base, there may be a real change in the concerns of governmental officials, issues debated, and funding allocations.

As the population ages, we also see an increase in the number of women due to longer life expectancy. Family changes from the extended to nuclear orientation may create some problems, particularly within families, as to the decisions made about living arrangements and geographic locations. How these issues are dealt with will depend in part on the orientation and attitudes of the family members, housing availability, health status and needs, and personal desires. There is no doubt that special concern and monies will be needed to provide services for the aging population.

Resources

The exact and direct relationship between population members and resource utilization is an extremely dynamic area of debate and concern. We are experiencing increasing levels of water and air pollution. Land use is often planned and implemented without a full assessment of the impact it will have on the environment. There is increased demand for and use of recreational land. Particularly during the summer, national parks and recreation areas are filled with people who have the opportunity to get out and see the land. Housing, transportation, recreation, and technology needs all influence the society and the resource reserves.

There are limitations on our natural resources. Regardless of how we use them, whether wisely or not, we will eventually be faced with the ultimate depletion of such resources. These include minerals, coal, trees, water, air, oil, and land. We are using them at a high rate and need to carefully evaluate this direction. Single housing is sought and land is used which is unsuitable. Examples are tracts set up in wet land areas or along geologic fault lines where earthquakes are possible. Wet land destruction has an unbalancing effect on our ecosystem influencing birds, insects, fish, and eventually man.

Technology has increased our ability to produce many products, however, this has been an area of increased concern. For as we have used resources to produce products of various kinds at a low cost, we have depleted resources and increased environmental refuse. Vast amounts of plastic and synthetic products are developed and manufactured which are nonbiodegradable meaning they cannot decompose when buried. If burned, air pollution is increased. Such products litter the entire land.

More people are requiring more products, technology, land, and resources. At one time in our history, there seemed little need for great concern over environmental pollution or depletion. Now, however, we know or at least are beginning to know the seriousness of the problem. The oil crisis of recent years is a prime example of such demand issues. Technology is highly sophisticated in this country. Changes could be made in such areas as car efficiency (both emission control and gas utilization), home fuel utilization, electricity production, food production and fertilizer usage, product packaging (so that it is bio-degradable), and other areas which would provide for a cleaner environment and shorten our rapid environmental decline and perhaps demise.

Education

As the numbers of children fluctuate, so do the needs for educational facilities and services. The decline of the early 40s followed by the baby boom of the late 40s and 50s created a demand on schools which we were unprepared to meet.

Full efforts were put into preparing teachers and constructing classroom space. Primary, secondary, and collegiate programs have been affected. Presently, though, the declining birth rate is creating another crisis in education and this is a decline in enrollment. Teachers are being laid off and teaching jobs are hard to find. Communities of all sizes are faced with a need to close schools, dismiss teachers, and seek ways of consolidating services.

Colleges have experienced great student crushes too, but this may be declining as a result of the lowered birth rate. As collegiate education is increasingly valued, though, there may be a trend to return to school at a later age, to obtain second career training, or attend school for personal growth without seeking a degree. Changes in student orientation will influence programs which schools will offer and will impact on the number of faculty used for such education.

Support for education at the primary and secondary levels will face increasing stress as the tax base shifts with the increasing age of the citizens and perhaps a reduction in total population. The property tax which has traditionally paid for education costs is already facing strain and may be totally unable to support such efforts in the future.

Political and Economic Concerns

As stated earlier, the increased life expectancy and declining birth rate will impact on the overall age distribution of the population. An increase in the number of aged may constitute a local, state, and national voting block. National voting may be changed as population migration takes increasing numbers of aged to the southern section of the U.S. Such change could result in electoral college changes and in a more conservative political stance.

Economic issues will be concerned with maintenance of the work force, possible change in retirement age, and Social Security benefits. Tax base changes will also result as there are increasing numbers of elderly renting residences rather than owning homes or giving up their homes. The Social Security tax may be increased so that the workers will be paying more to meet the needs of the elderly. The inflation rate will profoundly affect the status of those on limited or fixed incomes. Alternatives to Social Security and various private retirement and savings plans need exploration.

Health

Health care for all segments of the population will hopefully move more into a health maintenance-illness prevention model. With increasing numbers of elderly, there will be more need for special services to meet their needs. Since chronic diseases are of high incidence here, efforts in care, education, and research should be conducted to meet some of these needs. Likewise, there will be a changed need for health services for children. There will be fewer children but probably an increase in various physical, mental, and learning disorders which we have more ability to diagnose and now to treat.

Since health access and availability is essential, there may be an increase in satellite health services and facilities. Nursing homes of all levels will need to be more available. Hospice services hopefully will be available as people begin to take more active decision roles in their rites of dying as well as living. Fee schedules and payment plans for all services will require innovative approaches.

SUMMARY

The impact of population size/growth will be felt in every segment of our society and life. As nurses, we need to be sensitive to the changes that various fertility and mortality practices/rates will have on the population we provide services for both in the short and long run.

Changes in resource utilization, education, and health services can have a direct bearing on the quality of life we all enjoy. Community health nurses, because they are so familiar with the needs, desires, and orientation of their population of care, can have a direct input into policy debate and changes which are made. They can also provide information to citizens to help them in the formulation of opinions on such policy matters.

We cannot at this time predict the absolute population number or character we will encounter in the future. We can, however, anticipate increases in total numbers, increases in the elderly, and either stabilization or perhaps a decline in the birth rate. Scrutiny of trends will aid in identifying areas of future need. Flexibility and futuristic vision and planning can help to anticipate and meet some of these needs.

REFERENCES

1. Morris, William (ed.): *The American Heritage Dictionary of the English Language.* Houghton Mifflin Company, Boston, 1976.
2. Westoff, Charles F., and Parker, Robert, Jr. (ed.): The Commission on Population Growth and the American Future. *Demographic and Social Aspects of Population Growth.* Government Printing Office, Washington, D.C., 1972.
3. U.S. Department of Commerce, Bureau of the Census: *Statistical Abstract of the United States, 97th Annual Edition.* Government Printing Office, Washington, D.C., 1976.
4. Spingler, Joseph J.: *Population and America's Future.* W.H. Freeman and Company, San Francisco, 1975.
5. Gray, Virginia, and Bergman, Elihu: *Political Issues in U.S. Population Policy.* Lexington Books, Lexington, 1974.
6. Speryler, Joseph J.: *Population and America's Future.* W.H. Freeman and Company, San Francisco, 1975.
7. Ehrlich, Paul, and Holdren, John: "Impact of Population Growth," in Marden, P.G., and Hodgson, D. (eds.): *Population, Environment and the Quality of Life.* AMS Press Inc., New York, 1975.
8. Commoner, Barry, Carr, Michael, and Stamler, Paul: "The Causes of Pollution," in Marden, P.G., and Hodgson, D. (eds.): *Population, Environment and the Quality of Life.* AMS Press Inc., New York, 1975.
9. Cohen, Wilber J., and Westoff, Charles F.: *Demographic Dynamics in America.* The Charles C Moskowitz Memorial Lecture No. XVIII. Macmillan Publishing Co., New York, 1977.

BIBLIOGRAPHY

Hanlon, John J.: *Public Health Administration and Practice,* 6th ed. The C.V. Mosby Company, St. Louis, 1974.
Marden, Parker G., and Hodgson, Dennis: *Population, Environment and the Quality Of Life.* AMS Press, Inc., New York, 1975.
Pennycuick, Roy A.: *People, Pollution and Payment.* Acco, Leuven, Belgium, 1973.
U.S. Statistical Atlas: Prepared by Joe B. Williams, Elinwood, Nebraska, 1973.

CHAPTER 34
SAFETY AND ACCIDENTS

LINDA L. JARVIS, M.S.N., R.N.

Accidents injure and kill thousands of people of all ages every year. Accidents ranked as the fourth cause of death with a rate of 49.5/100,000 estimated population in 1974.[1] Accidents can occur at any time and in any situation—home, school, work place, highway, recreation area. Most accidents are the result of carelessness or ignorance and most could and should be prevented. Therefore, safety education and enforcement is paramount to reducing the frequency and seriousness of accidents.

Accident can be defined as "an unexpected and undesirable event, a mishap; anything that occurs unexpectedly or unintentionally."[2] Safety is defined as "freedom from danger, risk, or injury; any of various devices designed to prevent accident."[2] As nurses in a variety of community health settings, our focus needs to be directed toward the reinforcement of safety enhancing activities and the extinguishing of accident promoting activities for the individual, family, and community. This requires active assessment of environmental conditions in the home, school, occupational setting, health care sites, recreational areas, and community sites and resources of all kinds. Accidents can be prevented or reduced in frequency through vigorous educational activities, safety inspection visits, and enforcement of safety laws and regulations.

STATISTICS AND SCOPE OF PROBLEM

It is difficult to estimate the exact number of accidental injuries which are sustained each year. This happens partly because many accidental injuries do not require emergency room or physician visits for treatment, and there is no consistent, systematic program for reporting accidents. It is easier to determine death rates due to accidents because the cause is reported on the death certificate and is available for tabulation. Such information provides data on specific accident frequency and can become a focus for educational and preventive efforts.

The distribution of accident frequencies throughout the age span of the population provides some interesting findings. The rate between males and females remains approximately the same until about age 15 years when males outrank females and continues until about age 65 when females then outrank males in accidental death rate.[3] In age groups, accidents are the major cause of death in the following spans: 1 to 4 years, 5 to 14 years, 15 to 24 years, and 25 to 34 years.[3] In terms of income levels, females have the highest rate of home accidents in low income groups, and males have the highest home accident rate in high income groups.[3] The kitchen is the site of the most frequent number of home accidents, while the bedroom is the site of most fatal home accidents.[3] Accidental injuries result in restriction of activities temporarily or permanently, hospitalization, and death. The financial impact is experienced through increased insurance premiums, hospital and ambulatory care costs, workmen's compensation expenditures, sick leave benefits, and income losses from not being able to return to one's former job and salary rank or being unable to complete educational programs due to injuries. The impact of accidental injury and death is felt by all segments of the society in direct and indirect financial, rehabilitation, and social terms.

Since accidents can happen to anyone at any time, some attention needs to be given to the kinds and sites of accidents which can occur. In the home, injuries result from such causes as falls, fires, particularly in the kitchen and bedroom, poisoning, particularly for children from such sources as household cleaning products and various drugs, including aspirin, and various lacerations, abrasions, and fractures from tools, lawn care equipment, and various cutting equipment such as scissors and knives.

At the work place, the type of accidents and injuries will depend on the kind of activities carried on. Falls are a source of injury regardless of site and may be due to water or other liquid on the floor, improperly positioned extension cords, and objects in travel ways such as corridors and stairs. Lacerations, abrasions, and various eye injuries may be due to unprotected equipment and machinery, failure to use safety equipment such as gloves and goggles, improper use of equipment, and failure to follow accepted safety protocols. Additional injuries may result from high noise levels and from various inhalants such as asbestos, coal dust, and cotton mill dust. The last mentioned injuries may be due to long exposure and their impact will be delayed. Job stress may cause mental health problems which can be linked to various accidents and injuries.

Vehicular accidents account for a large number of injuries and fatalities. They are particularly dramatic because of the severity of injuries and the number of people and vehicles involved. Vehicular accidents include those involving cars, bicycles, tricycles, motorbikes, motorcycles, snowmobiles, trains, buses, and airplanes. Highway safety is a major source of concern at the local, state, and national levels. Who does not recall the grim fatality statistics which are predicted and then confirmed at the approach and passing of each holiday?

Each vehicular accident requires an investigation as to cause. Safety factors are investigated and recommendations are made to prevent such accidents in the future. As a result of such investigations, speed limits have been established. Airports have established flight control procedures and various safety equipment has been installed in planes to help prevent accidents. Rail travel is regulated by a variety of safety regulations in an effort to prevent derailments and various train collisions. Unfortunately, it often takes a major tragedy to obtain full implementation of some safety standards for our commercial transportation system.

Auto and other motor vehicles also are subject to various safety regulations. Among them are highway speed limits, safety belt usage, roadway signs to alert the driver to such hazards as hills, curves, and no passing zones. As a result of auto accident investigations, increasing pressure is being placed on auto manufacturers to produce safer autos. Among the concerns are bumper impact safety, placement of rear end gas tanks, and seat and safety belt stabilization. It is important to note, though, that all the safety equipment and measures pertinent to highway travel will be to no avail if the driver is not cautious in his driving habits and practices.

Motorbikes, motorcycles, bicycles, and tricycles are involved in many roadway accidents. Proper navigation of such vehicles on the road is paramount to safety. Speed limits are applicable to all motorized vehicles. Bicycles should obey all travel patterns on the road including movement with the flow of traffic. Tricycles should be used in fenced or confined areas because the riders tend to be young, under age 5, and are prone to travel without thinking of dangerous situations. Safety equipment is vital and includes the use of protective head gear and proper clothing to reduce the severity of accidents which do occur.

Recreational accidents are often the result of poor physical conditioning, overexertion, failure to observe safety regulations, faulty equipment and sites, and inattention to the activity underway. Playgrounds, parks, campgrounds, swimming pools, tennis courts, athletic fields, and backyards are all sites for recreational activities. Because of the variety of activities, the kinds of injuries vary but can generally be classified as falls, head injuries from various causes, abrasions, lacerations, and fractures. Accidents can be prevented by adhering to safety rules. Equipment should be sturdy and in good working order. Playgrounds should be free of glass, tin cans, and other debris which could cause injury. Fencing of the area will reduce the incidence of children running into the street. Adherence to regulations about use of fires and storage of food stuff at campgrounds is important. Signing in at ranger stations when hiking and camping in mountainous terrain is good common sense and will increase chances for safe search and rescue should it become necessary. Movement of spectators at various athletic events should be limited in order to prevent injuries from accidental contact with equipment such as baseball bats.

The health site should be hazard free and serve as an example of a safe environment. Furnishings should be sturdy and free of splinters and exposed tacks or springs. Lighting should be adequate and properly placed. Extension cords should be avoided and safety plugs placed in unused electrical outlets. Toys should be clean, appropriate for the age level of the children, and free of hazardous parts. Floors should be free of liquids, objects, and scatter rugs or other floor coverings which could cause a fall. Building access and egress should be clearly marked and maintained in a safe manner. All stairs should have railings and steps should have safety treads. Equipment in the setting used for delivery of health services should be hazard free. Safety education can be an integral part of the entire program. Teaching can be particularly effective at the time of injury but caution must be taken not to produce guilt or enhance guilt in such efforts.

From the preceding, it should be clear that accidents can occur anywhere, any time and to anyone. The importance of education in accident prevention and safety measures and enforcement of safety regulations can aid in the reduction of accidents. It is the individual who carries a major responsibility for engaging in activities in a safe manner and in seeking correction of hazardous conditions.

ACCIDENT IMPACT AND SAFETY MEASURES

The exact impact of any accident will depend on such factors as age of individual, extent and type of injury, disability as result of injury, and role in family structure. There may be loss of skill, decreased activity participation, loss of income, hospitalization, rehabilitation effort, and death as a result of any accident.

For the individual, the injury will probably result in some degree of pain or discomfort depending on severity, a visit to an emergency room or physician, the need to treat the injury in some manner, a dependent state in terms of activity level and activities of daily living such as feeding, dressing, and personal hygiene, and potential loss of time from school, work, or play. There will be a cost for any injury in terms of funds, time, and/or discomfort. If one survives an accident, it is hoped that efforts will be made to avoid such situations in the future. Efforts in handling the accident should be directed toward prevention, education, and treatment.

For young children, particularly from neonate through about age 5 to 6, special preventive efforts, observation, and activity limitation must be the responsibility of adults who care for the child. The initiation of safety oriented behavior should begin at this age through example and education. Since toddlers are particularly prone to falls, efforts toward providing a safe environment and proper clothes and shoes for the child are paramount. This means that floors should be clean, dry, and free of hazardous coverings. Toys should be in safe repair and have a special place to be stored. Shoes and slippers and pajamas must have skid-proof soles. Clothing should fit properly and long pant legs should be shortened by sewing rather than rolling up. Access to stairs can be protected by closed doors or a variety of guards. All household cleaning supplies should be placed out of the child's reach in all areas of the house—kitchen, bathroom, cellar. Since many mothers carry medication such as aspirin in their purses, care needs to be taken that they are put in a safe place out of the way of exploring fingers. Outside play areas need to be free of glass and other objects which can cause injury, supplied with safe play toys and equipment, and supervised by responsible persons. For this age group, minor falls and scrapes may be inevitable as a result of their developmental stage, but serious, debilitating injuries can be avoided.

As children enter the school age and adolescent years, they will spend increasing amounts of time away from the home and in activities which may have the potential for accidents. Safety teaching through a variety of educational means as well as examples can increase safety awareness and hopefully safe behavior. As the use of bicycles and motorbikes and motorcycles increases, usage rules and regulations need frequent review and reinforcement. Individuals at this age also engage in an increased number of individual and group sports of both a supervised and unsupervised nature. First aid measures need to be taught as well as the variety of safety measures required. Safety education needs priority attention.

The adult years through retirement see an increase in home, occupational, and recreational accidents. They vary in degree from mild to fatal. Environmental safety in all areas of activities should be of prime concern. Obstacle free home, work, and play settings, adherence to safety rules and regulations, and thought before action can reduce the number and severity of accidents encountered. Severe injuries leading to disability can have lasting economic and family integrity impact at this time of life. A little caution can often avoid these consequences.

The impact on the family will depend on the member's role in the family and factors mentioned previously. If the wage earner is permanently disabled, economic issues may become paramount. Injury to either parent may result in those responsibilities being taken over by the other parent and/or children. Family goals and educational pursuits may have to be postponed or forgotten. If insurance does not cover the cost of health care, another financial crisis may be encountered. Rehabilitation demands may change home life routine on a temporary or permanent basis. The emotional stress, both from the accident and the realization of its meaning, can cause much disequilibrium. Guilt may aggravate reactions to the accident. Accidents generally stimulate much soul searching and need to explain or justify the injuries incurred. Such activity can be experienced by all family members.

Community responsibility to prevent accidents is shared at the governmental and citizen levels. Hazards from traffic, fire, recreation areas, industries, and home sources need to be sought, investigated, and corrected. Environmental safety actions can be carried out through voluntary citizen groups, the police and fire departments, the public health department, and public and private schools. Increased awareness and sensitivity to hazards as well as community based procedures for correcting them will aid in the prevention of accidental injuries and fatalities.

COMMUNITY HEALTH CONCERNS

Because of the large numbers of people injured and killed from accidents each year, this is a major area of concern for health practitioners in community health. Nurses in such settings are in a prime position to do home and community assessments, education, and case finding. Environmental assessment should be an ongoing activity of the community health nurse regardless of her work site. Prevention and correction activities can reduce the frequency and severity of accidents encountered. Because the nurse is generally considered a trusted visitor in the home, much teaching can take place here to improve environmental safety and safety behaviors. Reinforcement for safety behavior and activities should be openly provided. Community hazards can be reported to the proper authorities and citizen action groups. Schools are an arena for educational activities through didactic measures as well as example. Nurses in such settings can aid teachers and students in recognizing hazards and taking steps to correct them. Occupational nurses can aid in supporting on the job safety and accident prevention.

Educational efforts can be conducted for school children, health care providers, fire and police department personnel, and the general public. Efforts should be directed toward personal, home, and community safety. Since accidents are so frequent, the need for health departments to carry on active health education programs in this area is great. The impact of such efforts can be seen in accident rate changes, need for emergency room visits, and in increased participation in safety activities by the general public.

Research continues to be needed in areas such as product safety, environmental safety, vehicular safety, pedestrian safety, and others. We need more data on both the site of accidents as well as the cause of such accidents. From this data, efforts can be made to correct hazardous situations. Research into methods of first aid treatment can aid in the prevention of additional injuries at the site or during transfer to care facilities.

Also needed is additional research into modes of therapy in the physical and mental rehabilitation of accident victims. Such research can open new doors for the disabled.

The most important step we can take at this time, though, is accident prevention. All of us have a role in this activity. With thought, planning, and constant awareness, hazardous conditions can be decreased and accidents will follow suit. In the final analysis, the individual always has a major role in accident prevention.

REFERENCES

1. U.S. Department of Commerce, Bureau of the Census: *Statistical Abstract of the U.S. 97th Annual Edition* Government Printing Office, Washington, D.C., 1976.
2. Morris, William (ed.): *The American Heritage Dictionary of the English Language.* Houghton Mifflin Company, Boston, 1976.
3. Hanlon, John J.: *Public Health Administration and Practice,* 6th ed. The C.V. Mosby Company, St. Louis, 1974.

BIBLIOGRAPHY

Boeriche, Peter H.: "Emergency." *Nursing 75,* March 1975, pp. 40-47.

Cramer, Kathleen A., et al. "Botulism Nursing Care in an Epidemic." Nursing Grand Rounds. *Nursing 78,* November 1978, pp. 63-69.

Delgado, Cheryl, et al.: "Epidural Hematoma." Nursing Grand Rounds. *Nursing 75,* March 1975, pp. 34-38.

Dershewitz, Robert A., and Williamson, John W.: "Prevention of Childhood Household Injuries: A Controlled Clinical Trial." *American Journal of Public Health,* 67(12):1148, Dec. 1977.

Farrell, Jane: "Costs, Your Patients and You." *Nursing 78,* November 1978, pp. 57-61.

Ford, Jack R., and Duckworth, Bridget: "Moving a Dependent Patient Safely, Comfortably," (Part I). *Nursing 76,* January 1976, pp. 27-37.

Ford, Jack R., and Duckworth, Bridget: "Moving a Dependent Patient Safely, Comfortably," (Part II). *Nursing 76,* February 1976, pp. 58-65.

Friedman, Bonnie Jones, and Knight, Katherine: "Running for Life, Health and Pleasure." *American Journal of Nursing,* April 1978, pp. 602-607.

Galton, Lawrence: "Drugs and the Elderly." *Nursing 76,* August 1976, pp. 38-43.

Hamrick, Ann, et al.: "Caring for the Totally Dependent Patient." *Nursing 76,* July 1976, pp. 38-43.

Kukuk, Helen M.: "Safety Precaution: Protecting Your Patient and Yourself," Part One. *Nursing 76,* May 1976, pp. 45-51.

Kukuk, Helen M.: "Safety Precaution: Protecting Your Patient and Yourself," Part Three. *Nursing 76,* July 1976, pp. 45.

Spiegel, Charlotte N., and Lindamon, Francis C.: "Children Can't Fly: A Program to Prevent Childhood Morbidity and Mortality From Window Falls." *American Journal of Public Health,* 67(12): 1143, 1977.

Spitz, Phyllis, and Sweetwood, Hannelore: "Kids in Crisis." *Nursing 78,* April 1978, pp. 26-30.

Wahl, Sharon: "Only a Concussion." *Nursing 76,* August 1976, pp. 44-45.

Williams, Jane, and Ziegler, Jerome B. "Why Did Annie Hate Us So?" *Nursing 78,* May 1978, pp. 70-73.

Williams, Marcelle, et al.: "Trauma Care." Nursing Grand Rounds. *Nursing 76,* June 1976, pp. 58-63.

CHAPTER 35
AIR POLLUTION

PARKER C. REIST, S.M. in HYG., Sc.D.

In recent years we have been besieged with facts and figures which suggest that this compound or that practice can be harmful to human health. Near the top of the list is air pollution, which can mean many things to many people, depending on their own personal perspectives. It may be unsightly smoke pouring from an apartment house chimney, exhaust fumes surrounding a diesel bus idling in heavy traffic, the faint blue haze of particulates coming from a power plant stack, or even to some the smell of manure spread over a farmer's field in the springtime.

Although each insult to our senses may be personally defined as air pollution, there are a number of substances which, if present in excessive amounts in the air, would be considered by anyone to be air pollution. Such things as sulfur dioxide, particulates, cancer causing materials, and carbon monoxide all fall into this category.

Air pollution is generally thought to come from man's industrial activities although in special cases nature could be blamed, as in the case of a volcanic eruption. In the past it was thought that the air pollution remained in the atmosphere virtually unchanged from the form in which it was released. We now know that this is not the case, and in at least one major group of pollutants, the photochemical oxidants, it is the atmospheric conversion processes which produce the potentially harmful compounds. This makes regulation of air pollution much more difficult and complex than originally thought.

Air pollution can affect people's health, it can damage their properties, and injure or kill their animals and their plants. This suggests immediately that air pollution is bad and

637

something we should not have. On the other hand, the control of air pollution costs money, money that might better be spent on some other preventive health strategy. People and the environment can tolerate some air pollution—we have tolerated some degree of air pollution almost from Adam's time and we will be exposed to some levels of air pollution in the future. The problem is not a question of air pollution or no air pollution, but a question of how much air pollution is a reasonable amount to tolerate. Low levels of air pollution may have effects which appear in only 1 out of 10 billion people, and these effects may in themselves be so slight as to be hardly perceptible. High levels, on the other hand, may produce immediate and dramatic effects, and in some instances have been known to cause death.

Standards must be set to limit air pollution levels to acceptable amounts. Here again there is a problem because we must define to whom the standards are to apply. Should they apply to the polluter at his smokestack, and if so, is this practical? Should each automobile be expected to meet a pollution standard? Or should standards be set to apply to air in general, the ambient air, and all emitters of pollution be responsible for seeing that these standards are not exceeded? In the following sections we shall explore some of these questions in more detail and attempt to develop a rationale for coping with air pollution.

HISTORICAL PERSPECTIVE

Air pollution has been a companion of man from the time he discovered fire and moved into his first cave. The dense, smoky air provided a sense of security although the need to control the smoke concentration through ventilation quickly became obvious. In the crowded towns and villages of medieval Europe, woodsmoke was the indicator of prosperity and life and the smoky outdoors was only a slight improvement over the smoky indoors.

With the widespread use of coal for home heating, previously acceptable woodsmoke became unacceptable coal smoke, mainly because the coal contained significant amounts of sulfur which, when burned, resulted in unacceptable levels of sulfur dioxide in the outside air and hugh quantities of sooty particles. Conditions in England became so bad that by the 19th century Charles Dickens could write in *Hard Times* (1854):

> "(Coketown) was a town of red brick, or of brick that would have been red if the smoke and ashes had allowed it; but as matters stood it was a town of unnatural red and black like the painted face of a savage. It was a town of machinery and tall chimneys, out of which interminable serpents of smoke trailed themselves for ever and ever, and never got uncoiled."

The industrial revolution was in full swing and development of the steam engine gave birth to sprawling factory towns where smoke issuing from chimneys was a sign of prosperity. A chimney without smoke represented a factory that was bankrupt, so smoke was always shown by contemporary artists. Interestingly, although large smokestacks are used today as a means of dispersing pollution into a large volume of air, their original function was to provide draft for the furnaces and emissions of pollution were not even considered. It was inevitable that eventually smoke pollution would become so excessive as to demand public action. In the 1930s the air in downtown Pittsburgh, Pennsylvania, for example, was so polluted that motorists needed to have their headlights on during the day, even at high noon. Public reaction to this extreme pollution was to establish smoke inspectorates and enact laws and regulations that limited the amount of soot and smoke that could be emitted from a smokestack. A number of municipalities, such as Cincinnati, Pittsburgh, Chicago, and St. Louis, passed ordinances limiting the discharge of smoke. Similar laws were enacted in other cities as well, but in all cases the laws only partially dealt with the problem because they did not focus on ways that emissions from small domestic sources could be controlled. Although of limited effectiveness, these laws do represent the initial efforts in the United States to control emission of noxious materials to the atmosphere.

In 1948, in the small Pennsylvania mill town of Donora, the combination of weather, topography, and emissions resulted in air pollution levels building up of over a period of several days to such an extent that people with pre-existing respiratory problems were affected and at least 20 people died as a direct result of the pollution. About 6000 became ill. This incident was similar to one which had occurred in 1930 in the Meuse Valley in Belgium. A heavy smog, a combination of smoke, gaseous impurities, and fog, lingered in the valley for four days causing the death of some 60 persons.

In London during the four days of December 5th to 8th, 1952, a similar acute air pollution episode occurred. Again, heavy smog blanketed the city affecting mainly those with some existing respiratory ailment and some 4000 people died as a direct result of the air pollution.

These incidents pointed out the serious nature of the air pollution problem and the need for a more sophisticated approach to its solution, as opposed to merely controlling smoke emissions. The circumstances surrounding the incidents also illustrated the role that topography and meteorology had, along with emissions, in determining the concentration of pollution in the atmosphere. It took a combination of events to create conditions where death could occur. Without specific weather conditions which allowed the pollution to accumulate, topographic features which served to trap the accumulated pollution, and a strong pollution source, these incidents would never have happened. Thus it was learned that in order to understand the nature of air pollution and its potential effect on man and his environment, it is necessary that all three of these factors be taken into account.

There also have been many instances where emissions from a specific source have resulted in a localized nuisance or health hazard. In these cases, however, the people affected are those living immediately downwind from the source and the effect is somewhat limited in scale. There are numerous examples such as sulfuric acid mists from chemical plants, iron and zinc oxide smokes from metal producers, hydrogen sulfide from paper mill effluents, and fluoride compounds from mining or smelting operations. For the people affected, however, the problem looms just as large as if it were another London smog epidemic, and in some cases death has resulted which could be directly related to the air pollution. Again, the three factors of emission concentration, meteorology, and topography all interact to determine the problem's severity.

For example, in the early 1940s emissions from a fluorescent lamp manufacturing plant resulted in a number of neighborhood cases of beryllium disease downwind from the plant, which were attributed to emissions from the manufacturing plant. This indicated the possibility of toxic effects from fairly localized sources of pollution.

THE ATMOSPHERE'S ROLE IN AIR POLLUTION

When one looks at pictures of the earth taken from space it is apparent that there is very little atmosphere surrounding the earth. If we drew the earth as a five foot diameter circle, the thickness of the pencil line would represent the thickness of the atmosphere.

The atmosphere represents a very small part of the total mass of the earth, a fact that is not immediately apparent when we gaze out of the window. Of the 12 mile thick atmosphere surrounding the earth, the lower portion, called the troposphere, contains most of the air mass. The troposphere is about 10 miles thick at the equator and 5 miles thick at the poles. Within this narrow zone resides the oxygen necessary to sustain life and into which all of man's pollution is discharged.

Air is a mixture of about 78 percent nitrogen, 21 percent oxygen, with the remaining 1 percent consisting of carbon dioxide (about 0.03 percent) and inert gases such as helium, argon, neon, and others. Air can also contain variable amounts of water vapor. All of these compounds are gases. Air can also contain, suspended in it, varying amounts of particulate material which can either be present in solid or liquid form. Examples of such particulate material are clouds of very small water droplets, dust, haze from chemical reactions in the atmosphere which produced small amounts of particulate material from gases, and smokes from forest fires, volcanoes, or man's activities. The particulate material remains suspended because it is essentially too small to settle out.

This atmospheric "soup" does not remain still but is constantly being stirred by the circulation of the atmosphere. This circulation is brought about by two factors, the energy received by the atmosphere from the sun and the rotation of the earth. In order to understand how this circulation takes place, and this understanding is fundamental to an understanding of air pollution, it is necessary to review how the sun's energy warms the earth.

Energy from the sun can be distributed at the earth's surface by three mechanisms, radiation, conduction, and convection. It is easiest to understand these mechanisms by envisioning heat as molecular motion—the greater the motion, the greater the temperature.

Energy is received from the sun in the form of radiant energy or *waves* of energy. The atmosphere is incapable of absorbing much of this radiant energy so it passes to the earth's surface where it is absorbed. The earth can reradiate some of this energy at a longer wavelength which is then more efficiently absorbed by such atmospheric components as water or carbon dioxide, giving rise to a so-called greenhouse effect. The air acts like glass in a greenhouse, permitting incoming radiation to enter while blocking the passage of radiation out of the greenhouse.

The earth's heated surface can also transfer energy directly to the air above it in much the same way that heat is transferred from a frying pan to a hamburger. This method of heat transfer is known as conduction. Conduction is important in heating air very close to the earth's surface—air itself is not a good conductor of heat.

The most important method of heat or energy transfer in the atmosphere is by convection. Convection is the circulation or mixing of warm air masses with colder air masses. Since warm air is lighter or less dense than colder air, heating of air near the earth's surface causes the warmed air to rise. Cold air flows in to replace the warmed air, thus setting up circulation cells. As the air flows it is mixed, bringing about heat transfer from warm air masses to colder ones. A typical convection cell produces the sea breeze that can be observed along the beach on a warm summer day. Strong heating of air over land warms the air and, as it rises, it is replaced by cooler air from the sea. This circulation results in a breeze coming in off the sea. At night the process is reversed.

Because of the heating and cooling processes continually taking place, the temperature of the atmosphere can vary markedly both with height and over a very short distance. The extent to which warm air at the earth's surface will rise and mix with colder air above it is known as the mixing depth. This essentially sets the upper boundary for pollution dispersion. During the winter months the mixing depth may be as little as a few hundred feet above the ground, whereas during the summer with more heating of the atmosphere the mixing depth will usually extend several thousand feet above the ground. With a small mixing depth, pollution concentrations can build up more rapidly in the atmosphere than with a large mixing depth. We would expect then the potential for serious air pollution incidents would be greater in the winter than in the summer, and this appears to be the case.

If a layer of warm air lies above cooler air near the surface of the ground, an atmospheric condition exists which is known as an inversion. Under these conditions, the atmosphere is said to be particularly stable. The surface air cannot rise so that pollution discharged beneath the inversion layer will be trapped there. This particular atmospheric phenomonon was one of the contributing factors in the buildup of high concentrations of pollutants during smog incidents in Donora, London, and the Meuse Valley, as well as being a commonly occurring factor influencing pollution levels in the Los Angeles basin. Inversions very frequently form at night as the earth's surface cools by radiation, but they are rapidly broken up as the morning sun heats the ground and enhances atmospheric mixing.

Cities tend to act as good absorbers of heat and do not lose it as rapidly as open rural areas. This results in air warmed in the center of the city rising, circulating to the edge of the city where it cools and then flowing back to the center along the ground. This so-called "heat island effect" produces a dome of grimy air which is not readily broken up since small particles or aerosols in the dirty air reflect sunlight back into the atmosphere before it is able to enhance mixing by reaching the earth's surface. These haze domes are a common sight to air travellers approaching almost any major city in the United States today.

It should be obvious that atmospheric circulation plays a major role in determining the extent and concentration of pollutants in the air. With good circulation and mixing, material discharged into the atmosphere is rapidly dispersed and dissipated; with poor mixing or a stable atmosphere, the pollutant material is trapped near where it is released and can build up in concentration, sometimes to disastrous levels.

Nature provides some air cleaning on her own. Particulate pollution or aerosols can be removed from the air by collection on surfaces such as leaves of plants and trees, sedimentation or fallout, or may be scavanged from the air by rainfall or other precipitation processes. Gases can be converted into aerosols by photochemical reactions in the atmosphere and subsequently removed by aerosol removal mechanisms, or they can be directly scavanged by particles or raindrops and removed by that mechanism. Sometimes these natural removal processes can result in other forms of pollution such as acid rain arising from the conversion of sulfur dioxide to sulfuric acid.

SOURCES OF AIR POLLUTION

If we define air pollution in its broadest sense, that is, the presence of some "foreign" material in the air, then we could classify air pollution as being either natural or man-made. Since there is little we can do about much of the natural air pollution, it is customary to define air pollution as that which arises as the result of man's activities. Man's activities usually involve burning something, thus a large majority of air pollution arises as a result of combustion. Power plants generating electricity form one large group of pollution sources, as do apartment houses with incinerators and any dwelling which provides its own heat. Many industrial processes rely on combustion. Each industry has its own specific forms of pollution which it emits to the atmosphere. Processes involving attrition of materials such as grinding or crushing can produce large quantities of airborne dust, and even the process of handling or transferring organic liquids can result in significant quantities of these materials getting into the atmosphere. The evaporation or vaporization of solvents also results in significant levels of air pollution.

Air pollution sources which are fixed in location are known as stationary sources. This classification would include power plants, factories, apartments, houses, and even burning refuse piles. A single stationary source or group of sources may produce air pollution problems which exist over only a relatively small area, or problems may arise from a widespread number of sources and affect a whole community or urban complex.

Mobile air pollution sources are sources which can move about and therefore will create few, if any, local air pollution problems since the source is providing its own dilution and dispersion. However, with large numbers of mobile sources, a significant air pollution problem can develop because the dilution air for one source is the contaminated air of another. The most ubiquitous mobile source in the United States today is the automobile, but it should be recognized that the automobile pollution problem is only important in urban areas where large numbers of automobiles are operating.

Air pollutants can be classed as particulate material (or aerosols), inorganic gases, or organic gases. Each class may include many different compounds, emanate from several different sources, or react with one another to form other pollutants. As an example, oxides of nitrogen (an inorganic gas) which could come from automobile exhaust could react with hydrocarbons (organic vapors) in the presence of sunlight to form a photochemical aerosol, also known as smog, and an inorganic gas, ozone. In this case, major concern may not be with the primary pollutants (those emitted by the source), but with the secondary pollutants which are those produced by chemical reactions in the atmosphere.

Sometimes, whole regions or urban areas are considered to be sources of air pollution for other regions or urban areas. Ozone levels in Boston appear to be influenced greatly by hydrocarbon emissions in the New York City area, and New Yorkers for years have complained about the pollution "from Jersey." Because in many cases it is difficult to pinpoint a single offending smokestack as the source of an air pollution problem, it is impossible to solve area-wide problems without far reaching and all inclusive controls.

EFFECTS OF AIR POLLUTION

Air pollution can affect humans directly or indirectly by damaging plants, materials, or other animals. We can look at each effect separately.

Short of an air pollution episode so severe that people "drop dead like flies," there are three methods for determining the relationship of human health to air pollution. One method is to carry out experimental studies on animals; a second method is to carry out experimental studies on humans; and a third method is to carry out epidemiologic studies on human population groups. Each approach has its advantages and disadvantages. Experimental studies on animals yield answers relatively quickly and offer no risk to humans, but provide data which may not be directly applicable to humans. Often exposure concentrations are required in order to develop an effect in a significant number of animals which are greatly in excess of any reasonable level to be expected in the atmosphere. Also, the response to the pollutant by the animals may not be the same as the response observed in humans.

Human exposure studies, on the other hand, must by necessity be limited to low concentrations of pollutants. The effect on humans of low concentrations of pollutants can be precisely determined but even these findings may not apply to the very young, very old, or very sick or even to the general population exposed to a complex mixture of pollution.

Epidemiologic investigations can study the effects of real life exposures in various population subgroups. However, it is often impossible to definitely establish cause and effect—a person may smoke or commute from a rural area or be exposed to high concentrations of pollutants at work and these effects are difficult to sort out of the data.

There are three major types of air pollution which have been associated with the adverse effects of air pollution on human health. Emissions from power plants and other fossil fuel burning installations give rise to sulfur oxide and particulate complexes, thought to be one major potential health threat. A second class is photochemical oxidants, such as ozone, perhaps with some hydrocarbons, oxides of nitrogen, and carbon monoxide mixed in. This class is largely related to motor vehicle emissions. Miscellaneous individual pollutants such as lead, hydrogen sulfide, asbestos, and so on make up the third class of air pollution. These materials generally are emitted by localized single sources such as factories, smelters, or refineries.

Effects which might be observed are increased mortality of a population group or various types of illnesses. Incidents where increased mortality can be directly associated with air pollution are rare. The air pollution episodes listed in Table 35-1 represent the best known instances of the past 50 years.

Excluding diseases which can be attributed to relatively high concentrations of specific pollutants, illnesses which have been thought to be related to air pollution include chronic respiratory disease, acute respiratory disease, cancer of the lung, heart disease, and increases in rates of asthma attacks. A number of studies tend to show an association between one or several of these illnesses but it is difficult if not impossible to show that air pollution is the single causative agent. Other things, such as smoking, occupation, place of residence, degree of mobility and climatic factors such as temperature and humidity may also show associations with these diseases. For example, cigarette smoking seems to be a much greater cause of illness than air pollution, but one's chance of illness is increased if one both smokes and is exposed to high levels of air pollution. That is, the effect of air pollution appears to be additive.

Several carcinogens have been found in urban air, most notably the polycyclic hydrocarbon benxo-a-pyrene, but based on current evidence, it is still not possible to say either that air pollution does or does not cause cancer.

The sulfur oxide-particulate complex is thought to contribute to a greater incidence of chronic respiratory disease in adults and acute respiratory disease in children, and in very high concentration this mixture seems to have been implicated in the acute air pollution

TABLE 35-1. Air pollution episodes

Date	Place	Attributed excess mortality
December 1930	Meuse Valley, Belgium	63
October 1948	Donora, Pennsylvania	20
December 1952	London, England	4000
November 1953	New York City	200
December 1962	London, England	700

incidents involving some mortality. Even so, hard evidence is lacking showing a specific cause and effect relationship. In many studies of health effects, pollution levels were not measured, or, if they were, the measurements were made at distances well away from the population being studied. It is not surprising that there is little agreement on the pollutant concentration that has increased risk associated with it.

Similarly, although photochemical oxidants in high enough concentrations can cause eye irritation, cough, and chest discomfort, particularly when exercising, there is little agreement on what constitutes a safe oxidant concentration.

Plants are extremely sensitive to air pollution. Sulfur dioxide emissions have turned many green valleys into barren wastelands, have ruined valuable crops and, even in low concentrations, have caused stunted growth and lower crop yields. Photochemical oxidants, and particularly ozone, can affect plant leaves and especially seedlings. Smog injury to plants has been found in at least half of the United States, and recently smog damage has been observed in remote forested areas, resulting from emissions produced over 100 miles away.

A number of other air pollutants have also produced plant damage. Fluorides in particular can be especially devastating. Some plants are so sensitive to fluorides that they can be damaged by extremely low concentrations.

Fluorides can affect man in another way, too. Fluorides that fall on feed crops can be taken up by the leaves and remain in the plant after harvesting, then, when fed to cattle, produce sickness in the animals. There have been a number of instances where animals died or had to be destroyed because of excessive fluoride poisoning caused by eating tainted feed.

There are many other instances where animals have died as a result of air pollution. In Seveso, Italy following the accidental release of dioxin, wild and domestic animals sickened and died when exposed to the released material, and dead birds dropped from the sky. In Utah, a large number of sheep died following exposure to what was thought to be a poison gas in the air.

Even if air pollution does not affect living plants or animals, it can have a significant effect on materials. Stone is eaten away by acids in the air, corrosion of metals is accelerated, paints can discolor, rubber can become brittle when exposed to ozone, and paper and cloth can become weakened or destroyed. It is said that Cleopatra's needle has suffered more in 100 years in New York City than it did in 3000 years in the Egyptian desert. A 1960 study estimated that the annual per capita cost of air pollution in a relatively polluted city was equal to about one week's wages ($84 in 1960), and that estimate did not include added health costs.

CONTROL OF AIR POLLUTION

Although a number of states have had air pollution control legislation on their books for many years, it was not until the Clean Air Act of 1963 that it was recognized in the law that air quality criteria should be developed by the Federal government for use by the states in setting air pollution standards. Air quality criteria are descriptions of the damage individual air pollutants can do to health and property. The thought was that the standards thus proposed would be reasonably uniform since they would be based on the same criteria.

Two types of standards were to be considered. One, *Ambient Air Quality Standards*, were to apply to outside air in a town, city, or other defined region. These standards were to be met by the imposition of *Emission Standards* on various industries. Emission standards apply to specific emission sources.

In 1967 the Air Quality Act was passed which mandated setting criteria for six major pollutants: sulfur oxides, total suspended particulates, hydrocarbons, carbon monoxide, photochemical oxidants, and nitrogen oxides. Amendments to this Act in 1970 mandated national ambient air quality standards and gave authority to developing these standards to the newly formed Environmental Protection Agency (EPA). EPA was also authorized to set standards for any hazardous materials emitted from stationary sources not already covered by the ambient air quality standards.

The Clean Air Act Amendments of 1977 strengthened EPA's ability to set stringent standards for emission sources, especially new-source standards. The amendments require EPA to set emission limits for any category of industry whose air pollution causes or contributes to the endangerment of public health or welfare. The standards are to reflect the degree of pollution control that can be achieved by using the best technologic system of pollution control available. In setting these standards, EPA is supposed to consider cost and energy impacts as well as health and environmental benefits.

This approach seems to back off from the notion of ambient air quality standards since it is becoming more apparent that it is difficult to predict the effect of source control on ambient air quality. Secondary pollution must be considered and the photochemical processes which take place in the atmosphere are so complex that we are still struggling with just the rudiments of understanding. Ambient air quality standards still remain a dream for the future.

How are controls achieved? Either by replacing processes or materials which give rise to pollution with those that do not or by installation of engineering devices that clean dirty air before it is emitted. In the late 1960s many power plants switched from sulfur-containing coal, which produced large amounts of particulate-sulfur dioxide pollution, to low-sulfur oil, which was relatively pollution free. This seemed like a logical solution until the Arab Oil Crisis of 1973 sent the price of oil skyrocketing. Since then, the trend for power plants has been to switch back to coal and look for more efficient pollution control devices. Process or material changes can be useful, though, for many industries.

Engineering controls can consist of such devices as air filters which remove particulate material in much the same way a vacuum cleaner bag does, electrostatic precipitators which can remove very small dust particles but are generally quite expensive, scrubbers or air washers, afterburners which destroy the polluting material by burning it, or any of a number of other devices. Engineering control is always expensive and as standards become more stringent there is always the concern that even with control the standard will not be met, to the embarrassment of all.

PROGNOSIS

The late 1960s and early 1970s were marked with a zeal towards air pollution which was both refreshing and frightening. All too often legislators and special interest groups considered air pollution something which could be eliminated merely by legislation, strict governmental controls, and the imposition of stiff fines. The fact that knowledge about atmospheric chemistry, transport, and control processes was imperfect was lost in the rush to do something. Thus pollution controls were required on all automobiles, regardless of the fact that on many they were superfluous, and added an unnecessary expense to the cost of the automobile. For some areas, ambient air quality standards were set which not only limited industrial growth but were unattainable even with controls by existing industry.

We are becoming more sophisticated in our approach to air pollution. It is now realized that the imposition of realistic and attainable standards means much more than setting impossible goals. Attention must be directed to those industries where the public hazard potential is greatest, and in consideration of the broad picture one must not forget the small localized pollution sources which, although they affect relatively few people, can affect them severely.

For the health worker concerned with air pollution, information becomes paramount. Questions, such as what is the complaint, what are the symptoms, how many people are affected, when and where are they affected, what is the polluting material, and how long has the situation existed, will help determine the magnitude and importance of a particular worry about air pollution. With knowledge the problem can be approached reasonably and dealt with accordingly.

BIBLIOGRAPHY

Bates, D.V.: *A Citizen's Guide to Air Pollution*. McGill-Queen's University Press, Montreal, 1972.
Brodine, V.: *Air Pollution*. Harcourt Brace Jovanovich, New York, 1973.
Connolly, C.H.: *Air Pollution and Public Health*. Dryden Press, Inc., New York, 1972.
Corman, R.: *Air Pollution Primer*. American Lung Association, 1974.
Health Effects of Air Pollution. American Lung Association, 1978.
Lynn, D.A.: *Air Pollution: Threat and Response*. American Institute of Physics, 1976.
Stern, A.C. (ed.): *Air Pollution*, 3rd ed. Academic Press, New York, 1976.
Williamson, S.J.: *Fundamentals of Air Pollution*. Addison-Wesley Pub. Co., Reading, Ma., 1973.

CHAPTER 36
NOISE POLLUTION

ROBERT D. BRUCE, S.M. ELEC. ENG., E.E.

If a tree falls on a deserted island, does the impact of the tree on the ground generate noise? This version of the classic philosophic puzzle about the nature of reality serves to focus our attention on the central problem in forming a definition of noise. Noise is often regarded as unwanted sound. Thus, for a sound to be classified as noise, an observer must make a value judgment that the sound is annoying or unwanted. Without an observer on the island, there is sound, but no noise! There are sufficient observers and sounds in contemporary society to confirm that we are surrounded by noise. Cars, buses, trucks, motorcycles, airplanes, trains, subways, boats, construction equipment, recreation equipment, and industrial plants all contribute to the noise in the environment. Home appliances, workshop power tools, lawn mowers, vacuum cleaners, snow blowers, television, radio, and next door neighbors all contribute to the noise exposure of an individual at home. At work, noise exposure is dependent on the type of job as well as the industry in which an individual works.

Noise can be described by its magnitude, its frequently content, and its time history. The magnitude of a noise is measured in units called decibels (abbreviated dB). The dynamic range of the ear (the difference between the greatest sound the ear can withstand and the faintest audible sound) is over 120 dB. Examples of sound levels are presented in Figure 36-1. Sound frequencies are measured in Hertz (abbreviated Hz), a unit of frequency representing cycles per second. The audible range of frequencies for the human ear is between 16 Hz and 20,000 Hz. Infrasonic is a term describing sounds with

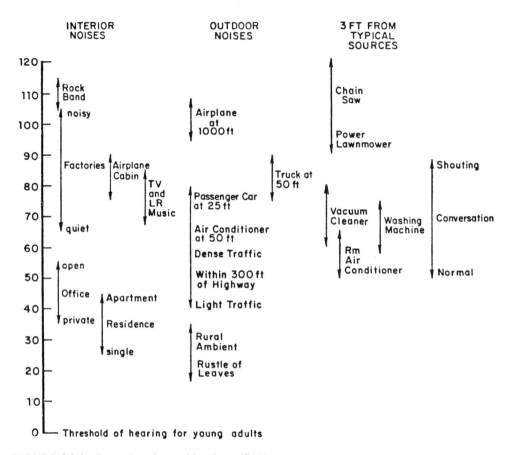

FIGURE 36-1. Examples of sound levels in dB(A).

frequency content below the audible range for human beings (usually lower than 16 Hz); ultrasonic describes sounds with frequency content above the audible range for human beings (usually 20,000 Hz).

A term or descriptor frequently used about a noise is the sound level, which is the frequency-weighted sound pressure level as measured in accordance with procedures suggested by the American National Standards Institute. Frequently, sound is weighted according to the A-weighing scale, which roughly corresponds to the way the human ear hears, by discriminating against low frequency sounds and emphasizing mid to high frequency sounds. When sounds are so measured, they are described as sound level in dB(A).

The major characteristic of environmental and occupational noise is that it is unsteady. The noise level at a particular location changes throughout the day. Thus, in order to discuss the noise exposure of an individual, it is necessary to select a suitable means of describing the variability of the noise over time. A single number descriptor is very desirable if there is a correlation between the single number and the impact of the variability of the noise. One such single number descriptor is the equivalent sound level, which is the noise level for an equivalent *steady noise* that in a stated time period would contain the same noise energy as the *time varying noise* during the same time period. This description has been selected by the Environmental Protection Agency (EPA) to describe levels of environmental noise.[1] Thus, the equivalent sound level (represented as L_{eq}) measured in dB(A) is a single number descriptor of a noise for which the details of the frequency content and the time variability have been sacrificed for simplicity. This approach is useful when describing the exposures of people to noise.

INDIVIDUAL NOISE EXPOSURE

An individual's noise exposure is determined in large measure by the individual's socioeconomic status, life style, and occupation. One way of determining a person's daily noise exposure is to have the individual wear an instrument called a noise dosimeter which can give a readout of the equivalent sound level for a specific time period, for example, an 8 hr period, $L_{eq}(8)$, or a 24 hr period, $L_{eq}(24)$. Another way is to describe each of the activities in which one engages, measure the noise level associated with that activity, and maintain a diary of one's activities.

Sociologists have analyzed how individuals spend time. Robinson and coworkers[2] have developed data on the average time spent by adults in 44 cities in 37 primary activities. Table 36-1 presents the time in minutes for each activity. Note that the authors have weighted the time "to ensure equality of days of the week and eligible respondents per household." In addition, a range of noise levels is shown for each activity and a typical L_{eq} is identified. An $L_{eq}(24)$ can be developed for this average exposure by selecting different values of L_{eq} (job), (combining main job and second job) as the variable.

$$L_{eq}(24) = 10 \log \left[\frac{\Sigma t_1 10^{(L_{eq1}/10)} + t_2 10^{(L_{eq2}/10)} + \cdots}{t_1 + t_2 + \cdots} \right]$$

where L_{eq1} is the equivalent sound level for time $t_1 + t_2 + \cdots$ equals 1440 min for an $L_{eq}(24)$. The following tabulation illustrates the dependency of the $L_{eq}(24)$ on the L_{eq} (job):

L_{eq}(job)	70	75	80	85	90	95	100	105
L_{eq}(24)	71.1	72.2	74.5	77.9	82.4	87.1	92.1	91.0

Note that the L_{eq} (job) has a significant influence on the $L_{eq}(24)$ because of the high noise levels and the extensive exposure. If the time spent on the job was 480 min (8 hr), then the impact would have been greater. The activity that results in the second greatest noise exposure is related to transportation. Naturally, individual differences in life style will result in different 24-hr L_{eq}s.

Several investigators have measured the $L_{eq}(24)$ of different categories of subjects. Schori and McGatha[3] measured the $L_{eq}(24)$ of 50 subjects in 5 occupational groups over 7 consecutive days. The groups were factory/commercial, office, homemaker, precollege, and college. The average $L_{eq}(24)$ for each group was:

Factory/commercial	74.9
Office	73.4
Homemaker	74.3
Precollege	76.2
College	73.5

TABLE 36-1. Activities and noise levels

Activity	Time in minutes	Range of noise levels	Typical L_{eq}
1. main job	225	70-95	
2. 2nd job	5	70-95	
3. at work other	12	70-80	80
4. travel to job	25		
via car		73-83	
public transportation		75-85	77
motorcycle		83-90	
walk/bicycle		75-82	
5. cooking	44	75-78	76.5
6. home chores	58	62-76	68
7. laundry	26	64-76	70
8. marketing	14	71-79	75
9. garden/pet care	3	67-75	71
10. shopping	18	70-80	75
11. other household care	24	68-72	70
12. basic child care	22	67-75	72
13. other child care	10	67-75	71
14. personal care	69	59-76	67
15. eating	81	65-74	69
16. sleep	470	40-50	45
17. personal travel	31	75-86	80
18. leisure travel	19	75-80	78
19. study	12	62-68	66
20. religion	10	75-85	80
21. organizations	6	68-73	70
22. radio	4	66-75	70.5
23. TV home	91	66-76	71
24. TV away	1	66-76	71
25. read paper	24	63-70	68
26. read mag.	6	63-70	67
27. read books	5	63-70	67
28. movies	3	75-80	78
29. social (home)	25	65-80	72
30. social (away)	38	65-80	74
31. conversation	18	70-80	73
32. active sports	6	78-82	80
33. outdoors	2	67-72	69
34. entertainment	5	66-80	68
35. cultural events	1	75-85	80
36. resting	9	60-70	65
37. other leisure	20	65-70	68
TOTAL TIME (in min)	1440*		

*1440 minutes is 24 hours.

Johnson and Farina[4] report the $L_{eq}(24)$ for a single individual over a 31 day period. The lowest $L_{eq}(24)$ was 60 dB(A) and the highest was 84 dB(A). Variation from day to day is presented in Figure 36-2.

It can be inferred from these two sets of data and the activity analysis that many people

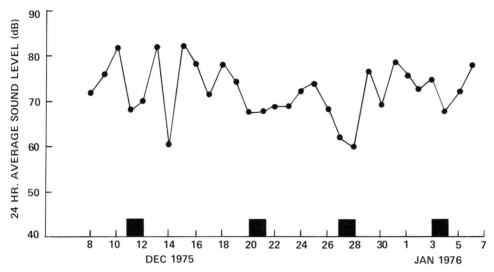

FIGURE 36-2. Variation in one individual's daily average sound level [L_{eq}(24)] over a 31 day period.

in the United States may have L_{eq} (24) exposures between 60 and 90, depending upon their life styles and occupations.

SCOPE OF PROBLEM

Noise is not only a public nuisance, it is also a significant health problem of contemporary society. All researchers in noise agree that the following problems are related to noise exposure: noise induced permanent threshold shift (NIPTS), speech interference, task interference, sleep interference, and annoyance.

Noise Induced Permanent Threshold Shift (NIPTS)

Noise induced permanent threshold shift (NIPTS) or hearing loss, as it is more commonly known, affects 10 to 20 million workers in this country alone. Exposure to high noise levels each workday for a working lifetime invariably results in permanent—irreversible— hearing loss. This continued loss of hearing among workers is inexcusable.

Under the Occupational Safety and Health Act of 1970, the Occupational Safety and Health Administration (OSHA), a part of the Department of Labor, is charged with protecting workers against material harm. With regard to noise, OSHA accepted the Walsh-Healey regulation of 90 dB(A) for an 8 hr exposure and a 5 dB increase in the noise level for each halving of the daily exposure. The EPA is charged with protecting the public with an adequate margin of safety under its enabling legislation. Because of the differences in the mandates issued by Congress to these agencies, they have developed different levels for exposure. Table 36-2 summarizes the existing OSHA regulation, the proposed OSHA regulation, and EPA's recommendation.

The basic differences between the recommendations of the two agencies concern the percentage of the population to be protected and the levels of noise they should be protected against. The OSHA regulation protects about 82 percent of the population

TABLE 36-2. Summary of existing and proposed regulations and EPA recommendations

Noise levels dB(A)	Maximum exposure time per day		
	Existing OSHA regulation	Proposed OSHA regulation	EPA recommendation*
70			
75			480 minutes
80			152 minutes
85		16 hr	48 minutes
90	8 hr	8	15 minutes
95	4	4	
100	2	2	
105	1	1	
110	1/2	1/2	
115	1/4	1/4	

*EPA has identified a yearly $L_{eq}(24)$ of 70 dB as the yearly sound level that protects the public with an adequate margin of safety. Thus, EPA recommends a 75 dB exposure for the 8 hours per day at work and not more than 60 dB for the 16 hours not at work. This places a severe restriction on the noise exposure of workers.

from incurring permanent hearing loss greater than an average of 25 dB at 500, 1000, and 2000 Hz. The EPA recommendation protects 90 percent of the population from incurring permanent hearing loss greater than 5 dB at 4000 Hz.

During the past four years, researchers have continued to discuss the merits and faults of these possible regulations. Two things are certain: Each individual accumulates hearing loss at his own rate; the higher the noise level and the longer the exposure time, the greater the probability of permanent hearing loss.

Speech Interference

Noise interferes with the understanding of speech. Individuals instinctively raise their voices whenever the noise level increases. Table 36-3 identifies the vocal effort required at several different noise levels, if the speaker and listener are separated by 3 feet. The quality of telephone communication in noisy environments can be estimated using the data in Table 36-4.

Task Interference

The effects of noise on job performance are not well understood. Practically the only generalization that can be made is that high intensity, intermittent, aperiodic noises impede efficient work more than low intensity, steady state noises. A few studies report improvements in performance attributable to noise exposure, and other studies have failed to uncover any effects. No criteria have been developed to assist industry in assessing the impact of noise on task performance. Thus, each suspected case must be evaluated by professionals capable of investigating the particulars of the case.

TABLE 36-3. Vocal effort required at various noise levels when speaker and listener are 3 ft. apart.

Vocal effort	Sound level dB(A)
Maximum	89
Shout	83
Very loud	75
Raised	66
Normal	57
Relaxed	50
Whisper	40

*Adapted from Webster, J.C.: "Effect of Noise on Speech," in Harris, C.M. (ed.): *Handbook of Noise Control*. McGraw-Hill Book Co., New York, 1978.

Sleep Interference

Noise interferes with sleep by delaying the onset of sleep and by shifting the stage of sleep from one level to another. As with the studies on task interference, there is insufficient evidence for an absolute criterion for noise exposure levels in sleeping quarters. As a rule of thumb, approximately 25 percent of the population has been known to be wakened by exposure to noise levels of 40 dB(A). About half of the population may be wakened by levels of 70 dB(A), and about half will have difficulty falling asleep when exposed to such levels.

Annoyance

All three characteristics of noise—level, frequency, and time history—are important in analyzing the annoyance created by a noise source. The responses of a random selection of individuals to a specific noise source are diverse. Current technology is not developed to the point where we can predict an individual's annoyance by a noise if the noise is not interfering with speech communication. However, the response of a community to a specific source of annoyance is somewhat more predictable. In general, a community's response to a noise source will depend on: noise level; frequency content—presence of pure tones or multiple tones; and time history—fluctuations in noise level, impulsiveness of the noise.

If there are no socioeconomic and political connections between the owner of the

TABLE 36-4. Telephone communication in noisy environments

Noise level dB(A)	Quality of communication
50 dB(A)	Good
50-70 dB(A)	Satisfactory to slightly difficult
70-90 dB(A)	Difficult to unsatisfactory

TABLE 36-5. Community response to increased noise levels

Increase in octave band noise levels dB	Anticipated response of community
0-5	Acceptable
5-10	Sporadic complaints
10-15	Complaints threatening legal action
15-20	Legal action

source and the community, Table 36-5 can be used to obtain a rough estimate of the community's response to an increase in the noise level.

If the noise source operates most of the time and the noise is impulsive in character, or if it contains pure tones in the frequency spectrum, serious complaints may occur with an increase of only 5 dB. However, if the noise source seldom operates, or if it operates only during the day, the increase in noise level can be greater than that shown for the same response.

In addition to the problems previously discussed, some researchers report the following:[5]

1. Noise may produce high blood pressure, faster heart rates, and increased adrenaline.
2. Noise may contribute to heart and circulatory disease.
3. Noise can cause regular and predictable stress in the human body.
4. Noise may aggravate existing disease.
5. Noise may threaten fetal development.
6. Noise has been linked to low birth weights.
7. Noise can cause extreme emotions and behavior.
8. Noise can obscure warning signals, causing accidents to occur.

METHODS OF NOISE CONTROL

Noise can be controlled. Perhaps the simplest way to analyze a noise problem is to use the source-path-receiver concept. The source may be the machine, the highway, or even the neighborhood dog that is generating the noise. The path is the way noise travels through air and solid structures to reach the receiver. The receiver is the individual who is exposed to the noise and who objects to it. Noise control can be accomplished by treating the source, the path, or the receiver.

Source controls include: replacement of source with quieter equipment, control of operating conditions, relocation of source, and better maintenance of existing equipment. Examples of these controls are shown in Table 36-6.

Path controls include: barrier—a solid section of material located so that the line of sight is broken, it is usually large in comparison to the source; enclosure—a structure that encloses the source; wrapping/lagging—a covering of the source; muffler—a device used in the intake or exhaust opening of a noise source; room absorption—acoustical absorbing materials that can be used to reduce the noise levels in a space at a distance far from the source; vibration isolator—an isolator used to reduce the vibrations transmitted from a source to some other structure; and surface damping—a coating applied to lightweight

TABLE 36-6. Examples of noise controls at the source

Source control	Type of source		
	Aircraft noise	Highway noise	Industrial plant
Replacement of source with quieter equipment	Quieter airplanes	Quieter cars, trucks, motorcycles	Quieter industrial machines and processes
Control of operating condition	Restrictions on flight plan	Restrictions on truck traffic	Operation at night restricted
Relocation of source	Restrictions on flight plan	Generally not applicable	Relocation of exhaust system to location away from neighbors
Better maintenance of source	Generally not applicable	Replacement of mufflers	Repair of steam leaks

panels to reduce the noise radiated from the panel. Table 36-7 contains examples of these controls.

Receiver controls include: relocation of the receiver, use of hearing protectors in related occupational situations.

Naturally, all of these controls require proper design in order to accomplish the full potential of the treatment.

RESEARCH NEEDS

Additional research is needed in two primary areas: Noise effects and noise controls. Research is needed in both the auditory and the nonauditory effects of noise. The Second Federal Interagency Noise Effects Research Panel[6] reviewed federal sponsored research programs related to effects of noise. In the report of their findings, the following topics were singled out as needing additional research.

TABLE 36-7. Examples of control of noise along the path

Path Control	Environmental/Home	Occupational
Barrier	Alongside highway to reduce noise radiated to neighbors of highway	Alongside aisle through noisy factory space
Enclosure	Housing on home appliances	Enclosure for automatic punch press
Wrapping/lagging		Of piping systems in process plants
Muffler	Cars, trucks, motorcycles, ventilation system	Intake of exhaust of large fans
Room absorption	Used inside the hood of cars	Placed on ceiling and walls of certain spaces
Vibration isolation	Isolators on washing machine, carpet on floor	Isolators on machines
Surface damping	Undercoating on cars*	On conveyers

*Primary use is rust proofing.

Noise Induced Hearing Loss

Effects of noise on children.
Effects of impulsive and intermittent noise.
Longitudinal studies of hearing in normal and noise exposed populations.
Relationship between temporary and permanent threshold shift.
Possible high risk and susceptible populations.
Social and economic impact of noise induced hearing loss.

Nonauditory Health Effects

Cardiovascular and other physiologic changes caused by noise (short term) in the general population.
Worker safety and health.
Long term nonauditory health effects.
Nonauditory health effects of impulse noise.

Effects on Sleep

Effects of chronic sleep interruption by noise.
Effects of sleep interruption on special populations (ill, aged).

Communication Interference

Prediction of speech intelligibility in noise.
Everyday communication in lifelike noisy environments.
Effects of noise on speech and message production.

Community or Collective Response

National baseline data bank on environmental noise exposure levels.
Sociologic effects of noise in relation to quality of life.

Noise Environment Determination

Development of standard methodologies to measure and characterize the effects of noise.
Audiometry (standardized methods and calibration).
   Fundamental research and development is needed in controlling noise sources by design considerations rather than by retrofit solutions. The programs should include demonstration programs in field operations. Areas needing such research support (funded by industry and/or government agencies) include: aviation (quieter aircraft), surface transportation (quieter trucks), machinery (quieter processes and machines), and construction equipment (quieter paving breakers). In general, much can be done to reduce noise of sources, but additional research and development will enable us to learn how to maximize noise control and minimize the cost of accomplishing it.

EDUCATION

The impact of noise on health is often unrecognized or misunderstood. For example, hearing loss has long been accepted in some occupations as just one of the things that happens, without any hope of prevention. The public needs to be informed of the effects of noise on health.

Consumers are frequently unaware that noise control is possible. For example, many consumers of noisy products (from motorcycle owners to housewives) assume that more noise means more power. This lack of understanding about the potential for noise control often prevents the consumer from requesting quiet products.

Education about the effects of noise and the potential for quieting is desirable. Eventually, this information will be incorporated into junior high and high school textbooks. In the meantime, such information will be disseminated by government agencies, such as the following:

Environmental Protection Agency
Department of Health and Human Services (NICHHD, NIEHS, NIMH, NINCDS, NIOSH)
Department of Labor (OSHA, MSHA)
Department of Interior (BOM, BOR)
Department of Agriculture
Department of Commerce (NBS)
Consumer Product Safety Commission
Department of Defense (Air Force, Army, Navy)
Energy Research and Development Administration
National Academy of Sciences
National Aeronautics and Space Administration
National Science Foundation
Department of Transportation
Veterans Administration

In addition, labor unions, private interest groups, and industry groups will communicate information on issues of noise and noise control.

NURSING IMPLICATIONS

From the preceding information, it is clear that noise is an issue of concern at home, work, school, and play. As we encounter it in all segments of our lives, it is necessary for the nurse to become more sensitive to the interpretation of noise and the impact it has on the health and well being of the client population. The time has long since past when we accept noise levels as inevitable.

Interventions are needed to meet immediate and long range noise control goals. Previously mentioned charts identify sources and intensities of some common noises, pointing out that exposure levels can vary with and between individuals depending on lifestyle, occupation, and recreation patterns. Since noise sources are universal, the community health nurse can use these data to establish rough estimates of noise sources and levels.

The exact extent of noise related health problems is still being determined. However, deafness, stress, sleep interference, and task completion interference are certainly high on the list of potential health problems caused by noise. In dealing with noise problems, the nurse may work in a collaborative relationship with the client, governmental officials and groups, occupational/school officials, and consumer groups. The activities will include assessment, documentation, various long and short term interventions, education, legislative activities, and research participation.

In this, as in other environmental pollution efforts of wide spread proportions, progress will likely be slow and painstaking. However, through goal directed activities, communities, singly and collectively, can modify the noise levels which they must endure. From household appliances to machinery in factories and the work place to transportation vehicles such as planes, trains, and cars, efforts at noise control can and should be a priority. Community health nurses, because of their widespread roles and contacts in the community, can help educate and sensitize people to the extent and impact of the problem as well as directions to take in order to resolve it.

SUMMARY

This chapter has briefly reviewed the effects of noise and the chief methods of controlling it. Noise affects all of us. Noise can be controlled. In order to control noise and reduce its adverse effects, the public must be educated to realize the effects of noise and the possibilities for its control. To develop cost effective noise controls, additional research is needed.

REFERENCES

1. EPA: "Information on Levels of Environmental Noise Requisite to Protect Public Health and Welfare with an Adequate Margin of Safety." Document 550/9-74-004, March 1974.
2. Robinson, J.P., Converse, P.E., and Szalai, A.: "Everyday Life in Twelve Countries," in Szalai, A. (ed.): *The Use of Time*. Mouton and Co., The Hague, 1972.
3. Schori, T.R., and McGatha, E.A.: "A Real-World Assessment of Noise Exposure." *Sound and Vibration*. Vol. 12, No. 9, September 1978.
4. Johnson, D.L., and Farina, E.R.: "Description of the Measurement of an Individual's Continuous Sound Exposure During a 31-Day Period." *Journal of the Acoustics Society of America* 62(6): 1431, Dec. 1977.
5. EPA Publication: "Noise: A Health Problem." Aug. 1978.
6. EPA Publication: "Federal Noise Research in Noise Effects." Document 550/9-78-120, Feb. 1978.

BIBLIOGRAPHY

Jensen, Paul, Jokel, Charles R., and Miller, Laymon N.: *Industrial Noise Control Manual*. Bolt Beranek and Newman Inc., Cambridge, Mass., 1978, Report No. 3959.
Harris, C.M. (ed.): *Handbook of Noise Control*, 2nd ed. McGraw-Hill Book Co., New York, 1978.
Beranek, L.L. (ed.): *Noise and Vibration Control*. McGraw-Hill Book Co., New York, 1971.
Burns, William: *Noise and Man*. J.B. Lippincott Co., Philadelphia, 1969.
Henderson, Donald, Hamernik, Roger P., Dosanjh, Darshan S., et al.: *Effects of Noise on Hearing*. Raven Press, New York, 1976.
Kryter, Karl D.: *The Effects of Noise on Man*. Academic Press, New York, 1970.
Olishifski, J.B., and Harford, E.R. (eds.): *Industrial Noise and Hearing Conservation*. National Safety Council, Chicago, 1975.

CHAPTER 37
WATER POLLUTION

DAVID P. SPATH, Ph.D. AND
JAMES CROOK, Ph.D.

The pollution of water through the activities of man has been a problem for centuries. Water has always been the most convenient vehicle into which human waste could be discharged and carried away. As populations increased, the need to dispose of greater quantities of wastes resulted in a transformation of many rivers, lakes, streams, and bays into bodies of water that more resembled open sewers than pristine waters. At the same time, man was being subjected to plague and epidemics as a direct consequence of his poor sanitation practices and polluted water supplies. The great typhoid epidemics that swept London in the mid 19th century underscored the peril of water pollution and launched the first organized steps to combat it. Until very recent times the emphasis has been placed on preventing the transmission of waterborne disease.

With the advent of the chemical revolution, a new and more sophisticated concern has materialized. The increased use of long lived, toxic chemical compounds in industry, agriculture, and even within the individual home leads to the deposition of these substances throughout our waterways. The effects of these chemicals on humans and other life forms have sometimes been very subtle or not evident until years after the exposure has occurred.

Today our appreciation for the effects of water pollution on human health has expanded to embrace a variety of concerns beyond the traditional transmission of disease. Modern health practice is concerned with the whole individual and the positive aspects of health implied in the concept of "quality of life." This is a more appropriate and comprehensive view of health and gives a better appreciation of water pollution as it affects the state of complete physical, mental, and social well being.

EFFECT OF WATER POLLUTION

Achievements in the control of water pollution and reduction in waterborne disease have been significant in this century. The epidemics due to contaminated drinking water are largely a part of history. The most significant waterborne disease historically, typhoid fever, has been almost eliminated in the United States. At the turn of this century, the typhoid fever death rate for the entire country was 31.3 per 100,000 population. Today the death rate is almost zero. The morbidity changes are also significant. The United States morbidity for typhoid fever in 1930 was 12.6 per 100,000 and in 1971 there were less than 0.2 cases per 100,000 population.[1] This reduction in disease incidence can be attributed to several factors. The most important factors have been the improvement in water treatment, particularly disinfection, and the treatment of human wastes and the corresponding elimination of raw waste disposal.

In terms of total numbers, waterborne disease outbreaks reached an average annual low of 10 during the period 1951-55.[2] Table 37-1 indicates that there has been an increase in outbreaks over the last two decades. Outbreaks such as that experienced in Riverside, California[3] in 1965 where an estimated 18,000 persons in a population of 130,000 were affected by gastroenteritis (etiologic agent: *Salmonella typhimurium*) also serve to remind us that water pollution and drinking water contamination still pose a serious potential danger.

Studies on waterborne disease outbreaks have also consistently shown that the greatest number of outbreaks occur in small communities as well as at institutions, resorts, and rural places. An investigation by Wolman and Gorman[4] indicated that between 1930 and 1939 the largest number of outbreaks occurred among population groups of 1000 and under and among groups from 1000 to 5000. Weibel[5] reported the greatest number of outbreaks and cases between 1946 and 1960 were in communities of 10,000 population or less. The most recent survey[2] covering the period 1971 to 1974 indicated that approximately 69 percent of the outbreaks occurred in small communities, at single residences, or locations where the public has access to drinking water (e.g., camps, parks, resorts, and institutions). This information emphasizes the fact that, in general, water pollution control and drinking water treatment are less reliable in small communities and

TABLE 37-1. Waterborne disease outbreaks, 1938-1974

Year	Annual average outbreaks
1938-40	45
1941-45	39
1946-50	23
1951-55	10
1956-60	12
1961-65	12
1966-70	14
1971-74	25

rural areas. Typically, this results from less sophisticated treatment and a lower level of operator training and awareness than are provided at larger communities.

As previously mentioned, the problem of small amounts of toxic chemicals in water represents a serious concern not only to human health but to other forms of life. Mercury is an important example of a water pollutant that was discharged for years in small concentrations from industrial and agricultural sources into waterways throughout the world. Mercury increases in concentration as it accumulates in the food chain. Large, toxic amounts of mercury were found in shellfish and food fish such as tuna and swordfish in the late 1950s and throughout the 1960s and the early 1970s. The consumption of these mercury laden foods resulted in serious, even fatal, poisonings, neurologic disorders, and birth defects. Mercury poisoning is sometimes referred to as "Minimata disease" named after a well documented outbreak that occurred in Minimata, Japan. [6]

Mercury pollution has affected the livelihood and well being of many commercial fishermen in the United States. The Federal government placed bans on the sale of several marine and freshwater food fish taken from certain waters until mercury concentrations were found to be within acceptable levels.

A similar example of contamination of a food supply by a toxic pollutant also occurred in Japan and involved high concentrations of cadmium in water used to irrigate rice fields. The cadmium accumulated in the rice which was consumed by the local population. The resulting effect was a long and debilitating illness, named "ita-ita" disease, that caused over 100 deaths within a 20 year period. [7]

Other examples include DDT, Kepone, and many of the other chlorinated pesticides and herbicides that accumulate in the food chain and exhibit long term health effects, including cancer.

Recently concern associated with water pollution and drinking water has centered around low concentrations of organic chemicals that have been found in drinking water supplies throughout the United States. The U.S. Environmental Protection Agency, along with numerous researchers, has conducted several studies which have identified more than 200 organic chemical compounds in public drinking waters. Most of these chemicals were from industrial and municipal discharges and agricultural runoff. Others were chlorinated organic products resulting from the reaction between organic material in the water and chlorine used for disinfection in the water purification process. Some of the compounds identified, such as chloroform and benzene, are also suspected carcinogens, while others are toxic in large amounts.

There is very little known about the effect of these contaminants at the low concentrations in drinking water. Epidemiologic studies have been carried out in an attempt to determine if a relationship exists between organic compounds in drinking water and increased incidence of cancer. Results from investigations on the consumption of Mississippi River water by the Environmental Defense Fund[8] and several studies[9] on chlorinated water supplies suggested that a positive relationship may exist. The studies, however, were only suggestive and did not establish a cause and effect relationship.

The impact on health of water pollution has not been limited solely to contamination of drinking water supplies. A large percentage of the population takes advantage of the recreational opportunities of our water resources. Water pollution from inadequately treated sewage from municipalities and runoff from agricultural areas can adversely affect these recreational activities.

Where recreation involves swimming in contaminated waters, the potential for disease transmission is obvious. There are examples of increased incidences of gastrointestinal disease among swimmers in waters that were affected by sewage discharges.[10,11] In many situations, bacterial counts reach unacceptable levels and public health authorities are forced to close bathing waters. Aside from increasing disease potential, pollution of recreational waters can have an adverse effect on the psychological well being of the community.

Similarly, contamination of shellfish growing areas can lead to serious health problems among the consuming public. Contaminated shellfish have been well established as a source of transmission of infectious hepatitis. As in the case of bathing waters, shellfish growing areas are immediately closed when bacterial contamination occurs. This not only deprives the public of an enjoyable food source but places a burden on the economic and mental well being of those individuals dependent on commercial shellfishing for their livelihood.

CONTROL OF WATER POLLUTION

Water pollution has been reduced significantly in this century with the assistance and direction of the Federal government. Federal water pollution control legislation has provided funding to municipalities to build sewage treatment plants in order to reduce or eliminate pollutants from going into our waterways. In 1910 barely 10 percent of the sewage from sewerage systems was treated, by 1940 the percentage rose to 55 percent and by 1970 to 95 percent.[7] Today, almost all sewage receives some form of treatment. The national goal as defined in the 1972 water pollution control legislation is to eliminate the discharge of pollutants by 1985.

Federal and state authorities have worked in concert to develop and impose stringent water quality requirements to insure that sewage treatment facilities are operating properly and water resources are protected. Federal efforts have also been directed at industrial and agricultural sources of pollution and significant gains have been made at reducing and, in some cases, eliminating them.

The water supply industry has concurrently upgraded and improved the methods of drinking water treatment. In particular, strong efforts have been made to provide adequate treatment to remove any pathogenic microorganisms that could cause disease.

In small communities and rural areas of this country there is a continuous drive to improve on water pollution control measures. Small communities, where possible, provide sewer systems and sewage treatment plants for their residents. In rural areas local county authorities have had good success in educating homeowners as to the importance of proper sewage disposal practices and the problems associated with contamination of water supplies.

CURRENT PROBLEMS AND OUTLOOK

A progressive upgrading of sewage treatment at the municipal level should continue with aid from the Federal and State governments. Federal and state water quality requirements are also expected to become more restrictive and vigorous and effective enforcement of the requirements should encourage compliance. The combination of the two should result in an overall reduction in general water pollution.

Historically, there has been a shortage of well trained sewage treatment plant operators. The consequence has been sewage treatment of varying quality and reliability. Along with marginal operation, sewage treatment facilities have a propensity for physical breakdowns.

Although the physical reliability of these facilities has improved with requirements for backup systems, alarms, and so forth, there are still far too many examples of breakdowns and untreated sewage discharges. The most important health effect will continue to be the significant disease potential from discharges of infectious agents to drinking water supplies, recreational waters, and shellfish growing areas.

In recent years, there has been a concerted effort to dispose of wastewater on land and eliminate the discharge of treated sewage to streams, lakes, or other waters. Land disposal of sewage utilizes natural purification processes, and a great deal of research is being devoted to this and other alternative methods of treatment.

Treated wastewater is being used as a supplemental water supply for various purposes in water-short areas of the United States and many other parts of the world. For example, there are over 200 wastewater reclamation plants in California that produce treated sewage effluent for such uses as crop and landscape irrigation, recreational impoundments, and industrial cooling water. Strict controls are placed on both the producers and users of the reclaimed water, and water quality regulations require complete destruction of pathogenic organisms for uses where public contact with treated wastewater is possible. As population increases and fresh waters become scarce, the beneficial reuse of sewage will play an important role in helping meet future water demands.

As mentioned earlier in this chapter, sewage may contain a myriad of chemical compounds which, if ingested, could result in acute or chronic adverse health effects. In addition, domestic sewage is likely to contain the range of disease organisms present in the community served by a treatment plant. In view of these factors and the well documented unreliability of most sewage treatment plants,[12] reuse for domestic purposes (i.e., drinking) would present unacceptable health risks and should be deferred until necessary research has been carried out.

Water pollution from industrial sources should see continued reductions. Over the last decade most industries have made considerable investments in waste treatment equipment and designing production processes that minimize waste. Many other industries (e.g., food processing) have wastes that can be treated efficiently (after pretreatment in some cases) by municipal sewage treatment facilities and have used this approach with good success. New federal standards directed at pollution from toxic organic chemicals should result in more effective control of these substances.

There are many organic chemicals, however, that may produce long term harmful effects (e.g., cancer, mutation, fetal abnormalities) at low levels of exposure. Although treatment can substantially reduce organic chemical concentrations in industrial discharges, residuals remain and are being found in drinking water supplies.

Solutions to this problem are difficult. Only through future research will there be an eventual answer to the health effects question. Because initial evidence suggests that a health problem exists, preventive measures are now being considered. These include limiting or prohibiting the use of certain organic substances or special treatment methods to remove them from wastewaters. In all cases these measures will probably be expensive.

Control of agricultural water pollution has improved over the last decade. Emphasis is being placed on preventing runoff from irrigation lands where waters high in organic matter and pesticide and herbicide residues have caused serious water pollution problems. Strict measures are being placed on runoff from dairies and feedlots which also carry a significant amount of organic material as well as high levels of bacteria, some of which are pathogenic.

Regulatory requirements are becoming more stringent and monitoring to ensure compliance is increasing. With the improvements in procedures for screening of pesticides for potential human health effects, the use of safer pesticides will diminish the threat to human health from occasional runoff into water supply sources.

Small communities and rural areas have been struggling for many years with water pollution problems. As mentioned earlier in this chapter, the largest number of waterbone disease outbreaks have historically occurred in these locales, and to a great degree these outbreaks are the result of sewage contaminated drinking water supplies.

Many small communities still rely on the use of individual home sewage treatment systems, such as septic tanks, while others have only small central treatment facilities. With increasing pressure from state and federal regulatory agencies over the past decade, many small communities have attempted to build sewers and sewage treatment plants. Other communities have tried to upgrade and enlarge existing sewage treatment facilities to accommodate increases in population and meet stricter water pollution control requirements. The skyrocketing rise in construction costs of conventional sewage treatment facilities, however, has placed many small communities in a difficult situation. Even with federal and state assistance, they are unable to afford these costs while many others appear unwilling to make the investment. The overall effect will be marginal situations where potential water pollution and health problems continue to exist.

Recently, emphasis has begun to turn away from costly conventional treatment facilities to less expensive alternatives. The Federal government and many states are beginning to look favorably toward new approaches which avoid the large, initial capital costs yet will provide efficient, reliable treatment. Many of these alternatives involve the application of partly treated sewage to land where the natural (soil and vegetation) process effectively removes pollutants. This approach provides an inexpensive, suitable source of water and nutrients for crop irrigation, particularly animal feed crops. Land use planning and growth control measures also appear to be tools that will be increasingly employed to control population and will serve to reduce water pollution problems.

Rural areas are generally so remote that the only means of sewage disposal has been the use of individual home systems. Drinking water supplies are also usually restricted to individual well water or nearby creeks and streams. There have been numerous examples of septic tank sewage disposal systems failing to operate properly and contaminating drinking water supplies.

The present trend is to be more selective when employing septic tank sewage disposal systems. Local county and state regulatory agencies have become more sensitive to the problems that these systems can create. Local counties are also placing more emphasis on homeowner education and awareness of the potential health and water pollution problems.

Future approaches to rural sanitation appear to be directed toward alternative sewage disposal systems and reuse of sewage. Of particular interest is the use of dry toilets and greywater disposal systems. Dry toilets are used to compost fecal matter. The composted material eventually being employed as a fertilizer or soil conditioner. Greywater systems treat wastewater from dishwashing, baths, showers, clothes washing, etc. The treated water has potential as irrigation water.

Although many alternative approaches show promise, their ultimate success will depend on the homeowner. Careful selection of a disposal system is important. It should be suitable for use under the specific environmental conditions (e.g., soil, water table, and climate) and be operated properly. The homeowners should be made aware of the importance of proper operation and maintenance of their systems and the health and water pollution problems that can result from a system failure.

NURSING IMPLICATION

The community health nurse seeks to aid the individual and the community in controlling water pollution. Whether working in a rural or urban area, she or he must be concerned about and aware of potential water pollution problems. Improper sewage and chemical disposal has been the source of many water borne disease outbreaks. Within the work setting and through close colleagueship with rural and urban sanitary engineers, the nurse can provide peer and lay education, environmental assessment for potential problems, and referral of data to the appropriate agencies.

SUMMARY

Water pollution has been and will continue to be a major public health problem. Sanitary engineering and preventive medical practices have combined to reach a point where waterborne disease outbreaks of epidemic proportions have, to a great extent, been controlled; however, the potential for disease transmission through the water route has not been eliminated. With a few exceptions, the disease organisms of epidemic history are still present in today's sewage, and the status of control is one of severance of the transmission chain through proper sanitation practices rather than total eradication of the disease agent.

In recent years there has been a demonstrated need to control chemical pollutants. As was the case with waterborne disease, development of these control measures will require the combined efforts of the sanitary engineering and medical professions.

REFERENCES

1. "Salmonella Surveillance Annual Summary—1969." National Communicable Disease Center, Atlanta, July 1970.
2. Craun, G.F., McCabe, L.J., and Hughes, J.M.: "Waterborne Disease Outbreaks in the U.S. 1971-74." *J.A.W.W.A.* 68:8, 1976.
3. Ross, C.R., and Creason, H.L.: "The Riverside Epidemic." *Water and Sewage Works* 113:128, 1966.
4. Wolman, A., and Gorman, A.E.: "Waterborne Outbreaks in the United States and Their Significance." *J.A.W.W.A.* 31:225, 1939.
5. Weibel, S.R., Dixon, F.R., Weidner, R.B., et al.: "Waterborne Disease Outbreaks, 1946-60." *J.A.W.W.A.* 56:8, 1964.
6. Takeuchi, T.: "Biological Reaction and Pathological Changes in Human Beings and Animals Caused by Organic Mercury Contamination," in Hartung, R., and Dinman, B.D. (eds.): *Environmental Mercury Contamination.* Ann Arbor Science Publishers Inc., Ann Arbor, Mich., 1972.
7. Hodges, L.: *Environmental Pollution,* ed. 2. Holt, Reinhart and Winston, New York, 1977.
8. *The Implications of Cancer-Causing Substances in Mississippi River Waters.* Environmental Defense Fund, Washington, D.C., 1974.
9. *Statement of Basis and Purpose for an Amendment to the National Interim Primary Drinking Water Regulations on Trihalomethanes.* U.S. Environmental Protection Agency, Washington, D.C., 1978.

10. Rosenberg, M.L., Hazlet, K.K., Schaefer, J., et al.: "Shigellosis from Swimming." *J.A.M.A.* 236:1849, 1976.
11. Cabelli, V.J., Haberman, P.W., Levin, M.A., et al.: "The Impact of Pollution on Marine Bathing Beaches: An Epidemiological Study." *Limnol. and Oceanog. Spec. Symp.* 2:424, 1976.
12. Crook, J.: *Reliability of Wastewater Reclamation Facilities.* California State Department of Health, 1976.

CHAPTER **38**
SOLID WASTE MANAGEMENT

EMIL T. CHANLETT, M.S.P.H., M.S.S.E.

The P game which describes the exponential growth and concentration of people, energy use, production, places, and pollutants has had an inevitable effect on the quantity and quality of solid wastes we produce. The exponential characteristic began about 100 years ago when energy from electricity and oil became increasingly available. The exponential curves of power use, production, and pollution have risen sharply in the last 30 years not only in the United States and Western countries but throughout the world.

The characteristic curves for solid wastes are shown in Figure 38-1. Both the upper and lower curves are only postconsumer solid wastes. That is the material collected from our homes, stores, and small industrial operations. The two curves illustrate the difficulties and divergencies of solid waste data, which varies by as much as 100 percent for postconsumer sources. The upper curve places the United States collection at a little over one ton per person per year. The lower curve places that number at 0.8 ton per person per year. On a daily basis the range is from 1.5 to 3 kg (3 to 7 lb) per person.[1]

Table 38-1 shows that the wastes with which we are most familiar and for which we are immediately responsible, the postconsumer category and street and road litter, total 300 million tons per year. The collection and disposal of these materials is a substantial cost whether by a local government or by a private contractor. For the postconsumer waste, the cost is about $25 per ton and rising. Eighty percent of that money is for collection and transportation to some means of disposal. Disposal costs about $5 per ton. Very few urban

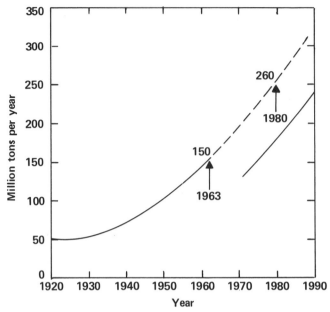

FIGURE 38-1. Postconsumer solid waste production, United States, 1970 to 1985. (Source: "Solid Waste Handling in Metropolitan Areas." U.S. Public Health Service Publ. 1554, 1968. Data for lower curve, 1971–1990, from "Resource Recovery and Waste Reduction," 4th Report to Congress, U.S. EPA 1977.)

or suburban dwellers wish to handle their own solid wastes for what amounts to $20 to $30 per year per person.

Table 38-1 indicates that industrial solid wastes amount to about 260 million tons per year. Some is salvaged and recycled on site. Some is sought by salvagers as it is relatively clean, homogeneous, and predictable in quantity and makeup. Much is dumped on site rather carelessly. Most serious has been the unregulated disposal of wastes containing hazardous substances. Such materials have been dumped without records of the contents and in some instances without identification of the location. Furthermore there is the possibility of continued reactions producing new products of unsuspected properties. The results of 23 years of burial from 1930 to 1953 of chemical wastes in the Love Canal area of Niagara Falls, N.Y., were not evident for another 20 years. In 1978, the site with 100 homes and a school was declared a Federal emergency area to provide help to families forced to evacuate their homes.

Fortunately about one-half of the prodigious quantities of agricultural wastes and animal manure remain at their point of origin, the farmland. The total quantity is 2.7 billion tons per year. The half that does not originate on farms is generated on animal feed lots for cattle and hogs, in the confinement feeding houses for chickens, and large centralized food processing plants. In each of these the pattern is one of increasing size and capacity, although in the case of animal feed lots the total number is decreasing. Mining wastes usually stay at the point of ore concentration. The troubles are with injudicious uses such as radioactive uranium tailings for fill or building materials and unstable coal wastes for dam construction. The disposal of taconite ore wastes into Lake Superior has introduced levels of asbestos fibers in the public water system of Duluth, Minn. Wind disperses dust from mine waste piles. Smouldering fires go on for years in some coal waste dumps.

TABLE 38-1. Solid wastes generated in the United States, 1976 estimates, by origin in total weights per year and per capita per day

Origin	Million tons/year	Allocated per capita per day	
		kg	lb
Postconsumer	150	0.7	1.5
Street and road litter	150	0.7	1.5
Industrial	260	1.2	2.6
Agricultural and crop residues	700	3.0	7.0
Animal manure	2000*	9.0	20.0
Mining and refining	1800	8.0	18.0
Total	5060	23.0	50.0

*Animal manure not stated in the Congressional report source.
Source: House Subcommittee on Transportation and Commerce. "Materials Relating to the Resource and Recovery Act of 1976." U.S. GPO, 1976.

OUR CONCERNS FOR SOLID WASTE HANDLING

There are five reasons for striving to manage solid wastes effectively:

1. The hazards of increasing pathogen transmission.
2. The hazards of discarded toxic and infectious materials reaching us.
3. The esthetic offense of irresponsible discard with consequent property depreciation in value and usefulness.
4. The recovery of materials or their energy content to conserve the world's resources.
5. The costs must be kept at acceptable levels.

Pathogen Transmission

In a literature search that encompassed over 1000 items, Thrift G. Hanks concluded that there was not enough data to permit a quantitative estimate of any direct soil waste-communicable disease relationship.[2] Pathogen transmission starts with garbage which is very attractive food for flies and rats. For flies the garbage is also good breeding material. Garbage is the food waste component; the rubbish and trash components of paper, cans, glass, and plastic provide harborage. Thus solid wastes provide the maternity wards, free lunch counters, and housing for flies, rats, and roaches. The role of flies and rats in communicable disease transmission is well established.

Where animal manure, another solid waste, is near dwellings, large fly populations are usual unless well chosen control measures are applied. These conditions have occurred where suburban development approaches cattle feed lots and poultry breeding houses. Similarly, in the Middle East where animals are housed integrally with families, dense fly populations are common. High incidences of trachoma and gastrointestinal infections among children occur in these circumstances. In open dumps mosquitos breed in water accumulated in bottles, cans, plastic containers, and discarded tires. *Aedes aegypti*, a clean water breeder, is the vector of yellow fever and dengue. Culex mosquitos breed in dirty water pools. Some Culex species transmit hemorrhagic fever. The cry of health hazard during solid waste collector strikes is usually premature. Rats are likely to make their first appearance by night if they are in nearby buildings. Flies will respond to the availability of food wastes. Fly reproduction will require 7 to 10 days with favorable moisture and temperature conditions. Such conditions are more likely to be found on open dumps and poorly operated land fills. Poor drainage from such sites results in mosquito breeding.

Toxic and Infectious Materials

It is only in the last 5 to 7 years that hazardous wastes are receiving serious attention in the United States. These are solid wastes which are injurious to human health, sometimes immediately, other times after long periods of exposure or storage. These wastes include poisons, infectious contaminants, flammable substances, explosives, and radionuclides.[3] Table 38-2 states the gross annual tonnage of wastes containing the indicated contaminants. The tonnage number includes the wastes accompanying the contaminants such as containers, inert materials, and diluents. Estimates are that the hazardous materials per se make up about 10 percent of the industrial waste output. As much as 90 percent may be

TABLE 38-2.   Types, quantities, and sources of hazardous wastes in the United States

Types	Tons/year	Sources
Toxic Metals		
Arsenic	40,000	Smelting copper, lead and zinc
Chromium	30,000	Metal finishing
Lead and mercury	—	Battery making, chlorine making, alloying of metals
Synthesized organics	750,000	In solid form organics
Pesticides	5,000	250 million containers discarded each year
Herbicides	15,000 in storage	Department of Defense holding
Explosives	150,000 in storage	Department of Defense holding obsolete bullets, bombs, and shells
Infectious wastes	170,000	Hospital wastes potentially infectious, from bandages to syringes: animal, culture, and human tissue
Radioactive elements		Weapon production data restricted
Nuclear power	2,000	40 million curies of low-, medium- and high-level radioactive wastes
Radionuclide users	22,000	200 thousand curies of low-level wastes
Uranium mine wastes	4,000,000	9 thousand curies. Should be stored strictly on sites. None to water. None moved.

Source: Report to Congress: "Disposal of Hazardous Wastes." SW-115, EPA, Washington, D.C., 1974.

in liquid or semiliquid form in containers ranging from barrels to storage tanks and ponds. Disposal of such wastes is difficult and hazardous in itself. Some forms can be neutralized chemically. Burning can be used for some with a usual fuel or by incineration. Combustion products must be known and controlled. Distillation and absorption recovery processes can be applied to some. Burial is in use but will have to be more carefully managed. National depositories are in use in the United Kingdom and Denmark. Burning well out to sea in a specially equipped incinerator ship has met success in northern Europe and in carefully observed trials for United States wastes in the Gulf of Mexico.

Cases of human injury thus far have been few. The remainder of a lead arsenate grasshopper poison was buried near Perham, Minn., in 1934. In 1977 a construction crew drove a shallow well 15 m (50 ft.) away for a temporary water supply. Thirteen were poisoned. At Hughes, Arkansas, a 2½ year old child played among a pile of drums the town had stored 15 m (50 ft.) from his home. He came down with organophosphorous poisoning. The drums contained residues of several pesticides. In another case, 15 men in northern California suffered gas poisoning while working in a drum reclamation plant.

The conditions at Love Canal, Niagara Falls, N.Y., are more severe. A rising water table, caused by a few years of high rainfall, moved the chemical wastes to the surface or near surface. The site is about one mile long following an old canal which was used as a chemical dump for some 20 years. The area was filled and used for a school and 100 homes. In early August 1978 problems peaked and gained nationwide press attention. There are no certainties on human injury except children being burned on contact with the oozing liquid. Alleged human damages are: a miscarriage rate of nearly 30 percent, 4 instances of birth defects among 24 births, and a number of cancer deaths in the neighborhood. Dogs with foot burns were reported and early death by age 3 claimed. Tests identify 82 chemicals in the wastes of which 11 are on the suspected carcinogen list. Air samples show evidence of these chemicals in basements and in houses. By mid August 1978 the families with pregnant women or children under 2 years had been evacuated from the area. This amounted to 40 of the 100 in the area. The alleged human injury may never be firmly established. Their economic loss is quite certain as the area and the houses will depreciate and be decidedly unattractive to others. The incident has a strong likelihood of speeding up the implementation of the Resource Conservation and Recovery Act of 1976.

Irresponsible Discard

The esthetic offenses of the irresponsible discard of solid wastes are to be seen in clandestine roadside dumps and road and street litter. Suburban and rural nonfarm families without collection services and without sufficient area to dispose of their wastes on site are regular patrons of dumps along drainage canals, streams, roadways, and bridge abutments. In the 1960s it was estimated that 25,000 clandestine dumps were the disposal facilities for 6 percent of our population who have to find a place for 17,500 tons of wastes each day. There has been a vast improvement in counties in which the "green box" system has been introduced. The green box is a large metal box with a capacity of 4 to 12 cubic yards located at road intersections or near service station-grocery stores. The contents of the green box is picked up by a packer truck for transport to a county or multicounty sanitary landfill. In the southeastern United States, this disposal and collection method has reduced clandestine dumps by 70 to 75 percent.

Litter dropped at the careless conveniences of people on streets, roads, beaches, parks, drive-ins, public gathering places of every sort (except places of worship) is particularly offensive and costly to remove. The answer to the advertising question, "Litter makes you sick. Are you sick enough to stop?" is all too frequently answered by a large silent "No." The cost of cleanup in our urban areas is more than $2 per person per year. $500 million dollars is spent annually to pick up litter from our 6 million kilometers (4 million miles) of streets and roads. The cost per mile for state maintained highways averages $60 per year, ranging from $9 in North Dakota to $400 in Massachusetts. The makeup of the litter is familiar. By item count 65 percent is paper and plastics. Beverage containers make up 20 to 30 percent by item count and 40 to 60 percent of the volume.

Resource Conservation

The recovery of materials or energy from solid wastes is gaining ground in the United States. A large share of salvage and recycling takes place at the point of processing, fabrication, and manufacture. Twenty-five percent of the 200 million tons of major metals, paper, rubber, glass, and textiles processed each year are recycled materials. Most sought after are copper, stainless steel, nickel, aluminum, lead, steel, and zinc.[1] These are high value metals and increasingly their ores must be transported long distances. The low cost of the raw materials and market fluctuations place paper and glass in less favorable positions for profitable salvage; we recycle about 25 percent of our paper. That is annually equivalent to the trees that could be harvested from an area equal to New Hampshire and Vermont.

Postconsumer recovery of home and commercial solid wastes has been more modest, but there are projections of increases. In 1978 the recovery from this category of wastes was as follows: corrugated paper board 22 percent; newspaper 21 percent; aluminum containers 16 percent; other paper 13 percent; rubber tires 13 percent; paper packaging 11 percent; steel cans 5 percent; glass containers 3 percent; plastics 0 percent. The projections for these recoveries are an increase from 8 million tons per year in 1975 to 35 million tons in 1985 and to 58 million tons in 1990. Municipalities have been hesitant to undertake recovery from their collections because of high capital costs for sorting equipment and facilities, existing mixed collection methods, imperfect separation methods, high maintenance and energy input costs, and marketing uncertainties. Then, having recovered all possible products, there remains 50 to 60 percent of the original material, by weight, which requires disposal.[4]

There are several federally supported recovery projects in the United States. Separate collection of paper and beverage containers in Somerville and Marblehead, Massachusetts for resale is proving workable and profitable. The separation and recovery of paper fiber, glass, and metal from mixed collections is successful in Franklin, Ohio. An adjacent roofing paper factory is the ready market for the paper fiber.[1] Private initiative has raised the recycling of aluminum cans through 1300 recycling centers to 1 million per year of the 4 million cans made. These are worth $300 per ton as the electricity required to reprocess the cans is only 5 percent of that needed to refine bauxite ore. The Oregon mandatory deposit on beverage containers has increased the percentage returned to 90 percent. The Vermont beverage container law has reduced the container portion of highway litter by two-thirds.

The use of solid waste as an energy source has had successes and some disappointing failures. The best established method is to equip incinerators with heat recovery equipment to generate steam which may then be used for heating or for producing electricity. Examples are found in Braintree, Mass.; Hempstead, N.Y.; Chicago, Ill.; the Norfolk Navy Yard, Va.; and Nashville, Tenn. This direct method of heat recovery from burning the solid waste prevents the heat from being largely dissipated up the stack. There has been limited experience with a promising method of burning separated shredded municipal solid wastes in the fire boxes of electric generating stations. Metal, glass, grit, and as many noncombustibles as possible are removed and given separate disposal. After shredding, the refuse derived fuel (RDF) is blown into the fire box along with the pulverized coal. The installation with the longest operating record is in St. Louis at the Union Electric Meremac Plant. The solid waste provides about 10 percent of the fuel value and is equivalent to 150 tons of coal per day. A similar installation at Ames, Iowa, is getting underway. Projects in study or planning are in Monroe County, N.Y., with the Rochester Gas and Electric Company, New York City with the Consolidated Edison Company, and Madison, Wis.

Pyrolysis is an oxygen starved combustion which produces gas, combustible liquids, and char. It is basically the process by which people have been making charcoal for hundreds of years. The largest effort in the United States was a plant built to process 1000 tons per day of Baltimore's solid waste to produce methane gas. After two years of difficulties and shutdowns the plant was closed in 1977. A San Diego pyrolysis facility is designed to produce oil from solid wastes for use by the San Diego Gas and Electric Company; it is in start-up and shake-down. Projects are in study using pyrolysis in Knoxville, Tenn.; Charleston, W.Va.; Mt. Vernon, N.Y.; and Seattle, Wash. Refuse derived fuel use presents unpredictable variations in composition, moisture content, response to grinders, air classifiers, and metal separators. Such changes are different from fossil fuels which are supplied on rather definite specifications.[4]

Prepared solid wastes have about one-half of the heat content of coal on a weight basis. It is an attractive energy source, but it is not a panacea. If we were able to burn all of our solid wastes, the contribution to our total energy need would not exceed 10 percent. In the overall strategy of energy conservation, waste recovery by salvage and recycling and waste reduction can produce greater energy savings. That can be done by increased recycling of metals which require a lower energy input to reuse the scrap than to process virgin ores. Decreasing our extravagant packaging and returning to refillable beer, soft drink, and milk containers can produce a very large energy savings.

Cost Levels

The cost of collection which accounts for 80 percent of a municipal or private contractor's solid waste removal service has already been cited as between $20 and $30 per person per year. It is really a modest sum for the labor, equipment use, and transportation provided. The remaining 20 percent is for the first stage of disposal. This would bring the average cost to $25 per person or approximately per ton, per year. For a city of 50,000, the annual cost would then be $1,250,000, a sizeable sum. That would cover the handling of home, commercial, and small manufacturing wastes, and street litter. Private contractor service for the same wastes would be about the same. These services in the United States are very extensive particularly in suburban areas, and for such concentrated sources as shopping centers, factories, hospitals, and large housing developments. About 150,000,000 of our people have solid wastes service. At the average cost of $25 per year per person, the total approaches $4 billion annually. To this must be added the expenditures for handling the wastes from manufacturing, food processing, some portion of agricultural activities, and mining. Such a substantial economic enterprise requires management skills. In the past solid wastes handling did not receive much attention even in middle sized cities. The costs were not easily separated from the total public works budget. Equipment and people were moved and transfered without identification. That is changing. Collection routes are being studied to gain maximum use by trucks and laborers. Hauling time and distances are being examined to determine the usefulness of transfer stations where street route packer trucks discharge their collections for loading very large tractor trailer units. The entire matter of costs and means of financing solid wastes services is receiving more attention.[4]

SOME CHOICES FOR DISPOSING OF SOLID WASTES

Three options for the disposal of wastes are: "burn it," "bury it," or "hide it and forget it." Each of these is still in use. The latter was the open dump, the clandestine dump, and the farm site dump. We are just beginning to realize that the "hide it and forget it" method has been used extensively for hazardous solid wastes. Our increasing intensity of land use, our growing density of people, and our urban and suburban development have made the open dump, even with so-called controlled burning, a rarer means of disposing of municipal solid wastes.

The "burn it" option is much more frequently used for factory wastes than for post-consumer wastes. The number of municipal incinerators in the United States is decreasing. In 1977 there were less than 200. Some of the surviving facilities are quite large, requiring continuous firing for economy and process efficiency. Such large incinerators are still viable alternatives for big cities. Favorable answers are needed to these questions:

1. Can the stringent emission standards for air pollutants be met? The requirements by the Commonwealth of Massachussetts are at the limits of control technology, virtually ruling out incineration.
2. Will the combustion products of the changing composition of solid wastes damage the grates, the fire brick, breeching, and pollution control units? Plastics and coated paper produce acidic vapors and gases. Some burn with high heat outputs. Some plastics do not burn. They merely melt and hang as globs in the grate openings.
3. What should be done with the residues? There is about 20 percent by weight of noncombustibles including the ash. There is hot and dirty quench water. There are the materials cleaned from the gas stream in solid and liquid form. Incineration is not a complete disposal method.
4. Can the heat of burning solid wastes be recovered? Yes, several examples of success have been noted earlier in this chapter. The capital and operating costs for heat recovery on incinerators are high. Table 38-3 shows that for a 1000 ton per day incinerator capable of serving 0.5 million people, heat recovery for electricity generation doubles the cost of simple incineration. Steam generation and residue recovery increases the capital cost by nearly 50 percent. After taking the value of the energy recovery into account, incineration is the most costly method on a net per ton basis as shown in Table 38-3. As energy costs continue to rise these margins will shift. However, efforts to reduce the waste we generate would conserve more energy than heat recovery efforts.

TABLE 38-3. The costs and returns of alternate methods of handling postconsumer solid wastes after collection at a 1,000 ton/day facility serving about 500,000 people

Method	In millions of dollars			Net cost per ton in dollars
	Capital cost	Total operating	Returns	
Sanitary landfill, short haul	2.5	0.8	0	2.60
Fuel recovery (RDF)	7.6	1.7	0.9	2.70
Materials recovery	11.5	2.7	1.3	4.80
Sanitary landfill, long haul	2.8	1.8	0	5.90
Composting, mechanical	17.0	3.0	1.0	6.30
Incineration with steam and residue recovery	13.0	3.5	1.5	6.60
Incineration, simple	9.0	2.3	0	7.70
Incineration with generation of electricity	18.0	3.9	1.2	9.00

Source: Council on Environmental Quality: "Resource Recovery Processes for Mixed Municipal Solid Wastes," by M.R.I. Published by U.S. EPA, 1973, p. 56.

"Bury it" has been an alternative used by people for a long time for really obnoxious wastes such as dead animals, slaughter wastes, and dead fish swept ashore. Modern earth moving equipment, such as bull dozers, scrapper pans, and heavy compactors, have made sanitary landfill the most widely used disposal method in the United States. Table 38-4 shows its advantages and disadvantages among other alternatives. Not only is this means used for small towns but also for very large ones as long as sites are available. Landfill is used by New York City. The process is one of planned and controlled burial. The technique varies with the site and terrain. It is a process of getting earth for cover, of spreading and compacting the wastes, of covering thinly each day, and with a final cover of about 0.6 m (2 ft). Here are the principal requirements for sanitary landfill:

1. A site must be within economical hauling distance at a favorable acquisition cost. With very good compaction the area needed is about 0.4 hectare (1 acre) per 15,000 people per year. Less compaction will reduce the number of people served to 10,000. Greater depth of compacted waste will increase it to 20,000.
2. If any waterways or groundwater strata have actual or potential use for water supply or recreational use, the drainage and vertical movement of water from the fill must be controlled. A decomposing fill produces leachate high in dissolved solids, acids, organic residues, and possibly some traces of toxic substances.
3. During the first six months a completed fill is partially in aerobic decomposition. The gas production is largely carbon dioxide which is readily soluble in water. Thereafter anerobic processes produce increasing proportions of methane. Usually this inflammable, explosive gas vents through the earth cover to the atmosphere. Sites which have gravel formations or fissured rock do permit lateral gas movement. This must be prevented by impermeable barriers of compacted clay, plastic liners or vents. In 1968, a National Guard Armory on the edge of a fill in Winston-Salem, N.C., was damaged in a gas explosion that killed three guardsmen and seriously injured two.
4. The site choice should consider truck traffic and the noise of operations. These can

TABLE 38-4. First-stage disposal methods of solid wastes

Methods	Advantages	Disadvantages
Incineration	Combustion of breeding materials. Takes combined garbage and rubbish. Can be very efficient and run 24 h/day in large cities. Can recover heat and metallic wastes.	Final ash residue, cans, and bottles remain. High capital investment. High operational and maintenance cost. Particulates and odors from poor operation. Requires control of newly formed air and water pollutants. Often requires addition of combustibles for start up.
Open dumps	Hauling is only cost. Combined collection.	Optimum for rat and fly breeding. Neighborhood depreciation. Mosquito breeding. Air pollution from dump fires. Water pollution from leaching.
Grinding and adding to sewage	Gives garbage same handling as excreta. For home units, collection phase of food wastes is eliminated.	Takes only garbage. Requires proper sewer design if home units are used. Requires added sewage plant facilities for central grinding and treatment. Rats appear in sewers. Digested solids must be handled.
Sanitary landfill	Combined collection. Low capital investment. Moderate operational cost. Land reclamation for restricted use. Adapted to small towns.	Land requirement may result in long hauls in the future. Requires selected soil for cover. Requires standby fire control. Leaching adds pollutants to ground- and surface-water sources.
Composting	Conserves and recycles wastes. Provides humus for soil. Decomposition heat controls flies. Aerobic action free of odors. Sewage sludge can be combined.	Requires presorting and grinding and turning. High capital equipment and maintenance cost. Requires assured market for compost. Requires disposal of noncompostables. Requires carbon: nitrogen ratio of about 30:1.
Salvage by sorting	Recovery of usable and salable material. Conservation of resources. Defrays cost of waste handling.	Limited to special wastes and selected materials. At mercy of market. Special equipment required. Remainder must be managed.

be very disturbing to nearby families. Such conditions produce strong objections to locating future sites.

5. Drift fences are needed to control windblown paper and plastics. A tidy area and daily cover prevent complaints and help to control rats, flies and mosquitos. The benefits of these measures are not only immediate but make the acquisition of future sites easier. Poor operations give the sanitary landfill method a bad reputation.

There is one more option for the first stage disposal of solid wastes: "Transform it." That is the goal of composting. Table 38-4 states the advantages and disadvantages of composting. Unfortunately in the United States the disadvantages have outweighed the advantages. In the 18 operations for composting municipal solid wastes that were started in the United States and Puerto Rico from 1951 to 1969, only three were functioning in 1971. The most consistent has been a unit processing 45 tons per day of wastes from Altoona, Pa. It has been working since 1951. A Houston plant has been handling 360 tons per day since 1966. In San Juan, Puerto Rico, 150 tons of municipal collection has been composted per day since 1969. Springfield, Mass., has attempted composting garbage-only food wastes in 1954 and 1961. The plant was closed in 1962.

Composting is an aerobic process. Bacteria, primarily, and fungi feed upon the organic material. The same action goes on in the leaf cover on the ground of woodlands. A carbon to nitrogen ratio of about 30:1 is needed to provide the nitrogen for forming new protoplasm. The composting material has to be stirred to renew the oxygen supply which the pile needs. The pile can literally be that, a windrow on tamped earth or concrete. It must be turned every third or fourth day. The internal temperature of 60°C (140°F) or more for several days kills the pathogens and fly larva. Turning, that is, aeration, prevents anaerobic stinks. The windrow method requires 20 to 30 days to convert the material to a dark humus. The product is an excellent soil conditioner. It is not a balanced fertilizer. In fact it is a rather poor fertilizer. It is low in phosphorus and potassium and not particularly rich in nitrogen. Nearly a dozen mechanical means have been used to accelerate the turning and aeration of prepared solid wastes to reduce the composting time from 20 or more days to 4 or 5 days. These have shared in the failures and the successes in the United States.[4]

Composting has fared better in other parts of the world. Among these are Switzerland, Japan, Thailand, South Africa, Israel, West Germany, The Netherlands, England, Scotland, France, and Mexico. There are 100 plants in the world. Most of them serve cities with a population under 100,000. There are larger plants serving Bangkok, Edinburgh, Rome, Teheran, and Tel Aviv. Composting cannot accept solid wastes as is. The noncompostables must be separated. That includes metals, glass, and plastics in film form or shaped. That separation is labor intensive. Shredding follows to get a lot of surface area exposed for bacterial feed. The compost pile is another cafeteria and maternity ward which our wastes provide for bacteria and higher forms of life. The compost must have a market at least to recover costs. That has been a disastrously weak link in the United States applications. In The Netherlands and Israel the product has been used in land reclamation. In West Germany the compost maintains soil quality on steep sloped vineyards.

In the utilization of compost and in recycling salvage and reclamation, transportation costs determine success or failure. Solid wastes management is materials handling in which transportation comprises a high fraction of costs. It is a major factor in collection, in transfer to intermediate stations, and in further movement when salvage or transformation is used. Salvage has already been examined. Table 38-4 summarizes the advantages and disadvantages. Although it has failed in Baltimore, the pyrolysis process is also transformation of solid wastes with the potential to recover gas, combustible liquids, and usable char. Large scale technology may yet be developed. Another little used natural process is feeding solid wastes to the familiar earthworm. These worms produce a remarkable change. The results are castings and many more worms. Both can be harvested. The process is slow and requires control of pH and temperature. Large areas would be needed for earthworm or annelidic feeding of solid wastes. The area would be usable again and again after harvesting in contrast to sanitary landfill. Again a market for the casting and the worms would be needed.

CHANGES TO COME

The intent of waste reduction is to decrease the weight and volume now generated. Some specifics are:

1. Mandatory deposits on beverage containers to promote the return to refillable beverage bottles.
2. The redesign of packaging to reduce the volume of paper and plastics that are discarded.
3. The reexamination of manufacturing methods and materials selection to facilitate repair and to extend the useful life of hard goods.
4. The design, fabrication, and assembly of products and packaging to facilitate disposal and recovery.

The dedication of land and sea sinks for waste disposal for short and long terms must be done within the assimilative capacities of the particular environments within hygenic, ecologic, and esthetic bounds. Ocean dumping of solid wastes has ended in the United States. Exceptions may be necessary.

Laws and regulations must be modified to encourage salvage. Presently federally determined railway freight rates favor virgin iron ores over the cost of shipping scrap iron and steel.

Improvements in the management skills applied to solid wastes handling will continue.

The methods of financing solid waste collection and disposal will undergo changes. In some instances fees for service will replace funding from general tax receipts. This is not usually favored by elected officials, nor does it have merit for solid waste control among the poor. Disposal charges added to the initial cost of the product such as an automobile to provide for its ultimate disposal have been suggested. Six million cars per year are discarded in the United States, many haphazardly and clandestinely.

Materials and energy recovery may come to be so socially desirable that the requirement of profit from the operation will become secondary. Municipalities may then undertake recovery at a loss. The position would be that we are conserving materials or energy for a long term benefit and regaining something from our solid wastes without a financial profit being required.

EFFECTS AND CONSEQUENCES OF POOR HANDLING OF SOLID WASTES

Hazardous wastes pose real risks to human health. Poor burial methods of the past are exposing limited numbers of people to uncertain dangers. Sites have not been identified. Contents are an unknown mixture which go on to new reactions and products. Ground water pollution from old burials could affect larger numbers of people. Alternate means of incineration, transformation, and recovery require the protection of the workers and safeguards against air and water pollution. The putrescible contents of solid wastes attract and produce flies, rats, and to a lesser extent mosquitos and roaches. Large populations of these vectors of communicable diseases increase the number of human victims and the possibilities of outbreaks.

The esthetic responses of people to the careless handling of solid wastes are nuisance complaints to the local health department and public works agency. The causes are uncollected wastes; noise from collection, transfer station, and landfill operations; smokey unsightly open dumps; windblown debris and drainage from landfills; incinerator smoke and dust. Usually there is some speedy corrective action as elected officials are sensitive to frequent and widespread complaints.

The ecologic effects of solid wastes practices are often viewed as bad, but some are beneficial. Filling tidal flats and swampy areas certainly changes the plant and animal life in those areas. Many such places are not particularly attractive, producing their share of mosquitos, stinks, and water quality deterioration. Automobile bodies and other non-floating junk have been used to create artificial reefs to shelter marine life. Off the shore of Long Island, such reefs brought about the return of good fishing. A portion of our solid waste is food for other forms of life. Some animal manure is being processed for incorporation into animal food. Composting is ecologically beneficial when the product is used as a soil conditioner and to restore eroded land. Solid wastes practices have been less damaging than our liquid and airborne wastes. The processes in a landfill, for example, are slow and allow time for new regimens to come into being. There is a need for more imaginative use of our solid wastes for ecologic benefits, for example, the feeding and breeding of earthworms.

NURSING IMPLICATION

As community health nurses become more knowledgeable about the issues and problems in the control of solid wastes, they will be in a position to provide support and direct assistance in meeting this need. Through educational efforts for both lay and peer groups, thorough home and community assessments, and close working relationships with sanitary engineers, they will be able to provide direct intervention in dealing with this problem.

REFERENCES

1. Fourth Report to the Congress: "Resource Recovery and Waste Reduction." EPA, Washington, D.C., 1977.
2. Hanks, Thrift G.: "Solid Wastes/Disease Relationships." U.S. Public Health Service Publ. 999-UIH-6, 1967.

3. Report to the Congress: "Disposal of Hazardous Wastes." SW-115, EPA, Washington, D.C., 1974.
4. Tchobanoglous, George, Thiesen, Hilary, and Eliassen, Rolf: *Solid Wastes.* McGraw-Hill Book Co., New York, 1977.
5. General Electric Co.: *Solid Waste Management—Technology Assessment.* Van Nostrand Reinhold Co., New York, 1975.

39

IONIZING RADIATION AND COMMUNITY HEALTH

CAROL A. SILBERSTEIN, M.Ed., R.N., AND EDWARD B. SILBERSTEIN, M.D.

As you read this you are being exposed to a wide variety of radiation from natural and manmade sources. Radioactivity has been part of mankind's external and internal environment since the origin of our species. Within the last 35 or 40 years, however, additional types of exposure have been developed artificially which have increased this radiation and the potential for resultant harm. It is therefore important to understand the kinds of ionizing radiation bathing our environment and its origins, the relative amounts from each source, and the potential effects on the community.

PARTICLES AND RAYS

The ionizing radiation which we shall consider includes subatomic particles as well as the more energetic part of the electromagnetic spectrum. Alpha particles are nuclei of helium atoms that have a very short range in tissue, measured in fractions of a millimeter, so that an alpha particle cannot even penetrate your skin. Beta particles are very energetic electrons which have a normal path of no more than a few millimeters in living tissue before giving up all their energy. Neutrons and protons are other subatomic particles which can deliver radiation to tissue. The proton is the nucleus of a hydrogen atom and has a single positive charge. The neutron is approximately the same size but with no charge. X-rays and gamma rays are not particles, but electromagnetic waves which a physicist also views as *photons* or packets of energy. They have amplitude and wave length similar to that of ultraviolet or visible light but with much greater energy. X-rays are emitted from excited electrons circling about a nucleus, while gamma rays come from the nucleus of an atom which has an excess of energy for one of a variety of reasons. Gamma and x-rays pass through many centimeters of tissue before full absorption.

The effects of all of these kinds of radiation depend on the amount of energy delivered to the tissue by radiation. The term *rad* is a measurement of the amount of energy received by tissue. The definition of a rad is 100 *ergs* (a measurement of energy) delivered to a gram of tissue. The *roentgen* is a unit of exposure based on ionization of air. It is not an absorbed dose in air. The *rem* (roentgen equivalent man) provides an indication of the biologic effect of different kinds of radiation. The rem and rad are equivalent for gamma and x-rays. Other forms of radiation have a relative biologic efficiency (*R.B.E.*) greater than one, so that the rem value then equals the rads received multiplied by the R.B.E. of the quality of radiation received. Alpha particles and neutrons are more damaging than x-rays and gamma rays (higher R.B.E.), as there is a greater chance of these particles interacting with molecules near their path. Such interaction of any of the forms of radiation we have mentioned may lead to a temporary or permanent change in the structure of the molecule. Depending on the uniqueness of that molecule to the cell, the ability of that cell to repair the damage which has occurred, and the number of cells which are damaged in the radiating event, molecular and cellular structure and function may be immediately or eventually impaired.

SOURCES

Most of the radiation which we receive in a year comes from natural sources. The first kind is called cosmic radiation, emanating largely from within our own galaxy and in part from the sun, consisting of many kinds of particulate and electromagnetic radiation. The intensity of cosmic radiation is greatest at high altitudes and varies somewhat at different latitudes because the earth's magnetic field deflects some of the charged particles of this radiation back into space. Cosmic radiation increases during solar flares. The average dose from all components of cosmic radiation has been estimated to correspond to about 30 millirem (0.03 rem) per year.

A second component of natural background radiation comes from soil or any rock containing appreciable natural radioactivity and lying within a few centimeters of the surface. Radioactivity is low in most sedimentary rocks but high in those of volcanic origin. Radiation received by body tissues from these sources varies according to ground cover by moisture in the soil or by snow and is decreased by shielding caused by roads or buildings. However, building materials themselves may be radioactive or may release tiny amounts of radioactive gases such as radon. Living in a brick or stone house adds about 30 millirems per year of exposure over that received from living in a wooden home. The average exposure from natural, terrestial sources is between 40 and 50 millirem per year, although there may be large variations according to local geologic formation. Thus, in areas where the underlying rock is of volcanic origin, the average dose rate may be 80 to 150 millirem per year or higher.[1]

A third source of natural background radiation is internal in origin, due mainly to the existence of a naturally occurring radioactive component of normal body potassium, the radioisotope called potassium-40 which comprises about 0.01 percent of the potassium in the body. (A *radioisotope* has the same number of nuclear protons as a stable isotope, which, by definition, gives off no radiation but differs from it in the number of nuclear neutrons). We receive 15 to 20 millirem per year from potassium-40 and another small dose of about 0.7 millirem per year from a radioactive form of a carbon called carbon-14 formed within the atmosphere by the action of cosmic radiation and then incorporated in body tissues. There are small amounts of other radioactive materials normally occurring in the biosphere, such as rubidium, polonium, radon, and uranium, responsible for doses of about 8 millirems per year to the gonads and bone marrow, and about 35 millirems per year to the bone cells. The totals for internal radiation therefore are about 28 millirems for germinal (gonadal) tissues, 24 millirems for bone marrow, and 51 millirems for the endosteal cells of the bone.[2] Thus, natural sources of radiation will deliver about 100 to 120 millirems per year to your body on the average. The National Council on Radiation Protection has set a level of 500 millirems as the upper limit of acceptable radiation exposure per year for individuals not involved in occupational radiation exposure. For these latter the upper limit for total body irradiation is 5 rem per year (Table 39-1).

The first source of artificial or manmade radiation which we receive comes from the fallout from nuclear bomb tests. Some of the radioactivity does not enter the body. We have, or will, ingest small amounts of cesium-137 which is widely distributed through body tissues. Strontium-90 is concentrated and maintained in bone. The remainder of fallout is from carbon-14, and most of this exposure is delivered at an extremely low dose rate over a long period of time. For the world population, atomic bomb tests prior to 1971 involve, or will involve (since clouds of radioactivity are still in the stratosphere), total doses of 120, 180, or 160 millirems to germinal tissues, bone cells, or bone marrow

TABLE 38-1. National Council on Radiation Protection dose limiting recommendations

Maximum permissable dose equivalent for occupational exposure	
Combined whole body occupational exposure	
Prospective annual limit	5 rems in any one year
Retrospective annual limit	10–15 rems in any one year
Long term accumulation to age N years	$(N - 18) \times 5$ rems
Skin	15 rems in any one year
Hands	75 rems in any one year (25/qtr)
Forearms	30 rems in any one year (10/qtr)
Other organs, tissues and organ systems	15 rems in any one year (5/qtr)
Fertile women (with respect to fetus)	0.5 rem in gestation period
Dose limits for the public, or occasionally exposed individuals	
Individual or occasional	0.5 rem in any one year
Students	0.1 rem in any one year
Population dose limits	
Genetic	0.17 rem average per year
Somatic	0.17 rem average per year
Emergency dose limits—life saving	
Individual (older than 45 years if possible)	100 rems
Hands and forearms	200 rems, additional (300 rems, total)
Emergency dose limits—less urgent	
Individual	25 rems
Hands and forearms	100 rems, total
Family of radioactive patients	
Individual (under age 45)	0.5 rems in any one year
Individual (over age 45)	5 rems in any one year

respectively. Tests since 1971 are estimated to add about 10 percent to these figures. The estimated average dose rate from fallout over the northern hemisphere is about 6 millirems per year.[3]

Very small amounts of radiation are received by workers in specialized areas of medical and dental work, industrial radiography, and specific manufacturing processes. Radium in certain luminous watches distributes a tiny amount of radiation to the wearer. These are not significant sources to the population as a whole.

The radiation dose from diagnostic medical procedures ranges from slightly less than, to 50 times greater than, the annual dose from all other background sources. For example, the body receives a dose of about 50 millirems from a chest x-ray, but, without proper shielding, as occurs in some portable x-ray units used in community screening programs, that dose may be 500 millirems per chest x-ray. Serious consideration should be given to discontinuation of mass chest x-ray screening programs and employing intradermal tuberculin testing instead for case detection of tuberculosis. An intravenous pyelogram or kidney x-ray will give a total body dose of 400–800 millirems on the average, depending on the number of films taken, while an upper gastrointestinal series or barium enema with fluoroscopy (a constant beam of x-ray passing through the tissues involved) may give tissue doses of 1–5 rems.[4]

GENETICALLY SIGNIFICANT DOSE

In determining the meaning of this wide range of doses to a community, the concept of the "genetically significant dose" has been evolved.[5] If we know the average dose to the gonad per radiologic examination, frequency of every type of examination in a total population, and the size of the population, then the mean gonad dose per year can be estimated. The estimated radiation exposure of gonadal tissues, when combined with the values for the average number of children normally conceived after the ages at which the examinations were performed, gives the genetically significant dose because, as will be discussed further, mutations involving future offspring only occur in the gonads. Hence, for an average American community the genetically significant dose is about 35 millirems per year from radiologic procedures (diagnostic, therapeutic, and nuclear medicine), although many of us will not have had a radiologic procedure during that year. The increasing use of diagnostic x-rays and nuclear medicine in many developing countries will tend to raise these contributions to the average radiation exposure of the whole population in the future, although this increase may be offset by x-ray equipment requiring lower doses and radiopharmaceuticals delivering lower radiation doses which are now under active development. Finally, the average exposure from an extensive world program of nuclear reactor power production would add a few millirems per year to the average body exposure throughout the population.

RADIOBIOLOGIC CONSIDERATIONS

So far we have considered the kinds of ionizing radiation, i.e., radiation which can disrupt molecules within the body (this discussion excludes ultraviolet radiation, a known skin carcinogen), sources of radiation in the community, and the average quantities involved. Thus, some radiation exposure is seen to be inescapable.

Next we must consider the harm which may be caused by radiation. The delivery of energy to radiation sensitive body tissues may cause ionization of water molecules or directly damage nearby cellular molecules by splitting any of these into charged ions or very reactive chemical forms with unpaired electrons called radicals. These in turn give up their energy to neighboring molecules with potential disruption of chemical bonds. A large body of research has indicated that the primary target for damaging radiation in a cell is the nucleus, and specifically the desoxyribonucleic acid (DNA) molecules of the genes in the cell's chromosomes. The resultant change in the chemical structure of the DNA may alter the genetic information carried by the chromosomes in the cells.[4] What can this lead to? First, the cells may die, because the altered sequence of bases (purines and pyrimidines) on the DNA chain may no longer be a valid code for continued production of some protein or other essential substance of cells. However, we know that most organs can function even if two-thirds of their mass is removed. This is very unlikely except at very high radiation doses or with lower doses in a developing embryo with organs of microscopic size. Another effect of DNA damage by radiation from any source may be to cause failure of chromosomes to divide. The cell continues to function normally but may be unable to reproduce itself. With tissues in which cell division is normally rapid and the cell life span short, as in bone marrow or the lining of the gastrointestinal tract, tissue function may be rapidly altered. If the bone marrow stops producing cells, infection, bleeding, and, later, anemia may result. Life threatening diarrhea and vomiting may result from radiation of the gastrointestinal tract. However, such effects are again only important if large numbers of cells are irradiated with radiation doses a hundred or so times higher than those which we have discussed.

LONG TERM EFFECTS

Cells damaged by radiation but surviving the exposure may still be capable of producing viable but subtly altered daughter cells.[6] Cells from germinal tissues (of the gonads) following fertilization may transmit an abnormality in the coding sequence of the bases in DNA to the offspring which may appear as a mutation in the next generation of offspring if the mutation is "dominant" or in many generations if the mutation is "recessive."

Since 3 to 5 percent of live births carry some chemical or visible genetic defect, measuring additional mutations from radiation is very difficult. The percent of children with genetic disease has not increased in Hiroshima and Nagasaki. If, however, the damaged cell forms part of any of the other nongonadal body organs and tissues, such damage will not be expressed in the offspring, but mutations (abnormalities induced in the DNA sequence of the chromosomes) of such body cells may sometimes change the ability of that cell to divide, so that cell multiplication proceeds more or less unchecked, producing a benign or malignant tumor. The mechanism of this carcinogenic effect of radiation is not entirely certain and may involve not only somatic mutations in DNA sequence but possibly changes in the immunologic, surface, or other properties of the damaged cell and its environment. The amount of radiation which can cause a malignancy in an irradiated tissue varies greatly with the kind of tissue and quality of radiation. There is growing evidence that as little as 10 to 30 rads may cause malignancy of some organs, such as the thyroid gland.

There is currently a debate as to whether prenatal irradiation at low levels causes leukemia. There is no increased incidence of leukemia in children who were *in utero* at the time of the atomic bomb blasts in Japan. Other epidemiologists have found a 40 percent increase in leukemia in the children of mothers who received pelvic x-rays during the later stages of their pregnancies, however. An unanswered question is whether some of these mothers had underlying conditions related to the need for pelvic irradiation which might also be etiologic factors in leukemia. Nevertheless, this controversy is still with us. It does appear from animal studies that the fetus or newborn is more susceptible to the carcinogenic effects of radiation than the adult.

In some populations a nonspecific life shortening effect has been noted at higher dose rates, even when deaths due to cancer are excluded, perhaps by decreasing the number of mitoses possible in vital tissues.[6]

The final delayed effect of radiation overexposure is cataract. Growing cells in the lens of the eye which are hit by ionizing radiation in doses of about 200 rads slowly develop abnormal lens fibers. The increased density of the lens will show up many years after such exposure.[7]

DOSE AND EFFECT RELATIONSHIP

We have dealt with four long term effects of ionizing radiation on populations of a community, but the dose-effect relationship is highly controversial at the low levels of radiation caused by "natural" and manmade radiation which we have quantitatively discussed above. Figure 39-1 includes several possible relationships of radiation dose and the long term effects which we have discussed. Curve A shows a model in which effects (such as cancer) would occur even in the absence of radiation and are increased as radiation is introduced into the environment. Curve B is the "linear no-threshold" model upon which our most conservative current radiation protection standards are based. This linear no-threshold model implies that there is an effect linearly or directly proportional to dose, even at the very lowest radiation dose. Curve C is a nonlinear, no threshold model, in which the effect is seen to be less than that for the linear threshold model, at any given dose. Curve D indicates the theoretic model where there is a threshold for linear effect so that below a critical dose no effect is observed.

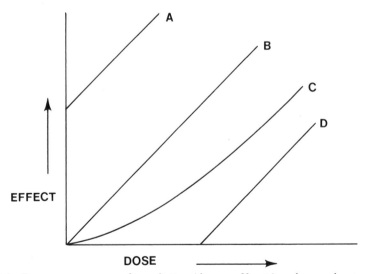

FIGURE 39-1. Dose-response curve for radiation (dose on X axis) and several potential radiation effects (Y axis). Curve A: Effects occur in absence of radiation. Curve B: Linear no-threshold model. Curve C: Nonlinear no-threshold model. Curve D: Theoretical model with threshold for linear effect.

With this background we can understand the controversy surrounding the effect of low levels of irradiation. It may well be that the low level of environmental radiation, about 120 millirems per year to each of us, is a factor in the prevalence of cancer in the community. However, for virtually all forms of malignancy, including leukemia, there are data in exposed populations to suggest some kind of threshold. For example, at Hiroshima and Nagasaki, sites of the two atomic bomb explosions during World War II in 1945, no case of leukemia has occurred in an individual who received less than 50 rems, with a followup in excess of 30 years. The threshold dose for carcinoma of the thyroid (in patients who have received external irradiation for a skin or neck condition in childhood) appears to be in the range of 10 to 30 rems. In fact, over a certain dose, which is about 2000 rems for the thyroid, carcinogenesis disappears as a radiation effect, probably because irradiated cells which would have undergone malignant transformation are prevented from dividing by the very radiation which caused the potentially malignant transformation.

The presence or absence of a threshold for carcinogenesis is not easy to determine. Unfortunately, the human data available provide inadequate numbers for rigid statistical analysis. Extrapolation from animal studies is always hazardous. There is evidence that the latent period before cancers develop increases with decreased exposure and for small exposures it may exceed life expectancy. Furthermore low doses of radiation cause types of molecular damage more easily repaired than higher doses, further bringing into question the linear, no-threshold hypothesis.[7]

ACUTE RADIATION SYNDROME

Acute illness may be caused if the acute radiation exposure is sufficiently high. There have only been six fatalities from acute radiation sickness in the United States. These include four criticality incidents (the last in 1964) and two caused by misadministration of Gold-198, a radioisotope no longer commercially available. Three other deaths at Idaho Falls, Idaho, were caused by explosion, despite the fact that the victims were heavily contaminated. None of these occurrences were related to nuclear power plants. At a dose of 10 to 100 rems, there are subtle changes in the lymphocytes of the body, but the exposed individual remains asymptomatic, with no changes in his granulocytes, platelets, erythrocytes, or blood chemistry. With doses from 100 to 250 rems received acutely, the incidence of nausea and vomiting rises from virtually zero to almost 100 percent. Bone marrow depression with resultant low circulating blood cell counts will also occur, raising the risk of bleeding or infection. These are treatable and reversible and so should not be lethal up to an acute radiation exposure of about 250 to 300 rems in a previously healthy person.

As the radiation dose received acutely rises, mortality increases, so that at doses of about 500 rems only 50 percent of an irradiated community would be expected to survive for a 2 month period despite excellent medical treatment. Very recent data on bone marrow transplantation for certain blood conditions has indicated that patients may survive a dose of 1000 rems of total body radiation if given bone marrow transplantation postirradiation to replace damaged blood cell precursors, and intravenous fluids for several days to replace fluid loss from nausea, vomiting, and diarrhea. Radiation doses received acutely in excess of 1200 to 1500 rems to the whole body are associated with death within a week, however. Remember that we have been discussing total body doses. A local radiation dose delivered therapeutically to a tumor will usually be in excess of 4000 rads, but the total body will receive very little (due to scattering or "bouncing" of some of the radiation used for treatment).

NUCLEAR POWER PLANTS

Nuclear reactors serve as giant water heaters, employing the energy released from uranium fission to warm water pumped through the reactor. As of June 30, 1977, 67 nuclear power reactors in the United States were licensed to operate, 89 were being built, and another 76 in the planning state, totaling a potential 232 nuclear power reactors.[3] There is continuing community concern about the safety of these reactors for several reasons. First, a typical nuclear power plant may produce as much as 500 pounds of plutonium per year, but only 20 pounds of plutonium are required to make a bomb of "blockbuster" size. Security measures are believed to be fairly effective in this area. There are serious concerns as well that a nuclear power plant accident may release amounts of radioactive material, much of it in gaseous form, which could expose the neighboring population to an acute radiation syndrome described above, or to later carcinogenic and mutagenic effects. This can only happen if the uranium dioxide fuel melts, at a temperature of over 5000°F. Every nuclear power plant has a safety system, an Emergency Core Cooling System. If a pipe breaks which carries water to the fuel, this system is supposed to provide emergency cooling water within 60 seconds to prevent overheating, melting, and subsequent release of radiation from the massive fuel "core" of the power plant.[3] Is the Emergency Core Cooling System a "fail-safe" system?

The experience at Three Mile Island (TMI) in Pennsylvania in 1979 has stimulated high degrees of concern about the safety of such plants. Congressional investigations are being developed to examine the extent of damage as a result of the Three Mile Island incident, to attempt to determine why the safety measures did not function as designed, and what role human error may have played in the whole event. Even at TMI the greatest whole body dose received by any one person in the neighboring population was about 180 mrem, while the maximum estimated average dose ranged from 10-15 mrem. All nuclear plants—ones being used and those on the drawing boards—are being reevaluated for design and functional safety.

Radioactive nuclear wastes created when nuclear fuel is used up include strontium-90, cesium-137, and plutonium-239. No proven method for long term safe storage or disposal of these radioactive wastes has been developed which is entirely risk free, although burial in earthquake-free areas with no ground water to leach out the material appears to be a reasonable solution. There have been radioactive waste leaks in several parts of the United States, although the amounts of radiation involved are not believed to be hazardous and no radiation injury has resulted.

The dose of radiation received from an accident at such a power plant would be delivered from both external sources (passing cloud, contaminated ground) and as an internal dose received predominantly during the first week after the accident from inhaled radionuclides. The current ability to evacuate American communities rapidly makes actual dose estimates very difficult, because distance from a radiation source and decreased time of exposure to radiation are two major factors which reduce exposure dramatically. However, the chances of a significant melt down occurring at a nuclear power plant are estimated at about once in 20 thousand reactor years (with 200 reactors, once in 100 years) by the massive Reactor Safety Study commissioned by the United States Nuclear Regulatory Commission.

An estimate has been made of the total of all fatal accidents and diseases and major nonfatal conditions resulting within one year in a population of 1 million people deriving 1 kilowatt per person of electrical energy from nuclear power. These estimates suggest that in a year in the population of 1 million this level of power production could lead to about 1 death from malignant disease, 1 case of malignant disease fully curable by operation, 1 fatal and 50 other disabling accidents, and, after some generations of operation, on the order of 1 to 1-1/2 genetic "effects" of greater or lesser severity.[3] The risk of fatal malignancies involved in some forms of industrial exposure to chemical agents which are known carcinogens, including benzene and asbestos, involve up to 10 to 30 deaths per 10,000 workers per year. Very similar estimates of death have been made for a year's production of coal, oil, and gas yielding 1 kilowatt per person for 1 million people. One must include the health hazard to the general population from sulfur dioxide, suspended particulates, polycyclic hydrocarbons, oxides of nitrogen, oxygen, and other secondary products in such calculations. Estimates of mortality to an 80 km. radius from such a power plant are 45 deaths annually from coal, 1.5 from oil, and 0.15 from gas (with 1.0 from nuclear power).[3]

NURSING IMPLICATIONS OF RADIATION EXPOSURES

The community health nurse needs to implement the nursing process in regard to possible radiation exposure within the community and to her clients. The first assessment should be made of the community at large. Radiation therapy within the hospital setting is a familiar activity, but what and where are the sources within this particular community setting? "Normal" background radiation differs within the continental United States; what is the background radiation in this area? Are nuclear power plants part of the community or are there facilities being planned? If so, what types of reactors are being contemplated? What health screening programs are being designed? What about disaster plans? What are the manufacturing industries in the community? Are there sources of radiation exposure within these industries? What percentage of the community work force is employed in these industries? Are both men and women represented in this exposed group? What kind of precautions are taken for these workers? These are important questions for the community health nurse to answer.

Once the nurse has these answers she can begin to plan and implement necessary health screening or education programs. Health care today emphasizes the concept of health promotion and disease prevention. In answering these questions and implementing appropriate nursing interventions, the nurse is dealing with health problems which have long latent periods, that is, the disease itself may not be manifested for 5 to 30 years. Health professionals can cope with infectious diseases which have incubation periods of 6 to 21 days. This is a short time period, and epidemiologic methods are employed to isolate the causative organism, identify exposed and/or susceptible individuals, and initiate immunization or protective programs. The latent period or incubation period for cancer caused by potential carcinogens, such as radiation, may be 5 to 30 years, so that the exposure to the carcinogen may be difficult to trace. Health programs designed to educate the community to potential health problems and assuage unnecessary fears are a major area of health promotion. Such activities might occur at science fairs, school curricula at all levels, museum exhibits, and in professional society projects.

Once the nurse is aware of the broad picture within the community, she can use this knowledge in caring for her particular patients. Some of the patients in the community will have had brachytherapy, that is, special implantations of radium, iodine, or cesium for cancer of the cervix, prostate, or pharyngeal area. These patients will remain in the hospital, closely monitored by a radiation safety officer. The nurse in the hospital will have taken special precautions regarding time with the patient and distance related to patient care. The family will have received special instruction as to the amount of time they can spend with their loved one. Once the implant is removed and the patient returns home, he and his family may need reassurance from the community health nurse that the individual is not radioactive and normal family relations may be resumed.

The nurse practicing in the community must be aware of which of her patients who have received radiation require isolation or special precautions and which ones need no special precautions. The patient who has received diagnostic x-ray or therapeutic external beam therapy (usually from a cobalt-60 unit or linear accelerator) of any sort is not radioactive and carries no traces of radiation. Such external beam diagnostic or therapeutic radiation is dissipated in energy deposited in the patient as soon as these photons interact with tissue. There is no radiation left over, and no hazard exists in these instances. These patients require no special precautions.

Family, coworkers, and friends of patients may need reassurance from you as the health professional that an individual who has received radiotherapy is not radioactive. There are many myths among the lay population as to the dangers of radioactivity. Family and friends may avoid contact with the patient because of these misconceptions. The patient undergoing radiotherapy has a great need for the comfort and support of his family and friends at this time. The community health nurse can facilitate this process by reassuring these groups (after patient consent, since he may wish the disease state or treatment not divulged) that radiation is not a danger.

Patients who have undergone diagnostic nuclear medicine testing similarly provide no radiation hazard for their home or community environment. This is because the amounts of tracer radioactivity administered are so small, and the half lives of the radiopharmaceuticals given (the time for a certain amount of radioactive material to decrease in activity by 50 percent) are so short that such patients do not provide a source of measurable radiation for those around them. Their urinary excretion of such materials contributes virtually nothing to the measurable background of radiation, and no urinary precautions need to be taken. Patients receiving these diagnostic tests are usually upset and fear they have cancer. Support from the immediate family will help them through a very stressful situation. The nurse can facilitate that process by providing the patient and family with the appropriate information.

Individuals who have a toxic nodular goiter or Graves' disease may be treated with radioactive iodine-131 on an outpatient basis. This individual is emitting small quantities of radioactivity. The community health nurse should reinforce the instructions received at the hospital. The patient should sleep in a single bed, ideally have separate bathroom facilities, and the bed clothing and personal garments should be washed separately. After urination, one ounce of a potassium iodide solution (4 gm per liter) should be added to the toilet bowl and allowed to stand for 2 minutes before flushing. This dilutes out any radioiodine which might be splashed about and blocks thyroid uptake of this material. There are no time or distance restrictions placed on visitors. In the case of both men and women, the conception of children should be avoided for 3 months after therapy is completed, but coitus is permitted.

Individual clients will frequently ask the advice of the community health nurse in terms of the appropriateness of a particular therapeutic or diagnostic procedure which involves some form of radiation exposure. It is the professional responsibility of the nurse to be able to answer these questions truthfully and accurately. As a member of the health team the nurse practicing in the community can utilize the informality of the home situation to identify and clarify the concerns which the patient expresses.

SUMMARY

Ionizing radiation is received from cosmic radiation, building materials, internal sources, and medical sources. These low doses may have genetic and/or carcinogenic potential from the energy deposited in cells, but dose-relationships are uncertain and a threshold for such effects may exist. Nuclear power plant risks appear to be less than those from current energy sources. The nurse should function as a source of information and reassurance in her community.

REFERENCES

1. Eisenbud, M.: *Environmental Radioactivity.* Academic Press, 1973.
2. "Natural Background Radiation in the U.S." National Council on Radiation Protection Measurements Report #35, Washington, D.C., November 15, 1975.
3. Pochin, E.E.: *Estimated Population Exposure from Nuclear Power Production and Nuclear Radiation Sources.* Nuclear Energy Agency, Organization for Economic Cooperation and Development, January 1976.
4. Chanlett, E.T.: "Ionizing Radiation and Its Control," in *Environmental Protection.* McGraw-Hill, 1973.
5. Lewis, E.B.: "Possible Genetic Consequences of Irradiation of Tumors in Childhood." *Radiology* 114:147, 1975.
6. Anderson, R.E.: "Longevity in Irradiated Human Population, with Particular Reference to the Atomic Bomb Survivors." *American Journal of Medicine* 55:643, 1973.
7. *The Effects on Populations to Exposure of Low Levels of Ionizing Radiation.* Report of the Advisory Committee on the Biological Effects of Ionizing Radiation. Division of Medical Sciences, National Academy of Sciences and National Research Council, November 1972.
8. Cohen, B.L.: "Impacts of the Nuclear Energy Industry on Human Health and Safety." *American Scientist* 64:550, 1976.

UNIT **VII**
PERSONAL EXPERIENCES IN COMMUNITY HEALTH NURSING ROLES

The chapters included in this unit focus on the sharing of work experiences by nurses functioning in these roles. They are meant to be personal accounts explaining the kinds of nursing care issues encountered and how interventions were provided. Hopefully, they will stimulate thinking on your part to explore a variety of community health nursing roles and to examine various nursing interventions used and their effectiveness.

These chapters represent real nursing experiences and identify real difficulties, problems, and issues which have been encountered and ways to use the nursing process to provide nursing care. Would you do the same thing?

CHAPTER **40**

AMBULATORY CLINICAL ROLE STUDY

MARYROSE CONDON, M.S., R.N.

Two or three babies out of every 1000 live births are born with serious congenital heart disease. Medical advances in recent years have dramatically changed the outlook for babies and children with congenital heart disease. Early detection, improved diagnostic tools, and early surgical intervention have made the field of pediatric cardiology and cardiac surgery an exciting and optimistic one. So much has been achieved in such a relatively short time. However, unless we deal with the infant and/or child as a total person within a particular family structure, we will not be giving our patients the best possible care.

I would like to discuss the role of the nurse within a pediatric cardiac center and what her major contributions might be. The clinical setting in which I function is a large teaching hospital. I am assigned as a nurse practitioner to the pediatric cardiology department. There are five cardiologists and four cardiothoracic surgeons with whom I work. I consider myself the pediatric generalist within a highly specialized group. I see the patients and their families during their regularly scheduled visits and maintain contact with them via telephone between visits.

My role includes interpreting the cardiac diagnosis to the parents, teaching administration of cardiac medications, helping parents deal with the day-to-day care of an infant or young child with a cardiac problem, assessing the child's level of development, preparing the child and/or parents for hospital admission for cardiac catheterization and cardiac surgery, and communicating with the inpatient nursing service regarding the specific patient. I spend considerable time with the parents, evaluating the child's growth and development, his daily activities, and family reactions and interactions. I also evaluate the parents' ability to cope with the cardiac problem, and what effect the cardiac child is having upon the other children and upon the marriage. The presence of a chronically ill child within a family can sometimes have a devastating effect on other members of the family. Early intervention by myself with the help of child guidance and social service is essential and may prevent long term damage to the family.

Once parents are told that their infant or child has a congenital heart defect, many aspects of normal routine care of the child at home become difficult hurdles for parents to overcome. Can I let my baby cry, and if so, how long? Should he have the usual baby shots? What should I do when he gets a cold? Will a cold be bad for his heart? Will he have a heart attack if he coughs too much? Should I let my toddler run around without restrictions? Should he be allowed to participate in sports? These are just a few questions that assail parents. The nurse, working closely with the pediatric cardiologists, has a unique opportunity to teach and guide the parent. Many times she should initiate discussion with the parents about various problems of day-to-day living and not wait for the parents to ask. The nurse should prepare a definite teaching plan which she can use with a number of parents with only slight variations. She should divide her plan into two areas: immediate problems and anticipatory guidance. In the next few paragraphs, I would like to discuss in more detail a few immediate and long term problems.

IMMEDIATE PROBLEMS

Feeding and weight gain

Babies with the more serious forms of congenital heart defects often gain weight at a slower rate. This is probably one of the most upsetting and disturbing problems that mothers must face and accept. They continually compare their baby with either their previous children or with the baby down the street who is the same age and is growing at the usual rate. They need constant encouragement that they are doing a good job. Both the cardiologist and the nurse should spend more time during each visit discussing the baby's weight, emphasizing that the slower rate is to be expected and is satisfactory.

The nurse can give the mother a few specific suggestions which may help. Since feeding is the most work that a baby does, the baby who has less cardiac reserve is going to tire more easily. Therefore the mother may have to feed the baby smaller amounts at more frequent intervals. The night feeding may have to be continued longer until the baby is taking a satisfactory amount at each feeding during the day for his size and weight. The nipple should be soft and fairly free flowing. It might be helpful if the nurse has the mother bring with her to clinic the bottle and nipple that she usually uses. The bottle should never be propped. This should be discussed at the first visit, because there is an increased danger of aspiration with the cardiac baby. Solids may be introduced earlier than usual because some of these babies do better with solids because chewing is less work for them than sucking. Even with these suggestions, feeding the baby with a serious congenital heart defect can be a very time consuming aspect of the baby's care. The nurse must try to keep the mother from becoming too discouraged or upset.

Many times the parent will benefit from discussing this problem with other parents who have gone through similar problems. The nurse can often be the catalyst in initiating this type of discussion with a group of parents. The nurse should also discuss with the parent how she is managing the rest of her household when the baby is taking so much of her time and energy. If possible both of the parents should be present during this discussion. The father may need some encouragement to take over some of the chores; many fathers need to be made aware of the problem before they offer to help. Relatives also can help, but many times the mother needs some urging before she can accept additional help. The use of home health aides often available through the Visiting Nurse Association is another source of temporary help.

Signs of congestive failure

The parents of infants who have large left to right shunts need to be made aware of the possibility of failure, occurring especially in early infancy and/or at times of acute infections. They need to know that this will develop over a period of a few days and that "heart failure" does not mean that the "heart will stop," which is a frequent misconception. We ask the parents to watch for certain specific changes, such as increased respirations of 80 to 100, especially when the baby is asleep, increased sweatiness, increased fatigue or irritability, and tiring more easily during feedings. The parents are told that if several of these symptoms occur, the parent should check with the pediatrician, cardiologist, or nurse, whichever is more easily contacted. If the doctor feels that these symptoms are serious, then he will usually want to check the baby. The mother may be told to watch for another 24 hours and if the symptoms persist, to bring the baby in for a visit. Parents should be reassured that the situation, if it does occur, can be treated successfully with medication. Parents should be told not to start watching the baby constantly. The development of congestive failure is a slow process and the baby will give them clues that he is not feeling well.

Use of digitalis preparation

When the infant or child is started on digitalis (usually the pediatric digoxin preparation, Lanoxin), the parents need to be taught about the medication. They must know and understand all aspects of the medicine just as the nurse does when she gives the medication in the hospital. Digoxin is usually given with a specially calibrated dropper at 12 hour intervals once the child has been digitalized. It should not be added to the baby's formula but put directly into the baby's mouth or diluted with a very small amount of juice or formula. Most children take it without any problem. Because it has a pleasant taste and is a potentially lethal drug, the parent must be cautioned to keep it away from all their children. This is a warning that the nurse should repeat to the parent on subsequent visits. Parents sometimes leave this drug on a kitchen counter so they won't forget to give it. If the baby or child vomits within 30 minutes after giving the digoxin, it is generally best for the parent to repeat half the dose again.

When the digoxin dose is increased, as it usually is as he gains weight, the parent needs to be alert to signs of digoxin toxicity. Vomiting, increased irritability, or increased fatigue are the usual signs that parents can watch for. We do not usually have parents check the apical pulse except in a few cases. If signs of digoxin toxicity do occur, the parent should withhold the next dose and bring the child into the clinic for an electrocardiogram.

ANTICIPATORY GUIDANCE

Physical activities

From the time the young child is able to walk most cardiologist will tell parents that they should allow their child to carry on normal activities. The nurse should go into more specifics as to exactly what is meant by normal activities. Generally most young children with congenital heart defects can be allowed to carry on activities appropriate for their age to their level of tolerance. This is very easy for any member of the cardiac team to suggest, but some parents find it difficult to carry through, especially when the parent sees her cyanotic child get bluer or get more short of breath with fatigue. It must be constantly emphasized to the parent that the young child will stop and rest for a few minutes when he is tired. To impose restrictions on the young child will often cause havoc with the basic parent-child relationship. The child who fights taking naps and cries for an hour is really using as much energy as if he were running around.

The nurse should periodically discuss with the parent the child's typical day to make sure that the toddler's or young child's normal need for activity is not being frustrated or hindered, sometimes unconsciously, by the parent. If the 3 or 4 year old is spending most of the day in front of the T.V. set, this is not normal activity for his age. In discussing this problem with the parent, the nurse should try to discover if the mother is being urged by a grandparent or other relative to keep the child restricted. Sometimes it is necessary to get a grandmother in for a clinic visit to discuss the child's activities and to take some pressure off the mother.

When the child is ready for school, the question of participation in the school's physical education program and competitive sports should be discussed with nurse, cardiologist, and parent. Most of the children can be allowed to participate in the gym programs, again to their level of tolerance. This means specifically that the child should be allowed to drop out of any gym activity if he is tiring without being urged to continue by the teacher. Many times the doctor may ask that he not participate in competitive games or races where he may push himself beyond his limits for the sake of coming in first. The child may continue to join the usual afterschool activities where there is usually less pressure.

There are some cardiac conditions, such as aortic stenosis, that do require some limitations. Many of these children would not be allowed to take full physical education programs, nor would they be allowed to engage in competitive sports, probably throughout their school life. Parents need to know this very early, even before the children start to school. They need time to understand and accept this so that they can help their young school child to accept it. Their attitude and acceptance, especially the father's, will determine how well the child accepts the restriction. Parents need to be able to understand that the child who is being restricted from competitive or organized games can still participate in some physical play.

Preparing the child for hospitalization

The first step in preparing the child for hospitalization is to give him some understanding of why he is being seen by a cardiologist at specific intervals. Even the young child of 3 or 4 years can be taught why he goes to the clinic for a checkup on his heart. When he understands that he has a problem with his heart, we can then build on this knowledge when it comes time for admission to the hospital for catheterization or cardiac surgery.

Once the cardiologist decides that the child should have a catheterization, then the nurse and parent can work together in planning how to prepare the child. If the child is school age, then the nurse can direct her discussion to both parent and child. If the child is younger, then the first discussion, which may be weeks to months before the actual admission, should include only the parent. The catheterization should be explained, both how it is done and why it is being done to their child, the specific hospital routine, length of stay, accommodations, visiting hours (should be unlimited), and what the child should bring with him. The school age child should have an opportunity to ask questions and he should get nothing but absolutely honest answers. If he asks if he is going to have any needles, he should be answered truthfully. Because this may be the child's first experience as an inpatient, absolute honesty cannot be stressed too much. The parent can learn much by listening to the nurse as she explains the procedure to the child. This explanation should be repeated to the child on the day of admission and the child given another opportunity to ask questions. Once admitted the child should have each procedure explained to him before it is done. We usually take the children to see the catheterization laboratory on the preceding day. He then has a chance to meet the technicians and see the setup which looks a little like science fiction.

In preparing the young or preschool child for admission to the hospital, the nurse may have to work more through the parents than directly with the child. The young child may not be told about admission until a few days before the time, but they should not arrive at the hospital that day without having been told that they are going to stay overnight and sleep in a different bed. We encourage one of the parents to plan to stay with the young child during this hospitalization if at all possible. We have a family unit setup available for parent and child. I would say that about 80 percent of the parents of the young children stay with them during hospitalization. This is done even though there may be other children at home. Fathers take their vacation, grandmothers come for visits, or neighbors pitch in and help. The toddler, once he is settled in the room with his mother, can then be prepared step by step without too much difficulty. They will still cry and get very upset when they have blood tests and so forth, but they recover from the upset much faster if their mother is with them. If the mother is to stay, she must be prepared or she may get too upset to comfort her child.

Parents of children with congenital heart defects have many of the problems that parents of a child with any type of chronic health problems have. To help these parents bring up happy, well-adjusted children who will develop into mature, well-adjusted adults takes the combined efforts of the entire health team: pediatrician, cardiologist, nurse, social worker, school nurse, and nutritionist. I have tried to list some of the areas that the nurse can influence.

CHAPTER **41**

OCCUPATIONAL NURSING CLINICAL ROLE STUDY

MARY E. SCANLON, M.Ed., C.O.H.N., R.N.

Health care is currently a national issue in the United States. The American people are demanding premium health care delivery, and the cost of such programs is astronomical. For employees of the Gillette Company in Boston, Massachusetts, premium health care has been available at no cost to the employee for 26 years. Comprehensive occupational health programs are meeting health needs of workers which are not fulfilled by health care systems in the community. The health maintenance organizations of the future may be in an industrial setting.

Dr. William E.R. Greer, the Corporate Medical Director of the Gillette Company, is a pioneer in occupational health. In 1951 he convinced the executives of the Gillette Company that a comprehensive medical program would insure a healthier, more productive work force. The concept of preventive medicine 26 years ago was revolutionary. However, the program of quality health care has grown over the years and is constantly expanding.

I joined this health care team 20 years ago as the Visiting Nurse. My function was to provide continuity of care for the ill or injured employee and to assist in the rehabilitation and return to work of such employees.

My work experience had been in the field of public health with official and voluntary agencies. I had worked for the New York City Health Department, the Brooklyn Visiting Nurse Association, and the Lynn, Massachusetts, Visiting Nurse Association. My orientation to occupational health as practiced at Gillette was as revolutionary as the health program. My first month was spent working in every productive department of the facility. This experience gave me an opportunity to know the employees, the types of jobs, the physical demands of different job classifications, and the physical makeup of the plant. Looking back, I realize production must have hit rock bottom in each department upon my arrival. I can still vividly remember having motion sickness for three days while working on a razor assembly line. I did, however, acquire great respect for the manual dexterity of the workers and invaluable knowledge of job categories. This experience also introduced me to the safety program and the importance of observing safety regulations and performing each work assignment in a safe manner. For example, in certain areas of the blade production departments safety shoes are required. The steel for razor blade production comes in large coils, weighing approximately 30 pounds. In the event that a coil slipped, the employee could suffer fractures or possible amputation of the feet. In many areas safety glasses are mandatory to protect employees in high speed machinery departments. One of the intangible benefits of this experience is getting to know employees as healthy, productive people. This is a decided advantage for occupational health nurses because we have a great basis for comparison when an employee is ill.

After my rotation in the production departments, I was assigned to the medical department. As a member of the health team I learned the routine of the clinic, the responsibilities and duties of the nurses, as well as the philosophy of the medical program. Essentially, that was and still is occupational health as preventive medicine. The goal of the medical program is to maintain employees at optimum health. To achieve this goal the medical department had at that time three registered nurses on the day shift, an afternoon nurse who covered 2:30 p.m. to 11 p.m., a registered x-ray technician, and a registered laboratory technician. The medical staff consisted of four internists, two surgeons, a dermatologist, and an allergist. A complete eye program including examination by an ophthamologist and followup with prescription glasses by an optician was also part of the medical program. Almost any health need of an employee could be met at no cost to the employee, on company time. Over the years the program has continued to grow and expand to meet the needs of the expanding Gillette work force.

At the present time the medical department in the South Boston facility has been enlarged and completely remodeled. This was necessary to satisfy the health needs of a three shift work force of 3800 employees. The total visits to the South Boston clinic for the year of 1979 were 46,309, a figure substantially higher than some of the outpatient departments of hospitals in the Boston area. The medical staff includes three internists, a hematologist, and an endocrinologist who visit daily. Two surgeons come on a rotating basis, as well as an allergist, dermatologist, three ophthamologists, and an optician. A gastroenterologist visits weekly. A complete x-ray department, clinical laboratory, surgical unit, and physiotherapy facility are also included in the South Boston clinic.

I made reference earlier to the advantages of occupational health personnel in knowing employees as normal healthy adults. We also have medical documentation of this status via the medical record. Applicants for employment at Gillette must pass a preplacement physical. The company policy has always been to hire for a particular job rather than establish a rigid set of physical standards. Occupational health personnel in our company are expected to know the job categories and be able to discriminate wisely and fairly whether an applicant is capable of performing in the specific labor skill for which he or she is making application. The preplacement physical includes a detailed medical and occupational history, complete blood profile, urinalysis, electrocardiogram (if 35 years of age or older), chest x-ray, pulmonary function tests, hearing test, and a complete physical examination by a doctor. The occupational history is becoming increasingly significant since some diseases are definitely job related (i.e., asbestosis, mesothelioma, byssinosis).

We offer an annual physical examination which is voluntary and is probably our best key to the door of preventive medicine. This perodic examination is the same as the preplacement exam with an interval health and occupational history and also includes papilloma screening for females and proctoscopic examination for males. This type of a routine physical in the presumably well employee may uncover abnormalities in early stages. More important, it helps to overcome the fear of physical examinations. One of the ways this is accomplished is to have the employee personally choose the physician of his choice. This private patient approach rather than the company doctor image is very important and provides great opportunities to establish the rapport necessary to health maintenance programs and effective living habits. Confidentiality of medical records is assured since no medical record is subject to management or personnel review. Change of job because of medical conditions or stress related job situations is discussed on a physician-nurse-management basis. All of our doctors are on staff at the University Hospital in Boston. One internist is on call 24 hours a day, 7 days a week.

At the present time we have a full-time manager of rehabilitative services at Gillette who is responsible for our alcoholic program. He has the full support of top management but reports only to the corporate medical director. His records are completely confidential, and the company maintains an outside telephone answering service for him to further ensure confidentiality. His success rate is 85 percent, and the rate is measured on one year's sobriety.

The nurses are responsible for the initial assessment when an employee reports to the clinic. There are established protocols for treating respiratory infections, gastrointestinal complaints, strains and bruises, as well as primary first aid. Nurses can order routine x-rays or laboratory tests. Actually, this type of nursing function gives maximum service to the employee and is very helpful in utilizing the physician's time. For example, if an employee falls on his way to work and reports to the clinic with a swollen wrist, it makes good sense for the nurse to have x-rays taken, have the patient soak in cold water, and try to make him as comfortable as possible until the physician arrives. The physician reads the x-ray and can promptly treat the condition. The doctors at Gillette realize that the nurses know the employees on a more personal basis because of more frequent exposure. In my own role as a visiting nurse, I have the secure feeling that I am only a phone call away from expert medical care. If when visiting an employee at home I feel medical help is necessary, I phone the clinic and such assistance is always available. Recently while visting an employee with a fractured tibia, his chief complaint was a sore throat. On examination his throat was inflamed and there were several white patches. His temperature was 101.4°. I telephoned the clinic and gave this report to the internist who follows him medically. The physician contacted the pharmacist of the employee's choice and ordered medication. The employee called in the next day and reported he was afebrile and feeling much better. I believe the team concept of medical care has been completely acceptable to the Gillette working population.

The benefit program at Gillette is excellent. Master Medical Blue Cross/Blue Shield is offered to all employees with the company paying 65 percent of the cost. Life insurance, tuition refund, savings plan, loan program, a subsidized cafeteria, full recreation program, income tax assistance—all are included as benefits. However, the cornerstone of the benefit program is the salary plan. Any permanent employee who is ill or injured receives his full salary as long as he is expected to return to his job. Every employee is covered under this plan whether he is a janitor or a vice-president. We are all aware of the fact that financial anxiety can complicate or delay convalescence. This source of anxiety, as well as threat of job loss, is removed for Gillette employees. Their job is secure. Their paycheck is mailed every week.

I try to see all of our employees when they are hospitalized. The purpose of these visits is primarily to let the employee know the company is interested in him and his progress. I assist in discharge planning with hospital personnel and the families of employees.

Last year I was involved with discharge planning that was extremely difficult for me, primarily because I felt it was wrong. One of our employees had been admitted and a diagnosis of bone cancer had been made. His condition was deemed inoperable. He was treated with radiation and chemotherapy, but the progression of the disease was rapid. He had been born and raised in Italy and had been in the United States for 15 years. He had become a citizen. He had been a Gillette employee for eight years. His hospitalization was prolonged (three months) and during this period I got to know him and his wife intimately. Their marriage had been "arranged." Their relationship was beautiful and an inspiration to all of us. Maria was at the hospital from 10 a.m. to 8 p.m. Tony was a complete bed patient and required intensive, constant nursing care. Maria assisted the floor nurses and learned quickly how to bring comfort to her husband. The time came when it was decided that Tony should be transferred to a level I nursing home, because all treatment for his condition had been stopped. Tony wanted to go home and die and Maria wanted to grant this request. I had visited the home with Maria and she demonstrated how she could make the adjustment to care for a full-time bedpatient. There were three children—14, 12, and 10 years old. Maria prepared breakfast for the children, got them off to school, and then went to the hospital. After school the children went to their maternal grandparents who lived across the street. The children had their evening meal with their grandparents, then went to their own home to do their homework and await the arrival of their mother. This had been a grueling schedule for Maria for three months. The children visited their father on Saturday and Sunday for brief periods. Tony had been the dominant figure in this household. He made all the decisions and had been a strict disciplinarian. He did not like his children seeing him in bed—physically dependent on others and in constant pain. He limited the childrens' visits to him in the hospital. Maria had planned to remove their double bed and install two twin beds. She intended to rent a wheel chair and, with assistance from Tony's brother, let Tony spend part of every day in the sunporch (his favorite room in their home). She felt that with the help of the local visiting nurses and my weekly visits she could cope. I admired her courage and devotion but tried to convince her that her husband required 24 hour nursing care at this point. I felt that physically she could not do this. I also felt that the children and their needs were being overlooked completely. I had so many of my own uncertainties in this regard that I felt I was not being objective. I decided to talk this situation over with one of our staff nurses who had recently lost her husband. He, too, had been terminally ill with cancer and had died at home. He was also of Italian descent. Pat did convince me that Maria was absolutely correct. It was the Italian way. Tony should be allowed to die at home. She assured me that the children could cope with this experience and that Maria would have help from all the family members. On a Friday morning I met with Maria, the physician, the nurse clinician, and the social worker at the hospital. All the details were worked out. Tony was to be discharged and taken home by ambulance the next morning. The physician, a Gillette internist, was as totally involved as I was. He knew the family and had been most supportive to all, especially the three children. He volunteered to make a house call on a weekly basis. That night Tony developed pneumonia. He was critically ill all day Saturday. All of his family were at his bedside when he died Saturday night.

As a followup to this case I visited the home two weeks later. One of my seemingly unrelated nursing duties is making deceased calls. I visit the family and explain insurance benefits, medical coverage, and assist in making application for benefits under Social Security or Veterans Administration. Most deaths of employees are preceded by a period of illness. During this period I have direct contact with the employee and his family. The red tape involved in dying in our society can be frustrating for a family in a grief situation. Having someone they know, myself, to assist at this time can be helpful and supportive. When I made the call to Tony's family, the three children took me to the sunporch and showed me a new recliner chair, complete with a "Welcome Home, Dad" gold ribbon. They had bought this as a surprise for their father. Somehow, I think no one has yet sat in that chair.

All of us in occupational health like to think every visit to the clinic can be an opportunity to do health teaching. On occasion we have scheduled teaching programs done on a one-to-one basis. Recently during a routine physical examination one of our employees was diagnosed a new diabetic. He had no complaints at the time of his annual physical but he had a 4 + sugar in his urine, a blood sugar of 700, and abnormal liver function tests. He had no family history of diabetes. He was admitted to the hospital for workup and regulation. I visited him in the hospital and have yet to see anyone more apprehensive. This was his first hospitalization in his 35 year old life and he was terrified. Routine hospital procedures for diagnostic purposes were a series of frightening experiences for him. I tried to allay some of his fears and visited him three times in his five day stay. He was comfortable with me only because he knew me. The nurse clinician spoke with me on one of these visits and said that he was having great difficulty in learning how to test his urine and would not attempt to learn to give his own insulin. I talked with him about this, and he said he couldn't remember because he had a different nurse every day and each had her own approach. I talked with the Gillette internist involved, and we agreed he could be taught in our clinic. He was discharged from the hospital on Sunday and reported to the Gillette clinic Monday morning at 7 a.m. One nurse was elected to teach him. He tested his own urine and was taught how to administer his insulin. He went to the cafeteria for breakfast and then to his job. He knew if he had any adverse symptoms, his nurse was waiting for him in the clinic. By Friday, the nurse felt he was doing reasonably well, but that his sister (with whom he lived) should also be taught. The sister came in with him on Saturday and the nurse had two students. While teaching these procedures, the nurse included many other aspects of health care in relation to diabetes, such as personal hygiene, foot care, and physical activities. She developed a great relationship with the sister who was bright and quick to learn. The patient now is well controlled and makes only social visits to the clinic and his teacher. He seems to have accepted his condition and is living with it.

I made the point earlier that those of us in occupational health get to know our patients as healthy, productive adults and how advantageous that can be. Early in November one of our third shift employees reported to the clinic complaining of an upper respiratory infection, some chest congestion, and a nonproductive cough. Our charge nurse did the initial assessment. She knew him and was aware of the fact that he worked the third shift so that he could attend day classes at a local college. His temperature was 99.0°—not alarming—his chest sounds negative, but he complained of extreme fatigue. She knew his schedule and how well he handled it, but was concerned with this complaint. She asked him to wait over until 8 a.m. and have a chest x-ray. Two days later he was admitted to the hospital with a diagnosis of tuberculosis. The nurse said at the time and still says, "He just wasn't right, he is never tired." A diagnosis of tuberculosis at Gillette triggers off a series of preventive measures. All of his coworkers in his department were contacted and each had a tuberculin test and/or a chest x-ray. Any employee on the first or second shift who had contact with him was included in this program. The tuberculin tests were ready in 48 hours. If an employee converts from a negative to a positive tuberculin test, he is started on medication (INH and Hexa-betalin). Liver function tests are also done at this time, with a repeat in one month, then every three months while on medication. The medication regimen is for a one year period. Family contacts are referred to their local health departments.

As nurses engaged in occupational health we feel a decided responsibility to keep up with the changes in health care, the involvement of government, and new concepts of preventive medicine. The passage of the Occupational and Safety Health Act by Congress in 1970 opened new areas of responsibility for occupational health teams. Noise conservation, environmental factors within and outside of the plant, industrial hygiene, and long term occupational exposures all have become targets for investigation and control. In January of 1975, the charge nurse and I were given the opportunity to enroll in an Occupational Nurse Practitioner program. The course was the first one of its kind in the United States and was sponsored by the Boston University School of Medicine, the Boston University School of Nursing, and the Massachusetts Department of Labor, Division of Occupational Hygiene. The course was divided into two main components: physical assessment and knowledge of occupational health. Our mornings were spent at the Jewish Memorial Hospital in Roxbury doing physical assessment under the direction of preceptors from the Peter Bent Brigham and University Hospitals. Afternoons were spent at the Boston University School of Medicine. These sessions included lectures on the following: epidemiology, toxicology, physical hazards in the occupational environment, ionizing radiation and principles of protection, industrial dust, accident prevention, human engineering, dermatology, environmental control and the principles of industrial hygiene, alcoholism, drug addiction, the legal aspects of the role of the nurse practitioner, screening programs, mental health in industry, health services in industry, and ethics in the field of occupational health and rehabilitation. The course was demanding but very rewarding to both of us. In June of 1975 we took the national examination for certification in occupational health nursing sponsored by The American Board for Occupational Health Nurses, Inc. In this era of specialization in nursing, our field has offered this examination on a national basis and has done a great deal for nursing by setting standards for national certification in occupational health nursing. It is our goal that in the next decade all nurses in occupational health will meet these requirements. The role of the nurse in occupational health is expanding rapidly. To meet the requirements and perform adequately nurses need specialized training. Conferences with safety engineers and industrial hygienists can be beneficial. Knowledge of the community agencies is most important and must be constantly updated.

I mentioned earlier that each visit to the clinic can be a health teaching experience. We have offered some formal teaching programs to employees. All of our managers and supervisors have taken the Multimedia First Aid Course as outlined by the Red Cross. This course is offered on company time. The course is offered twice a year to all employees on their own time. Recently, we offered the CPR course to our security people on Saturday. Nineteen members of the security force—all shifts—were certified. The plan is to offer this again in the spring. We show the Heimlich manuever film twice a year and also "Breast Self-Examination" produced by the American Cancer Society. We have continuing hypertensive screening programs and weight reduction plans on all three shifts.

For many years we have offered an orientation to occupational health for student nurses in the greater Boston area. The format is the showing of our orientation film which covers the fringe benefit program at Gillette, a tour of the Medical Clinic and an explanation of the duties of the occupational health nurse, a talk by our counselor for alcoholism, a tour of the production facility, and a talk by the manager of the safety program. We have about 18 schools of nursing (diploma as well as collegiate) participating in this program. We also offer a student nurse internship program in which the student comes daily to the clinic for a period of five to seven weeks. Contracts with the schools of nursing have been worked out which limit the student's involvement and responsibilities but are liberal enough to give him or her good experience in this specialized field.

The cardiac program at Gillette has served as a model for concerned occupational physicians. Any Gillette employee who suffers a myocardial infarction must be out of work three months. This period is still enforced at Gillette, even though the trend in this area is to return employees after an eight week period. Prior to the employee's return, an electrocardiogram, chest x-ray, and blood test (if on anticoagulants) are done at the Gillette clinic. We do not do stress test or exercise test as a routine—only in specific cases as ordered by our physician. The employee is examined by one of the Gillette internists. If all the physical and laboratory findings are negative, the internist evaluates the employee's job. All occupational health personnel at Gillette are expected to be aware of the physical and emotional demands of job categories. If a medical transfer is indicated there is no salary regression. The employee receives his same rate of pay, even though it may be a lower grade job. Since Gillette is considered a light, highly automated industry, very few medical transfers are indicated. The cardiac employee returns to work on a four hour basis, and the employee choses the hours most convenient to him. If rush hour commuting will be a problem, the employee may elect to work 10 a.m. to 2 p.m. Any third shift employee is transferred temporarily to the first shift during this work-rehab period. The employee is seen weekly in the medical clinic. His physical and psychological adjustments to his work assignment are evaluated carefully. Gradually his work day is increased until the full eight hour work day is attained. May I point out again how important our salary plan is in the success of this plan. Two important sources of anxiety—economic and job security—are removed for Gillette employees. Our program works. Our cardiac patients return to full-time employment to the same job held prior to a catastrophic illness. At the present writing we have 66 employees who have incurred myocardial infarction in our work force in South Boston. All are productive people who have coped with a major illness and have returned to their regular jobs. In my own role I feel very close to these employees and their families. I visit them briefly every other day when they are in the cardio-care unit. The interest and concern showed by the company in this out-of-plant followup is greatly appreciated by the employee and his family. Discharge planning is very important with these employees, as well as periodic visits to their home after discharge from the hospital. In these cases contact with me as a fellow worker has a positive influence. The goal of return to work is emphasized during the enforced inactivity during early convalescence. Each step of increased activity is a step toward return to work. Our cardiac patients are special people to all our medical staff. We encourage them to use the clinic for any kind of problem. Our overall impression is that our cardiac patients feel more secure at work than at home. In addition, these individuals have an excellent record of longevity and productivity.

The opportunity for professional growth is always rewarding to nurses in all fields. Part of our job satisfaction is self-motivation to improve patient care. Occupational health offers great growth potential. Nurses are required to provide primary care, monitoring of chronic disease, family counseling, knowledge of community resources, laboratory procedures, occupational diseases as well as injuries, rehabilitation, and the effects of social change. Indeed, health workers in industry are effecting social change. The health maintenance approach is a method to reduce medical costs by preventive measures and early detection of disease processes. Cooperation and communication with other health agencies in the community may prove to be part of the answer to spiraling health care costs. We in the occupational health setting are anxious to function optimally in our industrial environment, to be aware of the social problems in the community, and to participate in their solutions.

BIBLIOGRAPHY

Aquilera, Donna C., Messick, Janice III, and Farrell, Marlene S.: *Crisis Intervention: Theory and Methodology.* C.V. Mosby Company, St. Louis, 1970.

Bridges, Helen M.: "A Survey Report on the Expanding Role of the Industrial Nurse." *Occupational Health Nursing* pp. 22-26, Oct. 1976.

Miller, Frances H.: "The Right of the Employee as a Patient." *Occupational Health Nursing* 25 (12): 11-13, Dec. 1977.

Onyett, Helen P.: *Role of the Occupational Health Nurse.* U.S. Dept. of Health, Education and Welfare, Occupational Safety & Health Symposium, Center for Disease Control, Cincinnati, Ohio, 1976.

Serafini, B.: "Nursing Assessment in Industry." *American Journal of Nursing* 66:755, Aug. 1976.

Snyder, T.: "The Fringe Benefit Factor: An End to Business as Usual." *Modern Medicine* 45:17, 1977.

CHAPTER 42

SCHOOL NURSE PRACTITIONER

LEANNE P. HALFMAN, M.S., S.N.P., R.N.

In 1972 and after eight years of functioning within the policies of the Gary, Indiana Public School Corporation and laws of the State of Indiana as a traditional school nurse, I was becoming frustrated. I personally did not feel sufficiently adequate assessing children's health needs with a thermometer, flashlight, and present nursing knowledge and practices. The Gary school nurses routinely screened children at various grade levels for tuberculosis, visual acuity problems, and for sick child or first aid emergency intervention, but the majority of time was spent on clerical duties.

I wanted to learn complete assessment skills of children, become proficient administering and interpreting tests and measurements to children, understand norms of growth and development, and become more effective in communicating children's health needs to parents, teachers, and others and in determining how we could work together to meet identified needs.

The University of Colorado School Nurse Practitioner (S.N.P.) continuing education program in Denver and the expanded skills one would acquire seemed like the professional key to augment my expertise, understanding, and effectiveness in working with school aged children's health needs.

During the school year 1971-1972, the Gary Public School Board of Trustees became aware and convinced of the need for additional nursing services to the school population and began endorsing and supporting educational leaves for school nurses. During that academic year, full salaries were paid to the three school nurses who had applied to and were accepted at the University of Colorado 16 week S.N.P. course Phase I.

In August 1972, one other school nurse and myself were also paid full salaries and granted leaves to attend the S.N.P. program and upon our return to Gary, Indiana in January 1973, we began Phase II, which was eight months long, for our on-the-job internship with part-time work with a local pediatrician as our medical preceptor.

As of 1978, the Gary Schools have granted full salary and University of Colorado S.N.P. program study leaves to nine school nurses. Since 1976, there have been study leaves without salary reimbursement to three other staff school nurses who attended the Indiana University Family Nurse Practitioner program in Gary, Indiana.

EDUCATIONAL/CLINICAL PREPARATION

My basic nursing educational preparation was a Bachelor of Science Degree in Nursing from Indiana University School of Nursing in 1962 and a Master of Science Degree in Health and Safety Education from Indiana University in 1967. Following completion of the S.N.P. program and a course on psych-educational approaches for the emotionally disturbed child, I took post-graduate courses at Purdue University about learning disabilities.

From December 1976 to summer 1978, I have had the title of School Nurse Practitioner Coordinator of the Gary Community School Corporation Elementary School District III. I have helped coordinate health services in 13 elementary schools with an enrollment of approximately 8000 students. I have been a member of an interdisciplinary evaluation team, Basic Skills Support Team (B.S.S.T.) which does in-depth studies for District III students who are exhibiting learning, health, emotional, behavioral, or family dynamics problems. We evaluate approximately 350 new cases each year.

The S.N.P. comprehensive health assessment of these children includes a pediatric history taken from the parent, a physical examination, neurologic examination, and behavioral and developmental testing of the children referred.

In addition we are implementing an early identification program in the preschool aged group. We have done this to help identify and remediate as early as possible high risk learning problem students. Our school corporation is requiring the passing of a proficiency-competency tests in mathematics, language, and oral reading skills before students are awarded a high school diploma, thus the earlier intervention approaches by the B.S.S.T. concept hopefully will help the high risk learner.

Between September 1976 and December 1976 I functioned in the same job role as stated above, but was not given an administrative title and was considered a staff S.N.P. for District III. For the school year 1975-1976, I took a leave from the Gary Schools in order to gain collegiate teaching experience and sharpen my adult assessment skills by working at Purdue University Calumet Campus, Hammond, Indiana, Department of Nursing. I taught both theory and clinical aspects of physical assessment skills of children and adults to junior year baccalaureate nursing students.

From January 1973 to June 1975 I functioned as an S.N.P. in two elementary schools with 1600 students and then served as a resource person to 28 other elementary schools for children needing S.N.P. evaluations.

During 1962 through 1972 I had experiences as a staff school nurse, sickle-cell detection program and genetic counseling nurse, staff pediatric hospital nurse, Head Start program nurse, public health nurse, visiting nurse, parochial school nurse, and doctor's office nurse.

HEALTH ISSUE IDENTIFIED

When most lay persons as well as health professionals think of the traditional school nurse role, it is only in a first aid provider role. Even within personnel ranks of most public and private school systems, no one fully understands the role, functions, and responsibilities of the school nurse. This lack of understanding is due in part to the nurse being a health-oriented professional rather than an educator who has the primary task of imparting knowledge to children. We as a society assume that most children enjoy "good health" and that their parents take the responsibility of teaching good health behaviors by having routine annual physical examinations and following through with doctor's recommendations and orders. If nothing is abnormal in the child's health record when he enters school, he is probably able to enter into the learning process of our educational system. Health is often the least important factor considered in the educator's busy day when curriculum guides and recommendations for other learning experiences will possibly be shortchanged due to time.

Because of the educator's lack of understanding of the services a school nurse can provide, many school nurses are responsible for providing health services to pupil enrollment numbers varying between 125 to 4500 students. The larger the number of students the nurse must work with, the more limited her scope of nursing skills demonstrated and delivered to the students, parents, school personnel, and community. Without clerical assistance, the traditional school nurse often becomes an underutilized health professional who is primarily a record keeper.

Depending on nurse to student ratios, the health delivery services a school nurse can provide are the following: visual acuity screening; color blindness screening; hearing acuity screening; height and weight measurements which are plotted on the child's own growth chart; scoliosis and posture screening; blood pressure measurements; dental health screening; dip-stick urinalysis screening; immunization and tuberculosis skin test programs; gross fungal and parasite screening; first aid for emergencies; and sick child walk-in evaluations. Some of the other services the school nurse can provide are monitor and dispense students' chemotherapy at school when ordered by their physician; health education programs; provide health education resources to other school personnel; parent interviews and counseling; referrals to private and public health agencies within the community; continue to follow through on recommendations of children's unmet health needs; and maintain a cumulative health record for each child.

One recent major breakthrough in school children's unmet health needs has been the national immunization program. Educators have become aware of the lack of parent involvement in completing their children's basic immunization status and providing that proof to school personnel in order to comply with many of the state laws that now require complete immunization series for the children to remain in schools. School nurses across the nation are having to spend almost all of their time getting parents to comply with the requirements for their children's immunizations. This is but one area of health, yet it has been proven that children's families are not sharing the responsibility, nor are they as aware of their children's health needs as they should be.

NEED FOR SERVICE IN COMMUNITY

During the 1960s, no medical doctor or dentist was employed by the Gary schools to examine children and then provide treatment for problems found. In the mid-60s medical and dental consultant services were also eliminated. The 33 school nurses were, more often than not, unable to provide the necessary health assessments and management of health problems common to the 45,000 students of which 27 percent were medically indigent.

Gary, Indiana is an industrial community that once was called a "melting pot" of persons from almost every ethnic and cultural background. It still is a "blue-collar worker" community but it has experienced many population changes with much of the white community moving from the inner city to the suburbs during recent years.

The present school population numbers approximately 34,000 students of which three-fourths are black and about 26 percent qualify for reduced price school lunches. This reduction in school student population has also caused a reduction in the number of school nurses as attrition occurs.

Since 1970, when the city's population was 170,000, many of the medical and dental health care providers also relocated in the suburbs, thus limiting the professional health services available to the community. There are presently 72 physicians and 24 dentists within the city limits. The newly created Medical Center of Gary, Inc., has been able to recruit 11 new health care providers to the community in the last 18 months. This brings the pediatric specialists number to 4. A trend that became widespread in the 1970s was that many of the health care providers would not accept medically indigent patients in Gary.

At present the two hospitals, the city board of health, and the new Medical Center of Gary are developing more outpatient clinics to serve the previously unmet health needs of the community. The Gary Board of Health is proposing to implement National Health Service Corps physician provider services. These new plans are slowly turning around the decreasing number of professionals and the services provided to the citizens of Gary.

OBJECTIVES OF THE PROGRAM

The Gary Public School Board of Trustees endorsed short term school nurse practitioner preparation for the school nurses. This education would enhance the nurses' health assessment and management skills for the same type of clients they were already serving. The cost of the educational leaves for the school nurses was offset by the new services provided by the S.N.P.s and the changes in the utilization of the expanded skills.

As the various S.N.P.s returned to their preeducational leave assignment and re-oriented themselves and coworkers to their new role and the services they could provide, planning changes were necessary. It was found that students needed the S.N.P. services city wide rather than in a few schools. The creation of a reliable and necessary S.N.P. referral system was needed. S.N.P.s needed to be relieved of the traditional school nurse responsibilities to have sufficient time for comprehensive health assessments and follow through of the recommendations and plans for each child.

More importantly, though, was the fact that the S.N.P.s' augmented skills brought additional services not previously perceived or utilized in the school's educational program. The S.N.P. was to become an integral part of the "Basic Skills Competency Program."

The Gary Public Schools adopted a policy in 1974 requiring competency in basic written language, basic oral language, and basic mathematical computational skills at the second, fifth, ninth, and eleventh grade levels in order to earn a high school diploma. This policy was instituted due to the increasing number of students leaving the Gary schools without having sufficient skills to read, speak, or compute mathematics at a sixth grade level. Beginning with the graduating class of 1977, the high school diploma represented competency and proficiency of skills rather than just a certificate of attendance.

When a profile was gathered from all of the cumulative records, test scores, social worker files, health records, and teacher's comments for the seniors between 1974 and 1977 who were unable to pass the proficiency levels, it was found that they had been known to school personnel for many years. These students had faced from time to time many known and documented environmental, health, and socioeconomic obstacles that were not being monitored. There were no coordinated and long term intervention services implemented to help these proficiency test failures succeed in school.

Since several S.N.P.s were already trained and functioning in their schools but were not being utilized city wide nor where the greatest educational needs were being identified, it was decided to include them in the "Basic Skills Competency Program." In 1976, multidisciplinary "Basic Skills Support Teams" (B.S.S.T.) were created on the elementary school level to deal with early identification of high risk learning students and preschoolers entering kindergarten.

Each elementary B.S.S.T. consists of three permanent members: a school nurse practitioner, a psychologist, and an educational specialist with a background in learning disabilities. Due to the fact that it was impossible to address the entire school population, it was decided to begin evaluating kindergarten and first grade students with various developmental screening tools and the teacher's recorded observations.

Gathering pertinent materials for each case to be evaluated by the team is the responsibility of the school resource teacher, principal, classroom teacher, social worker, school nurse, speech therapist, and any other staff member who has valuable information to present. When the B.S.S.T. evaluates the cases with the individual school team members' data base materials, recommendations and educational prescriptions for the teachers and various team members are made. In addition, appropriate referrals both within the school system and to other community service agencies or private professional resources are made.

Scheduled initial evaluation and followup conferences are made for each of the 28 elementary schools so the B.S.S.T. can discuss the weaknesses and strengths as well as problems that the children are incurring at this early point of their education. The objective of the team approach is to help alleviate, remediate, and monitor factors that are obstacles to learning for 10 percent of kindergarten students and 10 percent of the first grade students identified as high risk learners.

Records of each case are kept in the child's cumulative record at the school as well as at the B.S.S.T. central office. After the initial evaluation, it is the support team's responsibility to follow up all of the recommendations.

When there are recommendations for the S.N.P. to see the child, her evaluation includes: review of materials presented at the evaluation including all group and individual test results, review of kindergarten registration information, review of the cumulative record, a conference with the classroom teachers and any special teachers, classroom observation of the child, conference with the parent(s) to obtain an up-to-date pediatric and social health history, physical and neurologic examination of the child with the parent present if possible, an S.N.P. impression or diagnosis, recommendations and plans for remediation of health and relevant educational problems, and a parent conference to explain the findings and recommendations to gain their support to follow through on the recommendations.

As the high risk learners progress through the various grade levels, followup evaluations, conferences, progress reports and special services support personnel intervention reports, and up-to-date curriculum prescriptions are suggested to help avoid school failure and hopefully promote success in school.

During the academic year 1978-1979, middle school and senior high school level Basic Skills Support Teams were created to address the high risk learners who have failed the competency examination.

CLINICAL PRACTICE SETTING

The clinical practice facilities of the S.N.P.s are the health services offices of the traditional school nurses based at each of the 41 Gary Schools. Because the S.N.P.s have more than one school to service, they each carry their own equipment consisting of stethoscope, sphygmomanometer, otoscope, ophthalmoscope, tuning fork, reflex hammer, charts and records, developmental tests, forms, manuals, kits, and other necessary assessment items.

Each of the B.S.S.T. S.N.P.s has an office at the elementary, middle, or senior high school level district offices she is assigned. There is a B.S.S.T. supervisor who coordinates the evaluation schedules, the district office central files, the evaluation report distributions, the statistical analysis of the evaluation findings, and helps to promote an understanding of the B.S.S.T. procedures and objectives.

ADMINISTRATIVE/AGENCY SUPPORT

One of the Gary community medical surgeons was on the School Board during 1970-1972 and it was his insight about the School Nurse Practitioner concept and program in Denver, Colorado that brought the Gary Schools to consider benefits school children could derive from such a project. Two pediatricians were included in the early planning stages and they visited the S.N.P. program in 1971 before any of the Gary school nurses attended the course. The University of Colorado program insisted that there be agency support for the S.N.P.s upon their return to their work setting. This required support became the bridge which brought the medical and educational community together.

As the various S.N.P. functions and roles were established and determined by the S.N.P.s and education administrators, the two pediatricians and surgeon provided consultation services for the direction of the S.N.P. role. These physicians served as medical preceptors without remuneration and approved standing orders for some common childhood problem management protocols the S.N.P.s use.

The impact realized by the utilization of S.N.P.s was not just a role model for Gary, Indiana. Several inquiries for more information about the Gary S.N.P.s from other local, state, and national nursing groups as well as authors of books on innovative primary health care delivery programs have been requested. Every effort has been made to cooperate with inquiries by allowing each of the S.N.P.s to speak at meetings or make presentations that explain the expanded nursing skills and services the Gary S.N.P.s now provide.

Membership in nurse practitioner organizations and active participation and attendance in nurse practitioner continuing education conferences are encouraged. The school superintendent keeps a continuing relationship with the University of Colorado S.N.P. program directors for short and long term planning.

FINANCIAL SUPPORT

The financial expenditures for S.N.P.s have not increased the budget of the health services department. The S.N.P.s were not paid any differently than traditional school nurses until the positions for the B.S.S.T. were created. The B.S.S.T. members are paid on the administrative salary schedule rather than on the teacher's salary schedule.

The school health services department budget remains constant at 1 percent of the total school budget per year. The cost of health services provided to the Gary school population is about $10.00 per child per year.

The administrative salaries for the B.S.S.T. nurse practitoners is offset by the fact that as attrition occurs, there is no need to hire additional nursing personnel due to declining pupil enrollments.

NURSING INTERVENTIONS IMPLEMENTED

The S.N.P.s were confronted with the fact that as they returned to the Gary school system with an expanded role and new services to provide, they were assigned to their preeducation leave schools. Already the traditional school nurse's role was not utilized to its fullest due to responsibility for so many students' health screenings and record keeping. Each S.N.P. was assigned a full-time health aide who was to assist her with much of the routine work and thus relieve the S.N.P. to do more in-depth comprehensive examinations.

The hiring of health aides worked well, but the S.N.P. was involved in training the health aide and was still not able to meet health needs of the high risk student population since multidisciplinary evaluation teams were not functioning city wide.

The relationship of the S.N.P. expanded role and services to improved student learning had to be shown before S.N.P. acceptance and greater utilization occurred. This proving period took exactly four years after the first S.N.P. graduates returned to Gary and the B.S.S.T. with an S.N.P. as a key member was developed.

The B.S.S.T. approach is an effective means of identifying children who are high risk learners and who show need for the S.N.P. evaluation and the necessary followup of plans, recommendations, and reevaluations each succeeding year. This new intervention also allows the S.N.P. to travel to all of the schools and provide each individual school access to her services.

Other nursing interventions which have been implemented since the return of the S.N.P.s to Gary in 1971 have been a city wide sickle cell anemia and trait detection and genetic counseling program, scoliosis and postural screening programs, hypertension screening programs, adolescent nutritional obesity programs, planned parenthood educational programs for adolescents, prenatal care educational programs for adolescent females, and the adoption of a city wide family life education curriculum coordinated by an S.N.P.

The S.N.P.s also helped develop limited size physical education classes for children identified as needing perceptual motor remediation in elementary schools, physical examinations of Head Start program students by S.N.P.s, administer Denver Developmental Screening Tests to prekindergarten students, further examination and testing of developmentally lagging prekindergarteners as early as possible, physical examinations for special education students participating in annual "Special Olympics" contests, physical examinations for participants in city wide elementary track meets, inservice programs presented by S.N.P.s for traditional school nurses, role model educational programs by S.N.P.s for local area general nursing and nurse practitioner students, and articles published in local newspapers about the S.N.P. role and services.

The S.N.P.s had to develop new record keeping forms for the various assessments of the children they served. Many changes and revisions were made when necessary to reduce the number of xeroxed copies for each child's comprehensive assessment. When a child is evaluated for the B.S.S.T. by the S.N.P., it was found that copies of this communication enhance followup if the S.N.P. file, the child's school health record, the child's cumulative record, the B.S.S.T. central file, and significant others all have copies of the evaluation.

At the end of this chapter are samples of record keeping forms which are used at present. These forms are used with permission.

PROBLEMS ENCOUNTERED

Some of the problems encountered with the S.N.P. role were that there was lack of understanding of the S.N.P. role by the traditional school nurses, lack of understanding by school personnel of the S.N.P. role at all of the elementary schools when the B.S.S.T. would evaluate the children, lack of understanding by school personnel of the B.S.S.T. procedures and objectives, and lack of a plan for record keeping and followup of recommendations, plans, and curriculum prescriptions from the B.S.S.T. evaluations. It was also found that of the high risk learner students who were evaluated, about 33 percent have changes in residence each year and record keeping and a continuum of B.S.S.T. services become interrupted. Furthermore, the S.N.P.s are unable to see all of the children referred to the B.S.S.T. each year, there is a lack of understanding of S.N.P. skills and services by parents of the high-risk learner students, and there is a lack of cooperation or compliance with the S.N.P. recommendations and referrals to various private and community agencies by parents of the high risk learner students.

The local community physicians and dentists did not have a good understanding about the B.S.S.T. objectives and its relationship to attempting to help the academic achievement potential of high risk learning students, and a large number of the community physicians and dentists were not accepting medically indigent or medicaid recipients as patients. Continuing education resources within the community for S.N.P.s were nonexistent except for the medical preceptor relationship that continued without payment for the preceptor.

HOW PROBLEMS WERE RESOLVED

These problems have been a challenge and many of them still exist, but to a lesser degree. There have been consistent planning sessions, linkage strategies, and various approaches and techniques implemented to eliminate or avoid problems as they became apparent.

We have increased the understanding of the S.N.P. skills and services by the traditional school nurses by assigning the B.S.S.T. services to evaluate children in all of the city schools. Since the creation of the B.S.S.T., most school personnel have had an opportunity to become familiar with the S.N.P. services since the assessments are done in each child's own school. S.N.P. findings and recommendations are explained to the parent, child, teacher, and significant others so they will understand the child's problem, how she determined the findings, and why the necessary recommendations were made.

The B.S.S.T. procedures and objectives are much clearer to all who participate through the utilization of resource teachers and because a Coordinator of Special Services was implemented to promote an understanding about the B.S.S.T. The coordinator also schedules evaluations, maintains district office central files, gathers evaluation information, and prepares statistical analysis of all of the various team members' findings.

Because so much preparation of information before evaluations can occur and so many children change residences each year, the school resource teachers were assigned to coordinate the records, follow through on all recommendations, and help teachers with curriculum prescription needs for each child evaluated. It is the resource teacher's responsibility to keep the Coordinator of Special Services apprised of all followup progress, problems, and the actual transferring of records if the child moves to another school.

Since the S.N.P. cannot see all of the children who are evaluated, the traditional school nurse is becoming more involved in working with the high risk students and the S.N.P. sees only the priority cases.

Parents are becoming more aware and knowledgeable about the S.N.P. role when they are present for the assessment of their child and receive a personal explanation and demonstration of their child's deviations from normal and guidance in remedying the condition.

There is continual followup by the S.N.P. and school nurses with parents of children evaluated who have unattended or unresolved problems. Each succeeding year, the children who were evaluated earlier are discussed and seen again if necessary to monitor their progress and present status.

All of the local physicians and dentists have received letters of explanation of the B.S.S.T. purpose, objectives, S.N.P. skills and services available, and the various special education programs and the services the schools provide.

Many of the local professional agencies are accepting S.N.P. referrals as a basis of actual health need for the medically indigent or medicaid recipients. The Medical Center of Gary, Inc., has promoted and actually secured many new physicians and dentists to the community for service in the newly created outpatient health care delivery clinics that accept patients regardless of their ability to pay for services rendered. Drawing board plans are being looked at to create school based medical clinics in collaboration with the city board of health if they are successful in securing National Health Service Corps physicians.

The school board and administrators have been approving of most requests for the S.N.P.s to attend conferences, seminars, workshops, and programs that will provide continuing education. Educational leaves for graduate course work and other practitioner experiences and medical preceptor learning experiences have been granted. Most requests for S.N.P. presentations to the Gary staff school nurses and other interested nursing groups and schools of nursing have been addressed.

IMPACT OF THE ROLE

The impact of the S.N.P. skills and services is now reaching all of the Gary school students. Through the B.S.S.T. findings, it has been shown that one-third of the children assessed are found to have health problems which interfere with their learning. In order to remediate learning problems, we must consider health as an integral part of the child's learning potential.

In the past, as children entered kindergarten, few attempts were made to monitor the progress or provide educational plans for the child who had significant pediatric health histories and problems. We are now looking at children who present with histories that might include: maternal-prenatal complications, labor or delivery complications, congenital or inherited defects, inherited mental ability deficiencies, delayed developmental milestones, acquired health problems, environmental and family unit problems, mental depression or other mental health problems, unresolved or unidentified chronic health problems, or nutritional problems.

The task we have undertaken is to remediate the child's health or learning problems as soon as possible and to adjust the child's educational program to meet his or her needs.

RECOMMENDATIONS

The Gary, Indiana schools are convinced of the value of the School Nurse Practitioners as well as Family Nurse Practitioners for improving school aged children's health. It would be ideal if all school nurses had these expanded skills, but presently this is not foreseen.

My recommendations for improved school health care and services delivery are that: each child have an individual computerized school health record which he or she helps to maintain from the fifth grade until he or she graduates from high school, computerize all of the B.S.S.T. records, prepare statistical analysis of health services information annually, and plan the school health services program from the yearly analysis.

We should strive to have more school nurses prepared as nurse practitioners. Those nurse practitioners should be required to successfully complete "entry to practice" national nurse practitioner certifying examinations and the proposed subsequent recertifying examinations.

Hopefully the plans for school based health clinics serviced by S.N.P.s and the proposed city board of health National Health Service Corps physicians and possibly dentists will come to fruition.

Audiovisual materials in the form of slides or filmstrips should be prepared about the B.S.S.T. and the S.N.P. role as a part of the Basic Skills Competency Program.

Traditional school nurses should be provided inservice and extracurricular workshops on assessing children. Implementation of the family life education program as well as a kindergarten through grade 12 sequential health education program would improve the school population's understanding of health.

I think a one-half time position should be created for the investigation and planning of programs or proposals for grant funding, investigation of state or federal funding reimbursement through "Early and Periodic Diagnosis and Screening Tests" programs for the nurse practitioner health assessments to medicaid recipients as some school corporations are presently doing, and investigation of funding reimbursement through the new Public Laws regarding Rural Health Services Act or Public Health Services Act for S.N.P. services rendered or the role model demonstration projects they now provide.

CONCLUSION

The school nurse practitioner role has been a rewarding and dynamic change agent to the health services rendered to the Gary public school children. Even though the role is in the early and pioneering stages, I know it has changed my personal professional nursing career and I believe it has been worth all the additional effort. Without support from the local school administration and community health agencies, the Gary school health program would not have enjoyed these benchmarks. School aged children are going to be tomorrow's adults and we must address the influential role that health and being an informed health consumer plays in molding these individuals to their optimal potential.

GARY COMMUNITY SCHOOL CORPORATION

From: Dr. Frank Wade
        Director Special Services

Subject: Authorization Permit for School Nurse Practitioner Services

Child's Name _____ B.D. _____
Address _____Telephone _____
School_____

I, _____ parent or guardian of
        (Parent's Name)
_____ give my permission
        (Student's Name)
to the Gary Community School Nurse Practitioner
to do a developmental assessment and physical examination on my child
in accordance with our Special Services Division. I understand that I
will be notified of any significant findings.

Date_____Signature _____
                              Parent or Guardian

GARY COMMUNITY SCHOOL CORPORATION
HEALTH SERVICES
KINDERGARTEN AND ELEMENTARY PUPIL ENROLLMENT FORM

This form is confidential and your response will be shared only with school personnel. Please fill out the form IN FULL. Ask the school nurse if you have any questions about your child's health status.

Registration Date_____ Entry Date_____

School_____ Grade_____ Class_____

I. GENERAL INFORMATION:

Child's Name_____ Sex: M____ F____ Birthdate:_____
                Last   First   Middle

Address_____ Telephone_____

PERSONS LIVING IN GARY TO NOTIFY IN CASE OF AN EMERGENCY OTHER THAN HOME PHONE:

1st Choice: Name_____ Phone_____
               Address_____ Relationship to child_____

2nd Choice: Name_____ Phone_____
               Address_____ Relationship to child_____

Child's Doctor's Name:_____ Address_____ Phone_____
Family Doctor's Name _____ Address_____ Phone_____

Father's Name_____ Age_____ Work Hours_____
Occupation:_____ Where employed_____ Phone_____

Mother's Name_____ Age_____ Work Hours_____
Occupation_____ Where employed_____ Phone_____

Who does child live with?_____ Relationship:_____

Number of brothers_____ Number of sisters_____

II. FAMILY HEALTH HISTORY:

                                            (Circle One)

Is father in good health?   Yes   No
  If no, explain_____
Is mother in good health?   Yes   No
  If no, explain_____

IF A MEMBER OF YOUR IMMEDIATE FAMILY HAS A HEALTH PROBLEM, CHECK AND IDENTIFY THE MEMBER BY THEIR RELATIONSHIP TO THE CHILD.

Asthma_____	Kidney problems_____
Alcoholism _____	Mental illness_____
Allergies_____	Mental retardation_____
Anemia _____	Overweight_____
Breathing problems_____	Parkinson's Disease_____
Cancer_____	Seizures_____
Cerebral Palsy_____	Sickle cell disease_____
Convulsions_____	Sickle cell trait_____
Diabetes_____	Skin problems_____
Epilepsy_____	Speech problems_____
Hearing loss_____	Thyroid problems_____
Heart problems_____	Tuberculosis_____
High blood pressure_____	Vision problems_____
Hyperactivity_____	OTHER_____

III. MOTHER'S PREGNANCY AND BIRTH HISTORY WITH THIS CHILD:

How many months pregnant were you before seeing a doctor?_____

What doctor cared for you during your pregnancy?_____

A. PREGNANCY PROBLEMS THAT YOU HAD WITH THIS CHILD: (PLEASE CHECK)

____ABO incompatibility	____Kidney problems
____Accidents	____Malnutrition
____Anemia	____Medications
____Bleeding or spotting	____Rh Factor
____Diabetes	____Swelling
____Excessive vomiting & weight loss	____Syphilis or gonorrhea
____German measles (Rubella or 3 day)	____Toxemia or pre-eclampsia
____Heart problems	____Toxoplasmosis
____High blood pressure	____Trauma
____Hospitalization during pregnancy	____Weight gain of more than 35 lbs.
____Illnesses	____ X-rays
____Infections	____Other_____

B. LABOR AND DELIVERY PROBLEMS THAT YOU MIGHT HAVE HAD WITH THIS CHILD: (PLEASE CHECK)

____Abnormal bleeding	____Number of months pregnant at delivery
____Blood transfusion	____Delivery outside of hospital
____Breech birth	____Long labor -- No. hours_____
____Caesarean delivery	____Short labor -- No. hours_____
____Forceps delivery	____OTHER_____

C. CONDITION AND PROBLEMS OF BABY WHILE IN THE HOSPITAL (PLEASE CHECK)

Birthweight: Lbs_____ Oz._____

____ABO incompatibility	____Jaundice (yellow color)
____Birth defects/birth injuries	____PKU test results positive
____Blood clot on head	____Rh Factor
____Cyanosis (blue color)	____Thyroid problem
____Difficulty breathing	____Surgery - Explain_____
____Incubator -- How long?_____	____Stayed in hospital more than 3-5 days
	If yes, how long?_____
	____Twin birth or multiple birth?_____
	____First or second delivered?_____

IV. CHILD'S EATING HISTORY:

	Please	Circle
Did you bottle feed your baby?	Yes	No
Did you breast feed your baby?	Yes	No
Did your baby have any unusual feeding problems during the first 3 months of life (excessive spitting up, colic, food allergies, or milk allergies)?	No	Yes
If yes, please explain_____		
Is your child's appetite usually good?	Yes	No
Are your child's eating habits regular now?	Yes	No
Does your child eat paste,cornstarch, dirt, paint, plaster, pencils, crayons, hair or other objects often?	No	Yes
If yes, explain_____		
Is your child able to use a fork and spoon without help?	Yes	No

-2-

V. <u>CHILD'S GROWTH AND DEVELOPMENTAL HISTORY</u>:   <u>Circle One</u>

Did your child have a poor weight gain during the first 6 mo. of life?	No Yes
Did your child sit alone by 7 months of age?	Yes No
Did your child walk alone by 12 months of age?	Yes No
Was your child toilet trained by 18 months of age?	Yes No
Does your child wet the bed at night now?	No Yes
If yes, how often_____	
Does your child wet and soil clothes during the day?	No Yes
If yes, how often_____	
Does your child have sleeping problems, fears, or nightmares?	No Yes
Does your child snore frequently at night?	No Yes
Does your child have poor relationships and fight with siblings or peers?	No Yes
Does your child bang his/her head?	No Yes
Does your child have tempter tantrums?	No Yes
Does your child have a short-attention span?	No Yes
Does your child have any special interests?	No Yes
If yes, explain_____	
Were either parents separated from the child during the first year?	No Yes
If yes, explain_____	
Were either parents separated from the child during any other time?	No Yes
If yes, explain_____	
Is this child as quick to learn as your other children?	Yes No
Is this child as quick to develop as your other children?	Yes No

Do you think your child's learning potential is:
(check one) Slow ____ Average____ Fast_____

Do any of your other children have problems with behavior, grades or emotional adjustments?	No Yes

If yes, explain_____

Which hand does your child prefer to use most often? Right___Left____

Does your child have difficulty dressing himself?	No Yes
Did your child say single words by 12 months of age?	Yes No
Did your child say simple sentences by 18 months of age?	Yes No
Does your child mispronounce certain speech sounds?	No Yes
Does your child use "baby talk"?	No Yes
Does your child stutter?	No Yes
Does your child often lose his balance, fall easily, have difficulty going up or down stairs, injure himself a lot, or is extremely clumsy?	No Yes
Is your child hyperactive or overactive?	No Yes

VI. <u>ILLNESSES HISTORY</u>: (Please check any of the illnesses your child has had or has now)

____Aches or pains frequently	____Epilepsy	____Rheumatic Fever
____Anemia	____Fainting spells	____Sickle cell disease
____Bronchitis	____Fevers Frequently	____Sickle cell trait
____Canker sores in the mouth	____German measles(3 day)	____Sore throats
____Chickenpox	____Hayfever	____More than 6 per/yr.
____Colds -- more than 6 per yr.	____Headaches frequently	____Stomachaches
____Cold sores	____Heart problems	____Strep throat
____Constipation frequently	____Hives	____Surgery--Explain_____
____Convulsions or seizures	____Impetigo	____Tuberculosis
____Diabetes	____Lead poisoning	____Urinary or kidney
____Diarrhea frequently	____Measles (10 day)	problems
____Ear infections - 3 or more	____Meningitis	____Wheezing
____Eczema	____Mumps	____Whooping Cough
____Encephalitis	____Pneumonia	____OTHER_____

2nd of 2

VII. INJURIES HISTORY: (Please check any of the injuries your child has had):

____Amputation of body part (s)	____Serious burn (s)
____Fractured bones	____Sprains
____Head injuries or concussion	____Stitches
____Knocked out teeth	____Unconsciousness
____Serious accidents	____OTHER_____

VIII. HEALTH PROBLEMS HISTORY (Please check any of the health problems your child has had or has now):

____Abnormal spinal curvature	____Skin problems
____Cerebral palsy	____Stayed in hospital 1 day or more.
____Contact with a person having	____Takes medication now
active tuberculosis	____Takes vitamins and/or minerals now
____Crossed eyes	____Underweight
____Dental problems	____Vision problems
____Emotional problems	____Wears glasses - Eye doctor_____
____Food allergies	____Surgery scheduled now or to be scheduled
____Hearing problems	in the future.
____Medication allergies	If so, explain_____
____Nosebleeds frequently	_____
____Orthopedic braces	____OTHER_____
____Orthopedic shoes	_____
____Overweight	
____Physical defects or handicaps	
____Sinus problems	

The Indiana State law (P.L. 103, Acts of 1972) requires that parents or guardians of all children entering school for the first time shall declare whether such children have been tested for lead poisoning or sickle cell anemia

Tested for Lead Poisoning: No____ Yes ____ Results_____

Tested for Sickle Cell Anemia: No____ Yes ____ Results_____

Signature_____Relationship_____

Date_____

Parent and child interviewed by:_____ R.N

Date_____

LH/JT

HS Rec-2
Revised 2/77

-4-

SCHOOL CITY OF GARY
HEALTH SERVICES DEPARTMENT

PEDIATRIC HISTORY

DATE _____

NAME _____ ADDRESS _____

BIRTHDATE _____ SEX _____ TELEPHONE _____

INFORMANT _____ PARENT OR GUARDIAN _____

INTERVIEWER _____ FAMILY DOCTOR _____ SCHOOL _____ GRADE _____

SCHOOL PROGRESS AND REASON FOR REFERAL

What did the school tell you about your child? _____

What is it about your child that concerns you the most? _____

When was it first noticed? _____
Whom have you seen when and what were you told with regard to the problem? _____

IMMUNIZATIONS-TYPE AND DATE

DPT	POLIO VACCINE (type)	
SMALLPOX	RUBELLA	RUBEOLA
TBC (type and result)	SICKLE CELL TEST	LEAD POISONING

PREGNANCY AND BIRTH HISTORY   PRENATAL PHYSICIAN:

Gestation	Labor (length)	Transfusion
Bleeding	Birth Weight	Comments:
Infection	Spontaneous Crying	
Medication	Oxygen	
Toxemia	Resuscitation	

EATING HABITS & SLEEPING PATTERN AS INFANT

GROWTH AND DEVELOPMENT

Sat Alone _____ Sentences _____
Walked Alone _____ Dressing Self _____
Words-Single _____ Toilet Trained _____
Compare to Siblings _____
Temper tantrums or breath holding? _____
Sleep disturbances? _____
Discipline Problems? _____
Enuresis? _____ Nail Biting-Thumb Sucking? _____
Happy? _____ Irritable? _____ Easily Upset? _____
Rapid Mood Changes? _____ Peer Relationship? _____
Does he present any problems at home? _____

In the neighborhood? _____

ILLNESSES, OPERATIONS, AND INJURIES: (List dates and complications)

_____

_____

_____

_____

Any Drug or Food Sensitivities? _____

Any History of eczema, asthma, or hay fever? _____

Is student receiving any medicine?   Yes _____   No _____

If Yes, explain why and name of drug _____

_____

FAMILY HISTORY (Parents and Siblings)

Name   Birthdate   Occupation   Health Status-Stature _____

_____

_____

_____

_____

_____

_____

_____

_____

_____

Give academic history of parents and any school problems of siblings: _____

_____

Were there any fetal deaths or miscarriages? _____

Allergy _____   Cancer _____

Diabetes _____   Renal _____

Cardiovascular _____   Mental retardation _____

Hearing disorders _____   Congenital anomalies _____

Learning problems _____

GENERAL SYSTEMS REVIEW

Eyes _____   Genito-Urinary _____

Ears _____   Skin _____

Nose & Throat _____   Muscles _____

Teeth _____   Bones & Joints _____

Lungs & Chest _____   Menstrual _____

Cardiovascular _____

Nurse's Summary _____

_____

_____

_____

                              Signature _____

Student's Cumulative Folder Information _____

_____

_____

_____

GARY COMMUNITY SCHOOL CORPORATION
Health Services Department

NEUROLOGICAL EXAMINATION FORM

DATE_____

NAME_____
BIRTHDATE_____
EXAMINER_____

I. CEREBRAL FUNCTION

GENERAL

1. General Behavior_____
2. Level of Consciousness_____
3. Intellectual Performance: Immediate memory_____
                              Calculation_____
                              Orientation_____
4. Emotional Status_____
5. Thought content_____

SPECIFIC

A. Cortical Sensory Interpretation
B. Cortical Motor Integration
C. Language

Test for:	How Performed:
1. Sound recognition:	Pts. eyes closed, identify sounds_____
2. Aud.-Verbal comprehension	Does he answer & follow instructions_____
3. Recog. body parts & sides	Know L from R, recog. body parts_____
4. Perform motor acts	Drink from cup; open safety pin_____
5. Visual object recognition	Know object: pen, watch, shoe_____
6. Visual-verbal comprehen.	Read sentence & explain_____
7. Motor speech	Imitate sounds: la-la; me-me_____
	puh-tuh-kuh_____
	this is a good book_____
	Note abnormal verbage_____
8. Automatic speech	Repeat know series: days, months_____
9. Volitional speech	Answer questions relevantly?_____
10. Writing	Write name:_____
	Write address_____
	Write sentence_____
	Write one word with eyes closed_____
	Write one word with eyes open_____
	Write the name of an object_____

II. CRANIAL NERVES

I. Olfactory: identify familiar odors with eyes closed (ea. side)_____
II. Optic: visual acuity each eye_____
        visual fields each eye with tests vertically 60°_____
            "   "   "   "   "   tests laterally 100°_____
            "   "   "   "   "   tests nasally 130°_____
        visual extinction with simultaneous fingers moving in opposite sides of
            fields_____

Revised 1/21/77
Page 1 of 3

-2-

III. Oculomoter; IV. Trochlear; VI. Abducens: Extra-ocular muscles_____
                                       Pupils equal, react to light
                                          and accommodation_____
                                          Nystagnus_____
                                          Ptosis_____

V. Trigeminal: Light touch with cotton to forehead, cheeks, jaws_____
              Sensitivity with eyes closed to pinpricks_____
              Sensitivity with eyes closed to warm & cold objects_____
              Corneal reflex with cotton cornea_____
              Palpate masseter and temporal muscles with jaws clamped_____
              Tap mid chin with hammer for jaw jerk_____

VII. Facial: Imitate looking at ceiling, wrinkling forehead,
                  frown, smile, raise eyebrows_____
              Eyes closed while you attempt to open them_____
              Identify taste of sugar & salt on tongue bilat._____

VIII. Acoustic: Hearing by moving ticking watch till pt. cannot hear_____
              Lateralization by Weber test with fork atop skull_____
              Air & bone conduction by Rinne test with fork on
                  mastoid process till no more sound, then
                  place vibrating portion next to ear_____

IX. Glossopharyngeal; X. Vagus: Gag reflex by touching ea. side of pharynx_____
                        Palatal reflex by stroking ea. side of uvula_____
                        Vagus by swallow & speech without hoarseness
                        and soft palate movements with "ah"_____

XI. Accessory: Palpate strength trapezius muscle with shoulders
              shrugged against resistance_____
               Palpate sternocleidomastoid muscle for strength_____

XII. Hypolossal   Note lateral deviation of tongue when protruded:
              check atrophy or tremor, strength moving
              side to side against depressor_____

III. CEREBELLAR FUNCTION

BALANCE AND COORDINATION

1. Eyes open touch finger to nose with alternate hands. Repeat eyes closed_____
   Eyes open touch finger to nose, then to examinser's finger as examiner
      changes positions_____
2. Pronate and supinate hands_____
   Rapidly move each different finger to the thumb_____
3. Run heel down shin; point to examiner's hand with each big toe_____
   Make a figure "8" with the whole foot_____
4. Without shoes, stand with feet together with eyes open and then closed_____
   Eyes open, walk naturally; eyes closed, walk naturally; walk heel to toe_____

MOTOR SYSTEM

1. Muscle size: inspect and palpate size with tape for consistence and/or atrophy_____
   Tap muscles for irritability _____
   Note symmetry of posture, muscle contours and outlines_____
2. Muscle tone: palpate at rest, passive movement resistance_____
   Note spasticity, rigidity for flaccidity_____
3. Involuntary movements: twistings, irregular jerkings, tics_____
4. Muscle strength: by extension, flexion & other movements of major joints with
           resistance and then the examiner offering resistance. Compare
           corresp. muscles of each side_____

-3-

IV. SENSORY SYSTEM

PRIMARY FORMS OF SENSATION

1. Superficial tactile sensation: cotton one side with corresponding opposite
    side, proximal to distal of hands, forearms, upper arms, trunk, thighs,
    lower legs, feet, perineal and perianal:_____
2. Superficial pain: above procedure with a pin_____
3. Sensitivity to temperature: various parts of body with test tubes containing
    hot and cold water_____
4. Sensitivity to vibration: tuning fork to bony prominences comparing side to
    side, proximal and distal portions of wrist, elbow, shoulder, hip, knee,
    shin and ankle_____
5. Deep pressure pain: squeeze the Achilles tendon, calf and forearm_____
6. Motion and position: fingers and toes moved passively and pt. indicates position____

CORTICAL AND DISCRIMINATORY FORMS OF SENSATION

1. Two point discrimination: eyes closed, body touched with 2 pins_____
2. Point localization: eyes closed, pt. point to spot where touched_____
3. Texture discrimination: recognize cotton, wool by touching_____
4. Stereognostic function: identify familiar objects placed in hand_____
5. Graphesthesia: recognize letters and numbers written on palms with blunt point_____
6. Extinction phenomenon: eyes closed, 2 points touched simult. on opposite
    sides of body_____

V. REFLEXES

Scoring: 0 = absent   3 = normal very active
           1 = diminished but present   4 = hyperactive
           2 = normal active   5 = clonus

Deep Reflexes

1. Biceps
2. Brachioradialis
3. Triceps
4. Patellar
5. Achilles

Superficial Reflexes

1. Upper Abdominal   Pathological Reflexes
2. Lower Abdominal
3. Cremasteric   1. Babinski
4. Plantar   2. Chaddock
5. Gluteal   3. Oppenheim
                                       4. Gordon
IMPRESSION:

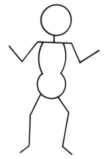

PLAN OF ACTION:

_____
School Nurse Practitioner

GARY COMMUNITY SCHOOL CORPORATION
PHYSICAL EXAMINATION

Principal/Cum folder _____
S. N. P. copy _____
Curric. team/Psych. _____
Nurse _____

Child's Name _____ School _____ Date _____
Address _____ Telephone _____ Birthdate _____
Parent's Name(s) _____ C.A. _____
Teacher(s) Grade _____ Class _____

Date }
Eyes _____
　　Eye tracking _____
　　EOM's _____
　　Cover test _____
　　Vision Rt. _____
　　Vision Lt. _____
　　Vision with glasses _____
Ht. _____ %ile

Wt. _____ %ile
Head Circum. _____
Nutrition _____
Speech _____
Ears _____
　　Rt. _____
Date　Lt. _____
Hearing test: Rt.　Lt. _____
Skin _____
Nose _____
Teeth _____
Teeth Temp. _____
Teeth Perm. _____

Mouth Br. _____

Mouth _____

Oral Hygiene _____

Tonsils _____
Attendance _____

Special Considerations: _____

Pediatric History: _____
_____
_____

Birth Order: _____

Lymph Nodes _____

Thyroid _____

Chest _____

Breasts _____

Lungs _____

Heart _____
_____
　Apical Pulse _____
　Radial Pulse _____

B/P _____

Genitalia _____

Kidney _____

Extremities _____
　Rt. _____
　Lt. _____

Spine _____
Gait _____
Posture _____
_____

Hernia _____

Abdomen _____

Nervous System _____
　Neurological _____
　Appearance _____
I. Cerebral Function _____

　General _____
_____
　Specific _____
_____
II. Cranial Nerves _____
_____
III. Cerebellar Function _____
　Laterality _____
　Balance/Coord. _____
_____
　Rt. _____
_____
　Lt. _____
_____
Motor System _____
_____
IV. Sensory System _____

　Primary Forms _____
_____
　Discrim. Forms _____
_____
V. Reflexes _____

Deep _____
_____
Superficial _____
_____
Pathological _____
_____

Impression: _____
_____
_____
_____
_____

Recommendations: _____
_____
_____
_____
_____

_____ S. N. P.

43

PUBLIC HEALTH NURSING CLINICAL ROLE STUDY

LAURA NELSON TRENT, B.S.N., R.N.

As an employee of a public health agency, the baccalaureate nurse has opportunities to experience different facets of nursing and to apply the principles learned in her college education. I am a staff nurse with the Metropolitan Health Department of Nashville and Davidson County and have found that my educational background, coupled with the desire to work with a diverse group of patients, has made public health nursing very rewarding.

Several discoveries stimulated my interest in the public health field. After choosing public health as my senior elective in school, I found that working with a variety of patients was important in increasing my confidence and competence as a nurse. Since a public health nurse is not limited to a single specialty, I was able to work with entire families, addressing their psychological and social as well as physical needs. My interest was increased by the opportunities for patient counseling which are more frequent in the community where interaction is enhanced by forming a long term relationship with the patient. I also enjoyed the independence and responsibility of managing my own case load. The public health nurse is often the primary link between the patient and the community and must be creative as well as knowledgeable in making nursing decisions. Another positive factor was the contact with other professionals, agencies, and health related organizations. I have gained an awareness of public policy and health care trends as well as a sense of involvement when working in the community daily.

I have been especially pleased by the discovery that community nursing is a special challenge because the nurse must always be able to adapt to the patient's environment.

731

In home care, family numbers, culture, tradition, and economic resources are crucial factors in devising a practical care plan. These factors directly influence the patient's attitude about his health care and his degree of cooperation. The nurse must care for the patient without the benefit of the structure of the hospital system where the patient's therapy is carefully controlled and his progress is monitored daily. Thus, home care is successful only when the nurse utilizes her knowledge of the patient's life style and incorporates this understanding into a unique plan of care.

My educational and clinical preparation for public health work, in addition to enrollment in the senior clinical elective, included part-time employment as a student nurse which improved my basic nursing skills and understanding of medical terminology. As a student it is invaluable to participate in community organizations. Indeed, my first exposure to many public health issues stemmed from working with retarded and emotionally disturbed children. I also have a B.S. degree in psychology and have found this background to be helpful both in terms of patient counseling and in increasing my sensitivity to the non-physical needs of the patient.

OVERVIEW OF NURSING PROGRAM

The Metropolitan Health Department is organized into 11 divisions with a director in charge of each division. One such division is nursing, which is further divided into six groups of nurses with a supervisor for each group. It is important to note that the health department is recognized as an official home health agency, licensed by the State of Tennessee to perform home care.

Every division within the health department has a philosophy which sets forth the general purpose of each program. The nursing division philosophy declares that it is the

> ... obligation of the nursing profession to provide that quality of nursing care which gives consideration to the mental, spiritual, physical, and social needs of every individual. This encompasses promotion of health, prevention of disease or disability, and nursing care during sickness and rehabilitation.[1]

The philosophy also states that nursing personnel are encouraged to grow professionally by active membership in professional organizations, participation in continuing education and formal education programs, and involvement in community affairs.

The nursing division sets objectives for itself and for its home health program. The primary objective of the division is to provide skilled, comprehensive patient care. This includes promotion of the patient's potential, well-being, dignity, and autonomy, as well as encouraging continuity in care and preventive care. Other division objectives are promoting proper interpretation of our nursing services in the community, implementing personnel policies which contribute to employee satisfaction and growth, contributing to scientific advancement of health services through research, and participating in community planning for better health facilities. Another objective is to improve the nursing division's functions through cooperation with the administration and by incorporating new developments into our policies and procedures.

As a licensed home health agency, there are also objectives for this component of the program. These objectives are specific in stating that skilled nursing services will be provided to 100 percent of the patients referred who meet the criteria of acceptance by the agency. These include medical therapy, enterostomal therapy, physical therapy, speech therapy, and home health aide services. Our goals also include providing homemaker services for those patients eligible, maintaining close contact with the patient's physician, and increasing our referrals through utilization of a hospital coordinator. Finally, we strive to provide support and instruction for the patient and family, as well as to improve our services through continuous reassessment of patient needs, innovation in delivery of health care, and improved knowledge and skills. The nursing philosophy and objectives provide the framework by which the division plans, implements, and evaluates its programs and policies and by which ultimately the staff nurse performs her duties.

There are many reasons why the services of our agency are needed in the community. The health department is the only agency which sees homebound indigent patients who cannot afford private care. The demands of a growing population in the metropolitan Nashville area are reflected in our increasing referrals and expanded clinic services. Our clinics are unique in the community, both in terms of the broad segment of the population they serve and in their dual function of treatment and counseling. With the escalating costs of institutionalized care, there is a trend to home care for the chronically ill patient. Our visiting nurse service enables many of these patients to remain at home, gaining psychological as well as economic benefits. One of our most important functions in the community is serving as a source of referrals. A health department nurse is often the first person to discover an individual with a health need and will refer him or her to the appropriate agency for assistance. With a fragmented health care system, we provide the vital link in the community between the patient and his or her physician and the wide array of social and medical services.

As a district nurse I am responsible for a specific case load of patients who live in one geographic area. My case load is composed primarily of patients who meet certain criteria for our "visiting nurse service" (VNS). These patients must be homebound and require skilled nursing or related health services. I see my VNS patients on a regular basis with specific orders for care from their physicians. The remainder of my case load is composed of "public health" patients who are seen as often as their condition warrants. These include prepartum and postpartum, child health, adult health, crippled children, rheumatic fever, and communicable disease cases.

In addition to my case load of patients, I supervise the health care in a school. My school program includes conducting vision, blood pressure, and scoliosis screening programs, following up on immunization deficiencies, and handling various student health problems. District nurses also substitute for regular clinic nurses in the immunization, venereal disease, and tuberculosis clinics. Many district nurses additionally manage general practice or well baby clinics in the community several days a week.

The population of patients I work with in these various settings is very broad. The majority of my VNS cases are at least 65 years of age, and I encounter all ages in public health and school work. Although most of my patients are members of middle income families, I have patients at all levels of the economic strata. My district has no identifiable ethnic group and is mixed racially.

In organizing my work week, I plan a schedule for each day realizing that often a new case or an emergency will arise and the whole day will have to be rearranged. I check each day to see which VNS cases need to be seen and then fill in the time with public health cases who are due for a followup visit. I also budget time for my school program, for charting, and for meetings. My VNS cases usually take priority over public health or school work because they require a specific procedure to be performed which cannot be postponed (catheter changes, injections, dressing changes, and so forth).

District nurses are given feedback and support from several sources within the nursing division. Our work is formally critiqued by an audit committee which reviews our patient records for proper utilization of services. A nurse's supervisor also offers suggestions and solutions to problems as well as regularly evaluating the nurse's job performance. Weekly group meetings provide another forum for discussion and announcements of changes in policies and procedures. I have found my peer group to be very supportive, and it certainly plays a large role in my development since information and ideas are exchanged freely.

As a staff nurse I have access to extensive health department facilities. Within the nursing service are administrative offices, meeting rooms, supply rooms, and the consultant offices. Our consultants include a social worker, nutritionist, speech therapist, home health aide coordinator, and several physical therapists. Each nurse has a semiprivate cubicle with telephone connections. We also utilize the health department library and the health education division to provide educational material for our patients. Clinical facilities for immunizations, tuberculosis, venereal disease, family planning, and primary care are available. There are also physical therapy facilities for the ambulatory patient.

Funding for nursing services is derived from a variety of sources. Local taxes are the primary financial support, although we receive federal grants for special programs such as influenza immunizations. Certain salaried positions, consultants, supplies, and equipment are funded by the state government, but this is not a constant source of revenue. Financing for our VNS program comes from third party payments (Medicare and Medicaid), patient fees on an ability to pay basis, and veterans' benefits for certain services.

NURSING PROCESS

The nursing process is probably universally taught to baccalaureate nursing students, and, I thought, probably universally forgotten when they actually practice! I was, therefore, amazed to discover when gathering material for this paper that I use the nursing process every day. Most of the time I am not conscious that I am applying a formal way of thinking to my interactions with patients, and certainly the components of the process continually overlap. Nevertheless, the process of assessment, planning, intervention, evaluation, and revision is applied to every problem I encounter. The nursing division encourages the use of the nursing process by supplying us with forms to systematically collect data on each patient. I also follow a written guide when opening or summarizing patient records which includes a statement of my assessment, treatment regimen, goals, and the patient's progress. Using this outline shapes my thinking when writing a plan of care and reinforces my mental use of the process. The remainder of this chapter will be devoted to illustration of the use of the nursing process in five case histories.

Whenever I open a VNS case I use a "Chronic Illness Record" form to collect vital data on the patient. The information gathered is used to prepare a treatment plan and to state goals. I began accumulating information on Mr. G., a 65-year-old male who had experienced a cerebrovascular accident, by recording a complete narrative of his current illness—dates, systems, treatment, prognosis, and so on. I then asked Mr. G. to recount his medical history and any significant family medical history. Information was then recorded about Mr. G.'s vital signs, medications, mental state, activity level, functional limitation, his ability to communicate, diet, and fluid balance. I also noted who was in the home to give care, and the family's and patient's attitude toward his illness. At the time of my assessment, Mr. G. had only partial left sided hemiparesis. He was able to walk unassisted but had poor use of his left arm. Mrs. G. was very supportive and happily assisted Mr. G. with most activities. Mr. G. had a good appetite and a normal fluid balance but complained of occasional constipation. Social and economic data revealed that Mr. G. had been physically active before his illness maintaining a full time job as a carpenter to support his wife and a granddaughter. The drastic change in body image he had suffered helped to explain why he cried easily when discussing his illness.

My plan for Mr. G. included referring him to our physical therapist for an evaluation and requesting a home health aide to assist him with his personal care. The aide would also assist Mr. G. with his exercises after the therapist prepared an exercise routine. Goals included increasing Mr. G.'s strength, mobility, and ability to perform activities of daily living, maintaining personal hygiene, maintaining a normal bowel function and preventing constipation, and improving Mr. G.'s emotional status.

The physical therapist instituted an exercise routine after evaluating Mr. G. He is currently performing these exercises with the therapist's supervision and his family's assistance. As he progresses, the therapy plan will be changed to accommodate his needs. The therapist also assisted the family in choosing some special equipment to enable Mr. G. to have more independence in his home. The home health aide has begun working with Mr. G. and assists him with his exercises twice a week. With my supervision she is also assisting him with his bath and other personal needs. Our goal now is to get Mr. G. into the bathtub since this will contribute to his comfort as well as cleanliness. Intervention with this patient has included discussion of good bowel habits with Mr. and Mrs. G., and I have found Mrs. G. to be most receptive to my suggestions. I believe that a willingness to accept Mr. G. as he is and then support and encourage his efforts to recover is, perhaps, the most potent intervention that our health team can use in our therapeutic plan.

Every time I visit Mr. G. I evaluate his progress. He is very cooperative and appears to be improving. If he was not improving, the therapist and I would discuss ways to alter our plan. I feel that the good relationship between Mr. and Mrs. G. and the health department personnel is indicative of their acceptance of our intervention. Our work with Mr. G. will be evaluated by my supervisor and possibly by the nursing audit committee which reviews records randomly. After six months I will write a summary of our work with Mr. G. and his progress for the purpose of evaluating the rationale and effectiveness of our therapeutic plan. This summary is written on all VNS patients and provides the opportunity to systematically use the nursing process in written form.

Mrs. J. is a 78-year-old woman with a diagnosis of chronic brain syndrome. She has been on our service for four years, and I have cared for her for a year and one-half. Mrs. J. is confined to her bed, is incontinent of bowel and bladder, has a foley catheter, and is dependent for all aspects of care. She is aware of little in her environment and speaks a word only occasionally with prompting. Mrs. J.'s husband is 81 and is devoted to her. He has employed an attendant to care for Mrs. J. during the day and cares for her himself at night.

Mrs. J.'s condition was stable until she developed a sacral decubitus ulcer while her attendant was on vacation. Mrs. J. is a heavy woman, and the ulcer had developed quickly. Mr. J. was very upset about the ulcer and could not understand how this could happen after all these years with no skin problems. However, in talking with Mr. J. I found that he resisted turning his wife because she disliked lying on her side. Her nutritional status had also declined prior to the appearance of the pressure sore because her appetite was poor. My assessment revealed a wound the size of a half-dollar with thick, green drainage. The surrounding skin was very irritated, and the wound emitted a foul odor.

My plan for Mrs. J.'s care included cleaning and protecting the wound as well as reviewing the basics of skin care for the bedridden patient with the attendant and Mr. J. Goals included promoting the healing of the wound, preventing further skin breakdown, and improving Mrs. J.'s general health status.

Intervention began with obtaining orders for an antibiotic from Mrs. J.'s physician since the wound was obviously infected. While cleaning and covering the wound with a sterile dressing, I decided a consultation with the health department's enterostomal therapist would be helpful. After she made a home visit, the therapist recommended using a karaya procedure on the ulcer. This procedure was taught to the attendant to facilitate regular dressing changes. To prevent further skin breakdown, I discussed at length the importance of turning the patient regularly with both Mr. J. and the attendant. We reviewed proper positioning, and Mr. J. purchased a new flotation mattress. Mrs. J. was too rigid to employ passive range of motion exercises, but I encouraged her attendant to massage her skin after every bath. We also discussed the importance of keeping her skin clean and dry and of protecting all bony prominences. We began spraying reddened areas with a protective plastic chemical which prevented new areas of breakdown from appearing. I encouraged Mr. J. to give his wife fluids and then obtained recipes for high protein dishes from our nutritionist to improve the patient's nutritional status.

The evaluation of these measures is ongoing. The karaya procedure has been successful in reducing the sacral ulcer to the size of a one-half inch slit. However, the wound has not healed completely largely due to occasional irritation caused by urine when Mrs. J.'s catheter leaks. This problem has also been dealt with, and it appears that her sacral decubitus ulcer will eventually heal. Mrs. J. is kept scrupulously clean. She has remained infection free, and her fluid intake is excellent. Her diet is high protein and well balanced and her appetite is good. Mrs. J. had no further skin breakdown for six months after the initial ulcer appeared. Then she was once again left in one position for too long and a fresh decubitus formed on her right hip. This occurred, as before, when the attendant was away, so I must judge my intervention with Mr. J. unsuccessful. He still does not understand some of the basic principles of skin care despite repeated discussions. Therefore, my plan must be revised to find another way to enlist Mr. J.'s cooperation. As always, the nursing process remains flexible to meet the challenge of altered circumstances.

The nursing process is employed by public health nurses when visiting public health patients as well as VNS patients. I will illustrate my use of the process with three examples, Ms. W., a maternity case, Baby W., a newborn case, and Mrs. S., an adult health case.

After receiving a referral on Baby W. from a local hospital I made a home visit. Ms. W., the child's mother, was friendly, cooperative, and had many questions to ask. She had begun breastfeeding her child with no instruction and was particularly anxious about this, so I answered her questions first before proceeding with collecting data. Of course, observation of the home environment, Ms. W.'s reactions to my teaching, and her attitude toward her child were noted in my general assessment.

When Ms. W. felt more confident about breastfeeding, I proceeded with my assessment. To aid me in gathering information on public health patients I use a check list. For example, I questioned Ms. W. about her general health, prenatal history, labor and delivery, anesthesia, and complications. I also collected information on her lochia, breasts, sutures, diet, elimination, emotional status, and family planning measures. The checklist, along with the adult health form where the information is recorded, helps me to gain a complete picture of the patient's history, life style, and needs. Information collected on Baby W.

included his neonatal history, birth weight, feeding and sleeping habits, status of cord and circumcision, and description of stools and urine. I also performed a physical inspection of the baby to add to my data. The assessment is completed after gathering social information on the patients including family support, finances, work experience, and living accommodations.

My assessment revealed that Ms. W. was an intelligent, articulate woman who held a graduate degree in teaching. Although she was not married, the baby's father visited regularly and was very supportive. Ms. W. stated they planned to be married in six months. Baby W. was a well-developed, active, week old baby boy with a normal physical assessment. My plan for Ms. W. included a great deal of teaching since this was her first child, and because she expressed an interest in many aspects of baby care. Since she was an avid reader, I collected pamphlets on postpartum care and child care for her from our health education department. I also planned to refer her to La Leche League, an organization which promotes breastfeeding. Goals for Ms. W. were to continue normal recovery from childbirth, to prevent complications, to promote safe, comfortable breastfeeding, and to provide alternatives for family planning. For Baby W. the goals were to promote normal growth and development, prevent complications, and maintain a regular immunization schedule. A comprehensive goal for both mother and child was to foster a nurturing relationship between them, so that a strong, emotional bond develops.

Achieving the stated goals is even now an ongoing process which will stop only when the public health record is closed. My initial intervention with Ms. W. included discussion of breast care, perineal care, diet, activity, and birth control. We also reviewed several pamphlets on newborn care and discussed cord care, bathing, skin care, feeding and sleeping schedules, and the need for a PKU (phenylketonuria) test. I also enjoyed discussing the child's reflexes with his mother and encouraging her to touch and talk to her child. As the child grows, I will observe for developmental milestones and assist Ms. W. with any problems which may develop. Assuming she has no other health problems, Ms. W. will be discontinued as a patient when lactation ceases.

I am continually evaluating my work with this family, and often find it difficult to be objective since there is no formal tool to measure success. Perhaps mother and child would have followed a normal, healthy course without my intervention. However, on my fourth home visit I observed a definite change in Ms. W.'s demeanor. She was secure, confident, and cared for her child with ease. She agreed with my observation that she seemed very happy and truly enjoyed being with her child. Baby W. was gaining weight and following a normal developmental course. Perhaps the most accurate evaluation of the effectiveness of my intervention was Ms. W.'s receptiveness to future public health nurse visits. This is a positive step since it indicates that the patient felt she benefited from past interactions.

My assessment of Mrs. S. began with reading the public health record, which had been opened six months before I took over the case. The record revealed a 79-year-old widow who lived alone and was generally able to care for herself. Her only son, stationed with the Navy in Japan, had become alarmed and notified the Red Cross when he received a letter from his mother with the statement, "I have a terminal illness," and no other explanation. The record further revealed that Mrs. S. had a breast mass and had refused the pleas of friends and our health department social worker to seek medical attention.

My initial visit revealed a pleasant, talkative woman who was eager for company and enjoyed talking about everything but her health. She did permit me to examine her breast, and I was quite shocked to see that the entire upper outer quadrant of her right breast was a weeping ulcer where the tumor had broken through the skin. The tumor was hard and the size of a small orange, but Mrs. S. denied having pain. She dressed the wound herself and told me it would go away soon. Despite this seeming denial of the problem, Mrs. S. spoke of her impending death, stating that she was glad because she was of "no use to anyone anymore."

My long range goal was to convince Mrs. S. to seek medical care. Since earlier attempts to get her to see a physician had failed, my immediate plan was to gain her trust and confidence. When she asked why I had come, I replied that I wanted to check on her and see if she needed help with anything. Mrs. S. was very independent and declined my offer of an aide to help with her personal care or a homemaker to help with housework. She did, however, want me to visit again.

For two months I visited Mrs. S. She enjoyed telling me stories of her life as a young woman on a ranch in Texas. She spoke often of her only son, and the bond between them that had led her to following him from base to base when he had joined the Navy. She also told me of his marriage to a Japanese woman which she had opposed and had led to a break in their relationship. This greatly saddened Mrs. S. and grossly affected her will to live. It also explained the strange letter to her son. She desperately wanted his attention but paradoxically did not want him to know her true condition for fear he would not be concerned. Despite her problems, Mrs. S. maintained a strong religious faith and enjoyed a support system in the form of neighbors and close church friends.

During this two month period Mrs. S.'s general health remained good, and I felt my intervention had been successful. Mrs. S. trusted me and felt free to talk about anything. However, since the tumor was probably malignant, I judged it time to revise my plan and take concrete steps toward urging Mrs. S. to obtain medical help. Thus ensued discussions about Mrs. S.'s future and her fear of losing control over her life. We talked about her right to refuse surgery or any other extraordinary means of treatment. Although Mrs. S. expressed no fear of dying, she was afraid of a lonely, painful death in a hospital. She finally agreed that if she postponed treatment too long her illness might prevent her from remaining at home.

My plan then shifted to making specific arrangements for her to see a physician. I offered to make an appointment at a hospital clinic for her and arrange transportation. At this point I became very frustrated because Mrs. S. continually made excuses not to see the doctor while asking me to help her. It seemed that Mrs. S. wanted to be assured that her life still had meaning and that she would not be forgotten. I then included her support system in my plan, asking her friends, especially her minister, to comfort Mrs. S. and alleviate her loneliness. With the help of her friends, Mrs. S. finally found the courage to allow me to make an appointment. The mass had begun bleeding, also, and the discomfort had convinced Mrs. S. of the urgency of the situation. Four months after my first visit to Mrs. S., she made the trip to the hospital clinic. I judged my intervention to be successful since the patient had sought medical attention but more importantly had arrived at the decision herself.

Shortly after her clinic visit, Mrs. S. had a simple mastectomy for carcinoma of the breast. When her son came from Japan, Mrs. S. was overjoyed and relieved that he was there to handle her affairs. Her wishes for no extreme medical measures were respected and she returned home. My plan was then revised to address the needs of a terminal cancer patient with the goals of maintaining comfort and continuity of care. My role became one primarily of assistance and support since her church congregation took over complete care of the patient. I continued to visit Mrs. S., maintaining the trusting friendship we had established, and was saddened to see her gradually weaken. Three months after her surgery, Mrs. S. died surrounded by her friends. I was glad to know that in her final days she had been loved and cared for, and that my nursing had played a large role in easing her loneliness.

The nursing process can be applied to a group of patients as well as an individual. Such is the case when investigating an outbreak of pediculosis, commonly known as lice. Epidemics of lice, especially among school children, have become quite common in recent years, and my referrals usually originate in a school.

When I receive the message from a school that a child is suspected of having lice, my first step is to collect data on the problem. I list the children known to have lice and note if they are in one or more classrooms. I also note if they have siblings in the school, and if any lice has been found in their classrooms. Information is collected on whether the children identified with lice have been treated, what treatment was used, and whether they are back in school. Teachers are questioned on the amount of contact between children, where the children hang their coats, and if the small children use sleeping mats. Teachers are also asked to report any child observed to be excessively irritable or scratching.

The goal in treating an outbreak of lice is always to eradicate the existing cases and prevent reinfestation. To achieve these goals, I screen the classrooms with the reported cases of lice and the classrooms of their siblings. I always explain to the children what the screening procedure is for to alleviate apprehension and increase their understanding of the problem. I also plan to teach school personnel facts about lice and distribute educational material. The actual classroom screening is accomplished on my first visit to the school, and notes are sent home to parents of children found to be infested. In the meeting with the school personnel questions are answered, and a demonstration of the screening procedure is given so that the teachers can learn to identify lice. I also discuss ways to disinfect the school and home and leave the literature on lice to reenforce my teaching.

The best measure of the effectiveness of my intervention is when the school has no new cases of lice after three to four weeks. I usually find several cases in my screening, and most schools will not allow these children back in school until they have been treated and no longer have any nits (eggs). I also feel successful when the school faculty or administrative staff feels competent enough to rescreen the infested children themselves rather than have me recheck the children. The evaluation is completed by comments from the school personnel and children which reveal their attitudes toward the problem of lice, and if they understand how to avoid reinfestation.

Sometimes my plan is revised and I rescreen infested children myself, especially if there is a problem with one family or the teacher is still unsure of her ability to identify the lice. I have also telephoned parents when there was a question about disinfection in the home. Whatever specific problems may arise, the nursing process provides an orderly means by which the lice can be identified and eradicated.

Public health nurses are a vital force in our community, and, I believe, will acquire new roles and greater responsibilities in the health care system in the years to come. Our contribution to the protection of the public from disease is unquestioned, and the support we give to families in a crisis is invaluable. Although the number of patients we encounter is large, our concern for the health and welfare of the individual is always the primary focus of our work. Our patients are very special to us, and the relationships we establish enrich our personal lives as well as our careers. Public health is a dynamic field of nursing and will always welcome the nurse who is willing to combine knowledge and clinical skills with creativity, patience, and a genuine affection for people.

ACKNOWLEDGMENT

I wish to acknowledge the assistance of Mrs. Marjorie Hester, R.N., in the preparation of this chapter.

REFERENCES

1. Metropolitan Health Dept.: *Home Health Agency Manual*, 1977.

CHAPTER **44**
COMMUNITY HEALTH NURSING: ONE NURSE'S PRACTICE

BARBARA B. BECKER, M.S., A.N.P., R.N.

I have written this chapter so that you who are new to nursing or have experience in other areas of nursing will be able to learn from a colleague about a different aspect of community health nursing. I will show how I was able to implement my philosophy of wellness into my practice with senior citizens. Therefore, I will explore my framework of practice and how it evolved, and how my framework affects my association with the Denver Visiting Nurse Service/Association and the development and supervision of a new program. Nursing is both rewarding and frustrating, and a framework helps to keep progress and problems in perspective.

BACKGROUND

I graduated from Loyola University in Chicago in 1967 with a Bachelor of Science in Nursing. This program instilled in me the fundamental belief in the dignity of man and how he can and should be respected at all times. After graduation I worked one year as a staff nurse at a Veterans' Hospital where I could not handle the constraints of that system. When unable to talk with a dying patient because of all the other pressures I felt, I decided to leave. From there I went into a geriatric community experience with Hull House, one of the oldest social work agencies in Chicago. In that experience I saw what poverty can do to the elderly and how my caring and intervention could improve a life, even in a small way. This brought immense satisfaction, but anger at a system that allowed such poor treatment of the aged.

Because of many frustrations with this agency that I felt could not be changed, I left. From this experience I went into a public health agency with a heavy emphasis on maternal-child nursing. After moving to Denver, I continued in public health nursing and moved into coordination, i.e., arranging home nursing care following discharge from Children's Hospital.

During graduate school at the University of Colorado School of Nursing in 1974-1975, I developed my framework of practice. Graduate school also helped me to formalize my framework for working with families. During this time I enrolled in the nurse-practitioner program. I started out with pediatrics but, because of a conflict between departments, I had to switch my emphasis to adult medicine. My preceptorship and place of employment for one and a half years after graduation was in family practice in a rural setting, so that I evolved into a Family Nurse Practitioner. It may seem incongruous to switch from pediatrics to adults to geriatrics; however, my framework of enhancing self-esteem carries into all age groups. I do not like to see people slighted, and I feel this has been a problem with our aged population. Also, each age group has different health needs that can be somewhat satisfied through health education and prevention. Another very important component has been the warmth that so many seniors express to the nurse. Senior citizens are a truly needy and appreciative group.

After trying my hand in emergency medicine for one year, I decided the constraints of the hospital system were not for me. An opportunity arose for me to become a supervisor of a new program in geriatrics. The emphasis was to help the senior *stay well* in his/her own home. This philosophy was in accordance with my beliefs. The details of this program will be described later.

Another important influence in my becoming involved with senior citizens was my family. In my family, respect of the elderly was indoctrinated. I had older parents and many family friends were older. My mother was reared in a generation where the elderly were respected and remained a part of the family. Being around the old folks gave me a real feel for some of their problems. Because of this family background, it was even more frustrating to buck a health care/social system that demeaned older people.

SERVING SENIORS PROGRAM

The program, Serving Seniors, grew out of a philosophy of helping seniors *stay well* in their own homes. Hospital costs are escalating and identifying problems early decreases costs both in patient care and nursing home placement. Also, many seniors do not seek appropriate preventive care because they feel no need, they lack money, or they are unable to travel, but seniors have many questions about their health and they need frequent reassurance. Many of the elderly are willing to take positive steps to maintain their own health.

The program was originally started by the Denver Visiting Nurse Service (VNS) in 1974 in six congregate living sites and the services were well received. Funding was through the agency but later there were budget cuts and only two sites remained. The remaining sites were staffed by two public health nurses and the sites paid for the nurses' time through fund raising projects. As word spread of the service offered, many other areas requested the same service but the agency was unable to provide the service because of lack of funding. Mile High United Way had been donating to the Visiting Nurse Association of the Denver Area, Inc., for many years but felt that a specific program was now needed for their funds. This was the Serving Seniors Program which was fully operational by April of 1978.

What is unique about this program? To date I believe that no other agency is serving well seniors in quite the same manner. We travel to our sites (38 in the City and County of Denver), congregate living areas, recreation centers, and churches. There is a staff of four nurse practitioners—two adult, one geriatric, and one pediatric. Nurse practitioners were chosen because of their ability to physically assess a client, knowledge of when to refer a client based on these findings, and the ability to manage chronic illnesses. As the supervisor, I have a dual role of staffing clinics and supervising the program. This dual role is frustrating with all of its responsibilities and the role will be evaluated. At present, 40 percent of my time is supposed to be spent on supervision and 60 percent in the clinical area. With the present number of clinics that I have (six) and all the followup required on the seniors, I find that supervision slips. Supervision includes staff, sites, public relations, development of new sites, problem solving, setting and meeting objectives, evaluation of the program relating to administration, and development of forms, protocols, job descriptions. In the future, there will be evaluation for expansion and establishment of a consistent volunteer program. I feel that I could not supervise if I had not experienced some of the same problems that my staff encountered. There is also a clerk typist, but no program aide or screening technician. The only other help we may have at the site is a volunteer. The amount of equipment, records, and so forth is enough to fill a shopping cart which the nurses use to unload the equipment for their care. Equipment carried includes centrifuge, scale, blood pressure cuffs (medium and large), stethoscope, diagnostic set, reflex hammer, tuning fork, public health nurse's black bag, cups for urine, Dextrostixs, urine Multistix, *Physician's Desk Reference*, blank records, patient education materials, and other varied items.

The goal of the program is to help people *stay well* in their own homes. This goal is accomplished through health screening, health education, and health maintenance services to City and County of Denver residents who are 55 years of age and older. Based on the 1970 census, it is estimated that there are 85,000 people over 60 years of age, with a higher proportion of women.

Health screening services offered are blood pressure and weight measurement, hematocrit, urine and hemaoccult testing, health screening questionnaire, and a partial physical examination. Hearing and vision screening are being developed.

Health maintenance is monitoring of a chronic problem, e.g., hypertension, COPD, or diabetes, in conjunction with the client's medical care source. This requires frequent consultation with the physician, nurse practitioner, or physician's assistant, and proper interpretation of findings or what is normal for that client.

To me, the uniqueness of nursing is health education. Because of my nursing background which emphasized the total patient and his family and my philosophy of wellness, health education is an important part of the program. In order for a client to stay well, he or she has to understand the disease process, medications, need for proper diet, and exercise. Seniors have many questions about staying well and most are willing to take an active part in their health care. However, many clients first come to the nurse to have their blood pressure taken, and by either the health screening questionnaire or open-ended questions, the nurse practitioner frees the client to ask other questions. With appropriate questioning many problems can be uncovered and dealt with by either the nurse or a referral to the appropriate source.

We work on an appointment system, usually every 15 minutes, but longer if necessary. Drop in clients, especially if ill, are evaluated and an appropriate care plan is instituted. The nurse will also do a one time home visit for ill clients and make an evaluation and appropriate referral. The nurse will render first aid while at the site.

Because we are in 38 sites that are not meant to be clinics, we all work and adapt to different situations. Some of us have small private rooms with a cot, table and chairs, an electrical outlet, running water, bathroom(s), and telephones nearby. Other clinics are conducted in noisy corners of a gym, dining area, or stuffy kitchen. Clients range from the very poor, lonely, isolated senior living in a one room apartment in a hotel to the residents of a model retirement community. As we all learned, nursing care can be adapted to any situation.

Even though all has gone relatively well, there have been minor and major problems to contend with. Some minor problems have been choice of equipment and supplies, protecting materials from hot/cold damage, and development of forms and a data collection system. Maintaining appointments and working with a forgetful population has been difficult and not fully solved at present.

Some major problems encountered have been preparation of the medical community to receive the program, public relations to inform people of the program and what we do, and the development of the influenza immunization program for 38 different sites as well as visual, glaucoma, and hearing screening programs. Choice of future sites will depend upon program analysis after the first six months of operation. Even though our objective is to provide continuity of care with the same nurse at a site, this will have to be re-evaluated according to volume of usage at the sites.

As with any new program, new staff had to be oriented to the program. Their input was invaluable as to handling of clients, working with volunteers, development of forms, discussion of how to handle certain problems encountered with clients and/or equipment. As a new supervisor, it was difficult to begin to anticipate all the possible problems. I had to deal with a new nursing role and return to the agency after a four year absence, the development of a new program, working with a new staff, lack of office space, and dissemination of information regarding the program. Functional job descriptions and protocols, unfortunately, have not been developed, but will be shortly. Staff has been asked to write their own job descriptions and to codevelop new protocols if present published ones are inadequate.

Denver VNS has been most supportive of this program. Even though the main source of funding has been through Mile High United Way funds, the Visiting Nurse Association also made a modest contribution. The Director of Nursing has been supportive and is helping us seek additional funds for research. (For a further description of this agency, see Chapter 45.)

By having the Visiting Nurse Association/Service behind the program, all the resources of the agency, the Neighborhood Health Program, and Denver General Hospital are available. Consultants in mental health, physical and occupational therapies, social work, and medical-surgical nursing, as well as statisticians, experienced administrators, a public information assistant, speciality clinics, and the field nursing program are readily available to our staff. At present, we do not have a medical consultant but we are arranging this backup. Because this is a nursing program and we are practicing within the confines of the Colorado Nursing law, medical consultation was not felt to be a priority.

The VNA Board had started a Serving Seniors Task Force in 1977. The task force was responsible for the broad objectives of the program and for seeking funding. The Administrator of Specialty Programs did most of the preplanning, initial assessment of the sites, drafting letters of intent, hiring of staff, and selection of equipment. Without this foundation, my implementation of the program would have been difficult.

The grant for our program is renewable each year. The budget request is submitted in August to be reviewed in October. Funds will be allocated after the fall campaign of Mile

High United Way. Even though this can be an unstable foundation, renewal does not seem to be a problem. The major concern is the amount of money to be allocated, and I feel our statistics will show the need for continued support of the program. Increased funding has been requested for professional education. To receive continued support our business manager, director, administrator, and myself will have to be looking at unit cost of service, and at different costs incurred for a first time visit, repeat visit, blood pressure check, health counseling, health education visit, and so on. This has to be done and even though it is frustrating to all of us; it is necessary. Health care dollars are becoming scarce, and therefore they have to be justified and spent wisely. We will also attempt to show how our early intervention saved health care dollars. From the financial analyses, new ways of meeting health needs will evolve, be tried, and be evaluated.

Because of a belief that people appreciate what they have to pay for, even a minimal amount, donations have been requested, but without a set amount being stipulated. At some sites, this has been successful; at others, no donations are received. A goal for next year is to obtain a 25¢ donation per client per site. Donations are used to help defray costs, particularly for laboratory work. For the influenza immunization program, vaccine has been obtained through the Colorado Department of Health at no cost. Therefore, donations have to be unsolicited.

NURSING INTERVENTIONS

Self-Esteem

In order to work with clients, I periodically have to sit back and reevaluate my framework of practice. There are two aspects of the framework: working with the individual and family and working with the health care system.

Working with individuals has made me realize the importance of self-esteem. When a person has a poor self-image, he or she has a decreased ability to cope with stress and to take a positive step towards self-help. The aged in America are relegated to a lower social position, may have decreased financial resources, may be alone, are losing friends through death, have decreased hearing and vision, and have a good chance of a chronic health problem. Family structure has changed, and the elderly person has diminished importance to the family. Any of these factors, let alone a combination, would depress a person. Depression leads to low self-esteem. An important function of the nurse is to increase self-esteem by caring and sharing. Caring is a genuine interest in another, taking time to point out the positive aspects of behavior or qualities of the person. Suggestions for changes are done in a nonthreatening, ego enhancing manner. The client is involved in all decisions that affect him or her personally. Feelings are explored and a client is allowed to express emotions. Many fears, health problems, and concerns can be expressed to the nurse and not to the physician. When the client experiences an increase in his or her self-esteem, positive health behaviors can be adopted. I have used this framework with my families, young mothers, and myself. As my self-esteem has increased, I am free to give more of myself to my clients and to see myself as a change agent. Current thought in self-growth is based on this premise.

Sharing of one's self will also increase client self-esteem. Because when you, the nurse, are able to share of yourself, you are saying that this other individual is worthwhile. Too often nurses do not share themselves and yet we expect our clients to share themselves with us. This caring and sharing is being human and a part of the development of a trusting relationship. When I was able to start sharing more with my clients, I felt a positive difference in their response to me. Positive health behaviors frequently followed.

The term "client" is used to refer to our patients because it implies that the individual makes a rational choice to come to and continue with the health care provider. The client has direct input into the health care plan. Health education is done under this concept of equal input to the decision.

Effecting Change

In being a change agent, a nurse must be able to influence the health care system. The framework that I developed for this involves theories on wellness, planned change, and power structure. The framework evolved from many frustrations with the health care system, and finally I accepted the fact that you cannot ignore the politics, but you must learn to deal with them. The following is an unpublished paper that elaborates on these concepts and meshes them into my framework of practice.

CONCEPTS

Wellness

Wellness is not only the state of being free from illness but "a state of complete physical, mental, and social well-being, and not merely the absence of disease and infirmity."[1] Dunn goes on to elaborate on his idea of wellness:

> High-Level (sic) wellness for the individual is defined as an integrated method of functioning which is oriented toward maximizing the potential of which the individual is capable. It requires that the individual maintain a continuum of balances and purposeful direction within the environment where he is functioning.[1]

As stated above, wellness takes in the whole person and is on a continuum. This philosophy underlies all nursing care given by me to patients and families.

In a community health nursing setting, nursing goals come from many sources. Short range goals usually come from the referral and are modified according to identified patient and family needs based on their strengths and weaknesses. Long range goals are based on Dunn's concept of high level wellness for the individual and family. A professional relationship has to be established and maintained through the use of interviewing skills. Nursing care to effect change is based on sound psychological, physiologic, and sociologic theories. These principles aid in the establishment of mutual goals of care between the nurse, the patient, and the family, and progress towards these goals is periodically checked.

Because the patient and the family are part of a community and often have unmet needs, especially during a crisis, they need to participate in the established community agencies. The role of the nurse is to help the patient and family understand the services offered and why they are needed, to determine how services can be obtained, to act as a liaison where indicated, and to evaluate patient and family satisfaction with the services received.

As my view of community health nursing evolved, the need to participate in community groups became obvious in order to learn about the group and to contribute expertise when indicated. The nurse is a part of the community, both work and home, and the nurse cannot be separated from it. But to effect change within community groups that would ultimately affect patient care, the ability to plan change and to work within the existing power structure has to be developed.

Planned Change

Planned change is important to accomplish goals and to allow continuous, harmonious progress. Lippitt defined planned change as a "decision to make a deliberate effort to improve the system."[2] Bennis defined planned change in a similar but more elaborate way. His definition is "a conscious, deliberate and collaborative effort to improve the opportunities of a human system, whether it be a self-system, social system, or cultural system through the utilization of scientific knowledge."[3] Planned change can also be seen as strategy to accomplish goals, and without this strategy actions do not fit into the larger plan. Therefore, effort and resources can be wasted.

Chinn[4] sees different types of strategies being employed in order to accomplish planned change. These strategies are 1) empirical-rational where one introduces change to meet needs which are based on a belief that man is a rational being and will respond to his unmet needs; 2) normative-reeducative where the change agent appeals to the attitudes and value systems of the individual and educates on the basis of these systems; and 3) application of power to effect change which could be either from the political system or from the informal system of power within the community.

Bennis[3] also sees planned change involving problems of identification of goals and values, collaboration and conflict, control and leadership, resistance and adaption to change, utilization of human resources, and communication. In effectively planned change, there must be problem solving and a way of assessing communities and outcomes.

There are several phases that occur in the process of planned change. These phases are 1) development of a model for change, i.e., unfreezing of ideas or values and now being able to see the idea of improvement; 2) establishment of a relationship with a change agent; 3) clarification of the problem which is a beginning move towards change after examination of alternate choices; and 4) generalization and stabilization of change where an individual or group can look at the change process and apply it to other areas.[2] This process is basically where an individual or group unlearns previous behavior before being able to learn new behavior.

Planned change is a process of moving forward or changing with a definite plan or objective. With definite objectives, change that has occurred can be measured in an objective way and only through some type of measurement can it be determined if actual change has occurred. By evaluating past accomplishments and failures, new objectives can realistically be planned.

Power Structure

In order to view how any community group functions or how it can accomplish its goals, one must look at the power structure that the group has to encounter and work with. Power has been defined by Max Weber as the "chance of man or a group of men to realize their own will."[5] Warren[6] sees community action as activating the horizontal power, i.e., the power within the group and the power within other groups on the same level. Community development is the strengthening of the horizontal power. However, in all systems, there also is power from above or vertical power. This is the government which is operating under a set of laws and has the authority to enforce these laws and allocate resources for the accomplishment of the goals established by the group.

Warren[6] has developed an action system for community development. His first three stages look at the available resources in the community, how to involve the needed element of the community in the planned change, and how to bring these additional elements or groups into the action system. These additional elements or resources would be from both the horizontal and vertical power structure.

Perlman[7] sees organizational tasks varying according to the purpose, composition, and power position and structure of the organization. Waehtel[8] also sees that any planned change is dependent upon the power structure within the community. This power structure can be either pluralistic which gives some of its power to others, or elite where power stays with only several people. When able to understand what power structure is existent within a community, then the community group can plan action to get through the political structure. Power rests where the resources and authority are,[7] and a group's power is increased if it is effectively able to gather some of these resources.

Power is not seen as a bad force, but a force that is existent in all areas and all cultures. It is through proper use and attainment of power that planned change can be implemented.

CONCEPTUAL FRAMEWORK

The previous concepts of wellness, planned change, and the power structure can be seen in a conceptual framework. This framework has, and will continue to be, the basis for my nursing intervention with patients.

Wellness is the goal of patient care, but in order to bring this about, nurses must plan strategy that will change the medical, or illness, model of patient care. In order to effect change in any system, change must be planned with knowledge of the existing power structure of the agency or government. Within these systems of power, which would be on the vertical plane, there also is horizontal power or power of peers, community groups, and other professionals who can bring pressure on the vertical power. Through knowledge of these power structures and effective planning and working within the power structure, nurses can make lasting changes for patient care (Fig. 44-1).

PROGRAM EVALUATION

At present, the main source of evaluation of the program is through the data gathered. Statistics are being kept on all sites, then totaled for the week and month. Eventually, quarterly, semiannual, and annual reports will be compiled. Data are gathered on ages, number of new and return visits, number of screening procedures, and type of problems encountered. Statistics are kept on the individual sites and then totaled for the whole program. Because statistics have not been kept for a full year, I am not including them because I do not feel they give a true picture of the health problems of seniors. Publication of this program and findings will be done in the future.

In response to the community and clientele, our program is a success. We are asked to expand the number of sites, and the usage in most sites is increasing. Another indicator we feel of the success of the program is the reception by the medical community. Physicians were prepared through an article in the medical society newspaper. Physicians have been receptive, encouraging their clients to return to us between office visits. This saves costs for the client, and most times it is more convenient for the client to see us. The nurse will con-

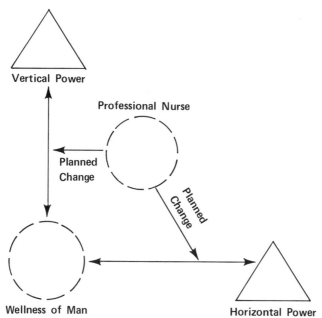

FIGURE 44-1. Power structure diagram.

tact the physician, if indicated, regarding the status of the client. An important emphasis in working with the client is health education, and this is seen as being very important by us, the client, and the physician. Many times we monitor a client to see how he or she is doing. Educational emphasis is placed on diets, e.g., high potassium or low sodium, exercise, and knowledge of the disease process. Clients are also encouraged to follow good health practices in order to stay well. Clients are reappointed according to need.

Outcomes of nursing interventions have not been developed, however, they are being considered. At present, the percentage of positive findings (which is averaging around 33 percent), is being used as an indicator of the success of screening procedures and nursing interventions (as the number of referrals to a physician or a medical care source). Positive findings are those findings which are abnormal to the client and warrant further evaluation by us or the client's source of medical care. On our newly revised Daily Log, there is an area next to the diagnosis that indicates condition of the client, and if he or she shows improvement, status quo and chronic, acute, deteriorating, or resolved condition. This will hopefully be correlated to nursing intervention.

Because of the newness of the program, its impact is not fully appreciated. Evaluation needs to be done on usage of sites, percentage of positive findings, positive outcomes, and cost of our service versus hospitalization or outpatient medical care. Another area that needs to be addressed is client compliance. We feel that we have a very high rate of compliance and speculate that it is due to the interest and education that the nurse practitioners give to a client along with caring and sharing.

Because of the size of our client population, there is great research potential. Empirically, I have observed that sound habits, moderate daily exercise, and an interest in life make for a healthier individual. Obviously, this and other observations and speculations need to be researched.

The program is expected to be funded next year, and I feel the program will definitely continue to prove its worthiness. Objectives have been written with projections of an increase in the number of new and return visits of clients, and an increase of one to two sites. My staff has said that I made the projection too low, so I will have to reexamine the objectives on a quarterly basis. In order to meet or exceed the objectives, public information will have to be ongoing. This can be accomplished through speaking engagements, meeting with community groups, resident councils, and articles in papers for seniors. Additional projects may be to have a major newspaper do a human interest story, explaining the program and following a client. These and other avenues will be pursued with our public information assistant. In the 1980 budget, hopefully, more monies will be allocated for public information.

In working with seniors, a constant reminder of our existence and services needs to be done. Even with much advanced publicity and with reminding people of the program through newspaper articles and bulletins, many of our people say they have never heard of the program. Others have heard of it but have felt they could only come if they did not have a physician. Also, many people may not need our care, or they are not sure of what we have to offer. So periodic reminders of the Serving Seniors Program will be done.

A great amount of work still needs to be done to fully develop the program and reach out to more seniors. Research is definitely a must for the future. With these exciting thoughts and all the positive strokes received from clients, my enthusiasm and excitement keep growing.

SUMMARY

In doing this chapter, I reflected on the impact of my education and life experiences and how these affected my nursing practice. My philosophies of wellness and working with the horizontal and vertical powers helped me to implement health care ideas. Using the internal power within the client and myself, the horizontal power of community groups, and the vertical power of the community health care agency and the board that influences the policy of the Serving Seniors Program, I am able to effect change. With all the frustrations of a new program, having a framework of practice helped me to keep a perspective on accomplishments and problems, and it provided a practical way to begin to solve these problems.

REFERENCES

1. Dunn, Halbert: *High-Level Wellness*. Beatty, Arlington, Va., 1973.
2. Lippitt, Ronald, Watson, J., and Westley, B.: *The Dynamics of Planned Change*. Harcourt, Brace and World, New York, 1958.
3. Bennis, Warren: "Theory and Method in Applying Behavioral Science to Planned Organizational Change," in Bennis, W., Benne, K., and Chin, R. (eds.): *The Planning of Change*. Holt, Rinehart Winston, New York, 1969.
4. Chin, Robert, and Benne, K.: "General Strategies for Effecting Changes in Human Systems," in Bennis, W., Benne, K., and Chin, R. (eds.): *The Planning of Change*. Holt, Rinehart and Winston, New York, 1969.
5. Presthus, Robert: "Community Power Structure: Theoretical Framework," in Cox, F. et al. (eds.): *Strategies of Community Organization*. F. E. Peacock, Itasca, 1970.
6. Warren, Roland: *The Community in America*. Rand McNally, Chicago, 1973.
7. Perlman, R., and Gurin, A. :*Organization and Social Planning*. John Wiley and Sons, New York, 1972.
8. Waehtel, Dawn: "Structures of Communities and Strategies for Organization," in Cox, F. et al. (eds.): *Strategies of Community Organization*. F. E. Peacock, Itasca, 1970.

CHAPTER **45**

COMMUNITY HEALTH NURSING: A PERSONAL PERSPECTIVE

PHEBE GOLDMAN, B.S.N., P.H.N., R.N.

This chapter describes a personal view of public health nursing. My feelings, perceptions, and philosophy have been derived from my own experience. It is this experience that I am sharing in the following pages.

I completed my Bachelor of Science Degree in Nursing in 1970 at Columbia University in New York. My first introduction to community health nursing or public health nursing was as a student in my senior year. I was assigned to a Visiting Nurse Association office in the South Bronx. Prior to that experience I had identified medical-surgical nursing and pediatric nursing as my two primary areas of interest. The four months I spent in the South Bronx served to reaffirm my decision to work in a hospital and to confine myself to a specialized area within nursing.

I found most of what I was exposed to during that student experience in public health to be overwhelming. For a small town New England girl, the poverty with all its social, emotional, and cultural facets was frightening. Although the patients who were serviced by the hospital where I worked as a student came from this geographic area, I had never fully comprehended where they were from or where they were going back to. I can vividly remember walking the streets of the South Bronx laden down with dressing sets, patient records, and my black bag. On one side of the street might be a ten story apartment building vacant and boarded up. On the other side of the street there would be school aged children engrossed in a game of stick ball. Doorways and stoops were crowded with young adults with little to do and no place to go. It seemed everyone was high on something. It was totally foreign to anything I had known about life.

This aura of unreality and my shock with all that I saw was compounded by what I was expected to do. It seemed to me that public health nurses were expected to know something about everything. They had to understand all the pathology of cardiac conditions, for example. They also had to know what to say to new mothers when asked about such things as diaper rash. Not only that, they had to do all this alone. There was no accessible physician or head nurse to query. The wealth of knowledge and independence required were terrifying to me. It seemed impossible to imagine that I would ever function in such a setting.

In spite of all my anxiety, I managed to do well. At least my instructor felt the outward manifestation of my performance warranted a good grade. Of the families that I followed during that clinical rotation, I remember two. It is the relationship that I developed with those two people that I recall most clearly. At the time, I failed to grasp the importance of those relationships to myself or to those two patients. When I moved into public health, the process of relationship formation became the fulcrum of my nursing philosophy. I was not to see that for several years.

When I graduated I went to work on an orthopaedic ward of the hospital where I went to school. It was fun. It was challenging. I was busy with the personal care of patients, with medications, with preoperative and postoperative teaching, and with planning discharges. I moved to the pediatric orthopaedic ward and learned more about bones and lots about children. I had become confident with my skills as a nurse. I knew a lot about orthopaedics and a great deal more about myself.

After three years in the same hospital, on the same service, I decided I needed a change. I moved to Denver, Colorado on somewhat of a whim and started looking for work. There was an opening for a field nurse with the Denver Visiting Nurse Service. I wish I could say that I now felt ready for that challenge, or that public health was something I had always wanted to do. I remember reflecting that many of my classmates who had chosen public health were people I had admired for their maturity and intelligence. Here now was an opportunity to find out what attracted them to public health and a chance to overcome a fear of seeming ignorant and dependent. I took the job.

It was hard for me to describe the impact that first year in public health had on me as a person. It was a remarkable time. I probably grew more that year than I had in all my 20 odd years up to that point.

The first major task that I needed to accomplish was to evaluate my life style in terms of why I was doing what I was doing. I needed to define and clarify how I made choices and decisions for myself. Within that process lay the heart of what I felt I needed to be a good public health nurse. Could I relinquish my expectations of others to do what was right as defined by my value system? Could I examine other peoples' lives without judgment? It was paramount for me to be able to rid myself of judgment and of expectations of others if I was to facilitate my patients' achieving the goals they had chosen for themselves.

I received a tremendous amount of guidance and support from my supervisor as I explored my feelings related to many issues. It seemed that I would never be helpful to a mother fearful of abusing her child if I believed such behavior was aberrant. I needed to achieve some understanding of how such feelings could exist and then with that understanding intervene in a helpful, positive fashion. There was little hope of my affecting change with a schizophrenic client if my agenda was to get him back to work when he could not even get on a bus. No mother would listen to my suggestions about nutrition if she sensed my aversion to her unwashed children. No alcoholic client was going to stop drinking because the public health nurse thought it would be good for him.

It was a long struggle, working daily to confront feelings and judgments I had made about behaviors. It was an ongoing process through which I am still learning. Towards the end of that first year, I found it easier to understand and to know my patients. Without the interference of judgment or expectations, I began forming relationships with my patients that were meaningful to me and, I believe, to them as well. It was through those relationships that I saw people make changes. This then for me was how I began to define public health.

I believe the single most important function of a public health nurse is to be that of a facilitator. If the nurse can facilitate the patient in identifying his or her goals for the nurse-patient relationship, she has done the best possible job to insure compliance with the physician's plan of care, as well as the nurse's plan of care. When the nurse and the patient agree on the goals for the relationship, learning can take place. Changes can be made as a direct result of that relationship. The nurse can then facilitate the patient's understanding of his illness, his compliance with his treatment plan, his communication with his medical care source and his support systems, and his achieving what he wants for himself.

Facilitating all of the above is vastly important. None of it can be achieved without knowledge. My fears were confirmed that the public health nurse needs a broad knowledge of pathophysiology, pharmacology, mental health, growth and development, and maternal and child health. The public health nurse is in fact a generalist. Without a current updated base of knowledge, the nurse cannot effectively give care. The depth of knowledge required, however, depends on where the nurse's interest lies. The nurse may know enough about diabetes to deliver quality care but may have a strong desire to know all about the management of the terminally ill patient in the home. Therefore that nurse may have more expert knowledge of that particular type of patient. This flexibility within public health, the ability of the field to absorb a variety of nurses skilled in particular areas, is fascinating. The job skill remains that of a generalist, however.

As a generalist with a broad base of knowledge of nursing care, the public health nurse by necessity needs a wide variety of physical care skills. The nurse needs to be competent in making complete, thorough physical assessments. The nurse needs to be comfortable with all aspects of medical-surgical nursing. One of the challenges in this is the creativity demanded in providing care in the home. How does one devise good lighting to insert a urinary catheter? How does one elevate a bed? How does one give a bed bath where the mattress is on the floor? Which is the best colostomy appliance? Do egg cartons make the best setup to remind a patient to take his medication? In summary, how can the nurse best use what is found in the home to deliver safe, quality care? I find that demand on one's creativity exciting and challenging.

The ability of the nurse to identify problems is another important skill. In trying to weigh where it should fall in the spectrum of necessary skills, I believe it ranks with the skill of facilitator. To me, the essence of nursing is the ability to identify problems quickly and accurately.

When asked to make a home visit to a mother whose child is not gaining weight and is missing clinic appointments, the nurse needs to first identify the problems of the patient's perspective. What is the mother's understanding of nutrition? How available is food? What is the child like when he feeds? How much time does the mother have for feedings?

What other demands does the mother have on her time? Once the problem is clearly defined a nursing intervention can be chosen. The process of problem identification is ongoing, since the problem needs to be redefined on each visit. The nurse must see this as a primary focus of each visit in order to deliver effective care.

The development of a helping relationship can occur if the nurse is flexible, that is, if she can incorporate the patient's agenda into her treatment plan. The nurse must have a variety of counseling skills in her repertoire as well as a variety of bedside nursing skills. In order to carry out the treatment plan, the nurse needs good, independent judgment.

After a most inauspicious start in public health, I find myself immersed in the field. I find that for me it is the most satisfying way to deliver nursing care. Where once the broad spectrum of cases seemed overwhelming, now there is challenge in the variety. There is opportunity to expand all but the most technical nursing skills. I find that the skills I have developed over my five years in public health have easily been incorporated into my personal life and that I am a much richer person for it.

I have had the opportunity to explore and develop specific areas of interest within my caseload. At several points I conducted a variety of groups. There was a remotivational group for chronic schizophrenics that I led weekly in a boarding home. There I learned about setting short term day-to-day goals. I learned to cope with my own frustrations in not being able to make sweeping changes in people's lives. Later, I held a weekly group for pregnant women in a motel. There I learned about group process. I learned that the group members were often their own best resources. My answers were not always the best or most helpful ones. I learned a lot about the financial aspects and most common problems of child care. The last group I conducted was a weekly teaching and health screening group in a senior citizen highrise. There I learned about the resistance older people have to dependency. I learned how very important it is to leave them in control of their own lives as often as is feasible. I learned that most older people have a vast repertoire of survival skills that have brought them through life, and that these strengths are too infrequently tapped. The opportunity to explore my interests within the framework of public health has been exciting.

I find it hard to imagine working without the independence I now have. Where once it was frightening, now it is a major attraction for me in what I am doing. The management of my caseload is dependent on how I see the needs of any given individual in any given day. Changes in medical care plans are recommended to the physician, and it is my assessment of the situation that in most cases dictates the disposition of any problem.

The Denver Visiting Nurse Service is one of 40 agencies in the county that delivers nursing services via the Visiting Nurse Association and the County Public Health Department. The structure is complex at times and cumbersome in some ways. However, the collaboration between public and private sectors has resulted in an excellent response to community needs for nearly a century.

The basic premises of the Denver Visiting Nurse Service are that:

1. The Denver Visiting Nurse Service serves the individual, family, and community and recognizes the interrelatedness of these systems. The goal of the service is to assist the individual, family, and community to achieve and maintain a functional equilibrium.
2. Health care, the scientific body of knowledge, and the artful application of the

knowledge in aiding the consumer to achieve a health equilibrium is a right and of primary importance to the individual, family, and community.

3. Visiting Nurse Service serves a community need and since its support is derived from the public, it is accountable to the community for its service.
4. Visiting Nurse Service best meets the needs of the community by:
    a. Providing a family centered approach to health needs and individualized service to assist with special problems.
    b. Using a multidisciplinary approach in the delivery of health care.
    c. Serving people without distinction as to age, sex, race, creed, nationality, or political association.
    d. Charging fees to third party insurors, where applicable, for therapeutic care in the home; requiring persons who are financially able to pay for therapeutic care in the home, either in whole or in part (based on their ability to pay); and providing funds through governmental and other community resources for care for those patients who cannot afford to pay. There is no distinction in service between those who can and those who cannot pay.
    e. Recognizing the agency has an expertise in community health service, the agency accepts the responsibility to facilitate student learning.
    f. Developing appropriate contacts with community agencies when it benefits the service.
    g. Involving consumer groups in planning health programs.
    h. Identifying gaps in service areas, promoting use of existing resources, and co-ordinating services given to individual patients.
    i. Assuming responsibility in helping identify new models for service and professional practice in response to evolving needs of the individual, family, and the community.
5. Visiting Nurse Service can render the most effective and efficient service by:
    a. Providing a generalized home health service.
    b. Providing generalized service in clinic settings focused on the needs of the ambulatory patient and family.
    c. Providing specialized service where depth of knowledge in a given clinical area is vital to quality service.
    d. Providing services as resources will allow to function safely.
    e. Committing resources to staff development.
    f. Initiating and participating in research.

Funding for the Home Visiting Program comes from a variety of sources. Operational financing comes from patient revenues, i.e., Medicare, Medicaid, other third party insurors, health maintenance organizations, and direct patient payment. Other revenues for operational financing include: grants from the United Way, the State of Colorado, the federal government, and private sector. Also included are endowments, contributions, and interest and dividends from capital investments. Capital financing comes from the federal government, reserves, contributions, tax exempt revenue bonds, FHA insured mortgages, public taxable bonds, and conventional mortgage financing.

The Home Visiting Program, or Field Program of the Denver Visiting Nurse Service is only one aspect of public health nursing within the agency and within Denver. Routine outpatient care is provided through a system of Neighborhood Health Centers and Stations. Specialty clinics provide services to patients with tuberculosis, venereal diseases, and hypertension. Well-Child Clinics, Head Start Nurses, and on site health screening for senior citizens offer care to specific population groups within Denver. The Rocky Mountain Poison Control Center is staffed by public health nurses and offers a regional service. A marketing team keeps the community updated on all programs and assesses the community's needs for additional services on an ongoing basis.

Requests for home visits can be made from any of the above programs, private physicians, all of the hospitals within Denver, social workers, patients' families, friends and neighbors, nursing homes, the police department, mental health workers, and public health nurses themselves. The referral is processed at the central office and forwarded to one of the six field offices. Each field office serves a specific geographic area within Denver. The staffing and caseload of these offices is reflective of the needs of the population within that geographic area.

A variety of nursing services is provided to patients in their homes. Nurses meet requests for home evaluations from any concerned party. Of the 3500 individuals receiving home nursing care from the Denver Visiting Nurse Service, approximately 1000 are individuals with a diagnosed illness. In these cases the nurse provides direct physical care, does teaching related to the patient's illness, monitors and evaluates the progress of the patient's disease, and coordinates other health related services such as home health aides, physical therapy, occupational therapy, and speech therapy.

The remaining 2500 individuals open to service at any one time fall into several categories, the overall group known as Public Health Cases. Within the broad heading of mental health counseling fall the victims of sexual assault, patients who have attempted suicide, families of sudden infant death syndrome children, and mothers having difficulty coping with parenting. Services are provided to identified high risk mothers and infants in the postpartum period. Individuals with reported communicable diseases are followed for purposes of identifying contacts and monitoring symptoms. Teaching is done related to the prevention of the spread of disease and control of symptoms. As the incidence of reported child abuse and neglect has increased, so has that component of the public health nurse's caseload. Nurses follow these cases in conjunction with the Department of Social Services. In these cases it is important that the nurse carefully assesses the parents' perception of the problem. At times the parents are able to identify the difficulties within their role as parents and can utilize the nursing interventions offered. Where this occurs the result is that the parent is able to maintain or develop a safe environment for his child. Sometimes the nurse facilitates the parents' decision to relinquish their child. It is challenging and exciting to work within an agency whose philosophy of care encompasses so much of the community it serves.

Community needs are assessed by all program areas. Several new programs have been developed through such assessments. Expanded hours for service to patients receiving care in their homes were made available, resulting in the provision of bedside nursing care to patients until 9:00 p.m., seven days a week. Nurse practitioners do general health screening in 40 senior citizen highrises responding to a stated need.

The public health nurse out in the community is a valuable person in identifying community concerns. That nurse is the person who makes contact with, and is aware of, the community resources within her catchment area. It is the public health nurse who is most sensitive to the gaps in service provided to her own patients.

As the cost of hospital care has increased over the years, the consumer has become less able to bear the burden of chronic, debilitating disease. The care of people in their homes has expanded to lessen this financial burden. This is reflected by the total number of people referred by hospitals to the Denver Visiting Nurse Service, which has increased markedly within this past year. As the total numbers have increased, so have the number of very ill people being cared for at home, many of whom are receiving intravenous therapy and hyperalimentation therapy. Neonates with multiple congenital problems are being discharged to their parents' care with supporting and instructional assistance provided by the visiting nurse. More terminal patients are requesting to die at home with their families around them. These changes have meant that the public health nurse expand her already diversified skills to meet the new demands of her caseload.

My office, located in the southwest area of Denver, services the large geographic area of Denver. Service is provided to all age groups within this area, although infants and mothers, preschool age children, school age children, and people over 55 make up the preponderance of the caseload. Adolescents and young adults make up only a small percent of the caseload, except in instances of sexual assault, diagnosed mental illness, or pregnancy.

The proportion of the cases by sex within the oldest and youngest population groups is fairly equal. There are more females receiving service within the adolescent and young adult groups.

The largest minority group within the southwest area of Denver is Spanish-American. There are few blacks and an increasing number of Vietnamese and Koreans. The caseload is reflective of this distribution.

Although income levels within this geographic area vary greatly from those who are destitute to the very wealthy, the majority of the population is low income. Most people live in single family dwellings. There are six senior citizen highrises. There is one public housing project and a large variety of rental housing.

The southwest office is housed in the basement of a small, private office building. Unlike many of the other field offices, there is no clinic facility on site. The office is comfortable and located in the center of our service area, facilitating travel to patients' homes.

When a case is referred to the southwest office, it is assigned to one of the two teams within the office. If the care requested is predominately counseling, it is then delegated by the team leader to one of the public health nurses.

The public health nurse makes an initial visit to assess the patient's physical, emotional, environmental, and social needs as she perceives them and as the patient perceives them. The nurse then establishes a care plan based on the identified problems. By negotiating with the patient, appropriate interventions for the most important problems are identified. On subsequent visits the nurse evaluates the effectiveness of each intervention suggested or implemented, and reassesses the status of each individual problem, resulting in revisions or additions to the original plan. The nurse and the patient examine and evaluate the effectiveness of their relationship on an ongoing basis. Progress towards the mutual goals is assessed on every visit. At the point when patient identified problems and nurse identified problems have been resolved, the process of terminating the relationship begins. During this phase the nurse assists the patient to maintain the progress achieved to date.

Patient progress as well as problems in making progress is communicated to the referring source. The decision to dismiss the patient from service is also relayed to the individual who requested the visiting nurse's involvement.

During the course of a patient's admission to the Visiting Nurse Service, the public health nurse establishes the frequency of visits needed to accomplish agreed upon goals. In setting the interval between visits, she takes into account the needs of her entire caseload. This fluctuates with the demands of the team's work. A public health nurse may have 45 to 90 families open to service at any one time.

When difficulties arise with identifying a patient's problems or establishing appropriate interventions, the case may be presented at the weekly team meeting. At these meetings conducted by the team leader, the most difficult or puzzling cases are discussed, with team members assisting the nurse presenting the case to clarify her concerns. Often role playing is utilized to assist the nurse in achieving a better understanding of the patient's problem. Once the problem is clearly identified, interventions are suggested by team members. In subsequent meetings, the team assists the nurse who presented the case to evaluate the progress toward her goals. As individuals within the team have a variety of strengths and areas of interest, this format can be particularly helpful in establishing a viable plan of care. Nurses also have the option to utilize their weekly individual conference time with their supervisor to accomplish the same thing. Clinical specialists in mental health nursing, medical-surgical nursing, maternal-child health nursing, occupational therapy, physical therapy, communicable disease, and social work are available to all staff. The clinical specialists provide in-service education for the general agency in their given specialty. They also utilize their expertise in making demonstration home visits with nurses where their knowledge, skills, and abilities add depth and quality to patient care. Through the team process, direct supervision, and the clinical specialist staff, there is a broad base of support and expertise available to the public health nurse making home visits.

I have learned something in each of the cases I have followed as a public health nurse, but I remember one case with particular fondness. Mr. C was referred to my office and assigned to me by my team leader. The referral from the local general hospital identified that Mr. C was an alcoholic with tuberculosis, chronic obstructive pulmonary disease, and a mass in his chest. The referring physician requested the patient return to the outpatient department for followup x-rays of his chest. He also requested that the public health nurse assist the patient in getting help for his drinking problem and difficulties with his finances.

On my initial visit I found Mr. C nervous and unable to maintain eye contact, but he responded easily to my questions. He looked tired with circles under his eyes. His breath smelled of alcohol. He explained to me that he was only drinking beer, and this wasn't the same thing as wine or hard liquor. He was receptive to help to stop drinking. He had stopped all of his tuberculosis medications and denied any respiratory symptoms. He was unaware of the reported chest mass. He was anxious to find work as he had many bills. He lived with his wife of 17 years and his 15-year-old stepson in a roomy attic apartment.

From that first home visit the problems broke down in order of priority to:

Nurse Identified Problems
1. Mr. C. unaware of lung mass.

2. Mr. C drinking with inaccurate information regarding alcohol content of beer.
3. Not taking tuberculosis medications.
4. Unemployed with financial stress.

Patient Identified Problems
1. No prior knowledge of lung mass with resulting fear.
2. Asking for help to stop drinking.

3. Wants to find job.

In light of the fact that Mr. C and I saw the problems in much the same way with the same order of priority, establishing the initial care plan was fairly simple. In order to handle his concern and the physician's concern about the undiagnosed lung mass, I instructed him where and when to go for followup treatment.

His drinking problem was more difficult to pin down. By providing him with information about the alcohol content of beer, we got closer to defining what "to stop drinking" meant to him. I described my role as a public health nurse, my willingness to help him, and the limitations of my job. I encouraged him to express and identify his concerns and supported his attempts to do so. I then set up our next visit for five days later.

During that first visit interventions consisted of:

1. Providing information.
   a. About his lung mass.
   b. About the alcohol content of beer.
2. Describing the public health nursing role.
3. Expressing concern and willingness to offer help.
4. Supporting and encouraging Mr. C to identify his own concerns.

Over the next several visits the process of defining the patient's problems continued. Mr. C's primary concern was his inability to stop drinking. In order for him to find work, take his tuberculosis medications, and to feel better about himself he needed to dry out. I visited weekly. I hoped to show him that my presence week after week was an investment in him as a person, and that I cared about what happened to him. I never stayed more than half an hour. We focused on what his life had been like without alcohol. He was able to identify some personal strengths that had helped him through difficult times in the past. If on any visit he was incoherent, I would leave telling him I would return.

During those first few weeks Mr. C tried to stop drinking on his own. It was a difficult time for him with many ups and downs. He was refusing help from Alcoholics Anonymous or from Medical Detoxification. After one month of making little headway when I visited Mr. C and found him drunk, I felt discouraged and depressed. My efforts to identify his strengths to support his efforts to stop drinking and to encourage him to explore the reasons for his drinking were getting us nowhere. I decided to try a different tactic. I explained to Mr. C that I cared about what happened to him. I told him it made me sad to see him this way. I stated that drying out was something he couldn't do alone, and that I was going to take him to the Detoxification Unit at the County Hospital. To my amazement he agreed and we got on the bus together and traveled the few blocks to the County Hospital where I delivered him to the Detoxification Unit staff.

I am not sure what I would have done had he refused my offer to take control. It did work, however. When he called me several days later to say he had been discharged, I went right out. When I saw him I found I was pleased and proud of what he had done. We talked about what it had been like for him and where he wanted to go now. Helping him to set realistic goals was my next task. He set several manageable short term goals:

1. Stay sober
2. Look for work
3. Get out of the house every day
4. Start taking tuberculosis medications

In order to stay sober he decided he needed more support than my weekly visits. Alcoholics Anonymous was something he was willing to try. In order to find work he decided he needed a specific skill. I helped him get into a vocational rehabilitation program. He liked to read the paper so that if he went out to buy it daily, he would get out of the house. He saw no problem in remembering to take his tuberculosis medications, but allowed me to make a chart to help him to not forget.

During the next month as I visited Mr. C, I kept reflecting on his overall progress. We talked about how he could identify situations that might start him drinking again. Drinking was his way of dealing with his anger. We would role play situations that before had led to his drinking. I would be Mr. C and he would play the other person. These visits were exciting for him. He would always be waiting for me, eager to tell me about a new situation that he'd thought of, wanting to see what possible solution I could come up with. We would always review what had gone on the visit before. Gradually he was able to think of his own solutions to the situations he presented.

It was fun to see Mr. C every week. I was pleased with how things were going. He had passed an exam and was now working as a T.V. repairman. He was attending Alcoholics Anonymous once a week, and going daily to get his Antabuse. He was neat and clean. He was taking his tuberculosis medications correctly. He was pleased with his own progress and was able to tell me on every visit what he had accomplished the previous week. Our visits were productive and positive. I boasted to my team mates of my success and started planning to dismiss Mr. C from my caseload.

It had been six months since my first visit when I climbed the familiar three flights to his apartment. I could hear banging around in his apartment. The sounds were unusual. Then I heard a crash. I stopped. It couldn't be possible that he was drinking again. When he opened the door and I saw him drunk and disheveled, it was all I could do not to cry! We talked briefly, and I told him I would come back when he was sober. I told him of my sadness at seeing him drinking and that things must be very bad for him.

I vividly remember my hurt and anger. It was difficult not to personalize what had happened. It seemed impossible to go back and start from the beginning. However, that is what eventually happened. I followed him for another six months going through the same process. It worked as well the second time around.

I chose to present Mr. C not only to show how I identified nursing interventions to deal with the presenting problems but also to show that personal involvement and investment in a relationship make that process happen. Disappointment, hurt, and frustration were my measures of investment in Mr. C, as much as my pleasure with his successes. Helping him to establish a trusting relationship with me made the process of identifying the problems easier and made selection and utilization of interventions simpler.

Community health nursing is the setting for me where this process can occur. An individual's chance for coping seems better in a familiar environment, where support systems in the form of friends, family, and community agencies are more readily accessible. When health care is taken to the patient, it is implied that he is important, that health care providers care enough to create a system sensitive to his needs. Outreach in the form of home visiting has the capacity to quickly identify illness, to prevent hospitalization, and to maintain general health.

CHAPTER **46**

THE AHEC NURSE AS A COMMUNITY EDUCATOR*

BARBARA JO McGRATH, M.N., R.N., AND THERESE G. LAWLER, M.S.N., R.N.

Little did we imagine that when we began functioning as faculty in Area Health Education Centers (AHEC) over three years ago that we would be forging out a possible new role for nurses. Challenge and innovation in the AHEC system initially attracted us to the outreach positions, this coupled with a budding belief in its potential. That potential has grown into a reality where nursing education plays a vital part, touching the professional lives of nurses heretofore isolated from academic support systems.

With the opening of an expansive new vista of opportunity comes not only challenge but also responsibility. So it was with AHEC. The challenge was, indeed, inviting and the responsibility awesome. We found ourselves assuming the office of change agents in a nursing milieu which was impoverished in many ways.

The nurses in the sandhills and coastal plains of North Carolina viewed themselves as isolated, as poor in resources, and as often divorced from collegial relationships and formal learning situations. This view becomes clear when one understands the geographic and demographic characteristics of the area. North Carolina is the third most rural state in the country. Per capita income is $3208 (1973), well below the poverty standard. Approximately 24 percent of the population is nonwhite.[1] As far as health care manpower is concerned, much of the state is underserved by poor physician and nurse to

*This paper is a result of work supported by the North Carolina Area Health Education Centers Program, 1978.

761

citizen ratios. The eastern part of North Carolina is even more disadvantaged when its health indices are compared to those of the more industrialized piedmont areas. Traditional problems of maldistribution of primary care providers and inaccessibility of medical services have placed a real burden on those who have been practicing in this region.

In nursing, these issues were accentuated by the provincial nature of an inbred educational system. Historically until the late 1960s, few educational and training initiatives were mounted in the regions served by the AHECs. Prior to the advent of the AHEC program, there had been gradual strengthening of the regional universities accompanied by a steady increase in the number of baccalaureate nursing graduates. It was into this setting that the Area Health Education Centers came to attempt to remedy the problems stemming from an indigenous weakness in nursing education which impacted on clinical practice.

Nothing in our background as nursing educators seemed to make us ideally suited for this new role as community outreach nurses or as advocates of our constituencies. We are products of generic baccalaureate programs, we practiced in the field of maternal-child health and then returned to pursue master's degrees. After completion of graduate studies we taught in two separate campuses of the University of North Carolina system. McGrath's background includes working as a staff nurse in various pediatric inpatient settings ranging from community hospital to medical center. She is the Director of Nursing Education in the Fayetteville AHEC. Lawler has worked in hospital and health department settings primarily in the area of maternal-child health and has been involved in the planning of the state's regional perinatal program. She was the Associate Director of Nursing Education in the Eastern AHEC and is currently on academic leave.

Fortified by the excitement of participating in making a new concept work and bolstered by confidence that only "old hands" wear, we began carving out new nursing roles. The need was great and one of the glories of AHEC was that it was freely a systems approach to meet that need. It is a flexible system and one that encourages experimentation.

HISTORY OF THE CONCEPT OF AHEC AND THE NORTH CAROLINA AHEC PROGRAM

The Carnegie Commission on Higher Education's 1970 report on medical and dental education recommended Area Health Education Centers (AHECs) as one means of providing specialized health care to those people not within reasonable reach of a university health science center. Each AHEC would revolve around a community hospital or group of hospitals, and the educational programs within the AHEC would be affiliated with a university health science center. The AHECs would train medical and dental students and medical residents on a rotational basis; provide continuing education opportunities for local physicians, dentists, nurses, and other health care personnel; cooperate with local health authorities and hospitals; assist community colleges and comprehensive colleges in training allied health personnel; and in other ways improve health care in the area.[2] In the Commission's view, the AHECs would thus bring most of the local advantages of a health science center into localities that were not large enough for full scale centers.

A year after the Commission's report, the Comprehensive Health Manpower Training Act of 1971 authorized Area Health Education Center contracts to educate health personnel at locations where health needs were greatest. In October of 1972, 11 medical schools and university health science centers contracted with the Bureau of Health Manpower Education at the National Institutes of Health (now the Bureau of Health Manpower, Health Resources Administration) to set up Area Health Education Centers.

The University of North Carolina School of Medicine at Chapel Hill was awarded a five year $8.5 million federal contract on October 1, 1972, to develop three AHECs in Charlotte, Wilmington, and Area L (Edgecombe, Halifax, Nash, Wilson, and North Hampton Counties). The potential for health manpower development demonstrated by these three centers led to the adoption of a statewide plan for health professional education by the Board of Governors of the University of North Carolina in October 1973. This plan called for a network of nine AHECs in partnership with the other medical centers in the state.

In 1974, the General Assembly accepted this plan and appropriated $28.5 million to strengthen and expand the AHEC program. The appropriation included $4.7 million for program operations and the development of new primary care residency positions and $23.5 million for the construction or renovation of health education facilities at each of the proposed nine AHECs. In 1975, the General Assembly reaffirmed its commitment to the long term security of the statewide network of AHECs by appropriating an additional $2.8 million for program operations.

Before the federal AHEC contract was received, 50 percent of the funding for the program came from the individual hospital in which the program was offered and state appropriations provided the other 50 percent. Now funding is roughly 75 percent state, 15 percent federal, and 10 percent local.

With a population of 5 million, North Carolina ranks 38th in per capita income and is one of the most rural states in the nation. Of the 100 counties, 34 are 100 percent rural and another 50 are at least 50 percent rural. There are only 4 towns with a population greater than 100 thousand. These are hardly the characteristics which attract young, enthusiastic, and energetic physicians, dentists, nurses, and other health manpower to a community to practice. In some areas of the state there is no physician within a 30 mile radius of a given community. In other areas physicians are available, but the ratio might be one physician per 3000 people. The statistics are similar for other health care personnel.

The North Carolina Area Health Education Centers (AHEC) program is a major statewide effort to decentralize medical, dental, pharmacy, and public health education, and to regionalize nursing and allied health education, residency training, and continuing education for all health practitioners in order to improve the geographic and specialty distribution of health manpower throughout the state. The North Carolina AHEC program is under the leadership of the School of Medicine of the University of North Carolina at Chapel Hill, in partnership with its sister schools of Dentistry, Nursing, Pharmacy, and Public Health, the Duke University Medical Center, the Bowman Gray School of Medicine, and the School of Medicine at East Carolina University.

The goals of the AHEC program are:

1. To improve the professional environment in each of the 100 counties of North Carolina by decreasing the professional isolation for practitioners through student, resident, and continuing education programs conducted on regional and local levels.
2. To train students, interns, and residents in community practice settings so as to increase the likelihood of their settling in the community.

4. To improve the coordination of training for nursing and allied health professionals on a regional basis so as to avoid duplication of training efforts while training manpower needed by the service institutions.

All nine AHECs mandated by the General Assembly of North Carolina are now operating as a statewide network. Each AHEC is a community hospital or a legally incorporated foundation representing one or more hospitals which agrees to accept the responsibility for health manpower development programs in a several county area. These programs span the continuum of education for a variety of health professionals in a manner which reflects regional needs while focusing on primary care. As such, the program represents a fundamental commitment by the community hospitals to work closely with health service and health educational institutions throughout their multicounty service area to develop educational programs for practicing health personnel, for university health science students on rotation, and for allied health and nursing students based in the region.

Each AHEC has a director and a cadre of university faculty. As of January 1, 1977, there were 50 full time medical school faculty based in the nine AHECs along with 30 full time faculty in other health disciplines. The AHECs are now supporting and training health personnel for nearly all counties in North Carolina.

From a geographic standpoint, the Eastern AHEC is the largest of the nine constituent AHECs comprising the North Carolina Area Health Centers Program. This AHEC, organized in mid-1974, serves the predominantly rural counties of Beaufort, Bertie, Camden, Carteret, Chowan, Craven, Currituck, Dare, Gates, Greene, Hertford, Hyde, Jones, Lenoir, Martin, Onslow, Pasquotank, Pamlico, Perquimans, Pitt, Tyrrell, Washington, and Wayne. (See Fig. 46-1).

The administrative offices are located adjacent to the Pitt County Memorial Hospital in Greenville, North Carolina, a tobacco town of approximately 30,000 people. Selected centralized services are provided by these offices, but most programming is accomplished on a decentralized basis throughout the region. Greenville is the seat of a young, growing East Carolina University, which is the primary affiliate for the AHEC. The University Division of Health Affairs with its Schools of Nursing, Medicine, and Allied Health serves as resource base.

The Fayetteville AHEC, also organized in mid-1974, serves nine counties in the south central region of the state: Bladen, Cumberland, Harnett, Hoke, Moore, Richmond, Robeson, Sampson, and Scotland. (See Fig. 46-1). The AHEC offices are located across the street from the largest of two county hospitals in the most populated county in the area, Cumberland County. The city is Fayetteville, often described as a military town because Fort Bragg, a large Army base, is located 10 miles away. The population of Fayetteville is approximately 60,000. The Fayetteville AHECs primary university affiliation is Duke University Medical Center which is 75 miles from Fayetteville.

CLINICAL PRACTICE – BEFORE AHEC

It seems necessary to set the stage for the reader by describing some elements apparent in clinical nursing practice in rural North Carolina in the decade between 1963 and 1973. By establishing a conceptual baseline, changes brought about by AHEC intervention may be clarified and more readily appreciated.

Diploma nursing programs had long served the region. They were based in small private and municipal hospitals. The programs were devoted to immediate community need.

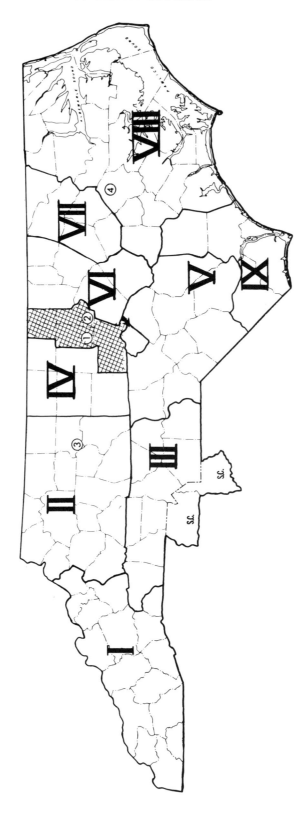

FIGURE 46-1. Counties served by the North Carolina Area Health Education Centers Program: I. Mountain; II. Northwest; III. Charlotte; IV. Greensboro; V. Fayetteville; VI. Raleigh; VII. Area L; VIII. Eastern; IX. Wilmington; ▦ affiliation undetermined. Location of University Medical Centers: 1. U.N.C. at Chapel Hill; 2. Duke; 3. Bowman Gray; 4. East Carolina University.

There was uneven quality among them, and they not only used the medical model for training, but also they were fairly well controlled by medicine. While vestiges of paternalism remained in the 1960s in other geographic locations, it was rampant in these isolated areas. Nurses were still viewed as servile, provincial, and dependent practitioners. One must remember that North Carolina did not even have a mandatory Nurse Practice Act on the books until 1965.

Students were socialized to fit the mold, reinforced by older nurses who had been trained in the same classrooms and on the same wards. Almost all the enrollees in a nursing program were indigenous to the community and never left home during their student days. Indeed there was an inadequate learning experience for a number of nursing students utilizing the traditional clinical models. Many faculty, also, within the programs were often ill prepared and had few resources to call upon.

There were few baccalaureate or master's prepared clinical models. Local health agencies did not understand the different levels of nursing practice, and even if it was understood there was great reluctance to pay for the difference. The universities which did have degree programs were far removed and had a dubious policy of keeping their students close to the scholastic breast. Few students left academe for field experiences. Never having been exposed to the pastoral delights of rural living, these graduates naturally did not elect to practice in the underserved communities. In addition there was a lack of attractive professional features to lure practitioners away from the cosmopolitan centers into the rural countryside to work.

There was as well little opportunity for continuing education aside from self-directed learning. Even inservice programming was weak or frequently nonexistent in the smaller hospitals and health departments. Although there began a gradual assimilation of nursing education programs by the community colleges and regional universities, activities by necessity centered on the generic curriculum. Continuing education offerings were sponsored by the health science centers which were 100 miles away or more. There was, too, essentially no consultation or technical assistance routinely available to the nursing administrators in the health agencies. No one helped with needs assessments, with problem solving, or with identifying suitable resources—unless a request was channeled to one of the large teaching centers. This frequently began a costly, time consuming process which yielded solutions more altruistic than pragmatic. Many of the nursing leaders in towns perhaps 20 miles apart did not even know each other, which certainly compounded their professional isolation.

The state of nursing practice suffered from a regional lack of coordination and cohesion. It suffered because no one fulfilled an advocacy role. It suffered because there existed no educational support system for the nurses who were providing health care for the citizenry of rural eastern North Carolina.

NURSING INTERVENTIONS AND CLINICAL PRACTICE NOW

To meet the long range goals of the North Carolina AHEC system, each of the nine constituent units has established objectives of decentralizing and regionalizing health personnel education. The central aspiration of the program is to change the ambience of the professional climate so that skilled practitioners in all the disciplines will be retained and additional personnel will be encouraged to move into these regions.

Nursing in our two AHECs set about the task of professional "climate control" by identifying expected program outcomes and by selecting appropriate methodologies to achieve the desired results. Specifically, programmatic endeavors have focused on continuing education, clinical education and technical assistance, and consultative activities. Objectives were formulated which address these issues:

1. To plan, promote, and conduct continuing education programs by means of lectures, symposia, workshops for all—based on assessed needs.
2. To assist health care agencies in delivering quality inservice educational programs to meet community needs.
3. To support and assist in the development of a Family Nurse Practitioner Program to be operated in concert with the existing North Carolina programs.
4. To develop training rotations for students in all levels of nursing education through use of community hospitals, physicians' offices, clinics, centers, and health agencies in the region as an integral part of their curricula.
5. To allocate funds and offer technical assistance for the planning and construction of additions, renovations, or alterations of community hospitals for educational purposes. These improvements might include conference rooms, classrooms, on-call rooms for students, libraries, offices for inservice education directors. They would then serve as community learning centers for interagency utilization.
6. To offer technical assistance and consultation to health care personnel.[3]

We decided immediately that it was necessary to have a high profile among our constituents. Increased visability of the AHEC nurses, accomplished by direct personal contact with the nursing leaders in the communities we served, established liaison between the practicing constituency and the educational institutions, especially the AHEC. We were most interested in forging strong linkages. Furthermore, we insured initial credibility by implementing continuing education offerings as quickly as possible after completion of the needs assessment. Programming was designed to be relevant to the perceived problems in patterns of care and nursing practice in the eastern regions.

Assessment of Educational Needs in the Fayetteville AHEC

Since the AHEC nurse is responsible for meeting the educational needs of *all* the nurses in a specified area, the assessment of these needs can be quite an undertaking. Many of the North Carolina AHEC nurses have assessed education needs through the use of a survey followed by selected interviews. I (McGrath) sent an assessment tool (Appendix A) to the director of nursing in each hospital, health department, and nursing home in my area. Upon receipt of the completed assessment tools, I made an appointment with each director of nursing and asked that the person responsible for inservice education be present if possible. I used this interview to learn more about the agency, the number of nurses employed, the extent of inservice and continuing education offered at the agency or nearby, and to give the director of nursing and inservice director an opportunity to expand the information given on the completed assessment tool. I was particularly interested in establishing priority of need and level of instruction.

I recognized that the needs expressed by the director of nursing for the nurses he or she directed might not be the actual felt needs of the staff nurses themselves. Therefore, I obtained a list of all licensed nurses in each region from the North Carolina Board of Nursing. The same survey tool was sent to a random sample of these nurses. It was encouraging to learn that the needs identified by the directors were similar to those identified by the individual nurses.

Once I had made an initial contact with each agency and once the nurses became familiar with the kinds of learning experiences available through AHEC, most of the nurses in the region voluntarily made their needs known. I soon had more requests for learning experiences than could be filled.

As can be expected, some nurses were more sophisticated in expressing their needs than others. Some agencies were also able to express their needs more clearly and precisely. It is much easier for the AHEC nurse to meet the expressed needs, but she must be careful not to use all the budgetary resources to meet the needs of only a select few. Some nurses and some agencies need considerable assistance in identifying learning needs and expressing them clearly. For example, in my AHEC region, one agency requested a workshop on patient teaching. Since there are numerous aspects of patient teaching which can be taught, I had to help the inservice instructor pinpoint the specific needs of the nurses she was serving.

Many needs were identified at once, but the meeting of needs began more slowly. I started in one or two counties. When some needs had been met there, I moved on to meet the needs in the other counties.

Each AHEC nurse has spent considerable time and energy explaining what AHECs can and cannot do. At first many hospital administrators and other health professionals thought that AHEC merely provided funds for whatever sort of education they decided to offer. AHEC funding for continuing education is extremely limited. The bulk of the funding is used to support primary care residencies in North Carolina. When funds are used for continuing education, it is only after a proposal has been submitted to AHEC and usually AHEC requires the requesting agency to invest either funds or other resources in the project.

Educational offerings are not provided free of charge. Most of the AHEC nurses believe that education is not free. We realize that although considerable funding was needed to propel the initial program, the continuing education aspect is to eventually become self-supporting. Registration fees are kept to a minimum, but the nurses are learning that they must be financially responsible for their own education.

Assessment of educational needs is kept current by periodic meetings with directors of nursing and inservice educators and by surveying nurses who attend the various education offerings. Each year each AHEC nurse writes a set of workstatements (Appendix B) or a proposal of work to be accomplished during the next year. A budget is then drawn to meet these workstatements and submitted with the rest of the AHEC budget. Each AHEC budget is reviewed, revised, and approved each year. The budget approval depends on the availability of state and federal funds.

Continuing Education in the Eastern AHEC

Programming across the specialties in continuing education in the eastern AHEC has been based on sound principles of adult education including the concepts of formal needs assessments, consumer planning input, and participative learning/teaching strategies. We (Lawler and other eastern AHEC faculty) have taken offerings out on a rotating subregional basis assuring accessibility even to the geographically remote health care agencies. Linkages between the AHECs and community professional and voluntary organizations have been encouraged through the mechanism of cosponsorship. We had a total of 37 other organizations or institutions closely involved in program implementation during the years 1975-77 and many of these units participated in more than one educational event. Faculty for the continuing education offerings have been recruited from a diversity of academic and practice settings. A substantial number of the guest presenters served as instructors for several workshops or short courses in their area of expertise. The eastern AHEC professional staff also contributed many hours of direct teaching time within each person's area of competence and concentration on topics of special interest.

Because of its flexibility, the AHEC system encourages experimentation to meet regional and disciplinary continuing education needs. Indeed, in nursing it has allowed the innovator in some of us to surface unfettered. We have had the opportunity to pursue nontraditional models of continuing education programming. Some of the new directions have included:

1. Establishing contractual arrangements with a specific university or school of nursing to serve as prime affiliate and academic support. East Carolina University Schools of Medicine, Nursing and Allied Health serve eastern AHEC. Duke University Medical Center serves the Fayetteville AHEC.

2. Replicating learning experiences on a rotating basis so that each participant group is small, dialogue is encouraged, and institutional needs can be met more efficiently. A young neonatologist from a teaching center and one of the AHEC nurses presented a program on newborn assessment, stabilization, and transport. It was $6^1/2$ hours in length and was repeated 9 times. Similar formats were used for "Hypertension Screening," "POMR and the Nursing Process," "Management of the Stroke Patient," and "Designing Patient Care Plans."

3. Utilizing the thematic vs. "one-shot" approach: Since many of the nurses are unable to leave their families or places of employment for more than a day at a time, offerings were designed to be broken into learning segments. Some ran in three four-hour blocks for eight weeks, e.g., "Introduction to Physical Assessment," "Patient Care Management." Others were structured for one full day a month for several months, e.g., "Leadership Skills for the Head Nurse," "New Concepts of Maternal Health."

4. Training local nurses to function as trainers in a specific competency area: One highly successful project was the 80 hour course for cardiovascular preceptors formulated by the North Carolina Task Force on Cardiovascular Nursing and sponsored by EAHEC and FAHEC. Sixteen experienced CCU nurses from community hospitals spent two weeks reviewing teaching methods and advanced care protocols. They in turn taught 40 hour Basic Coronary Care Courses, using a standardized curriculum, to staff members in their own and proximal hospitals. These basic courses have been repeated over a $2^1/2$ year span. This has provided the area with many more qualified coronary care nurses than ever before.

5. Designing self-instructional learning packages complete with audiovisual software to be passed on from community to community and shared by the staff of health departments, hospitals, and nursing homes. Nurses have been able to improve the quality of care delivered to patients even when a formal learning experience was not available.

6. Instituting out-reach or extension credit courses for nurses wishing to matriculate for a baccalaureate degree. This is still a large, unmet need which calls for an expansion of out-reach programming.

7. Building in quality assurance by channeling the offerings through the approval process of both the universities for the granting of Continuing Education Units (CEUs) and the North Carolina Nurses' Association for the granting of recognition points (CERPs). Standards set by both accrediting bodies are scrupulously adhered to. This also begins to pave the way should mandatory continuing education for re-licensing become a reality in North Carolina.

8. Setting up learning centers in each community to be used by all health disciplines and agencies. Many of the centers were constructed with AHEC funds, others were renovated and remodeled. All were given an extensive package of audiovisual hardware teaching models and library materials. Software is kept in a central repository on campus and can be requested by phone and available within two days. Student use of the learning center facilities has been strongly encouraged.

Clarification might be enhanced for the reader by an overview of descriptive data related to provision of Continuing Nursing Education through eastern AHEC in the year 1976. It may be well to keep in mind that prior to the advent of EAHEC (1975), little or no continuing education was available to eastern North Carolina nurses on a local basis. In 1976, however, there were 235 offerings, accounting for a full 19.4 percent of the state total. Instruction hours totaled 1037 and participants numbered 4438, which was 13.2 percent of the active nurses in North Carolina.[4] All of this was accomplished with one full-time and one-half time faculty and many borrowed faculty from affiliated schools and institutions.

Evaluations of continuing education programming have been largely subjective with some cognitive pretesting and posttesting and a smattering of instrumentation to measure effective change. Appraisal by our nursing peers has been honest, thoughtful, helpful, and overwhelmingly positive. AHEC indeed seems an ideal vehicle to deliver continuing education to nurses on a regional basis.

Nurse Practitioner Education in AHEC

The lack of sufficient primary care providers in the rural area stimulated the formation of the North Carolina AHEC system. The main thrust of the program is to remedy that problem. Medicine has taken the approach of setting up residencies for family practice physicians in small communities—hoping to keep the young doctors there. Nursing, too, has proposed a solution, that of training indigenous nurses to function in an expanded role coinciding with a prevalent trend. This approach is especially well suited for the Coastal Plains.

The Nurse Practitioner Program at East Carolina University was developed and implemented through the collaborative efforts of the School of Nursing and the AHECs. The program is designed to prepare nurse practitioners in the areas of family, pediatric, adult, obstetric-gynecologic, and emergency care. The program enrolled its first class on October 6, 1975.

The purpose of the program is to prepare the nurse to expand her role as a member of the health team in the delivery of primary care in eastern North Carolina. Students are expected to augment their nursing knowledge and skills with preparation in the areas of medical diagnosis and treatment in accordance with the rules and regulations adopted by the North Carolina Board of Medical Examiners and the North Carolina Board of Nursing.

The North Carolina Practitioner Task Force Programs have developed a working definition for the nurse practitioner which seems to suit our aims. "Nurse practitioners are registered nurses who have completed a formal program of study which qualifies them to function with a combination of traditional nursing skills, such as counseling and teaching, and newly acquired medical skills, such as diagnosis and treatment. They are prepared to provide primary health care to patients, chiefly in ambulatory settings in collaboration with designated physicians who supervise their medical activities within established protocols of care."

The practice of nurse practitioners is oriented to the needs and concerns of consumers and includes preventive health maintenance as well as medical management. They use knowledge of the complex interplay of health, social, and economic factors to make personal interventions on behalf of patients and families and to use appropriate community agencies. Their concerns extend to the identification of the health needs of the entire community, and they contribute to the development of needed resources and programs.

Admissions to the program are handled through a committee mechanism. The Admissions Committee is composed of Nurse Practitioners Program faculty and representatives from the AHECs. Individual members are called upon to interview applicants and make site visits. The decision about admission of each applicant is made by the Committee as a whole based on established requirements and priorities. Both requirements and priorities for the admission process have been delineated and speak to regional need and proper utilization of the nurse as a primary care provider.

Requirements for admission are as follows:

1. The applicant must be a registered nurse.
2. A physician sponsor must agree to accept primary responsibility for precepting the student within the framework of his clinical practice during the clinical practice and preceptorship phase and to submit periodic evaluations of the student's practice to the Nurse Practitioner Program Director.
3. The practice site, which may be with the sponsoring physician or the health system within which he or she works, must agree to the conditions required during the clinical practice and preceptorship phase and to employ the nurse practitioner upon completion of the program.

Priorities for admission include:

1. Rural settings and a consideration of the geographic distribution of nurse practitioners within eastern North Carolina.
2. Practice sites where the role for which nurse practitioners are prepared can best be realized, namely, where nurse practitioners are allowed, under the supervision of a physician and within written medical guidelines, to make the kinds of decisions for which they are prepared.
3. Nurses with several years of clinical experience.
4. Nurses whose applications indicate potential for future leadership as nurse practitioners.

The curriculum is arranged in specific courses or modules which include Physical Assessment, Common Health Problems, Pediatric Care, Obstetric-Gynecologic Care, Adult

Health Care, and a Role-Change Seminar. Students may elect to take all courses to become a Family Nurse Practitioner or may concentrate in pediatric, OB-GYN, or adult care.

All students are required to take three core courses or modules: Physical Assessment, Common Health Problems, and the Role-Change Seminar. Students then elect the course(s) related to their area of practice to become Adult Nurse Practitioners (ANP), Pediatric Nurse Practitioners (PNP), or OB-GYN Nurse Practitioners. Family Nurse Practitioners (FNP) must take all courses. In addition, courses in emergency care and geriatric care are available as further electives.

The program requires full time study over a period of two to three academic semesters (nine to twelve months). The program for FNPs is three semesters or twelve months; the program for the specialty NPs is two semesters or nine months. The program of study involves two days per week of classroom instruction and three days per week of supervised clinical practice. The last three months of the program are spent in preceptorship which includes full time supervised clinical practice.

Academic credit is given for each course successfully completed. Before the student is granted a Nurse Practitioner Certificate, he or she must pass comprehensive examinations developed by the Statewide Task Force for Nurse Practitioner Programs in North Carolina.

One of the most unusual features of the three Nurse Practitioner Programs in North Carolina is that they operate in consortium, or as the Associate Director for Nursing Education from Mountain AHEC (MAHEC) so aptly phrases it, "with controlled diversity." Linkages to the AHEC System are strong, and in the east and west quite direct. The parent program (1970) resides in the School of Nursing at University of North Carolina at Chapel Hill. The "offspring" are at East Carolina (EAHEC), and Asheville (MAHEC). The description of the evolution of the Statewide Task Force by the Dean at University of North Carolina, Chapel Hill School of Nursing seems the best precis of the process.

"North Carolina is unique in having a successful statewide effort in the planning, coordination and implementation of nurse practitioner preparation. In the summer of 1974, representatives of interested faculty of East Carolina University School of Nursing (ECU) and the School of Nursing at the University of North Carolina at Chapel Hill (UNC-CH) met as a task force to discuss the development of the Nurse Practitioner Program at ECU. Shortly thereafter, Mountain Area Health Education Center (MAHEC) and Western Carolina University Department of Nursing (WCU) joined the task force. Initial concerns focused on the need to assure a common base level of clinical competence for all nurse practitioners practicing in the state regardless of the program in which they were prepared. At subsequent meetings, a common core of concepts basic to the preparation of nurse practitioners was agreed upon. It was recognized, however, that diversity of modalities of implementation was necessary to maintain local autonomy and insure that the programs would meet regional needs and objectives.

Our work as a group has been consistent with the principles of the newly consolidated university mandate, and the AHEC system, i.e., decentralization of programs to achieve regional objectives and collaboration among regional centers. There has been consistent sharing of ideas, materials, and resources among the programs and we have found considerable strength in our informal task force. We have experienced collective achievement toward common goals in the development and conduct of regionalized nurse practitioner training."[5]

While there is diversity among the various programs, quality is the central theme. The product of these programs is the same, the nurse practitioner.

Besides contributing teaching time in various courses and committee work, the AHEC nurse has brokered many of the clinical matches between students and preceptors. This seems to be a natural role because of familiarity with manpower needs and possible resources. As a result of joint efforts the program has produced over 30 more primary care providers who live and work in eastern North Carolina. From that vantage point alone it has been a highly successful venture.

Clinical Education of Nursing Students

The clinical education component of AHEC activities focuses on placement of nursing students in varied field experiences from which mutual benefit for student and agency will accrue. AHEC faculty assist in coordination of placements and in efficient "matching" of student to clinical facility.

Clinical rotations in nursing occur on multivaried levels spanning associate degree community college based programs to graduate education programs. The primary affiliations in the eastern AHEC, again, are with East Carolina University and its School of Nursing (which has as its components not only a generic and graduate education but also a Family Nurse Practitioner Program, which is part of a statewide consortium) and Duke University School of Nursing, which sends both undergraduates and graduate students into the field.

The School of Nursing and the School of Public Health at Chapel Hill have also rotated students into preceptor sites in both eastern and Fayetteville AHECs.

It is hoped that experience away from the health science center will encourage the settlement and retention of health practitioners 1) whose reservations about practice in rural or small communities concerned isolation and the lack of colleague interaction and professional backup and 2) who were reluctant to go to areas which lack the resources to meet their professional needs.

Since one of the goals of the AHEC program is to attract health practitioners to the rural areas of North Carolina, it is AHEC's responsibility to make the area as attractive as possible to rotating university students. Medical students and residents were rotating to various areas of North Carolina before the advent of the AHEC program, but the concept is fairly new for nursing students.

In order to make the experience a pleasant one for both students and the agencies they are working in, the AHEC nurses act much as facilitators. For example, when the UNC-CH School of Nursing decided to send students on a rotation fairly far from the school, they asked me (McGrath) for suggestions of possible agencies they could use. Since there seemed to be several appropriate agencies in the Fayetteville AHEC, that is one of the AHECs being used for nursing student rotations.

The students who rotate through the Fayetteville AHEC are spring semester seniors who are involved in Advanced Clinical Nursing. At this level, they can function well with an agency clinical preceptor and a faculty member to help integrate the theoretical content. Since the faculty member may be responsible for 17 students, clinical supervision is not to be expected. In fact, the faculty believes that the student can learn more clinically from an expert in the field.

Initially, I contacted the appropriate agencies and learned of their receptivity to having students—especially students whose clinical learning would be the responsibility of some of the employees of that agency. If the agency required direct supervision by faculty at all times, either a local person was hired as a part time faculty member or the agency was not utilized. After learning of the agency's receptivity, I helped the faculty negotiate numbers of students in the clinical setting and particularly tried to avoid any conflict with students (associate degree, practical nursing) currently using the setting.

At first not all the university based faculty were sold on the idea of students rotating all over the state. They had concerns that the quality of the experiences might differ greatly and there seemed to be little control or even observation because the faculty-student ratio was so high. Opposition was such that some faculty were unwilling to group class days (taught in Chapel Hill) so that the students could spend a block of time in their clinical settings. The first students traveled a great deal between Chapel Hill and various settings in the Fayetteville AHEC. Surprisingly this did not dampen the feelings of the students. They believed that the experience gained in the rural settings far outweighed the travel inconvenience. When, finally, more faculty became convinced of the value of the experience, they grouped their class days so that students now travel only once a week. Since travel time varies anywhere from 45 minutes to $4\,1/2$ hours one way, the better the grouping of class days, the easier it is for the students.

Housing for students is another one of my responsibilities. When students are too far away from Chapel Hill to commute, they stay somewhere in the area in which they are practicing. Although living in the area has many advantages, there is one distinct disadvantage. The advantages are that the nursing student can get to know the people better, can learn what entertainment is available, can work more flexible hours (i.e., 12 hour shifts, attend emergency C-sections, etc.), and can venture out and see the area. The distinct disadvantage is that health science library facilities are not available. Each AHEC has a mini health science library in its central location, but these libraries may still be too far away from affiliating students to provide any kind of ready access.

Housing may be found in private homes, AHEC-leased apartments, or local motels. Some AHECs will lease apartments if they have students rotating constantly. The AHECs also negotiate reasonable rates for the students in private homes and local motels.

Some AHEC nurses become involved in the student teaching in addition to the administrative work necessary to ready the area for them. All of the AHEC nurses hold clinical appointments at their affiliating university. If they are interested and feel capable of teaching the students, they may do so. Both of us have been teaching students for the past three years. I currently serve as the faculty person for two students working in a pediatrician's office. The office nurses still serve as primary clinical preceptors. This works well as I have direct contact with the students and am able to relieve the university-based faculty person in charge of students practicing in AHEC areas of some responsibility. Relieving the faculty of two students may not sound like much, but it can be a big help when those two students are in a town 45 miles away from the other students.

Thus far the experience has been an overwhelming success for the students, faculty, and the staff of the various agencies. The student benefits in several ways. This experience provides a period of "weaning" which may make the transition to a new graduate an easier one. The university faculty person is actually in the agency only one of the three days per week the students are there. This gives the students the opportunity to negotiate directly with the staff and not through the instructor as is so often the case. The students negotiate their own working hours and choose their experiences, which gives them more commitment to their learning experiences. In the community hospital setting, the students often choose the evening and night hours, sometimes in order not to conflict with associate degree nursing student experiences, sometimes because these are the hours the preceptor is working, and sometimes because that is when they feel they can learn the most.

The university based faculty person responsible for these students finds this mode of teaching challenging. It is a new experience not being the person directly responsible for all the teaching. She fits in perfectly in the hospital setting where she might have had the greatest problem adapting to her role. She makes the preceptors and other members of the nursing staff comfortable in their new teaching roles. One of her biggest assets is that she does not claim to be an expert in any area of the hospital.

The staff in each agency has developed as a result of this particular student experience. The staff nurses are moving from an attitude of suspicion and mistrust toward learners (especially baccalaureate and master's nursing students) to one of confidence and trust. This new attitude is due partly to a broadening of their own learning opportunities. There is much more interest in continuing education and much more continuing education for these nurses to take advantage of. The staff is learning that one is not expected to know everything and it is all right to admit ignorance. The staff is discovering that they can learn from students and some have even been interested in reading student term papers. The staff is recognizing that their preparation for entry into practice in many instances is diverse and the baccalaureate students and the staff are sharing their different but valuable experiences and learning from each other.

The Director of Nursing in one community hospital setting is especially pleased about having baccalaureate students in his agency. He believes it helps the staff to have a more open mind about the different entry levels into nursing practice. The staff is more confident in their strengths and more willing to share these strengths with others and is more willing to admit weaknesses and work on them.

Recruiting these students to return and work in these communities is looking promising. After the first year when there were only two students in the Fayetteville AHEC area, one of these returned to work in her student clinical setting. After the second year, there were several students interested in returning to the community hospital for employment after graduation. They did not come because the starting salary was too low. The hospital must have learned something from this, as they have since raised the salaries, and new students have begun for the third year. It will be interesting to see what the recruitment possibilities are. We hope this approach to student clinical rotations will increase the number of baccalaureate nurses practicing in eastern North Carolina.

Clinical Preceptorship in the Fayetteville AHEC

Another statewide problem is that of bridging the gap between the student experience and the graduate nurse experience. Hospitals find new graduates unable to meet the job responsibilities which have been set for them. Hospitals have charged nursing schools with inadequate preparation of nurses for their job responsibilities. The nursing schools claim to prepare beginning practitioners, not practitioners ready to manage effectively the care of groups of patients utilizing various levels of personnel, which is usually what the hospitals expect.

I helped plan and conduct a clinical preceptorship for new graduates in one of the area rural hospitals. The FAHEC faculty was interested in helping solve the problem identified at this hospital and believed that if a solution could be implemented there, it could serve as a model for other hospitals in the state. The goals to be achieved in this experience included the improvement of patient care, the development of self-confidence, the practice of patient centered nursing, and the documentation of weaknesses.

The clinical preceptorship was designed to provide the new graduates supervision and assistance in facing the new problems certain to arise in their first work experience. An overall objective was written and specific subobjectives were written to correspond with the overall objective (Appendix C).

The experience was planned so that a preceptor would be available to the new graduate as a resource person. The preceptor was not defined as or viewed as an instructor. The appropriate times for the preceptor to assist the new graduate were limited to those sought by the new graduate or when the preceptor felt that the graduate was heading for unexpected trouble. The faculty hoped such guidance would be effective in strengthening self-confidence and responsibility and in encouraging initiative in the use of support resources.

Instead of hiring clinical experts from outside the hospital, the planning committee decided to select the preceptors from among the existing nursing staff. Since staff members would have already established credibility with the rest of the staff, the preceptors would not have to prove themselves before attaining the respect and cooperation of the nursing and medical staffs. The cooperation of the nursing staff was considered essential to the success of the program. The new graduate would have more chance of being successful in this experience as an accepted member of the staff.

It was expected that the responsibility for meeting the objectives rested with the new graduate, *not* with the preceptor. The new graduate was expected to initiate, pursue, and evaluate her own learning activities to meet the stated objectives and to demonstrate how these objectives were met. The graduate was expected to utilize a preceptor and a comprehensive variety of other people as consultants.

Twenty new graduates participated in the clinical preceptorship. All the new graduates were aware before they were employed that they would be participating in this clinical preceptorship. Since it was imperative that these new graduates be exposed to a real work situation, they were assigned to patient care areas just as they would have been had they not been in this supervised experience. The new graduates rotated shifts and worked weekends and the preceptors worked the same hours.

A rating form for ongoing and final evaluations was used. At the end of the second week the preceptors distinguished four new graduates who they identified as "of concern." These new graduates exhibited poor judgment, were unorganized, slow in their work, and had made medication and other errors. Three of these four later failed the licensing examination. One value of the clinical preceptorship was identifying weak new graduates early so that they could receive the extra help they needed to pass the licensing examination and become effective staff members.

At the conclusion of the preceptorship, all concerned, including preceptors, graduates, staff, administration, and physicians, subjectively evaluated the experience as being successful and thought it should be offered again. Most of the administrative people involved believed that giving the new graduates the responsibility for their own actions rather than the staff development instructors or individual head nurses taking the responsibility made the difference.[6] Patient care was improved since the new graduates became comfortable in the new role more quickly than they had in the past.

The clinical preceptorship has become an integral part of the orientation process at the hospital involved. In addition, several other hospitals across the state have since implemented a clinical preceptorship using this original demonstration project made available through AHEC as a model.

Baccalaureate Education for RNs

As the AHEC nurses across the state assessed the educational needs for the nurses they were serving, it became apparent that baccalaureate education was an important concern of many RNs. A majority of the RNs in North Carolina are prepared at the diploma and associate degree levels. In order to assess the interest in baccalaureate education among these nurses, a questionnaire was devised and distributed in a number of AHEC areas.

I distributed questionnaires to 1200 of the 1860 RNs in the FAHEC region. There were 606 usable returns. Approximately 45 percent of the respondents were from Cumberland County, with the remainder fairly evenly distributed among the other eight counties. This is not as skewed a sample as it may seem because approximately 50 percent of all RNs in the Fayetteville AHEC work in Cumberland County. Of the nurses responding to the questionnaire, 65 percent indicated a definite interest in a BSN degree and only 19 percent said they were definitely not interested. The analysis of the response also indicated that 80 percent of the nurses interested in pursuing a baccalaureate degree were married, and 62 percent indicated family responsibilities as a possible deterrent to further education.

Other deterrents to completing the requirements of a BSN degree included the following: degree could only be obtained by studying on a full time basis; residence requirements included spending from one to four semesters on campus; existing baccalaureate programs were not within commuting distance and therefore the nurses would have to move; lower division course work available in the rural areas was often not transferrable to the universities with BSN programs; and existing programs often lacked meaning for the RN student.

Proximity and economics seem to be the two strongest deterrents to the RNs in the FAHEC region. The closest university to these nurses offering the BSN degree is from 70 to 100 miles from their homes. Economically, the majority of nurses in the region come from middle class families. Most must work in order to assist in the support of their families. Economic and family constraints deter these nurses from spending one to four semesters pursuing their education on a university campus far from home.

All but a very small portion of resources in any BSN program in North Carolina are directed toward and tailored to the generic student. Spaces in existing classes need to be made available to those nurses within commuting distance of a BSN program or for those willing and able to spend one to four semesters in residence. For those unable to commute, nursing courses need to be offered on an outreach basis. Some of the AHEC nurses believe nursing in North Carolina may indeed reap a great reward by directing more resources toward the RN student. It is widely recognized that large numbers of persons newly educated in nursing either do not enter practice, practice for a short period of time before leaving, or have rather long periods of inactivity at one or more points in their career. Therefore, expending more resources for BSN education for RNs already working and committed to long term career goals would seem to be more cost effective than expanding generic baccalaureate programs.

Most RNs seeking a BSN have been employed for some length of time, and many are currently employed. Since most find nursing a rewarding profession, they are eager to continue their education in nursing. There is every reason to believe these nurses will remain employed and will greatly improve patient care since most have credibility and can effect change easier than a new graduate. Their interest in pursuance of the BSN degree speaks of their commitment to upgrading the quality of nursing care.

Data from the survey of the nurses in the FAHEC area indicate a long term career commitment on the part of the nurses surveyed. When asked directly of their long range career goals, over 70 percent of the respondents said they expect to continue working, regardless of their opportunity to pursue further education.

In North Carolina as in other states fortunate enough to have an AHEC system, a satellite or extension of an existing BSN program could be easily and appropriately administered from the local AHEC. The centers already have a mechanism for acquiring university faculty to teach in the community both in academic and continuing education programs. Some of the centers have classroom and audiovisual equipment.[7] Such advantages could make the adaptation of a university based BSN program to an outreach area easier.

Since the problem exists across the state, the AHEC nurses discussed the issue and arranged to meet with all the baccalaureate deans in the state. This provided an opportunity for the AHEC nurses to serve in their advocate role and speak to the deans on behalf of the practicing nurses in the state. Several of the problems involved in modifying existing programs to accomodate RN students were discussed. One of the major problems is money. No school has enough money to meet its existing commitments and branch out into innovative, outreach programs for RNs. Some of the AHEC nurses would like to develop a demonstration project which could be implemented to meet the need in a variety of settings across the state and then apply for grant funds. Hopefully, the project will be funded eventually through the state system. These efforts are currently in progress.

Technical Assistance and Consultation in the Eastern AHEC

Technical assistance and consultation are rather nebulous terms used to describe or categorize AHEC nursing activities not directly related to continuing education or clinical education. These activities fall under many guises.

Consultation efforts by the Eastern AHEC nursing faculty has incorporated many foci. Most activities have been predicated on response to direct requests for assistance from health care providers and institutions. The request-response format lends itself to the problem solving model for technical assistance, with AHEC staff serving as facilitators. Thus the AHEC faculty has played an increasingly important role as an educational community interface in establishing linkages between academia and the grass roots practitioners. Resources such as printed media, audiovisual software, and teaching models as well as guest lecturers from various educational programs are channeled through the eastern AHEC program. Mini-resource centers have been established in each hospital for informal teaching/learning contracts. Inservice education programming has been developed and sustained with staff support. Community liaisons among hospital, health department, technical institute, and other health organizations have been fostered by staff support. Recruiting in all the disciplines has been undertaken. Community based educational training has been strengthened by sharing curriculae and providing assistance in modifying educational strategies. All of these endeavors coalesce to form a support system and substructure for health care delivery in an otherwise rurally isolated region.

Three of these endeavors call for further elaboration: support of inservice programming, work with community colleges, and establishment of a nursing administrators forum.

INSERVICE SUPPORT

In its working commitment to the 16 hospital consortium, eastern AHEC operates under the premise that continuing education encompasses the traditional model of workshops, symposiums, seminars, and short courses designed and directed by the AHEC faculty. However, they also support inhouse staff development programming in each constituent institution to meet immediate needs. The faculty has found that personnel orientation training, specific skills training, and selected cognitive and affective learning is best accomplished through inservice education within the organizational structure of the various hospitals. A strong ongoing inservice program seems to stimulate improvement across a wide spectrum of hospital services.

When the nursing component in the Eastern AHEC became operational in March 1975, only 2 of the 16 hospitals had a concurrent inservice program with a specific individual identified as program coordinator. Two and one-half years later, much to the delight of the AHEC faculty, 15 of the 16 hospitals have an inservice director and the 16th is now actively recruiting an inservice director. One might speculate that multiple stimuli caused the health agencies to begin making an overt commitment to a viable internal educational component. Not only did AHEC play an apparently significant part in the encouragement of inhouse educational development but so too did the Joint Commission on Accreditation of Hospitals (with its well delineated accreditation standard), together with the North Carolina Hospital Association, and the Division of North Carolina Department of Human Resources, which have an impact on setting standards for inpatient facilities. Whether or not all this was merely chance, the results have been undeniably positive and certainly have led to a broadening of the educational opportunities for all who work in hospital situations.

Eastern AHEC currently supports a series of inservice programs in each of the participating hospitals featuring resource persons from the medical, nursing, and allied health hospital staffs as guest teachers, backed by library materials and audiovisual software from East Carolina University and AHEC's statewide pool.[8]

REGIONAL NURSING EDUCATION

The linkage with the nursing education programs in the coastal plain has produced very positive results. There are presently eight practical nurse programs, six associate degree programs, and one hospital based diploma program in addition to the baccalaureate program at East Carolina University. Directors from the educational institutions began meeting with me (Lawler) on a quarterly basis. Ostensibly, the motivating factor for bringing the group together was to enhance coordination of student clinical rotations to assist in identification, development, and coordination of clinical facilities for the use of faculty and students. However, two additional factors played a major role in the formation of the standing advisory committee structure the group took.

It was seen as vital that the Area Health Education Center not be perceived as yet another take over by the University, specifically by the School of Nursing. The integrity of the system had to be preserved and association with the University needed to be viewed as a partnership rather than authoritarian. Therefore, the Dean of the East Carolina School of Nursing from the beginning agreed to meet with the group, and I served as discussion leader. This proved to be a wise decision and brought immediate cohesiveness into the committee. The Dean has been a marvelous resource person for the other nursing program directors who have come to rely in some measure on her knowledge and experience. The territorial imperative has also been diminished by group process and for the first time clinical facilities have been shared by realistic planning and by consensus.

In addition, a moratorium on school enrollment expansion has been agreed to for a five-year period so that emphasis can be placed on upgrading the existing programs.

Improving faculty qualifications and the quality of instruction within the associate degree schools was really what stimulated the development of the directors group. Many of the programs were relatively new, and not one was similar to another in objectives or definitions of the product. Curricula working together has brought some standardization to the programs with constructive curriculum sharing.

Intensive instruction in teaching strategies and curriculum concepts has been offered to the faculty members of the Associate Degree in Nursing Programs through the educational resources of East Carolina University. By training the teachers of the basic programs, the AHEC faculty expects to strengthen these programs and therefore produce more knowledgeable and skilled nurses.

It is anticipated that the impact of such a program may be reflected in a higher percentage of passing rates on the State Board of Nursing Examinations in eastern North Carolina which will impact on improving the delivery of health care. It is projected that through AHEC involvement, some failure rates may be lowered by 20 percent by 1980.

NURSING ADMINISTRATION

To find out that many of the nursing administrators from the community health agencies did not even know each other came as a startling reinforcement of the fragmentation of nursing efforts and leadership in the region. The only exceptions to the pattern were the health departments whose nursing supervisors have met periodically in a loosely formed council.

Response, however, was immediate and affirmative to the suggestion that the nursing administrators meet with me. Provision of a forum, convening every 8 to 12 weeks, and concentrating on the aggregate needs of the group has proven most rewarding. Group process has involved brainstorming to identify common inhouse problems and so facilitate problem solving techniques. These techniques have been collectively applied to the areas of establishing staffing patterns, developing care plans, recruiting, compliance to the Joint Commission of the Accreditation of Hospitals (JCAH) standards, and setting up concurrent and retrospective quality assurance activities. Resources have then been sought to remedy the problems.

Learning about effective nursing audit programs within the hospital setting was a major project of the administration group. Under the expert tutelage of a JCAH consultant from Connecticut, progress has been quite gratifying. The audit committee membership began with workshops on the basics of the audit mechanism and the need for a viable method for quality assurance of patient care. Further workshops were held on advanced concepts and methodology after a period of six to eight months to allow for practice and development of skills. In the interim period audits were submitted for critique and resubmitted if necessary so that there was a continuing learning experience reinforced. The nurses have increased competence so markedly that many are utilizing the audit process to direct nursing research relating to practice on their care units. According to the nurses serving on the audit committees, the next step is an interdisciplinary one beginning with the socialization of physicians to the concept.

The nursing directors after having identified audit as a priority learning need committed themselves to supporting the efforts of their staff members as they increased their skills. Release time, tuition fees, resources, and backup relief were all provided. The change that resulted was not only behavioral but attitudinal as well. Enthusiasm and dedication for improvement were evidenced and spread from the audit project to others which would also improve patient care.

This process has been repeated in addressing other needs selected by the nursing administrators' committee. Many of the members have come to rely on each other as well as on the resources provided by the AHEC. At times there have been "hot potato" issues where no consensus has been reached. Reluctance to support membership in the State Nurses Association is an example of an attitude which continues to frustrate us. But in all, many benefits have accrued to those participating in this forum.

Clinical Practice by the AHEC Nurse

We believe that competency in a skill is necessary in order to be able to teach it. Therefore, we believe that it is vital that we maintain our clinical skills. While it is common for academic physicians to be vitally involved in their own clinical practice, this has not been the trend in nursing.

I (McGrath) happen to enjoy clinical practice and especially the care of sick children in the hospital. Throughout my career I have been involved in my own clinical practice. While teaching in a generic nursing program, my clinical practice was over and above my teaching load as time was not provided for it to be an integral portion of my position.

When I accepted my AHEC position, I realized that I would need to be involved in clinical practice more than ever, as I would be only minimally involved with supervising generic students. In the past that had been one source of maintaining and/or increasing my clinical skills and competencies.

Approximately a month after I began work, I realized that I could not be satisfied in my work if it did not involve some actual caring for patients. I also realized that my teaching could quickly become dull and totally academic. Therefore, I negotiated with my 'director to spend a day a week working as a staff nurse on the pediatric ward at one of the hospitals in my area. It has been an invaluable portion of my position.

I chose a hospital where I could be in closest touch with all the health care providers caring for the patients. I am there to learn as well as to provide whatever service I can. I arrange my clinical time at the hospital around my other commitments and around the staffing of the pediatric unit. I know that I can get more experience when the ward really needs another RN than when they are relatively well staffed. Sometimes my other AHEC commitments are too heavy for me to practice one day a week, but I try to stick to that schedule as closely as I can.

Professional Support System for the AHEC Nurse

One of the biggest problems facing the AHEC nurses in the truly rural areas of North Carolina is the feeling of professional isolation. Some of them are located very close to a university school of nursing and find professional support and collaboration in their relationship with that faculty. What do the rest of us do to overcome professional isolation?

The quarterly AHEC nurses' meetings partially solve the problem of isolation. All 11 AHEC nurses meet on a regular basis to relay information, discuss common problems, and meet and talk with invited guests, often people holding key health care related positions in the state. These meetings offer the opportunity for us to share a problem with the group.

Oftentimes another AHEC nurse has experienced a similar problem and can offer suggestions for a solution.

These meetings are also used to discuss "policy." The reason this word is placed in quotes is that even though a course of action may be agreed upon by the majority of the AHEC nurses, each AHEC is relatively autonomous and may go about its work in whatever way seems most feasible for that particular area of the state. Even so, it is helpful to discuss such things as registration fees, what sorts of programs AHEC can sponsor, and so forth. It is well known that on the AHEC borders, nurses from one AHEC area will talk to nurses from another AHEC area, and it is much less confusing to the population served if business is conducted similarly in all of the AHECs. The nurses were the first AHEC faculty group to meet on a regular basis. Other AHEC faculty quickly learned the value of regular meetings and many others meet regularly now.

The AHEC nurses' meetings also help each AHEC nurse to know the other AHEC nurses better. Since each of us has a different background and experience, the group as a whole is an invaluable resource. For example, when I (McGrath) became aware of a need of a hospital in my area to reorganize its nursing service, I first approached the resources at my affiliating university. Since the hospital in my area has less than 100 beds, the university resources suggested that I look for a consultant who could relate to a small hospital as the hospital at my affiliating university is almost 1000 beds. My thoughts quickly turned to one of my fellow AHEC nurses who was formerly a nursing administrator in a community hospital. I was hoping she would help me find an appropriate consultant. Fortunately this AHEC nurse offered to come and make the first consulting visit so that she could better evaluate the need. As it turned out, the AHEC nurse ended up doing all the consulting. In exchange I went to her AHEC area and helped her with some pediatric programs.

Since I am located in a very rural area of the state and since there is no baccalaurate nursing program in my area, I find myself needing professional encounters and stimulation at times other than AHEC nurses' meetings. My faculty appointments at two university schools of nursing come in handy here. I feel free to visit the schools, attend meetings and continuing education programs, and I schedule such visits regularly. Thus, I have come to know some of the faculty on a less formal basis. In some instances, I have been able to gather faculty support for some projects in the rural areas.

I make it a point to make good use of the time when I have faculty teaching or consulting in my area. I am eager to collaborate over lunch or in the evening if faculty members are staying overnight. I have found these encounters to be invaluable in keeping me professionally stimulated.

Finally, I have made an effort to become more involved in my professional associations on state and national levels. I have met and talked with many new people, always keeping in mind that I may someday be able to utilize the person as a resource for some program in my area. I also believe this gives me an opportunity to make health care providers more aware of the work of the AHEC program.

Evaluation of the AHEC Program

Evaluation is an integral component of the decision making process. Examination and documentation of processes and achievements are critical to the development, modification, and replication of a program. For these reasons, the North Carolina Area Health Education Centers Program began a systematic evaluation of its activities in 1976.

Furthermore, for evaluation purposes, AHEC must be viewed not only as a state and federal program, but as a demonstration of the concepts of decentralization of health manpower education and of regionalization of the health system, including health manpower distribution.

The approach that was proposed for the evaluation of AHEC was to begin to assess the three basic components of decentralized health manpower training: changes in the distribution of health manpower, modifications of the health manpower education system, and interorganizational relationships between health care providing and manpower training institutions. A fourth topic of focus is the utilization of money and other resources.

Regionalization is thought to contribute to the improvement of the health manpower situation in somewhat different ways than decentralization. Regionalization may be defined as the sharing of resources and expertise throughout a defined geographic area. Resource sharing may be done by institutions, professional organizations, schools, health care organizations, or professionals within a given geographic area and is done for the mutual benefit of those involved. Regionalization implies maximum utilization of scarce resources, in particular resources which depend upon a large population base for efficient and effective use. The power balance of those involved may take any of several forms, but participation and exchange are implicit.

With regard to the education of health personnel, regionalization implies educating students or personnel in a way which makes maximum utilization of educational resources of the region, and which also meets the region's needs for the numbers and types of personnel being educated.

Regionalization of nursing education programs implies cooperative efforts between the many community colleges, technical institutes, and hospitals which educate these personnel. These programs tend to be directed toward persons who are from and will remain in local areas, and tend to be for the production of types of manpower which are needed at local institutions. The basic hypothesis is that by working together, schools and training institutions within a region will focus on regional rather than individual needs, and regionalization of health manpower education should thereby contribute to a more even distribution of the various types of nursing personnel. Furthermore, educational resources should be used more efficiently, since not all institutions will be trying to train all types of personnel.

Regionalization of continuing education among health professionals is a way to enable health practitioners who may be few in number in an area of widely dispersed population to pool their resources and to develop learning experiences which are of common benefit. Furthermore, the interaction with colleagues which comes through regionalization of activities contributes to alleviating a sense of isolation that might be felt by health care practitioners in sparsely settled and rural areas, whether they are a solo physician or the single laboratory technician in a small hospital. The existence of a communications network is the first evidence of regionalization; participation and exchange of resources may then follow.

Other measures of regionalization include:

1. Location and number of continuing education programs sponsored by each AHEC.
2. Source of participants in continuing education programs.
3. Organizations cosponsoring continuing education programs with AHEC.
4. Committees with which AHEC staff are involved, and committee membership.
5. Local (regional) organizations with which AHEC is involved.

6. Exchanges of or distribution of resources within region, such as audiovisual network.
7. Location of student rotations and institutions involved.
8. Location of technical assistance activities of AHEC staff.
9. New personnel recruited, including new positions established.
10. Relationship of regional education activities of health personnel to changes in quantity or geography or specialty distribution of personnel.
11. Number of vacant positions, changes over time.
12. Number of graduates of regional training programs placed in positions within regions.
13. Number of graduates of regional training programs unable to find positions.
14. Attitudes of health personnel toward professional environment in region.
15. Attitudes of health personnel toward contribution of educational programs to professional environment in region.

Evaluation of the North Carolina AHEC system is conducted by the central staff team in Chapel Hill. The preceding description is based on their model.

EASTERN AHEC EVALUATION

Eastern AHEC from the outset has been committed to a broad multidisciplinary scope of educational activities. It was decided that all major health disciplines should be involved in order to have lasting impact, not only on the health care providers, but also on the rural delivery system itself.

Substantial anecdotal and some empirical evidence exists to document Eastern AHEC program impact. Priority emphasis has been placed on evaluation techniques and tools, beginning with the current program year. It is believed that the following accomplishments can be directly or indirectly attributed to programming initiated and maintained by the Eastern AHEC and other elements of the North Carolina AHEC network.

1. There has been a significant improvement in the numerical and specialty distribution of physicians in several eastern North Carolina locales.
2. A sizeable number (30+) of family nurse practitioners have chosen to practice in eastern North Carolina following training.
3. There has been an overt commitment to staff development by all hospitals and most community health agencies served by the Eastern AHEC. Little commitment or interest was in evidence three years ago.
4. There has been an increased regional compliance with the Joint Commission on Accreditation of Hospitals and Professional Standards Review Organization (PSRO) standards as a direct result of Eastern AHEC program activities.
5. Eastern AHEC has been designated and utilized as a central education clearinghouse by those institutions and agencies it serves.
6. Significant involvement has been initiated and is being developed with various regulatory and planning bodies such as the North Carolina Department of Human Resources and Health Systems Agency in the region with Eastern AHEC serving as a prime educational resource for those groups.

7. A wide range of educational print and nonprint media materials, equipment, and services is now available for local usage on request. Thus, all health interests, regardless of location, have ready and timely access to an entire range of learning resources. Usage has been steadily increasing through the eastern counties.

In its provision of continuing education offerings, the Eastern AHEC already uses a fairly sophisticated array of traditional evaluation tools including pretesting and posttesting. Cognitive, psychomotor, and affective assessment tools are developed and employed with regularity, and the results attest to the success of individual offerings and continuing education programming in general.

There was one recent anecdotal evaluation that perhaps was the most meaningful. It was spontaneous and quite unsolicited. During a lunch break at a small hospital at which an AHEC sponsored workshop was taking place, a young nurse spoke. She related what a culture shock she had suffered after moving from a metropolitan area in California. She also related that it was difficult and rather frightening to try to cope with a work situation so different from those she had grown accustomed to. Moreover, learning "to do" without multiple and varied resources was frustrating. But, she said, looking up and smiling, "AHEC is our lifeline." What more of an evaluation could one want?

ROLE INNOVATION

We AHEC nurses strongly feel that we have created a new role for community nurse educators, one which has evolved with the actual development of the AHEC system. Functioning within that system we have been involved in clinical education, continuing education, and consulting activities. Under these guises, roles and functions have progressed and slowly become delineated. Many hats have been worn, yet with the passage of time they began to blend and become of one style, just as the objectives of the AHECs themselves have merged so that they now form a network of support systems which blanket the state—this is the "lifeline."

Each of the North Carolina AHEC nurses has found herself playing the part of Gunga Din early in the game hauling overhead projectors, blackboards, and reference books to stage the first continuing education offerings often held, as has been said, in rather unusual settings. This, too, exposed us as teachers from the beginning—nontraditionally— away from the university. Also, since we offered technical assistance to the various hospitals and health departments we were seen as consultants. As relationships and ties developed among nurses in our regions and the health institutions began community interactions, we came to function as interface managers. Involvement with socialization of our constituents concerning current issues facing nursing and interpreting their response to the nursing leadership has made us into strong advocates.

We became resource coordinators for the identification, location, and channeling of human and learning resources. Because of our visibility in the nursing community we not only serve as role models but also often find ourselves acting as recruiters for all levels of personnel, problem solvers, career counselors, and frequently peacemakers. These are some of the ways we have been utilized as liaisons. The role that has been forged and repeatedly reinforced is new, exciting, and certainly challenging. It is one which epitomizes the community health nurse as an educator in the fullest sense.

IMPACT AND RECOMMENDATIONS

There is little doubt that the AHEC program has had dramatic impact on the nursing profession in North Carolina. It is a workable model, because it both increases the numbers and ditribution of care providers and it truly improves the ambience of the professional climate in previously underserved areas. AHEC has formed an education support system, therefore, it is indeed a "lifeline." By establishing linkages between community agencies and community nursing leaders, by providing a regional resource network, by facilitating decentralized education programming, and by electing and reinforcing a truly interdisciplinary approach, AHEC has fashioned, as well, a power base for nursing.

The AHEC nurses have as a consortium a considerable amount of clout in the nursing arena. Perhaps this system provides, too, the closest ties and the most direct channels between the grass roots and the bureaucratic decision makers. The impact of the AHECs has wrought changes which are believed to be for the betterment of nursing. Continued formal evaluation will more fully document the kind of changes wrought and the role definition of the AHEC nurse as a community educator.

The recommendations which flow from a review of these experiences are few and relatively simple. We, as AHEC nurses, believe that continued funding to the existing national AHECs, especially those which foster a multidisciplinary effort, is imperative. In North Carolina, the State General Assembly has underwritten an increasingly major portion of the AHEC budget. This is laudable. Efforts should also increase toward making the continuing education portion of the activities self-sufficient. Sufficient funds can be generated through registration fees to offset program costs so that needed monies can be diverted to support student clinical education.

Nursing should continue to demand equal footing with medicine and a collegial relationship with all the disciplines. The representative team functioning away from the university is the faculty core of AHEC and should be preserved. The nursing component also must strengthen its advocacy relationship with the community constituency. Herein lies its real strength.

Finally, we enthusiastically recommend that the AHEC nursing model be emulated and replicated in other locales. It is an effective outreach program and can be made operational on either an expanded or limited basis. Almost any university school of nursing might modify the system to its own needs and beneficially serve its community. The challenge and innovation drew us to the AHEC system, and the excitement of trailblazing has never left. The AHEC concept remains exciting, and we urge you to share it with us.

REFERENCES

1. Schafer, Donna: *Rural Family Nurse Practitioner Project Proposal, East Carolina University School of Nursing.* Division of Nursing, HEW: 5DIONUO1585-03, 1975.
2. Carnegie Commission on Higher Education: *Higher Education and the Nation's Health: Policies for Medical & Dental Education. A Special Report and Recommendations.* McGraw-Hill Book Company, New York, 1970.
3. *A Self Description of Nine North Carolina AHEC Programs.* A Report to the Bureau of Health Resources Development (HEW), 1978.
4. Explorers' Task Force: *Continuing Education for the RN and LPN: Issues and Implications.* North Carolina Board of Nursing, Raleigh, 1978.

5. Copp, Laurel: *Consortium Project for Psych-Mental Health Nursing.* NIMH 1-0401-4401-HA-388, 1977.
6. McGrath, Barbara Jo, and Koewing, J. Robert: "A Clinical Preceptorship for New Graduate Nurses." *Journal of Nursing Administration,* 8 (3):13, March 1978.
7. McGrath, Barbara Jo, and Bacon, Thomas J.: "Baccalaureate Education for the RN: Why Is It So Scarce? *Journal of Nursing Education,* 18 (6):40-45, June 1979.
8. Lawler, Therese: "Support of Inservice Programming—An AHEC Priority." *Journal of Continuing Education in Nursing,* 9 (4):3-7, July-Aug. 1978.

APPENDIX A. AHEC NURSING EDUCATIONAL NEEDS SURVEY

Name of Agency _____

Address_____

Telephone _____

Director of Nurses _____

Administrator _____

Number of Beds (if applicable) _____

Average Census or Caseload _____

Number of Nursing Supervisors [include Director(s)] _____

    Inservice Instructors _____

    Head Nurses _____

    Staff Nurses_____

    LPNs _____

    Nursing Assistants _____

Which are the best days for nurses to attend workshops? _____

_____

Other comments regarding times and places for workshops? _____

_____

_____

Who filled out this survey and what is the person's position? _____

_____

Instructions: The following are specific topics which could be dealt with in continuing education workshops. Please indicate by check (✔) which topics need more emphasis for nurses in your agency.

1. KNOWLEDGE OF DISEASE AND UNUSUAL CONDITIONS

____ Stroke

____ Cancer

____ Hypertension

____ Heart disease

____ Diabetes

____ Accidents

____ Renal disease

____ Tuberculosis

____Vascular disease

____ Liver disease

____ Gynecology

____ Allergic disorders

____ Problems of the eye

____ Communicable disease

____ Neurology

____ Neurosurgery

____ Orthopedics

____ ENT

____ Arthritis

____ Pregnancy

____ Pulmonary disease

____ Hematologic disorders

____ Gastrointestinal problems

____ Genitourinary disorders

____ Dermatologic disorders

____ Endocrine and metabolic disorders

____ Other

____ Other

____ Other

____ Other

2. METHODS OF ASSESSMENT AND INTERVENTION

____ History taking

____ Interviewing

____ Patient observation and assessment

____ Physical exam

____ Laboratory techniques

____ Reading EKGs

____ Charting

____ Radiation therapy

____ Acid base balance

____ Pacemakers

____ Postural drainage

____ Fetal monitoring

____ POMR

____ Fluids and electrolytes

____ Renal dialysis

____ Pharmacology

____ Identification of high-risk groups

____ Other

____ Other

____ Other

3. BEHAVIORAL SCIENCES

____ Child development

____ Family dynamics

____ Death and dying

____ Other

____ Crisis intervention   ____ Other

____ Process of aging   ____ Other

____ Interpersonal relationships   ____ Other

4. PROCESS

     ____ Nursing audit   ____ Evaluation

     ____ Leadership   ____ Other

     ____ Teaching-learning   ____ Other

     ____ Management   ____ Other

5. SETTING

     ____ Emergency care   ____ Intensive care

     ____ Coronary care   ____ Long term care

     ____ Rehabilitation   ____ Infection control

     ____ Ambulatory care   ____ Disaster nursing

Comments and/or suggestions:

APPENDIX B. SAMPLE WORK STATEMENTS – NURSING EDUCATION

1. Maintain Director of Nursing Education.
2. Maintain full time secretary for Director of Nursing Education.
3. Provide special programs in the following areas:
    a. Conduct the "Leadership for the Health Professional" course using the leadership tapes in two agencies in the AHEC service region.
    b. Conduct the "Assertiveness Training" course using the assertiveness training tapes in two agencies in the AHEC service region.
    c. Plan and conduct a series of four workshops for nursing home personnel.
    d. Plan and conduct a workshop for nurses on management of the patient with a pacemaker.
    e. Provide a learning experience for nurses caring for patients with renal disease who require dialysis.
    f. Provide a workshop on advanced nursing audit.
    g. Provide a followup workshop to the workshop held last year to assist nurses to deal with infection control problems.
    h. Provide a followup workshop to the workshop held last year to assist nurses to deal with problems related to discharge planning.
    i. Plan and conduct at least two workshops to meet the needs of faculty teaching in associate degree nursing programs and licensed practical nursing programs.
    j. Plan and conduct a workshop for nurses focusing on neurosurgical nursing.
    k. Plan and implement a continuing education experience on the Nursing Process for nurses in one agency in the AHEC service region.
    l. Provide a workshop for nurses involving the integration of psychiatric nursing concepts in all practice areas of nursing.
    m. Work with the Regional Perinatal Program to provide at least two workshops for the nurses working with patients in the Regional Perinatal Project.
    n. Provide a workshop for nurses including content on the nursing care of the patient with burns.
    o. Provide a workshop for nurses dealing with the concept of primary nursing.
    p. Provide a management workshop for nurses in administrative positions.
    q. Plan and conduct a workshop on nursing care of eye patients.
    r. Plan and conduct a diabetic workshop for pediatric office nurses.
    s. Plan and conduct a surgical nursing course for one agency in the AHEC service region.
    t. Plan and conduct an emergency nursing course for one agency in the AHEC service region.
    u. Provide two workshops for nurses on the subject of cancer.
4. Continue identifying educational needs of nurses in the AHEC service region and provide special programs to meet these needs.
5. Continue to serve as a link between the educational needs of nurses in the AHEC service region and the resources available to them locally, statewide, or nationally.
6. Coordinate clinical experiences of university nursing students who come into the AHEC area for a portion of their education.

7. Continue to work toward having BSN courses offered to RNs in the AHEC area on an outreach basis.
8. Attend AHEC nurses' meetings.
9. Continue to work with the Area Planning Committee for Continuing Education for Nurses to plan and cosponsor programs.
10. Increase the library materials and other resource materials available to registered nurses and nursing students in the AHEC service area.

APPENDIX C. OBJECTIVES FOR CLINICAL PRECEPTORSHIP

I. Overall objective:

Upon satisfactory completion of the clinical preceptorship, the graduate nurse will be able to demonstrate development of nursing skills, interpersonal relationship, patient care management, and leadership ability, which will meet the expectations of performance of a charge nurse at a minimum level.

II. Subobjectives:

A. Continuously evaluates the care given by self and other members of the health team.
   1. Identifies skills still requiring direct supervision (i.e., dosage calculation).
   2. Identifies resources available to assist with development of nursing skills.
   3. Uses available opportunities and experiences to acquire these skills.
   4. Evaluates skills, strengths, and weaknesses of assigned staff.
   5. Uses her knowledge to revise patient care as indicated.

B. Recognizes the need for plans and conducts patient and family teaching.
   1. Uses opportunities to talk with patients and families in an effective and purposeful manner (therapeutic vs. nosey).
   2. Identifies specific learning needs for patients and family.
   3. Implements patient and family teaching.
   4. Evaluates patient and family teaching.

C. Examines and copes effectively with feelings regarding patients, peers, coworkers, and supervisory personnel.
   1. Discusses the new graduate's role in the existing hospital system.
   2. Identifies discrepancies in the graduate's perception of self and the existing staff's perception of the graduate.
   3. Establishes methods to deal with these discrepancies and perceptions.
   4. Examines and copes effectively with feeling regarding relationships between self and other members of the health team (i.e., physician, dietician, etc.).
   5. Fulfills the role of patient advocate and expands her present knowledge by functioning in a colleague relationship with the physician and other members of the health team.
   6. Learns to recognize the social feelings (anger, hostility, jealousy, etc.) of patients, peers, coworkers, and supervisory personnel and relates them to the situation rather than personalizing them.

D. Utilizes all her nursing knowledge to relate the patient's characteristics (i.e., vital signs, lab results, etc.) to the patient's total condition and appropriately intervenes on these findings.
   1. Relates one patient's vital sign to his other vital signs and identifies the significance of these findings.
   2. Continuously assesses and evaluates the patient receiving IV therapy (i.e., site, rate of flow, and relationship of patient condition to fluid).
   3. Relates the patient's treatment to his signs, symptoms, and diagnosis.
   4. Assesses intake and output to be adequate or inadequate.
   5. Appropriately documents nursing activities.
   6. Relates the patient's medications (dosage, frequency, administration times, etc.) to his signs, symptoms, and diagnosis.
   7. Recognizes a patient's social feelings (crying, anger, hostility, etc.) and helps him to deal with these.

   E. Gains experience in the management of patient care for a group (5 to 7) of patients
      with increasing complexity of condition.
      1. Assesses the total situation.
      2. Sets appropriate priorities.
      3. Plans patient care for a select group of patients.
      4. Implements the plan of patient care for the select group of patients.
      5. Continuously assesses the total situation.
      6. Evaluates the patient care given to the select group of patients.
   F. Demonstrates effective leadership.
      1. Evaluates skills, strengths, and weaknesses of assigned staff.
      2. Makes assignments based on need and individual staff abilities.
      3. Delegates tasks appropriately.
      4. Supervises the tasks which have been delegated to the coworkers.
      5. Values staff and rewards them appropriately.
      6. Coordinates patient care in the patient's interest by taking into consideration
         the work schedules of the other hospital and educational departments.
      7. Determines that appropriate data are recorded and communicated to the nec-
         essary people.
      8. Evaluates care given in terms of patient need, cost, utilization of resources.
   G. Demonstrates a desire for continued growth through participation in team con-
      ferences, physician rounds, unit meetings, and continuing education programs.

CHAPTER **47**

A PREVENTIVE HEALTH PROGRAM FOR LOW INCOME WOMEN

MARGARET MATTHEWS SLOCUM, M.S., R.N.

There is a need for health professionals to look at the preventive health behaviors of low income, high risk families, particularly where young children are at risk, and to ascertain the most effective methods of health intervention and promotion for this population. There is a particular need for the nursing profession, which is committed to the quality of care received by all patients, to take the lead in establishing innovative ways of reaching these high risk families. Community health nurses, in particular, can take the initiative in exploring more appropriate and relevant ways to serve lower income families. While working in various communities as a public health nurse I began looking at specific nursing interventions which would best facilitate the delivery of preventive health information to urban poor communities. One such attempt at providing a more relevant form of health intervention to low income families was an educational project initiated by me as partial fulfillment of the requirements for my degree of Master of Science in Community Health Nursing. The objective of this program was to foster parenting skills and to stimulate preventive health behavior within a high risk population. The intent of this chapter is to provide a documentation of the processes involved in establishing a mothers' discussion group in a low income housing project.

My interest in low income, high risk families was developed mainly through my experiences as a public health nurse which, prior to completing my master's degree, included working for seven years as a community health nurse in several large cities in the northeast, southwest, and western United States. My functions encompassed many different

nursing roles in the community and were carried out in varied community settings including schools, drug abuse centers, well-child clinics, and home visits for a variety of
services. The majority of my clients were lower socioeconomic, urban families. Often
assuming the role of primary health care provider for these families, I developed an
interest in the preventive health practices of low income families and, particularly, those
single parent families where the woman assumes the role of head of the family.

In planning the design of the discussion program for the women of a low income
housing unit, I utilized some specific theoretic concepts taken from the motivational
theories of an existing public health formulation, the Health Belief Model. This theory of
motivation underlies an approach drawn mainly from Lewin[1] and formulated by Rosenstock.[2] The Health Belief Model postulates the belief that within the decision making
process there exists a particular combination of variables which influence a person's
decision to act by either promoting or inhibiting that action. These variables, which play
such a vital role in the decision making process, are rooted in deeply held social, cultural,
and religious beliefs. A person's beliefs about health and illness may therefore play a
major role in influencing a decision to take a particular health related action. This action
may be preventive in nature, as with yearly chest x-rays and pap smears, or may be
restorative, as in complying with a prescribed medical regimen once disease has been
diagnosed. There are a number of studies that have been done by Kosa,[3] Friedson,[4] and
others which support the conclusion that income and preventive health behavior are
positively related, with lower income persons tending to take asymptomatic health action
less often than those with a higher income. These studies further suggest that a certain
constellation of beliefs must be present before a person takes a preventive health action
and that these beliefs tend to be less prevalent among the lower income groups. One
reason for this may be that those with lower income possess less information about health
and disease than those of higher income. Nearly all available evidence supports the
proposition that knowledge of health matters and exposure to health information are
prerequisites to taking preventive health actions and are associated with income. Because
of these striking correlations between poverty, health beliefs, and health behavior, I
decided to use some of the concepts from the Health Belief Model as a basic theoretic
framework for planning a preventive health education program for low income women.

Through various studies done in project areas, Louis Kriesberg[5] found that a great
degree of social and physical isolation exists for lower income groups, particularly those
groups residing in public housing. He also suggests that compounding this isolation,
husbandless poor mothers are less likely to feel that parents are responsible for how their
children turn out and feel more of a sense of helplessness and frustration in their lives.
Subsequently, parental values, beliefs, and practices in childrearing of the poor may not
be conducive to the child's later independence and achievement and this can be compounded by the absence of a father. In the area of interpersonal influence, Friedson[4]
concludes that those on a lower socioeconomic level tend to use a lay referral system
rather than a professional referral system, thus recommending group support from peers
as a more motivating technique than straight information from professionals. These
studies formed the basis of my rationale for reaching lower socioeconomic groups of
people for the purpose of influencing health beliefs and behaviors and my rationale for
using a group discussion design as a useful health education tool. The underlying theory
of the Health Belief Model of behavioral prediction provided the theoretic concepts for
both the rationale and the design of the project. But the versatility of this theoretical

framework and the importance of applying this same motivational theory to the actual process of organizing the discussion group became apparent only after the project was underway. The specific motivational elements taken from the Health Belief Model, which were identified and manipulated to bring about the organization of the mothers' group, will be outlined in the following section.

PURPOSE OF PROGRAM

Pavenstedt[6] identifies five types of high risk families: fatherless homes where the mother encounters great difficulty in coping with raising her children alone; hard core poverty homes where one or both parents are emotionally bankrupt from stress, continual depression, and a feeling of helplessness and loss of control over their lives; homes where the child receives inadequate mothering, due to the mother's own emotional deprivation as a child which contributes to her inability to fulfill a nuturing role; families where the well-being of the members is compromised due to a real or potential threat of illness which is not dealt with in any preventive manner; and a family network where there does not exist a healthy relationship between parent and child which is based on the parent's knowledge of the developmental stages of children or on an understanding of the parental role.

Health information plays a major role in triggering a positive response to personal preventive health behavior. This triggering process can be initiated by the communication from a nurse to a patient of salient health information which is relevant to the patient's particular life style. This information can, in effect, raise a person's level of consciousness concerning his vulnerability to disease and can often play a vital role in changing beliefs and attitudes about health and illness. Most health attitudes and practices are influenced by social and cultural beliefs. The health practices of a family are often determined by the health beliefs and behavior of the mother. Pender [7] suggests that patterns of utilization of preventive health services, a measure of preventive health behavior in a family, are contingent on the mother as the major decision maker in the family in matters of health. Thus, it would seem imperative to reach mothers of high risk children as a first step in intervention.

Communicating health information on a one-to-one basis in order to influence health behavior has traditionally been a nursing role, but using peer group discussions in order to influence health beliefs and facilitate behavior change has not been effectively utilized by nurses. This technique has been effectively used in the area of parent education for years, but we need to look at it specifically in terms of its value in promoting positive preventive health behavior, particularly with lower socioeconomic groups of people. Because the economically deprived often have a present rather than a future orientation (having more concern for the problems of today than for the consequences of tomorrow), facilitated peer group support may be more influential than receiving advise from experts. Nurses are placed in an ideal position to influence their patients' health beliefs by manipulating the influencing factors which effect these beliefs. Access to knowledge available in the social sciences can provide nurses with certain guidelines in creating new and relevant preventive health services to the urban poor. With a solid grasp of theoretic rationales for health intervention, nurses have the opportunity to assess and initiate new programs for low income populations, a group which is often bypassed by our middle-classed system of health care.

Traditionally, community health nurses have dealt with modifying preventive health behavior via instruction on a one-to-one basis through home visiting or in talking with individual mothers during well-child clinic visits. Often the nurse's education efforts have been primarily patient centered and she feels comfortable working in a one-to-one relationship, but inadequate when dealing with groups. It is important to evaluate the effectiveness of one-to-one instruction in terms of effort expended and numbers of people reached in comparison to the effectiveness of working with groups of people. The group method not only provides more exposure for the same expenditure of time, but also allows the participants of the group to learn from one another as well as from the nurse, who can act as the professional with expertise as well as the facilitator of shared experiences for the group. Some group teaching by nurses does exist in settings where the potential participants are physically available and psychologically ready for instruction such as clinic waiting rooms, school classrooms, and Parent-Teacher Association group meetings. But the task is far more difficult for the nurse who is attempting to initiate a group as a tool for health education within a community setting where the potential participants are not readily available, may not recognize the value or purpose of the group, and have developed a chronic passive response to any outside initiative from a "helping" person. This person often represents a health system from which they feel alienated.

The community based nurse is in a unique position to initiate group intervention as a teaching tool and possesses such valuable qualifications as knowledge of the psychodynamics of group process; a preventive health orientation with a biologic basis and knowledge of public health principles; knowledge of referral systems within the community; knowledge of existing complementary health and other service agencies in the community and expertise in community liaison work among the different agencies as the patient advocate; a knowledge and understanding of growth and development, both individual and family; a role which has traditionally included aspects of teaching and role modeling; and the ability to assess a community's needs and interests for such a program.

Overview

In the community nursing project which is to be described, two areas of focus emerged which are important aspects of group organization in any type of community where nurses want to effect changes in health behaviors. Originally my major focus centered on using some of the motivational variables from the Health Belief Model as a framework in order to design a peer discussion group for low income women. This peer group format was to be used as the vehicle for communicating health information to the women in a relaxed atmosphere. With the emphasis on peer control, rather than professional dominance, these women might then influence one another to adopt more consistent patterns of preventive health behavior.

After the project was underway, a second area of focus began to emerge as the most important aspect of the project. This was dealing with the actual process of initiating the group. Accomplishing that first difficult step of forming the group itself soon involved applying those same motivational variables to the task of organization. This entailed identifying what the women perceived to be their most important and immediate needs. Once this was established, I was able to reorganize my original priorities for the group so that our mutual goals would be more consistent.

The Motivational Variables

The Health Belief Model attempts to explain preventive health behavior on the basis of certain motivational variables such as a person's perceptions of susceptibility to a disease, the perceived severity of a disease, and benefits and drawbacks associated with the actions taken to prevent the illness. A cue or triggering mechanism is also believed necessary to promote appropriate action. This cue often takes the form of health information which is received at a crucial point in the decision making process. From his research on why people use health services, Rosenstock[2] surmises that many lower socioeconomic groups of people are close to accepting such beliefs as susceptibility to illness and perceived benefits of taking certain preventive actions, and need only the proper information and stimulus to take such actions. He argues that efforts to increase response to preventive health actions should aim at minimizing barriers to action, increasing opportunity to act through education and awareness, and providing cues to trigger a certain response. In using this theory to establish a rationale for employing group education as a tool to promote health behavior, the variables identified as most relevant were interpersonal influence, which is enhanced by interaction with others via peer sharing, and perceptions of the effectiveness of preventive health behavior, which are altered through information input and providing acceptable cues to action. A group discussion method of providing health information was chosen as an effective technique for promoting personal influence in modifying health beliefs because of the combination of emotional appeal and group pressure. This same motivational formulation was then applied to the dynamics involved in actually establishing a group of this type in a low income community. The variables which were identified as providing a positive motivating force in this situation were the women's perceptions of their particular vulnerability, their perceptions of the severity of their situation, and their belief in the benefit of joining the group. Also necessary to identify were the particular barriers which were perceived to inhibit their decision to join the group and stay with the group. Although only selected variables were chosen from this theoretical model as a basis for intervention, action programs to modify or influence behavior can legitimately focus on any one or more of the model's motivational determinants.

Project Outline

In the planning stages of this project several steps were identified as crucial for the development of a successful community program. These steps then formed the basis for my actions in designing and implementing the program.

The first step involves an assessment of the needs of the population to be reached. This assessment must be in terms of the needs and interests of the consumer of the service. The service must also be designed for accessibility to the consumer, and the consumer must be involved in the initial goal setting and planning stages. I chose as my population a group of low income women who were each the single parent head of families with young children. My plan was to hold the discussion group within the immediate environment of the housing project in order to be physically accessible to the women tenants. I planned to articulate my goals to the women at the start but would encourage the group, once underway, to formulate their own goals and to participate in the planning of the discussions. Hopefully, this would provide a general framework for mutual goal setting and provide me with the opportunity to visualize their needs as they perceived them.

This first step also involves an assessment of the pertinent resources available to the people within their community. In this way, auxiliary resources may be tapped to support the program and duplication and fragmentation of services can be minimized.

The second step involves setting goals for the program, both immediate and long range. These goals give the nursing plan of action direction and purpose. The goals must be clearly understandable, realistic, desirable as a high priority of need, and consistent with what the recipients of this service perceive to be most relevant and beneficial to them. If the goals are not formulated in this framework of mutual priority setting between the nurse and her clients, the program may be destined to fail. It was on this important aspect of goal setting that the success of my project was determined.

OBJECTIVES

My long range goal was to establish a mothers' discussion group within a poverty level housing project in a low income community. The plan was for the mothers to meet once a week for approximately an hour or so to discuss various health related topics. The direction of the discussions was to be focused on two dimensions of preventive health care for families with young children. This would include the areas of parenting and of physical health maintenance of the child and the mother. Parenting is considered here as a dynamic process which is as preventive in nature as are the more concrete actions taken by parents to maintain the physical health of the family members. The parenting focus was to be placed on the difficulties associated with rearing children, expectations of the child at different stages of development, and those difficulties especially faced by low income mothers, most particularly when the family is fatherless.

On matters of physical health, the emphasis was to be placed on motivating the mother to incorporate preventive health behaviors in their daily lives. I hoped that the discussions could be facilitated to include such aspects of preventive health as nutrition, dental care, immunizations, lead paint poisoning, and accidents.

Four objectives were tentatively identified for discussion content.

1. To provide direct health information in order to stimulate preventive health behavior.
2. To increase knowledge of child development and thus increase confidence as a parent.
3. To provide an atmosphere of peer support as well as professional expertise in matters of parenting and preventive health measures.
4. To provide needed socialization for emotionally impoverished mothers who have few daily social contacts.

The socialization aspect of the group was not initially a motivating force, but once fear and suspicion had been overcome this aspect had a large influence on the development of the group and subsequent cohesiveness of the members.

The third step involves the actual implementation of the program. It is at this point that the nurse may want to involve key community representatives or specific people with power and influence in order to mobilize support for the program. In this case strategic persons having the most contact and influence with the women of the housing project were included in the planning and implementation phases of organizing the group. This was to enhance the credibility of the program and to broaden the base of support. These persons included teachers from the local elementary school, public health nurses from the district, the housing project social worker, and the tenants' representative. Key persons of power and influence who assisted in the implementation phase included several officials from the city's housing authority office. Their role will be defined in the description of the project.

Several different alternatives may be examined or evaluated in determining the best course of action for implementing a particular plan. This involves a fourth step which includes constant evaluation of the implementation phase of the project in order to determine the validity and effectiveness of the nursing plan of action in relation to the goals which were set. This may produce a reordering of priorities and goals. In this particular project it was the realization that the consumer community had a set of priorities and needs apart from those nursing needs that had been identified that produced the necessary reordering of my priorities and goals and subsequently led to a successful program. Even a skilled and experienced community worker is never completely safe in deciding for a people just how their needs can best be met, or even what those total needs may encompass. The greater the difference between the nurse and her patients— whether that difference is in education, ethnic background, or economic standard of living— the harder it will be for her to see their needs as they see them or to judge the acceptability to them of her way of meeting these needs. As part of this continual evaluation of a nursing plan, a nurse must make an honest assessment of her goals in terms of what the patient perceives as most important to achieve. Thus, an analysis of the combination of factors which would motivate a group of low income mothers to participate in a weekly discussion group proved to be more crucial to this project than the actual content and direction of the planned discussions. A description and evaluation of the difficulties associated with initiating such a project in this community has implications for nurses in all service oriented institutions and particularly those nurses in the public health service system who are involved with the planning and providing of health services to lower socioeconomic families.

PROJECT DESCRIPTION

The mothers' group project was initiated under the auspices of a storefront family information, education, and referral agency where I was working as a consultant in order to fulfill the clinical component of a community health master's program. Specifically, the discussion group was to provide a vehicle for communicating important health information to the women tenants of a 265 unit low income housing development on the outskirts of a large urban area. The ethnic background of the tenants was predominantly black, and the population included mostly single women with children who were receiving some type of government financial aid. There was particular interest in developing some type of program within this housing project as the poverty level was extremely low and apathy of the tenants and management was notoriously high. Several community service agencies had attempted to initiate various types of programs in this housing project, such as educational, recreational, and health screening, but had met with apathy, resistance, and subsequent failure.

After assessing the needs of my population and setting my goals for the project, I planned to meet with strategic persons who could best represent the interests of the people for whom the project was designed. I met with the housing manager, the social worker, and the community representative who worked full time at the housing project in order to present the idea of a mothers' group to them and to gain their support. The community representative's job was to act as liaison between the tenants and the management of the housing project. In this new capacity she had already met with large numbers of tenants and by now was familiar to most. Both the social worker and the community worker were black women with similar economic backgrounds to the tenants. The agreed upon first attempt by me at reaching the tenants was door-to-door knocking. This proved to be not only time consuming but produced poor results as well. The tenants were either not at home or they refused to open their doors out of fear and suspicion.

I also met with the public health nurse from the district which serves the housing project to obtain a list of families with young children. A list of children living in the project was obtained from the files of the public health well-child clinic. Addresses of several young families known to the information and referral agency and to the district children's mental health center were noted. A second attempt to selectively knock on doors was made but was met with the same negative results as the initial random attempts. Questions were sometimes asked, through closed and locked doors, concerning my identity and purpose. Responses to these inquiries opened few doors. Reaching the families by telephone was almost impossible as this convenience was not available to most of the tenants. Notices were printed and left in the manager's office announcing the formation of a mothers' group—a chance to socialize with other mothers, to discuss common problems of child rearing, and an opportunity to meet with a community health nurse to discuss good health practices for the family. There was still no response.

Evaluation of Nursing Interventions

At this crucial point in the implementation phase of any nursing plan, after repeated failures have occurred, it is time to reassess one's goals and evaluate the methods used to promote those goals which have failed to generate success. In this case, the reasons for the almost unanimous negative response had to be identified and examined, with alternative actions devised. Several factors were considered.

Through years of isolation, living alone in a tough ghetto climate, the women had defensively developed a strong fear and suspicion of one another. Thus, presenting the idea of a group discussion as a satisfying method of social interaction was not consistent with their past experiences. For the economically disadvantaged, general apathy and a depressed emotional outlook can be created by the hardships and frustration of coping with the day-to-day insults of poverty. This passivity and reluctance, particularly to making changes, is reinforced by a bureaucratic system which often deals with them in terms of disappointments and broken promises. The urban poor are not unfamiliar with government and local community programs whose goals are either inconsistent with the real needs of the people they wish to serve or are so unrealistic as to be destined to fail. This produces a pervasive suspicion of all assistance programs and those people connected with them. The most important aspect of the reevaluation phase of this project was to determine whether my goals were consistent with the needs of the women of the housing project. The answer to this question was supplied indirectly by the women, themselves, in subsequent home visits and provided the major framework for a reordering of my priorities.

In reassessing my approach, I realized that I had to gain the women's confidence in my commitment to them and not just to the idea of the group, itself. At the same time, I had to offer these women an opportunity to regain control over a portion of their lives. In light of this reassessment, I once again began knocking on doors, this time with the project community worker, a black woman and a resident of a similar housing development in the city. She was someone with whom the tenants were more familiar and who was trusted by them. With this new approach, more and more doors were opened and conversations with some of the tenants were initiated.

It was during these selected conversations that it became apparent that the issues of parenting and preventive health were not of primary concern to the women. They were most concerned with the degenerating physical conditions at the housing project, the lack of a safe place for their children to play, vandalism which was prevalent among the teenagers, and a feeling that they had lost any personal control over their lives. Often a passively flat affect changed to aggressive expressions of anger as these topics were discussed. I wondered if these common expressions of anger and frustration might not be the catalyst that was needed to motivate the women to organize, rather than the promise of obtaining preventive health information. It was also apparent that the preventive health information that these women most needed was how to provide an outlet for their anger and a constructive method of dealing with the source of this anger. This reassessment of goals in relation to need led to the design of an alternative plan of action in the form of a tenants' task force committee. In talking with a group of community organizers who were working at the project to develop a youth recreational program, I learned that several housing projects in the city had developed a task force organization as a form of tenant self-government. I contacted officials of the city's housing authority and also learned that city funds were available to subsidize certain activities of any viable tenants' task force which was formed in any of the city's housing units. This information, unfortunately, was not readily made available to the tenants of the various housing units. In most cases a great deal of organizational effort plus a determined and cohesive tenant population was necessary to formalize such a committee. However, a tenants' task force committee, if organized, would officially have the power to channel complaints to the main housing office. This committee could also demand that action be taken on certain complaints and could utilize housing money allotted to the projects to reopen the vandalized recreation center for the teenagers. Most importantly, a tenants' task force organization could give the tenants a representative structure through which they could realize control over their lives in the project. Once again, discussions were initiated with the community worker and the social worker at the housing project in order to formalize the plan and determine its feasibility.

Implementing the New Plan

The first step to implementing the new plan was, again, reaching the tenants. I was known to most of the teachers at the local elementary school. I had visited the school in my initial planning stages in order to obtain the names of some of the project families whose children attended the school. I had subsequently been asked to act as consultant for a health fair which the children and teachers were organizing that spring at the school. I now returned to the school to ask if I might speak at the parent-teacher meeting that week in order to present the idea of a tenants' action group to those parents from the housing project. I spoke at the meeting and afterwards to many of the housing project parents. The tenants' group idea was met with unexpected enthusiasm and support.

As a second step, some of the more vocal women in the project, who seemed willing to translate their anger into some viable form of action, were revisited. Five women committed themselves to attending an initial meeting the following week to formalize plans, but we had, as yet, no place to meet. This third step presented some problems, at first. Using the school auditorium was a possibility, but I thought that the first meeting place should be based in the housing project in order to include those mothers whose children were not of school age. Eventually, one woman's enthusiasm for the task force overcame her fear and she offered her apartment for the first meeting.

It was now necessary to provide a specific cue or stimulus which would motivate the other women in the project to participate in a first meeting. Again it was helpful to consider some of the major motivational components of the Health Belief Model in order to implement this second phase of action.

THE MOTIVATIONAL VARIABLES

The two influencing factors considered were "Perception of Vulnerability" and "Perception of Seriousness."

Perception of one's vulnerability or susceptibility to disease is one of the major variables or factors affecting health behavior motivation. Obviously, the area in which these women experienced the strongest sense of vulnerability transcended specific disease entities and encompassed their total physical environment. A feeling of powerlessness over their personal lives prevailed. Their lives were controlled by external events and other persons. I tried to capitalize on this vulnerability in preparing the fliers to be distributed to all of the tenants announcing a meeting for the purpose of forming a task force at this housing project. The fliers articulated the tenants' discontent, complaints, and feelings of powerlessness which were calculated to generate maximum emotional arousal. A cause around which to mobilize their vulnerability was what I hoped to provide. The fliers enumerated the visible deplorable conditions in the project such as broken windows, a general lack of security, missing locks on main doors and mailboxes, the vandalized and boarded youth center, and infestation of rats and roaches. This was followed by the announcement of a meeting of all interested tenants which would offer them a chance to mobilize their strength through the organization of a task force committee.

Perception of the seriousness of the situation is a variable which is influenced by the visibility of a threat, the immediacy of a threat, or an emotional arousal at the thought of a threat.[2] The women in this housing project had become passive, denying the severity of conditions in their lives and making compromises in order to cope. There might be more willingness to recognize the degree of severity of their situation if the women believed that there was a positive way in which to deal with and overcome the threat. The tenants' task force offered them a realistic approach to a solution and a reasonable opportunity to resolve the severity of their situation. The fliers were distributed to all of the apartments with the hope that a few tenants might attend. Fifteen women and three men came to that first task force meeting which was considered quite an accomplishment in view of the previous negative responses. Anger and hostility were the dominant emotions at that meeting, but with careful facilitation these labile emotions were channeled into tentative plans to form a task force committee.

During the initial planning of this meeting, a third motivational variable was considered for maximum effect and success. A person's perception of vulnerability and of the seriousness of a situation can influence his or her psychological state of readiness to act. In other words, these two factors provide the energy to act. A third factor which seems to provide the impetus to channel that energy into a specific action (in this case, joining the task force committee) involves weighing the benefits of taking an action against the barriers, whether they be real or imagined. A person may ask, "Is this action worth the effort I must expend and will it be successful?" People tend to choose an alternative with the least amount of threat and the highest probability of success. A related problem is that many persons of lower socioeconomic groups have not been exposed to various alternatives for improving their lives and are distrustful of those who might try to persuade them of the benefits of taking a certain action. Careful intervention at this point, in the form of how the task force alternative was presented, would be crucial to acceptance of the idea.

A TASK FORCE IS FORMED

As a caucasian nurse from an obviously middle-class background involved in what was viewed by these women as a nontraditional nursing role, my presence in this black ghetto was considered suspiciously at first. My mode of intervention at this point was two-fold. I invited the project community worker to that first meeting. She was not only black but familiar to and trusted by the tenants. Living in a housing project herself, where a task force had been in operation for several years, she was someone who had intimate knowledge of how a viable task force could improve conditions. She also could provide concrete information about the mechanics of activating a task force. Thus, she could influence their belief in the benefit of taking this action by citing task force successes in other housing projects, including her own. She was also able to reinforce their perception of vulnerability by fully empathizing with their anger but providing them with productive input as to how tenant control could effect a change.

Secondly, rather than becoming an active participant in the angry discussions, I saw my role as group facilitator, keeping the strong emotions at a manageable and constructive level, keeping the topics within the bounds of what could effectively be dealt with at this first meeting, and channeling these emotions into constructive plans to activate a tenants' task force. A second task force meeting was planned. All tenants again would be invited for the purpose of electing eight permanent task force members. A member of the official city housing authority was invited to specifically outline the rights and prerogatives of a tenants' task force committee. It was learned that once a task force committee was established, official tenant representatives from that task force would meet with the city housing authorities once a month. The tenants needed to hear from a city official precisely what rights they would exercise as an official task force committee. Fliers were again prepared and distributed to all apartments announcing this second meeting. To reinforce the paper announcements, a car cruised the housing project with a bullhorn on the day of the meeting announcing the time, place, and purpose. Teenagers from the project were recruited for that mission. The meeting was held at the elementary school auditorium in anticipation of a higher attendance. Forty tenants came to that evening meeting. The participants included both men and women from the project. The official from the city housing authority provided specific input as to the governing structure and influence of a task force. The community representative led the tenants through the procedure of electing eight temporary task force members who would eventually be voted upon as permanent task force officers by balloting within the entire project complex. Thus, an official community task force, the first one ever to be organized in this housing project, was established.

THE MOTHERS' GROUP IS FORMED

An outgrowth of these two task force meetings was a new feeling of closeness among the women of the housing project who had helped to organize the tenants. Having shared anger, frustration, and hopelessness in those first meetings and having channeled this anger into a workable solution had generated a new feeling of camaraderie and enthusiasm. It was while working together to formulate a task force that the women also realized that they shared other common concerns. Although the women would continue to work with the task force committee, several of them expressed a desire to meet as a separate women's group to share the common problems of being a single parent in an urban poverty community. The mothers' group was finally becoming a reality. We began meeting on Wednesday mornings from 10:30 A.M. until 12 noon with only four or five women attending each week. But word of our weekly discussion groups spread throughout the housing project and at times the number of women attending increased to 12 or 15. I encouraged them to set their own goals for the group at our first meeting. Enthusiastic discussion about the beginning work of the separate task force committee occupied the first part of the early meetings, but they soon restructured their discussions to include such topics as common problems of weight control and sharing ways of coping as a single parent. The women also wanted information regarding summer camps and recreation facilities in the community which I was able to provide, along with information about the new health center in the area. Not all of the women attended each time, and from week to week the attendance would vary from 3 to 15 or more. Some of the barriers which were identified as inhibiting attendance and the methods which were used to minimize these barriers should also be mentioned, as these factors must be considered in any community action program where participation is voluntary.

THE BARRIERS

Three types of barriers which seemed to influence the stability of participation in the weekly discussions were identified.

Physical

The main physical barrier was in finding a place to meet which was convenient and accessible to all the women. An apartment in the housing project would be the most convenient and centralized place to meet. However, it was still difficult for most of the women to open up their homes to one another. Only two women felt comfortable enough to offer their apartment to the group and we alternated each week. This arrangement seemed to work out satisfactorily in the beginning, but it was recognized that more space would be needed in the future as attendance increased. A neutral area which all of the women could consider as their group meeting place would be ideal. We utilized the new tenants' task force to help us with this problem. A viable task force committee in existence at any city housing project was entitled to the use of one empty apartment as an office area. In discussing our need for space with the new task force committee we were promised the use of this apartment for our weekly meetings. Securement of the space from the housing authority would be a longer term goal for both the mothers' group and the new task force committee to work toward.

Situational

Two types of situational deterrents were observed—weather and children. The presence of snow or rain was always directly related to a low group attendance. No successful way was found to avoid this, other than peer pressure. The women were encouraged to walk to the meetings in pairs or groups. The problem of children could be handled more directly. Meetings were held in the morning hours so that the older children would be in school. The number of preschool children never became a problem for us as most of the children were at least of kindergarten age and attended school for a half day. In a different situation where more preschool children are involved, it might be possible to design a program whereby nursing students or early education majors from local colleges could fulfill their child development clinical responsibilities by supervising the children in a play group.

Psychological

If a psychological barrier exerts a strong enough negative influence at a time when a person's readiness to act is also strong, that person may remove herself psychologically or physically from the conflict.[7] The fear and suspicion that many experienced at first caused at least one woman to terminate, complaining that her privacy would be destroyed. This fear and suspicion, experienced at different levels by all of the women, were not easy to overcome after years of reinforcement. Vacillating attendance was viewed as an attempt at emotional manipulation of the others as the women came to look forward to the meetings and to chatting with one another. This pattern of attendance occurred with two women, both of whom eventually stopped coming altogether. Either their needs were not being met by the group or they were feeling threatened by an invasion of their privacy as the group explored more personal feelings. This phenomenon was also seen in one woman who constantly committed herself enthusiastically to the task force committee as well as the mothers' group and then always managed to miss a crucial task force meeting. But the interpersonal influence that each began to exert on the others in the group and the support that this provided, along with a slowly developing bond of trust among the women, were the most influencing factors in modifying this psychological barrier. Passivity, another great psychological barrier to overcome, was counteracted mainly by providing the women with an opportunity to take responsibility for their lives through uniting, thus giving back to them some rational control over their lives.

EPILOGUE

The weekly mothers' group meetings with this author as facilitator continued for seven weeks following the initial task force meeting. Our weekly discussions ranged from children's issues, such as bedwetting, discipline, nutrition, immunizations, and when to take a child to the doctor, to women's issues such as coping alone, self-breast exams, the need for regular pap smear exams, nutrition, and weight control. This latter topic generated such enthusiasm that an exercise group was formed as an adjunct to the regular group. This group the women would manage on their own. I arranged to have an instructor from the YWCA come to one of our meetings to demonstrate specific exercises which the women could do on their own and as a group. Those women who were interested then met weekly to form their own exercise support group. Other issues the group began to discuss were as diverse as creating a summer craft program for the children of the housing project and discussing legal alternatives for low income single parents. Speakers were often provided by the family service agency which had much influence in the community. The women even discussed the possibility of swimming together one day a week at the local YMCA.

By the end of this seven week period, my clinical experience at the family service agency was completed and I had to terminate as facilitator of the group. Although I was viewed by the women as a professional with expertise, our relationship had evolved into one of trust and friendship. Although I facilitated the discussions, I was also considered a member and active participant of the group. Hopefully, this type of relationship will have an influence on their perception of community nurses and community professionals and programs in the future. The women wanted to continue meeting. I felt a strong commitment to maintain the cohesiveness of the group and did not want my termination to have a negative effect on the structure of the group. The director of the family service agency where I had been associated for these four months had experience in working with groups in this community. Most importantly, she wanted the opportunity to facilitate a women's discussion group in this housing project. A psychiatric social worker from the mental health satellite clinic in this community had heard of my success in forming this women's group and became intrigued with the idea of organizing lower income women into self-help groups. Eventually, she became cofacilitator of the group. Their mutual goals for the group were more mental health related, but plans were made to have public health nurses from the community agency come to the group meetings as guest discussion leaders to continue the emphasis on family preventive health. At this writing, two years later, the women are still meeting as a group.

The task force organization is now an independent functioning unit, separate from the mothers' group, supported by a majority of the tenants (both men and women), and assuming responsibility for all tenant action within the housing project. There was suspicion at first on the part of housing management to be overcome, but the tenants' frustration had been channeled into determination and action. The community worker at the project provided the needed continuity of leadership and stability for the tenants' action group. The people of this housing project now have a legitimate voice in determining their day-to-day affairs.

DISCUSSION

It is essential that we as nurses explore our role in promoting health maintenance and in providing health information particularly to the urban poor. We have not, as yet, found appropriate and relevant ways of serving many nonmiddle-class groups, but it must be recognized that there is no one ideal approach to use in reaching this population. It is our responsibility, however, to take the initiative in developing and providing innovative community based programs for the poor. The major emphasis of this chapter has been to target the population of low income women with children. But there is no reason why a group technique method of community education could not be used with other high risk and hard to reach groups such as adolescents and the elderly population of our urban cities. If group intervention can prove to be a more viable and practical method of reaching large numbers of people in the community, outside of the traditional primary care setting, then more nurses need to look at this method as a tool for health education in the community. When participating in the group is on a voluntary basis, however, then the emotional processes which motivate a person to participate in a group must be evaluated as closely as the content and rationale for the group. Awareness of knowledge available in the behavioral sciences can be beneficial when forming guidelines for an assessment of the population to be served. Again, this assessment must be in terms of the needs and interests of the people. Goals must be set in relation to what the participants perceive to be most relevant and beneficial to them, otherwise the program is destined to fail. Potential barriers to the program as well as motivating factors must be considered at the planning stage. Key community representatives should be consulted and involved. Financial backing, though not a consideration in this case, is often available through many community sponsored programs. The nurse must assume the role of political activist in promoting a particular program idea to the various community agencies whose support is essential.

An initial cue chosen to stimulate participation in a group may only indirectly relate to your long term goals for the group. As in this case, meeting the women's more immediate needs concerning shelter and safety and giving the women a sense of power or control over their lives were more effective as motivating cues than persuading them to see the benefit of long term preventive health behaviors. An initial cue, in whatever form it may take, must stimulate interest or a readiness to act and should provide proof of the effectiveness of that action as well. It is then that compliance with longer term health goals can be accomplished.

Though the task force formation may have been seen as nonhealth related at first, in a broader sense this aspect of the program may have been the most important for the women in terms of preventive health.

It is this type of nontraditional community action program in which nurses must be ready to participate. We must improve upon our traditional methods of community health nursing, but we must do so with careful planning and a theoretic basis for implementation. In utilizing peer group education as an intervention technique for attempting to modify health behavior, I attempted to apply a specific model of behavioral prediction in order to identify the unique factors which may determine a person's readiness to participate in a group setting. These predictor variables may be applied to many similar health education programs which seek to modify or influence health behaviors. Using sound theoretic rationale as a basis for designing and evaluating a program of health education, nurses can legitimately consider group intervention as a viable and effective health education tool.

REFERENCES

1. Lewin, K.: *A Dynamic Theory of Personality*. McGraw-Hill, Inc., London, 1935.
2. Rosenstock, I.M.: "Prevention of Illness and Maintenance of Health," in Kosa, J., Antonovsky, A., and Zola, I. (eds.): *Poverty and Health*. Harvard University Press, Cambridge, Mass., 1969.
3. Kosa, J., et al.: *Poverty and Health*. Harvard University Press, Cambridge, Mass., 1964.
4. Friedson, E.: *Patients' Views of Medical Practices*. Russell Sage Foundation, New York, 1961.
5. Kriesberg, L.: *Mothers in Poverty*. Aldine Publishing Company, Chicago, 1970.
6. Pavenstedt, E.: "An Intervention Program for Infants from High Risk Homes." *American Journal of Public Health* 63:393, May 1973.
7. Pender, N.J.: "A Conceptual Model for Preventive Health Behavior." *Nursing Outlook* 23:6, 1975.

CHAPTER 48

NURSE-MIDWIVES IN ACTION AT THE CHILDBEARING-CHILDREARING CENTER

SHARON SCHINDLER RISING, M.S.N., C.N.M., R.N.

Several years ago I experienced great frustration with the traditional medical care system. Women and couples coming to me for care were making very reasonable requests which required some deviations from the current care routines. Even though I was a nurse-midwife responsible for the management of their care, I was not able to negotiate such changes with those physicians, nurses, and administrators who controlled the system. At that point I felt I had three available options: continue in the system and hope consumer pressure would eventually effect change, leave that system and look for another which would be more supportive of my needs and of consumer demands, or leave the "system" and join the counterculture. I elected to search for a system that was a better fit for me.

My own base for practice developed most clearly following my exposure to several theories presented during my educational experience at the Yale School of Nursing. Most influential was Ernestine Wiedenbach, chairperson of the nurse-midwifery program, and author of *Clinical Nursing: A Helping Art.*[1] Besides providing me with a framework for my nursing care, it taught me to be reflective about my practice. The development of this framework allowed me a context out of which to evaluate consumers' needs and my ability to respond to them, clinically and philosophically. Gradually I began to see myself as a facilitator of care (growth) and the consumer as the central point in the determination of the care plan.

During this period I was also concerned with the fragmentation that existed within childbearing care and with the separation of childbearing and childrearing care. My own observations, coupled with the wants and needs brought to me by consumers, supported a conclusion that traditional medical care was basically inadequate for normal childbearing. Some of the consumer concerns were: having come control over their experience, assurance of relief from certain routines, minimal or no separation of mother and baby, and the option of early discharge. In addition, since the obstetrician usually said "goodbye" to the mother in the delivery room and the pediatrician "hello" at the two month visit, the new family frequently was quite abandoned by the system during the crucial transition period. Some were fortunate to have one or more visits from the public health nurse, but little continuity in overall care was given. Since the father seldom was integrated as a member of the care team, he frequently did not see himself as a *primary* caregiver during the early postpartum period. Certainly he had few role models to help him with transition from man/husband to father. What should have been one of the most joyous and growth producing experiences for the mother/father/family too many times turned into a depressing chain of failed expectations and doubts about self-adequacy.

The system was all too slow in responding to consumer demands. It was unprepared for the effects of parent education. Couples, through education, began to expect active participation in care. Once women started refusing medication and fathers insisted on being present for labor *and* delivery, it was a whole new world. Many professionals felt threatened by this invasion into the realm of decision making and had extreme difficulty in defining their roles. Many times I heard, "I just don't understand why a woman would elect to feel pain during labor when she could go through the whole thing pain-free."

During my teaching/clinical years following my educational experience at Yale, I had time to listen, observe, and solidify my own philosophy of care. It was this experience that led me to design the type of center that now exists in Minnesota.

EARLY INTRODUCTION

The University of Minnesota was interested in nurse-midwifery from two perspectives. The chairperson of the Obstetrics-Gynecology Department felt nurse-midwives brought an additional quality service to the total complex of obstetric care. The School of Nursing was eager to develop a graduate maternal-child program and felt that nurse-midwives would fit well into that framework. The program, then, started with an academic base within an institution that easily supported innovative programs. At that time, only one other nurse-midwife was providing care within the community, and that was outside the University.

The year for this beginning was 1972. That was about the time when the media was starting to broadcast the existence of nurse-midwives. It was well before Suzanne Arms' *Immaculate Deception*[2] was published (1975) but coincided with the increasing popularity of *Our Bodies, Ourselves*[3] (1973), one of the first self-help books to reach the popular market.

Since the program was located within an academic environment it was immune to some of the normal community scrutiny. We had much discussion related to childbearing care with community agencies. Many were helpful in the early planning stages; most needed education regarding the role and responsibilities of a nurse-midwife. The State Health Department also participated in early planning stages. Many community physicians quite honestly felt the program would not last long and so did not get involved.

The University itself does not have a readily identified obstetric population outside of its students. University personnel are given several health insurance options including a health maintenance organization. It is extremely difficult to assess the need for a service that is nonexistent in a community. Because an educational program for nurse-midwives was being planned, that alone could dictate need for such a service.

Other input was obtained through:

1. Health professional knowledge of services which could be provided by a nurse-midwife which were now not available or costing considerably more.
2. Individual women in the community who contacted me to share their concerns for certain services.
3. Larger women's groups, many of which invited me to speak and subsequently urged me to move forward with plans.
4. Encouragement from the University itself as to the efficacy of the project. Some of the major support for the project came from the Office of the Vice President for Health Sciences. This office provided some needed financing as well as essential moral support.

The major objectives of the program were two-fold:

1. To develop a nursing model for the delivery of care to essentially healthy childbearing families.
2. To provide a nursing practice site for the basic education of nurse-midwifery students.

THE CHILDBEARING-CHILDREARING CENTER

In the spring of 1973 I was joined by a maternity nurse, Sr. Mary Meyer, who left her obstetric administrative job at a community hospital to help with the development of this innovative program. She possessed invaluable knowledge of the community and was well known by those involved in the delivery of childbearing care. She is still with the Center today and has had enormous influence on our growth and development.

My caseload initially developed from women I cared for in conjunction with the obstetrician in charge of the obstetrics division at the University. I billed directly for my professional services which allowed the recruitment of a "private" nurse-midwifery population. The first nurse-midwife deliveries were in 1973 with a total of 21 by the end of that year. A second nurse-midwife was added to the staff that fall.

That year, 1973, also saw the start of the nurse-midwifery educational program. Twelve students were admitted in the fall for a two year graduate program leading to a master's degree and certification in nurse-midwifery.

In 1974 we employed a part-time pediatric nurse practitioner (PNP) who was affiliated with the University's well-child clinic. She began providing care to our childbearing families who elected to remain in our system. We immediately began to see the benefits of this continuity of care.

Another core component of our service, support groups for couples delivering around the same time period, began early in 1974. These groups, for four to six couples, were facilitated by our professional staff and dealt with the critical issues of childbearing and early childrearing. The groups formally organized one month prior to due dates and continued for approximately two months postpartum. The first support group that we had is still meeting occasionally now some six years later!

The Center developed very independently within the University setting. The Obstetric Department gave its support through professional backup and varying amounts of salary support. The School of Nursing, while not involved in direct care services, did view the Center as important for its educational program. The Office of the Vice President for Health Sciences was pleased to see such an innovative program and gave critical financial support, especially to the childrearing aspect, in those early years; and University Hospitals like the freshness of the approach and hoped it would add important numbers to the obstetric population.

In 1975 the Center became an outreach clinic of University Hospitals. The Hospital assumed responsibility for the salaries of the nurse-midwives and temporarily took over the billing for our professional services. This move to the Hospital gave the Center stability and has continued to be a satisfactory arrangement. We have been fortunate in working with a group of hospital administrators who are futuristic in their thinking.

One of our early goals called for an out of hospital setting for our service. The Hospital's General Director readily saw the need for a wellness service such as ours located outside of the hospital. It is extremely difficult not to take on the role of patient when you are receiving care in the "ill" institution. Once the Obstetric Department was also comfortable with that need, a move of our offices and clinic space occurred rapidly to a home which met our criteria: warm and homey, adequate parking, near the University. This move was in the summer of 1976 and was really the start of a clearly identified Childbearing-Childrearing Center (CCC). Now all activities were under the same roof and the childrearing component looked definitely connected to the whole. Even hospital business office people came to the Center so our consumers would not have to negotiate the difficult hospital registration process.

The house has space for a reception area, two exam rooms with a third available when needed, a living room/waiting room (fireplace included), large meeting space/children's play area in the basement, a small laboratory, kitchen, and four office rooms. It is a ten minute walk from University Hospitals and very accessible by bus. This has proven beneficial for students, consumers, and personnel alike. Since the Center has some evening hours for clinics and parent education, the space is well used but rapidly becoming inadequate as new programs develop.

The Center, then, from the start developed as more than a nurse-midwifery service. I feel that it is very important to integrate childbearing care within a total system of *health* care. One of our original goals, that of a *family* health center, is only now being seriously studied. So, although the actual operations may be added in pieces, the overall design needs to be clearly defined early in the development.

Who Is Our Population?

Initially the service started with women who were already seeking care at the University. In our latest survey over 66 percent stated they would not have come to the University if it had not been for the availability of nurse-midwifery services. Now approximately 12 percent of our consumers are repeaters with us. Some women have driven several hundred miles from their homes to receive service at our Center. In the future, we hope that similar services will be available throughout the state.

Tables 48-1, 48-2, and 48-3 provide the exact numbers and percentages of the total number of women serviced by us from 1973 through June of 1978. These three tables show that the majority of our women are married, primiparas in the 18 to 29 year age

TABLE 48-1. Age of CCC consumers

Age	N	%
Under 18	20	3.8
18–24	186	35.3
25–29	249	47.2
30–34	68	12.9
35 +	4	0.8
Totals	527	100.0

TABLE 48-2. Marital status of CCC consumers

Status	N	%
Married	433	82.2
Single	94	17.8
Totals	527	100.0

TABLE 48-3. Parity of CCC consumers

Parity	N	%
Primipara	333	63.2
1–2 children	167	31.7
more than 2 children	27	5.1
Totals	527	100.0

range. In addition, most of our women are white. One recent determination showed that women of color comprised 7.7 percent of our total. These women include native American, Oriental, Spanish, and black.

As is shown in Table 48-4 the majority of women in our service have spontaneous deliveries. Since 1973 our forceps rate has been dropping, probably due to our increasing competence regarding positions for pushing and coaching strategies. We do not screen out population for possible pelvic problems, and with such a large number of primiparas this spontaneous delivery percentage is excellent. Of a recent group of 130 women, only 16 percent used an analgesic during labor. In this same population, 21 percent had internal monitoring, 3 percent needed a pitocin induction, and another 13 percent needed pitocin augmentation. Over 33 percent had an intact perineum and another 7 percent just a minor laceration. Fifty-three percent needed intravenous therapy and 15 percent were classified as having a postpartum hemorrhage. Most of the babies needed little resuscitation; 5 percent had Apgars of under 7 at 5 minutes.

It also is not surprising that most of the women utilizing our service breast fed their infants, many for prolonged periods (Table 48-5). They get a lot of support from the entire staff, including the Center's pediatrician.

TABLE 48-4. Type of delivery of CCC consumers

Delivery	N	%
Spontaneous	403	76.5
Forceps	67	12.7
Caesarean	57	10.8
Totals	527	100.0

TABLE 48-5. Feeding method chosen by CCC consumers

Method	N	%
Bottle	52	9.9
Breast	472	90.1
Totals	524	100.0

Table 48-6 shows the educational level of the CCC consumers in 1977. This population is reflective of what one would expect in a University setting. It also supports the cross mix of people from the community at large. This is important if one is to evaluate the appropriateness of the Center concept for the population at large.

A few other statistics may help to further define our population and the outcomes of care. Our service does not accept women for care after 36 weeks gestation (Table 48-7). Approximately 40 percent of these 129 women transferred to us during their pregnancy from another care source. The average number of visits with us was 11, with the greatest frequency being 12 visits. Some of the outcomes of good prenatal care should be reflected in lower rates of toxemia and prematurity. Medical consultation for pre-eclampsia was needed for 9 percent (N = 12) of the women with 2 percent (N = 3) needing hospitalization. Six babies or 4.6 percent weighed under 2500 grams at birth; 16 or 12.5 percent weighed over 4000 grams! There were two cases of fetal/newborn demise out of the 130 deliveries.

How and why do women select our program? Consistently women say they hear about us from their friends. This, we feel, is the strongest publicity we can have. Others hear about us through our public relations efforts or through another agency. We have always been interested in why they chose us over other care providers. In an evaluation questionnaire we ask them to rank the importance of several reasons for choice according to those most important to them (Table 48-8). The strongest reasons consistently are wanting to have some control over their experience, not wanting to have routine procedures applied to them, and wanting their family involved to the greatest extent possible. These desires are in accord with the usual nurse-midwifery practice at the Center and tend to lead to a very satisfied outcome.

We feel that having our consumers highly involved in their care has led to a high degree of satisfaction with our service (Table 48-9). The consumers have been very instrumental in helping to change the hospital system to allow for labor room deliveries, early

TABLE 48-6. Mother's and father's education level

Years of Education	Mother's		Father's	
	N	%	N	%
12 or under	34	29.8	21	20.6
13-16	56	49.1	46	45.1
17-20	23	20.2	29	28.4
over 20	1	0.9	6	5.9
Totals	114	100.0	102	100.0

TABLE 48-7. Registered for care

Number of weeks	N	%
12 and under	55	42.6
13-19	39	30.2
20-27	16	12.4
28 and over	19	14.7
Totals	129	100.0

TABLE 48-8. Top three priorities for choice of CCC for childbearing care of consumers in 1977

Priority	N	%	Total N
Control over my experience	97	80.8	120
Family involvement	72	60.0	120
No routines	60	50.4	119
Second best to home birth	20	16.8	119
Lower costs	10	8.4	119
Woman to woman care	29	24.4	119
Continuity of care	35	29.4	119

TABLE 48-9. Satisfaction of care of CCC consumers

Satisfaction	N	%
Highly satisfied	343	85.5
Satisfied	49	12.2
Neutral	8	2.0
Dissatisfied	1	0.3
Highly Dissatisfied	0	0
Totals	401	100.0

discharge, and sibling visiting. Currently they are assisting our efforts to allow siblings to be present for labor, delivery, and early postpartum.

A brief report on other services at the Center shows a total of over 100 well woman visits last year, 120 new childrearing children enrolled, and a total of 632 visits made to the Childrearing Clinic.

Financial Support

Monetary support for this service has come directly from the University. Income from patient fees helps to offset this expense but the Center still is not self-sufficient. Many third party payers, including Medicaid, reimburse directly for our services. An article written by Rising and Houde[4] further outlines reimbursement strategies. Recently the Center has received money from the city and county for a teenage mother's education/ support program. This program provides early and late pregnancy and early parenting education for small groups of teens.

As new positions have been added to the staff, efforts have been made to predict extent of income to be generated. I would term this "responsible expansion." Hopefully it will help to lead us to a more secure financial base.

THE NURSING MODEL

As the Center continues to evolve we are further expanding and modifying our concepts as needed. We have viewed the Center as a professionally directed, consumer oriented service that sees the consumer as an equal partner in assessing, implementing, and evaluating the care.

From the beginning, this service has attempted to provide a type of care that will fulfill basic goals of safety and satisfaction for each consumer and, hopefully, for the care provider.

Implied in this basic goal are these beliefs:

1. The present system of sickness care does not adequately address itself to health care needs.
2. Consumers are becoming more health oriented as basic medical problems are being controlled and as basic human needs such as clothing, food, and shelter are being met.
3. Nursing is just emerging as a leader in the area of health. Health care is at the core of the nursing profession, but nurses have been stifled in their ability to deliver such care. It is imperative, therefore, to demonstrate alternative patterns of health care in which nursing leadership is clear.
4. As alternatives to present medical systems are available, consumers will be able to find viable systems of response to their clearly articulated needs for personalized health care. If such new systems are found responsive by the consumers, free enterprise will support the growth and continuance of the system. Power today ultimately rests with the consumer, and it is she or he who will decide on directions for the future.
5. As nursing is allowed to develop fully, the gap between the ideal and the real will be much smaller, and more nurses will be able to tolerate the work setting. This should directly reduce the nursing dropout rate and, furthermore, will increase the

nurse's own credibility. It is becoming more difficult for the thoughtful, consumer oriented nurse to answer the patients' expressions of dissatisfaction and still maintain her own integrity.[5]

6. Childbearing is an essentially healthy activity and is a family affair. It involves the total community and care should be closely related to the community. In addition, childbearing and childrearing are inextricably linked within the family. That principle should be reflected in the organization of our care system.

7. Nurse-midwives and pediatric nurse practitioners are potentially ideal care providers to bring health oriented care to healthy individuals within the scope of childbearing-childrearing.

Fortunately, those in positions of authority at the University agreed with these basic statements and allowed us the freedom to proceed with an operationalization of a model based on these statements. Some components were obvious almost immediately: visits should be of adequate length for sharing of concerns (approximately 30 minutes); contact with numbers of care providers throughout pregnancy should be limited; an education/support program for consumers would be essential for their full participation; written statements by consumers of their expectations for care would be helpful; and full participation of consumers in their care would be essential.

One rather unexpected outcome was the spontaneous requests by women for continuing involvement in the life of the Center after their childbirth. This grew to such proportions that we had to hire a consumer to coordinate the consumer activities! We now have a newsletter, clothing exchange, library, and periodic education/social sessions, all of which benefit the Center.

Recently, we have further defined our nursing model. I will share components of it and, as appropriate, further describe our service.

Philosophic tenets in our nursing model include the following:

1. Childbearing-childrearing are basic family functions.
2. These functions are essentially healthy and contain potential for growth.
3. Individuals are essentially capable of assessing their own state of health and, indeed, have potential for knowing themselves better than does anyone else.
4. The health care system embraces both an illness and a wellness care system.
5. The health care system is only beginning to develop an approach that facilitates the delivery of both illness and wellness care.
6. A dynamic union of health care provider and consumer holds the greatest potential for personal growth of both.
7. The repeated contacts with the wellness/illness system during pregnancy and early childrearing and the intrinsic stress of these periods make them ideal times to foster personal growth.

An honest attempt to operationalize these tenets leads to the development of a truly different system for the delivery of childbearing care. Let us develop the tenets in more depth.

1. Childbearing-childrearing are basic family functions.
   a. The basic care unit is the woman and whomever she defines as her family support unit.

    b. Opportunities must be provided for family members to be included in all aspects of care to the greatest extent that they so desire.

    c. All family members need opportunity for education that includes the varied aspects of childbearing and childrearing.

The Center has evening hours to encourage full family participation. Children are actively included in the visits and their questions encouraged. Grandparents and friends are also welcome. We are continuing to work on a policy to liberalize sibling participation in the birth experience. At present, our women give birth at University Hospitals; over half of these births occur in the labor room with a minimum of procedure.

  2. These functions are essentially healthy and contain potential for growth.

    a. Emphasis in care is on personal growth needs. Women and children, once accepted into the service, are considered healthy until evidence to the contrary is observed.

    b. Orientation of care facilitators is toward supporting the woman's basic capability to make satisfactory decisions for herself.

Wiedenbach's theory of capability encourages us to first help women to draw on their own resources before relying on the judgments and suggestions of others. Our practice is sharply contrasted to that of the new student who is full of information and so eager to share "expertise!"

  3. Individuals are essentially capable of assessing their own state of health and, indeed, have the potential for knowing themselves better than does anyone else.

    a. A program of education and support is essential to teach new skills to prepare individuals for assuming greater responsibility for their own health.

    b. Consumers are encouraged to respond to their body signals in an effort to increase their level of wellness.

Increasingly we are realizing the necessity for developing a health promotion model that will assist with these goals. We have consciously worked on not fostering provider-consumer dependence. Now we feel a need to go further with the development of self-awareness and self-care activities that will encourage consumers toward greater responsibility.

  4. The health-care system embraces both an illness and a wellness care system.

    a. This health system is tied to a medical system that can provide care if pathology does develop and to a wellness system which usually emphasizes health maintenance and health promotion.

    b. Women who have no medical problems properly may receive care in a wellness system.

Our Center has a pediatrician and an obstetrician each of whom spends about four hours/week at the Center for consultation and direct care. All of the services at the University are available to us and our consumers. This is essential to help assure safety. For most women and children, these services are not needed but the skills of the nurse are critical for healthy family functioning.

  5. The health care system is only beginning to develop an approach that facilitates the delivery of both illness and wellness care.

    a. We still do not know what the potential is for health promotion during the childbearing and childrearing period.

    b. It is essential that a variety of approaches to illness-wellness care be employed and carefully studied.

We feel that no ideal model has been developed for health promotion. As such, we are proposing an openness to new ideas and hope for an increased sensitivity on the part of foundations and state and federal governments to the need for funding of many pilot programs.

6. A dynamic union of health care provider and consumer holds the greatest potential for personal growth of both.
    a. The consumer is viewed as an equal provider in care and works actively with the care provider to develop goals and appropriate means to reach those goals. The provider initiates intervention only when such goals are not being met.
    b. The care provider has a unique opportunity for personal growth as she or he participates actively in the experience of the consumer.
    c. Evaluation of goals is continual and is the joint responsibility of the consumer and care provider.

The Center takes the evaluation process seriously and encourages its consumers to be honest about the care they have received. We are working on the development of more tools that will assist consumers and providers in determination of goals, health state, and needs-for-help.

7. The repeated contacts with the wellness/illness system during pregnancy and early childrearing and the intrinsic stress of these periods make them ideal times to foster personal growth.
    a. Patterns for care established by the medical care system can be used to advantage in the continued development of the wellness system.
    b. Studies show that many people learn best in groups from their peers. Alterations in the care system might include more group interactions and less scheduled individual visit time.
    c. Consumer and care provider work together to identify needs and to develop a care plan that will best address those needs.

Perhaps this model would work best with much of the care being given in groups. I am hoping that we will soon have a pilot program of self-care and group interaction that will span both childbearing and childrearing. Topics for group discussion could include: nutrition, body conditioning, sexuality, communication, blood pressure determination, stress reduction, parenting, values clarification, recognition of illness in self and child, growth and development. We are also developing a well-woman program that includes annual reproductive health exams. This program has the potential for many group experiences in wellness care.

I think it is critically important that we remember that the consumer is at the center of all that we do, that our responsibility is to respond first to consumer needs and second to our needs and those of other professionals and the institutions with which we work.

FLOW CHART

As a summary of all of the pieces of care previously described in this chapter, I would like to take you on a "flow" tour of care at the Center. The first contact with the Center usually comes over the phone when information is requested and registration is handled. The woman or couple then attends our orientation session where she receives an overview of total Center activities, basic nutrition information, financial counseling, laboratory work, and referral to social service, as indicated. Her history and present concerns are also gathered at that time. She returns a few days later for a physical examination and meets the Center's obstetrician if any findings warrant physician review. She then returns at specified intervals for assessment of progress both physically and in areas outlined by her for personal growth. Her family usually comes with her, participating actively in the care. These visits are all conducted by the nurse-midwife.

Her partner and she then enroll in a series of parent education classes and meet weekly with six other couples for eight weeks, continuing with these couples in a support group that formally meets through two months postpartum but may, in fact, continue informally for years. These group sessions prepare the couple to handle the stress of labor and delivery and also provide them with a group with which to share their feelings.

When this woman is in active labor she meets the nurse-midwife at the hospital and, if all goes well, labors and delivers in the same room. The family unit is kept together as much as possible during the early postpartum hours. If she leaves the hospital within 48 hours, postpartum home visits will be made by the nurse-midwife and pediatric nurse practitioner. Both of these individuals are readily available by phone for the many questions that arise during those early weeks.

At the postpartum visit, and over 90 percent of the women make such a visit, a birth control method is implemented. Often this is foam and condoms to be followed by a diaphragm fitting at three months postpartum. The Center continues to follow these women for their ongoing reproductive health needs. Approximately 85 percent of our first time parents enroll their baby in the childrearing component of the Center and so continue to have contact with our philosophy of care. The first well-baby visit is 2 weeks after birth and the visits continue at regular intervals thereafter.

If the woman happens to be a teenager or older single mother there are individual and group activities at the Center in which she can participate. Other groups, such as a postpartum mothers' group, form as there is demand for such an activity.

THE FUTURE

The Center continues to grow and expand its impact on the community. It is viewed as a resource for students from many disciplines, as a source of information on health care alternatives, and as a site for exploration of many new ideas. Within the past year it has supported the development of a teenage support/education program, a well-woman program open to the community, a large parent education program, and a breast diagnostic center utilizing the Sar-B technique.

Plans for the future include the development of an adolescent health care component, conduction of deliveries in an out of hospital birth home, and the exploration of a family health component. A recent survey of our population showed that 26.5 percent do not have a primary health source and 62 percent would be interested in supporting a wellness care model.

In 1978 there were over 20 people formally affiliated with the Center: nurse-midwives, pediatric nurse practitioners, maternity nurse practitioner, adult health nurse practitioner, parent educators, social workers, physicians, consumer coordinator, laboratory technician, and several support personnel. In addition, many professionals and consumers serve on our advisory board.

Obstetric care within the University and community has also been affected by nurse-midwifery activities. For example, the University's obstetricians are flexible in their care plans often supporting labor room deliveries, no episiotomy, and extended mother-baby contact. The Center staff has been extremely active in presenting workshops and talks at professional organizations, lay women's groups, consumer groups, and in the public schools. Childbirth Education Association has supported the development of nurse-midwifery; two of our staff have been active on its professional advisory board. There are now four nurse midwifery services in the metropolitan area and the demand for those services is increasing rapidly.

After continued reflection on our Center, I am convinced that it should have two primary functions:

1. To assess the state of health of women and children coming for care and to provide an atmosphere in which a healthy state has maximum potential for continued growth.
2. To provide an education/support program that will equip women/couples to better understand and care for themselves physically, psychologically, and socially.

This puts some very real demands on the care providers (nurses and others) who function in this setting. The care providers must:

1. Honestly believe in the capability of consumers.
2. Basically believe in the essential normalcy of childbearing-childrearing.
3. Recognize that physical, social, and psychological deviations often do exist requiring intervention based on recognition of a need for help.
4. Be skilled in assessment factors that enable the facilitation of growth and identify the basic limits of safety.
5. Feel personally rewarded when growth parameters are met.
6. Utilize other care providers as appropriate to complement care as needed for physical, social, psychological, and spiritual deviation.

There is no question in my mind about the need for more such programs or about the difficulty in implementing them. What would it take?

1. Some changes in nursing education programs probably are needed. Nursing students must be filled with a sense of purpose and professional identity. They must have a clear concept of health and be exposed to health maintenance and health promotion models. They must have positive interdisciplinary experiences in which differences and similarities of professionals are identified and valued.
2. Funding must be available to support innovative programs, at least in their initial stage. This money must be available for basic service needs as well as for evaluative studies. Historically, nursing has received minimal federal money for service. That needs to change.
3. More nurses need to take risks in establishing new models. For some this will mean independent practice, for some it will mean free-standing centers, for others it will mean serious changes within the institution.

In an era of increasing cost-consciousness as well as new insight on wellness and illness, nursing cannot afford not to be in the forefront of innovation.

SUMMARY
With this well approach to care, what can one hope to achieve for outcome? What is the overall goal of such a Center?

Although there are many outcomes one could list I am convinced that such a model should lead to increased personal growth and sense of self-esteem within all people participating: care providers and consumers alike. And, if one is really concerned with successful living, successful parenting, and success as a professional, then this is the most important goal of all. We are currently designing a research project to attempt to measure this. Perhaps our data eventually will support this belief; I hope so.

REFERENCES

1. Wiedenbach, E.: *Clinical Nursing: A Helping Art*. Springer Publishing Company, Inc., New York, 1964.
2. Arms, S.: *Immaculate Deception*. Houghton Mifflin Company, Boston, 1975.
3. Boston Womens Health Collective: *Our Bodies, Ourselves*. Simon and Schuster, New York, 1973.
4. Rising, S.S., and Houde, R.J.: "Reimbursement for Nurse-Midwifery Services." *Journal of Nurse Midwifery* 22(2):6-8, 1977.
5. Rising, S.S.: "A Consumer-Oriented Nurse-Midwifery Service." *Nursing Clinics of North America* 10(2):251-262, June 1975.

CHAPTER 49

INDEPENDENT NURSING PRACTICE IN DEVELOPMENTAL DISABILITIES

SALLY M. O'NEIL, Ph.D., R.N.

As nursing has evolved as a profession, the problems of role diffusion and confusion have been evidenced in the various kinds of educational programs and the types of practice seen in different settings. While this lack of role establishment within nursing allows the creative implementation of roles, it fosters further confusion about the identity of nursing.

In my personal development as a nurse I have come to share the belief that "nursing as a profession should establish its identity by asserting its unique role, not by assuming those functions and responsibilities which pertain to the profession of medicine."[1]

This belief is, in part, based upon the following conception of the nursing process through which nursing emerges as an intellectual, interpersonal, and technical process by which the professional nurse identifies client problems, plans and implements interventions which are designed to solve them, and evaluates the degree to which the intervention program was effective in resolving the identified problems. The nursing process is essentially a problem solving approach which is characterized by the general goals of 1) assisting the individual client and family with the maintenance of optimal health and development, 2) coping with the stress of illness and/or disability, 3) providing care until the client is able to assume responsibility for the fulfillment of his basic needs, and 4) providing compassionate assistance with dying. The purpose here is to assist the client in meeting all basic needs. This involvement with the total person is in contrast to the goals of other health professionals whose focus is on one or two specific aspects of the individual's needs. The process of nursing practice is a combination of operational components—stages and phases—which must be integrated to insure therapeutic outcomes.

For purposes of this presentation, the term *stage* refers to the problem solving aspects of nursing which rely on skills in critical thinking and inquiry. These four stages are: assessment, planning, implementation, and evaluation. The term *phase* refers to the relationship aspects of nursing which rely on skills in interpersonal communication. As the nurse applies the stages of the problem solving approach, she or he and the client move through the orientation, maintenance, and termination phases of their relationship. It is the degree of interdependence between the stages and phases which determine the extent of the therapeutic outcome of the nursing process. Unless the problem solving stages are applied within a framework of effective interpersonal skills, they remain depersonalized and meaningless. Similarly, when emphasis is placed exclusively on interpersonal aspects, tasks and goals may be forgotten. In these instances, relationships are undirected and ultimately of little therapeutic value.

In the field of developmental disabilities, the clinical nurse specialist is known as "the generalist among the specialists." A broad background in the social and biologic sciences provides the nurse with the knowledge of the needs of individuals and families within the context of a variety of settings and a multiplicity of problems, as well as the awareness of the contributions of a wide variety of disciplines to the client's and family's well being. This knowledge places the nurse in a pivotal role within the interdisciplinary team providing services to the developmentally disabled child and his family. Although the nurse's specific involvement with children and families may change from setting to setting, the stages and phases of the nursing process can be identified and the central concern of nursing "the total client" remains constant. Nursing roles in developmental disabilities vary, as in other fields of nursing. However, as roles become defined, it is crucial that they not only be appropriate to the practitioner but to the public served. My personal motivation to function in independent practice is to delineate more specifically the needs of the developmentally disabled and their families and to define practice roles to meet these needs. The remainder of this chapter describes how one role is operationalized within the specialty of nursing in developmental disabilities.

NURSING ROLE

In addition to applying nursing concepts to clinical practice, it is essential to have a thorough knowledge of the specialty in which one chooses to practice and to be able to operationalize that knowledge into day-to-day problem solving strategies.

A multitude of overwhelming feelings, dilemmas, and problems is imposed upon the family with a developmentally disabled child. "What's wrong with my child?" "Is it my fault?" "How do we find out what is wrong with our child?" "What can we do about it?" "How do we tell our relatives?" "What kind of future can we plan for?" "What kind of school placement is there?" "How much can my child learn?" "Will my child outgrow this?"

Regardless of the specific diagnosis a child might receive (mental retardation, cerebral palsy, autism, epilepsy, learning disability, blindness, deafness, or any combination of these), the most difficult aspects with which parents must learn to cope are the constancy of the problem and the grief surrounding it. Although many disabled individuals will learn to work and to live independent lives, a large number will continue to be dependent on family or others for some degree of nurturance and support their entire lives. Parents are constantly reminded by other children of what "might have been" if their own child were not handicapped, and their grieving is nearly continuous.

There is a continual demand from the time that a parent suspects that something is "wrong," through assessment, diagnosis, and a lifetime of habilitation, for someone to assist families as well as the disabled individual in making the best use of their own resources and in bringing as much equilibrium into their existence as possible. This is not a one time task. The outcomes of developmentally disabling conditions are still unpredictable and idiosyncratic, and the individuals are too complex to be viewed simply. To be effective, services need to be available within the health care system at every contact, as adaptation is a continuous, evolving process. This is where I see the role of the nurse— as the facilitator of the disabled individual's and family's physical, emotional, and behavioral adaptation to the disability, regardless of where they are on the continuum of mental, physical, or behavioral disturbance. The nurse is in the unique position to provide the continuity necessary in carrying out such care. Emphasis can shift with each contact so that priorities in both child and parent development can be facilitated. For example, my contacts may include assisting a family in requesting services from a local office of the Bureau of Developmental Disabilities; another may involve implementation of a behavior management plan for development of self-feeding skills; while another may focus on discussion of respite care or group home placement so that the parents can experience some relief from their child's care for a short period of time. Nursing the individual who is developmentally disabled and his or her family is a continual dynamic process of assessment, intervention, and evaluation.

A continuity of community services for the developmentally disabled through their lifetime is, of course, at the present time only a figment of one's imagination. Generic services, those which are available to a community at large, are often exclusionary to developmentally disabled individuals since they frequently do not have staff who know how to deal with the mentally retarded or those with behavioral disorders. In addition, architectural barriers still exist in many buildings which may automatically exclude persons with physical handicaps.

While a multitude of specialized health, educational, and recreational programs do exist, many of these are forced to be exclusionary by virtue of categorical funding. For instance, a preschool may take children who have a combination of handicaps, however, the child must have the "right" combination to be admitted. A program for the deaf-blind child may not take deaf-blind children who also have cerebral palsy; a program for autistic children may not take children who appear to be more "retarded" than autistic; a program for cerebral palsied children may exclude retarded children who exhibit only mild motor disturbances; recreation programs for young developmentally disabled children may require that they be toilet trained in order to participate.

Health care services are equally exclusionary. Generic health services frequently do not have staff knowledgeable about working with clients and families with mental retardation or other developmental disabilities. Inpatient nursing and medical staffs are usually unable to handle effectively a scared mentally retarded child who presents behavior problems. They frequently do not know or find out the child's level of development in order to foster behavioral expectations similar to those of the child's parents when at home.

Even when comprehensive interdisciplinary evaluations of the disabled child and family are carried out, very often families are referred to community agencies which in reality cannot meet their needs for continuity and coordination of services. This, again, is usually because of limitations of financial resources of both the evaluation agency and those agencies attempting to provide treatment in the community.

Involvement in independent practice allows me to provide the continuity necessary to assist families to better identify and utilize the continuum of services which are available and to assist them in adapting other strategies during periods when no agency exists which can meet their needs. It also allows me to better identify needs in staff education as much as possible as I accompany parents through the various aspects of health care and to offer inservice programs as a part of my practice.

APPROACHES TO PARENT COUNSELING

If I were to specify a purpose to my practice it would be to increase parental competence or to increase their positive perceptions of their competence. Generally, when parents seek help they express feelings of incompetence, discouragement, or failure. My basic goal is to assist them in examining the problems and difficulties, discovering new options, techniques, and strategies. Gradual success with this process increases their skills and their positive perceptions of their competence.

The concepts which have been of considerable usefulness in increasing parental competence are those related to the socialization of parents to their role, and those related to behavior analysis and modification. The following section is a brief overview of these aspects of my conceptual framework for parent counseling.

It has been said that "no parent is ever prepared to be the parent of a handicapped child."[1] The socialization to this role is indeed "a transition to an unwanted and distasteful status for most if not all who find themselves in this position."[3]

Meadow and Meadow[3] utilize two broad categories to characterize the role of parent of a handicapped child. The first is the emotional aspects of the role to be assimilated: learning to cope with feelings of guilt, shame, and sorrow; learning to cope with responses of pity, rejection, and avoidance from neighbors; learning to cope with the urge to overprotect or underprotect the child; learning to cope with the disequilibrium within the family unit; learning to cope with additional situational crises associated with family functioning.

The second category includes the technical aspects of the role to be learned: learning how to assist the child to achieve developmental skills; learning to assist the child in using adaptive devices such as hearing aid, crutches, special braces, chairs, or utensils.

These two aspects of the parent role are closely interwoven as the parents' ability to resolve successfully the expressive components of the role will profoundly affect their perception of their child and the ease with which they can carry out technical tasks. A parent counselor must deal with both expressive and technical aspects of the parent role if she or he is to be effective in contributing to the parent socialization process.

One approach which offers a useful methodology for analyzing the expressive and technical aspects of the parenting role is that of *behavior analysis and modification*. This approach allows for the systematic analysis of the very complex interactional systems which occur between parent and child. Not only does this analysis lead to more specific and effective intervention, but it is easily integrated into nursing process. The following section is a brief overview of a behavioral framework for assessment and intervention.

Behavioral Concepts

The central focus of any behavioral approach is *operant behavior*. This is voluntary behavior which operates on the environment, causing consequences. These consequences, in turn, affect the recurrence of the specific operant which caused them: operant behavior→consequences→recurrence or nonrecurrence of operant behavior. Operant behavior is distinguished from respondent or reflex behavior as shown in Table 49-1. The process by which an individual learns the extent to which he can control and be controlled by his environment is termed *operant conditioning*.

Consequences are defined by the concepts reinforcement and punishment. *Reinforcement* is the process in which consequences (reinforcers) occur which *increase* the behaviors they follow. *Punishment* is the process in which consequences (punishers) occur which decrease behaviors they follow. Reinforcers and punishers are always operationally defined by their effect on an individual's behavior. Reinforcers increase behavior they immediately follow. If they do not increase an individual's behavior, then they are not reinforcing for that individual. Similarly, if punishers do not decrease the behaviors they follow, then they are not punishing for that individual.

There are two types of reinforcers: *Positive reinforcers* are desirable consequences which are added to the environment as a result of a specific operant behavior. Positive reinforcers include 1) primary reinforcers—those which answer biologic needs such as food, water, warmth, sex, and 2) secondary reinforcers—those which become reinforcing because they were paired with a primary reinforcer(s) during an individual's reinforcement history. This includes toys, tokens, money, praise, attention, and so on. *Negative reinforcers* are defined as the removal or absence of something aversive to an individual. Negative reinforcers increase behaviors which avoid or terminate something aversive. These include the absence of noise after a mother stops her baby from crying by putting a pacifier in his mouth; the absence of the noise will reinforce her for whatever she did which terminated the crying.

It is important here to view reinforcers in a mathematical sense, i.e., the addition (+) or absence (−) of consequences rather than to place a "good" or "bad" value judgment on positive or negative reinforcers. Think of positive reinforcers as R+ —the addition of a consequence that is viewed as desirable by the individual who receives it. Think of negative reinforcers as R− —the consequence here is the absence of something aversive which the individual has been able to remove or subtract from the environment.

There are also two types of punishers: *Punishment* is the *addition* of an aversive consequence as the result of a behavior. Such punishers include spanking, yelling, nagging, angry looks. *Extinction* is the *removal* or subtraction of a positive reinforcer, such as ignoring a behavior which has previously received attention (Table 49-2).

TABLE 49-1. Operant behavior vs. respondent behavior

Operant behavior	*Respondent behavior*
Voluntary behavior	Reflex activity, i.e., knee jerk, eye blink
Controlled by stimulus that follows it—technically termed stimulus consequences—commonly called consequences or contingencies.	Controlled by stimulus preceding it

TABLE 49-2. Types of punishers

	Addition	Subtraction
Desirable consequence	Positive reinforcement	Extinction
Aversive event	Punishment	Negative reinforcement

CONSEQUENCES VIEWED AS INTERACTIVE PROCESSES

Reinforcers and/or punishers can be identified in any interaction between family members. Although the examples presented here are those typical of parent-child interactions, the same kind of consequences occur between adults as well. The important consideration is that each family member provides consequences for every other family member.

Parent-child interaction is a reciprocal process. This process includes parents' expressions of attitudes, values, interests, beliefs, and their care taking behaviors as well as children's individual growth patterns, learning potentials and abilities to incorporate increasingly complex experiences into their current stages of thinking and functioning.

Events occur in sequence on an interaction continuum between parents and children in which each response to an action can become the cause of future behaviors. It is by this interactive process that both parents and children learn new behaviors.[4] Behaviors are both the cause and effect of other behaviors. Consider the following examples:

Situation 1. A mother takes her child to a friend's house. The child starts crying for a cookie. Mom is embarrassed by the crying but says "No." The child screams and Mom immediately gives her a cookie. The child stops crying. In this situation, the child was positively reinforced for crying by receiving a cookie. Mom was negatively reinforced for giving the cookie because the crying stopped. Mom was negatively reinforced for stopping the crying.

Situation 2. Another time this mother took her child to a friend's house, and the child cried for a cookie. Mom went on about her talking and ignored the crying. After a short while the crying stopped. This time the child's crying was extinguished (received no positive reinforcement). Mother was again negatively reinforced because the crying stopped.

Situation 3. A third time this mother took her child to a friend's house, and the child cried. Mom became angry and spanked her. The child screamed for a few seconds, then stopped crying. Here, the child was punished for crying (spanked). Mom was, once again, negatively reinforced (this time for spanking) because the crying stopped.

In each situation the mother was negatively reinforced for stopping the crying, regardless of which method she used. However, the child received a variety of consequences for her crying behavior. Among these consequences was an occasional positive reinforcement (cookie) for crying. This occasional or intermittent positive reinforcement can exert very powerful control over the maintenance of her crying behavior. In addition, because each method mother uses seems to work some of the time, mother is negatively reinforced to be inconsistent in her approach. In order to further analyze why this pattern of mother-child interaction could be maintained over such a long period of time it is important to consider how reinforcers may be scheduled and the effect of these schedules on behavior.

Continuous reinforcement is used when teaching a new behavior or when increasing the rate, duration, or intensity of an existing behavior. Reinforcement follows *every* occurrence of the desired behavior. Following this period of continuous reinforcement, a schedule of intermittent reinforcement is used to maintain the desired behavior. An *intermittent reinforcement schedule* involves the gradual increase in the number of behaviors which are required in order for reinforcement to occur. Thus, the number of reinforcers is gradually decreased. Intermittent scheduling is important to strengthen behaviors and to ensure their resistance to extinction. The greater the interval between reinforcers, the less likely it is that a behavior will decrease if reinforcers are discontinued, the more likely it is that a behavior will be maintained.

It is important to note that intermittent reinforcement is equally effective for both desirable and undesirable behaviors. In the previous example, the intermittent reinforcement that the child received (cookie) for crying at the friend's house can maintain her crying behavior during many visits.

In order to understand why family interaction patterns have long term stability it is important to consider that in all exchanges, both parents and children receive reinforcers, ignoring, and punishers from each other. The intermittent scheduling of reinforcers to parents as well as to children may well account for much of the long term maintenance of disruptive and/or ineffective parent-child interactions. Consider the following parent-child exchange:

1. Mother pours milk into a glass saying "Here's your milk."

2. Child starts crying "I want soda."

3. Mother says, "You can't have soda, now drink your milk."

4. Child cries louder, pushes glass of milk away.

5. Mother pushes milk toward child. "Drink your milk, it's good for you."

6. Child screams, throws milk to floor.

7. Mother says, "OK, you can have soda now, but you must drink your milk later." Gives child soda, then cleans up mess.

8. Child stops crying, drinks soda.

In this situation the child responds to the parent initiation by crying for soda and not drinking milk; mother reciprocates (punishes) by insisting child drink milk; child reciprocates (punishes) by crying louder and pushing glass away; mother reciprocates (punishes) by pushing glass toward child and coaxing the child to drink; child reciprocates (punishes) by screaming and throwing glass; mother reciprocates (positively reinforces) by giving child soda; child reciprocates (negatively reinforces) mother by stopping crying. (Remember—negative reinforcement is the absence or removal of a punisher.)

Obviously the child was reinforced for crying by getting soda, and mother was reinforced for giving the soda because the crying stopped. But, not only were they both reinforced for the final behaviors which immediately preceded the reinforcers, they were also reinforced for enduring the sequence of punishing interactions which occurred prior to the reinforcement. In other words, they get reinforced for engaging in and maintaining the whole exchange. In addition, as a result of the reinforcement, they are both likely to engage in similar exchanges in the future.

Assessment of parent-child interactions must necessarily 1) define the family's goals— both long and short term goals which are specific to a given family's life styles and which consider the needs of each member; 2) identify and specify the problems which inhibit the achievement of family goals; 3) identify and specify exchange patterns (behavior and consequences) which support ineffective behaviors; and 4) determine and specify treatment goals. Treatment then becomes a matter of assisting family members in becoming aware of their interactions and assisting them to actively modify the reinforcement contingencies that perpetuate their present exchange patterns.

Intervention involves assisting parents in becoming aware of where they are in their role as parents. Their understanding of the emotional aspects of the role in general can assist them in identifying their coping strengths as well as the degree of additional emotional support they may need. At the same time, they need to have techniques and strategies to care for their child successfully. In many instances, other family members and/or friends may be able to meet some of these needs for parents, and it is important to identify whatever supportive network may be available. My role then becomes one of assisting parents in determining how and by whom their needs can be met and identifying additional support and techniques they may need from me. Intervention requires developing and implementing simple and easy strategies parents can employ which produce immediate results, as well as longer term plans to achieve lasting parental competence. Optimal interaction would be that by which family members frequently reinforce each other for behaviors that are supportive of a happy, healthy family constellation and is the general goal toward which parents strive and for which they seek help.

These concepts related to role socialization and behavior analysis have been useful to me as I evolve a framework for parent counseling and have served here to describe a portion of the conceptual basis of my independent practice. As previously alluded to, additional components of practice relate to parent education about available services and strategies to utilize these services, serving as advocate for parents in securing services they have difficulty obtaining for themselves, and assisting families with decision making issues around institutionalization and deinstitutionalization, respite care, educational programs, health care, and job training and placement.

IMPLEMENTATION OF INDEPENDENT PRACTICE

In addition to being academically and experientially ready to undertake this endeavor, it is important to know how to establish a business. The first step is to determine the legality of establishing independent practice. This means that the Nurse Practice Act in my state must cover my activities. A check with the State Nurses' Association determined that this was true. The second step is to give the business a title (in my instance Parent Counseling Services), and to apply to the State Department of Internal Revenue for a tax or business number. This gives one the dubious honor of paying a Business and Occupation tax to the state, but it also duly registers and recognizes the business.

A very important consideration before starting practice is to determine the type and scope of services to be provided. I decided I would focus on parent counseling for parents who expressed most any kind of child rearing concern including difficulties with children who might be gifted, as well as those who have disabilities. I would refer to colleagues those children whom I felt needed mental health assessments and therapy, as well as any parents whose needs I could not meet. I determined that I would provide home visits to evaluate parent-child interactions and behavior management programs or to see parents who would not be able to come to my office at my home. In addition, I would make school and agency visits for observations and conferences and accompany parents as necessary. I anticipated, correctly, that a large part of my practice would be that of family advocacy in assisting them through the health care and educational systems.

The next issue to consider in setting up practice is that of financial support. At the present time in my state, I am not eligible for third party payments from insurance companies or Medicaid unless I were to become licensed as a psychologist. However, I prefer to keep my nursing identity and to work toward third party payment for nursing services.

Fortunately, the state of Washington has established a regional system of Bureau of Developmental Disability (B.D.D.) offices which are currently mandated to identify and follow all developmentally disabled individuals. They have established a contract system with individuals and agencies who will provide assessment and intervention services to clients and their families. This contract system serves as third party payment for my services to some families.

I also chose to remain as a part-time faculty member in the University school of nursing. This provides continued access to colleagues and students and library resources, as well as a financial base. In addition, my part-time practice brings rich clinical experiences to my course content.

Once third party payments are explored (usually their fees are set), fees must be established for direct payment by families who are not covered by third party sources. In this instance, I established a fee schedule on an hourly rate using the B.D.D. contract as a top rate with a sliding scale which was then individually negotiated. In addition, parents are able to earn discounts by achieving mutually agreed upon program goals (either related to their own development in communication with each other, with appropriate assertiveness with agencies, or in assisting their child with the acquisition of developmental skills).

The next concern is to let referral sources know when one is prepared to receive referrals. This can be accomplished by sending an announcement, by visiting agencies or physicians' offices, by telephone contact, or by word of mouth. It helped considerably in my instance to have carried out family counseling within the University affiliated child evaluation center prior to establishing independent practice. This enabled me to have many referral contacts around the community. These contacts plus those resulting from my attending staff meetings at the local B.D.D. offices provide me with all the clients I can currently handle on a part-time basis. As might be expected, the referrals I received were those families who had "stumped" the previous staffs. Once I was able to deal effectively with these, referrals came rapidly.

Another consideration which is important is the confidentiality of information, and therefore the need to develop forms which parents and/or clients sign to give permission to share information among the professionals with whom they are involved. I find two forms are useful. One can be sent to other agencies for information (Fig. 49-1). The second form is one which gives permission to care for the family and transmit information to other professionals (Fig. 49-2).

In summary, I have found a role in which I have been able to function in a collaborative, cooperative relationship with other professionals and hope that this is a step toward a larger goal for nursing. I realize, however, that until we can bill insurance carriers such a goal cannot be reached. If nursing had such access to billing, a nurse could then join group practices working for a percentage of the income she or he generates. This would allow families to utilize comprehensive nursing services to better meet their needs.

```
Developmental                                    Child Rearing
Disabilities                                         Concerns
                PARENT COUNSELING SERVICES
                    Sally O'Neil, R.N., Ph.D.
        15238    12th AVE. N.E.     Seattle, WA.    98155
                        (206) 365-8142


        TO:
        _____ NAME
        _____ ADDRESS
        _____
                                ZIP _____



                            CONSENT FORM


            I hereby give my full permission to the above named
        individual (institution) to furnish Parent Counseling
        Services any and all information regarding the medical
        history, diagnostic and treatment records and similar
        information from its records of:



        _____ Birthdate _____
        Signature of Parents _____
                                _____

            Date _____
```

FIGURE 49-1. Information release form for agencies.

CONSENT FOR CARE AND AUTHORIZATION
FOR RELEASE OF INFORMATION

I hereby grant permission to Dr. Sally O'Neil, of Parent Counseling Services, to employ such procedures as deemed necessary and which I agree to carry out in the treatment of my family.

I hereby authorize Dr. O'Neil to give any information deemed relevant to the following named individuals/agencies:

_____

_____

_____

_____

_____

_____   _____
Witness   Person giving consent

_____   _____
Date   Relationship

FIGURE 49-2. Permission for family care and relevant information release.

REFERENCES

1. Van Scoy-Mosher, C.: "The Oncology Nurse in Independent Professional Practice." *Cancer Nursing* Feb. 1978, pp. 21-28.
2. Barsch, R. 2d.: *The Parent of the Handicapped Child: The Study of Childrearing Practices.* Charles C Thomas, Springfield, Ill., 1968, p. 9.
3. Meadow, K.P., and Meadow, L.: "Changing Role Perceptions for Parents of Handicapped Children," *Exceptional Children* 38:21, Sept. 1971.
4. O'Neil, S., McLaughlin, B., and Knapp, M.E.: *Behavioral Approaches to Children with Development Delay.* C. V. Mosby Company, St. Louis, 1977.

CHAPTER 50
GERONTOLOGY CLINICAL ROLE STUDY

**LYNNE BIGELOW M.S., R.N.,
NANCY BINNER M.P.H., R.N., AND
EILEEN KIRK M.S., R.N.**

Although nursing has always been concerned with the care of the aged, the role of the gerontologic clinical nurse specialist is a relatively new one. Rationale for the emergence of this role lies mainly in the rapid increase in numbers of persons over the age of 65 during this century. Statistics from 1900 indicate that slightly more than 3 million elderly persons inhabited our country at that time; the numbers of persons over the age of 60 exceeded 20 million by 1970.[1] The 1970 census revealed that persons over 65 years of age constituted approximately 10 percent of the total population. While our population of persons under age 45 increased 30.5 percent, those over 65 increased 63.1 percent.[2]

In addition, it is undeniable that the process of aging brings with it greater risks related to the maintenance of health, economic solvency, and significant interpersonal relationships. The old tend to have more chronic illnesses than do the young. They tend to be poorer, and they often suffer social isolation.

These factors, combined with modern technologic and therapeutic advances influencing the care of our aged population, have set the stage for the creation of the role of the gerontologic clinical nurse specialist. The study and practice of this role offer the practitioner opportunities available in no other specialty. Although the aged share many of the same problems, they are far from a homogenous group. The gerontologic nurse specialist must combine theoretic knowledge from each of the nursing specialties and from the science of gerontology. She or he must be flexible, patient, creative, and always ready to meet a challenge. These challenges are many, but the rewards, particularly those related to our understanding of life, are even greater.

In 1969, the ANA adopted the position that "the major purpose of graduate study in nursing should be the preparation of nurse clinicians capable of improving nursing care through advancement of nursing theory and science."[3] Nurse educators acknowledge that graduates of baccalaureate programs are generalists, and that specialization in specific areas is offered at the graduate level. The clinical nurse specialist is not a single role, but an encompassing one, including components of practitioner, teacher, consultant, researcher, and change agent. It is our belief that the gerontologic clinical specialist must be first and foremost a practitioner who assumes direct and continuous responsibility for her patients. She accepts direct responsibility for her decisions and for the quality of care delivered by those under her direction. In addition, she works collaboratively with other health disciplines involved in total care of her patients. The nurse prepared to function at this level must, by necessity, be educated at the master's level. The graduate program selected must be well rounded in nursing science and accompanied by thoughtful, well-planned clinical role experiences.

The role of the geronotologic clinician in the community is a relatively new one. Until the last decade, chronically ill elderly persons were most often relegated to institutional care. The development of a home care program such as the one we work in, with its goal of allowing each client, regardless of disability, the option to spend their remaining days at home, is seen as an exciting challenge. We function in different roles, one as the nurse coordinator and the other two as nurse clinicians. We found these roles to be natural extensions of the community health practice that we had been involved with in previous work experiences. They offered a chance to utilize specialized skills in an independent, multidisciplinary framework.

THE PROGRAM

In the early 1970s, the Medical Director of Upham's Corner Health Center, an affiliate clinic of a teaching hospital, was concerned about the elderly people seeking care at the health center which is located in Dorchester, a community within Boston. Their numbers were disproportionately low considering the number of people over 65 living in the community surrounding the health center. Examination of statistics from the U.S. Department of Health, Education, and Welfare revealed that 80 percent of people over 65 have one or more chronic conditions, 17.6 percent have mobility limitations, and 5.2 percent are completely homebound.[1]

The following questions were considered. Are the homebound elderly in our community receiving ongoing medical care? If they are receiving medical care, are the services comprehensive enough to deal with the complexities of the social and environmental problems that are an integral part of health problems for all ages, but especially for low income, chronically ill, or disabled people? Also, do the services provided impact in any way to allow people to remain in their own homes rather than being repeatedly hospitalized or being placed in a chronic care facility?

A two month study conducted at the Boston City Hospital which surveyed all patients over the age of 65 showed that 80 percent of the patients admitted had no identifiable source of medical care, that the risk of hospitalization correlated significantly with the degree of difficulty in exiting the home, and that 40 percent of readmissions were because of complications of unmonitored or untreated chronic disease. Some patients had been admitted six to ten times during a one year period, and often the deterioration of their condition which led to their current hospitalization began shortly after the previous discharge. Primary care followup was either absent or inadequate given the patient's complex array of problems. Often, community resources were too limited to provide the necessary support services, the patients were unable to return home, and placement in a chronic care facility was necessary.[4]

In the latter part of 1973, a home care pilot project was started by Upham's Corner Health Center. Included in the planning of this project were administrators, physicians, nurse clinicians, and social workers from three other health centers in the community. Representatives from the health center's community board and from the Continuing Care Department of Carney Hospital provided ongoing feedback. The program began with a staff of one nurse clinician and two physicians. Initially, much time was spent doing case finding and introducing the program to people who would be the major sources of referrals: community agencies, community residents, and hospital personnel. The major struggle was establishing policies, procedures, and protocols that met the needs and goals of the home care program while still fulfilling the requirements for certification by the Department of Public Health. The program has grown slowly, but consistently. There are currently 120 people receiving services. The staff now includes four part-time physicians, a nurse coordinator, two full-time and one part-time gerontologic nurse clinicians, five home health aides, a physical therapist, and a part-time social worker.

The objectives of the program are:

1. To make high quality health care accessible to those people whose diseases or disabilities prevent access to ambulatory services.
2. To provide a community based alternative to both repeated hospitalizations and institutionalization.
3. To bring nursing and other ancillary support services, in addition to medical care, into the home.
4. To involve clients and their families completely in the planning and implementation of care.

People followed in the home care program have a broad spectrum of diseases and disabilities with a varying range of problems and needs. At one end of the spectrum are the medically fragile, who are most at risk for admission to an acute or chronic hospital. They are homebound because of their acute medical diseases such as recurrent congestive heart failure, advanced pulmonary disease, severe cardiac decompensation, and terminal cancer. It is this group of patients who usually require the greatest amount of medical and nursing input and monitoring. At the other end of the spectrum are people who require, mainly, the support of services such as home health aides/homemakers, delivered meals, and chore services to enable them to remain in their own homes. These people are often homebound because of physical disabilities resulting from a stroke, from advanced arthritis, or from sensory impairments. The health status of this group is by no means static, and at times an illness such as pneumonia will necessitate more intensive medical and nursing intervention.[4]

When a person is referred to the home care program, the nurse coordinator visits the patient and his family to explain the way the program functions, to assess the person's appropriateness for home care, and to begin, if indicated, the plan of care, e.g., initiating home health aide services. If the person does not want to be involved with the program or if admission is not appropriate, for example, if the person is not truly homebound, the nurse coordinator helps him locate the resources and services he needs.

The gerontologic nurse clinician is the primary agent in providing care to each person admitted to the program. She is responsible for implementing and coordinating the plan of care. She is also responsible for the ongoing management of the patient's health status. Consistent with the family focus of the program, the importance of the relationship between the patient and his family and the importance of their involvement with his care are always primary considerations in planning the care for an individual.

Every person admitted to the program receives the following evaluation by the nurse clinician: complete history and physical examination (see Appendix 1), psychosocial assessment, laboratory work and electrocardiogram.

In addition to the initial evaluation, the nurse clinician is responsible for:

1. Ongoing management of patient's health status—monitoring current physiologic/psychosocial status, delivering direct nursing care, updating and revising health care plans, determining need for laboratory studies and evaluating results.
2. Coordination of patient's care—scheduling monthly case conferences, ongoing discussions with multidisciplinary team, participating in the inservice programs for home care staff, providing community consultation and health education.

Within approximately one week (sooner if indicated) after the initial evaluation is completed, the physician visits the patient in his home. During this visit, the physician and the nurse clinician develop a plan of care which is discussed with the patient and his family. A copy of the patient's record is kept in the home to be used by the patient, his family, and the home care staff. This consists of narrative reports written in the problem oriented format, completed by each provider at the time of the visit. The physician, from this point on, provides ongoing consultation to the nurse clinician, making additional followup visits if indictated. A decision matrix has been developed (Fig. 50-1) which describes the process involved in making a nursing diagnosis and judgment. Guidelines for many of the more common problems, e.g., congestive heart failure, diabetes, fever, and urinary tract infections, have been developed to guide but not restrict the nurse clinician. The physician is also involved with the 24-hour on-call service and follows the patient in the hospital if admission there is necessary.

The nurse clinician works closely with the nurse coordinator in all aspects of home care. The nurse coordinator's responsibilities include the following activities:

1. Day-to-day administration of the program—monitoring the paper flow, making initial assessments for all referrals, answering telephone inquiries, responding to billing questions from third party payers, rescheduling staff, preparing narrative reports for grant funding, and scheduling and attending staff and professional advisory meetings.
2. Orientation, education, and supervision of the home health aides—an orientation program is conducted yearly to certify homemakers/home health aides. The course includes 65 hours of clinical and didactic experience. The nurse coordinator supervises homemaker/home health aides every two weeks during a home visit and arranges a monthly inservice program.
3. Planning inservice education program. This is done in conjunction with the health educator in the clinic. Some programs, such as CPR, are done cooperatively. In addition

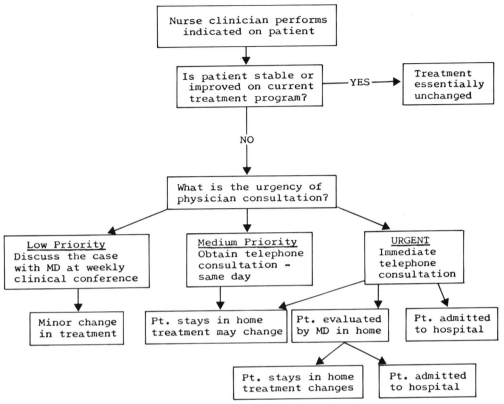

FIGURE 50-1. Decision matrix. (From Master[4] with permission.)

to planning inservice education, the nurse coordinator posts educational offerings of interest to the entire staff.

It has been implied throughout this chapter that the gerontologic nurse clinician is the spearhead of the home care program. She is the planner, practitioner, and catalyst, but because we take pride in a holistic assessment of the family and because our goal is to provide comprehensive care to the homebound, our interventions are naturally multi-disciplinary in nature. As stated previously, the actual home care staff consists of nurse clinicians, physician specialists in internal medicine, physical therapists, medical social workers, and home health aides. These providers are individually and/or collectively able to meet the majority of our clients' needs. However, we actively collaborate with many other agencies in our attempt to provide comprehensive care. Some of the most commonly called upon community sources of help are:

1. The Counsel of Elders, who provide transportation, friendly visitors, and delivered meals.
2. Senior Home Care Office, which provides homemakers.
3. The Greater Boston Legal Aide Society.
4. The mental health centers which, in some instances, provide day care for area elders.
5. Numerous religious organizations or groups, which provide their special type of support and reassurance.

CLINICAL PRACTICE SETTING

Description of Population

The home care program services homebound clients and their families in the Dorchester area. The area is a low income, working class community with a high incidence of chronic illness. The home care program is open to all ages but serves a predominantly elderly one. The mean age of the clients is 77.5 years, and the median age is 78 years (n = 168). Statistics compiled from January 1976 to July 1977 covered 1127 patient months and a total of 170 clients. Table 50-1 is based on these statistics and provides the age breakdown. The sex ratio and minority breakdown are detailed in Table 50-2.

The five major limiting conditions of the 170 clients were: 1) cardiopulmonary, 2) neurologic, 3) cancerous, 4) musculoskeletal, and 5) psychological.

Descriptions of Clinical Facilities

The health center is located in a municipal building with a library, city offices, and a vacated gymnasium. It is convenient to the shopping area and public transportation and, therefore, accessible to the community at large. The center occupies approximately 12,292 square feet—half of which was a 1977 addition. The home care office is located in the basement of the new addition and is wheelchair accessible by ramp and elevator. This is the home base for the program which is affiliated with three other neighborhood health centers—Little House Health Center, Dorchester House Health Center, and Bowdoin Street Health Center. Under this arrangement, the home care client is followed by the same physician who knew him or

TABLE 50-1. Client age breakdown

Age	No. of clients	%
40-49	3	1.8
50-59	7	4.2
60-69	20	12
70-79	62	36.5
80-89	58	34.7
90-99	18	10.8
Unknown	2	

TABLE 50-2. Client sex and ethnic group breakdowns

Sex	No. of Clients	%	Ethnic group	No. of Clients	%
Male	49	28.8	White	145	86.3
Female	121	71.2	Black	20	11.9
			Spanish	3	1.8
			Unknown	2	

her in the health center. Referrals are also made by consumers from the affiliate health centers for neighbors who need home care services in their area. These three health centers were involved in the original planning for a home care program for Dorchester.

Administrative/Agency Support

The home care program is governed by a Board of Directors composed of consumers. One of the subcommittees of the Board is the Home Care Committee, who interview all home care applicants and advise on policy matters. The Executive Director of the Upham's Corner Health Center is also the administrator of the home care program. The administrator spends approximately 10 percent of his time on home care responsibilities. These responsibilities include reviewing contracts, writing proposals, preparing the budget, recommending staff to the home care committee, and interpreting monthly financial statements.

The home care program is fiscally sound because of the abilities and commitment of the administrator. The deficits that accumulate due to free service and inadequate reimbursement fees are covered by the grant from the City of Boston.

A full-time secretary handles phone calls, filing, and typing duties. A part-time (20 hours per week) clerk prepares invoices for Medicare, Medicaid, private insurance companies, and self-payers. In 1977, the health center leased an IBM System 32 computer for processing the billing and for compiling statistics. The system allows for increased accuracy over the hand billed system and for current information on which to base management decisions. The medical records department maintains the security and privacy of the clinic's medical records. The home care clients' records are filed in the same area of the record room for accessibility. The ending digits are in the 97-98-99 range and easily returned for chart review or filing. All records are numbered by family and use a problem oriented system.

Financial Support

The home care program is a department of Uham's Corner Health Center which is one of seven neighborhood health centers affiliated with the Boston City Hospital. All aspects of health care that can be efficiently and economically handled at the neighborhood level are provided, while program components of a larger scale are handled centrally at the Boston City Hospital in order to realize increased economics. If a program is funded by the city, the joint budget is reviewed by the Board of Directors of the health center and of the hospitals. The budget for the health center is separate, however, and approved by the Board of Directors. The home care program budget is approximately $100,000 per year. In addition to billing third party payers such as Medicare, Medicaid, and private insurance companies, the program has a contract with the Senior Home Care Corporation to provide homemaker service. The homemaker services are billed to Medicaid or Title XX and Title III funds. A Community Development Block Grant provides additional funding for nursing care, medical services, physical therapy, social services, and homemaker/home health aides. The grant is funded through federal revenue sharing and monies dispersed at the local level in the Department of Housing and Urban Development. The City of Boston then holds hearings for citizens to set priorities. Programs are varied and include physical, economic, and housing improvement projects. The Home Care Program is just one of the projects which receives funds through this grant.

NURSING INTERVENTION

The nursing process utilized by the home care team is essentially an eclectic one, with concepts, assumptions, and theories drawn not only from nursing science but also from the varied social and medical disciplines. The family as the recipient of health care planning and services then becomes the focus of our nursing practice. The family is viewed as an open living system with each member considered a subsystem. The entire system interacts continuously with its environment and with the greater society, its goal being the maintenance of a steady state. Stresses with which the family must cope can be seen as input to the system. Characteristics of the family such as their group identity, authority scale, interpersonal relationships, and values determine the ways in which they deal with these stresses. Nursing assessment, diagnosis, intervention, and reassessment are based on the identifiable positive or negative feedback (output) resulting from the family's interaction with the stressor(s). Our ultimate goal is to assist the family in maintaining or regaining their steady state.

In addition to viewing the family structurally, the nurse clinician must be cognizant of humanistic factors which influence interpersonal relationships between family members and among the family and society. We are aware that the role of each individual is interdependent with other members of the family. With this in mind, we strive to understand each individual within the family as a whole and in his or her individuality. Man is viewed as a rational being who directs his life toward the realization of goals. His nature is seen as innately good, friendly, and constructive, but his ability to be adaptable or creative in dealing with life's stressors is dependent upon the positive or negative nature of his self-concept.

Our interpretation of this humanistic perspective defines fulfillment as the ultimate goal. The growth which the individual and family must attain in order to achieve this sense of fulfillment comes through mastery of developmental tasks. It is generally accepted that individual and family development tend to follow definite schedules. During each state of development, there are certain tasks which the individual and family must master. If these tasks are not mastered at the appropriate times in the life cycle, certain incompetencies place the individual and family at a disadvantage in adjusting at later developmental levels. Since our clinical practice deals mainly with old persons who are facing disengagement and dissolution of their families as systems, it is particularly important that we are able to assess developmental competencies in order to help our clients work toward that sense of fulfillment.

Summarizing to this point, then, our eclectic approach to client and family assessment 1) is aware of the history and development of the family, 2) sees each family member as an individual in interaction with all other members of the group, 3) watches how the group as a whole system interacts with the environment and greater social structure, 4) takes into consideration the individual effect on the family and the family's influence on personality development, 5) determines critical periods of personal and family growth and realizes these as ideal times in which to plan interventions, 6) evaluates effectiveness of family coping methods in terms of positive and negative feedback, 7) is aware of cultural influences on family life, 8) is aware of similarities and differences between families and individuals, and 9) provides a productive approach to the evaluation of family processes at a given period in the life cycle.

Continuing on this vein, the theories for our interventions are also drawn from a variety of sources. The humanistic approach forms the consistent thread in the entire nursing process. By its nature, the helping approach gives the support and encouragement necessary for families to work through their problems, the end result being progress toward a certain level of fulfillment.

Of equal importance is our ability to understand why people do or do not seek health care services. We have found that the classifications delineated by the Health Belief Model seem to offer the most valid insight into this question. The variables of this model "deal with the subjective world of the behaving individual."[5] It is through these perceptions that we can understand an individual's current health behavior and can then, if necessary, plan interventions to alter these perceptions. The major tenets of the model state that in order for an individual to take action to avoid a disease, he must believe that he is susceptible to it; that if he were to contract the disease, it would have at least moderate severity on some part of his life; and that taking action would benefit him by either decreasing susceptibility or reducing severity.[6] The model further addresses the importance of our awareness of barriers which might prevent action, such as cost, inconvenience and pain, and the necessity of cues—instigating events which are capable of setting the action process in motion.

Factors which influence an individual's perception of susceptibility and seriousness are variables referred to as modifying factors. These fall into three categories: demographic, including such factors as age, sex, race, and ethnic groups; sociopsychological, including personality, social class, peer and reference group pressures; and structural, including such factors as prior contact with or knowledge of the disease.[6]

Because of its subjective orientation, this model is easily compatible with the humanistic philosophy underlying our practice. It gives direction to the nurse by allowing her to assess specific family perceptions—those related to susceptibility and severity. Once these are determined, the model offers effective guidelines for the development of nursing intervention. For example, an approach with a specific family who were aware of their susceptibility might be directed toward the removal of barriers or the establishment of cues (help with enrollment in Medicaid due to worry over cost).

Thus far, we have discussed our foundation as that of a humanistic approach to relationship building and health care intervention. Secondly, we have delineated guidelines by which we assess families' willingness to take health directed action and have offered a model suggestive of intervention techniques.

The following case study demonstrates the application of the theory discussed thus far.

Mr. H is a 64-year-old man who was admitted to the home care program approximately eight months after he had a laryngectomy and radiation for a squamous cell carcinoma of the larynx. Tests showed no evidence of metastasis. During the time period between his surgery and admission to the home care program, he was followed at a neighborhood clinic by his primary physician and at home by another nursing agency. He did not do well during this span of time and required three hospital admissions for treatment of pneumonia, congestive heart failure, and stress gastritis. He was depressed; he spent the greater portion of the day in bed, lost weight, and was lax about his pulmonary hygiene. During his last hospitalization, there was much concern that he could not be adequately cared for at home. His condition had deteriorated to the point where he was physically dependent on oxygen all the time and was resistive to doing his own tracheostomy care. In spite of this, Mr. H wanted to return to his home, and plans were made to have him admitted to the home care program.

In retrospect, Mr. H's year after surgery was more complicated, more difficult than is probably true for many people who have undergone the same surgery. He had to cope with the overwhelming fears and frustrations all people with laryngectomies experience when they no longer are able to communicate verbally, when they must find new ways of maintaining their independence and control, and when they must live with the fear that cancer will recur.

In addition, though, Mr. H had to cope with the fact that his wife was, in many ways, more handicapped than he was. Mrs. H was eight years older than her husband. She had diffuse cerebellar degeneration and moderate cerebral atrophy. She had a very unsteady gait, which was only minimally improved with the use of a walker. She tended to be forgetful, had at times an inappropriate affect, and required careful and patient instruction and direction. She found it almost impossible to understand anything her husband said. Consequently, his communication was written, which proved lengthy and tedious. They were childless. One of Mr. H's brothers was as helpful as he could be, but he also had a disabled wife and much responsibility at home. Mrs. H's cousin helped with the shopping and the errands.

Their relationship was sustained and strengthened by the fact that they cared very deeply for each other. Their ultimate concern was the other's welfare. Their life before they became disabled was traditional in many ways. Mr. H worked in the Navy Yard most of his adult life until he retired early at the age of 58 because of a leg injury. He was responsible for the maintenance of the house, yard, and car. She, as the housewife, was responsible for the cooking, cleaning, and shopping. They were not active in community affairs; their social life centered around a few friends and the neighbors. After Mrs. H was no longer able to manage all the housework, Mr. H assumed responsibility for much of it. He had symptoms of hoarseness and throat pain for almost one year before seeking medical attention—he was fearful of the possible diagnosis of cancer because of the potential devastation for himself but was equally concerned about who would take care of his wife if his fears were proven true.

When we received the referral on Mr. H, we were hopeful but not overly optimistic that our interventions could significantly impact to help the H's adapt to their stress laden situation. Given his history of negative responses to previous health workers who visited him at home, we were pleasantly surprised by his openness and receptiveness to us. He welcomed our help and encouragement. Initially, the nurse clinician visited at least weekly and sometimes more frequently. She monitored his physical status but was more concerned about how well he and his wife were coping with their many responsibilities. She found that by being supportive without being dogmatic, Mr. H unfailingly followed through with our mutually developed plan of care, e.g., he suctioned his tracheostomy consistently and with good technique, he cleaned his equipment correctly, and he ate a well-balanced diet. We did not hesitate to help him with his care if he asked—occasionally, he would ask a nurse to suction his tracheostomy. Mrs. H had more difficulty following through with some of her responsibilities although she had been very conscientious about preparing nutritious food. A home health aide/homemaker spent several hours two to three times a week with the H's. Initially, she helped Mr. H with his personal care and with the care of his equipment, but eventually he did this himself, and she mainly helped his wife with her care and with household tasks. Mr. H also had assumed helping with the housework.

We now direct our attention to the process of adaptation—that method by which a family interracts with a constantly changing environment. Adaptation is an integral part of living. It is a process we must constantly address as our growth proceeds through life. However, one is not always able to adapt unaided. Significant others and health professionals are often called to help during difficult adaptation periods related both to health and illness.

The need for adaptation is precipitated by a stimulus impinging upon the individual or the family as a whole. Since we view man as a biopsychosocial being, we realize that the stimulus might be biologic, psychological, or social in origin. Sr. Callista Roy[7] has developed a model which helps us to assess a client's ability to adapt to five stimuli. The model delineates three classes of stimuli, the combined effect of which determines man's adaptation level. These are:

1. Focal stimuli: those which immediately confront the client (e.g., pain, secondary to malignancy).
2. Contextual stimuli: all other stimuli present (e.g., need to climb stairway to bedroom, ability to do so inhibited by weakness or pain).
3. Residual stimuli: beliefs, attitudes, and traits which have an indeterminate effect on the present situation (e.g., patient with terminal disease who had developed long term goals for future).

In addition, Sister Roy alerts us that man's adaptation level is comprised of a zone indicating the range of stimulation which will lead to a positive response. This zone is much like a threshold: if the stimuli fall within that zone, the individual can respond favorably; if not, the client will need help to make a positive response. Sister Roy guides us in nursing interventions by supporting manipulation of the variables effecting the three types of stimuli. Examples of nursing's ability to intervene are considered in the following discussion.

Focal Stimulus Manipulation

Initially, Mr. H was admitted to the respiratory ICU for total respiratory support. After the critical phase ended, he was transferred to a medical floor on continuous oxygen. Sequential arterial blood gasses supported his subjective statements that he needed oxygen. He was discharged home on oxygen and used it continuously. The setup allowed for ambulation throughout the home. Some time after he was decanulated, he had repeat arterial blood gasses drawn. They revealed that after 30 minutes without oxygen, he maintained normal oxygen tension. He was advised to remain off the oxygen for one half hour periods four times a day to start. If he felt that his breathing was not compromised, he could gradually increase the duration and frequency. Mr. H was reticent about beginning this treatment. The assessment of the nurse clinician was that his cognitive field was inadequate to serve as a guide for action. Interventions were directed towards education regarding the meaning of arterial blood gasses. Reassurance was provided initially by the nurse clinician and the home health aides' presence during weaning. As the client became more comfortable, he was able to continue the treatment independently.

Contextual Stimulus Manipulation

Mr. H's equipment was disorganized. His suctioning apparatus was stored in the bathtub, and each time he needed to use it, he had to lift it from the tub to the toilet seat. He stood in front of the bathroom mirror to perform the procedure. When he felt the need for suctioning, he first had to gather the sterile equipment from the living room, walk 20 feet to the bathroom, lift the suction machine from the bathtub, and strain to align himself with the mirror. The nurse helped him move all his equipment into the sitting room where he spent most of his time. He found a light and mirror, and arranged the supplies so that they would be easily accessible.

Residual Stimulus Manipulation

During one of his hospitalizations, it was determined that Mr. H had significant neurosensory hearing loss. However, he refused to be fitted for a hearing aide at this time. After his discharge, his hearing deteriorated even further, but he continued to be reluctant to accept an assistive device. His unwillingness to acknowledge this as a problem was consistent with his previous health related behavior. (He did not seek health care for his hoarseness and pain for more than a year after the onset of symptoms). The nurses' encouragement towards acceptance of a hearing aide was consistently unsuccessful. However, when the problem was approached in terms of speech rehabilitation, he was able to see the necessity of improved auditory acuity.

In further consideration of the process of adaptation, we remain cognizant of man's need to use defenses in his coping responses. Although defense mechanisms have taken on negative meanings to many, if not overused, we see them as favorable responses, allowing the individual to step away from the situation temporarily in order to better mobilize resources for adaptation. The recognition of defenses also gives us another method by which to assess a client's zone of adaptability. Observations by the nurse clinician of the types of coping strategies used by the family help her to assess whether the stimulus has fallen within their zone of adaptability. If the family's anxiety level remains inordinately high, or if they continue to use defense mechanisms over a prolonged period, she may assume that the combination of stimuli have fallen outside the range in which the family is able to make a positive response. It is likely, then, that interventions will need to involve other disciplines.

Other variables of adaptation which are considered in our assessment are those developed by Robert White: 1) that the cognitive field have adequate information about the environment to serve as a guide for action, 2) that satisfactory internal conditions be maintained both for action and the processing of information, and 3) that autonomy be maintained.[8] It is possible that positive adaptation may result through a nursing manipulation of only one stimulus or variable. However, since we are constantly assessing the status of the family through identification of positive or negative feedback, and since we are aware of the stimuli, strategies, and variables of adaptation, we are constantly able to alter and refine our interventions.

IMPACT AND RECOMMENDATIONS

The home care program is currently serving 120 clients. Because of the available comprehensive services, the program has been able to offer this select population an alternative to institutionalization. The primary benefit of the program is that the client can make a real choice about remaining at home for health care. The client receives the psychosocial supports that family and friends can provide on an ongoing basis. The family can assess the quality of care since it is performed under their auspices. This can allay many fears of both family and client regarding the amount and intent of care by exercising direct control over the therapy. During the three years in operation, we have found that with adequate supports, most elderly clients can be maintained in their homes. The contributions made by family members and/or friends to the daily care of the physically or psychologically dependent client have proven to be critical factors in our ability to maintain these individuals at home.

The role for the clinician is an innovative one. The nurse clinician is the primary agent of care, who manages and coordinates an individual panel of clients. The physician in this model acts as a consultant and willingly relinquishes management responsibilities to the clinician. The nurse clinician is the logical team leader. She coordinates the various services needed at home in order to deliver comprehensive care. She participates in the 24-hour on-call system and provides her home phone number for the terminally ill clients and their families. The clinician role is crucial to the functioning of this home care model, since she is the pivotal point.

As the elderly population continues to increase, more programs will need to be developed to meet their needs in a comprehensive fashion. Programs are needed in rural and urban areas and will necessitate a concomitant act by the government to invest attention and monies. Nursing must take an active role in determining the process and direction of growth and must support the development of programs to educate the gerontologic nurse clinician. Finally, nursing must contribute to the research regarding home care, especially in the area of cost effectiveness.

Nursing needs to participate in controlled studies that evaluate both the quality and quantity of home health care. Cost effectiveness research should preview variables such as reimbursement schedules, quality of life issues, and client/family preferences. Nursing research could expand the data base and answer current questions on home health care.

REFERENCES

1. United States Department of Health, Education and Welfare, Vital and Health Statistics, Estimates from National Health Interview Survey, U.S. 1972 Series 10, No. 85, 1973, as cited by Robert J. Master, M.D. in "A Comprehensive Home Care Alternative to the Hospital and Nursing Home," Boston, June, 1976.
2. Burnside, Irene Motorside: "Gerontology and Geriatric Nursing," in Burnside, I.M. (ed.): *Nursing and the Aged.* McGraw-Hill Book Company, New York, 1976.
3. Donley, Sister Rosemary, Jepson, Virginia, and Perloff, Evelyn: "Graduate Education for Practice Realities." *Nursing Outlook* 21 (10): 646, Oct. 1973.
4. Master, Robert: "A Comprehensive Home Care Alternative to the Hospital and Nursing Home." Boston, June 1976.
5. Rosenstock, Irwin M.: "Why People Use Health Services." *Milbork Fund Quarterly* 44:98, 1964.
6. Rosenstock, Irwin M.: "Historical Origins of the Health Belief Model," in Becker, Marshall H. (ed.): *The Health Belief Model and Personal Health Behavior.* Charles B. Slack, Inc., Thorofare, N.J., 1974.
7. Sr. Callista Roy: "The Roy Adaptation Model," in Roy, Callista and Riehl, Joan P.: *Conceptual Models for Nursing Practice.* Appleton Century-Crofts, New York, 1974.
8. White, Robert: "Strategies of Adaptation," in Coelho, George V., Hambert, David A., and Adams, John E. (eds.): *Coping and Adaptation.* Basic Books, Inc., New York, 1974.

UPHAM'S CORNER HOME HEALTH CARE PROGRAM   **INITIAL ASSESSMENT**
500 Columbia Road, Dorchester, Mass. 02125

Patient's Record # _____

FROM: _____

PATIENT
NAME _____

Unit/Clinic _____

ADDRESS: _____

ADDRESS _____

_____ TEL. _____

TEL. _____

| FLOOR | APT. # | BIRTHDATE |

| ADM. DATE | DISCH. DATE | AGE | SEX M F | MARITAL STATUS S M W D SEP. | RELIGION |

TO: _____

RELATIVE OR
GUARDIAN: _____

ADDRESS: _____

ADDRESS: _____

TEL. _____   TEL. _____

| MEDICARE NO. & LETTER | PLAN A B | BLUE CROSS NO. | SOC. SEC. NO. | OTHER |

| CLINIC APPOINTMENTS | DATE | TIME | AGENCY WORKER, OFFICE ADDRESS, TELEPHONE |

DIAGNOSIS(S) Surgery Performed and Date, Allergies or Infections

Is Patient ___ Family ___ aware of diagnosis?   Date of last physical _____

PHYSICIAN'S ORDERS: (include specific orders for Diet, Lab Tests, Speech, and O. T.)

| MEDICATION | STRENGTH AND FREQUENCY |

TREATMENTS & FREQUENCY: _____

DIET: _____

PHYSICAL THERAPY   Restrict Activity ☐ Yes ☐ No   Sensation Impaired ☐ Yes ☐ No

Precautions   Weight Bearing Status - Non-Weight ☐   Partial-Weight ☐   Full-Weight ☐

SPECIFIC TREATMENT & FREQUENCY: _____

ANTICIPATED GOALS: _____

REHABILITATION POTENTIAL IS: _____

HOME HEALTH
SERVICES: ☐ NURSING   ☐ OCC. THERAPY   ☐ SPEECH THERAPY   ☐ SOCIAL WORK   ☐ H.H. AIDE   ☐ OTHER-SPECIFY

CERTIFICATION: ★(when applicable)
Services above needed to treat condition for
which patient was hospitalized ☐ Yes ☐ No
I certify that the above named patient is: (check one)
   ☐ Under my care (or has been referred to another
physician having professional knowledge of patient's
condition); is home bound except when receiving outpatient services; requires skilled nursing care on
an intermittent basis or physical or speech therapy
as specified in the orders.
   ☐ Requires skilled nursing care on a continuing
basis for any of the conditions for which he/she
received care during this hospitalization.

_____ M.D.
Signature

_____ M.D.
Print Name

_____

ADDRESS: _____ TEL. _____

HISTORY

Check (✓) indicates a normal finding or the absence of abnormality. Make no mark if no observation is made. ENCIRCLE abnormalities and describe in detail.

FAMILY HISTORY

cancer	heart disease
tuberculosis	hypertension
diabetes	kidney disease
endocrine	allergy
arthritis	obesity
anemia	bleeding
jaundice	migraine
epilepsy	psychosis
gout	alcohol

SOCIAL HISTORY

Birthplace, residence
Marital status
Pregnancies
Social and Economic status
Occupation
Day's activities
Diet—type and adequacy
Drugs, alcohol, tobacco

PAST HISTORY

a. General Health
   Weight (date)
   Weight change
   Life insurance exam.
   Military service
   X-ray studies

b. Infections

scarlet fever	diptheria
rheumatic fever	chorea
German measles	pleurisy
pneumonia	tuberculosis

c. Admissions to hospitals

d. Operations and injuries without
   hospitalization

SYSTEMIC REVIEW

1. SKIN

rash	sweating
itching	bleeding tendency

2. BONES, JOINTS, MUSCLES

pain	swelling
trauma	

3. LYMPH NODES

enlargement	discharge
pain	

4. HEAD

headache	syncope
trauma	vertigo

5. EYES

vision	scotoma
glasses	inflammation
diplopia	pain
blurring	

6. EARS

pain	tinnitus
deafness	mastoiditis
discharge	

....
....
....

7. NOSE, THROAT, RESPIRATORY

sinusitis	hemoptysis
epistaxis	cough
sore throat	fever
hoarseness	night sweats
pain	x-rays
wheezing	

....
....
....
....

8. BREASTS

lumps	discharge
pain	

....
....

9. CARDIOVASCULAR

palpation	cyanosis
pain	fatigue
dyspnea	blood pressure
orthopnea	claudication
edema	treatment
anemia	

....
....
....
....

10. GASTRO-INTESTINAL TRACT

teeth	pain
tongue	hematemesis
swallowing	melena
appetite	jaundice
indigestion	constipation
gas	diarrhea
nausea	hemorroids
vomiting	cathartics

....
....
....
....
....

11. GENITO-URINARY TRACT

dysuria	retention
nocturia	frequency
oliguria	urgency
hematuria	incontinence
pyuria	pain

....
....
....

a. Venereal History

chancre	epididymitis
blood tests	bubo
gonorrhea	treatment

....

b. Menstrual History

age onset	amenorrhea
cycle	menorrhagia
duration	dysmenorrhea
amount	last period
irregularity	menopause
discharge	spotting

....
....

12. ENDOCRINE SYSTEM

goiter	sterility
exophthalmos	impotence
glycosuria	treatment

....
....

13. ALLERGIC AND IMMUNOLOGIC

sensitivity to allergens	serums or vaccines
eczema	hay fever
hives	asthma
skin tests	drug sensitive

....
....

14. NEUROPSYCHIATRIC

cranial n.	sensation
paralysis	anxiety
convulsions	hysteria
gait	affect
coordination	

....
....
....
....

History (Cont.)

Check if Pertinent: (describe at right) ▷

DISABILITIES
- ☐ Amputation
- ☐ Paralysis
- ☐ Contractures
- ☐ Decubitus
- ☐ Other

IMPAIRMENTS
- ☐ Speech
- ☐ Hearing
- ☐ Vision
- ☐ Sensation
- ☐ Other

COMMUNICATION
- ☐ Can Write
- ☐ Talks
- ☐ Understands Speaking
- ☐ Understands English
- ☐ If no, Other Language?
- ☐ Reads
- ☐ Non-Verbal

BEHAVIOR
- ☐ Alert
- ☐ Forgetful
- ☐ Noisy
- ☐ Confused
- ☐ Withdrawn
- ☐ Wanders
- ☐ Other

REQUIRES
Mark "S" if sent; "N" if needed

- ☐ Colostomy Care
- ☐ Cane
- ☐ Crutches
- ☐ Walker
- ☐ Wheelchair
- ☐ Other
- ☐ Dentures
- ☐ Eye Glasses
- ☐ Hearing Aid
- ☐ Prosthesis
- ☐ Side Rails

NURSING: Self Care Status Check Functional Level	Inde-pendent	Needs Assist-ance	Unable
Ambulation — Bed-Chair			
Walking			
Stairs			
Wheelchair			
Crutches			
Walker			
Cane			
Activities — Bathe self			
Dress self			
Feed self			
Brushing teeth			
Shaving			
Toilet			
Commode			
Bedpan/Urinal			

Bowel & Bladder Program ☐ Yes ☐ No

Incontinence: Bladder ☐ Bowel ☐

Catheter: Type
Date last changed:

Weight   Height   Date

Anointed Yes ☐ No ☐   Date

NUTRITION

Special Diet

Nutrient Adequacy

Food Shopping

Meal Preparation

ENVIRONMENTAL FACTORS & FAMILY ADJUSTMENTS

Household Management

Housing

Safety Hazards

Family Dynamics/Interaction

Response to Illness

_____
Signature of Nurse

Date _____

PHYSICAL EXAMINATION　　date _____

Check (✓) indicates a normal finding or the absence of abnormality.

Make no mark if no observation is made.

ENCIRCLE abnormalities and describe accurately in detail.

	Temp.	Pulse	Resp.	Blood Pressure	Weight

General appearance _____

_____

_____

_____

_____

1. INTEGUMENT

temperature	hair
texture	nails
color	lesions

2. LYMPH NODES

cervical	axillary
occipital	epitrochlear
supraclavicular	inguinal
	femoral

3. HEAD

a. skull:　　scalp
　　nits　　defects

b. eyes:　　fundi
　　vision　　ocular tension
　　fields　　movements
　　sclerae　　pupils-size, shape
　　corneas　　　equality, reactions
　　eyelids　　lenses
　　conjunctivae

c. nose:　　mucosa
　　obstruction　　polyps
　　discharge　　sinus
　　septum　　　tenderness

d. ears:　　tophi
　　canals　　hearing
　　discharge　　　air
　　ear drums　　　bone
　　mastoid　　　Weber

e. mouth:　　breath
　　lips　　gums
　　tongue　　mucosa
　　teeth

f. throat:　　color
　　exudate　　pharynx
　　tonsils　　uvula

4. NECK

　　masses　　supple
　　thyroid　　trachea
　　　　vessels

5. BREASTS

　　development　　nipples
　　masses　　discharge
　　　　tenderness

6. CHEST WALL AND LUNGS

shape   diameter
symmetry   diaphragms
expansion

describe abnormal pleural,
   mediastinal and pulmonary
   findings

_____
_____
_____
_____
_____
_____
_____
_____
_____
_____
_____

7. CARDIOVASCULAR SYSTEM (Describe)

a. pulses: B.P. arms
   radial   Rt.
   femoral   Lt.
   d. pedis
   p. tibial

	MSL	MCL.......cm.
1		
2		
3		
4		
5		
6		

b. heart:
   rhythm
   deficit
   thrill
   sounds
    A2 P2
frict'n rub
gallop
murmurs
(describe
and
diagram)

_____
_____
_____
_____
_____
_____
_____
_____
_____
_____
_____

8. ABDOMEN (Describe)

shape   liver
scars   kidneys
vessels   spleen
peristalsis   masses
tenderness   herniae
spasm   shifting dullness
costovertebral fluid wave
   tenderness urinary bladder
sacral edema

_____
_____
_____
_____
_____
_____
_____
_____
_____
_____
_____
_____
_____
_____
_____
_____

9. GENITALIA

  a. male:
     penis   scars
     scrotum   swelling
     testes   discharge

  b. female:
     introitus   adnexa
     urethra   perineum
     cervix   tenderness
     uterus   discharge

10. RECTUM

  hemorrhoids   masses
  fissures   prostate
  pilonidal cyst   feces
  sphincter   bleeding

11. BONES, JOINTS, MUSCLES

  spine: nodules
    mobility   muscle bulk
    tenderness   joint: motion
    long bones   deformity

12. EXTREMITIES

  color   edema
  temperature   clubbing
  varicosities   tremor

13. NERVOUS SYSTEM

  cranial nerves   gait
  motor system   stiff neck
  sensory system Kernig
  coordination   Brudzinski
  Romberg   tremors
  Reflexes   Rt. Lt.
    biceps
    triceps
    radial
    abdominal
    cremasteric
    knee
    ankle
    ankle clonus
    Hoffman
    plantar

14. MENTAL STATUS

  orientation   content of
  mood   thought
  behavior   insight
  memory   speech
              intelligence

Summary _____

_____

_____

_____

_____

_____

_____

_____

_____

_____

_____

_____

_____

_____

_____

_____

_____

_____

_____

_____

_____

_____

_____

_____

_____

_____

Diagnostic Impression _____

_____

_____

_____

_____

_____

_____

_____

_____

Signature, Title

Date

MEDICATION SHEET

ALLERGIES: _____   PT. NAME: _____

            _____   #: _____

MEDICATION	BEGUN	DATE D/C	DOSE	COMMENTS

PROBLEM INDEX

Problem No.	Problem - Active	Date Onset	Problem - Resolved	Date Resolved	

UPHAM'S CORNER HOME HEALTH CARE PROGRAM
PATIENT CARE AND TREATMENT PLAN

Patient's Name _____ Chart No. _____ Date _____

Date	Prob. No.	PLAN AND ACTIONS TO BE TAKEN

Progress, estimated time to reach goals and recommendations:

6/76   signature   title

CHAPTER 51
COMMUNITY MENTAL HEALTH CLINICAL ROLE STUDY

JOAN STACK KOVACH, M.S., R.N.

The following is a description of my practice as a community mental health nurse. Perhaps one could start with the formal job description presented to me when I assumed the position. However, this will not prove helpful in describing the role and the reasons why suggest two factors which will be discussed in this section. One is the rapid pace of change and development in the area of community mental health programming. Another is the opportunity for nursing in this area to creatively develop an expanded role.

I was hired as a head nurse. The description that goes with my job applied to the functions of a registered nurse in an adult inpatient setting. The requirements were licensure and experience and the salary was relatively low. At the time I was hired, I was a master's level psychiatric nurse, hired to function in an outpatient setting for children and their families. The discrepancy between the official job title and description and the functional assignment of the position was not uncommon. (In fact, a video technician was hired into a "barber's position"!) The reason for these discrepancies is that this state system requires legislation to change the title and job description of a position and this is a lengthy process. In the meantime, the community mental health movement demands that services reach out into the community (thus the establishment of outpatient clinics away from the state hospital); and that services be available to children as well as adults (thus the development of the children's service). These newly developed programs are staffed by transferring positions from the state hospital inpatient units to the outpatient setting. This causes an unusually high ratio of nurses in the outpatient department staff, as compared to other outpatient mental health settings.

This situation does not provide any serious obstacles in the performance of my role as a community mental health nurse. In fact, it provides an opportunity for my colleagues and me to create a role in community mental health nursing.

Because, technically, the position does not require advanced education and because master's level nurses are recruited for these somewhat ill defined and decidedly low paying positions, there was an expectation on my part that there would be a good deal of autonomy and on-the-job training. Initially, this was quite true. As the mental health center has grown, there has been an emphasis on procedure and standardization which results in less autonomy. However, the opportunities for inservice education and future training have been plentiful and continue to be so. During my employment, I have been able to participate in a two year Family Therapy Training Program, a two year seminar in Bioenergetics and Newer Therapies, as well as attend weekly or twice weekly case conferences. Supervision by senior clinicians is always provided and through this a variety of skills is learned. In addition, working at the agency makes it easy to hear about lectures, seminars, courses, and conferences that are presented in the area because notices are sent here. Essentially, then, the position is in state employment and it has a balance of assets and liabilities.

I came to this position with a background in community health, pediatric, psychiatric, and general medical nursing and a recently acquired master's in psychiatric mental health nursing. These experiences influence my philosophy of practice. Community health nursing has provided me with the broad, epidemiologic perspective of health problems. I feel that health care problems had to be looked at in terms of the larger systems affecting individuals. Thus, if three of my ongoing cases had to do with children having psychosomatic responses to unresolved grieving for the loss of an important person in their lives (a parent or grandparent), I would recognize the need for a parent education group in the community to address the issues of death and bereavement and their effect on children. Public health nursing also contributes to my understanding of the wellness-illness continuum. It helps me to recognize that patients in different situations require different levels of intervention. A psychotic or self-destructive teenager needs the safety and total care of an inpatient hospital. The same client, who later has returned home and is working and attending school, may only require bimonthly outpatient contact with her therapist. I am able to see that outpatients may be inpatients and vice versa. This is a result of my community health nursing experience.

My pediatric nursing experience provided me with an understanding of children as self-directed, autonomous beings who exist outside of their families as well as within. I feel that the child advocate approach is not as helpful to my work in a children's clinic as an approach which accepts the child, as well as the parents, as responsible members of the system in which they function. Pediatric nursing experiences have helped me understand the strength and resilience of children and their capacity for progress and regression in their efforts to change and grow emotionally and physically.

The psychiatric nursing experience provided me with familiarity with the forms of expression of emotional disorders and the effectiveness of nursing interventions. I know that directive intervention is an appropriate intervention during extreme stress, and that patient, supportive reality testing can best assist clients in their efforts to work out long term disorders.

My graduate studies in psychiatric-mental health nursing prepared me to function as a clinical specialist in this field. Added to my basic nursing education is a body of knowledge about psychiatric disorders, their diagnosis and treatment, some familiarity with the mental health care delivery system, and some beginning skills as a psychotherapist. The graduate program was two academic years. This provided me with the opportunity for one year of work with chronically ill clients in a state hospital setting and one year of work with emotionally and behaviorally disturbed children and their families in a community setting. An exposure to systems theory in graduate school and an opportunity in the community placement to observe family systems in distress and interventions which helped these systems to return to an equilibrium were especially important experiences for me.

Personally, I feel particularly interested in the challenge of using myself, my mind, presence, and personality as the primary tool of nursing interventions and in helping clients in an outpatient setting where they can call upon their own resources to a great extent. I feel particularly interested in parent intervention and education, in both the prevention and treatment of childhood emotional disorders.

I had graduated from a bachelor's degree nursing program which emphasized the psychological aspects of patient care. Like many new graduates, I doubted my competence as a skilled nurse, especially in the medical-surgical setting. I did maintain some sense of confidence in my psychiatric nursing skills, but at graduation time I doubted these skills too and worried if I could really go out there and work as a registered nurse! Initially, I worked in a general medical setting, suffering through that painful new graduate experience *wanting* to know everything and do well and *feeling* like I knew nothing and did horribly. Probably the experience is universal and a good one. Eventually, by working in a medical-surgical area, I did gain some confidence in my nursing skills and knowledge. The emphasis on the psychological care of the patient offered by my undergraduate program strongly influenced me and I continued to look forward to an opportunity to increase my knowledge in psychiatric nursing.

Another important influence is the fact that I come from a very large family. This influenced my professional philosophy in many ways. I can recall being surprised to learn that all families were not big families. Gradually, I took an interest in the differences between families, the different ways adults assumed the parenting role, the different characters that emerged from within the same family. I watched how my family worked as a system and took notice of how others did, and when another style was advantageous and when it was not. I became comfortable in dealing with families and in sitting with large groups of related people. I learned the value of the perspectives of children and the necessity for including them in observations about families. Thus, my interest in child-parent and family-society interactions has drawn from my primary life experience—that of being a member of a family. Influenced in all these ways, I began a job as a community mental health nurse in the children's service of an outpatient mental health clinic.

DESCRIPTION OF THE AGENCY

In order to describe the agency and my role it seems necessary to do so historically, dynamically, and politically. Community psychiatry is a young concept and the nursing role in this field is constantly evolving, just as the clinic in which I work is ever growing and changing. It seems important to mention that when I first came to the agency, I was one of three full-time nurses in a small (seven member) staff. Within three years, the staff expanded to include 21 people and the equivalent of 14 full-time members. Another important fact is that during my employment at the clinic, there were a series of three directors—a psychiatrist who started the program and who used broad based systems theory interventions to establish a network of community mental health services; a psychologist who was acting director while the search continued for a physician director; and finally, a child psychiatrist with a traditional, psychoanalytic frame of reference who was interested in the principles of community mental health. The agency changed significantly each time the leadership changed and this affected the experience of the staff and the patient care which was delivered.

Another event which influenced the workings of the clinic was the mental health center's application for accreditation as a community mental health center. Some aspects of patient care needed development and, thus, became a priority in order to meet accreditation guidelines. Other programs were abandoned so that staff energy could go into meeting the criteria for accreditation. Of course this meant the loss of some services, and, to me, the loss of some of the opportunities for spontaneous creativity in my role. However, to be an accredited agency meant an increased possibility of receiving federal and other grants for programming. These changes could be considered a short term loss toward the goal of a long term gain.

Two more factors which are ongoing influence my experience of being a community mental health nurse in a children's outpatient clinic. The first is that the clinic seems to have two separate and sometimes conflicting mandates. One is the mandate of the state, that the clinic care for the residents of the geographic (catchment) area which it serves. The state wants to reduce the incidence of, and the progression of, mental illness. To that end, sometimes services are court ordered such as mandatory hospitalization of a patient who is dangerous to himself or others known as "commitment." The second mandate comes from the nonprofit community based organization which is responsible for part of the funding and all of the community representation for the clinic. (All grants and private funding go through the community organization. The remainder of the funding is from the state or income generated by the clinic through third party payments which also is handled through the nonprofit agency.) This organization and its advisory board mandates that the clinic be responsive to its consumers in the community and provide them with the services they seek. Thus, if the community does not want sex education or birth control facilities in the area, the clinic is under some pressure not to provide or seek such services for clients, even though they are deemed essential to carrying out the state mandate of reducing the problems of the area.

The conflict created by these separate mandates is mostly a subtle, unseen, but strongly felt factor and certain situations bring this conflict into the open. In one situation, a community resident who was on the staff of the mental health center became involved with the politics of the local health center. When the issue of the health center's position on abortion referral and birth control came up, her participation became problematic. If she spoke *for* abortion referral and birth control information services, she might cause the community to see the mental health center as representing a pro-abortion viewpoint. If she spoke *against* these services, the community was unlikely to get a much needed service. She was asked to withdraw her involvement in order to protect the agency's standing in the community. Essentially, the conflict is between the ethics of the community and the philosophy of the mental health system.

The second ongoing factor has to do with the nature of the work in a children's service. Such a clinic services patients, male and female, under the age of 18. Therefore, in all the work we do, help is sought for someone under the age of 18 who is considered the identified patient. Often the "identified patient" does not have a mental disorder but serves the function of a "calling card" for their parents, siblings, or the entire family who needs help. Thus, services often are provided to patients who cannot or do not consider themselves in need of help but who come to our attention indirectly as family members. Frequently, it is the family, as a unit, which needs intervention. Often, a parent is in difficulty but cannot see the situation that way. Parents are often treated for their difficulties through "child focused work" in which the parent and the nurse or other therapist agree to meet in order that the parent can better help the child. This special characteristic of a children's clinic means that a sophisticated, holistic approach is always demanded.

Describing the nursing role in the community mental health center without describing the many facets of the center, its growth and changes, its attempts to define and refine itself, its idiosyncracies, would have been inadequate. This being done, I will now focus on a description of the day-to-day aspects of this job to provide an example of the expanded role of the nurse.

CLINICAL PRACTICE SETTING

I will start with a description of the facility. The clinic is located on a main street in a residential section of a large New England city. The community is part of the city and shares the schools, transportation, police department, and other city services with areas that are not at all similar. This section of the city has many small town aspects: a local deli, a local shoe store, and bakery.

There are two large Catholic churches with active parish organizations, as well as churches of a number of Protestant denominations, a Greek Orthodox church, and a Jewish synagogue. Ethnically, there is a mix of people of Irish, Italian, and Middle Eastern heritage.

The clinic is located on the second floor of a two story building which also houses a tailor shop and a shoe store. It is a former dentist office and many of the offices still have sinks. The physical setting is sparce and outmoded and, at times, disheveled but business thrives and from time to time there is a new coat of paint or a new plant or a new piece of furniture.

Until recently, most of the improvements to the physical plant have been initiated by staff members. The addition of an assistant director who has some responsibility for the facility's appearance and functioning has resulted in a new coat of paint and some additional phones for the agency. These events complement the ever present sense of change in the agency.

The children's clinic is part of a larger network which makes up a growing rambling community mental health center. This network consists of an inpatient unit (located on the state hospital grounds but possibly moving out into the community in the future); an adult outpatient rehabilitation center; a geriatric program; a community residence program for the retarded; an outpatient drug treatment program; an adolescent recreational program; an outpatient group treatment program for children; a small school for emotionally disturbed children; and a storefront information and referral agency.

What the children's clinic does is provide evaluation and treatment services to anyone under 18 in the catchment area who seeks mental health services. Among the services provided are play therapy for children, supportive therapy, couples therapy for parents, child guidance, psychological testing, school consultation to teachers both in general and on behalf of specific children who are clinic patients, consultation to other agencies in the network or in the community, case advocacy, and the training and supervision of students from many disciplines including nursing, medicine, social work, psychology, counseling, occupational therapy, art and movement therapy, and education.

The children's clinic is located in one of the three communities contained in the catchment area. The adult clinic (the component of the mental health center providing parallel services to those over 18) is in a second community, three miles away. The third community, which lies in between the children's and adult clinic, has three of the many other mental health center programs within its boundaries so there are facilities in each of the three communities and patients may be seen in their own community. One result of the expansion of the agency is a need for more space and, as yet, there has been no decision about whether to purchase one large building and offer all services from it or continue to rent small, separate spaces where satellite clinics can be set up. Within the clinic and its administration, philosophies differ, and so the preferences on how to handle the space problem differ. Presently, the children's clinic is quite inconspicuously located in the center of the business and shopping district. Parents often do errands while their children are in therapy. Some parents, perhaps fearful or embarrassed to tell their children that they are going to a mental health center, will suggest a trip to the ice cream parlor or department store and then at the last minute bring them to the clinic. This strategy is not encouraged, but it happens and the location seems to facilitate the clinic and its services being integrated into other errands of life.

NURSING INTERVENTIONS

The scene being set, we can move on to a description of the expanded role of the community mental health nurse in the children's clinic of a community mental health center. Basically, the job is to meet the needs of the patients. So simple a task can get quite confusing when patients themselves are uncertain about what their needs are and, often, uncertain about *who* the patient is. In most situations, referral to the mental health center is made because someone is in pain. It is in attending to this pain that the role of the nurse and her colleagues is actualized.

As a community mental health nurse, I function as one of a number of staff members who provides direct service to patients in the form of one of the therapies mentioned earlier. In many ways, the disciplines of social work, psychology, and psychiatry overlap with nursing in the field of mental health. While psychologists are mainly those who administer psychological testing, nurses and other professionals incorporate many aspects of psychometry in their work. For instance, I will often ask a child I am evaluating to "draw a person" or for their "three wishes." These questions are part of some psychological testing protocols. Many aspects of a mental status exam (an assessment of one's present mental functioning), which as a nurse I administer both to children and adults, are derived directly from intelligence tests. Some of my colleagues in nursing have studied psychometry and themselves administer psychological tests, but for the most part this is a function of the psychologists in this clinic.

Psychopharmacology is often considered an area mastered only by nurses and physicians. In the field of mental health, many social workers and psychologists are informed about and familiar with psychopharmacologic medications, and while they cannot prescribe or administer medication (a function of the physician and nurse, respectively) they do share somewhat in that particular body of knowledge.

Often in this clinic, the nurses are considered the resource persons for psychopharmacologic as well as physiologic data. Nurses are often asked to interpret medical reports or explain the meaning of certain medical terminology. For example, a case may be presented in which the mother has reported, as part of the child's developmental history, that the baby was "born with diarrhea." The birth records may state there was meconium staining. Members of the staff who are nurses may be asked to explain what this means and suggest what it might indicate about the child and his family at the time of birth. For instance, if a parent correlates the encopresis (fecal soiling) their nine year old son is experiencing with the "diarrhea" they feel the child had at birth, the nurse will be relied upon to state whether or not this is a realistic physiologic possibility or a distortion on the part of the parent. In this case, the nurse could help her colleague understand that there is no known or likely connection between these two conditions. The colleague might want to explore the child's medical history further to understand how realistically the parent has approached it, or to see if the parent has made other assumptions about their child's health, or if the encopresis has gone on for a long time, untreated, because the parents felt guilty about the child's difficulty at birth. Most of the mental health professionals at this clinic are fairly sophisticated about medical and growth development issues but the nurse is often the resource for these questions.

Another area in which the nurses on the staff have demonstrated a particular interest and expertise is the mother-child interaction. Six years ago, a program called "Mothers and Kids Groups" was started by a psychologist and a community mental health nurse. The psychologist, along with the public health nurse in the area, met weekly for one and a half hours with local mothers who had not sought help at the mental health center but who were interested in meeting other mothers and enjoying a break from their children. Often these were high risk mothers with problematic mother-child relationships who did not experience their situations as a mental health problem and would never seek help at a mental health center. While the mothers met and had coffee (provided by the group leaders), the community mental health nurse, with the assistance of some high school students, met with the children, mostly preschoolers since the group was held during the day. At this time, the children were provided with structure, consistency, an opportunity to do a project (usually a very simple arts and crafts activity), and a snack. The children were screened for developmental or emotional problems and behavioral interventions were made accordingly. (An example of such an intervention will be provided later in this chapter.) When stressful mother-child interactions were noted at the drop-off (beginning) or pick-up (ending) time of the group, the nurse would intervene by talking with the mother about her child, validating her feelings, and suggesting other ways of dealing with the child. These groups were considered preventive programs since the consumers were not care seeking patients of the clinic. For some reason, as the staff changed and the original "Kids Group" nurse moved on, the program, or one like it in the next community, would continue, usually because a new *nurse* on the staff expressed an interest in taking over the program. Because the program is a preventive one and because the clinic is mandated to treat primarily the care seeking clients, there has been little support for continuing these groups in recent years and the last of them is likely to end this year, when the nurses presently involved in the program leave the clinic. It is not clear why there has always been a nurse involved in the program. Perhaps it is related to the fact that the nurse's education includes opportunities to be involved in prenatal, labor and delivery, neonatal, and postpartum care. Unlike my non-nurse colleagues, I have a familiarity and comfort with the mother-child interaction and perhaps a stronger interest in working in this area.

Now you may have an idea of how the nurse works along with other mental health professionals and compliments the staff composition. I will explain further how the clinic functions. Children are referred to the clinic from many sources and for many problems. Parents refer unhappy or unruly children; schools refer unresponsive, hyperactive, or unsuccessful children; courts refer delinquent children; confused and depressed children sometimes refer themselves.

Most of the time, referrals are made via phone call. Occasionally, a patient or parent will walk in and request services. Clinicians (any of the mental health staff) take turns being on "intake" which means being available for any phone calls or "walk-ins." A full time clinician is assigned a half day (4 hour) block of time during which she or he must be at the clinic and "interruptable." The clinician usually does not schedule appointments for the hours spent on intake as the session may be interrupted by an intake call. The time is usually spent providing or receiving supervision, doing paperwork, or making phone calls. Prospective clients who call or walk in are greeted by the intake worker and asked to explain why they are calling. If there is an emergency, they are asked to come right in and are seen by the intake worker. An assessment is done and if medication, hospitalization, or temporary placement is needed, the intake worker contacts a physician on call, the hospital, or the welfare department respectively, as deemed appropriate. If there is no emergency situation but a request for the services provided by this agency, the client is given the name of a clinician and told they will be called by this person in the next day or two. The clinicians are assigned on a rotating basis and are provided with whatever basic information was gathered on the phone. Typically, a parent may call and report that a previously well behaved child is stealing from his mother's purse or a generally quiet and withdrawn adolescent has run away from home or a smiling six year old hasn't smiled once since his mother remarried. The clinic, through the assigned clinician, offers the child and their parents an evaluation of the current difficulty and a treatment plan.

As a staff member, I am involved in evaluating children and their families and in developing and providing many different types of treatment. Some children are seen alone in play therapy; some in groups; some in the context of their families; some are serviced indirectly, that is, the nurse provides consultation to the school, day care center, or parents regarding how to help a child with special problems, in his environment. Sometimes parents are seen in therapy without their children.

Thus, this nurse's role is a composite of providing evaluations and treatments as well as assessing the needs of the community and the agency. I provide consultation to other providers such as a social worker in the welfare department or a community worker who runs a mothers' group. I also provide supervision to other staff and to students from graduate programs in counseling and nursing who have placements at this agency. In addition, I receive supervision as well as ongoing training. The way this comes about will become more clear as a work day is described.

Monday begins with my participation as a co-leader in a preschool group for 11 children aged 3 months to 6 years old. This group is one of the Mothers and Kids Group described previously. The group meets for an hour and a half which is arranged to include a free play time, a project time, an outdoor or gross motor play time, a quiet or story time, and a snack and goodbye time. The children's mothers meet simultaneously in another room with another nurse-therapist who facilitates their group therapy experience, thus, the name of the program is the Mothers and Kids Group. Mothers and children have been referred to this program because the mothers experience problems with their parenting or because they were concerned about the behavior of their children. Many have referred themselves. A few have been referred by the welfare department or Children's Protective Service. In general, these are not mothers who would seek help at a mental health clinic.

The program provides parents and children with an opportunity for support, clarification, and growth. My role in the Kids Group is to help provide a stable, consistent environment where the children can express their concerns and act out their difficulties. Having co-led the group for three years, I find my role to be beyond that of group leader (or "teacher" as the children call us), and I feel more like a familiar visiting aunt who loves them, disciplines them, watches them grow, and knows them from regular weekly contacts. The group has many family traits. Often a child in the group who is having trouble with a sibling uses the group not to aggravate his annoying younger sister but to interact (sometimes aggressively) with another group member the same age as the antagonistic sibling. With the help of one of the "teachers," children learn that anger is okay but hitting is not. The child has not been able to successfully vent his anger toward his sibling at home because the parents have, appropriately, protected the sibling. The child may try to vent it on another child in the group who reminds him of his sister. The group leaders redirect the anger to a game of bean-bag toss or beat the drum thus helping the child to deal with feelings that might otherwise cause behavior problems. Some of the children have been in this group (which has been running for five years) all their lives. Some were "born into the group," in fact, their mothers attended the program throughout their pregnancy, and some have "graduated from the group" into kindergarten. Once in a while, these alumni return to the group. They can experience a sense of mastery when they hang their coat on the hook they once were not able to reach, and when they see younger members struggling to color a paper as they once did.

The group is co-led by a mental health worker. A mental health worker is a staff member without formal training in one of the mental health disciplines but with recognized skills fostered by a considerable amount of on-the-job training. Often mental health workers are community residents and understand the mental health needs of an area in a way a professional does not. Our mental health worker was hired to drive a van for the agency. When we did not get the van, he became a video technician assistant. Eventually, he began participating in clinical activities (such as the Kids Group) and began seeking out supervision and educational opportunities on the job. By the time the agency secured a van, he was a valuable clinician well integrated into his job as a mental health worker. (Someone else was hired to drive the van.) Other professionals staff the group from time to time in order to gain experience with groups of young children. Presently, a master's level community worker and a child psychiatrist attend because of their interest in working with small children. Together this staff assesses the needs of a child, proposes interventions, and evaluates the response. An example of this intervention is provided by the following story of Tony.

Tony is a 6-year-old boy who, along with his younger brother, has been a group member for three years. He frequently fell down while playing. His clumsiness was observed and discussed with his mother who said she had seen this behavior often and was also concerned. His mother checked with his pediatrician and he was evaluated for physiologic problems related to the falling and found to have none. The problem was considered one that could be treated behaviorally in the group. We hypothesized that Tony, the oldest group member, was being overlooked for his assets and noticed more regularly for his problems. The more often and dramatically he fell, the more attention he received from the staff. In general, we felt we probably gave more attention to the younger, more helpless members and provided few incentives for Tony to demonstrate his age 6 abilities.

Tony was told that if he could go through free time without falling, he could be in charge of the ball at outdoor time. The intervention was planned so that instead of running to him when he fell so frequently, we would acknowledge his ability to spend a half hour without falling and his ability to do an older child task, be in charge of the ball, and praise him for this. Tony's clumsiness declined with this intervention and efforts were made to share this with his mother so he could experience support for his growth at home too.

The leaders of the Kids Group meet with mothers as needed before or after the one and a half hour program. In this instance, I met with Tony's mother and told her our assessment of the problem and our intervention. She felt that she, too, did not support Tony's age 6 accomplishments and said she thought it would be good to do that but she felt badly when she did not respond to his falls. I supported her position to let her know that sometimes mothers feel they are not doing a good job if they do not rush to a child who has fallen. We discussed ways to check with Tony to see if he was injured without paying a lot of attention to each fall. The problems demonstrated by other children were dealt with similarly through the use of the nursing process.

In addition to specific interventions for specific symptoms, the group experience itself provides the members with healthful interventions. Most of the children remain in the group until they begin first grade. Through the group experience, they practice separating from their mothers, and their mothers practice separating from them. They also learn the beginning aspects of negotiating with peers and following rules. Their ego development (sense of self) is supported through their receiving recognition as group members at snack time when each member is named and greeted by the others and through their creating something of their own at project time when they make something which they can take home. The group has provided preventive intervention for high risk children. It facilitates their entrance into school and, therefore, their ability to gain from what school can offer. In addition, along with the other staff members, I meet with the parents periodically to discuss the children and support the parents' efforts at caring for the mental health needs of their children.

After the group meeting, the leaders of the Kids Group and the leaders of the Mothers Group meet to discuss the program. The themes of both groups are elicited and reported and program planning is done. Often the tone of the Kids Group is excited and anxious. This may be on a day when the mothers in their group are dealing with an especially anxiety provoking situation such as the loss of a parent. The summary of the two groups allows us to make a correlation of the themes and to design optimum interventions. The Mothers Group leader can validate for a mother that children can be hardest to handle when a mother is already upset about other things. The Kids Group leaders can make a point of "talking to the feelings" the children are having in order to relieve them. Such an intervention might be to say at project time when the children are gathered together: "Last week everyone seemed jumpy and this week they are calmer. Maybe everyone was worried because Diane was gone and relieved because today she's back."

As mentioned earlier, this program is likely to be discontinued because the leader of the Mothers Group is leaving.

The next appointment of my workday is with the two leaders of another mothers group. This group was started by me last year in a housing development in the community. The recreation worker for the development invited representatives from community agencies such as this agency to come to a luncheon, meet the residents of the area, and offer our services. Some of the women in the development expressed a desire to meet regularly and talk and a Mothers and Kids Group was developed, using this nurse, the community health nursing instructor, the recreation worker, and a community resource person in the Mothers Group. The community health nursing students and a community mental health worker lead the Kids Group. The program ran well for six months and was terminated at the end of the school year. It was started up again this year using the community resource person and a parent group leader from another agency as the two leaders for the Mothers Group and local volunteers for the Kids Group. Scheduling made it impossible to use the community health nursing students again but efforts are continually being made to reinvolve them in this program as a learning experience.

I now meet with and consult to the Mothers Group leaders. As they present the data from their group meetings, I provide ideas on what needs are being expressed by the mothers and suggestions for how these group leaders can meet these needs. In addition, we discuss the future programming for the Mothers and Kids Groups throughout the tricommunity area and what impact the financial and political situation of the mental health center will have on these needs. Of course, all administrative decisions are made by the clinic administration but ideas for program planning may come from the providers, the community mental health nurse, and her colleagues who can be invaluable for their ideas, experience and familiarity with the issues.

After this meeting, I join my co-leader, the community mental health worker with whom I do the Kids Group, this time for a one hour therapy group for boys. The boys are aged 7 to 10 and all have parents who are separated due to divorce, death, or temporary marital discord. All of the boys were referred to the clinic by their mothers for behavioral problems and have been evaluated and determined candidates for group therapy. Three of the members have individual therapy as well. This group therapy hour is divided differently from the Kids Group, since the purpose is different. The first 20 minutes is gross motor activity, a time when the boys invent and perform activities that call upon their strength, coordination, and sense of competition. Since all the boys have difficulty with impulse control, such games as "Simon Says" and "Bean Bag Toss" are incorporated. The second 20 minutes is expression activity. During this time, drawing, acting, or writing are used as a means to help elicit data about the members' life experiences which are shared and discussed. The goal is to provide an opportunity for sharing and support among group members. The next 10 minutes is for discussion of the expression activity and the final 10 minutes is for snack.

After this session, I meet with my co-therapist to discuss the group, the data presented by each member, possible ways to respond to the needs identified, and program planning in general. During this time, we may plan to meet with a member's parent to attempt to enhance support and concern for the member, or to understand what factors of family life are affecting the group member. Group members seem to benefit from the opportunity to explore, recreate, and master their family experiences within the context of a group co-led by a male-female team. The skills of the nurse and those of the community mental health worker (communication and support) complement each other in this task.

The next hour is generally spent doing family therapy. Since most of the families using the service are working class families, family treatment is often done in the early evening so that working fathers can attend. One advantage of the community mental health nursing position in this agency is an opportunity to participate in a two year family therapy training program. This program emphasized a systems theory approach to family intervention. Exposure to systems theory in my graduate nursing program facilitated my ability to understand and use the training provided. In doing family therapy, I assess the needs of the family and make interventions, sometimes verbal sometimes nonverbal, with the goal of helping the family change problematic behaviors. The nurse, as well as her non-nursing colleagues, may be a family therapist. Some states require special licensure or certification for the title "family therapist" but at this time most do not. I consider myself a family therapist because of my additional training. I also consider family therapy to be that specific situation in which the family experiences a need for change and makes a commitment to work toward that change. I do family therapy, but more often in my role as a community mental health nurse, I am called upon to do *family work*, which I distinguish from family therapy. Family work is done when a mental health professional decides that the best way of treating the problems presented by the child or parents is to meet with some or all members of the family for exploration or clarification. Sometimes one meets with the parents and child, the child and his siblings, the child and his parent and grandparent, the entire family, or any combination of family members that seems relevant. Often this is provided in addition to individual or group therapy for the child. The difference between family therapy and family work is that in the latter situation, the family has not made a commitment to work for change but has agreed to participate in the clarifying and exploratory sessions offered by the professional. Family work is also referred to as "providing support for the family."

Family therapy with the Jackson family, whom I usually meet on Monday evenings, is focused on helping the family adjust to the changes brought about by the growth and development of their only son, Jimmy, who is approaching 18. The family feels there are problems and has agreed to work on changing their way of doing things. Jimmy has a history of social and school problems. The family has been involved with social service agencies for many years and now the son, whose problems have been the reason for all of their connections with helping agencies, is about to graduate from high school and has already secured a job. Jimmy has been diagnosed as retarded, emotionally disturbed, and learning disabled. He is presently working toward ending his use of special classes and spending his entire school day in regular classes. His mother, a housewife who has not worked since Jimmy's birth, and his father, who is presently unemployed but constantly job hunting, seem unable to support Jimmy's gains because they pose the need for role changes within the family. The family seems to create and recreate crises to deter themselves from the tasks at hand. As their family therapist, I pointed out these tasks and wonder with the family what disadvantages there may be to Jimmy's progress. When the family comes into a meeting wanting to talk about a recent father-son fight and wanting me to decide for them who is right, we talk about the factors in the current family situation that may have caused the need for a fight as a distraction. The family therapy session lasts one hour. When it is over, I spend a short time jotting down notes that will help me to track the progress of the meetings and refocus our efforts at change.

This ends the work day for Monday. The remainder of the week consists of some similar activities; I usually see three or four families each week; I have two other groups, one adolescent group for young women aged 14 to 17 and one adult women's group for mothers who have sought help at the clinic; and there are some other activities such as intake meetings with new clients, participation in the staff meeting, presentation or participation at diagnostic conferences, attendance at supervision sessions where my work is reviewed by another more senior nurse clinician, and individual psychotherapy sessions.

I presently am treating children (ages 8 and 11), adolescents (ages 13, 14, and 17), and an adult (age 47) in individual psychotherapy.

On the average, I spend 15 to 17 hours providing direct clinical service to clients, meet with 17 to 25 clients per week, either individually or in groups. The psychotherapy I do is a treatment which relies heavily on the nursing process. For each client, no matter what the ongoing treatment may be, there is a constant need to identify problems, develop interventions, implement these interventions, evaluate their effectiveness, and make changes in the interventions as necessary. With the Jacksons, for instance, a problem developed with Jimmy's constantly being late for the meetings. I decided to begin on time with whomever was present, and Jimmy, concerned that he would miss something, began to be on time for the family meetings. This was a change in my original plan which was to postpone the start of any meeting until all members were present. This was done to emphasize the need for full family participation. It became clear that the family needed and wanted full participation and would all be present. I was then able to change my approach to help Jimmy attend on time. This is treatment of patients in which the nursing process is used. Each week, as a community mental health nurse, I provide patient care on many different levels.

A program which has not yet been discussed is the "Parent Orientation Group," an innovation used for two years at the clinic in order to handle the large numbers of weekly referrals to the clinic. The Parent Orientation Group was a group meeting which gave parents who had called the clinic an opportunity to come into the clinic within a week, meet two staff members, and meet other parents who were in the similar situation of seeking help. The meetings originally were an event where parents came together, had coffee, and shared, to the extent that they felt comfortable, some of their difficulties as parents. At the end of the meeting, the clinicians would describe how the clinic worked and ask parents to fill out application forms if they wished evaluations for their children.

As a staff member, I participated in the design and implementation of this program. Although the program allowed for a warm, nonthreatening entrance into the mental health system, it did not provide for immediate screening and assessment of the child and was discontinued in favor of an individual intake system. This change reflected both the philosophy of the new director, who felt that intakes should be done individually, and the requirements of the accreditation guidelines which suggested that the "identified patient" (identified patient is an expression used to specify that person the care seekers have identified as in need of service) be seen within a week of the initial phone call. It is important to understand how, in a community setting, agencies must respond to many different forces and factors. New developments affect the role of the nurse, and one must appreciate the community mental health nursing role as an ever changing position.

IMPACT AND RECOMMENDATIONS

The children's clinic and the mental health center as a whole have been growing and changing to keep up with the mental health needs of the community. My work as a community mental health nurse provides nursing care for children, parents, and entire families who experience difficulty in coping with their life situations. It is difficult to evaluate the benefits of work done in the area of mental health because the tools of measurement are yet imprecise and unreliable and because agencies like this one are often totally consumed in providing services and unable to take the time and money necessary to do followup studies on patients.

Patients do return now and then to tell us about their lives and the effect our services may have had on them. One teenage client I worked with for two years returned seeking a letter from me, as a mental health professional, to the court to allow her to marry her boyfriend prior to their 18th birthdays. She had sought help for herself at the clinic when she was stressed over a volatile family situation. Her widowed mother had remarried a young immigrant who provided well for the family but could not tolerate the adolescent behavior demonstrated by this young woman. Without the support of her mother, who sided with her new husband, Suzanne acted out her pain and confusion by drug and alcohol abuse and sexually precocious behavior. When she first came in to the clinic, she was upset because she was drinking nine cans of beer at night and her mother did not even notice. She used the clinic to find someone to talk to and she used her relationship with me to get some validation for her feelings and test out her understanding of herself. I did not focus on her behavior or expect behavior changes but instead tried to understand with her why she felt so lonely and why she took steps that were ultimately self-destructive to her. During the course of treatment, she responded by withdrawing from the conflicted relationship with her stepfather, establishing what seemed to be a positive and nurturant relationship with a new boyfriend whom she brought in to meet me, and ceasing her use of drugs. She returned with a request which could be interpreted as an endorsement from me for the work she has done.

One of my colleagues, also a community mental health nurse, told me of a patient who initially presented herself at the clinic as a deprived, depressed woman who was a negligent and abusive parent. She worked with my colleague for five years and, with the help of many agencies, especially the welfare department which provided a homemaker, this woman created some order in her life and improved greatly the care of her children. She returned to the clinic employed as the driver of one of the vans which brings children to the clinic for therapy. These events suggest to us that the services provided by a community mental health center meet the needs of the community residents. In a community where "I'll put you away!" is often the final threat of an overwhelmed parent who feels helpless about managing his child, many people are now aware that an ever expanding helping agency exists which can assist them in handling their life difficulties.

The mandate to service the care seeking population has resulted in less emphasis on the preventive aspects of community mental health. My role has changed in response to many things and is now a more narrow direct service provider role. The move to separate the clinic from the state hospital and the development of third party payment reimbursement as a source of income has rendered preventive programs such as parent education groups, Mothers and Kids Groups for noncare seeking clients, and community consultation as economically impractical. Many of the nurses' skills, especially those of the nurse with community mental health training, go underutilized. For instance, in the direct service model, there seems no place to use skills in case finding and preventive intervention. The nurses' understanding of the physical/psychological interplay in patients' symptoms and dynamics provides her with knowledge about preventive psychiatry and skills in helping patients through a *normative* crisis. Teenaged mothers, who experience the normative crisis of adolescence compounded with the normative crises of pregnancy and parenting, are candidates for the preventive intervention of a community mental health nurse. Limitations on financial resources demand that their care is not a priority unless they initiate a referral to a mental health center or experience some symptoms of stress and are referred by others.

Recommendations for the future development of the agency need to address this situation. Perhaps independent grant monies from government or private agencies can be secured to promote these programs. In addition, a means of evaluating the effectiveness of both the preventive and direct service programs must be further developed so that there is a basis for recruiting ongoing funding.

In summary, the potential for the utilization of the community mental health nurse is unlimited in today's health care situation. Reality issues of program politics, funding, community needs, and the growing understanding about a community's mental health needs and how to meet them can influence the direction which the nurses' roles may take. While there are opportunities to use the many skills the nurse has available, there are also many impediments to the development of programs. What matters most is that the nurse continue to call upon her nursing knowledge of problem solving to assess the needs of herself as a professional, her agency, and her community in order to develop a role of maximum satisfaction and effectiveness.

CHAPTER **52**

CONTINUING CARE CLINICAL ROLE STUDY

PAULA GANNON, B.S., R.N.

For many months when I first began as a continuing care nurse, the physicians, nurses, and social workers with whom I worked frequently commented that they would never want my job. Most of these people saw me as someone whose primary role was facilitating transfers of patients to nursing homes and chronic care hospitals. Because the idea of needing care in these facilities created so many negative images, it seems that arranging for that care is considered an unpleasant task at best. Over the past year, as my colleagues and I have approached a better understanding of the scope of my role, the comments have taken an entirely different direction. Recently, a staff nurse requested a meeting with me to discuss her career goals and how she might prepare for a community health or continuing care nursing role.

Since we are in the early stages of constructing an educational framework for continuing care, there is only slight evidence of specific preparation in my educational and clinical background. After graduating from a baccalaureate program, I worked as a staff nurse in a large innercity general hospital, as an instructor of fundamentals and medical-surgical nursing in a diploma school of nursing, and as a public health nurse in two large suburban communities. I have also taken postgraduate courses in counseling and interviewing, educational philosophy and methods, and curriculum development. These combined experiences have helped me identify skills and areas of special interest.

My position as a continuing care nurse allows me a type of synthesis of these personal and professional interests. I have always enjoyed the acute care setting because of the exciting opportunities to learn new and innovative medical and nursing management. I find the atmosphere dynamic and fascinating. As a staff nurse years ago, I can recall the frustration of having little influence over the patients' care beyond the crisis of hospitalization. My position affords me an appealing educational atmosphere and a chance to direct and coordinate care after discharge.

Community health nursing experience sparked my interest in liaison work, interagency communications, and a coordinated approach to hospital discharge planning. On occasion when a plan of care broke down, it was due, in part, to the failure of the referring hospital to see health care as a continuum or to assume responsibility to initiate and followup on the discharge plan. When the patient's needs extended beyond the agency's resources, a hospital based person to assist in examining and revising the plan would have been invaluable.

The relationship between my experience in nursing education and continuing care nursing might seem remote, but education is one of our most important tasks. The nature of the role and the setting provide countless opportunities for formal and informal teaching. The continuing care nurse who shares my responsibilities comically refers to our curbside consults—those many instances when we are stopped in the hospital halls, cafeteria, or parking garage to counsel, explain, or simply reassure staff, patients, or family members. I have respect for the learning process, particularly the influence of attitude and social thought on behavior outcome. My work allows me to continuously test and develop skill in interpersonal relationships and insight into behavior.

CLINICAL PRACTICE SETTING

Tufts New England Medical Center is an incorporation of Tufts University Schools of Medicine and Dental Medicine and a 450 bed hospital which includes the Boston Floating Hospital for Infants and Children. Located near Boston's Chinatown and South End, it serves as a teaching facility for many students of allied health professions. The inpatient unit is unique for its 25 bed Rehabilitation Institute, 10 bed psychiatric unit, and Clinical Study Unit funded by the National Institute of Health. Of the 14,000 patients admitted annually, approximately 26 percent are pediatric admissions and 21 percent are Medicare admissions. About 50 percent of our patient population is 50 years old and over with slightly more women than men. Almost one third are residents of Boston, and many of these live in the South Boston and Dorchester areas which have a significant Irish ethnic composition. In terms of occupational distribution, many of our patients are women at home and unemployed or retired persons.

The Continuing Care Program was developed in accordance with the 1971 Massachusetts Department of Public Health Regulations. Today, the objectives of the program are essentially the same: to improve the quality of care by providing a comprehensive plan which extends beyond hospitalization, and to reduce the patient's length of stay and number of readmissions. In August of 1977, administrative responsibility was transferred from the Department of Nursing to the Department of Social Service.

At present our continuing care team is comprised of an acting coordinator who is a social worker, two continuing care nurses, an administrative aide, and a part time office worker/secretary. In addition, a nurse from the Boston VNA Coordinated Home Care Program works with us and in the hospital two days a week, and a nurse liaison from the Laboure Health Center in South Boston visits two afternoons a week. Although salaried by their agencies, these two nurses are considered a vital part of our team.

It is important to note that the people with whom I work on the team are competent and deeply dedicated individuals. I attribute a considerable amount of my personal job satisfaction to the respect, trust, and affection I feel for them as people devoted to the right of patients to quality care.

There are unique features to being a nursing member of a social service department. The most obvious is the psychosocial orientation of its members. Social workers at the Medical Center are primarily involved in psychosocial diagnosis and treatment of patients and their families. We have many patients in common and work closely with the social workers. Their availability and valuable input has enhanced the comprehensiveness of our continuing care plans.

There is a feeling among people in nursing that the placement of a continuing care program within a department of social service is somehow an abdication of responsibility on the part of nursing administration. Although the Department of Nursing at the Medical Center is large and sophisticated, I do not feel less effective as a member of Social Service. Perhaps I am forced to wear two hats, but I find it comfortable. I have a professional responsibility to the Department of Nursing, and I have the unusual freedom to take advantage of educational programs in both departments. In some ways our conspicuousness as nurses in Social Service allows a license which would not be possible otherwise. I have realized that on a few occasions health team members have seemed to assign me certain powers because of my unusual position. Although it has seldom been a real power, it has nevertheless been useful in formulating and implementing some plans of care.

NURSING INTERVENTION

Generally, the plan for continuing care is implemented by making referral to home care agencies, rehabilitation facilities, and extended care facilities. The Continuing Care Team receives consults from a variety of sources. We use weekly patient care or discharge planning conferences on the hospital units as one method of early screening. These are attended by the continuing care nurse, the primary nurses, and occasionally social workers and physicians. We also accept incidental and formal consultation requests from any member of the health team, other agencies, patients, and family members. As many as a dozen people within and outside of hospital might be contacted in gathering information and formulating the plan.

To best depict the complexities of continuing care nursing, I would like to share an experience with one of my patients that is representative of the variety of nursing interventions employed in continuing care.

I met Ms. C for the first time on the morning of her discharge from the hospital. Her primary nurse had contacted me and explained that she had some concerns about the patient's ability to manage alone at home. Ms. C is a 75-year-old single woman who had been admitted several days before with anemia, cachexia, and severe dehydration. She lived alone in a second floor apartment in a low income area of Boston. She was dressed and anxious to go home when I arrived at her room. I recognized her niece, Mrs. M, as the daughter of a patient I had followed months earlier. Ms. C's impending discharge limited me to a rather cursory assessment.

She was alert, oriented, and independent in activities of daily living. She was obviously poorly nourished and her niece expressed concern about her eating habits and meal preparation. The patient explained that, although her landlady bought her groceries, she seldom felt like cooking and often ate crackers with tea. Mrs. M had tried but could not send her aunt meals every day. Even though she seemed to be independent, Ms. C struck me as a lonely lady whose socialization was limited to brief visits by her niece. She also had a severe hearing loss which made communication difficult, and she complained of poor vision.

We faced the following problems: providing good nutrition, her vision and its effect on her health and safety, her hearing loss and accompanying social isolation, and financial assistance as her fixed income and Medicare would not cover some services. She had no interest in getting meals at a local seniors' center, but her niece and I persuaded her to accept a low cost home meal program. Mrs. M and the primary nurse arranged for eye and hearing evaluations at the clinics, and I collaborated with the primary nurse in completing a VNA referral for home assessment. The patient's niece agreed to continue to visit Ms. C regularly, to assist her in submitting a Medicaid application, and to contact me in the event of any problems. When Ms. C was discharged, I was left with the uneasy feeling that what we had accomplished was patchwork, and that I would see her again, perhaps in crisis.

During the following two weeks I called Mrs. M and the visiting nurse. Both reported that Ms. C was managing marginally, and that she had refused homemaker-home health aide assistance. Her visit to the eye clinic precipitated an emergency admission for acute glaucoma. Her physician planned surgery if laser treatments proved unsuccessful. During this admission I visited the patient regularly, although I had no formal request for consultation. She seemed to recognize me as a friendly face, and I hoped that in establishing a better relationship I might help her to accept more assistance at home. Communication was extremely difficult, but in time I learned more about her and began to appreciate her need to be able to manage alone. She confided that she had considered going to live in a nursing home but did not feel she was disabled enough.

The crisis occurred when it became evident that surgery was necessary to prevent blindness. Ms. C refused. Her physician contacted me and the primary nurse to discuss approaches which might make surgery more acceptable to the patient. In our initial discussion, I learned that Ms. C had expressed some unusual, if not superstitious, perceptions of anesthesia and surgery. When our efforts at some basic teaching failed, the physician requested a psychiatric evaluation to rule out dementia and determine her competence to make an informed decision. The psychiatrist found Ms. C entirely competent but also reported what I had feared all along—that perhaps only by allowing herself to become blind could Ms. C justify and accept nursing home care or extended home services. In the patient's words, she would then "need to be taken care of" and would "not be lonely anymore." She was discharged the following day and her previous home services were resumed.

Within two weeks Ms. C returned to the hospital for eye surgery. She has never told me how or why she reversed her previous decision. A few days after surgery she greeted me with a request to find her a nursing home. With a tremendous sense of relief, I met with the patient and her niece to identify preferences and priorities. The most important was that she remain in Boston near her niece.

We began the task of locating a vacancy in an appropriate nursing facility. A basic part of my role is to determine the level or type of care required and to match that with the ability of the facility to provide for those needs. With one eye patched and very poor vision in the other, Ms. C needed more assistance in activities of daily living. She also needed help with the administration of eye drops and continued observation and management of her nutrition. I enlisted the help of Mrs. M in visiting those facilities which might have a vacancy.

At the present time, much of the burden of locating vacancies falls upon the administrative aide in our office. Using a written nursing assessment and care plan, we contacted more than two dozen facilities. At the end of two weeks, we found a vacancy in a nursing home which seemed to suit the patient's and family's needs perfectly. We arranged for her transfer the following day.

While we were searching for an appropriate nursing facility, the patient and Continuing Care Office were notified by the hospital Utilization Review Committee that it was necessary for the Committee to terminate her Medicare benefits for the current hospitalization. P.S.R.O. monitors, in routinely reviewing the charts of patients with Medicare and Medicaid had determined that Ms. C no longer needed an acute care setting. The patient was spared the cost of additional hospital days for two reasons: first, the continuing care notes in the patient's chart reflected an ongoing need and search for an extended care facility, and secondly our office had notified the Committee and financial office that a Medicaid application was pending. Under these circumstances and a regulation which governs administratively necessary days, the hospital continues to receive reimbursement for additional hospital days.

We evaluate our nursing interventions by periodic phone contact with the patient, home care agency, or extended care facility. Weekly meetings with our coordinator are designed to discuss problems and develop new interventions. In addition, we use part of our daily staff meeting to review patient care plans and share ideas. We find our contact with the visiting nurse liasons extremely valuable in examining the effectiveness of the plans for patients discharged home.

In reviewing my involvement with Ms. C, I feel several changes might have improved the plan of care. Seeing Ms. C early during her first admission might have reduced the rather frantic character of our initial assessment and plan. It is conceivable that arranging an eye examination during the hospitalization might have altered the course of events.

As a result of her first admission, Ms. C had already been identified as a patient at risk. A primary team conference early in the course of her second admission might have helped to better coordinate the interventions of the primary team.

It is also unfortunate that we did not request the assistance of a social worker to explore Ms. C's attitudes regarding health, hospitalization, and nursing home care. A supportive therapeutic relationship might have eliminated some of the stress associated with her decision about surgery.

IMPACT AND RECOMMENDATIONS

We are in the process of developing better statistical data and we do not, as yet, have a tool which effectively measures the objectives and benefits of the Continuing Care Program. Statistics shared at the monthly Utilization Review Committee meetings indicate that patients at the Medical Center have an average or slightly less than average length of hospital stay in comparison with other area hospitals. We rely heavily on the feedback we receive in followup from patients, family members, agencies, and facilities. The response of the hospital staff is generally positive.

In examining our program the staff has identified problem areas and made recommendations for new projects. Our most immediate problem is one of staffing. At the present time the responsibility to provide for the continuing care needs of approximately

100 patients per month falls upon two nurses and an administrative aide. As a result we are not able to assure quality of service to many patients. The Social Service Department and its leadership have created an atmosphere that is entirely supportive and cooperative in this developmental phase of our program. In the very near future, the department will hire a Continuing Care Nurse Coordinator who, based on our needs and recommendation, will have some responsibility for direct patient assessment and planning in addition to the responsibility as coordinator.

Working in an acute hospital can be an insular experience. The emphasis is unmistakably that of diagnosing and treating the patient's immediate problems. We see ourselves as having an important role in ongoing staff education. Our hospital staff needs and wants to know more about continuing care, external resources, and the medical, nursing, social, and economic factors involved in providing care after hospitalization. We are already involved in giving small conferences to staff nurses on the patient floors, but we would like to expand them to include other members of the primary team. We are now working with the Department of Nursing to design a tool and method of assisting new primary nurses in making referrals to visiting nurse agencies. In the future we also hope to become more actively involved in the orientation program for nurses new to the Medical Center.

We need to increase our knowledge of community resources and develop a method of more regularly contacting, visiting, and evaluating agencies and facilities. By working with the area Continuing Care Association, we might organize, compile, and share this information.

The problems of bed availability in extended care facilities and the availability of homemaker-home health aides raises important issues for the patient, the hospital, and the health care system. Some of our patients have had to remain in the hospital for weeks awaiting a nursing home vacancy or, less frequently, for home health aide assistance. Recognizing the stressful circumstances in deciding to go to a nursing home or in waiting for care to be arranged, we have discussed the creation of a group composed of these patients and possibly their family members. The purpose of the group, led by a social worker, would be to explore the difficulties and to assist the members in finding mechanisms to reduce or cope with the stress.

We are deeply concerned about the painful issue of choice for patients in need of nursing home care or chronic care. Under present P.S.R.O. policy, once we locate a vacancy in an appropriate facility, arrangements should be made to transfer the patient to that facility. If the patient refuses to be transferred for reasons such as distance from the family, location of the facility, or an unfavorable impression at the family's visit to the facility, the patient risks absorbing the cost of additional days in the hospital while searching for an alternative. As health care professionals and consumers, we need to examine the health care system and work toward changes in the meaning of quality assurance that include respect for the patient's right to choose.

SUMMARY

I cannot deny that there is a high degree of difficulty in the nature of my position. Despite the magnitude of the work and its pressures, I find it exciting and challenging. Some of my deepest satisfactions arise out of that part of my role as patient advocate. I treasure many special experiences with patients whose strength, wisdom, and love have contributed to my professional and personal growth.

INDEX

ACCIDENTS
  age distribution of, 632
  community health concerns and, 635-636
  health site and, 633
  impact and safety measures for, 634-635
  recreational, 633
  safety and, 631-636
  statistics and scope of problem and, 631-
    634
  vehicular, 632-633
  work place and, 632
Accountability
  community mental health nursing and, 335
  developmental disabilities and, 286-287
Accreditation in home health care, 213
Adolescent
  family with, 527-528
  mental health and, 346
  nutrition of, 580-583
    boys and, 582
    girls and, 582
    interfering factors in, 581-582
    intervention in, 582-583
    psychosocial needs and, 580
  pregnant, 585

Adult
  death perceptions of, 613
  young unmarried, 522-525
Advocates
  developmental disabilities and, 274-275
  gerontology and, 316
Aging. See also Elderly; Gerontology.
  blood chemistry and, 307
  blood levels and, 308
  blood volume and, 307
  bone marrow and, 306
  cardiovascular system in, 303
  emphysema in, 304
  endocrine system in, 306
  functional-structural changes in, 297-301
  gastrointestinal tract in, 304-305
  hemopoietic system and, 306-307
  lymphoid system and, 307
  musculoskeletal system in, 299-300
  nervous system and, 300-301
  nutrition and metabolism in, 307-308
  nutritional assessment in, 309-311
  organ-body weight ratio in, 308
  personality changes and, 301
  reproductive organs and, 306

Aging—*Continued*
  respiratory system in, 303-304
  skin and subcutaneous tissues in, 298-299
  special senses in, 301-303
    hearing, 302
    smell and taste, 302
    speech, 302
    tactile, 303
    vision, 301-302
  temperature maintenance in, 308, 312
  urinary tract and, 305
Air pollution, 637-646
  atmosphere and, 639-641
  chronic obstructive lung disease and, 481
  control of, 644-645
  effects of, 642-644
  historical perspective on, 638-639
  prognosis in, 645-646
  sources of, 641-642
  standards, 644-645
  types of, 643
Alcohol
  abuse, 537-554. *See also* Substance abuse.
  pregnancy and, 585
Alternative housing, 348
Ambulatory care
  defining role in, 114
  educational preparation for, 117-118
  emerging trends in, 118-119
  historical development of, 115-117
  legal considerations in, 120
  legislative impact on, 120-121
  nursing role in, 113-122
  scope of service in, 114-115
Ambulatory clinical role study, 695-699
  congenital heart disease and, 695-699
    congestive failure and, 697
    digitalis preparation in, 697
    feeding and weight gain in, 696-697
    hospitalization in, 698-699
    physical activities in, 698
American Association of Industrial Nurses, 128
Amphetamines, 539
Anemia in infants, 574
Angiopathy, 438
Ankylosing spondylitis, 512
Area Health Education Centers
  assessment of educational needs in, 767-768
  baccalaureate education for RNs and, 777-778
  clinical education of nursing students in, 773-775
  clinical practice before, 764-766
  clinical practice in, 781
  clinical preceptorship in, 775-776
  clinical preceptorship objectives and, 793-794

  continuing education in, 768-770
  educational needs survey and, 788-790
  evaluation of, 782-785
  history of, 762-764
  impact and recommendations for, 786
  nurse as community educator in, 761-794
  nurse practitioner education in, 770-773
  nursing interventions and clinical practice now, 766-784
  professional support system and, 781-782
  role innovation in, 785
  sample work statements-nursing education and, 791-792
  technical assistance and consultation in, 778-781
Architectural barriers, 605-606
Arthritis, 497-517
  ankylosing spondylitis, 512
  dermatomyositis and polymyositis, 511-512
  gout, 513-515
  juvenile rheumatoid, 509-511
  osteoarthritis, 515-516
  rheumatoid. *See* Rheumatoid arthritis.
Associate degree programs, 223
Asthma, 475-476
Atmosphere, 639-641
At-risk indices, 9-19
Audits, 104, 185-197

Barbiturates, 539
Behavior modification, 270
  cardiac and circulatory disease and, 387
Biostatistics, 106
Birth rate, 13-14
Black bag, 105
Blood chemistry and aging, 307
Blood levels and aging, 308
Blood volume and aging, 307
Bone marrow and aging, 306
Boston Industrial Nurses Club, 127
Boston Instructive District Visiting Nurse Association, 202
Bottle feeding, 570-571
Boundaries, community, 6-7
Breast feeding, 570-571
Breathing
  coordinated, 490-491
  intermittent positive pressure, 491
Brompton's cocktail, 415
Bronchiectasis, 476
Bronchitis, 483-487
Budgeting, food, 590

Cancer, 393-421
  community attitude toward, 403-404
  community health nursing and, 411-419

Cancer—*Continued*
  community services in, 419
  family involvement in, 416–419
    nutrition and, 416
    terminal care and, 417–419
    waste elimination and, 417
  individual in, 411–416
    nutrition of, 412–413
    pain control for, 414–416
    terminal care of, 414–416
    waste elimination by, 413–414
  definition of, 393
  diagnosis of, 405–406
  education about, 419–420
  etiology of, 394–396
    carcinogens in, 394
    genetic factors in, 394
    hormonal factors in, 394
    immunologic factors in, 395
    psychologic factors in, 395–396
  family and, 401–403
    adaptation of, 401–402
    financial burdens on, 403
    grief and, 403
    roles and relationships in, 402–403
  impact of disease in, 397–403
  individual with, 399–401
    adaptation of, 399
    coping mechanisms of, 401
    fear of death and, 401
    fear of pain and, 401
    self-concept and body image of, 400–401
  prevention of, 404–405
  prognosis in, 410–411
  research and, 420
  scope of, 397
  statistics in, 396–397
    age and, 396
    cultural background and, 397
    economics and, 397
    ethnic background and, 396
    politics and, 397
    sex and, 396
  treatment of, 406–410
    chemotherapy in, 407–409
    immunotherapy in, 409
    quackery in, 409–410
    radiation therapy in, 406–407
    surgery in, 406
Carcinogens, 394
Cardiac and circulatory diseases, 371–392. *See also* Cardiovascular disease.
  adaptation to illness in, 378–382
    attitudes and behavior in, 379–382
      coronary prone personality and, 379–381
      preadmission, 381–382
    individual, 382

normative adult life cycle and, 379
  family life cycle and, 379
  marital life cycle and, 379
normative developmental life cycles and, 378
  systems model and, 378
adaptation of spouse and family to, 382–384
community implications of, 383
current treatment modalities in, 377–378
impact on individual and family of, 382
primary prevention of, 384–386
  community health appraisal in, 384–385
  family health record in, 386
  risk modification in, 385–386
role of community health nurse in, 384–389
secondary prevention of, 386–387
  behavior modification in, 387
  early diagnosis and treatment in, 386
  exercise and physical fitness in, 387
  limiting disability in, 386–387
  relaxation techniques in, 387
significant life changes and, 383–384
tertiary prevention of, 387–389
  cardiac rehabilitation in, 389
  client health appraisal in, 387–389
  community resources for, 389
Cardiac screening, 161
Cardiovascular disease. *See also* Cardiac and circulatory disease.
  clinical characteristics of, 375–377
  dimensions of, 371–377
  epidemiologic data in, 372–373
    coronary artery disease and, 372–373
    hypertension and, 372
    rheumatic heart disease and, 373
    statistics and, 372
    stroke and, 373
  etiologic factors in, 373–375
    cerebrovascular accident and, 375
    coronary artery disease and, 373–374
    hypertension, 374–375
    rheumatic heart disease, 375
Cardiovascular system and aging, 303
Carrier states, 455
Cataract, senile, 301–302
Cerebrovascular accident, 375
Certification
  community mental health and, 334–335
  developmental disabilities and, 285–286
  home health care and, 212–213
  school health nursing and, 149–151
Chemotherapy, 407–409
Child(ren)
  adolescent. *See* Adolescent.
  couple without, 525–526
  death perceptions of, 613
  developmentally disabled. *See* Developmental disabilities.

Child(ren)—*Continued*
  grown, 528-529
  nutrition of
    school age, 579-580
    toddler and preschooler, 579
    young, 526-527
Child abuse, 345, 561-563
  incidence of, 561
  parent in, 562
  treatment of, 562-563
  victimology and, 561-563
Child Labor Law, 125
Childbearing-childrearing center, 813-818
Children's Charter of 1930, 142
Chronic obstructive lung disease
  air pollution and, 481
  asthma as, 475-476
  bronchiectasis as, 476
  etiologic factors in, 479-483
    air pollution as, 481
    allergic responses as, 482
    genetic predisposition as, 482-483
    smoking as, 479-481
  nursing intervention in, 487-493
    breathing coordination and, 490-491
    medications and, 492-493
    physical rehabilitation and, 488-490
    secretion clearance and, 491-492
  pathophysiology of, 483-487
  prevalence and predisposition of 476-479
Circulatory diseases, cardiac and, 371-392
Client centered health care system model, 48
Client services, 101-106
  black bag in, 105
  community assessment and, 103-104
  community resource file and, 104
  health screenings and, 105
  nursing audits and, 104
  nursing peers and, 106
  nursing process in, 102-103
  record keeping and, 104
  referral and, 105
  telephone and, 104-105
Collegiate nursing programs, 221-222
Community, 5-23
  assessment of, 103-104
  boundaries of, 6-7
  culture of, 7
  definition of, 5-8
  fertility differentials and, 13-14
  health action of, 16-20
    community resources in, 19-20
    consumer participation in, 18
    environmental issues in, 19
    health planning in, 16-18
  health care in, 1-110
  migration and, 15-16

nursing role in, 20-21
occupational health nurse and, 137-139
population of, 8-13
resources of, 19-20
Community after-care programs, 347-348
Community health and major social issues, 567-620
Community health nurse, roles and functions of, 44-46
Community health nursing, 39-51. *See also* Public health nursing.
  a personal perspective, 751-760
  American Nurses' Association definition of, 40
  categories of, 45
  current issues in, 46-50
  health concept and, 26-27, 36
  health education and, 98-99
  history of, 70-72
  nursing theory and, 41-44
  one nurse's practice in, 741-750
    background in, 741-742
    concepts in, 746-748
    conceptual framework of, 748
    nursing interventions in, 745-746
    program evaluation in, 748-750
    seniors program and, 742-745
  roles in, 111-368
    ambulatory care, 113-122
    community mental health, 319-353
    continuing care, 355-368
    developmental disabilities, 257-293
    education, 219-238
    gerontology, 295-317
    home health care, 199-218
    midwifery, 239-256
    occupational health, 123-140
    public health, 175-197
    school health, 141-174
  views and definitions of, 40-41
Community mental health, 319-353
  accountability and, 335
  center for, 348-350
  clinical nurse specialist in, 330-333
  clinical role study, 861-875
    agency description in, 863-865
    clinical practice setting in, 865-866
    impact and recommendations in, 873-875
    nursing interventions in, 866-873
  financial aspects of, 336-339
  historical development of, 320-323
  legal considerations in, 333-335
    certification and, 334-335
    licensure and, 334
  legislation and, 350-351
  level I nurse in, 327-329
  level II nurse in, 329-330

Community mental health—*Continued*
nursing
development of, 323-325
levels in, 327-333
personal identity and clinical skills in, 326-327
role in, 325
President's Commission on Mental Health and, 350-351
primary prevention and, 340-341
mental health education for, 341
preventive programs for, 340-341
psychotherapy in, 331-332
scope of services for, 339-350
secondary prevention and, 342-347
adolescence and, 346
child abuse and, 345
crisis intervention in, 342-343
developmental crisis and, 342
diagnostic evaluation and, 343
elderly and, 347
identification and case finding in, 342
liaison and referral and, 343-344
mental health consultation and, 344-345
middlescence and, 346-347
situational crisis and, 342
sudden infant death syndrome and, 345-346
suicide and, 346
treatment and, 343
victim crisis and, 342
tertiary prevention in, 347-348
alternative housing and, 348
community after-care programs and, 347-348
Community resource file, 104
Composting, 677-678
Congenital heart disease. *See* Ambulatory clinical role study.
Consumer movement
health care legislation and, 89
health planning and, 18
Continuing care
case study in, 362-365
clinical role study, 877-882
discharge planning and, 360
educational preparation in, 359
historical development of, 355-357
Massachusetts rule and regulations concerning, 358-359
Medicare in, 356-357
nursing role in, 355-368
objectives of, 360
scope of service in, 359-362
specific skills in, 360-362
Coronary artery disease, 372-373
cigarette smoking and, 374
diabetes and, 374

lipid abnormalities and, 374
stress and, 374
Coronary prone personality, 379-381
Counseling
developmental disabilities and, 273-274
school health, 162-164
Crippled children's clinics, 284
Culture, community, 7
Curing and caring cults, 76-79

DATA collection, 152-156
Death
adult perceptions of, 613
children's perceptions of, 613
dying and, 611-620
life cycle and, 613-616
nursing interventions in, 617-619
euthanasia and, 616
funeral services and, 615-616
geriatric persons and, 614
Kübler-Ross' theories on, 612
legal criteria of, 616
phases of, 612
terminal illness and, 614-615
types of, 611
Delivery system, health care, 53-67
Demography, 10
birth rate and, 13-14
data collection and, 10
gerontology and, 296
migration and, 15-16
mortality rate and, 11-13
Dental caries, 574, 578
Dentists, 61
Denver Developmental Screening Test, 266
Dermatomyositis, 511-512
Developmental disabilities. *See also* Disabilities.
advocating and, 274-275
assessment in, 262-267
background history and, 262-263
Denver Developmental Screening Test in, 266
Developmental Profile in, 266
Developmental Screening Inventory in, 266
Fels Behavior Rating Scales in, 264
Home Inventory for Infants in, 263-264
independence in self-help skills and, 266-267
parenting process and, 263-265
physical, 265-266
physical environment in, 267
case history of, 275-280
advocating in, 280
assessment in, 276-277
coordinating in, 279
counseling in, 280

Developmental disabilities—*Continued*
   supporting in, 279
   teaching in, 277–279
  coordination of services and, 272–273
  counseling and, 273–274
  crippled children's clinics for, 284
  diagnostic and evaluation clinics for, 284
  educational preparation and clinical experience in, 259–262
  evaluating and revising nursing interventions in, 275–285
  health department clinics for, 284–285
  history of nursing care in, 258–259
  independent nursing practice in, 825–835
  infant and preschool programs for, 282
  institutional care for, 283–284
  legal considerations and, 285–287
   accountability in, 286–287
   certification in, 285–286
   financial structure/funding and, 287
   licensure in, 285
  legislation and, 288–290
  master's and post-master's programs in, 261–262
  national associations and foundations for, 285
  nursing role in, 257–293
  planning and implementing nursing interventions for, 267–275
  school age programs for, 282–283
  service providers in, 280–282
   support personnel as, 281–282
   team members as, 280–281
  supportive nursing and, 271–272
  teaching and, 267–271
   basic health skills in, 270–271
   behavior modification in, 270
   child management in, 269–270
   facilitating development in, 268–269
   Portage Guide to Early Education in, 268
   self-help skills in, 270
  university affiliated centers for, 284
  where services are provided for, 282–285
  types of service in, 262
  undergraduate specialization in, 260–261
Developmental Profile, 266
Developmental Screening Inventory, 266
Diabetes insipidus, 424
Diabetes mellitus, 423–449
  classification of, 423, 426–427
  community impact of, 431
  coronary artery disease and, 374
  education and, 443–448
   complications and, 446–447
   meal planning and, 447–448
   record keeping in, 447
   self-injection in, 445

   teaching outline in, 444–445
   urine testing in, 446
  etiology of, 426
  family impact of, 430–431
  history of, 424
  individual impact of, 430
  insulin in, 424–425
  nursing concerns in, 439–441
   community and, 440–441
   family and, 439–440
   individual and, 439
  prevention-treatment approaches to, 431–435
   community in, 435
   family in, 434–435
   individual in, 431–434
  prognosis of, 435–439
  research on, 441–443
  scope of problem of, 429–430
  statistics in, 427–429
  treatment of, 436–439
   angiopathy in, 438
   chronic complications in, 438–439
   complications in, 437
   diabetic ketoacidosis and, 436
   hyperglycemia in, 436
   hypoglycemia in, 436
   illness and, 437–438
   neuropathy in, 438
   pregnancy and, 438
   surgery and, 437
Diets
  fad reducing, 596–599
  vegetarian, 595–596
  Zen-macrobiotic, 596
Disabilities, 603–610
  architectural barriers and, 605–606
  attitude barriers and, 606
  crisis situation and, 604–605
  definition of, 603
  developmental. *See* Developmental disabilities.
  educational barriers and, 606
  legislation and, 607
  nursing intervention in, 607–609
  occupational barriers and, 606–607
  personal barriers and, 607
Discharge planning, 360
Disease control, 107–108
  education and, 108
  immunization programs and, 107–108
  treatment plans in, 108
  vector control in, 107
Drug abuse, 537–554. *See also* Substance abuse.
Drugs and pregnancy, 586
Dying. *See* Death.

ECONOMIC concerns and population issues, 629
Education
    ambulatory care and, 117-118
    cancer and, 419-420
    community health nursing, 224-225
    continuing care and, 359
    developmental disabilities and, 259-262
    diabetes mellitus and, 443-448
    disabilities and, 608-609
    disabled persons and, 606
    disease control and, 108
    gerontology nursing and, 315-316
    health. See Health education.
    historical development of, 220-224
        associate degree programs and, 223
        Civil War and, 220
        collegiate programs in, 221-222
        community health nursing and, 222-223
        Goldmark Report in, 221
        schools of nursing and, 221
    home health nursing and, 204-206
    infectious diseases and, 471-472
    legislation and, 225-226, 237-238
    mental health, 341
    midwifery and, 242-243, 248-250
    noise pollution and, 657
    nursing organizations and, 235-236
    nursing role in, 219-238
    people and events in, 228-238
    population issues and, 628-629
    programs for, 231-233
    public health nurse generalist, 224
    public health nurse specialist, 224
    public health nursing and, 179
    rheumatoid arthritis and, 500-501, 509
    school health nursing and, 147-149, 164-
        169
    special reports and studies in, 233-235
Elderly. See also Aging; Gerontology.
    crisis intervention for, 347
    death perceptions of, 614
    family with, 529-530
    nursing homes for, 347
    outpatient group psychotherapy for, 347
Emotional disorders, 521-536
Emphysema
    aging and, 304
    pathophysiology of, 483-487
Endocrine system and aging, 306
Environmental
    health problems and, 35
    infectious diseases and, 453-454
Environmental issues
    health planning and, 19
    in community health, 621-691
Epidemiology, 11, 107. See also Infectious
        diseases

Ethnic food practices, 590
Euthanasia, 616
Exercise
    physical fitness and, 387
    rheumatoid arthritis and, 501-502

FAMILY
    cancer and, 401-403, 416-419
    dysfunctional, 530
    emotional disorders and, 521-536
    substance abuse and, 543
        treatment for, 550-551
Family health record, 386
Family life cycle, 522-530
    community health nursing practice and, 530-
        535
        help-seeking populations and, 531-534
        intervention guidelines in, 533-535
        nonhelp-seeking population and, 534-535
    couple without children and, 525-526
    family process, situational events and, 530
    family with adolescents and, 527-528
    family with elderly and, 529-530
    family with grown children and, 528-529
    family with young children and, 526-527
    young unmarried adult and, 522-525
Family therapy, 331
Farsightedness, 301
Feeding, infant, 570-578. See also Infant,
        feeding of.
Fels Behavior Rating Scales, 264
Fertility
    community and, 13-14
    population impact of, 625-627
    rates, 10-13
Fetal alcohol syndrome, 585
Financial structure/funding, 287
Financing of health care, 83-92
Folk politicians, 75-76
Food
    budgeting for, 590
    ethnic practices and, 590
    faddism and, 591-595
    labeling of, 591
    processing of, 591
Frontier Nursing Service, 246
Functions and Qualifications of School Nurses,
        147
Funeral services, 615-616

GASTROINTESTINAL tract, 304-305
Geneogram, 531
Genetic factors in cancer, 394
Genetic predisposition for chronic lung disease,
        482-483

Gerontology. *See also* Elderly; Aging.
  clinical role study, 837–860
    administrative forms in, 850–860
    clinical practice setting in, 842–843
    impact and recommendations in, 848–849
    nursing intervention in, 844–848
    program in, 838–841
    stimulus manipulation in, 847–848
  demographic factors in, 296
  functional-structural changes and, 297–301
  health maintenance-disability prevention in, 312–315
  health services system for, 315
  needs and services in, 296–297
  nurses as advocates for, 316
  nursing preparation for, 315–316
  nursing role in, 295–317
Glaucoma, 302
Goldmark Report, 221
Gout, 513–515
Greenhouse effect, 640
Grief
  cancer and, 403
  dying and death, 611–620
Group psycotherapy, 331
Guidelines for School Nursing, 143

HALFWAY houses, 348
Hallucinogens, 539
Hashish, 538
Health
  concept of, community health nurse and, 26–27, 36
  health behavior and, 31–36
  illness and, 25–38
  population issues and, 629
Health Belief Model, 32
Health care
  client centered model of, 48
  delivery system of, 53–67
  home. *See* Home health care.
  in community, 1–110
  legislation and financing of, 83–92
  organization of, 53–59
    federal, 58–59
    local, 54–57
    state, 57–58
  people in, 76–77
  politics of, 77
  providers of, 59–63
    dentists, 61
    doctors, 60–61
    nurses, 60
    nutritionists, 61
    pharmacists, 62
    physical or occupational therapists, 62
    podiatrists, 61

    psychologists, 61
    sanitarians and, 62
    veterinarians, 61
  resources of, 65–66
  setting of, 63–65
    community, 64
    drug treatment programs, 64
    Home Health Agency, 64
    hospices, 65
    hospitals, 63
    nursing homes, 65
Health education
  community health nursing and, 93–100
  definition of, 93–94
  evaluation of, 97–98
  impact of, 95–98
  learner and, 95–96
  learning needs in, 96
  learning objectives in, 96–97
  media in, 97
  scope of, 94–95
Health and Human Services, Department of, 58–59
Health-illness continuum, 29–31
Health Information for International Travel, 468
Health maintenance-disability prevention, 312–315
Health planning
  community, 16–18
  steps in, 17
Health Revenue Sharing and Health Services Act of 1975, 216
Health screenings, 105
Health Services Bill, 89–90
Health services system, 315
Health status, 151–152
Hearing in aging, 302
Hearing loss, 651–652
Hearing screening, 159–160
Hemopoietic system, 306–307
Home Health Agency, 64
  accreditation of, 213
  certification in, 212–213
  licensure, 211
Home health care
  agencies for, 64, 207–209
    accreditation of, 213
    certification of, 212–213
    combination, 208–209
    licensure of, 211
    official, 208
    proprietary, 209
    voluntary, 208
    Health Revenue Sharing and Health Services Act of 1975, 216
  historical development of, 200–204
    Social Security Act, 203
  legal and quality control in, 211–213

Home health care—*Continued*
  legislation and, 213-217
  Medicaid, 215
  Medicare, 214-215
  Medicare-Medicaid Anti-Fraud and Abuse
      Amendments, 216-217
  nursing role in, 199-218
  preparation for practice in, 204-206
  Rural Health Clinics Bill, 216
  scope of, 206-211
  team members in, 209-211
  Title III Grants For State and Community
      Programs on Aging, 216
  Title XX, 215
  types of, 199-200
  types of services provided, 207
  where services are provided, 206-207
Home Inventory for Infants, 263-264
Homemaker-home health aide, 209-210
Homocide, 565-566
Hope, death and, 612
Hospices, 65
Hospitals, 63
Hormonal factors in cancer, 394
Hyperglycemia, 436
Hypertension, 372, 374-375
Hypoglycemia, 436

ILLNESS, health and, 25-38
Immunity, 452
  active, 463
  cancer and, 395
  passive, 463-465
Immunization, 456
Immunization programs, 107-108
Immunotherapy, cancer and, 409
Independent nursing practice in developmental
      disabilities, 825-835
Industry
  health programs and, 84
  treatment of substance abuse and, 551
Infant. *See also* Child(ren).
  feeding of, 570-578
    breast feeding vs. bottle feeding in, 570-
        571
    nursing intervention in, 578
    solid foods and, 571, 574
    vitamin supplementation and, 571
  nutrition intervention for, 578
  nutritional problems of, 574-578
    dental caries and, 574, 578
    iron-deficiency anemia and, 574
    obesity and, 574
  preschool programs for developmentally dis-
      abled, 282
Infectious diseases, 451-473
  agent and, 452-453
  carrier states in, 455

community impact of, 459-461
definitions in, 451
education about, 471-472
environment and, 453-454
family impact of, 458-459
host in, 452
immunity in, 452
immunization and, 456
incidence and prevalence of, 460
individual impact of, 457-458
interaction in, 454-455
mutant strains in, 456
prevention and treatment of, 461-468
    community in, 466-468
    family in, 465-466
    individual in, 462-465
    primary prevention and, 462-463
    secondary prevention and, 465
    tertiary prevention in, 465
prognosis in, 469-470
research on, 470-471
scope of problem in, 455-457
surveillance for, 460
Institutional care, 283-284
Insulin, 424-425
Insurance benefits, 86
Ionizing radiation
  acute radiation syndrome and, 687-688
  community health and, 681-691
  dose and effect relationship of, 686-687
  genetically significant, 684
  long term effects of, 685-686
  nuclear power plants and, 688-689
  nursing implications and, 689-691
  particles and rays in, 681-682
  radiobiologic considerations in, 684-685
  roentgen and rem in, 682
  sources of, 682-684
    artificial or manmade, 683-684
    natural background, 682-683

JUVENILE rheumatoid arthritis, 509-511
  etiology in, 510-511
  pauciarticular, 509-510
  polyarticular, 510
  prognosis in, 510
  systemic, 509

KETOACIDOSIS, 436
Kübler-Ross, Elisabeth, 612

LACTATION, 586-587
Legal considerations
  ambulatory care and, 120-121
  community mental health and, 333-335
  developmental disabilities and, 285
  midwifery and, 251-252

Legislation
  community mental health and, 350
  developmental disabilities and, 288-290
  disabled persons and, 607
  education and, 225-226, 237-238
  midwifery and, 252-253
  of health care, 83-92
    bureaucratic factors in, 87
    case analysis of, 85
    consumer movement and, 89
    Health Services Bill and, 89-90
    insurance benefits and, 86
    jurisdictional framework for, 85
    other national issues and, 89-91
    political factors and, 87
    provider community and, 87-89
    topical perspective on, 85
Licensure
  community mental health nursing and, 334
  developmental disabilities and, 285
  home health care and, 211
Life cycle, 613-616
Life expectancy, 627-628
Lipid abnormalities, 374
Local health organizations, 54-57
Lung disease. *See* Chronic obstructive lung disease.
Lymphoid system, 307

MACRODEMOGRAPHY, 10
Marijuana, 538
Maternity Center Association, 246
Meal planning in diabetes mellitus, 447-448
Media and health education, 97
Medicaid, 215, 357
Medicare, 214-215, 356-357
Medicare-Medicaid Anti-Fraud and Abuse Amendments, 216-217
Menopause, 306
Mental health. *See* Community mental health.
Metabolism and aging, 307
Microdemography, 10
Middle years and nutrition, 587
Middlescence, 346-347
Midwifery. *See also* Nurse-midwife.
  childbearing-childrearing center and, 813-818
  definitions of, 239-240
  educational and clinical preparation for, 248-250
  historical development of, 240-247
    education and, 242-243
    Frontier Nursing Service and, 246
    male physicians and, 241
    Maternity Center Association and, 246
    nineteenth century, 245
    organizations in, 246-247
    twentieth century, 246

legal considerations in, 251-252
  legislation and, 252-253
  nursing model and, 818-821
  nursing role in, 239-256
  preparation for, 247-252
  scope of services in, 250-251
  personal experiences in, 811-824
Migration, 15-16
Morbidity care, 200
Morbidity and Mortality Weekly Report, 467
Morbidity rates, 10-13
Mortality rates, 10-13
Musculoskeletal system, 299-300

NARCOTICS, 539
National Institute for Occupational Safety and Health, 126
National Organization for Public Health Nursing, 203
Natural resources, 628
Nervous system and aging, 300-301
Neuropathy, 438
Nightingale, Florence, 201-202
Noise induced permanent threshold shift, 651-652
Noise pollution, 647-658
  annoyance and, 653-654
  characteristics of, 648-649
  control of, 654-655
  descriptors for, 647-648
  education and, 657
  hearing loss and, 651-652
  individual exposure to, 649-651
  noise induced permanent threshold shift, 651-652
  nursing implications and, 657-658
  research needs and, 655-656
  scope of problem of, 651-654
  sleep interference and, 653
  speech interference and, 652
  task interference and, 652
Nuclear power plants, 688-689
Nurse-midwives in action, 811-824. *See also* Midwifery.
Nurse Practice Acts, 333
Nursing audits, 104, 185-197
Nursing bottle syndrome, 574
Nursing homes, 65, 347
Nursing organizations, 235-236
Nursing preparation levels, 60
Nursing process, 102-103
Nursing role in community, 20-21
Nursing theory, 41-44
Nutrition
  adolescent and, 580-583
  aging and, 307
  basic principles of, 570
  cancer family and, 416

Nutrition—*Continued*
  cancer patient and, 412-413
  community, 569-601
  counseling, 599
  economics-food budgeting and, 590
  ethnic food practices and, 590
  fad reducing diets and, 596-599
  food faddism and, 591-595
  food labeling and, 591
  food processing and, 591
  infant feeding and, 570-578
  influences on food practices and, 590-599
  lactation and, 586-587
  middle years and, 587
  pregnancy and, 583-586
  school age child and, 579-580
  science of, 569-570
  senior years and, 588-590
  toddler and preschooler and, 579
  vegetarian diets and, 595-596
Nutritional assessment for elderly, 309-311
Nutritionists, 61

Oakland County Public Health Nursing Audit
      Tool, 185-197
  coordination of services, 186-187
  evaluate total situation, 185-186
  family data continuation sheet, 194-197
  family folder summary sheet, 197
  implementation of nursing plans, 186
  observation of situation, 185
  procedures and guidelines for audit commit-
      tee, 189-192
  recording format, 187
Obesity, infant, 574
Occupation, disabled persons and, 606-607
Occupational disease, 123
Occupational health
  history and legislation in, 124-127
  nursing role in, 123-140, 701-708
  nursing roles and functions in, 134-137
    assessment and, 135
    community and, 137-139
    evaluation and, 136
    planning and, 136-137
    record keeping and, 136
    retirement planning and, 135
    screening and preventive programs and,
      135-136
  response of nursing profession to, 127-129
  team work in, 129-134
Occupational nursing clinical role study, 701-
      708
Occupational Safety and Health Act, 125
Occupational Safety and Health Administra-
      tion, 125-126
Occupational therapy, 503-504

Opium, 544
Organ-body weight ratio in aging, 308
Organizations
  midwifery, 246-247
  nursing, 235-236
Osteoarthritis, 515-516

Parent
  child abuse and, 562
  disabled child and, 263-265
Pathogen transmission, 669-670
Personal experiences in community health nurs-
      ing, 693-882
Personality
  aging and, 301
  coronary prone, 379-381
Pharmacists, 62
Physical or occupational therapists, 62
Play therapy, 331-332
Podiatrists, 61
Politicians, folk, 75-76
Politics
  cancer and, 397
  health, 72-76
    folk politicians and, 75-76
    mandates in, 73-75
    trends in, 72-73
  health care and, 77
  nurses and, 78-79
  population issues and, 629
  practitioners and, 69-81
Pollution
  air, 637-646
  noise, 647-658
  water, 659-666
Polymyositis, 511-512
Population
  at-risk characteristics of, 9-10
  biologic characteristics of, 8
  community, 8-13
  definition of, 8-9
  health status of, 151-152
  mortality, morbidity, fertility rates of, 10-13
  social characteristics of, 8
  target, 94
Population issues, 623-630
  impact of, 625-629
    education and, 628-629
    fertility and, 625-627
    health and, 629
    life expectancy and, 627-628
    political and economic concerns and, 629
    resources and, 628
  statistics and terminology in, 623-625
Portage Guide to Early Education, 268
Pott, Percival, 125
Practitioners and politics, 69-81

Pregnancy
  diabetes mellitus and, 438
  nursing intervention in, 586
  nutrient needs in, 583
  nutrition and, 583-586
  risk factors in, 585-586
    adolescence, 585
    alcohol, 585
    drugs and, 586
    smoking and, 585
  sodium in, 585
  vitamin supplementation in, 584-585
  weight gain in, 583
Presbycusis, 302
Presbyopia, 301
Preschooler and nutrition, 579
President's Commission on Mental Health, 350-351
Prevalence, 11, 460
Preventive health program for low income women, 795-809
  project description in, 801-807
  purpose of program, 797-801
Preventive health services, 35
Primary care in school health nursing, 164
Professional Standards Review Organization, 74
Program planning in school health nursing, 156-157
Proprietary agencies, 209
Providers of health care, 59-63
Psychologic factors in cancer, 395-396
Psychologists, 61
Psychotherapy, 331-332
  elderly and, 347
  family, 331
  group, 331
  play, 331-332
  psychoanalytic, 331
  short term, 331
Public health nursing. *See also* Community health nursing.
  clinical role study, 731-740
    nursing process and, 734-740
    nursing program in, 732-734
  educational preparation for, 179
  generalist in, 41, 224
  historical development of, 177-179
  levels of prevention in, 180
  Oakland County Public Health Nursing Audit Tool, 185-197
  record keeping and, 183
  nursing role in, 175-197
  scope of service in, 179-184
  specialist in, 41, 224
  team approach in, 182
Public Health Service, 58

Pulmonary disease. *See* Chronic obstructive lung disease.

QUACKERY and cancer, 409-410

RADIATION, ionizing, 681-691
Radiation syndrome, 687-688
Radiation therapy, 406-407
Ramazzini, 124-125
Rape
  avoiding, 558
  DES and, 560
  emergency room examination in, 559-560
  friends and family and, 560
  impact of, 558
  incidence of, 557
  nursing role in, 559
  reporting, 557
  victimology and, 557-561
Rape trauma syndrome, 557-558
Record keeping, 104
  public health, 183
Referral, 105
Relaxation techniques, 387
Rem, 682
Reproductive organs and aging, 306
Research, 108-109
  cancer and, 420
  diabetes mellitus and, 441-443
  infectious diseases and, 470-471
  rheumatoid arthritis and, 509
  substance abuse and, 553-554
Resources
  health care, 65-66
  tools and, 101-110
Respiratory system and aging, 303-304
Retirement planning, 135
Rheumatic heart disease, 373, 375
Rheumatoid arthritis, 497-509
  community health nursing concerns in, 507-509
  definition and etiology of, 497-498
  diagnostic criteria in, 498
  education and, 509
  family impact of, 500
  individual impact of, 500
  juvenile, 509-511
  prevention and treatment of, 500-507
    education in, 500-501
    exercise in, 501-502
    family and community in, 506-507
    heat in, 501
    immunosuppressive drugs in, 506
    individual in, 500-506
    occupational therapist in, 503-504
    reconstructive surgery in, 505-506

Rheumatoid arthritis—*Continued*
 rest in, 502
  salicylates in, 502-506
 prognosis in, 506-507
 research on, 509
 rheumatoid factor in, 498
 rheumatoid nodules in, 498
 scope of problem in, 499
 sex and, 499
 statistics in, 499
Rocky Mountain spotted fever, 453-454
Roentgen, 682
Roles in community health nursing, 111-368
Rural Health Clinics Bill, 216

SAFETY
 accident impact and, 634-635
 accidents and, 631-636
Salicylates, 502-506
Sanitarians, 62
Sanitary landfill, 675-677
School age programs for developmental disabilities, 282-283
School health nursing
 assessment in, 151-156
  data collection and, 152-156
  need for, 151
  population health status and, 151-152
 certification for, 149-151
 counseling and, 162-164
 determining roles and activities in, 151-169
 educational preparation for, 147-149
 health education and, 164-169
 historical view of, 141-143
 implementation of, 157-167
 primary care and, 164
 program evaluation and, 167-169
 program planning in, 156-157
 role ambiguity and conflict in, 143-146
 role clarity and, 169
 role in, 141-174
 scope of service in, 143
 screening tests and, 158-162
School nurse practitioner, 709-729
 administrative/agency support and, 714
 administrative forms in, 719-729
 clinical practice setting in, 714
 community need for, 711-712
 educational clinical preparation for, 710
 financial support and, 715
 health issue identified and, 711
 nursing intervention and, 715-716
 problem resolution and, 716-717
 problems encountered and, 716
 program objectives for, 712-714
 recommendations and, 718
 role impact and, 717-718

Schools of nursing, 221
Scoliosis screening, 160-161
Screening tests, 158-162
 cardiac, 161
 hearing, 159-160
 scoliosis, 160-161
 strep throat, 161-162
 vision, 158-159
Sedatives, 539
Self-concept of cancer patient, 400-401
Self-help skills, 270
 independence in, 266-267
Senile cataract, 301-302
Senior years
 food intake and, 588
 nursing intervention in, 590
 nutrient needs in, 588
 nutrition and, 588-590
 special diets in, 589
Serving Seniors Program, 742-745
Short term psychotherapy, 331
Skin and subcutaneous tissues in aging, 298-299
Sleep and noise pollution, 653
Smell and taste in aging, 302
Smoking
 chronic obstructive lung disease and, 479-481
 coronary artery disease and, 374
 pregnancy and, 585
Social issues in community health, 567-620
Social readjustment rating scale, 384
Social Security Act, 203
Sociocultural patterns in substance abuse, 540
Solid waste management, 667-680
 agricultural, 668
 changes to come in, 678
 concerns for, 669-674
  cost levels in, 673-674
  irresponsible discard and, 671-672
  pathogen transmission in, 669-670
  resource conservation and, 672-673
  toxic and infectious materials and, 670-671
 disposal of, 674-678
  burning and, 674
  burying and, 675-677
  composting in, 677-678
  sanitary landfill and, 675-677
 industrial, 668
 nursing implications of, 679
 poor handling of, 679
Somogyi effect, 446
Specialized generalist, 114
Speech
 in aging, 302
 noise pollution and, 652

Standards of Community Health Nursing Practice, 46
State health organizations, 57-58
Statistics, 106-107
  accidents and, 631-634
  population issues and, 623-625
  vital, 106
Strep throat screening, 161-162
Stress in coronary artery disease, 374
Stroke, 373
Substance abuse, 537-554
  age in, 540
  alcohol, 538, 549-550
  amphetamines, 539
  barbiturates, sedatives, tranquilizers and, 539
  commonly abused drugs and, 538-539
  community health nursing approaches to, 552-553
  current trends in, 545-546
  definitions in, 538
  educational patterns and, 542
  etiology of, 546-547
  family life and, 543
  geographic patterns and, 542
  hallucinogens, 539
  historical perspectives on, 543-545
  impact of, 547-549
    community, 548-549
    family, 548
    individual, 547-548
  incidence of, 539-540
  marijuana and hashish, 538
  narcotics, 539
  occupations and, 542
  opium, 544
  peers and, 543
  preventive approaches to, 552
  race in, 540
  research in, 553-554
  scope of problem of, 539-543
  sex in, 540
  sociocultural patterns in, 540
  socioeconomic patterns and, 542
  treatment approaches to, 64, 549-551
    alcohol and, 549-550
    drugs in, 550
    family in, 550-551
    industry and, 551
Sudden infant death syndrome, 345-346
Suicide, 346
  victimology and, 565-566

TACTILE sense in aging, 303
Target population, 94
Teaching and developmental disabilities, 267-271

Telephone usage, 104-105
Television, 75-76
Temperature maintenance, 308, 312
Terminal illness, 614-615
Title III Grants for State and Community Programs on Aging, 216
Title XX, home care and, 215
Toddler and nutrition, 579
Tools and resources
  client services as, 101-106
  community health nurse and, 101-110
  disease control as, 107-108
  research as, 108-109
  statistics as, 106-107
Toxic and infectious materials, 670-671
Toxic Substance Control Act, 127
Tranquilizers, 539

URINARY tract in aging, 305
Urine testing in diabetes mellitus, 446

VECTOR control, 107
Vegetarian diets, 595-596
Vertical client, 113
Veterinarians, 61
Victimology, 555-566
  child abuse and, 561-563
  rape and, 557-561
  suicide and homocide and, 565-566
  wife abuse and, 563-565
Vision in aging, 301-302
  glaucoma and, 302
Vision screening, 158-159
Visiting Nurse Service of Philadelphia, 202
Vitamin supplementation
  infant feeding and, 571
  pregnancy and, 584-585
Voluntary agencies, 56-57, 208

WASTE elimination
  cancer and, 413-414, 417
Water pollution, 659-666
  control of, 662
  current problems and outlook on, 662-665
  drinking water and, 661
  effect of, 660-662
  food supply contamination and, 661
  nursing implications and, 665
  recreation and, 661-662
  shellfish and, 662
  waterborne disease and, 660-661
Waterborne disease, 660-661
Wellness, measurement of, 31
Wife abuse, 563-565

ZEN-macrobiotic diet, 596